THIRD EDITION

Clinical Guidelines for Advanced Practice Nursing

AN INTERPROFESSIONAL APPROACH

Edited by:

Geraldine M. Collins-Bride, MS, RN, ANP-BC, FAAN
Health Sciences Clinical Professor
Adult Nurse Practitioner
University of California, San Francisco
Department of Community Health Systems

JoAnne M. Saxe, DNP, MS, RN, ANP, FAAN
Health Sciences Clinical Professor
Adult Nurse Practitioner
University of California, San Francisco
Department of Community Health Systems

Rebekah Kaplan, MS, CNM, RN
Health Sciences Associate Clinical Professor
Nurse Midwife
University of California, San Francisco
Department of Family Health Care Nursing and
Department of Obstetrics, Gynecology, and Reproductive Sciences

Karen G. Duderstadt, PhD, RN, CPNP, PCNS, FAAN
Health Sciences Clinical Professor
Pediatric Nurse Practitioner
University of California, San Francisco
Department of Family Health Care Nursing

Associate Editor:

Lewis D. Fannon, MS, RN, ANP-BC
Health Sciences Assistant Clinical Professor
Adult Nurse Practitioner
University of California, San Francisco School of Nursing
Department of Community Health Systems

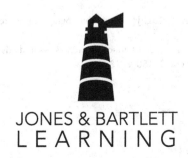

JONES & BARTLETT
LEARNING

World Headquarters
Jones & Bartlett Learning
5 Wall Street
Burlington, MA 01803
978-443-5000
info@jblearning.com
www.jblearning.com

Jones & Bartlett Learning books and products are available through most bookstores and online booksellers. To contact Jones & Bartlett Learning directly, call 800-832-0034, fax 978-443-8000, or visit our website, www.jblearning.com.

Substantial discounts on bulk quantities of Jones & Bartlett Learning publications are available to corporations, professional associations, and other qualified organizations. For details and specific discount information, contact the special sales department at Jones & Bartlett Learning via the above contact information or send an email to specialsales@jblearning.com.

Production Credits

VP, Executive Publisher: David D. Cella
Executive Editor: Amanda Martin
Associate Acquisitions Editor: Rebecca Myrick
Editorial Assistant: Lauren Vaughn
Production Manager: Carolyn Rogers Pershouse
Associate Production Editor: Juna Abrams
Senior Marketing Manager: Jennifer Scherzay
Product Fulfillment Manager: Wendy Kilborn

Composition: Cenveo Publisher Services
Cover Design: Kristin E. Parker
Rights & Media Specialist: Wes DeShano
Media Development Editor: Troy Liston
Cover Image: © Eliks/Shutterstock, © donatas1205/Shutterstock
Printing and Binding: Edwards Brothers Malloy
Cover Printing: Edwards Brothers Malloy

Library of Congress Cataloging-in-Publication Data

Collins-Bride, Geraldine M., editor. | Saxe, JoAnne M., editor. | Duderstadt, Karen, editor. | Kaplan, Rebekah, editor.
Clinical guidelines for advanced practice nursing : an interprofessional approach / [edited by] Geraldine M. Collins-Bride, JoAnne M. Saxe, Rebekah Kaplan, and Karen G. Duderstadt.
Third edition. | Burlington, MA : Jones & Bartlett Learning, [2017] | Includes bibliographical references and index.
LCCN 2015048813 | ISBN 978-1-284-09313-1 (pbk.)
MESH: Advanced Practice Nursing | Nursing Care—methods | Clinical Protocols—standards | Guideline LCC RT82.8 | NLM WY 128 | DDC 610.73—dc23 LC record available at http://lccn.loc.gov/2015048813

6048
Printed in the United States of America
20 19 10 9 8 7 6 5 4

DEDICATION

To our patients and students, we appreciate the many lessons that we have learned from you and the trust that you have given us over the years. We are privileged to have been your healthcare provider and/or mentor.

GCB, JMS, RK, KD, and LF

To my "boys" (Bob, Patrick, & Brendan) who have stopped asking when I'll be coming home! I appreciate all your support, love, and most of all, your patience and humor.

GCB

To my mother, Patricia, father, John, husband, Noel, daughters (Kelly, Jocelyn, and Lydia), son-in-law, Benny, granddaughter, Mícara, and all of my wonderful brothers and sisters for your years of support, love, and laughter. Thank you for all that you are and do!

JMS

To my husband, Chris, who is constantly patient and respectful of my work. Thank you for the love and support! And to the children and families I serve with humility and respect for what they have taught me over the years!

KD

To my husband, David, and sons, Ezra and Emmet. You make my world go round. Thanks for all you give me and for always making me laugh, even when faced with writing deadlines.

RK

To my wonderful family and friends who have been extraordinary in their support during the production of this text. Thank you for putting up with me! Also, a huge note of gratitude to Gerri, JoAnne, Rebekah, and Karen for allowing me to be part of something so special!

LF

A SPECIAL DEDICATION

To a dear friend and colleague **Barbara Boland, RN, MS, ANP-BC, CDE,** *who was a contributing author to all three editions of this book, one of the best NPs on the planet and a wonderful friend who always made us laugh. We miss you, Barbara!*

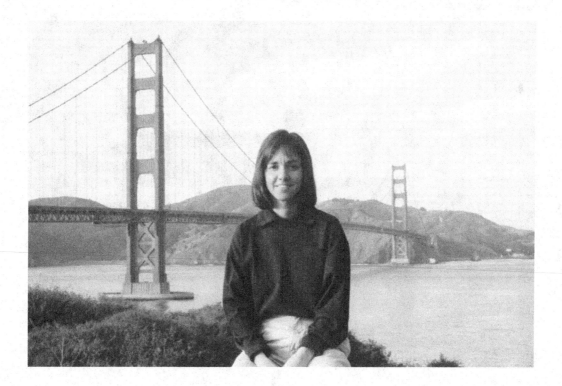

CONTENTS

Acknowledgments xv
Contributors xvii
Introduction xxvii

1 Legal Scope of Advanced Nursing Practice 1
Brian Budds and JoAnne M. Saxe
Introduction and General Background 1
Overview of Scope of Practice Legal Framework 1
Issues Related to Collaborative Practice
    and Documentation 4
Concluding Remarks 5

SECTION I Pediatric Health Maintenance and Promotion

2 First Well-Baby Visit 7
Annette Carley
I. Introduction and general background 7
II. Database 8
III. Assessment 9
IV. Goals of first well-baby visit 9
V. Plan 10
VI. Resources and tools 10

3 Care of the Postneonatal Intensive Care Unit Graduate 12
Annette Carley
I. Introduction and general background 12
II. Database 15
III. Assessment 16
IV. Goals of clinical management 16
V. Plan 16
VI. Resources and tools 17

4 0 to 3 Years of Age Interval Visit 18
Ann Birenbaum Baker
I. Introduction and general background 18
II. Database 18
III. Assessment 20
IV. Plan 20

5 3 to 6 Years of Age Interval Visit 23
Mary Anne M. Israel
I. Introduction and general background 23
II. Database 23
III. Assessment 24
IV. Plan 24

6 6 to 11 Years of Age Interval Visit 27
Bridget Ward Gramkowski and Ann Birenbaum Baker
I. Introduction and general background 27
II. Database 27
III. Assessment 29
IV. Plan 29

7 The Adolescent and Young Adult (12–21 Years of Age) Interval Visit 32
Erica Monasterio
I. Introduction and general background 32
II. Database 33
III. Assessment 36
IV. Plan 36
V. Self-management resources 38

8 Preventive Immunizations for Children and Adults 40
Lucy S. Crain
I. Introduction: Overview of vaccine-preventable diseases 40
Recommended U.S. Immunization Schedules and Catch-Up Schedules for Ages Birth Through 18 Years 42
I. Recommended pediatric vaccine schedule 42
II. Adult immunization recommendations 44

III. Immunization modalities 45
IV. Active and passive immunizations 46
V. Herd immunity 46
VI. Adverse event reporting 46
VII. Current concerns and vaccination rates 47

9 **Developmental Assessment: Screening for Developmental Delay and Autism 48**
Abbey Alkon

I. Introduction 48
II. Developmental surveillance and screening algorithm 49
III. Screening instruments 57
IV. Psychometrics 57
V. Conclusion 58
VI. Clinician resources 58

SECTION II Common Complex Pediatric Presentations

10 **Childhood Asthma 61**
Nan Madden and Andrea Crosby Shah

I. Introduction and general background 61
II. Database 61
III. Assessment 62
IV. Goals of clinical management 65
V. Plan 65
VI. Resources 68

11 **Atopic Dermatitis in Children 70**
Karen G. Duderstadt and Nan Madden

I. Introduction and general background 70
II. Database 70
III. Assessment 72
IV. Goals of clinical management 72
V. Plan 73
VI. Self-management 78
VII. Psychosocial and emotional support 79

12 **Attention-Deficit/Hyperactivity Disorder in Children and Adolescents 80**
Naomi Schapiro

I. Introduction and general background 80
II. Overview 80

III. Database: History 81
IV. Physical examination 83
V. Assessment 84
VI. Plan 84

13 **Childhood Depression 90**
Damon Michael Williams

I. Introduction 90
II. Database 92
III. Assessment 94
IV. Plan 94
V. Self-management resources 98

14 **Failure to Thrive During Infancy 99**
Annette Carley

I. Introduction and general background 99
II. Database 100
III. Assessment 101
IV. Goals of clinical management 102
V. Plan 102
VI. Resources 103

15 **Child Maltreatment 104**
Naomi Schapiro

I. Introduction and general background 104
II. Database 106
III. Assessment 110
IV. Plan 111
V. Resources 112

16 **Childhood Overweight and Obesity 114**
Victoria F. Keeton

I. Introduction and general background 114
II. Database 115
III. Assessment 118
IV. Plan 118
V. Helpful online resources 121

17 **Urinary Incontinence in Children 124**
Angel K. Chen

I. Introduction and general background 124
II. Database 126
III. Assessment 128
IV. Goals of clinical management 130
V. Plan 131
VI. Resources 134

SECTION III   Common Women's Health Presentations

18   Abnormal Uterine Bleeding   140
Pilar Bernal de Pheils
I.   Introduction and general background   140
II.   Database   145

19   Amenorrhea and Polycystic Ovary Syndrome   156
Pilar Bernal de Pheils
I.   Introduction and general background   156
II.   Database   158
III.   Assessment   161
IV.   Goals of clinical management   161
V.   Plan   161
VI.   Self-management resources and tools   169

20   Screening for Intraepithelial Neoplasia and Cancer of the Lower Genital Tract   171
Mary M. Rubin and Lynn Hanson
I.   Introduction and general background   171
II.   Database   176
III.   Assessment   177
IV.   Goals of clinical management   178
V.   Plan   179

21   Female and Male Sterilization   188
Janis Luft
I.   Introduction and general background   188
II.   Database   190
III.   Assessment   190
IV.   Plan   190
V.   Self-management resources   190

22   Hormonal Contraception   192
Lynn Hanson
I.   Introduction and general background   192
II.   Database   204
III.   Assessment   205
IV.   Goals of clinical management   205
V.   Plan   205
Appendix 22-1: Comparison of Hormonal Contraceptive Methods   209

23   Menopause Transition   217
Priscilla Abercrombie
I.   Introduction and general background   217
II.   Database   219
III.   Assessment   220
IV.   Goals of clinical management   220
V.   Plan   221
VI.   Self-management resources and tools   226
VII.   Clinical practice guidelines   226

24   Nonhormonal Contraception   230
Kimberley Chastain
I.   Introduction and general background   230
II.   Database   234
III.   Assessment   235
IV.   Goals of clinical management   235
V.   Plan   235
VI.   Self-management resources and tools   236

25   Urinary Incontinence in Women   237
Janis Luft
I.   Introduction and general background   237
II.   Initial evaluation   238
III.   Assessment   239
IV.   Goals of clinical management   240
V.   Plan   240
VI.   Self-management resources and tools   244

SECTION IV   Obstetric Health Maintenance and Promotion

26   The Initial Prenatal Visit   246
Rebekah Kaplan
I.   Definition and background   246
II.   Database   246
III.   Assessment   248
IV.   Goals of clinical management   248
V.   Plan   248
VI.   Internet resources   252

27   Prenatal Genetic Screening and Diagnosis   253
Deborah Anderson
I.   Introduction and general background   253
II.   Database   256

III. Assessment 256
IV. Goals for clinical management 256
V. Plan 257
I. Prenatal genetic diagnosis:
Introduction and general background 257
II. Database 258
III. Assessment 258
IV. Goals for clinical management 258
V. Plan 258

28 The Return Prenatal Visit 260
Rebekah Kaplan and Margaret Hutchison
I. Definition and background 260
II. Database 260
III. Assessment 262
IV. Goals of clinical management 263
V. Plan 263

29 The Postpartum Visit 268
Jenna Shaw-Battista and Holly Cost
I. Introduction and general background 268
II. Database 269
III. Assessment 271
IV. Goals for clinical management 271
V. Plan 272

30 Guidelines for Medical Consultation, Interprofessional Collaboration, and Transfer of Care During Pregnancy and Childbirth 277
Jenna Shaw-Battista
I. Introduction and general background 277

SECTION V Common Obstetric Presentations

31 Birth Choices for Women with a Previous Cesarean Delivery 282
Rebekah Kaplan
I. Introduction and general background 282
II. Risks and benefits of TOL versus repeat cesarean delivery 282
III. Data collection 284
IV. Goals for clinical management/assessment 284
V. Plan 284

VI. Internet resources for providers, clients, and families 288

32 Common Discomforts of Pregnancy 290
Cynthia Belew and Jamie Meyerhoff
I. Introduction to common discomforts of pregnancy 290
II. Poor quality of sleep 290
III. Musculoskeletal 291
IV. Gastrointestinal tract 294
V. Heartburn 298

33 Gestational Diabetes Mellitus: Early Detection and Management in Pregnancy 304
Maribeth Inturrisi
I. Introduction and general background 304
II. Database 305
III. Goals of clinical management 306
IV. Plan 306

34 Hypertension in Pregnancy: Preeclampsia–Eclampsia 313
Kim Q. Dau and Jenna Shaw-Battista
I. Introduction and general background 313
II. Database 315
III. Assessment 316
IV. Goals of clinical management 317
V. Plan 317

35 Preterm Labor Management 320
Mary Barger
I. Introduction and general background 320
II. Database 320
III. Assessment 321
IV. Goals of clinical management 321
V. Plan 321

36 Urinary Tract Infection Prevention and Management in Pregnancy 323
Mary Barger
I. Introduction and general background 323
II. Database 323
III. Assessment 324
IV. Goals of clinical management 324
V. Plan 324

SECTION VI Adult Gerontology Health Maintenance and Promotion

37 Adult Health Maintenance and Promotion 326
Helen R. Horvath and Hattie C. Grundland
I.   Introduction and general background 326
II. Individualizing screening decisions in the geriatric population 326
III. Database 331
IV. Assessment 333
V.   Goals of clinical management 333
VI. Plan 333
VII. Self-management tools and resources for health professionals 333

38 Healthcare Maintenance for Adults with Developmental Disabilities 345
Geraldine Collins-Bride and Clarissa Kripke
I.   Introduction and general background 345
II. Database 348
III. Assessment 351
IV. Plan 352
V.   Self-management resources and tools 362

39 Healthcare Maintenance for Transgender Individuals 365
Melissa Wong and Kathryn Wyckoff
I.   Introduction and general background 365
II. Database 366
III. Assessment 367
IV. Plan 367
Appendix A: A Guide to Common Gender-Neutral Pronoun Choices Among the Trans Community 374

40 Postexposure Prophylaxis for HIV Infection 375
Barbara Newlin and Brooke Finkmoore
I.   Introduction and general background 375
II. Database 380
III. Assessment 383
IV. Plan 383
V.   Clinician and patient resources 383

41 Preexposure Prophylaxis for HIV 385
Barbara Newlin and Brooke Finkmoore 385
I.   Introduction and general background 385
II. Database 386
III. Assessment 388
IV. Goals of clinical management 388
V.   Plan 388
VI. Resources for clinicians 389
Appendix 41-1: Behavioral Risk Assessment Questions 391
Appendix 41-2: Screening Tool for MSM 392
Appendix 41-3: Summary of Guidance for PrEP Use 393
Appendix 41-4: Provider Checklist 394

SECTION VII Common Complex Adult Gerontology Presentations

42 Abscess Management 395
Rosalie D. Bravo
I.   Introduction and general background 395
II. Database 395
III. Assessment 396
IV. Goals of clinical management 396
V.   Plan 397

43 Anemia 401
Michelle M. Marin and Laurie Jurkiewicz
I.   Introduction and general background 401
II. Database 405
III. Assessment 407
IV. Goals of clinical management 410
V.   Plan 410
VI. Self-management resources and tools 413

44 Anticoagulation Therapy (Oral) 415
Fran Dreier and Linda Ray
I.   Introduction and general background 415
II. Patient education and safety 421
III. Target-specific anticoagulants 424

45 Anxiety 428
Esker-D Ligon
I.   Introduction and general background 428
II. Database 429

III. Assessment 431
IV. Plan 432
V. Special populations 434
VI. Self-management resources and tools 435

46 Asthma in Adolescents and Adults 436

Susan L. Janson

I. Introduction and general background 436
II. Database 437
III. Assessment 438
IV. Goals of clinical management to control asthma 438
V. Plan 439
VI. Future update topics in asthma 446

47 Benign Prostatic Hyperplasia 449

Jean N. Taylor-Woodbury

I. Introduction and general background 449
II. Database 450
III. Assessment 451
IV. Goals of clinical management 451
V. Plan 451
VI. Self-management resources and tools 454
Appendix 47-1: The American Urological Association (AUA) Symptom Index for Benign Prostatic Hyperplasia (BPH) and the Disease Specific Quality of Life Question 456
Appendix 47-2: Benign Prostatic Hyperplasia (BPH) Impact Index ("Bother" Score) 457

48 Cancer Survivorship in Adult Primary Care 458

Tara D. Lacey and Sheila N. Lindsay

I. Introduction and background 458
II. Database 459
III. Assessment 460
IV. Goals of clinical management 462
V. Plan 463
VI. Self-management resources 466

49 Chronic Obstructive Pulmonary Disease 468

Lynda A. Mackin

I. Introduction and general background 468
II. Database 469
III. Goals of clinical management of stable COPD 471
IV. Plan 471
V. Care from a population health perspective 475

50 Chronic Nonmalignant Pain Management 477

JoAnne M. Saxe, Nicole Una, and Kellie McNerney

I. Introduction and general background 477
II. Database 478
III. Assessment 480
IV. Goals of clinical management 481
V. Plan 482
VI. Patient education 491
VII. Chronic pain support resources and tools 492

51 Chronic Viral Hepatitis 494

Miranda Surjadi

I. Introduction and general background 494
II. Database 495
III. Assessment 498
IV. Goals of clinical management 498
V. Plan 499
VI. Self-management resources and tools 503

52 Dementia 504

Jennifer Merrilees

I. Introduction and general background 504
II. Database 505
III. Assessment 509
IV. Goals of clinical management 509
V. Plan 509
VI. Assessment and management of concomitant conditions 512
VII. Assessment of the status of the family caregiver 512
VIII. Resources and tools 512

53 Depression 514

Matt Tierney and Beth Phoenix

I. Introduction and general background 514
II. Database 516
III. Assessment 518
IV. Goals of clinical management 519
V. Plan 521
VI. Self-management resources and tools 527

54 Diabetes Mellitus 529

Carolina Noya and Maureen McGrath

I. Introduction and general background 529
II. Database 529
III. Assessment 531
IV. Goals of clinical management 532

V. Plan 532
VI. Self-management resources and tools 537

55 Epilepsy 539

Maritza Lopez, Paul Garcia, and
M. Robin Taylor

I. Introduction and general background 539
II. Database 539
III. Assessment 540
IV. Goals of clinical management 541
V. Plan 545
VI. Self-management resources 546

56 Gastroesophageal Reflux Disease 547

Karen C. Bagatelos, Geraldine Collins-Bride,
and Fran Dreier

I. Definition and overview 547
II. Database 548
III. Assessment 549
IV. Goals of clinical management 550
V. Plan 550
VI. Self-management resources 553

57 Geriatric Syndromes 554

Courtney Gordon

I. Introduction and general background 554
II. Database 556
III. Assessment 560
IV. Goals of clinical management 562
V. Plan 562
VI. Online resources for clinicians, patients,
and caregivers 564

58 Heart Failure 566

Lisa Guertin and Barbara Boland

I. Introduction and general background 566
II. Database 567
III. Assessment 568
IV. Goals of clinical management 568
V. Plan 568
VI. Self-management resources and tools 574

59 Herpes Simplex Infections 575

Hattie C. Grundland and Geraldine
Collins-Bride

I. Introduction and general background 575
II. Database 577
III. Assessment 577
IV. Goals of clinical management 578

V. Plan 578
VI. Self–management resources and tools 581

60 Hypertension 583

Judith Sweet and Steve Protzel

I. Introduction and definition 583
II. Database 584
III. Assessment 587
IV. Goals of clinical management 587
V. Plan and management 587

61 Intimate Partner Violence
(Domestic Violence) 594

Rosalind De Lisser, Deborah Johnson,
JoAnne Saxe, and Cecily Reeves

I. Introduction and general background 594
II. The focused IPV assessment
and database 598
III. Assessment 600
IV. Goals of clinical management 601
V. Plan 601
VI. Self-management resources and tools 601

62 Irritable Bowel Syndrome 605

Karen C. Bagatelos, Geraldine Collins-Bride,
and Fran Dreier

I. Introduction and general background 605
II. Database 606
III. Assessment 607
IV. Goals of clinical management 607
V. Plan 607
VI. Self-management eResources 612

63 Lipid Disorders 613

Caitlin Garvey

I. Introduction and general background 613
II. Database 614
III. Assessment 615
IV. Goals of clinical management 615
V. Plan 615
VI. Self-management resources and tools 618

64 Low Back Pain 619

H. Kate Lawlor

I. Introduction/general background 619
II. Database 619
III. Assessment 625
IV. Plan 626
V. Self-management resources and tools 633

65 **Obesity 634**

Sherri Borden, David Besio, and Geraldine Collins-Bride

I. Introduction and general background 634
II. Database 636
III. Assessment 638
IV. Goals of clinical management 638
V. Plan 642
VI. Self-management resources 647

66 **Primary Care of HIV-Infected Adults 649**

Suzan Stringari-Murray and Christopher Berryhill Fox

I. Introduction and general background 649
II. HIV screening and testing 657
III. Database 661
IV. Assessment 663
V. Goals of clinical management 663
VI. Plan 663
VII. Resources 668

67 **Smoking Cessation 672**

Kellie McNerney and Lewis Fannon

I. Introduction and background 672
II. Database 675
III. Assessment 676
IV. Goals of clinical management 676
V. Plan 677
VI. Self-management resources 679
VII. Consultation 680

68 **Thyroid Disorders 682**

JoAnne M. Saxe

I. Introduction and general background 682
II. Database 683
III. Assessment 687
IV. Goals of clinical management 687
V. Plan 687
VI. Self-management resources and tools 690

69 **Upper Back and Neck Pain Syndromes 691**

Rossana Segovia

I. Introduction and general background 691
II. Database 695
III. Assessment 699
IV. Goals of clinical management 700
V. Plan 700
VI. Self-management resources and tools 703

70 **Upper Extremity Tendinopathy: Bicipital Tendinopathy, Lateral Epicondylitis, and de Quervain's Tenosynovitis 705**

Barbara J. Burgel

I. Introduction and general background 705
II. Database 706
III. Assessment 708
IV. Goals of clinical management 709
V. Plan 709
VI. Self-management resources and tools 711

71 **Wound Care 713**

Cynthia Johnson and Patricia McCarthy-Horton

I. Introduction and general background 713
II. Database 714
III. Assessment 718
IV. Goals of clinical management 718
V. Plan 718

Index 722

ACKNOWLEDGMENTS

The editors would like to acknowledge the following individuals for their contributions to the publication of this book:

- Lou Fannon, our fabulous colleague and associate editor for this text, who provided exceptional support to authors, reviewers, and the publisher through timely and thoughtful communications, constructive editorial feedback, and *meticulous* attention to timelines and publishing details. It has been a pleasure and honor working with you!

- Our colleagues at UCSF in the Schools of Nursing, Medicine, Pharmacy, and Dentistry; the Department of Physical Therapy; the UCSF Medical Center; and community organizations and other universities/colleges who contributed much time and expertise as authors and reviewers of this manuscript. We are grateful for having such an esteemed team.

CONTRIBUTORS

Priscilla Abercrombie, RN, NP, PhD, AHN-BC
Founder, Women's Health & Healing
Healdsburg, CA

Abbey Alkon, RN, PNP, PhD, FAAN
Professor
Department of Family Health Care Nursing
University of California, San Francisco, School of Nursing
San Francisco, CA

Deborah Anderson, MS, CNM
Health Sciences Clinical Professor
School of Medicine & Department of Family Health Care Nursing
University of California, San Francisco
Department of Obstetrics, Gynecology & Reproductive Sciences
San Francisco General Hospital
San Francisco, CA

Karen C. Bagatelos, RN, MSN, FNP
Assistant Clinical Professor (volunteer)
Department of Community Health Systems
Family Nurse Practitioner
Department of Medicine, Division of Gastroenterology
University of California, San Francisco
San Francisco, CA

Ann Birenbaum Baker, RN, MS, CPNP
Pediatric Nurse Practitioner
Newborn Nursery, Department of Medicine, Division of Neonatology
University of California San Francisco
San Francisco, CA

Mary K. Barger, RN, CNM, MPH, PhD
Associate Professor
Hahn School of Nursing and Health Sciences and Beyster Institute for Nursing Research
University of San Diego
San Diego, CA

Cynthia Belew, CNM, WHNP-C, MS
Health Sciences Associate Clinical Professor
Department of Family Health Care Nursing
University of California San Francisco, School of Nursing
San Francisco, CA

Pilar Bernal de Pheils, RN, MS, FNP-BC, FAAN
Health Sciences Clinical Professor
Department of Family Health Care Nursing
University of California, San Francisco, School of Nursing
San Francisco, CA

David Besio, MS, RD
Senior Clinical Dietitian
UCSF Adult Weight Management Program
Nutrition and Food Services
University of California, San Francisco Medical Center
San Francisco, CA

Barbara A. Boland, RN, MS, ANP-BC, CDE
Adult Nurse Practitioner
Edward S. Cooper Practice
University of Pennsylvania Health System
Philadelphia, PA

Sherri Borden, RN, MS, ANP-BC, CNS
Adult Nurse Practitioner & Psychiatric Clinical Nurse Specialist & Assistant Clinical Professor (volunteer)
Department of Community Health Systems
University of California San Francisco, School of Nursing
San Francisco, CA

Rosalie D. Bravo, RN, MS, ACNP-BC
Health Sciences Associate Clinical Professor
Adult/Gerontology Acute Care Nurse Practitioner Program, Department of Physiological Nursing
University of California, San Francisco, School of Nursing
San Francisco, CA

Brian Budds, RN, MS, ANP, JD
Adult Nurse Practitioner/Attorney at Law
Associate Clinical Professor (volunteer)
Department of Community Health Systems
University of CaliforniaSan Francisco, School of Nursing
San Francisco, CA

Adjunct Professor
University of San Francisco, School of Law
San Francisco, CA

Assistant Professor and Vice-Chair
Health Leadership and Innovation Department
University of San Francisco, School of Nursing and Health Professions
San Francisco, CA

Barbara J. Burgel, RN, ANP-BC, PhD, FAAN
Clinical Professor & Certified Occupational Health Nurse
    Specialist
Department of Community Health Systems
University of California, San Francisco, School of Nursing
San Francisco, CA

Annette Carley, RN, DNP, NNP-BC, PCPNP-BC
Health Sciences Clinical Professor
Coordinator, Advanced Practice Neonatal Nursing (APNN)
    Specialty
Department of Family Health Care Nursing
University of California San Francisco, School of Nursing
San Francisco, CA

Kimberley Chastain, MSN, ARNP-BC
Clinician III
Planned Parenthood
Seattle, WA

Angel K. Chen, RN, MSN, CPNP
Health Sciences Associate Clinical Professor and Vice Chair
Department of Family Health Care Nursing
University of California San Francisco, School of Nursing
San Francisco, CA

Geraldine M. Collins-Bride, RN, ANP-BC, MS, FAAN*
Health Sciences Clinical Professor & Vice Chair of Faculty
    Practice
Department of Community Health Systems
Adult Nurse Practitioner, Division of General Internal Medicine,
University of California San Francisco, Schools
    of Nursing and Medicine
Faculty, Office of Developmental Primary Care
Department of Family and Community Medicine
University of California San Francisco
San Francisco, CA

Holly Cost, RN, MS, CNM
Associate Clinical Professor (volunteer)
Department of Obstetrics, Gynecology & Reproductive Sciences
San Francisco General Hospital
University of California San Francisco, School of Nursing
San Francisco, CA

Lucy S. Crain, MD, MPH, FAAP
Clinical Professor of Pediatrics, Emerita
University of California San Francisco

Adjunct Professor
Stanford University
Palo Alto, CA

Kim Q. Dau, RN, MS, CNM
Health Sciences Assistant Clinical Professor
Director, UCSF Nurse-Midwifery/WHNP Education Program
Family Health Care Nursing
University of California San Francisco, School of Nursing
San Francisco, CA

Rosalind De Lisser, MS, RN, FNP-BC, PMHNP-BC
Health Sciences Assistant Clinical Professor
Co-Director Psychiatric Mental Health Nurse Practitioner
    Program
Department of Community Health Systems
University of California San Francisco, School of Nursing
San Francisco, CA

Fran Dreier, RN, MHS, FNP
Associate Clinical Professor (volunteer)
Department of Community Health Systems
University of CaliforniaSan Francisco, School of Nursing

Family Nurse Practitioner, Urgent Care and Anticoagulation
    Clinics
San Francisco, CA

Karen G. Duderstadt, PhD, RN, CPNP, PCNS, FAAN*
Health Sciences Clinical Professor
Director, Pediatric Nurse Practitioner Program
Department of Family Health Care Nursing
University of California San Francisco, School of Nursing
San Francisco, CA

Lewis D. Fannon, RN, MS, ANP-BC*
Health Sciences Assistant Clinical Professor
Department of Community Health Systems
University of California, San Francisco School of Nursing
San Francisco, CA

Brooke Finkmoore, RN, MS, MPH, AGPCNP-BC
Adult-Gerontology Primary Care Nurse Practitioner
Mission Neighborhood Health Center
San Francisco, CA

Christopher Berryhill Fox, RN, MS, ANP-BC
Health Sciences Assistant Clinical Professor
Department of Community Health Systems
University of California San Francisco, School of Nursing
San Francisco, CA

Paul A. Garcia, MD
Professor of Neurology
Associate Dean for Academic Affairs, School of Medicine
University of California, San Francisco
San Francisco, CA

Caitlin Garvey, RN, MS, AGPCNP-BC
Adult-Gerontology Primary Care Nurse Practitioner
U.S. Department of Veterans Affairs
San Francisco VA Medical Center
San Francisco, CA

Courtney Gordon, DNP, GNP-BC, MSN
Assistant Clinical Professor of Nursing (volunteer)
Geriatric Nurse Practitioner UCSF Care at Home
Division of Geriatrics
University of California San Francisco
San Francisco, CA

Bridget Ward Gramkowski, RN, MS, CPNP
Pediatric Nurse Practitioner
Almaden Pediatrics
San Jose, CA

Hattie C. Grundland, RN, MS, ANP-BC
Associate Clinical Professor (volunteer)
Department of Community Health Systems
University of California San Francisco, School of Nursing
San Francisco, CA

Adult Nurse Practitioner
Department of Public Health
San Francisco, CA

Lisa Guertin, RN, MS, ACNP
Health Sciences Assistant Clinical Professor
Department of Physiological Nursing
University of California San Francisco, School of Nursing
San Francisco, CA

Lynn Hanson, RN, MS, WHNP
Women's Health Nurse Practitioner
Department of Obstetrics, Gynecology Faculty Practice
University of California San Francisco
San Francisco, CA

Helen R. Horvath, RN, MS, ANP-BC, PHN
Health Sciences Assistant Clinical Professor
Department of Community Health Systems
University of California San Francisco, School of Nursing
San Francisco, CA

Margaret Hutchison, RN, MS, CNM
Leadership Council Chair, Nurse–Midwives of San Francisco
    General Hospital
Health Sciences Clinical Professor
Department of Obstetrics, Gynecology & Reproductive Sciences
University of California, San Francisco
San Francisco, CA

Maribeth Inturrisi, RN, MS, CNS, CDE
Certified Diabetes Educator
Sweet Success Program
Sutter Pacific Physician Foundation
San Francisco, CA

Mary Anne M. Israel, RN, MS, PNP
Health Sciences Assistant Clinical Professor
Department of Family Health Care Nursing
University of California, San Francisco, School of Nursing
San Francisco, CA

Susan L. Janson, PhD, RN, ANP-C, CNS, FAAN
Professor Emerita of Nursing and Medicine
Department of Community Health Systems
University of California San Francisco, School of Nursing
San Francisco, CA

Cynthia Johnson, MS, GNP-BC, FGNLA
Geriatric Nurse Practitioner
Integrated Soft Tissue Infection Service Clinic (ISIS)
San Francisco General Hospital
San Francisco, CA

Deborah Johnson, MSN, APRN, PMHNP-BC
Health Sciences Assistant Clinical Professor
Department of Community Health Systems
University of California San Francisco, School of Nursing
San Francisco, CA

Laurie Jurkiewicz, RN, MS, CNM
Assistant Clinical Professor (volunteer)
Department of Obstetrics, Gynecology & Reproductive Sciences
San Francisco General Hospital
University of California San Francisco, School of Nursing
San Francisco, CA

Rebekah Kaplan, RN, MS, CNM*
Health Sciences Associate Clinical Professor
Department of Family Health Care Nursing & School of
    Medicine
University of California, San Francisco
Department of Obstetrics, Gynecology & Reproductive Sciences
San Francisco General Hospital
San Francisco, CA

Victoria F. Keeton, RN, CPNP, CNS
Pediatric Nurse Practitioner
Children's Health Center
San Francisco General Hospital
San Francisco, CA

Clarissa Kripke, MD, FAAFP
Clinical Professor
Director, Office of Developmental Primary Care
Department of Family and Community Medicine
University of California San Francisco, School of Medicine
San Francisco, CA

Tara Lacey, RN, GNP-BC, AOCNP
Geriatric Nurse Practitioner
UCSF Comprehensive Cancer Center
University of CaliforniaSan Francisco
San Francisco, CA

H. Kate Lawlor, RN, MS, ANP-BC
Associate Clinical Professor (volunteer)
Department of Community Health Systems
University of California San Francisco, School of Nursing
San Francisco, CA

Instructor
Foundations of Patient Care
University of California San Francisco, School of Medicine
San Francisco, CA

Esker-D Ligon, RN, MSN, ANP-BC
Assistant Clinical Professor (volunteer)
Department of Community Health Systems
University of California San Francisco, School of Nursing
San Francisco, CA

Adult Nurse Practitioner
Kaiser Permanente Medical Center
Vallejo, CA

Sheila N. Lindsay, MS, RN, ANP-BC, OCN
Adult Nurse Practitioner
UCSF Helen Diller Family Comprehensive Cancer Center
University of California San Francisco
San Francisco, CA

Maritza Lopez, RN, MS, CNS
Epilepsy Clinical Nurse Specialist
UCSF Epilepsy Center
University of California San Francisco
San Francisco, CA

Janis Luft, RN, MSN, WHNP
Associate Adjunct Clinical Professor (volunteer), Department of
    Family Health Care Nursing
University of California San Francisco, School of Nursing

Women's Health Nurse Practitioner
UCSF Women's Health
Behavioral and Non-surgical Treatment Specialist, UCSF
    Women's Continence Center
Department of Obstetrics, Gynecology & Reproductive Sciences
San Francisco, CA

Lynda A. Mackin, RN, PhD, AGPCNP-BC, CCNS
Health Sciences Clinical Professor
Department of Physiological Nursing
University of California San Francisco, School of Nursing
San Francisco, CA

Nanette Madden, RN, MS, PNP
Health Sciences Associate Clinical Professor
Department of Family Health Care Nursing
University of CaliforniaSan Francisco, School of Nursing
San Francisco, CA

Former Clinical Director, Pediatric Asthma Clinic
Children's Health Center
San Francisco General Hospital
San Francisco, CA

Michelle M. Marin, RN, MS, ANP-BC
Assistant Clinical Professor (volunteer)
Department of Community Health Systems
University of California San Francisco, School of Nursing
San Francisco, CA

Patricia McCarthy-Horton, MS, ANP-BC, WOCN
Adult Nurse Practitioner
San Francisco General Hospital
San Francisco, CA

Maureen McGrath, MS, PNP-BC, BC-ADM
Health Sciences Associate Clinical Professor
Coordinator, Diabetes Minor
Department of Family Health Care Nursing
University of California San Francisco, School of Nursing
San Francisco, CA

Kellie McNerney, RN, MS, FNP-BC
Family Nurse Practitioner
Department of Community Health Systems
University of California San Francisco, School of Nursing
San Francisco, CA

Jennifer Merrilees, RN, PhD
Health Sciences Associate Clinical Professor
Clinical Nurse Specialist
UCSF Memory and Aging Center
University of California San Francisco
San Francisco, CA

Jamie Meyerhoff, CNM, WHNP
Women's Health Nurse Practitioner
Tigerlily Women's Health & Midwifery
Carmel Valley, CA

Erica Monasterio, MN, FNP-BC
Health Sciences Clinical Professor
Director, Family Nurse Practitioner Program, Department of
    Family Health Care Nursing
Nursing Faculty, Division of Adolescent and Young Adult
    Medicine
University of California San Francisco, Schools of Nursing and
    Medicine
San Francisco, CA

Barbara Newlin, RN, MS, ANP-BC
Assistant Clinical Professor (volunteer)
Department of Community Health Systems
University of California, San Francisco, School of Nursing
San Francisco, CA

Carolina E. Noya, FNP-BC, MS
Health Sciences Assistant Clinical Professor
Department of Family Health Care Nursing
University of California San Francisco, School of Nursing
San Francisco, CA

Beth Phoenix, PhD, RN, FAAN
Health Sciences Clinical Professor
Co-Director, Psychiatric Mental Health Nurse Practitioner
    Program
Department of Community Health Systems
University of California San Francisco, School of Nursing
San Francisco, CA

Steven Protzel, PharmD
Health Sciences Associate Clinical Professor
Department of Community Health Systems
University of California San Francisco, School of Nursing
San Francisco, CA

Linda Ray, RN, MSN, ANP-BC
Adult Nurse Practitioner
Anticoagulation Clinic, UCSF Medical Center
San Francisco, CA

Assistant Clinical Professor (volunteer)
University of California San Francisco, School of Pharmacy
San Francisco, CA

Cecily Reeves, RN, MSN, PhD, FNP-C, PA-C, DFAAPA
Professor
Samuel Merritt University, School of Nursing
Oakland, CA

Mary M. Rubin, RN-C, PhD, CRNP, FAANP
Certified Registered Nurse Practitioner
Clinical Professor (retired)
Women's Health Care Specialist
Department of Obstetrics, Gynecology & Reproductive Sciences
University of California San Francisco
San Francisco, CA

JoAnne M. Saxe, RN, ANP-BC, MS, DNP, FAAN*
Health Sciences Clinical Professor
Director, Adult Gerontology Primary Care Nurse Practitioner
    Masters Specialty Program
Department of Community Health Systems
University of California San Francisco, School of Nursing
San Francisco, CA

Adult Nurse Practitioner and Faculty
San Francisco VA Medical Center
Center of Excellence in Primary Care Education
San Francisco, CA

Naomi A. Schapiro, RN, PhD, CPNP
Health Sciences Clinical Professor
Department of Family Health Care Nursing
University of California San Francisco, School of Nursing
San Francisco, CA

Rossana Segovia, RN, MS, ANP-BC, COHN-S
Associate Clinical Professor (volunteer)
University of California San Francisco, School of Nursing
San Francisco, CA

Administrative Nurse Manager
Primary Care Services
University of California San Francisco Medical Center
San Francisco, CA

Andrea Crosby Shah, RN, FNP
Assistant Clinical Professor (volunteer)
Department of Family Health Care Nursing
University of California San Francisco, School of Nursing
San Francisco, CA

Family Nurse Practitioner
Children's Health Center
San Francisco General Hospital
San Francisco, CA

Jenna Shaw-Battista, RN, PhD, NP, CNM
Health Sciences Associate Clinical Professor
Department of Family Health Care Nursing
University of California San Francisco School of Nursing
San Francisco, CA

Certified Nurse Midwife
Communicare Health Services
Davis, CA

Suzan Stringari-Murray, RN, MS, ANP-BC
Health Sciences Clinical Professor, Emerita
Department of Community Health Systems
University of California San Francisco, School of Nursing
San Francisco, CA

Miranda Surjadi, RN, MS, ANP-BC
Health Sciences Assistant Clinical Professor
Department of Community Health Systems
University of California San Francisco, School of Nursing
San Francisco, CA

Judith Sweet, MS, FNP-C, NC-BC
Adjunct Associate Professor
California Institute of Integral Studies
San Francisco, CA

Associate Clinical Professor (volunteer)
University of California San Francisco, School of Nursing
San Francisco, CA

M. Robin Taylor, MSN, FNP
Clinical Research Manager
Department of Neurology
University of California, San Francisco
San Francisco, CA

Jean N. Taylor-Woodbury, RN, MS, ANP-BC
Assistant Clinical Professor (volunteer)
Department of Community Health Systems
University of California San Francisco, School of Nursing
San Francisco, CA

Adult Nurse Practitioner
Department of Public Health
San Francisco, CA

Matthew Tierney, RN, ANP, CNS, MS
Health Sciences Associate Clinical Professor
Department of Community Health Systems
University of California, San Francisco, School of Nursing
San Francisco, CA

Nicole Una, RN, ANP-BC, MS
Adult Nurse Practitioner
Tenderloin Health Services
San Francisco, CA

Damon Michael Williams, RN, PMHNP-BC, MS
Family Psychiatric Nurse Practitioner
Portland, OR

Melissa Wong, RN, MS, AGNP-BC
Adult Gerontology Nurse Practitioner
Petaluma Health Center
Petaluma, CA

Kathryn Wyckoff, RN, MS, AGNP-BC
Adult Gerontology Nurse Practitioner
Harborview Downtown Clinics
Seattle, WA

Reviewers

Brian Alldredge, PharmD
Professor of Clinical Pharmacy & Neurology
Vice Provost, Academic Affairs
University of California San Francisco, Schools of Pharmacy and
   Medicine
San Francisco, CA

Ryan Anson, RN, MS, AGPCNP
Adult Gerontology Primary Care Nurse Practitioner
East Bay AIDS Center
Alta Bates Summit Medical Center
Oakland, CA

Amy (Meg) Autry, MD
Professor
Director of Graduate Medical Education
Department of Obstetrics, Gynecology & Reproductive Sciences
University of California San Francisco, School of Medicine
San Francisco, CA

Jessica Axelrod, RN, MS, PNP
Pediatric Nurse Practitioner
Children's Health Center
San Francisco General Hospital
San Francisco, CA

Assistant Clinical Professor (volunteer)
Department of Family Health Care Nursing
University of California San Francisco, School of Nursing
San Francisco, CA

Robert B. Baron, MD, MS
Professor of Medicine
Associate Dean for Graduate and Continuing Medical Education
University of California San Francisco, School of Medicine
San Francisco, CA

Douglas Bauer, MD
Professor
University of California San Francisco, School of Medicine
San Francisco, CA

Lisa Benaron, MD
Medical Director, Far Northern Regional Center
Board Certified in Internal Medicine, Pediatrics and
   Neurodevelopmental Disabilities
Chico, CA

Peter Berman, MD, MPH
Assistant Clinical Professor (volunteer)
Department of Family and Community Medicine
University of California San Francisco, School of Medicine
San Francisco, CA

Judith Bishop, CNM, MPH
Clinical Professor
Department of Obstetrics, Gynecology & Reproductive Sciences
University of California San Francisco, School of Medicine
San Francisco, CA

Certified Nurse Midwife (volunteer)
Department of Family Health Care Nursing
University of California San Francisco, School of Nursing
San Francisco, CA

Aaron B. Caughey, MD, MPP, MPH, PhD
Professor and Chair
Department of Obstetrics and Gynecology
Associate Dean for Women's Health Research & Policy
Oregon Health & Science University
Portland, OR

Tonya Chaffee, MD, MPH
Clinical Professor
Department of Pediatrics
University of California San Francisco, School of Medicine

Medical Director
Child and Adolescent Support Advocacy and Resource Center
  Director
Teen Services, San Francisco General Hospital
San Francisco, CA

Angelique Champeau, RN, MN, CPNP
Pediatric Nurse Practitioner
University of California San Francisco Children's Hospital
Division of Pediatric Urology
University of California San Francisco
San Francisco, CA

Jyu-Lin Chen, RN, PhD, FAAN
Associate Professor
Department of Family Health Care Nursing
University of California San Francisco, School of Nursing
San Francisco, CA

Linda Chin, MS
Consultant
Harvard T.H. Chan School of Public Health

Former President/Executive Director
Asian Task Force Against Domestic Violence
Boston, MA

Doranne Donesky, RN, PhD, ANP
Associate Adjunct Professor
Department of Physiological Nursing
Acute Care Nurse Practitioner Program
University of California San Francisco, School of Nursing
San Francisco, CA

Susannah Ewing, RN, WHNP
Women's Health Nurse Practitioner
Department of Obstetrics, Gynecology, and Reproductive
  Sciences
University of California San Francisco
San Francisco, CA

Rena K. Fox, MD
Professor of Clinical Medicine
Division of General Internal Medicine
University of California San Francisco
San Francisco, CA

Michelle S. Franklin, MSN, APRN, FNP-BC, PMHNP-BC
Family Nurse Practitioner
Life Enhancement Medical Services
Principal Investigator, Nurse Practitioner Education in
  Developmental Disabilities
Faculty, UNC-CH Carolina Institute for Developmental
  Disabilities
Chapel Hill, NC

Roxanne Garbez, RN, PhD, ACNP, CNS
Health Sciences Clinical Professor
Director, Acute Care Nurse Practitioner Program
Department of Physiological Nursing
University of California San Francisco, School of Nursing
San Francisco, CA

Courtney Giraudo, RN, MS, CNS, CPNP
Pediatric Nurse Practitioner
Whitney NICU Follow-Up Clinic
California Pacific Medical Center
San Francisco, CA

Richard Goldwasser, MD
Private Practice (specializing in child, adolescent, and adult
  psychiatry)
Mill Valley, CA

Psychiatrist Consultant
Redwood Coast & North Bay Regional Centers

Josephina T. Gomez, MSN, FNP-BC, WOCN
Family Nurse Practitioner,
Benign Pancreas Program
Stanford Digestive Health
Stanford Hospital and Clinics
Stanford, CA

Juan M. González, MD, PhD, FACOG
Assistant Professor
Division of Maternal-Fetal Medicine
Department of Obstetrics, Gynecology & Reproductive Sciences
University of California San Francisco
San Francisco, CA

Caitlin Hildebrand, MSN, AGPCNP-BC, MS-HAIL
Director of Patient Care Services for Home Health and Hospice
American Care Quest
San Francisco, CA

Nurse Practitioner & Electronic Health Record Specialist
On Lok Senior Health
San Francisco, CA

Gail Hornor, RNC, CPNP, DNP
Pediatric Nurse Practitioner
Center for Family Safety and Healing
Nationwide Children's Hospital
Columbus, OH

Kathryn Johnson, MSN, RN, PMHNP-BC
Associate Clinical Professor (volunteer)
Department of Community Health Systems
University of California San Francisco, School of Nursing
San Francisco, CA

Katherine Julian, MD
Professor of Clinical Medicine
Division of General Internal Medicine
University of California San Francisco Medical Center
San Francisco, CA

Henry Kahn, MD
Clinical Professor of Medicine
Division of General Internal Medicine

Health Sciences Clinical Professor
Department of Community Health Systems
University of California San Francisco, School of Nursing
San Francisco, CA

Steven R. Kayser, PharmD
Professor Emeritus
Department of Clinical Pharmacy
University of California, San Francisco, School of Pharmacy
San Francisco, CA

Christopher M. King, RN, MS, AGPCNP
Adult Gerontology Primary Care Nurse Practitioner
San Mateo Medical Center–Edison Clinic
National HIV/AIDS Clinician's Consultation Center
San Francisco General Hospital
University of California San Francisco
San Francisco, CA

Sharon Knight, MD
Clinical Professor
Department of Obstetrics, Gynecology & Reproductive Sciences
University of California San Francisco
San Francisco, CA

Abner Korn, MD
Professor
Director of Gynecology
San Francisco General Hospital Division
University of California San Francisco
San Francisco, CA

Charlotte Kuo, APRN-BC, ANP, CDE
Adult Nurse Practitioner
Diabetes Clinic
San Francisco General Hospital
San Francisco, CA

Catherine Lyons, NP, MSN, MPH
Nurse Practitioner (retired)
University of California San Francisco AIDS Program
San Francisco General Hospital
San Francisco, CA

Andrea Marmor, MD, MSEd
Associate Professor
Department of Pediatrics
University of California San Francisco, School of Medicine
San Francisco, CA

Erin Mathes, MD
Assistant Professor
Departments of Dermatology and Pediatrics
University of California San Francisco
San Francisco, CA

Mary Mays, FNP, CNM, MS
Health Sciences Associate Clinical Professor (volunteer)
Department of Family Health Care Nursing
University of California San Francisco, School of Nursing
San Francisco, CA

Michelle Melisko, MD
Associate Clinical Professor
Department of Medicine
University of California San Francisco, School of Medicine
San Francisco, CA

Aaron Miller, RN, MS, PMHNP
Health Sciences Assistant Clinical Professor
Department of Community Health Systems
University of California San Francisco, School of Nursing
San Francisco, CA

Carol A. Miller, MD
Clinical Professor
Department of Pediatrics
Advisory College Mentor
Miller College
University of California San Francisco, School of Medicine
San Francisco, CA

Gina Moreno-John, MD, MPH
Clinical Professor of Medicine
Division of General Internal Medicine
University of California San Francisco Medical Center
San Francisco, CA

Rebecca S. Neuwirth, RN, MSN, NP-C, WHNP-BC
Adult Nurse Practitioner and Women's Health Nurse Practitioner
Golden Gate Community Health
San Francisco, CA
Kaiser Permanente
Redwood City, CA

Don C. Ng, MD
Clinical Professor of Medicine
Medical Director, General Medicine Clinic at Osher
Division of General Internal Medicine
University of California San Francisco
San Francisco, CA

Lynn O'Brien, FNP-BC
Associate Clinical Professor (volunteer)
Department of Community Health Systems
University of California San Francisco, School of Nursing
San Francisco, CA

Family Nurse Practitioner
VA Medical Center
San Francisco, CA

Sarah B. Pawlowsky, PT, DPT, OCS
Associate Clinical Professor
San Francisco State University
Core Faculty in the UCSF/SFSU Graduate Program in Physical
Therapy
San Francisco, CA

Susan Penney, JD
Director of Medical Risk Management
University of California San Francisco Medical Center
San Francisco, CA

Yvonne Piper, MLIS, MS, RN, FNP-C
Family Nurse Practitioner
San Francisco Department of Public Health, STD Prevention and
Control (City Clinic)
San Francisco, CA

Michael S. Policar, MD, MPH
Clinical Professor of Obstetrics, Gynecology & Reproductive
Sciences
University of California San Francisco, School of Medicine
San Francisco, CA

Patricia Purcell, RN, MS, FNP
Family Nurse Practitioner
Southeast Health Center
Department of Public Health
San Francisco, CA

Neal L. Rojas, MD, MPH
Associate Clinical Professor of Pediatrics
Department of Pediatrics
University of California San Francisco, School of Medicine
San Francisco, CA

Ronald J. Ruggiero, PharmD
Pharmacist Specialist in Women's Health
Clinical Professor
Departments of Clinical Pharmacy and Obstetrics, Gynecology &
Reproductive Sciences
University of California San Francisco
San Francisco, CA

George Sawaya, MD
Professor
Department of Obstetrics, Gynecology & Reproductive Sciences
University of California San Francisco, School of Medicine
San Francisco, CA

Allyson Scott, MS, LGC
Genetic Counselor
Department of Obstetrics, Gynecology & Reproductive Sciences
University of California San Francisco Medical Center
San Francisco, CA

Suzanne Seger, CNM, MSN, MTS
Health Sciences Associate Professor (volunteer)
Departments of Obstetrics & Gynecology & Family Health Care
Nursing
University of California San Francisco
San Francisco, CA
Nurse Midwife
Tiburcio Vasquez Health Center
Hayward, CA

Dominika Seidman, MD
Associate Physician
Department of Obstetrics, Gynecology & Reproductive Sciences
University of California San Francisco, School of Medicine
San Francisco, CA

Carlin Senter, MD
Assistant Clinical Professor
Primary Care Sports Medicine
Departments of Medicine and Orthopedics
University of California, San Francisco
San Francisco, CA

Vicki Smith, RN, MS, FNP-BC, PMHNP
Assistant Clinical Professor (volunteer)
Family and Psychiatric Mental Health Nurse Practitioner
Department of Community Health Systems
University of California, San Francisco, School of Nursing
San Francisco, CA

Mari-Paule Thiet, MD
Professor and Vice Chair
Director, Division of Maternal–Fetal Medicine
Department of Obstetrics, Gynecology & Reproductive Sciences
University of California San Francisco
San Francisco, CA

Stephanie Tsao, MSN, ANP-BC
Adult Nurse Practitioner
Healthy San Francisco Asthma/COPD Program Director
San Francisco General Hospital
San Francisco, CA

Juan Vargas, MD
Professor of Clinical Obstetrics, Gynecology & Reproductive
Sciences
Professor of Clinical Radiology
University of California, San Francisco

Carol S. Viele, RN, MS, OCN
Associate Clinical Professor (volunteer)
Department of Physiological Nursing
University of California, San Francisco School of Nursing
San Francisco, CA

Laura Wagner, PhD, RN, GNP, FAAN
Assistant Professor
Department of Community Health Systems
University of California San Francisco, School of Nursing
San Francisco, CA

Sharon Wiener, RN, MPH, CNM
Health Sciences Clinical Professor
Department of Obstetrics, Gynecology & Reproductive Sciences
University of California San Francisco
San Francisco, CA

Elisabeth Wilson, MD, MPH
Professor
Department of Family and Community Medicine
University of California San Francisco, School of Medicine
San Francisco, CA

Allen Wong, DDS, EdD
Professor and Director, AEGD Program
Director, Hospital Dentistry Program
University of the Pacific Dugoni School of Dentistry
San Francisco, CA

Mary Wong, RN, MSN, ANP-BC
Adult Nurse Practitioner
Division of Cardiology
University of California San Francisco Medical Center
San Francisco, CA

---

* Indicates they are both an author and a reviewer.

INTRODUCTION

Welcome to the third edition of our clinical guidelines text for advanced practice nurses and other clinicians in primary care. This new text, *Clinical Guidelines for Advanced Practice Nursing: An Interprofessional Approach, Third Edition*, builds upon the pioneering work of nurse practitioners, certified nurse–midwives, and clinical nurse specialists that began over 35 years ago in the Ambulatory Care Center at the University of California, San Francisco. The initial clinical guidelines work focused on meeting regulatory requirements for practice, targeting across the lifespan health promotion and common health problems seen in primary care settings.

In the second edition, the editors and contributing authors wrote evidence-supported clinical guidelines on common, *complex chronic health problems* and included chapters on health promotion for select vulnerable populations (adults with developmental disabilities and transgendered individuals).

In *this edition*, we have continued to focus on *complex chronic health problems* and have scrubbed and revised all the chapters with the most current evidence-supported information. Based upon feedback from a select group of readers of the second edition, we enthusiastically added several new chapters that address prevalent and often problematic chronic issues in primary care: childhood obesity, HIV PrEP, cancer survivorship, geriatric syndromes, and lipid disorders. Many of the previous edition chapters have undergone extensive revision: abnormal uterine bleeding, hormonal contraception, prenatal genetic screening, and immunizations to name a few.

Our text strives to integrate an interprofessional approach to clinical decision making and thus is a collaborative effort with contributions from a rich variety of disciplines: nursing, pharmacy, medicine, dentistry, nutrition, physical therapy, genetic counseling, and the legal profession. This text includes:

- Sections on pediatrics, women's health, obstetrics, and adult medicine
- S-O-A-P (Subjective-Objective-Assessment-Plan) formatting for easy reference
- Client/patient educational resources to enhance self-management efforts
- Recommendations for situations when advanced practice nurses should consider physician or specialty consultation
- Access to online decision support and patient self-management resources and tools via the Jones & Bartlett Learning web-based library
- Section on legal scope of practice for advanced practice nurses

Our hope is that this text will provide a substantial and timely resource for a variety of busy clinicians. We also anticipate that this text will be an important addition to decision support toolkits that clinicians rely upon for providing individualized, patient-centered, team-based care.

"Let us always be open to acknowledge, respect, and learn from great leaders in any field or discipline. Let us always be able to critique the work of any leader to move forward ideas and substantive knowledge for the betterment of humanity. For, indeed, great progress is largely contingent upon thoughtful reflections, critiques, and the creative use of worthwhile ideas."

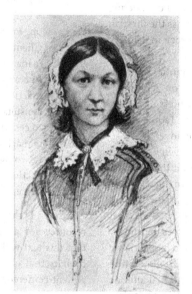

Courtesy of U.S. National Library of Medicine.

—Florence Nightingale

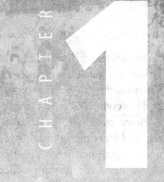

LEGAL SCOPE OF ADVANCED NURSING PRACTICE

CHAPTER 1

Brian Budds and JoAnne M. Saxe

▌INTRODUCTION AND GENERAL BACKGROUND

Nurses, like all healthcare professionals, must act within the scope of practice as outlined in statutes and regulations. Failure to comply with this by exceeding the permissible scope of practice could result in professional discipline or even criminal prosecution. Advanced practice nurses (e.g., clinical nurse specialists, nurse anesthetists, nurse midwives, or nurse practitioners) frequently encounter issues related to the scope of their practice.

These issues may arise as part of the individual nurse's ethical and professional concern or as a result of professional "friction" between nursing and other healthcare professions. This is especially so when the advanced practice nurse's scope overlaps with areas that have traditionally been viewed as the practice of medicine. Regardless of what may trigger such concerns, it is imperative that advanced practice nurses and practice managers know how to ascertain what is and is not part of their scope of practice and what actions they may need to take to be in compliance with the applicable law or regulation. Clear understanding of one's scope of practice, which may in some states be defined by protocols or procedures, can lead to enhanced collaboration among professionals, decreased professional tension, and safer, more effective provision of health care in clinical settings.

Two key questions emerge when considering the issue of advanced practice nursing and scopes of practice. The first is the extent of what one, by virtue of being an advanced practice nurse, can do. Thus, the advanced practice nurse—or perhaps the clinical manager of a setting in which the advanced practice nurse is working or a collaborating physician—wants to know the duties an advanced practice nurse may legally perform. Second, one must understand what constitutes the outer boundaries of a clinician's scope of practice. For example, one must know if there needs to be a supervisory relationship and, if so, of what nature and how it should be documented.

Of course, it would be wonderful if those answers were always clear, concise, and readily available. Although that may occasionally be the case, it is not the rule. As such, this chapter outlines for advanced practice nurses and those responsible for the management of advanced nursing practice in the clinical setting how to approach these questions and where to begin to find the information necessary to properly understand the limits of one's scope of practice and what steps need to be taken to ensure that one's practice is consistent with the appropriate legal framework.

In a number of states, it is necessary for nurses to develop written documentation to support their expanded practice. Different states use different terms to describe these documents and require different specific elements be addressed. In most cases, the specific requirements for each state can be found in statutes or regulations, as discussed later. An explanation of practice guidelines, such as *Standardized Procedures* that are used in California, can be viewed at http://www.rn.ca.gov/pdfs/regulations/npr-b-20.pdf.

▌OVERVIEW OF SCOPE OF PRACTICE LEGAL FRAMEWORK

▌*State Regulation of Professional Practice*

Control of the scope of practice of healthcare professionals rests at the level of state government. Although there are some areas of professional practice—including those relating to the advanced practice nursing roles—for which federal regulations have an impact, the basic definitions and limits of professional practice are determined at the state level.

This can sometimes lead to confusion. For example, some federal regulations dealing with reimbursement requirements for federally funded programs, such as Medicare and Medicaid, do address what can or should be done by advanced practice nurses. One such example is found in the Medicare Conditions of Participation for Rural Health Clinics (2013).[1] The regulations require that

---

[1] 42 CFR 491 et seq. This citation is to the Code of Federal Regulations. This particular chapter of the code addresses the regulations applied to healthcare providers who participate in the Medicare Program. These regulations can be accessed at the website of the Centers for Medicare and Medicaid, https://www.cms.gov/Medicare/Provider-Enrollment-and-Certification/CertificationandComplianc/RHCs.html

participating rural health clinic staff include one or more physician assistants or nurse practitioners. They further require that the physician assistant or nurse practitioner work with the physician on staff to develop and review clinic policies.

However, although compliance with these federal regulations is required for reimbursement for services, the individual healthcare practitioner's practice is directly regulated by the state in which she or he is licensed to practice. Thus, although the Medicare Conditions of Participation (2013) may not require that advanced practice nurses work with physicians in these settings, the rules governing who can become a nurse practitioner and what scope of practice the person has are set by the individual states and are subject to significant variation from state to state.

The Patient Protection and Affordable Care Act (PPACA) and its approach to accountable care organizations (ACO) demonstrate how this federal role continues to develop. The law identifies nurse practitioners among the provider types who can be considered ACO professionals, a designation that permits Medicare patients to receive care under this program and providers to share in savings. In enacting PPACA, Congress anticipated an extraordinary increase in the number of persons covered by the act and also predicted that there would be a shortage of physicians to care for these patients. Accordingly, the PPACA contemplated the expanded role of nurse practitioners. However, the initial assignment of particular Medicare beneficiaries to specific ACO entities has been limited to those beneficiaries who receive care from physicians. (Kendig, 2014).

In response to input from many sources, the Obama Administration has proposed new federal rules to address, among other things, the assignment of beneficiaries to these ACOs even if the beneficiary receives primary care from a nonphysician provider (Medicare Program, 2014). Though not yet resolved, this issue reminds us that federal rulemaking can have an impact on our local practice. Although states clearly retain the right to define and regulate professional scope of practice in their jurisdiction, the federal reimbursement rules can have a pragmatic, indirect role in determining what each provider may do.

Sources: Statutes

There are several sources of authority for the regulation of professional practice within states (and other jurisdictions within the United States). The most basic and important of these are statutes. Statutes are laws or acts passed by the legislative body of a particular jurisdiction. As such, statutes represent the voice of the people's elected representatives with regard to permissible activities.

Each state enacts a professional practice act addressing the specific health professions within the jurisdiction. In general, these statutes define the training requirements of healthcare professionals and what behaviors are allowed in the practice of the profession. For example, the State of California sets the basic legal framework for the practice of nursing in its Business and Professions Code (Nursing Practice Act, 2012). Similarly, the provisions for the practice of medicine, physical therapy, dentistry, and so forth are found in other sections of the Business and Professions Code.

Although not universally the case, most of these laws—known as practice acts—are relatively easy to locate. Most states have some board or agency charged with the regulation of each of the specific healthcare professions. Using California as an example, the statutes governing the practice of nursing authorize the Board of Registered Nursing to manage the practice of nursing within California. This state agency has a website (http://www.rn.ca .gov) on which it makes available links to the specific statutes relating to the practice of nursing within California (California Board of Registered Nursing, 2013). An interactive list allowing one to link to boards of registered nursing throughout the country can be found at the website of the National Council of State Boards of Nursing (2014) at https://www.ncsbn.org/115.htm.

When looking at state statutes to understand issues relating to scope of practice, it should be kept in mind that statutes may be written in fairly general and expansive language rather than in point-by-point details. One can think of the statutes as setting out the broad parameters of a professional practice without spelling out each particular specific aspect of the practice. Accordingly, statutes may be subject to interpretation, which could lead to differing opinions as to what conduct is within or outside the scope of practice. Examples of the broad language include this excerpt from the Washington State statute defining advanced practice nursing:

> *Advanced registered nursing practice* means the performance of the acts of a registered nurse and the performance of an expanded role in providing healthcare services as recognized by the medical and nursing professions, the scope of which is defined by rule by the commission. Upon approval by the commission, an advanced registered nurse practitioner may prescribe legend drugs and controlled substances contained in Schedule V of the Uniform Controlled Substances Act, chapter 69.50 RCW, and Schedules II through IV subject to RCW 18.79.240(1)(r) or (s).
>
> Nothing in this section prohibits a person from practicing a profession for which a license has been issued under the laws of this state or specifically authorized by any other law of the state of Washington.
>
> This section does not prohibit (1) the nursing care of the sick, without compensation, by an unlicensed person who does not hold himself or herself out to be an advanced registered nurse practitioner, or (2) the practice of registered nursing by a licensed registered nurse or the practice of licensed practical nursing by a licensed practical nurse. (Revised Code of Washington, 2000)

Sources: Regulations

Another authority for the control of advanced nursing practice can be found in regulations, which like statutes have the force of law. Regulations are not the result of the legislative process but rather rules or orders issued by an arm of government, such as a particular agency. The process of developing regulations typically involves those who have particular expertise in an area drawing up specific rules, making them available for public comment, and then promulgating or issuing them publicly.

Because regulations are often developed by the agency or arm of government closest to the actual profession, they often are more detailed and specific than statutes. Regulations often spell out the details of how to implement the vision of the legislature as stated in the statutes.

State health boards often provide links to scope of practice regulations. However, it is easier to find these links in some states than in others. Should it be difficult to find a direct link to an individual state's law and regulations, the reader may choose to do an Internet search on such terms as "advanced practice nursing statutes" or "nursing regulations" and the particular state's name. Should this not help, one could always call the particular licensing agency and ask how to access the statutes and regulations governing nursing or the specific aspect of advanced practice nursing in which one is interested.

Like statutes, regulations are readily available to the public. For example, in California, regulations addressing the practice of nursing are found in the California Code of Regulations (California Legislative Information, n.d.). Regulations in Title 16 address details relating to the practice of health professions, whereas those in Title 22 regulate how health care is provided in licensed institutions. Both require specific language. An example is the regulation describing what must appear in a "standardized procedure" document, required to allow registered nurses to practice beyond their usual scope of practice.

The website of a particular state's agency charged with the regulation of healthcare professionals often has links to the state regulations surrounding a particular profession available on that website. For example, the Commonwealth of Massachusetts Board of Registration in Nursing has its website as part of the larger Health and Human Services Agency's section of the state government website (www.mass.gov). Selecting "Nursing" from the "A-Z Topic Index," one can choose the link to "Statutes, Rules and Regulations" (Commonwealth of Massachusetts, 2014).

Sources: Statements of Regulatory Agencies

Unfortunately, even a thorough reading and analysis of all pertinent statutes and regulations may not yield a definitive answer to all questions regarding one's scope of practice. The issue in question may be complex enough that a simple answer may not be available in the statutes and regulations. For example, it may not be precisely clear what an advanced practice nurse may do in a very specific clinical setting under specific circumstances.

When this is the case, the governing body (e.g., Board of Registered Nursing) may issue an advisory statement or some sort of information addressing the specific concern. These statements can be extremely helpful in allowing clinical practices and individual practitioners to understand what is permissible or required in a particular circumstance.

For example, the California Board of Registered Nursing makes multiple documents and sources of information about these issues available on its website (California Board of Registered Nursing, 2013). Among the documents listed, the board has made available a statement helping to explain the statutes and regulations in regard to the roles of nurse practitioners and certified nurse specialists working in long-term-care settings (California Board of Registered Nursing, 2011).

Although this kind of statement can be extremely helpful in understanding the complexities of the statutes and regulations, it does not of itself have the force of law. Even so, should a practice issue ever come to the point of being litigated, courts may be inclined to give deference to the statement of specific regulatory agencies. In professional disciplinary actions, a licensing board may attempt to use such advisory statements as a basis for establishing gross negligence and incompetence.

Sources: Attorney General Opinions

In some circumstances, issues are very complex and even contentious. Sometimes these situations result in an agency or some member of government seeking an official opinion from the state's attorney general to clarify issues. This may often be the case when there has been substantial change in existing statutes and regulations that has led to confusion or even turf battles between organized medicine and advanced practice nurses.

One example of this can be found in an opinion of the State of Michigan Attorney General (1980) about the ability of physicians to grant "unlimited authority" to advanced practice nurses to prescribe medications. One can see in reading this opinion the evolution of Michigan law that led to confusion about just how much authority may be delegated and under what circumstances.

In this example, a member of the state legislature asked the attorney general to issue an opinion. As is often the case, the opinion carefully lays out what the issues are and what the history has been that has led to the question. Then, the attorney general issues an opinion as to how she or he understands the law.

Like the statements of the regulatory agencies, an attorney general's opinion does not carry the force of law. That is to say, such an opinion does not necessarily fully resolve the issue at controversy. However, courts routinely grant "great respect" or "great weight" to the opinions of attorneys general in cases that come before them. Thus, such opinions often have the power to effectively resolve a particular issue within a jurisdiction.

Sources: Statements of Professional Organizations

Professional organizations that represent the interest of advanced practice nurses may issue statements or information about a particular topic related to scope of practice. As with the other opinions cited here, these opinions or statements, although often very helpful, do not carry the force of law. One thing to keep in mind is that often these statements may be issued by the organization in its role as an advocate for the particular profession or advanced practice role. These position papers may occasionally be at odds with practice guidelines issued by physician advocacy groups and be a source of controversy in a medical legal case. Thus, within any treatment setting, it is important to consider a wide range of sources in developing standards, protocols, or policies.

A particularly helpful service offered by many professional organizations is a regular legislative update. These updates often review legislation that has been passed or proposed within a year and that affects the particular area of practice covered by the organization. These updates, rather than clarify specific issues, are intended to inform readers of new laws and regulations and potential trends within the states. For example, a 2014 American Association of Nurse Practitioners report provides notes on the practice environment by each state (full practice, reduced practice, and restricted practice) along with legislative alerts.

▌ *Other Sources*

There are other sources available to help understand scope of practice issues as they relate to advanced practice nursing. Two deserve at least a brief mention as part of this discussion.

The Center for the Health Professions is part of the University of California, San Francisco. The center engages in numerous activities to improve health care through research and development projects. Among their efforts has been research into scope of practice of health professionals. Their publication, *Overview of Nurse Practitioner Scopes of Practice in the United States—Discussion*, is a very valuable tool for understanding the state of scope of practice regulation and for accessing particular information (Christian, Dower, & O'Neill, 2007).

Another valuable tool is a textbook devoted to issues relating to nurse practitioner practice and legal issues. Carolyn Buppert's (2015) *Nurse Practitioner's Business Practice and Legal Guide* addresses, among other topics, details about state regulation of nurse practitioner practice. It is hoped that this discussion orients advanced practice nurses to the resources for determining and understanding their particular scope of practice.

▌ ISSUES RELATED TO COLLABORATIVE PRACTICE AND DOCUMENTATION

Once the advanced practice nurse has been able to identify the resources for understanding scope of practice, it is imperative to determine the level of independence with which she or he can practice and the level of collaboration that is required by her or his jurisdiction. Furthermore, if there are requirements related to collaborative practice, one needs to be able to determine how to meet and appropriately document those requirements.

It has been widely noted that there is significant disparity in the terminology used to describe advanced practice nursing. For example, statutory language describing the nature of the required relationship between advanced practice nurses and physicians can include such terms as "supervise," "collaboration with," "delegate,"

and even "collegial working relationship" (Ritter & Hansen-Turton, 2008). Furthermore, we have already seen that the nature of this relationship can lead—as it did in Michigan—to repeated changes in legislation and regulation that, in the end, required an attorney general opinion to sort it out.

Although not a comprehensive list, the following issues are offered as a guide for understanding the possible requirements and methods of documenting compliance. Practitioners should consider each of these areas when attempting to set up practice or understand the extent of their scope of practice.

▌ *Fully Independent Practice*

As of 2014, 19 states and the District of Columbia allowed nurse practitioners to practice independently of physicians (American Association of Nurse Practitioners, 2014). That is, in such states, the nurse practitioner is permitted to diagnose, treat, and prescribe medications without supervision by or collaboration with a physician. Alaska, Oregon, and Washington are examples of states that have this kind of broad scope of practice.

▌ *Some Collaboration, Supervision, or Delegation Required*

Most states require documentation of some sort of relationship with physician colleagues for the advanced practice nurse to practice within that scope of practice. The nature of the "collaboration," "supervision," or "delegation" may vary significantly from state to state.

Many states with this kind of requirement also require that there be a written agreement that sets forth the terms under which this relationship is defined. California's requirement of standardized procedures is an example of this need.

▌ *Collaboration or Supervision or Delegation Necessary for the Advanced Practice Nurse to Prescribe Medications in Most States*

Apart from the other elements of advanced practice nursing, such as diagnosis, ordering of diagnostic tests, and ordering of treatments, the issue of prescribing medications can be particularly difficult. The history of political and legislative difficulties in approaching this issue has been well documented elsewhere. The key issue here is that the advanced practice nurse wishing to have prescribing as part of her or his practice needs to be sure that all particular scope of practice requirements are met.

In some states, advanced practice nurses' prescriptive/drug authority is delegated by a physician (e.g., Texas [Texas Board of Nursing, 2013]). Other states (e.g., California) require advanced practice nurses to have signed prescriptive agreements to prescribe, order, or furnish drugs (California Board of Registered Nursing, 2013). An example of this is found in the Texas legal framework, which allows for advanced practice without a written prescriptive agreement but requires one for the advanced practice nurse to be able to prescribe (Texas Board of Nursing, 2013).

Precise Nature of the Supervision or Collaboration Required

In situations in which a supervisory or collaborative relationship is required, advanced practice nurses and physicians need to understand the precise nature of what is required. Furthermore, when that relationship requires documentation, as in a collaborative practice agreement or a standardized procedure, the nature of the relationship should be spelled out in the agreement. It is advisable to review the agreement on a regular basis to ensure continued understanding of the respective roles and responsibilities.

State regulations may spell out what needs to be included in such an agreement and can be very helpful in drafting such an agreement. North Carolina's regulations are an example of how one can find excellent guidance in translating the statutes and the regulations into a workable document (North Carolina Board of Nursing, 2014). Issues that may arise or need to be documented properly include the following:

1. On-site supervision requirements: Only a few jurisdictions require that a physician supervisor be physically present. When practicing in those states, advanced practice nurses should be aware of and document regulations relating to:

   ▶ Length of time (i.e., percentage of working day) that the supervisor must be on site

   ▶ What precisely constitutes "on site" within that jurisdiction

   ▶ Whether there exist any exemption or modified requirements for working in a particular area, such as remote rural setting or medically underserved setting

2. Chart review: A small number of jurisdictions require some level of advanced practice nurse chart review by collaborating physicians. In those states, attention should be paid to:

   ▶ The precise number or percentage of charts required to be reviewed in a specific period of time

   ▶ What constitutes a need for review and how it is to be documented

   ▶ Whether there is a particular type of chart (e.g., one involving an adverse outcome) that requires review

3. Limitations on oversight for the collaborating physician:

   ▶ In jurisdictions and settings that require some sort of physician oversight, the question necessarily arises as to how many practitioners may be supervised by a particular physician. These issues may arise in terms of the number of nurse practitioners with whom a physician may enter into a collaborative relationship, the number of individual practitioners who may be supervised at one time in an on-site situation, and other settings. For example, the question arises in those jurisdictions that require anesthesiologist supervision of certified nurse anesthetists.

   ▶ Advanced practice nurses and those physicians with whom they enter into collaborative relationships should be clear about the specific limitations and requirements of the oversight required. In those jurisdictions and situations that require documentation of this relationship, it should be made clear in the practice agreement how many individuals are to be supervised and in what manner.

CONCLUDING REMARKS

From this discussion, the reader should appreciate three important themes about the legal scope of advanced nursing practice and clinical guidelines:

1. The advanced practice nurse must have a thorough understanding of the respective state's nurse practice act. There are several sources that provide context for one's professional scope of practice.

2. The advanced practice nurse must be able to clearly communicate with other registered nurses, physicians, healthcare administrators, and healthcare consumers their scope of nursing practice.

3. The advanced practice nurse must communicate, often in writing, the legal scope of their practice in a clear, concise, and flexible manner that is in keeping with regulatory law and community standards.

REFERENCES

American Association of Nurse Practitioners. (2014). *State practice environment*. Retrieved from http://www.aanp.org/legislation-regulation /state-legislation-regulation/state-practice-environment.

Buppert, C. (2015). *Nurse practitioner's business practice and legal guide* (5th ed.). Burlington, MA: Jones and Bartlett Learning.

California Board of Registered Nursing. (2011). *Nurse practitioners in long-term care settings*. Retrieved from http://rn.ca.gov/pdfs/regulations /npr-b-22.pdf.

California Board of Registered Nursing. (2013). *Nurse practitioner practice information*. Retrieved from http://rn.ca.gov/regulations/np.shtml.

California Legislative Information (n.d.). Retrieved from http://leginfo .legislature.ca.gov/faces/codes.xhtml.

Christian, S., Dower, C., & O'Neill, E. (2007). *Overview of nurse practitioner scopes of practice in the United States*. Retrieved from http:// futurehealth.ucsf.edu/Public/Publications-and-Resources/Content .aspx?topic=Overview_of_Nurse_Practitioner_Scopes_of _Practice_in_the_United_States.

Commonwealth of Massachusetts. (2014). *Nursing licensing; Statutes, rules, regulations and policies*. Retrieved from http://www.mass.gov/eohhs /gov/departments/dph/programs/hcq/dhpl/nursing/nursing-regs/.

Kendig, S. M. (2014). Moving toward accountable care: A policy framework to transform health care delivery and reimbursement. In K.A. Goudreau & M. C. Smolenski (Eds.), *Health policy and advanced practice nursing: Impact and implementations* (pp. 273–286). New York, NY: Springer Publishing Company.

Medicare Conditions of Participation, 42 C.F.R. §§491 et seq. (2013). Retrieved from https://www.cms.gov/Medicare/Provider-Enrollment-and-Certification/CertificationandComplianc/RHCs.html.

Medicare Program; Medicare Shared Savings Program: Accountable Care Organizations, 79 Fed. Reg. 72760 (proposed December 8, 2014).

National Council of State Boards of Nursing. (2014). Retrieved from https://www.ncsbn.org/115.htm.

North Carolina Board of Nursing. (2014). *Collaborative practice agreement—A guide for implementation.* Retrieved from http://www.ncbon.com/dcp/i/nursing-practice-nurse-practitioner-collaborative-practice-guidelines.

Nursing Practice Act, Cal. Bus. & Prof. Code §§2700 et seq. (2012). Retrieved from http://leginfo.legislature.ca.gov/faces/codes.xhtml.

Revised Code of Washington §18.79.050. (2000). *Advanced registered nursing practice defined—Exceptions.* Retrieved from http://apps.leg.wa.gov/rcw/default.aspx?cite=18.79.050.

Ritter, A., & Hansen-Turton, T. (2008). The primary care paradigm shift: An overview of the state-level legal framework governing nurse practitioner practice. *The Health Lawyer, 20*(4), 21.

State of Michigan. Op. Att'y Gen. No. 5630. (1980, January 22). Retrieved from http://www.ag.state.mi.us/opinion/datafiles/1980s/op05630.htm.

Texas Board of Nursing. (2013). *Texas Board of Nursing Bulletin, 44*(4).

FIRST WELL-BABY VISIT

CHAPTER 2

Annette Carley

I. Introduction and general background

The birth of a child creates new challenges for a family. The initial outpatient visit affords the provider an opportunity to establish an ongoing relationship with the infant and family, follow up on residual issues from birth, and individualize and prioritize healthcare needs. For healthy infants, the American Academy of Pediatrics recommends that this initial visit occur within the first week following discharge, dependent on the duration of the initial hospitalization (Hagan, Shaw, & Duncan, 2008).

A. Follow-up of healthy infant after vaginal or cesarean delivery

1. For vaginal delivery, discharge typically at 48 hours: follow-up should occur within 48 hours of discharge (Benitz & Committee on Fetus & Newborn, 2015).

2. For cesarean delivery, where discharge typically occurs at 96 hours, follow-up should occur within 1 week of discharge (Hagan et al., 2008).

B. Follow-up of infant after early discharge

1. Early discharge (i.e., hospital discharge between 24 and 48 hours) may be offered to healthy singleton infants, born at 37–41 weeks gestation, who are appropriately grown for gestational age, have no abnormal physical findings, and who were born vaginally after an uncomplicated prenatal course. Family, environmental, and social risks should be identified and addressed. Before discharge, the infant must have completed a minimum of two successful feedings, had such issues as jaundice (if present) adequately addressed and demonstrated adequate voiding and stooling (Committee on Fetus & Newborn, 2010; Benitz et al., 2015). However, normal newborns may not void or stool within the first day of life. If discharge of the otherwise normal infant who has not voided or stooled is being considered, a documented plan for follow-up must be ensured and parents instructed about findings that warrant immediate follow-up (e.g., vomiting, inconsolability, or abdominal distention).

2. Plan for follow-up care should be confirmed and documented before discharge (Benitz et al., 2015; Hagan et al., 2008).

C. Follow-up of premature and late premature infant after discharge

1. Premature infants less than 37 weeks gestational age are commonly discharged at or near their due date. At discharge, they should demonstrate cardiorespiratory, hemodynamic, and thermal stability and adequate weight gain. Exact standards for discharge are lacking but most centers consider discharge after completion of the 35th to 37th postconceptual week and stabilization of weight at 1,800–2,000 g.

   a. Those with a complicated clinical course or birth weight less than 1,500 g are typically also followed by a specialty clinic versed in premature infant care and outcome.

2. Late preterm (i.e., 34–37 weeks gestation), also known as "near-term" infants, are frequently discharged using the same guidelines as term infants; however, this may underestimate some ongoing needs because of their immaturity or small size. Although no clear recommendations exist for timing of follow-up, the initial outpatient visit should occur no later than the first week following discharge.

3. Enhanced risks in this population that may complicate the early neonatal period or result in rehospitalization after discharge include hyperbilirubinemia, poor feeding, dehydration sepsis, and respiratory and thermal instability (National Perinatal Association, n.d.; Whyte & Canadian Paediatric Society, Fetus & Newborn Committee, 2010).

II. **Database** (may include but is not limited to)

A. Subjective

1. History and review of systems
   a. Parental concerns including feelings of readiness, stress, adequacy, and support
   b. Birth and health history to date
      i. Maternal age, gravida, and parity
      ii. Pregnancy complications, including substance exposure, infections, hypertensive disorders, gestational diabetes, and poor prenatal care
      iii. Duration of labor, delivery method, complications, use of anesthesia, timing of umbilical cord clamping
      iv. Birth complications, including premature rupture of membranes, meconium, need for resuscitation, and low Apgar scores at birth
      v. Birth date
      vi. Gestational age
      vii. Birth weight
      viii. Review of pertinent maternal and newborn lab work, including blood type and Coombs testing and bilirubin (if indicated)
      ix. Discharge weight and age at discharge
      x. Nursery complications, including jaundice
   c. Family, social, and environmental history
      i. Mother's age, health, occupation, level of education and literacy
      ii. Father's age, health, occupation, level of education and literacy
      iii. Siblings' age and health
      iv. Family history including such conditions as asthma, allergies, atopic dermatitis, chronic lung disease, diabetes, renal dysfunction, mental health disorders, heart disease, hematologic disorders, and tuberculosis
      v. Social or environmental concerns, such as unemployment, marital problems, physical abuse, substance exposure, and adjustment to newborn in home
      vi. Family source of support and religious affiliation
   d. Nutrition history
      i. Bottle-feeding infants: type, frequency, and volume of feedings; proper preparation of formula; strength of suck; burping
      ii. Breastfeeding infants: frequency; duration; perceived satiety; strength of suck; one versus two breasts used for feeding; maternal breast fullness before and after feeding; use of breast pump; use of other devices, such as breast shields or supplemental nursing systems; care of milk including labeling, storing (refrigerator vs. freezer), and rewarming
   e. Review of systems and clinical findings

B. Objective

1. Physical examination findings
   a. Skin: turgor, color, perfusion; note presence of rashes, birthmarks, dermal breaks, skin tags or pits, or jaundice
   b. Head–eyes–ears–nose–throat–mouth
      i. Assess size, shape, symmetry of head and fontanels; note presence of cephalohematoma, caput, or cranial molding
      ii. Assess red reflex, ocular mobility; note scleral color and presence of ocular opacification, drainage, and dacryostenosis
      iii. Assess nares patency, drainage, and symmetry of septum
      iv. Assess placement of ears, external shape/contour, patency of canals. Note natural accumulation of vernix may obscure assessment of tympanic membranes in the early neonatal period.
      v. Assess intactness of palate, strength of suck, presence of natal teeth, inclusion cysts
   c. Chest and thorax
      i. Assess character of respirations; respiratory rate (normal 30–60 breaths per minute); shape and contour of thorax; breast size and shape; note presence of chest asymmetry, nipple discharge, or tenderness. Assess for increased work of breathing, including retractions and abnormal lung sounds on auscultation.
   d. Cardiovascular
      i. Assess heart rate (normal 100–180 beats per minute), rhythm, perfusion, quality of pulses; note presence of arrhythmias or murmurs
   e. Abdomen and rectum
      i. Assess symmetry, tone, presence of bowel sounds, anal patency, timing of first stool, stage of umbilical healing; note presence of distension and tenderness
      ii. Assess liver size and note presence of hepatomegaly
   f. Genitourinary
      i. Assess appearance of external genitalia, timing of first void, voiding pattern, kidney size by palpation (normally 4–5 cm in size);

note presence of ambiguous genitalia or abnormal kidney size

    g. Musculoskeletal

        i. Assess extremities, presence of digits, intactness of spine, movement and stability of hips; note presence of deviation of gluteal cleft, hair tufts, or sacral dimple; note presence of click or clunk with hip exam

    h. Neurobehavioral

        i. Assess activity, tone, state regulation, and symmetry of movements; note presence of clonus, irritability, inconsolability, or excess sleepiness or difficulty awakening (Hagan et al., 2008; Tappero & Honeyfield, 2015)

2. Establish a growth trend, including comparative measurements of head circumference, weight, and length from birth, and adjust for gestational age as indicated (Hagan et al., 2008). The Centers for Disease Control and Prevention (CDC) recommend World Health Organization (WHO) growth records to be used for infants up to 2 years of age (Centers for Disease Control & Prevention, 2010).

3. Observe parent–child interactions, including holding, comforting, responsiveness, confidence, and mutual support. Assess for evidence of parental depression including use of Edinburgh Postnatal Depression Scale (EPDS) (Earls & Committee on Psychosocial Aspects of Child & Family Health, 2010).

4. Review supportive data from relevant diagnostic tests including:

    a. Results of neonatal screening. All states require newborn blood screening and screen for at least 26 of the 31 recommended conditions including organic acid disorders, fatty acid oxidation disorders, amino acid metabolism disorders, hemoglobinopathies, and others, differing by state (March of Dimes, 2012).

        i. Phenylketonuria (PKU) screening should occur after 24 hours of age, but less than the seventh postnatal day. If done before 24 hours of age, the infant must be rescreened to eliminate erroneous results (U.S. Preventive Health Services Task Force, 2014a).

        ii. Sickle cell screening should occur before discharge, with confirmation of positive results before 2 months of age (U.S. Preventive Health Services Task Force, 2014b).

        iii. Congenital hypothyroid screening is done at the second to fourth postnatal day or immediately before discharge if discharge occurs before 48 hours of age (U.S. Preventive Services Task Force, 2008).

    b. Hearing screen recommended, although not mandated, for all infants within the first month of age (American Academy of Pediatrics, n.d.) and ideally before discharge (Centers for Disease Control & Prevention, 2015).

    c. Screening for the presence of a critical congenital heart defect (CCHD) using pulse oximetry recommended, though not mandated, to improve early detection in the early newborn period (Mahle et al., 2012).

    d. Ongoing monitoring for the development of jaundice. All newborns who develop jaundice within 24 hours of birth should have direct serologic or transcutaneous bilirubin assessment and a management plan established (Muchowski, 2014; Subcommittee on Hyperbilirubinemia, 2004). The National Perinatal Association further recommends that preterm/late preterm infants have direct bilirubin assessment (serum or transcutaneous testing) at 24 hours of age and prior to discharge (National Perinatal Association, n.d.; Phillips, 2013).

    e. Immunizations deferred until 2 months postnatal age, except hepatitis B vaccine, which is recommended for all infants before 1 month. If immunization is received at birth, follow CDC recommendations for subsequent dosing found at: http://www.cdc.gov/vaccines/schedules/ (Centers for Disease Control & Prevention, 2015).

III. Assessment

A. Determine the diagnosis

Determine client's current health status, and identify general health risks based on gender, age, ethnicity, or other factors.

B. Motivation and ability

Determine caregiver and family willingness and ability to follow through with treatment plans.

IV. Goals of first well-baby visit

A. Screening or diagnosing

Choose a practical, cost-effective approach to screening and diagnosis, while abiding by mandated screening protocols.

B. Treatment

Select a treatment plan that achieves appropriate growth and development, is individualized for the caregiver and child, and maximizes caregiver compliance.

V. Plan

A. Screening

Elicit a thorough history and perform a thorough physical examination, with growth and development assessments at the initial and all well-child visits.

B. Diagnostic tests

1. Newborn screening as required by individual state but must include assessment for congenital hypothyroidism, phenylketonuria, and sickle cell.

2. Hearing screen recommended though not yet mandated (American Academy of Pediatrics, n.d.; Centers for Disease Control & Prevention, 2015).

C. Client education and anticipatory guidance (Hagan et al., 2008)

1. Nutrition
   a. Support the mother's nutritional needs for calories, liquids, adequate rest, and emotional and social support.
   b. Encourage breastfeeding or support bottle feeding as indicated.
   c. Milk intake considered adequate if baby has five to eight wet diapers and three to four stools per day and is gaining weight appropriately (15 g/kg/day) (U.S. National Library of Medicine, 2013). Initial stools with breastfeeding may be loose and after each feeding.
   d. Healthy infants should need no extra water, because both breast milk and formula provide adequate fluid for the newborn.
   e. Exclusive breastfeeding considered the ideal source of nutrition for the first 4–6 months; for formula feeders, always use iron-fortified formula, and provide 2–3 oz. every 2–3 hours; increase if infant seems hungry.
   f. Counsel about safety with milk preparation and storage.

2. Growth and development

3. Safety, including use of car seats; exposures, such as tobacco; back-to-sleep; cardiopulmonary resuscitation; when to call the provider; and illness prevention.

4. Referrals as indicated, including encouraging mother to seek appropriate postpartum follow-up for herself.

5. Women, Infants, & Children (WIC) referral should be initiated for eligible families.

6. Family transition to parenthood and well-being, including obtaining adequate rest and developing routines.

VI. Resources and tools

A. Patient and client education

1. The American Academy of Pediatrics website contains a variety of links of interest to parents, including the *Healthy Children* resources. https://www.healthychildren.org/English/Pages/default.aspx.

2. The American Academy of Family Physicians sponsors a website called Family Doctor.org, which provides resources and links of interest to parents. www.familydoctor.org.

3. The National Institutes of Health sponsors a website, MedlinePlus, that contains infant and newborn care resources for parents. http://www.nlm.nih.gov/medlineplus/infantandnewborncare.html.

REFERENCES

American Academy of Pediatrics. (n.d.). *Early hearing detection and intervention* (EHDI). Retrieved from http://www.aap.org/en-us/advocacy-and-policy/aap-health-initiatives/PEHDIC/Pages/Early-Hearing-Detection-and-Intervention.aspx.

Benitz, W., & Committee on Fetus & Newborn. (2015). Hospital stay for healthy term newborn infants. *Pediatrics, 135*(5), 948–953. doi: 1-.1542/peds.2015-0699

Centers for Disease Control & Prevention. (2010). *WHO growth standards are recommended for use in the U.S. for infants and children 0 to 2 years of age.* Retrieved from http://www.cdc.gov/growthcharts/who_charts.htm.

Centers for Disease Control & Prevention. (2014). *Recommended immunization schedule for children from birth through 6 years old.* Retrieved from http://www.cdc.gov/vaccines/parents/downloads/parent-ver-sch-0-6yrs.pdf.

Centers for Disease Control & Prevention. (2015). *Hearing loss in children. Screening and diagnosis.* Retrieved from www.cdc.gov/ncbddd/hearingloss/screening.html.

Committee on Fetus & Newborn. (2010). Policy statement: Hospital stay for healthy term newborns. *Pediatrics, 125*(2), 405–409. Retrieved from http://pediatrics.aappublications.org/content/113/5/1434.full.pdf.

Earls, M. F., & Committee on Psychosocial Aspects of Child & Family Health. (2010). Clinical report: Incorporating recognition and management of perinatal and postpartum depression into pediatric practice. *Pediatrics, 126*(5), 1032–1039. doi: 10.1542/peds.2010-2348

Hagan, J. F., Shaw, J. S., & Duncan, P. M. (2008). Supervision: First week visit. In J. F. Hagan, J. S. Shaw, & P. M. Duncan (Eds.), *Bright futures: Guidelines for health supervision of infants, children, and adolescents* (3rd ed., pp. 289–302). Elk Grove Village, IL: American Academy of Pediatrics.

Mahle, W. T., Martin, G. R., Beckman, R. H., & Morrow, W. R. (2102). Section on Cardiology and Cardiac Surgery Executive Committee: Endorsement of health and human services recommendations for pulse oximetry screening for critical congenital heart disease. *Pediatrics, 129*(1), 190–192. doi: 10.1542/peds.2011-3211

March of Dimes. (2012). Newborn screening. Retrieved from http://www.marchofdimes.org/baby/newborn-screening-tests-for-your-baby.aspx.

Muchowski, K. R. (2014). Evaluation and treatment of neonatal hyperbilirubinemia. *American Family Physician, 89*(11), 873–878.

National Perinatal Association. (n.d.). *Multidisciplinary guidelines for the care of late preterm infants.* Retrieved from http://www.nationalperinatal.org/Resources/LatePretermGuidelinesNPA.pdf.

Phillips, R. M. (2013). Multidisciplinary guidelines for the care of late preterm infants. *Journal of Perinatology, 33*(S2), S3–S4. doi: 10.1038/jp.2013.52

Subcommittee on Hyperbilirubinemia. (2004). Management of hyperbilirubinemia in the newborn infants 35 or more weeks of gestation. *Pediatrics, 114*(1), 297–316. doi: 10.1542/peds.114.1.297

Tappero, E. P., & Honeyfield, M. E. (Eds.). (2015). *Physical assessment of the newborn: A comprehensive approach to the art of physical examination* (5th ed.). Petaluma, CA: NICU INK Publishers.

U.S. National Library of Medicine. (2013). *Medline Plus. Neonatal weight gain and nutrition.* Retrieved from https://www.nlm.nih.gov/medlineplus/ency/article/007302.htm.

U.S. Preventive Services Task Force. (2008). *Final recommendation statement: Congenital hypothyroidism: Screening.* Retrieved from http://www.uspreventiveservicestaskforce.org/Page/Document/RecommendationStatementFinal/congenital-hypothyroidism-screening.

U.S. Preventive Services Task Force. (2014a). *Final recommendation statement: Phenylketonuria in newborns: Screening.* Retrieved from http://www.uspreventiveservicestaskforce.org/Page/Document/RecommendationStatementFinal/phenylketonuria-in-newborns-screening.

U.S. Preventive Services Task Force. (2014b). *Final recommendation statement: Sickle cell disease (hemoglobinopathies) in newborns: Screening.* Retrieved from http://www.uspreventiveservicestaskforce.org/Page/Document/RecommendationStatementFinal/sickle-cell-disease-hemoglobinopathies-in-newborns-screening.

Whyte, R. K., & Canadian Paediatric Society, Fetus & Newborn Committee. (2010). Safe discharge of the late preterm infant. *Paediatrics & Child Health, 15*(10), 655–660.

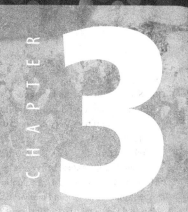

CARE OF THE POSTNEONATAL INTENSIVE CARE UNIT GRADUATE

CHAPTER 3

Annette Carley

I. Introduction and general background

Greater numbers of recuperating infants, shorter hospital stays, and complex health demands have increased the need for comprehensive postneonatal intensive care unit (NICU) care. Survival to discharge has improved across all gestational ages, although many survivors have residual disabilities requiring specialized care, expertise by providers versed in the needs of the fragile infant, and a provider who can intervene early (Carley, 2008; Kelly, 2006a). The American Academy of Pediatrics (AAP) has identified four categories of post-NICU infants who are considered high risk at discharge: (1) premature infants, (2) those with special health needs or who are dependent on technology, (3) those at risk because of social or family issues, and (4) those for whom early death is anticipated. Essential elements at discharge include physiologic stability, active caretaker involvement and preparation to assume care, and an integrated plan for follow-up care and management (AAP Committee on Fetus & Newborn, 2008).

A. Common issues for the post-NICU population include

1. The infant who is premature at discharge

   Premature infants constitute over 11% of births, and late preterm infants (of gestational age 34 0/7 to 36 6/7 weeks) comprise nearly three-quarters of preterm infants and account for most of the recent increase in numbers of preterm infants. With decreasing gestational age, the incidence of neonatal complications increases; however, even late preterm infants are at risk for complications such as impaired thermoregulation, poor feeding and nutrition, gastroesophageal reflux and other gastrointestinal issues, late-onset sepsis, jaundice, or neurodevelopment impairment. These infants are also at risk for rehospitalization in the early postnatal period (Darcy, 2009; Loftin et al., 2010). For successful transition, the post-NICU premature infant must be physiologically stable, feeding sufficiently well to support appropriate growth, able to maintain thermal neutrality in the post-NICU environment, and capable of sustaining mature respiratory system behavior (Barkemeyer, 2015; Centers for Disease Control & Prevention [CDC], 2014a; AAP Committee on Fetus & Newborn, 2008; Whyte, 2012).

2. Chronic lung disease (CLD)

   CLD is the leading cause of pediatric lung disease occurring secondary to pulmonary system immaturity or dysfunction and the additive effects of therapies, such as oxygen or mechanical ventilation support. Also referred to as "bronchopulmonary dysplasia" (BPD), CLD commonly affects the premature infant, and despite overall improved survival and advances, such as gentler postnatal ventilation strategies and exogenous surfactant therapy, it affects more than 25% of infants born weighing less than 1,500 grams (Jensen & Schmidt, 2014). The rate of CLD/BPD increases with decreasing gestational age at birth, and more than two-thirds of infants born ≤ 25 weeks gestation compared to 37% of those born between 26 and 30 weeks gestation develop this condition (Farstad, Bratlid, Medbo, Markestad, & Norwegian Extreme Prematurity Study Group, 2011). Infants with CLD/BPD are at increased risk for adverse health outcomes including chronic pulmonary morbidity, pulmonary infections, long-term growth failure, sensory deficits, developmental delay, and mortality (Jensen & Schmidt, 2014).

   a. Postdischarge therapies that may be used to optimize pulmonary function and growth include supplemental oxygen or ventilation, cardiorespiratory monitors, diuretics, and bronchodilators as well as enhanced nutritional strategies (Kelly, 2006b).

   b. Supplemental oxygen aims to optimize growth and stamina, and prevent development of cor pulmonale. For those discharged on supplemental oxygen, adequate caretaker training and team planning for weaning should be assured (Andrews, Pellerite, Myers, & Hageman, 2014; Barkemeyer, 2015)

c. Home mechanical ventilation, although rarely needed, may be used for those infants unable to wean from mechanical ventilation before hospital discharge. Careful caretaker training and establishment of outpatient supports is essential (AAP Committee on Fetus & Newborn, 2008; Andrews et al., 2014).

3. Apnea

Apnea is a serious condition for the neonate and may result from pulmonary disorders; infection; brain injury; or metabolic derangements, such as hypoglycemia. Apnea is also a common complication in the preterm population, caused by immature central regulation of respiratory effort, and may be managed with oxygen or ventilator support, respiratory stimulants (e.g., methylxanthines), and cardiopulmonary monitoring. Although typically resolved by 36–40 weeks postconceptual age, apnea caused by immaturity in some infants or "apnea of prematurity" may persist until the time of discharge. It is recommended that infants be free of significant apnea for 3–7 days prior to discharge (Andrews et al., 2014).

4. Gastroesophageal reflux disease (GERD)

Infants born prematurely, those whose early course included structural or functional disorders of the gastrointestinal tract, those with pulmonary conditions requiring surgical intervention, and those with neurologic compromise are at risk for GERD. GERD may lead to erosive esophageal injury and may be associated with serious conditions, such as apnea, bronchospasm, aspiration, or long-term growth failure.

a. Physiologic reflux is common in infants; up to two-thirds of all infants less than 4 months of age exhibit regurgitation.

b. Pathologic reflux, also known as GERD, is associated with complications including apnea, bronchospasm, esophagitis, esophageal strictures, and failure to thrive. It may be managed conservatively with small, frequent feedings; upright positioning; and medications to optimize gastric emptying; or it may necessitate surgical management for intractable cases. The use of thickened feedings has shown variable results, and this practice may carry risks for the immature gastrointestinal tract. In otherwise healthy infants beyond their due date it may be cautiously considered (Andrews et al., 2015; Horvath, Dziechciarz, & Szajewska, 2008).

5. Postnatal growth restriction

Premature infants are at increased risk for poor feeding and growth failure and at discharge typically are below their healthy term counterparts in weight. Growth risks are compounded by the effects of chronic illness and genetic potential. Premature infants frequently need higher calories and nutrients than their healthy term counterparts. Diligently applied nutritional support plays a key role in supporting adequate long-term growth and optimal neurologic development.

a. Human milk is the ideal food for all infants regardless of gestational age. However, an exclusive human milk diet may contribute to nutritional deficiencies in the recuperating post-NICU infant who has not attained adequate prenatal stores and has robust growth and recuperative needs. It is often necessary to supplement calories, protein, sodium, and calcium in these infants (Barkemeyer, 2015).

b. If human milk is not available, premature formula and postdischarge formula may be indicated to optimize catch-up growth (Greer, 2007).

c. Premature infants may require additional supplementation to support nutrient requirements for protein; calcium; phosphorus; sodium; vitamins, such as B_{12}, B_6, D, E, and K; and trace minerals, such as zinc, copper, magnesium, selenium, and carnitine (Greer, 2007; Shah & Shah, 2009).

d. Recuperating infants, especially preterm infants need up to 130 kcal/kg/d to achieve adequate growth (Billimoria, 2014). Those born small for gestational age or those attempting to achieve adequate catch-up growth may require up to 165 kcal/kg/d. Chronic health issues creating increased nutritional demands, such as CLD or growth failure, may warrant increased caloric goals.

e. Structural or functional comorbidities, such as orofacial anomalies or altered tone, may complicate the nutritional plan (Kelly, 2006b).

6. Neurobehavioral and sensory deficits

Infants recovering from the effects of initial illness or prematurity and the NICU environment may have residual neurobehavioral challenges. This risk increases with decreasing gestational age (Billimoria, 2014) and may include developmental delays, learning disabilities, hyperactivity, and cerebral palsy. Additionally, sensory deficits may include hearing or vision loss, auditory processing disorders, or language delay.

a. Hearing screening is recommended universally for all infants and indicated for the NICU infant before discharge. Hearing loss occurs in as many as 1.5% of all post-NICU infants (Andrews et al., 2014) and up to 50% of abnormal infant hearing screening occurs in NICU graduates (Kelly, 2006b). Special risks for the NICU population include a history of assisted ventilation, use of ototoxic pharmaceuticals, hyperbilirubinemia, infection, and craniofacial disorders (Andrews et al., 2014; Billimoria, 2014). Early intervention (i.e., at age < 6 months) enhances language development (Kelly, 2006b). Those with risks should have ongoing assessment including formal audiology evaluation by 30 months of age, even in cases with a normal initial hearing screen (Billimoria, 2014).

  b. Vision screening is recommended for preterm infants less than 1,500-g birth weight (or < 30 weeks gestation), those with a complicated medical course, and those exposed to supplemental oxygen. Severe retinopathy occurs in approximately 7% of infants born between 24–28 weeks gestation. Even without established retinopathy of prematurity. NICU infants are at risk for impaired visual acuity, refractive errors, and strabismus (Andrews et al., 2014). The first examination typically occurs at 31–34 weeks postconceptual age, with regular follow-up until vascular maturity is ensured at 3–6 months (Billimoria, 2014; Kelly, 2006b).

  c. Formal developmental assessment is indicated for all at-risk infants including those born preterm or with a complicated clinical course.

  d. Goals of developmental follow-up include optimizing growth and development to maximize long-term potential, integrating the infant into family and community, and providing early intervention to reduce medical, social, and emotional burden (Kuppala, Tabangin, Haberman, Steichen & Yolton, 2012).

7. Dependence on technology

Infants with unresolved cardiopulmonary issues, such as apnea, chronic hypoxia, or growth failure, may require technologic support in the home after discharge.

  a. Pulmonary support may be achieved with supplemental oxygen, cardiopulmonary monitoring, or the use of mechanical ventilation.

  b. Weaning from ventilatory support is dictated by the infant demonstrating normal oxygen saturation, resolution of apnea or bradycardia, and showing appropriate growth.

  c. Use of in-home technology requires vigilant attention to safety and hygiene, consistent education, and support of caretakers. Mechanical

ventilation requires dedicated personnel and ongoing caregiver support including respite care.

  d. Nutritional support may be achieved with complementary enteral feedings or parenteral nutrition. In-home use of intermittent orogastric gavage or gastrostomy feedings requires vigilant attention to safety, hygiene, and education and support of caregivers. Efforts should concentrate on encouraging oral feeding skills.

  e. Weaning from supplemental nutritional support can be considered when the infant demonstrates consistent appropriate growth, under the supervision of a nutrition specialist (Barkemeyer, 2015; Kelly, 2006b).

  f. A plan for emergency management in the case of equipment malfunction must be in place (AAP Committee on Fetus & Newborn, 2008).

8. Postnatal infection

Convalescing post-NICU patients, especially preterm infants, are at risk for complications related to infections, including respiratory syncytial virus (RSV) and influenza virus. Their increased vulnerability to infections may result in acute decompensation and the need for rehospitalization. At-risk infants discharged during peak RSV transmission seasons (i.e., October through March in the United States) should receive RSV prophylaxis in addition to routine immunizations given at recommended intervals (AAP Committee on Infectious Diseases & Bronchiolitis Guidelines Committee, 2014; CDC, 2014b; Kelly, 2006b).

B. Additional issues for the post-NICU population may include

1. Social and environmental risks

The AAP identifies premature birth, need for hospitalization, presence of birth defects, and infant disability as risks for family dysfunction and child abuse. These risks are compounded by family and environmental risks, such as low socioeconomic status, lack of social supports, substance exposure, and lack of family involvement during the infant's hospitalization. Identifying strategies to enhance infant safety and family functioning before discharge is encouraged (AAP Committee on Fetus & Newborn, 2008).

  a. Vulnerable child syndrome is recognized as a potential outcome caused by the effects of protracted neonatal hospitalization, parental anxiety or depression, impact of the illness on the family, or lack of social supports. This has been associated with excessive healthcare use and risk of impaired infant developmental outcome (Kokotos, 2009).

b. A posttraumatic stress disorder has been reported in parents of infants in the NICU, caused by ongoing stress of the hospitalization and uncertainty of neonatal outcome that may have a negative impact on the quality of interactions with the infant as well as between the parents (Hynan, Mounts, & Vanderbilt, 2013; Shaw et al., 2009). It is especially important to identify stress and depression in fathers whose degree of dysfunction may be overlooked because of a primary focus on the mother.

2. Infant with anticipated early death

To enhance the quality of remaining life, infants with terminal disorders may be discharged to the home for hospice care. Discharge planning and follow-up care attend to family needs and concerns and occur with the involvement of home nursing. Necessary elements include creating a plan for management of infant pain and discomfort, securing arrangements for equipment or supplies, and providing ongoing support to parents, siblings, or extended family members (AAP Committee on Fetus & Newborn, 2008).

II. Database (may include but is not limited to)

A. Subjective database

1. History and review of systems
    a. Parental concerns including feelings of readiness, stress, adequacy, and support.
    b. Birth and health history to date.
        i. Birth history, including gravida and parity, pregnancy complications, delivery method and birth complications, Apgar scores
        ii. Infant birth date, weight, and gestational age (AGA, LGA, or SGA/IUGR status)
        iii. Neonatal course including complications
    c. Family, social, and environmental history.
        i. Maternal age, health, occupation, and level of education
        ii. Paternal age, health, occupation, and level of education
        iii. Sibling ages, health, and history of prematurity
        iv. Family history including chronic conditions
        v. Parental head circumference and stature to compare with infant measurements
        vi. Social or environmental concerns, such as unemployment, abuse, marital problems, and lack of support
    d. Nutrition history.
        i. Date feedings initiated, formula versus breast milk, nipple versus gavage, feeding tolerance, complications
        ii. Parenteral nutrition support, use of hyperalimentation, peripheral versus central vascular access
    e. Review of systems and clinical findings.
        i. Dysmorphic features, which may suggest a genetic syndrome
        ii. Skin, including rashes, birthmarks, scars, or jaundice
        iii. Head, ears, eyes, nose, and throat including
            a. High arched palate caused by oral intubation
            b. Nostril distortion caused by feeding tube
            c. Head circumference: poor head growth in the premature infant strongly predictive of impaired cognitive function, academic performance, and behavioral issues
            d. Head shape may be transiently distorted as a consequence of NICU care practices that create positional deformities such as dolichocephaly (Billimoria, 2014).
        iv. Chest and thorax, including character of respirations, respiratory rate, and shape and contour of the thorax; findings may include
            a. Hyperexpansion caused by air trapping
            b. Tachypnea caused by chronic hypoxia
            c. Hypercarbia
        v. Cardiovascular, including presence of murmurs, perfusion, and quality of pulses
        vi. Abdomen and rectum, including stool pattern, distention, and inguinal or umbilical hernias
        vii. Genitourinary, including voiding pattern
        viii. Musculoskeletal, including symmetry of movements, strength, and tone
        ix. Neurobehavioral, including activity, tone, state regulation, and tremulousness
        x. Immune, including immunizations received before discharge
            a. Follow Centers for Disease Control and Prevention recommendations for dosing by chronologic age (CDC, 2014b).
        xi. Supportive data from relevant diagnostic tests including
            a. Results of neonatal screen (phenylketonuria, sickle cell, and congenital hypothyroidism screening mandated in all states)

b. Hearing screening
c. Vision screening
d. Developmental screening
e. Laboratory studies including baseline blood gas, oxygen saturation, electrolytes
f. Imaging studies including most recent chest radiograph, cranial ultrasound, or other cranial imaging study

B. Objective

1. Physical examination findings
   a. Establish a growth trend including comparative measurements of head circumference, weight, and length from birth. Plot and adjust for gestational age until 2 years of age.
   b. Thorough physical examination including vital signs and blood pressure.
   c. Essential to take into account size at birth (**Table 3-1**) and to use growth charts corrected for gestational age for accurate assessment of postnatal growth.
   d. The Fenton growth chart available at http://peditools.org/fenton2013/ is most commonly used in the NICU and remains appropriate until the infant reaches 50 weeks postmenstrual age. Beyond that age the World Health Organization chart is recommended for all infants (Billimoria, 2014).

2. Observation of parent–child interactions, including holding, comforting, responsiveness, confidence, and mutual support.

3. Laboratory studies as clinically indicated, such as blood gas, electrolytes, or complete blood count.

4. Chest radiograph as clinically indicated.

III. Assessment

A. Determine the diagnosis
Determine client's current health status and identify general health risks based on gender, age, ethnicity, and other factors.

TABLE 3-1 Birth Weight Classifications

Extremely Low Birth Weight (ELBW)	Very Low Birth Weight (VLBW)	Low Birth Weight (LBW)
< 1,000 g at birth	< 1,500 g at birth	< 2,500 g at birth

Data from Allen, M. D. (n.d.). *Development and follow-up of premature and low birthweight infants.* Retrieved from http://mchb.hrsa.gov/chusa13/perinatal-health-status-indicators/pdf/lbw.pdf%3E.

B. Severity
Assess the severity of illness, as indicated.

C. Motivation and ability
Determine family willingness to understand and comply with the treatment plan.

IV. Goals of clinical management

A. Screening or diagnosing
Choose a practical, cost-effective approach to screening and diagnosis, while abiding by mandated screening protocols. Post-NICU infants need careful, ongoing assessment related to neurobehavioral and growth risks and individualized screening based on clinical findings.

B. Treatment
Select a treatment plan that optimizes growth and development, is individualized for the caregiver and child, and maximizes caregiver acceptance.

V. Plan

A. Screening
Elicit a thorough history and perform a thorough physical examination, including growth and developmental assessment at all visits.

B. Diagnostic tests
If not already performed before discharge, these should include

1. Newborn screen as required by individual state.
2. Hearing screen.
3. Vision screen.
4. Developmental assessment, often done by referral to a specified neonatal follow-up clinic facility. Premature and at-risk infants may be seen as frequently as four to five times in the first year of life and are followed to school age. Typical criteria for follow-up includes birthweight, gestational age, acute illness during the NICU hospitalization, and referral request from an outpatient provider. However, there are no standardized guidelines for high-risk follow-up care (AAP Committee on Fetus & Newborn, 2004; Kuppala et al., 2012).

C. Management
A primary provider should be identified and accept responsibility for orchestrating care. Post-NICU patients may be managed cooperatively with a variety of consultant and subspecialty services, including but not limited

to nutrition services, dysmorphology and genetics, pulmonary, cardiology, gastroenterology, hematology, neurodevelopmental, and surgery. Specific intervals vary dependent on the complexity of the infant's history and current condition (AAP Committee on Fetus & Newborn, 2008).

D. Client education

1. Concerns and feelings

   Assist the family with expressing concerns and feelings about having a complex neonatal patient in the home and coping with uncertainties related to the infant's health status or anticipated development.

2. Information

   Provide verbal and written information related to
   a. Health maintenance
   b. Nutrition
   c. Growth and development
   d. Safety
   e. Anticipated referrals and follow-up plans

VI. Resources and tools

A. Parent–client–provider tools

1. The AAP website contains resources for caregivers, including information about high-risk neonatal growth, development, and health needs: http://www.aap.org.

2. The March of Dimes provides multiple neonatal and perinatal resources for providers and parents: http://www.marchofdimes.com.

3. AAP Section on Developmental & Behavioral Pediatrics. Provides recommendations for screening and assessment: https://www2.aap.org/sections/dbpeds/screening.asp.

4. Ages and Stages Questionnaire; Brookes Publishing Company: http://agesandstages.com/.

REFERENCES

Allen, M. D. (n.d.). *Development and follow-up of premature and low birth-weight infants.* Retrieved from www.hrsa.gov/.

American Academy of Pediatrics. Committee on Fetus & Newborn. (2004). Follow-up care of high-risk infants. *Pediatrics, 114*(5), 1377–1397.

American Academy of Pediatrics. Committee on Fetus & Newborn. (2008). Hospital discharge of the high-risk neonate. *Pediatrics, 122*(5), 1119–1126.

American Academy of Pediatrics. Committee on Infectious Diseases & Bronchiolitis Guidelines Committee (2014). Updated guidance for palivizumab prophylaxis among infants and young children at increased risk of hospitalization for respiratory syncytial virus infection. *Pediatrics, 134*(2), 415–420. doi: 10.1542/peds.2014-1665

Andrews, B., Pellerite, M., Myers, M., & Hageman, J. R. (2014). NICU follow-up: Medical and developmental management age 0 to 3 years. *NeoReviews, 15*(4), e123–e132.

Barkemeyer, B. M. (2015). Discharge planning. *Pediatric Clinics of North America, 62*(2), 545–556. doi: 10.1016/j.pcl.2014.11.013

Billimoria, Z. C. (2014). A pediatrician's guide to caring for the complex neonatal intensive care unit graduate. *Pediatric Annals, 43*(9), 369–372. doi: 10.3928/00904481-20140825-11

Carley, A. (2008). *Beyond the NICU: Can at-risk infant patients be better served?* Retrieved from http://nursing.advanceweb.com/Article/Beyond-the-NICU-2.aspx.

Centers for Disease Control & Prevention. (2014a). *Reproductive health. Preterm birth.* Retrieved from http://www.cdc.gov/reproductivehealth/maternalinfanthealth/pretermbirth.htm.

Centers for Disease Control and Prevention. (2014b). *Recommended immunization schedule for children from birth through 6 years old.* Retrieved from http://www.cdc.gov/vaccines/parents/downloads/parent-ver-sch-0-6yrs.pdf.

Darcy, A. E. (2009). Complications of the late preterm infant. *Journal of Perinatal & Neonatal Nursing, 23*(1), 78–86.

Farstad, T., Bratlid, D., Medbo, S., Markestad, T., & Norwegian Extreme Prematurity Study Group. (2011). Bronchopulmonary dysplasia: Prevalence, severity and predictive factors in a national cohort of extremely premature infants. *Acta Paediatrica, 100*(1), 53–58. doi: 10.1111/j.1651-2227.2010.01959.x.

Greer, F. R. (2007). Post-discharge nutrition: What does the evidence support? *Seminars in Perinatology, 31,* 89–95.

Horvath, A., Dziechciarz, P., & Szajewska, H. (2008). The effect of thickened-feed interventions on gastroesophageal reflux in infants: Systematic review and meta-analysis of randomized, controlled trials. *Pediatrics, 122*(6), 1268–1277.

Hynan, M. T., Mounts, K. O., & Vanderbilt, D. L. (2013). Screening parents of high-risk infants for emotional distress: Rationale and recommendations. *Journal of Perinatology, 33*(10), 748–753. doi: 10.1038/jp.2013.72.

Jensen, E. A., & Schmidt, B. (2014). Epidemiology of bronchopulmonary dysplasia. *Birth Defects Research. Part A, Clinical & Molecular Teratology, 100,* 145–157.

Kelly, M. M. (2006a). The medically complex premature infant in primary care. *Journal of Pediatric Health Care, 20*(6), 367–373.

Kelly, M. M. (2006b). Primary care issues for the healthy premature infant. *Journal of Pediatric Health Care, 20*(5), 293–299.

Kokotos, F. (2009). The vulnerable child syndrome. *Pediatrics in Review, 30*(5), 193–194.

Kuppala, V. S., Tabangin, M., Haberman, B., Steichen, J., & Yolton, K. (2012). Current state of high-risk infant follow-up care in the United States: Results of a national survey of academic follow-up programs. *Journal of Perinatology, 32,* 293–298. doi: 10.1038/jp.2011.97

Loftin, R. W., Habli, M., Snyder, C. C., Cormier, C. M., Lewis, D. F., & DeFranco, E. A. (2010). Late preterm birth. *Reviews in Obstetrics & Gynecology, 3*(1), 10–19.

Shah, M. D., & Shah, S. R. (2009). Nutrient deficiencies in the premature infant. *Pediatric Clinics of North America, 56*(5), 1069–1083.

Shaw, R. J., Bernard, R. S., Deblois, T., Ikuta, L. M., Ginzburg, K., & Koopman, C. (2009). The relationship between acute stress disorder and posttraumatic stress disorder in the neonatal intensive care unit. *Psychosomatics, 50*(2), 131–137.

Whyte, R. K. (2012). Neonatal management and safe discharge of late and moderate preterm infants. *Seminars in Fetal & Neonatal Medicine, 17*(3), 153–158. doi: 10.1016/j.siny.2012.02.00

0 TO 3 YEARS OF AGE INTERVAL VISIT

Ann Birenbaum Baker

CHAPTER 4

I. Introduction and general background

The 0–3 years of age pediatric visit encompasses a wide range of physical and developmental growth. Infants go through dramatic physical growth while constantly developing gross and fine motor, language, and social skills that allow them to respond to their environment. As infants reach early childhood, their physical growth slows as they begin an intense exploration of their environment (Hockenberry & Wilson, 2010). This developmentally and physically diverse patient population requires additional consideration at each visit.

The physical examination of infants and toddlers aged 0–3 years may need a different approach than for other age groups because they do not consistently respond to verbal instruction and developmentally may have stranger anxiety. Infants and toddlers may adjust to an examiner if they first watch the interaction between the examiner and their parent during the patient interview (Duderstadt, 2014). During this time, respecting a toddler's personal space and avoiding eye contact may help the toddler become comfortable before the examination. Instead of a head-to-toe examination, a more system-focused approach may be necessary with some patients. For example, auscultation can be completed first in infants before they become more active as the examination proceeds. Indirect examination can be a useful strategy in this age group. Breathing patterns, skin characteristics, symmetry of movement, and musculoskeletal integrity are examples of assessments that can be performed noninvasively. Infants up to 6 months of age can usually be examined on the examining table, whereas infants older than 6 months and toddlers may feel more comfortable being examined in their parent's lap (Hockenberry, 2013). In addition to assessing the child, it is also important to observe the parent–child interaction (Duderstadt, 2014). These interactions can give the provider clues to the parent–child dynamic, which is an important element of an overall assessment.

Health maintenance is a mutual goal for the patient and health provider and is aimed at potentiating the patient's state of well-being. During periodic scheduled visits, a complete history is taken, an examination is performed, and potential health risks are identified. Counseling and guidance are provided in the areas of physical, behavioral, and emotional development. Cultural considerations, such as language barriers, cultural values, folk health practices, recognizing one's own personal values, and working to eliminate health disparities related to race or ethnicity, are important to incorporate into each visit (Duderstadt, 2014). For children with special needs, promoting self-empowerment and self-esteem as well as maximizing development and function are also important considerations.

II. Database (may include, but is not limited to)

A. Subjective

1. Parental concerns
2. Interval history (if new patient include birth, patient and family medical history, and review of symptoms)
   a. Frequency and type of illness since last visit
   b. Medications
   c. Trauma or hospitalizations
   d. Status of any chronic illness management
3. Immunization status
4. Family and social history
   a. Changes from previous visit including new stressors
   b. Family planning
   c. Emotional support
   d. Means of financial support
   e. Childcare arrangements
   f. Peer or social interactions including siblings, other children and adults, parents
5. Review of systems (Duderstadt, 2014)

Maternal infections or drug use, prenatal history, history of preterm birth, birth history, neonatal history (including congenital anomalies and hospitalizations), and family medical history are important elements of the review of symptoms for this age group

a. Skin: birth skin trauma, skin tags, dimples, cysts, extra digits, birthmarks, hair, nails, diapering habits, clothing habits, behavioral history related to potential skin trauma, rashes, eczema, or skin allergies

b. Head: head growth, head trauma

c. Eyes: focusing, eye discharge or swelling, infant history of being shaken, vision, abnormal head positioning

d. Ears: newborn hearing screening results, infant reaction to sound, infant vocalization, and history of recurrent otitis media or effusion

e. Nose, mouth, and throat: difficulty sucking or feeding, mouth sores or lesions, tooth eruption, breastfeeding, bottle use, mouthing habits, language acquisition, sucking on finger or pacifier, daycare, dental care

f. Respiratory: respiratory infections, reactive airway disease or asthma, daycare attendance, frequent colds, breathholding, mouthing habits

g. Cardiovascular: heart murmur, cyanosis, failure to thrive

h. Gastrointestinal: stooling and voiding patterns, vomiting or reflux, weight gain and growth, constipation, toilet training, rectal bleeding

i. Genitourinary: urinary stream, urinary tract infections, dysuria, hematuria, testes descended, vaginal discharge

j. Skeletal: motor milestones, toe-walking, deformities, gait, bowing of legs, injuries or trauma

k. Neurologic: difficulty feeding, tongue thrust, developmental milestones, toe-walking, hand dominance, feeds self, poor coordination, seizures, staring spells, loss of consciousness, speech development, muscle tone

l. Lymph and endocrine: newborn screening results, weight gain, linear growth pattern, lymphadenopathy

6. Activities of daily living

a. Nutrition

  i. Milk

    a. Type: breast milk, formula, cow's milk

    b. Amount in 24 hours

    c. Method: breast, bottle (held or propped), cup

  ii. Type and amount of foods

  iii. Self-feeding: use of utensils

  iv. Meal routine: number of meals per day, where eaten and with whom

  v. Vitamins, iron

b. Oral health (American Academy of Pediatric Dentistry [AAPD], 2014)

  i. Brushing teeth and wiping gums with moist rag

  ii. Parental oral health

  iii. Dental visit

  iv. Fluoride supplementation as indicated depending on level of fluoride in community

c. Sleep patterns

  i. Daytime and nighttime sleeping: hours and routine

  ii. Where sleeping: cosleeping, crib, separate bed, own room

  iii. Sleep positioning

  iv. Nightmares and night terrors

d. Elimination pattern and, if age appropriate, toilet training history

e. Developmental and behavioral assessment (LaRosa, 2015)

  i. Evaluate at each well-child visit for early identification of developmental or behavioral disorders

  ii. 9 months: evaluate child's vision, hearing, motor skills, early communication skills

  iii. 18 months: evaluate motor, communication, and language skills; complete M-CHAT autism screening available at https://www.m-chat.org/

  iv. 24 or 30 months: evaluate motor, language, and cognitive skills plus autism screening

  v. Standardized developmental screening tools (see Chapter 9, Developmental Assessment: Screening for Developmental Delay and Autism)

f. Behavior

  i. Crying

  ii. Temper tantrums

  iii. Head banging

  iv. Body rocking

  v. Pacifier use

  vi. Thumb sucking

  vii. Stranger anxiety

  viii. Approach to discipline

B. Objective

1. Physical examination (Duderstadt, 2014)

a. Height, weight, and head circumference through 36 months of age—refer to the following link for Centers for Disease Control and Prevention

(CDC) growth charts: http://www.cdc.gov/growthcharts/charts.htm

b. Vital signs and pain assessment: heart rate, respirations, temperature, blood pressure (in children who are at risk or have chronic conditions), assess pain score

c. General appearance: state of alertness, nutrition

d. Skin: hydration, rash, birthmark, scar, bruises, signs of trauma

e. Head: anterior fontanel size, sutures, condition of hair and scalp, asymmetry

f. Eyes: eyelids, discharge, reactivity of pupils, corneal light reflex, red reflex, focus and follow, cover–uncover test (perform with infant sitting in parent's lap beginning at 9 months to 1 year of age), strabismus, nystagmus

g. Ears: external ear, external canal, tympanic membranes, pneumatic otoscopy

h. Nose: patency, discharge, turbinates

i. Mouth and throat: presence and number of teeth, caries, occlusion status, tonsils

j. Neck: supple, rigid, palpable lymph nodes

k. Chest: work of breathing, auscultation of lungs, chest wall shape, symmetry

l. Heart: rhythm, quality of heart sounds, presence of murmur, gallop or click, pulses, precordium, perfusion, color

m. Abdomen: umbilicus, palpate liver and spleen, any masses, quality of bowel sounds

n. Genitalia
   i. Male: urethral meatus, foreskin, testes, inguinal canal, anus
   ii. Female: appearance of perineum, clitoris, vaginal introitus, hymen, discharge, anus

o. Musculoskeletal: muscle strength, range of motion, joints, extremities, spine, Ortolani and Barlow maneuvers for infants

p. Neurologic: motor function, symmetry, tone, gait, language, social development, primitive reflexes, and postural reflexes

III. Assessment

A. *Identify the child's general health risks based on age, gender, ethnicity, and specific health risks.*

B. *Determine the child's current health status.*

C. *Determine parent's or caregiver's motivation to promote and maintain positive health behaviors.*

D. *Assess the child's developmental milestones and ability to accomplish and master skills.*

IV. Plan

A. Diagnostics

A periodicity schedule for preventive pediatric health care and screening and secondary prevention tests is available through the American Academy of Pediatrics (AAP) at http://pediatrics.aappublications.org/content/133/3/568.full?sid=84c54f2b-f79a-4830-80ca-2fdaf5c3b471 (AAP, 2014a)

1. Hearing risk assessment (Hagan, Shaw, & Duncan, 2008; Harlor & Bower, 2009)
   a. Auditory skills monitoring
   b. Developmental surveillance
   c. Assessment of parental concern
   d. Starting at 12 months, if risk factors are identified by review of symptoms or risk assessment children should be referred for diagnostic audiologic assessment.

2. Vision screen (Hagan, Shaw, & Duncan, 2008; Kelly, 2014)
   a. Detection of strabismus
   b. Vision
      i. Indirect assessment of vision in infancy and early childhood as noted previously
      ii. Direct assessment of visual acuity in early childhood to comply with vision screening test (AAP, 2014a)

3. Iron deficiency (AAP, 2014a; Kelly, 2014)
   a. Risk assessment screening at 4, 15, 18, 24, 30, and 36 months of age
      i. At 4 months, risk assessment includes history of prematurity, low birth weight, and diet.
      ii. After 1 year, risk assessment includes socioeconomic status, limited access to food, diet low in iron, and exposure to lead.
   b. Hemoglobin or hematocrit at 12 and 24 months of age

4. Lead poisoning (CDC, 2015; Kelly, 2014; Wengrovitz & Brown, 2009)
   a. Follow state screening plan
      i. State-specific links can be found through the CDC: http://www.cdc.gov/nceh/lead/programs/default.htm
   b. If no plan for state screening in place, consider universal screening
      i. Blood lead level at 12 and 24 months of age
      ii. Universal screening also recommended for recent immigrants, foreign adoptees, and refugee children between 6 months and 16 years
   c. Targeted screening; see state-specific questionnaires for suggested screening questions

5. Oral health screening (AAP, 2014b; AAPD, 2014)
   a. Risk assessment starting at 6 months of age using a caries risk assessment tool available at http://www.aapd.org/media/Policies_Guidelines/G_CariesRiskAssessment.pdf
   b. Dental referral to establish a dental home at 12 months of age

6. Tuberculosis (AAP, 2014a; Kelly, 2014)
   a. Risk assessment at 1, 6, 12, and 24 months of age, then annually
   b. Targeted screening with positive risk screening

7. Lipid profile (Ferranti & Newburger, 2014; Kelly, 2014)
   a. Risk assessment at age 2, 4, 6, 8, and 10 years
   b. Risk factors: family history of premature coronary artery disease, disease states associated with cardiovascular disease, significant tobacco smoke exposure, hypertension, elevated BMI (> 95% for children between 2 and 8 years of age)
   c. Hyperlipidemia screening if known risk factors

B. Treatment

1. Immunizations appropriate for age are available at http://www.cdc.gov/vaccines/schedules/

2. Oral fluoride (if primary water source is deficient in fluoride)

3. Vitamin D supplementation: breastfed infants and all children > 1 year old

C. Patient and family education (Hagan, Shaw, & Duncan, 2008)

1. Discussion of the following
   a. Presenting concerns
   b. Nutrition appropriate for age
   c. Safety and injury prevention
   d. Toilet training appropriate to age
   e. Available parent and community resources
   f. Childcare arrangements and preschool plans
   g. Growth and development appropriate for age with review of growth chart, physiologic development of lower extremities (bowed legs, knock knees)
   h. Age-appropriate behavior of infant or toddler (including separation anxiety, fear of strangers, and sleep patterns)
   i. Tantrums and limit setting
   j. Vaccine promotion
   k. Possible reactions to immunizations

D. Expected parent outcomes

1. Parents are able to:
   a. Be reassured about their concerns
   b. Verbalize knowledge of nutritional requirements appropriate for age—variable appetites, food fads, bottle habits (sleeping with bottle, juice in bottle, starting cup use), label reading
   c. Verbalize safety precautions appropriate for age
   d. Verbalize age-appropriate toilet training
   e. Verbalize available community resources
   f. Verbalize available childcare arrangements and preschools and the appropriateness for their child
   g. Verbalize understanding of age-appropriate growth and development including physiologic development of lower extremities
   h. Verbalize understanding for age-appropriate behavior including sleep patterns and separation anxiety
   i. Verbalize understanding of tantrums and limit setting in relation to development
   j. Verbalize understanding of immunizations and grant informed consent. Understand possible reactions to immunizations and treatment of possible fever including temperature taking.
   k. Verbalize the importance of timely immunizations

REFERENCES

American Academy of Pediatric Dentistry. (2014). *Guideline on infant oral health care.* Retrieved from http://www.aapd.org/media/Policies_Guidelines/G_InfantOralHealthCare.pdf

American Academy of Pediatrics. (2014a). *Recommendations for pediatric preventive health care.* Retrieved from http://pediatrics.aappublications.org/content/133/3/568.full?sid=84c54f2b-f79a-4830-80ca-2fdaf5c3b471

American Academy of Pediatrics. (2014b). Maintaining and improving the oral health of young children. *Pediatrics, 134*(6), 1224–1229.

Centers for Disease Control and Prevention (CDC). (2015). *CDC's Childhood Lead Poisoning Prevention Program.* Retrieved from http://www.cdc.gov/nceh/lead/about/program.htm

Duderstadt, K. G. (Ed.). (2014). *Pediatric physical examination: An illustrated handbook* (2nd ed.). St. Louis: Mosby, Inc.

Ferranti, S. D., & Newburger, J. W. (2014, July 3). *Definition and screening for dyslipidemia in children.* UpToDate. Retrieved from http://www.uptodate.com/contents/definition-and-screening-for-dyslipidemia-in-children?source=see_link

Hagan, J. F., Shaw, J. S., & Duncan, P. M. (Eds.). (2008). *Bright futures: Guidelines for health supervision of infants, children, and adolescents* (3rd ed.). Arlington, VA: National Center for Education in Maternal and Child Health.

Harlor, A. D., & Bower, C. (2009). Hearing assessment in infants and children: Recommendations beyond neonatal screening. *Pediatrics, 124*(4), 1252–1263.

Hockenberry, M. J. (2013). Communication and physical assessment of the child. In M. J. Hockenberry & D. Wilson (Eds.), *Wong's essentials of pediatric nursing* (9th ed., pp. 86–184). St. Louis, MO: Mosby.

Hockenberry, M. J., & Wilson, D. W. (2010). Communication and physical assessment of the child. In M. J. Hockenberry & D. Wilson (Eds.),

Wong's nursing care of infants and children (9th ed., pp. 117–226). St. Louis, MO: Mosby.

Kelly, N. (2014, August 27). *Screening tests in children and adolescents.* UpToDate. Retrieved from http://www.uptodate.com/contents /screening-tests-in-children-and-adolescents?source=search_result&s earch=screening+tests+in+children+and+adolescents&selectedTitle =1%7E150#H16

LaRosa, A. (2015, January 8). *Developmental-behavioral surveillance and screening in primary care.* UpToDate. Retrieved from http://www .uptodate.com/contents/developmental-behavioral-surveillance-and -screening-in-primary-care?source=search_result&search=developme ntal+screening&selectedTitle=2%7E18#H11

Wengrovitz, A. M., & Brown, M. J. (2009). Recommendations for blood lead screening of Medicaid-eligible children aged 1–5 years: An updated approach to targeting a group at high risk. *MMWR: Recommendations and Reports, 58,* 1–11.

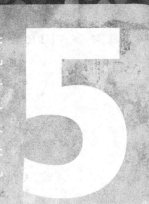

CHAPTER 5

3 TO 6 YEARS OF AGE INTERVAL VISIT

Mary Anne M. Israel

I. Introduction and general background

Health supervision and well-child visits are opportunities for the healthcare provider to assess a child's growth and development and to promote wellness in the child and family. In addition, the provider needs to address disease detection and prevention and offer proper anticipatory guidance during the visit (Hagan, Shaw, & Duncan, 2008a).

Children between 3 and 6 years of age experience an explosion of language, mastery of physical skills, sense of self and peers, an increase in independence, and endless curiosity, all in preparation for a successful school entry milestone (Hagan, Shaw, & Duncan, 2008b). They cross from early childhood into the beginning stages of middle childhood.

The approach to early childhood during the well-child visit is twofold: although most of the history may still be provided by the parent or caretaker, children at this age may now participate in some of the interview and actively engage with the provider. Careful observation of their behavior in the examination room is also useful, including their interaction with the parent or caretaker, the environment, and the provider (Duderstadt, 2014). Healthcare maintenance visits in this age range include comprehensive history, physical examination, screening tests (as appropriate), immunizations, anticipatory guidance, counseling at a yearly basis, and follow-up as needed.

II. Database (may include but is not limited to)

A. Subjective

1. Parental and child concerns (chief complaint)
   a. History of present illness
2. Interval history
3. Past medical history
   a. Birth history
   b. Trauma, surgeries, or hospitalizations
   c. Dental home: date of last examination (if any); caries or dental work
4. Medication (include homeopathic or herbal supplements and vitamins)
5. Allergies (medication, environmental, and food)
6. Immunization status
7. Family history
8. Social history
   a. Daycare or preschool attendance; kindergarten
   b. Household members
   c. Means of financial support in family
9. Environmental health history (National Environmental Education Foundation [NEEF], 2015)
   a. Indoor exposures: smoke, mold, cockroaches, rodents, damp walls, strong odors, broken windows, lead exposure, and parental occupation
   b. Outdoor exposures: sun, industrial smokestack, and housing proximity to heavy traffic
10. Nutrition
    a. Foods—intake of fruits, vegetables, lean meat/beans, iron-rich foods, whole grains; calcium sources: milk, cheese, and yogurt; and juice and water intake (source of water and fluoride)
    b. Eating habits, mealtime behavior, and family meals
11. Elimination
    a. Potty training process and status; voiding habits
    b. Stooling patterns
12. Sleep (quality and quantity): bedtime routine
13. Developmental (see Chapter 9, Developmental Assessment: Screening for Developmental Delay and Autism); evaluate overall school readiness
    a. Socioemotional: self-care skills, typical play, and description of self
    b. Language (expressive and receptive)

    i. 3–4 year-old: speech is usually fluent and clear, talks about experiences and understands who, what, where questions

    ii. 5–6 year-old: communicates easily to adults and children, long imaginative stories, enjoys stories and understands everything that is said

  c. Cognitive

    i. 5–6 year-old: increases memory capacity, follows directions, able to listen and attend, advances pretend play

  d. Physical

    i. 3-year-old: builds tower of cubes, throws ball, rides tricycle, walks up stairs, draws, and toilet training progress

    ii. 4-year-old: hops on one foot; balances for 2 seconds; copies crosses; dresses and undresses with minimal assistance; and pours, cuts, and mashes own food

    iii. 5–6 year-old: balances on one foot, hops and skips, ties a knot, grasps a pencil, draws a person with six body parts, recognizes letters and numbers, copies squares and triangles, and dresses and undresses without assistance

14. Review of systems

  a. General

  b. Skin, hair, and nails: birthmarks, rashes

  c. Head–eyes–ears–nose–throat: headaches; ocular history (vision, eyes straight, eyelid droop, eye injury); hearing and history of otitis media; nasal congestion, allergies, and nosebleeds; oral health, dental brushing, and flossing; and sore throats and difficulty swallowing

  d. Chest and lungs: history of asthma or reactive airway disease, croup, bronchitis, or persistent cough

  e. Cardiac and heart: history of heart murmur, cyanosis, shortness of breath, and energy level

  f. Abdomen and gastrointestinal: appetite, diet, abdominal pain, constipation, vomiting, and diarrhea

  g. Genitourinary: incontinence, enuresis, urinary tract infections, dysuria, frequency, hematuria, vaginal discharge, and phimosis or balanitis

  h. Musculoskeletal: deformities, limb pains, injuries, and orthopedic appliances

  i. Neurologic: seizures, fainting spells, loss of consciousness, headache, and gait

  j. Endocrine: recent weight gain or loss and linear growth patterns

B. Objective

1. Physical examination

  a. Weight, height, and body mass index (BMI)

  b. Pulse, respiratory rate, and blood pressure

  c. General: state of alertness and quality of interaction with parent and staff

  d. Skin, hair, and nails: hydration; rashes; birthmarks; scars; nail and hair health; and infestations (lice)

  e. Head–eyes–ears–nose–throat: symmetry of head; external inspection of eyes and lids, extraocular movement assessment, pupil examination, red light reflex examination, corneal light reflex, cover–uncover examination, ophthalmoscopic examination of optic nerve and retinal vessels (in 5- and 6- year-olds); tympanic membrane description and mobility; nasal septal deviation, nasal discharge and turbinate status; dental condition, dental caries, gingival inflammation, and malocclusion; throat and tonsils

  f. Neck: supple, note palpable lymph nodes

  g. Chest and lungs: symmetry of chest, auscultation of lungs

  h. Cardiac and heart: rhythm, murmur, gallop, click, pulses, and capillary refill time

  i. Abdomen: liver, spleen, masses, palpable stool, and bowel sounds

  j. Genitourinary: external genitalia and rectal status; for males, circumcision or retractable foreskin, meatus midline, testes descended bilaterally; for females, inspect urethra, vaginal introitus, labial condition

  k. Musculoskeletal: muscle strength, range of motion, inspect spine and back, and gait

  l. Neurologic: cranial nerves II–XII; deep tendon reflexes; symmetry, tone, gait, strength; observe fine and gross motor skills;

  m. Developmental: assess language acquisition, speech fluency, and clarity; thought content and ability to understand abstract thinking

III. Assessment

A. Summary of health, growth, and development

1. Identify general health risks based on age, gender, past history, and ethnicity

2. Determine child's and caregiver's motivation to promote and maintain positive health behaviors

3. Identify ability to accomplish and master developmental milestones

IV. Plan

A. Screening (Hagan, Shaw, & Duncan, 2008c); see resources and screening questions from http://www.brightfutures.org

1. Vision screening

2. Audiometric screening

3. Lead screening and risk assessment (see Chapter 4 for lead screening recommendations)

4. Anemia screening and risk assessment

5. Tuberculosis screening and risk assessment

6. Dyslipidemia screening and risk assessment

7. Urinalysis (one time between 3 and 5 years of age)

B. Treatment

1. Immunizations appropriate for age are available at http://www.cdc.gov/vaccines/schedules/

2. Oral fluoride (if primary water source is deficient in fluoride)

3. Iron supplementation: consider for children from low-income families (American Academy of Pediatrics, 2010)

4. Vitamin D supplementation: breastfed infants and all children > 1 year old (Institute of Medicine, 2010)

C. Anticipatory guidance and family education (Hagan et al., 2008b)

1. Address child and parental–caregiver concerns

2. Family support and routine
   a. Family decisions, sibling rivalry, work balance, and discipline methods
   b. Temperament

3. Reading literacy and comprehension, speech and language skills

4. Peers
   a. Interactive games, play opportunities, social interactions, and taking turns

5. School readiness
   a. Preschool: structured learning experiences; friends; socialization; and able to express feelings of joy, anger, sadness, fear, and frustration
   b. Kindergarten and elementary school: establish routine, after-school care and activities, parent–teacher communication, friends, bullying, maturity, management of disappointments, and fears

6. Physical activity
   a. Limit screen time (television, computer, mobile device) to 2 hours per day of appropriate programming; no television in child's room
   b. Encourage 60 minutes of physical activity per day (5–6 year-olds)

7. Personal health habits
   a. Daily routines including bedtime routine
   b. Oral health: daily brushing and flossing, adequate fluoride intake

c. Discuss proper nutrition for age: well-balanced diet, breakfast every day, three servings of fruits and two servings of vegetables per day, increased whole-grain consumption, two cups of milk or equivalent calcium intake per day, 3–4 oz. protein daily—lean meat/beans/soy; limit high-fat and low-nutrient foods and drinks.

8. Safety
   a. Car safety: seat or booster and safety helmets
   b. Pedestrian safety: falls from windows, outdoor safety, swimming safety, smoke detectors and carbon monoxide detectors, and guns and weapons in the home
   c. Stranger safety: reinforce rules about talking with and going with strangers if approached
   d. Sexual abuse prevention—review appropriate touching

D. Expected outcomes

1. Reassure child and parents about health concerns

2. Promote optimal health for children and their families

3. Promote family support and acceptable discipline approach

4. Promote social development

5. Encourage literacy activities

6. Empower parents to provide healthy eating habits and encourage physical activities; limit amount of television and computer time

7. Promote safety parameters at home, in the car, and in the neighborhood

8. Support school readiness

E. Consultation and referral

1. Dental home if not already established

2. Further developmental testing if indicated

3. Subspecialty referral if indicated

F. Resources for families

1. Healthy Children (American Academy of Pediatrics): www.healthychildren.org (includes special section on preschoolers in "Ages and Stages")

2. Kids Health (Nemours Center for Child Health Media): www.kidshealth.org

3. Bright Futures for Families: www.brightfuturesfor families.org

G. Resources for providers

1. National Association of Pediatric Nurse Practitioners: www.napnap.org

2. American Academy of Pediatrics: www.aap.org

3. Bright Futures: www.brightfutures.org

REFERENCES

American Academy of Pediatrics. (2010). *First AAP recommendations on iron supplementation include directive on universal screening.* Retrieved from http://aapnews.aappublications.org/content/early/2010/10/05/aapnews.20101005-1.full?rss=1

Bowen, C. (2014). *Ages and stages summary: Language development 0–5 years.* Retrieved from http://www.speech-language-therapy.com/

Duderstadt, K. (2014). Approach to care and assessment of children & adolescents. In K. Duderstadt (Ed.), *Pediatric physical examination: An illustrated handbook* (2nd ed., pp. 1–8). Philadelphia, PA: Elsevier.

Hagan, J. F., Shaw, J. S., & Duncan, P. M. (Eds.). (2008a). Introduction to the bright futures visits. In American Academy of Pediatrics, *Bright futures: Guidelines for health supervision of infants, children, and adolescents* (3rd ed., pp. 203–219). Elk Grove Village, IL: American Academy of Pediatrics.

Hagan, J. F., Shaw, J. S., & Duncan, P. M. (Eds.). (2008b). Early childhood: 3 year visit. In American Academy of Pediatrics, *Bright futures: Guidelines for health supervision of infants, children, and adolescents* (3rd ed., pp. 439–481). Elk Grove Village, IL: American Academy of Pediatrics.

Hagan, J. F., Shaw, J. S., & Duncan, P. M. (Eds.). (2008c). Rationale and evidence. In American Academy of Pediatrics, *Bright futures: Guidelines for health supervision of infants, children, and adolescents* (3rd ed., pp. 221–250). Elk Grove Village, IL: American Academy of Pediatrics.

Institute of Medicine. (2010). *Dietary reference intakes for vitamin D and calcium.* Retrieved from http://www.iom.edu/Reports/2010/Dietary-Reference-Intakes-for-Calcium-and-Vitamin-D/Report-Brief.aspx

National Environmental Education Foundation (NEEF). (2015). *Pediatric environmental history primer.* Retrieved from http://www.neefusa.org/pdf/primer.pdf

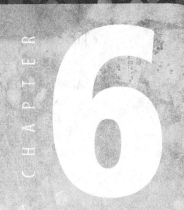

6 TO 11 YEARS OF AGE INTERVAL VISIT

Bridget Ward Gramkowski and Ann Birenbaum Baker

CHAPTER 6

I. Introduction and general background

Children in middle childhood spend less than half as much time with their parents as they did in early childhood. Although parents are still the most important influence in their child's emotional and physical development, teachers and peers become increasingly important as the child approaches adolescence. Opportunities for mastery and early identification of learning issues are critical to promoting self-esteem and academic success (Gonida & Cortina, 2014). Screening at well-child visits should include assessing peer interactions and bullying victimization in addition to academic performance and classroom behavior (Espelage & De La Rue, 2011). The influence of media in middle childhood is also increasing, with "screen time" for children ages 6–11 years averaging more than 28 hours a week (Gold, 2009). The timing of puberty varies widely between different racial and ethnic groups and genders and can start as early as 6 years in African American girls (Zuckerman, 2001). Early maturing girls are more likely to have internalizing behavior problems and exhibit more risk-taking behaviors (Zuckerman, 2001).

Health maintenance is a mutual goal for the parent or guardian and healthcare provider. During periodic well-child visits, a complete history is taken, an examination is performed, and potential health risks are identified. Counseling and guidance are provided to the child and parent in the areas of physical, behavioral, and emotional development. Cultural considerations, such as language barriers, cultural values, folk remedies, recognizing child's cultural identity and values, and working to eliminate health inequalities related to race or ethnicity, are important to incorporate into each visit (Duderstadt, 2014).

II. Database (may include but is not limited to)

A. Subjective

1. Parent and child concerns

2. Interval history (American Academy of Pediatrics [AAP], 2014a)
   a. Frequency and type of illness since last visit
   b. Chronic illnesses: current status and treatment plan
   c. Medications
   d. Trauma, hospitalizations, or emergency room visits
   e. Dental care status

3. Immunization status

4. Family and social history
   a. Changes from previous visit: emotional support, means of financial support/parental employment status, childcare arrangements, and changes to family medical history
   b. Sibling rivalry, parental stress, living arrangements, and childcare
   c. Safety: screen for domestic violence, substance abuse in home, neighborhood safety, school bullying, Internet use, personal, and weapons in home
   d. Environmental risk factors: cigarette smoke, sun exposure, pollution, lead, and allergens

5. Developmental and behavioral history
   a. Problems or concerns
   b. Appraisal of coping styles: anxiety, anger, frustration, fear, and happiness
   c. Interaction with peers, teachers, adults, and family
   d. Amount and type of screen time per day and per week, supervised versus alone, academic versus entertainment purposes
   e. Child's strengths and self-esteem
   f. Child's socialization skills and peer activities
   g. Parent's approach to sexuality and pubertal development
   h. Exposure to trauma, tobacco, alcohol, and drug use, history of physical or sexual abuse

6. Activities of Daily Living
   a. Nutrition
      i. Calcium: type and amount in 24 hours
      ii. Meal routine: 24–48 hour dietary recall, number of meals per day, at home and at school; frequency and type of snacks, family meal, any family meals, eating or snacking while watching TV
      iii. Attitude toward body image and food
      iv. Sugar sweetened beverages intake, caffeinated beverage intake
      v. Fast food or snack food frequency and type
   b. Physical activity: frequency, type, duration, and safety (American Heart Association [AHA] et al., 2006)
   c. Sleep patterns
      i. Amount of sleep, scheduled bedtime, sleep hygiene (routines and sleep-promoting habits), sleep environment (cosleeping, TV in room, cellphone charging next to bed)
      ii. Sleepwalking
      iii. Teeth grinding, snoring, apnea, and daytime sleepiness
      iv. Nocturnal enuresis
      v. Nightmares
   d. School
      i. Name of school, teacher, and grade; new or continuing at previous year's school
      ii. Scholastic achievement or grades, other areas of achievement, changes in performance, attention concerns
      iii. Attitude toward school, teachers, favorite subject, and future goals
      iv. Peer relationships
      v. School attendance and participation in activities
      vi. Reading, writing skills (have child demonstrate)
      vii. Learning differences, disabilities, and delays, Individual Educational Plan (IEP) or special education classes
7. Review of systems
   a. Skin: birthmarks, rashes, abrasions, and bruising
   b. Head–eyes–ears–nose–throat: headaches, head injuries, vision, corrective lenses or glasses, hearing, history of otitis media or effusion, nasal allergies, frequent colds, snoring, nose bleeds, dental hygiene, dentist visit, orthodontics, difficulty swallowing, hoarseness, and sore throats
   c. Respiratory: reactive airway disease or asthma, bronchitis, persistent cough, cough at night or with exercise
   d. Cardiovascular: heart murmur, cyanosis, shortness of breath, syncope, chest pain, energy level
   e. Gastrointestinal: appetite, food restriction, weight gain or loss, abdominal pain, vomiting, diarrhea, or constipation
   f. Genitourinary: polydipsia or polyuria, enuresis, urinary tract infection, dysuria, frequency, hematuria, penile discharge, vaginal discharge, and menstrual history
   g. Skeletal: deformities, scoliosis, limb pains, injuries, orthopedic appliances, and linear growth
   h. Neurologic: seizures, fainting spells, loss of consciousness, gait, and cognitive disorders
   i. Lymph: lymphadenopathy, enlarged tonsils or adenoids, and enlarged spleen

B. Objective
   1. Physical examination
      a. Height, weight, and body mass index (BMI)—chart on Centers for Disease Control and Prevention (CDC) growth charts: http://www.cdc.gov/growthcharts/charts.htm
      b. Vital signs and pain assessment: Blood pressure, heart rate, pulse, and respirations, assess pain score
      c. Vision/hearing—AAP (2014a) guidelines
      d. General appearance: state of health and alertness, mood
      e. Skin: hydration, lesions or rashes, scars, nevi, and birthmarks. Assess for bruising and/or signs of nonaccidental trauma (NAD).
      f. Head: hair growth and distribution, asymmetry
      g. Eyes: reactivity of pupils, red reflexes, fundus, extraocular movements, and cover–uncover test
      h. Ears: tympanic membrane description and mobility, cerumen, and external canal
      i. Nose: presence or absence of discharge, color of turbinates, and swelling
      j. Mouth: number of teeth, caries, occlusion, orthodontics, and lesions
      k. Neck: palpable nodes and presence of nuchal rigidity
      l. Chest: presence of rhonchi; coarseness; wheeze or diminished breath sounds in lung fields; breast development (females); Tanner stage
      m. Cardiac: rate, rhythm, pulses; presence of murmur, gallop, or click
      n. Abdomen: palpable organs, masses, tenderness, and guarding
      o. Genitalia: Tanner stage; circumcision, foreskin retractability, and testes (males); general description of vaginal introitus, clitoris, labia (females)

p. Musculoskeletal: muscle strength, range of motion, and scoliosis

q. Neurologic: mental status examination; cerebellar testing; sensory, motor (fine and gross) status; deep tendon reflexes; and cranial nerves II–XII

III. Assessment

A. *Determine the child's current health status*

B. *Identify the child's general health risks based on age, gender, and ethnicity and specific health risks*

C. *Determine child and caregiver's motivation to promote and maintain positive health behaviors*

D. *Delineate the child's ability to accomplish and master milestones of middle childhood*

IV. Plan

A. *Diagnostics (screening and secondary prevention tests)*

A periodicity schedule for preventive pediatric health care is available through the AAP (AAP, 2014b) available at http://pediatrics.aappublications.org/content/133/3/568.full.pdf.

1. Hearing risk assessment (Hagan, Shaw, & Duncan, 2008; Harlor & Bower, 2009). Auditory skills monitoring annually or if indicated by parental or teacher concerns

2. Vision screen (Hagan et al., 2008; Kelly, 2014). Assess for defects in visual acuity annually or if indicated by parental or teacher concerns

3. Oral health screening (AAP, 2014b; Kelly, 2014)
   a. Assessment for caries, gingival health, and orthodontic needs
   b. Recommend routine dental visit every 6 months

4. Lead poisoning (AAP, 2014a; Kelly, 2014) for recent immigrant, foreign adoptee, and refugee children between ages 6 months and 16 years

5. Tuberculosis (TB) screening (AAP, 2014a; Kelly, 2014)
   a. Targeted screening by purified protein derivative annually for children with the following
      i. Contacts with persons with active TB
      ii. Those who are foreign born; those who travel to or have household visitors from a country with a high TB prevalence, such as Mexico, Central America, the Philippines, Vietnam, India, and China
      iii. Contacts with high-risk adults, including those who are in homeless shelters, incarcerated, infected with HIV, or intravenous drug users; and those with chronic conditions, such as diabetes mellitus, renal failure, malnutrition, or other immunodeficiencies

6. Dyslipidemia risk assessment (AAP, 2014a; Kelly, 2014)
   a. Risk assessment at ages 2, 4, 6, and 8 years
   b. Risk factors
      i. Family history of dyslipidemia, premature cardiovascular disease, or diabetes, or if family history is unknown
      ii. Children with disease states associated with cardiovascular disease
      iii. Body mass index ≥ 85th percentile for age and gender, hypertension, or insulin resistance
   c. If risk factors are present, test with fasting lipid profile; repeat testing in 3–5 years if results are within normal limits
   d. Screen all children once between ages 9 and 11, regardless of risk factors (AAP, 2014a)

7. Depression: begin screening age 11 (Hagan et al., 2008)
   a. See Chapter 13, Childhood Depression, for screen recommendations and available screening tools

B. *Therapeutics and treatments*

1. Immunizations appropriate for age are available at http://www.cdc.gov/vaccines/schedules/

2. Oral fluoride supplementation (if primary water source is deficient in fluoride)

3. Vitamin D supplementation-consider for all children 6 to 11 years of age

C. *Patient and family education (Figure 6-1)*

1. Discussion of parent and child concerns

2. Discussion of nutritional requirements, physical activities appropriate for age, and limitation of entertainment screen time to 2 hours per day

3. Child–parent discussion of safety: helmet use, car (booster seats, seatbelts), protective sports and recreational equipment, water safety, pedestrian safety, exposure to bullying through school, texting, or social media

4. Discussion of approaches to discipline within the family

5. Discussion of middle childhood needs for peer interaction and socialization

FIGURE 6-1 Safety, Nutrition, and Activity Guidelines for Your School-Aged Child

- *Recreational activities* should always be supervised and full protective sports gear used. Helmets should be used with any wheeled devices. Pedestrian safety reviewed; bicycle, scooter, and skateboard safety and protective equipment; and water safety including sun exposure and protection reviewed.

- *Teach* your child to think carefully about his or her surroundings, particularly around new animals or people. Review the use of 911 and what to do if a child gets lost or separated. Model safe habits, such as seatbelt use, and instruct your child to wear his or her seatbelt appropriately for age and weight.

- *Prepare and practice* for emergency situations in the home, such as fire or natural disaster. Make sure you have a planned reunification point (a school, firehouse, and so forth) in the event of a catastrophe. Have emergency supplies for at least 3 days. Have an emergency "go bag" with essential items if you are forced to leave home quickly. Include in the bag any medical needs, emergency instructions, and contact information. Instruct all your caregivers regarding the emergency plan and location of the go bag.

- *Computers/tablets/cellphone use* or any other device allowing online access should be closely monitored. Computer use should be supervised and parents should review clear limits and enact parental controls on media as indicated. Review recommendations for limiting entertainment screen time to 2 hours daily.

Nutrition Tips (U.S. Department of Agriculture, 2010):

- *Make at least half your grains whole:* whole-wheat bread, oatmeal, brown rice
- *Vary your veggies:* go dark green and orange with your vegetables
- *Focus on fruits:* fresh, frozen, canned, or dried, and go easy on the fruit juice
- *Get your calcium-rich foods:* low-fat and fat-free milk products several times a day
- *Go lean with protein:* eat lean or low-fat meat, chicken, turkey, fish, and dry beans
- *Change your oil:* fish, nuts, and liquid oils, such as corn, soybean, canola, and olive oil
- *Avoid:* Sweetened-sugared beverages and foods. Encourage water daily.

Activity (CDC, 2010):

- *60 minutes or more EVERY day!*
- *Limit* "screen time" (includes television, video games, and computer time) to 2 hours a day.
- *Vigorous exercise* at least 3 days a week including outdoor activity—running; bicycle riding; jumping rope; swimming; organized sports including soccer, basketball, baseball, tennis, martial arts, or gymnastics.
- *Strengthen muscles* by participating in sports or gymnastics or using outdoor recreational equipment at least 3 days a week.
- *Strengthen bones* with activities such as jumping rope or running at least 3 days a week. Some examples of bone strengthening activities include such games as hopscotch, hopping, skipping, jumping, jumping rope, and running and such sports as gymnastics, basketball, volleyball, or tennis.

Data from Centers for Disease Control and Prevention. (2010). *Physical activity for everyone.* Retrieved from http://www.cdc.gov /physicalactivity/everyone/guidelines/children.html; U.S. Department of Food and Agriculture, Food and Nutrition Service. (2010). *Team nutrition: My pyramid for kids.* Retrieved from http://www.fns.usda.gov/TN/kids-pyramid.html.

6. Discussion of child adjustment to classroom and school setting

7. Discussion of opportunities for skill mastery and self-esteem building

8. Ages 8–11 years: discussions of child's pubertal development, hygiene, and body image

9. Discussion of child's relationship with peers, school, and family

D. Expected child–parent outcomes

1. Anticipatory guidance and reassurance when indicted in relation to parent and child's concerns

2. Nutrition and physical activity: understands nutritional and physical activity recommendations appropriate for age

3. Safety measures understood for helmet use, car boosters, sports and recreational equipment, pedestrian safety, social media exposure, texting, bullying and personal safety

4. Discipline and behavior: parents agree on an approach to discipline and implement it with consistency; address any behavioral problems in home and school setting

5. Developmental needs: parental understanding of child's need for peer interaction, socialization, and opportunities for skill mastery

6. Education: parents assess child's performance in school and adjustment to current teacher/class; address parental concerns and provide anticipatory guidance

7. Sexuality: developmentally appropriate discussion and anticipatory guidance on pubertal developmental stages and body image

8. Ages 8–11 years: encourage child able to verbalize "body concerns" and understanding of puberty; review available adult to talk with about issues with peers, family, teachers, and sports performance and participation

REFERENCES

American Academy of Pediatrics. (2014a). 2014 Recommendations for pediatric preventive health care. *Pediatrics, 133,* 568. Retrieved from http://pediatrics.aappublications.org/content/133/3/568.full?sid=84c54f2b-f79a-4830-80ca-2fdaf5c3b471.

American Academy of Pediatrics. (2014b). Maintaining and improving the oral health of young children. *Pediatrics, 134*(6), 1224–1229.

American Heart Association, Gidding, S., Dennison, B., Birch, L., Daniels, S., Gilman, M., Lichtenstein, A., et al. (2006). Dietary recommendations for children and adolescents: A guide for practitioners. *Pediatrics, 117*(2), 544–559.

Centers for Disease Control and Prevention. (2010). *How much physical activity do children need?* Retrieved from http://www.cdc.gov/physical-activity/everyone/guidelines/children.html.

Duderstadt, K. G. (Ed.). (2014). *Pediatric physical examination: An illustrated handbook* (2nd ed.). St. Louis: Elsevier.

Espelage, D. L., & De La Rue, L. (2011). School bullying: Its nature and ecology. *International Journal of Adolescent Medicine and Health, 24*(1), 3–10.

Gold, M. (2009, October 27). Kids watch more than a day of TV each week. *Los Angeles Times.* Retrieved from http://articles.latimes.com/2009/oct/27/entertainment/et-kids-tv27.

Gonida, E. N., & Cortina, K. S. (2014). Parental involvement in homework: Relations with parent and student achievement-related motivational beliefs and achievement. *British Journal of Educational Psychology, 84,* 376–396.

Hagan, J. F., Shaw, J. S., & Duncan, P. M. (2008). *Bright futures: Guidelines for health supervision of infants, children, and adolescents* (3rd ed.). Elk Grove Village, IL: American Academy of Pediatrics.

Harlor, A. D., & Bower, C. (2009). Hearing assessment in infants and children: Recommendations beyond neonatal screening. *Pediatrics, 124*(4), 1252–1263.

Kelly, N. (2014, August 27). *Screening tests in children and adolescents.* UpToDate. Retrieved from http://www.uptodate.com/contents/screening-tests-in-children-and-adolescents?source=search_result&search=screening+tests+in+children+and+adolescents&selectedTitle=1%7E150#H16.

U.S. Department of Agriculture, Food and Nutrition Service. (2010). *Team nutrition: My pyramid for kids.* Retrieved from http://www.fns.usda.gov/tn/team-nutrition.

Zuckerman, D. (2001). *When little girls become women: Early onset of puberty in girls.* The Ribbon. Retrieved from http://envirocancer.cornell.edu/Newsletter/articles/v6little.girls.cfm.

THE ADOLESCENT AND YOUNG ADULT (12–21 YEARS OF AGE) INTERVAL VISIT

Erica Monasterio

I. Introduction and general background

A. Developmental considerations

Adolescence, generally considered to encompass ages 12–21, is a time of enormous development and change in all domains of a young person's and a family's life. Bridging and overlapping childhood and young adulthood, adolescents experience the physical changes of growth and sexual maturation; continued developmental changes in both structure and function of their brains (a process not completed until the mid to late 20s); and cognitive, psychologic, and social changes related to both their physical changes and roles and expectations of the culture and society in which they live.

B. Adolescent consent and confidentiality

1. For the healthcare provider, the care of the adolescent may also be a time of transition, because it is the relationship that develops between the youth and the provider that becomes the key to the efficacy with which the provider can assess what services and interventions may be appropriate (Gilbert, Rickert, & Aalsma, 2014). The provider must develop an alliance with the youth, and addressing issues of confidentiality is the cornerstone of this alliance. Without assurances of confidentiality, the most vulnerable youth in need of attention and intervention, those who engage in behaviors that present a risk to their health, who are depressed or suicidal, and who report poor communication and lack of perceived support from their parent or caregiver, may avoid health care altogether (Lehrer, Pantell, Tebb, & Shafer, 2007). For these reasons, it is recommended that providers seeing adolescents be prepared to spend time in the visit with both the parent or caregiver and adolescent together and with the adolescent alone to get a full picture of the youth's strengths, risks, and overall physical and psychologic health status (Ford, English, & Sigman, 2004).

2. Although the involvement and participation of a caring adult in the provision of adolescent services is desirable, there are situations in which a young person may not feel able to involve their parent or in which parental involvement could impair the youth's ability to seek or receive services. All states give adolescents some rights to both consent to care and maintain privacy related to care for confidential issues (Klein & Hutchison, 2012). Laws vary significantly from state to state as to the services to which youth can independently consent; therefore, it is incumbent on the healthcare provider to be familiar with consent and confidentiality laws for minors in their state.

3. Effective communication with both youth and their caregivers about adolescent consent and confidentiality rights is essential to establishing rapport and eliciting pertinent information. A brief discussion of adolescent consent and confidentiality with youths and parents or caregivers, emphasizing the aspects of developing self-reliance and skills to manage their own health care, helps to set the stage. Assuring the parent or caregiver that youth are always encouraged to communicate with their parents and that their presence and participation is valued reassures them that they are not being "shut out" of their child's care. Additionally, it is important for youths to become more familiar with their own past health history as they transition into becoming the main source of their own health information. Both parents/caregivers and youths should be informed of the conditional nature of adolescent confidentiality rights because of obligations to protect adolescents in the event that they are a danger to themselves or others or have been subjected to any reportable

abuse. Once alone with the adolescent, it is helpful for the provider to elicit the youth's understanding of conditional confidentiality and provide a rationale for the personal nature of the questions that will be asked.

C. Rationale for the psychosocial assessment

1. The leading causes of morbidity and mortality in adolescents (accidents, homicides, and suicides) are rooted in behavioral risk that the astute provider can identify and in which they can attempt to intervene (Heron & Tejada-Vera, 2009). For this reason, the major consensus guidelines focused on the care of adolescents (*Guidelines for Adolescent Preventative Services* from the American Medical Association and *Bright Futures* from the Maternal-Child Health Bureau and the American Academy of Pediatrics [AAP]) concur that a psychosocial assessment, focused to determine the strengths and risks of the youth and guide the physical and psychologic assessment and intervention process, is recommended (Ford, English, & Sigman, 2004; Hagen, Shaw, & Duncan, 2008).

D. Periodicity and focus of well-adolescent care

1. Yearly well-adolescent visits are recommended, with an emphasis on prevention, education, and counseling for both youth and parents and guardians, screening for risk behaviors and their consequences, and counseling on healthy lifestyles. Healthy People 2020 identified 11 critical objectives for youth, focusing on the social determinants of adolescent health and their interactions with the core indicators, including reproductive health care, healthy development through engagement with parents, school and community, school completion, injury and violence prevention, mental health, substance abuse, sexual health, and prevention of chronic diseases of adulthood (Office of Disease Prevention and Health Promotion, 2015).

2. According to *Bright Futures*, priority areas to address in the well-adolescent visit include the following:
   a. Physical growth and development (physical and oral health, body image, healthy eating, and physical activity).
   b. Social and academic competence (connectedness with family, peers, and community; interpersonal relationships; and school performance).
   c. Emotional well-being (coping, mood regulation and mental health, and sexuality).
   d. Risk reduction (tobacco, alcohol, or other drugs; pregnancy; and sexually transmitted infections [STIs]).
   e. Violence and injury prevention (safety belt and helmet use, driving [graduated license] and substance abuse, guns, interpersonal violence [dating violence], and bullying) (Hagen et al., 2008).

II. Database (may include but is not limited to)

A. Subjective (to be obtained with both the youth and parent or caregiver present)

1. Client and parent or caregiver concerns
2. History of any presenting concerns
3. Past medical history
   a. Congenital or chronic conditions
   b. Surgery or hospitalizations
   c. Accidents or injuries, including injuries in sports activities that have required exclusion from play and head injuries resulting in loss of consciousness or memory loss
4. Medications inclusive of over-the-counter and complementary alternative medications
   a. Drug, dose, prescriber, and medication adherence
   b. Revisit topic of medications once alone with the youth to determine if using any medications to treat or suppress STIs or to prevent pregnancy
5. Dental
   a. Last dental visit
6. Communicable diseases
   a. Varicella (documented disease or vaccination)
   b. Hepatitis (travel to or recent emigrant from endemic areas, perinatal acquisition)
   c. Exposure to tuberculosis
7. Immunizations
   a. Completion of childhood immunizations
   b. Initiation or completion of adolescent immunizations—current schedule available at http://www.cdc.gov/vaccines/schedules/
8. Allergies
   a. Seasonal allergies
   b. Food allergies or intolerances
   c. Drug reactions
9. Family history
   a. First-degree relatives with a history of
      i. Hypertension

ii. Hyperlipidemia
iii. Cardiovascular disease
iv. Sudden cardiac or unexplained death
v. Cerebrovascular accidents
vi. Seizure disorder
vii. Diabetes
viii. Obesity
ix. Cancer
x. Mental health diagnoses
xi. Substance abuse
xii. Other medical or mental health problems

B. Subjective history (to be obtained only with the youth)

The psychosocial history, obtained after separating the youth and parent or caregiver, must be adapted to the age, developmental stage, and interactive style of the adolescent. The mnemonic HEEADSSS (for Home, Education/employment, Eating, Activities, Drugs, Sexuality, Suicide/depression/Self-image, and Safety) provides a flexible tool for guiding a discussion with an adolescent about the protective and risk factors in their lives (Klein, Goldenring, & Adelman, 2014). Another approach, SSHADESS (for Strengths, School, Home, Activities, Drugs/substance use, Emotions/depression, Sexuality, and Safety) ensures that the provider starts with a focus on strengths that can then be built on in the context of the assessment and counseling (Ginsburg, 2007).

1. Home
   a. Who lives in the home?
   b. How do family members get along?
   c. Connectedness and engagement with and monitoring by parents or caregiver
2. Education and employment
   a. School attendance
   b. School achievement (grades)
   c. School experience and connectedness to school (including direct queries about bullying)
   d. Concerns about school
   e. Attitude toward school: good, poor, or indifferent
   f. Work: type of work and how many hours
   g. Goals: academic and career
3. Eating
   a. Body image
   b. Recent changes in weight
   c. Nutritional intake
   d. Eating patterns
   e. Family meals
   f. Dieting and weight control
4. Activities
   a. Peers: same gender, opposite gender, relationship quality (friends or romantic partners)
   b. Peer relationships: close circle of friends or few friends or no close friends and often alone
   c. Outside interests: sports, music, dancing, hobbies, or organized club or church activities
   d. Amount of daily screen time (television, computer, tablet, video games, cellphone, texting)
5. Drugs and alcohol
   a. Tobacco, alcohol and drug use (quantify frequency, intensity, patterns, and context of use)
   b. Family and friends' substance use patterns
6. Sexuality
   a. Information appropriate for age
   b. Attracted to same, opposite, or both genders
   c. Romantic relationships
   d. Sexually active
      i. Age of sexual debut
      ii. Number of partners
      iii. Gender of partners
      iv. Contraception type and frequency of use
         a. Partner support or resistance to pregnancy and STI prevention efforts
      v. Type and frequency of protected or unprotected sex
      vi. Comfort or satisfaction with sexual activity
      vii. History of STIs
7. Suicide and depression
   a. Mood or energy level
   b. Stress and coping
   c. Depression
   d. Self-destructive behavior, cutting
   e. Suicidal thoughts or suicide attempts
   f. History of mental health services or experience with counseling
8. Safety
   a. Use of seatbelts
   b. Riding in or driving a car under the influence
   c. Use of protective equipment for sports activities
   d. Sense of safety, experienced bullying or violence or history of abuse in:
      i. Home
      ii. School (including being a target of or witnessing bullying)
      iii. Relationships (peer and romantic)
      iv. Community

C. Review of systems

1. General health: fatigue, fever, weight change, appetite change, mood change, and sleep problems
2. Skin: lesions, rashes, and acne
3. Hematology: excessive bleeding, bruising, and lymphadenopathy

4. Head–eyes–ears–nose–throat: headaches, head injuries, vision problems, wears glasses, ear pain, decreased hearing, allergies, frequent colds, snoring, dental hygiene, last dentist visit, difficulty swallowing, hoarseness, or sore throats

5. Respiratory: asthma, frequent colds or cough, wheezing, shortness of breath, and exercise-induced cough or wheezing

6. Cardiovascular: heart murmurs, chest pain, palpitations, syncope or near syncope, and shortness of breath on exertion

7. Gastrointestinal: abdominal pain, nausea, vomiting, diarrhea, constipation, and bloody stool

8. Genitourinary: enuresis, dysuria, frequency, hematuria, vaginal discharge, urethral discharge, testicular pain, vulvar lesions, and genital lesions

9. Skeletal: deformities or scoliosis, joint pain, joint swelling, injuries, and back pain

10. Neurologic: headache, seizures, syncope, dizziness, and numbness

11. Endocrine: polyuria and polydipsia

12. Female: menarche, last menstrual period, regularity and frequency, duration, dysmenorrhea, and premenstrual symptoms

13. Male: body hair and voice change

14. Psychologic and emotional: mood, stress, and emotional or mental health problems or diagnoses, behavioral or mental healthcare source if any

D. Objective

1. Physical examination
   a. Height and weight (measure and plot on growth chart if under 18)—refer to the following link for Centers for Disease Control and Prevention (CDC) growth charts: http://www.cdc.gov/growthcharts/data/set1clinical/set1color.pdf.
   b. Body mass index (BMI) (calculate and plot on BMI graph if under 18; underweight = age and gender-specific BMI at < 5th percentile; normal weight = age and gender-specific BMI at ≥ 5th to < 85th percentile; overweight = age and gender-specific BMI at ≥ 85th to < 95th percentile; obesity = age and gender-specific BMI at ≥ 95th percentile); refer to http://www.cdc.gov/growthcharts/data/set1clinical/set1color.pdf.
   c. Blood pressure, pulse, and respiration
   d. Vision (Snellen once in early, middle, and late adolescence—12, 15, and 18 years old; more frequently based on risk assessment)
   e. Hearing (audiometry only if positive responses to screening questions to determine risk for or evidence of hearing impairment)
   f. Mental status
   g. State of nutrition
   h. Skin: scars, tattoos, piercings, signs of self-injurious behavior, acne, and acanthosis nigricans
   i. Ears
   j. Eyes: include fundoscopic examination
   k. Nose: patency, adenoids, nasal mucosa, septum, piercings
   l. Mouth: teeth (gums, caries, and occlusion), piercings
   m. Pharynx: tonsillar size and quality
   n. Thyroid: size and quality
   o. Lymph nodes
      i. Cervical
      ii. Axillary
      iii. Inguinal
   p. Breasts: inspect for sexual maturity rating (SMR) or Tanner stage, clinical breast examination after age 20 in females; gynecomastia in males
   q. Lungs: wheezing and adventitious sounds
   r. Heart: murmurs (upright and supine), rate, rhythm, lower extremity pulses, and radial/femoral pulse delay
   s. Abdomen: masses and hepatosplenomegaly
   t. Genitalia
      i. Males: inspect for SMR, signs of STIs, palpation of scrotum and testes for masses, and presence of hernia
      ii. Females: inspect for SMR, signs of STIs and dermatologic conditions of the vulva; use noninvasive (urine-based or high vaginal swab) screening tests for gonorrhea and *Chlamydia* when possible
      iii. Pelvic examination indicated at 21 years of age to obtain first Pap smear or without a Pap smear if sexually active with signs and symptoms of STI, pregnancy, or pelvic infection or to evaluate abnormal pubertal development or abnormal vaginal bleeding
   u. Musculoskeletal
      i. Back: range of motion and presence of scoliosis
      ii. Extremities: joint pain, swelling, and stability; range of motion
      iii. Fourteen-point musculoskeletal screening (Rodriguez, 2014)
      iv. Neurologic: strength, deep tendon reflexes, coordination and gait, and cranial nerves II–XII

III. Assessment

A. *Identify the strengths and protective factors that will support the youth and family in successfully negotiating challenges in adolescence.*

B. *Identify the youth's specific health risks, based on family history, past medical history, and behavioral choices and activities in which the youth engages.*

C. *Determine the youth's current health status.*

D. *Determine the youth's motivation to modify health-damaging behaviors and promote and maintain health-promoting behaviors.*

E. *Determine the parent or caregiver's motivation to support the youth's behavior change plan as appropriate.*

IV. Plan

A. *Screening*

1. Psychosocial and behavioral assessment (annually) (Hagan et al., 2008).

2. Major depressive disorder screening when systems for diagnosis, treatment, and follow-up are in place, using such tools as the Patient Health Questionnaire for Adolescents or the Beck Depression Inventory–Primary Care Version (U.S. Preventive Services Task Force, 2009).

3. Alcohol and drug use risk assessment (annually), with follow-up in-depth assessment based on findings using a youth-specific alcohol and drug screening assessment tool, such as CRAFFT (Hagan et al., 2008).

4. Hemoglobin and hematocrit every 5–10 years starting in adolescence, more frequently if indicated based on risk (heavy or frequent menses, poor nutritional intake, limited dietary sources of iron, and history of iron-deficiency anemia) (AAP, 2014).

5. Dyslipidemia screening (fasting total cholesterol, low-density lipoprotein [LDL], high-density lipoprotein [HDL], and triglycerides)
   a. 12–16 years old: Selective screening using fasting lipid panel (FLP) two times (> 2 weeks and < 3 months apart), if family history of coronary heart disease (i.e., parent, grandparent, or aunt/uncle); parent with total cholesterol ≥ 240 mg/dL or known dyslipidemia; patient has diabetes, hypertension, BMI ≥ 85th percentile, or smokes cigarettes; patient has a moderate- or high-risk medical condition associated with cardiovascular disease (i.e., chronic kidney disease, recipient of a cardiac transplant, Kawasaki disease with current or regressed coronary artery disease, or chronic inflammatory disease)
   b. 17–21 years old: Universal screening once during this time period with a nonfasting lipid screening using non-HDL cholesterol levels; further evaluation if nonfasting non-HDL cholesterol level ≥ 145 mg/dL, and HDL < 40 mg/dL, FLP with LDL cholesterol ≥ 130 mg/dL, non-HDL cholesterol ≥ 145 mg/dL, HDL cholesterol < 40 mg/dL, or triglycerides ≥ 130 mg/dL (Daniels et al., 2012).

6. Tuberculosis testing based on risk assessment (family member or household contact with tuberculosis or positive TB test, born in tuberculosis endemic country, travel with > 1 week residence in tuberculosis endemic country), or annually if HIV positive, incarcerated youth or living in group home or shelter (AAP, 2007).

7. Chlamydia screening annually for all sexually active females ≤ 25 years old; screening of high-risk young men is a clinical option (U.S. Preventive Services Task Force, 2014).

8. Gonorrhea screening annually for all sexually active females ≤ 25 years old, young men who have sex with men, young men with multiple partners, and those seen in high-prevalence settings, such as adolescent clinics, correctional facilities, and STI clinics (CDC, 2010a).

9. Syphilis screening for all pregnant women, young men who have sex with men and engage in high-risk sexual behaviors, commercial sex workers, youth who exchange sex for drugs, and youth in adult correctional facilities (U.S. Preventive Services Task Force, 2014).

10. HIV screening once for all individuals between 13 and 64 years of age regardless of recognized risk factors (CDC, 2006). Repeat HIV screening should be discussed with all adolescents and encouraged in those who are sexually active or use injection drugs (CDC, 2010b) and all adolescents seeking screening and treatment for STIs (CDC, 2010a).

11. Cervical cancer screening (Pap smear) for all women at age 21 regardless of sexual history, then every 3 years if normal Pap smear (U.S. Preventive Services Task Force, 2012).

B. Immunization update

1. Immunizations for adolescents—current schedule available at http://www.cdc.gov/vaccines/schedules/.

2. Immunization lag: the following immunizations have commonly been missed in the adolescents and should be administered as "catch up" immunizations at the annual health visitor interval visit:
   a. Varicella #2
   b. Hepatitis A #2
   c. Tdap
   d. Meningococcal conjugate vaccine (MCV4) #1 and #2
   e. Human papilloma virus (HPV) series

C. Anticipatory guidance

1. Normative development and developmental progression (discuss with youth and parent or caregiver as appropriate)
   a. Adapt to youth's developmental stage and any concerns of youth or parent or caregiver
   b. Include counseling regarding physical and psychosocial development
   c. Address levels of stress in youth and family and discuss healthy versus dysfunctional coping mechanisms
   d. Use an approach that is dynamic, interactive, and inclusive of the youth, prioritizing behaviors that the young person is interested in modifying and developing a plan with the youth rather than for the youth (Erickson, Gerstle, & Feldstein, 2005)
   e. Address parenting issues, emphasize continued importance of parental support and control from parent or caregiver to youth

2. Nutrition and activity counseling (discuss with youth and parent as appropriate):
   a. Avoid skipping meals, particularly emphasize the importance of breakfast
   b. Drink adequate fluids, emphasize water and avoidance of high intake of soda, juice, sports drinks, and caffeinated drinks
   c. Increase intake of fruits and vegetables
   d. Avoid high caloric and low nutritional value snacks
   e. Build physical activity into everyday routine and limit "screen time"
   f. Refer overweight and obese patients to comprehensive moderate- to high-intensity programs that include dietary, physical activity, and behavioral counseling components (U.S. Preventive Services Task Force, 2010)

3. Safety, injury, and violence prevention counseling as appropriate to age and developmental stage and individual risk
   a. Use of protective gear for sports and leisure activities
   b. Automobile safety
      i. Seatbelt use
      ii. Counseling regarding alcohol and drug use and driving or riding with an impaired driver
   c. Nonviolent conflict resolution
   d. Dating and relationship safety and healthy relationships

4. Tobacco, alcohol, and other drug counseling as appropriate to age and developmental stage and individual risk (with youth alone, using a motivational counseling approach)
   a. Tobacco resistance and cessation
      i. Include discussion of "e-cigarettes" and risks of nicotine exposure in all forms
   b. Alcohol resistance and use modification
      i. Discuss binge drinking patterns, risks, and self-management
   c. Marijuana resistance and use modification
      i. Discuss impact of marijuana use on learning, school performance, goal setting, and decision making
   d. Other substances of abuse related to individual risk, individual use, and community use patterns

5. Sexual health and risk reduction as appropriate to age and developmental stage and individual risk (with youth alone, using a motivational counseling approach)
   a. Relationship quality and sexual decision making
   b. Encourage delaying onset of sexual activity with younger adolescents
   c. Contraception and pregnancy prevention
      i. Discuss access to emergency contraception with all youth regardless of current sexual activity
      ii. Counsel regarding contraceptive choice as appropriate to current and anticipated sexual activity, using an efficacy-based approach starting with the most effective, long-acting reversible contraceptives (LARC): implants and intrauterine devices (IUDs) (AAP Committee on Adolescence, 2014)
   d. STI and HIV risk reduction
      i. Discuss risk reduction approaches with all youth regardless of current sexual activity

V. Self-management resources

A. For adolescents

1. Interactive website with a question and answer format by and for teenagers by the Adolescent/Young Adult Center for Health at Goryeb Children's Hospital is available at http://www.teenhealthfx.com.

2. Centers for Disease Control and Prevention youth website with games and facts about health for middle school children and early adolescents is available at http://www.bam.gov.

3. Resource to increase teens' health awareness and empower young people to take an active role in their health by Nemours Children's Health Systems is available at http://kidshealth.org/teen.

4. Birth Control Method Explorer, an interactive website with medically correct contraceptive information by The National Campaign to Prevent Teen and Unplanned Pregnancy, is available at http://bedsider.org/methods.

5. Information and counseling about healthy relationships and unhealthy relationships and abuse including live chat and text to chat options hosted by the National Domestic Violence Hotline and Break the Cycle are available at http://www.loveisrespect.org/.

B. For parents or caregivers

1. Advice and tools for parents on how to talk to their teens about tough topics by the Office of Adolescent Health are available at http://www.hhs.gov/ash/oah/resources-and-publications/info/parents/get-started/.

2. Palo Alto Medical Foundation information for parents of teenagers and preteenagers about a variety of health and social issues is available at http://www.pamf.org/parents.

3. Basic information about talking with youth about challenging issues by Children Now and Kaiser Family Foundation is available at http://www.talkingwithkids.org.

4. Multimedia site for parents providing guidance on how to talk to teens about sexual decision making and pregnancy prevention by the National Campaign to Prevent Teen and Unplanned Pregnancy is available at https://thenationalcampaign.org/featured-topics/parents.

C. For healthcare providers

1. Parent information handouts on 15 adolescent topics ranging from vaccines to alcohol and drug use prevention by the American Medical Association are available at http://www.thefamilywatch.org/doc/doc-0113-es.pdf.

2. *Bright Futures: Guidelines for Health Supervision of Adolescents* (2nd edition), developed by the American Academy of Pediatrics and the Maternal Child Health Bureau, is available at https://brightfutures.aap.org/pdfs/Guidelines_PDF/18-Adolescence.pdf.

3. Adolescent Health Working Group's "Adolescent Providers Toolkit Series" available at http://www.ahwg.net/resources-for-providers.html includes five modules that contain screening tools, brief office interventions and counseling guidelines, community resources and referrals, health education materials for teenagers and their parents or caregivers, literature reviews, and Internet resources.

REFERENCES

American Academy of Pediatrics. (2007). Tuberculosis. In *Red book atlas of pediatric infectious diseases.* Elk Grove Village, IL: American Academy of Pediatrics. Retrieved from http://www.ebrary.com.

American Academy of Pediatrics. (2014). *Recommendations for pediatric preventive health care.* Retrieved from http://pediatrics.aappublications.org/content/133/3/568.full?sid=84c54f2b-f79a-4830-80ca-2fdaf5c3b471.

American Academy of Pediatrics Committee on Adolescence. (2014). Contraception for adolescents. *Pediatrics, 134* (4), e1244–e1256.

Centers for Disease Control and Prevention. (2006). Revised recommendations for HIV testing of adults, adolescents, and pregnant women in health-care settings. *Morbidity and Mortality Weekly Report, 55*(RR-14), 1–17.

Centers for Disease Control and Prevention. (2010a). *Sexually transmitted diseases treatment guidelines 2010. HIV infection: Detection, counseling, and referral.* Retrieved from http://www.cdc.gov.ucsf.idm.oclc.org/std/treatment/2010/hiv.htm#a1.

Centers for Disease Control and Prevention. (2010b). *Sexually transmitted diseases treatment guidelines 2010. Special populations.* Retrieved from http://www.cdc.gov.ucsf.idm.oclc.org/std/treatment/2010/special pops.htm#a2.

Daniels, S. R., Benuck, I., Christakis, D. A., Dennison, B. A., Gidding, S. S., Gillman, M. W., et al. (2012). *Expert panel on integrated guidelines for cardiovascular health and risk reduction in children and adolescents: Full report.* Bethesda, MD: National Heart Lung and Blood Institute. Retrieved from https://www.nhlbi.nih.gov/files/docs/guidelines/peds_guidelines_full.pdf.

English, A., & Ford, C. A. (2007). More evidence supports the need to protect confidentiality in adolescent health care. *Journal of Adolescent Health, 40*(3), 199–200.

English, A., Ford, C. A., & Santelli, J. S. (2009). Clinical preventive services for adolescents: Position paper of the society for adolescent medicine. *American Journal of Law and Medicine, 35*(2–3), 351–364.

Erickson, S. J., Gerstle, M., & Feldstein, S. W. (2005). Brief interventions and motivational interviewing with children, adolescents, and their parents in pediatric health care settings: A review. *Archives of Pediatrics & Adolescent Medicine, 159*(12), 1173–1180.

Ford, C., English, A., & Sigman, G. (2004). Confidential health care for adolescents: Position paper for the Society for Adolescent Medicine. *Journal of Adolescent Health, 35*(2), 160–167.

Gilbert, A. L., Rickert, V. I., & Aalsma, M. C. (2014). Clinical conversations about health: The impact of confidentiality in preventive adolescent care. *Journal of Adolescent Health, 55*(5), 672–677.

Ginsburg, K. R. (2007). Viewing our adolescent patients through a positive lens. *Contemporary Pediatrics, 24,* 6–76.

Hagan, J. F., Shaw, J. S., & Duncan, P. M. (Eds.). (2008). *Bright futures: Guidelines for health supervision of infants, children, and adolescents* (3rd ed.). Elk Grove Village, IL: American Academy of Pediatrics.

Heron, M. P., & Tejada-Vera, B. (2009). Deaths: Leading causes for 2005. *National Vital Statistics Reports, 58*(8), 1–98.

Klein, D. A., & Hutchinson, J. W. (2012). Providing confidential care for adolescents. *American Family Physician, 85*(6), 556–560.

Klein, D. A., Goldenring, J. M., & Adelman, W. P. (2014, January 1). HEEADSSS 3.0: The psychosocial interview for adolescents updated for a new century fueled by media. *Contemporary Pediatrics.* Retrieved from http://contemporarypediatrics.modernmedicine.com /contemporary-pediatrics/content/tags/adolescent-medicine /heeadsss-30-psychosocial-interview-adolesce?page=0,2.

Lehrer, J., Pantell, R., Tebb, K., & Shafer, M. (2007). Forgone health care among U.S. adolescents: Associations between risk characteristics and confidentiality concern. *Journal of Adolescent Health, 40*(3), 218–226.

Office of Disease Prevention and Health Promotion. (2015). *Healthy people 2020: Adolescent health.* Washington, DC: U.S. Department of Health and Human Services. Retrieved from https://www.healthypeople .gov/2020/topics-objectives/topic/Adolescent-Health.

Rodriguez, C. R. (2014). Sports medicine in children: Preparticipation physical evaluation. *FP Essentials, 417,* 30–37.

U.S. Preventive Services Task Force. (2009). Screening and treatment for major depressive disorder in children and adolescents: U.S. Preventive Services Task Force recommendation statement. *Pediatrics, 123*(4), 1223–1228.

U.S. Preventive Services Task Force. (2010). Screening for obesity in children and adolescents: U.S. Preventive Services Task Force recommendation statement. *Pediatrics, 125*(2), 361.

U.S. Preventive Services Task Force. (2012) *Final recommendation statement: Cervical cancer: Screening.* Retrieved from http://www.uspreventiveservices taskforce.org/Page/Document/RecommendationStatementFinal /cervical-cancer-screening.

U.S. Preventive Services Task Force. (2014). *USPSTF recommendations for STI screening.* Retrieved from http://www.uspreventiveservicestaskforce .org/Page/Name/uspstf-recommendations-for-sti-screening.

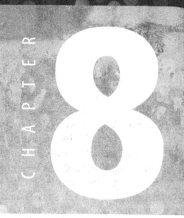

PREVENTIVE IMMUNIZATIONS FOR CHILDREN AND ADULTS

Lucy S. Crain

CHAPTER 8

I. Introduction: Overview of vaccine-preventable diseases

Simply stated, vaccines prevent disease, with their ultimate goal being to eradicate or eliminate preventable infectious diseases. Along with pure water and refrigeration, preventive vaccines are the most important public health development of the past century. Prevaccination era statistics support the remarkable impact of vaccinations. United States public health records document 48,164 annual cases of smallpox and 175,885 annual cases of respiratory tract diphtheria with high mortality in 1900–1904 and no cases of these diseases in the United States since 2003. Diphtheria is one of the vaccine-preventable diseases that remains endemic in the former Soviet Union and in Africa, Asia, Latin America, parts of Europe, and the Middle East where there are low diphtheria immunization rates (Centers for Disease Control and Prevention [CDC], 2015c).

A. Polio

There were 16,000 cases of paralytic polio reported in the United States annually during 1951–1954, a period 4 years before vaccine licensure, and no indigenously acquired cases of wild poliomyelitis since widespread use of the Salk vaccine. The oral polio live, inactivated vaccine (Salk vaccine) was replaced in the United States by killed polio (Sabin) vaccine in 1997–2000 in response to concerns about vaccine-acquired paralytic poliomyelitis (VAPP) and vulnerability of individuals with impaired immunity. The killed vaccine (Sabin) has been used exclusively in the United States since 2000 and is not associated with VAPP (Kimberlin, Long, Brady, & Jackson, 2015).

B. Measles

More than 503,000 cases of measles were reported in the United States in 1958–1962, a period 5 years before the first measles vaccine was licensed in 1963. Measles remains very common in the developing world and in Europe and Asia. Between 2001 and 2011, incidence of measles in the United States was low (37–140 cases per year), but

there were more than 600 cases of measles reported in the United States in 2014 (CDC, 2014a). Since the passage of personal belief and religious exemption legislation in several states, measles has again become a public health issue in the United States. Also called "10-day measles" or rubeola, measles is commonly thought of as an infectious disease of childhood. If uncomplicated, it is a benign viral infection with fever, cough, coryza (runny nose, upper respiratory illness-like symptoms), conjunctivitis, and a maculopapular rash that is erythematous in appearance. Koplik spots (white spots on the buccal gingival mucosa) in the mouth are pathognomonic. Measles may occur in adolescents and adults who are not immune or have not been vaccinated. Less well known to healthcare professionals who may never have seen cases of measles are the complications of this disease. These include otitis media, bronchopneumonia, croup (laryngotracheobronchitis), and diarrhea with dehydration in young children. Acute measles encephalitis occurs in approximately one of 1,000 cases in the postvaccine era and results in permanent brain damage and convulsions. Since the advent of vaccines, deaths occur in 1–3 of 1,000 cases, most commonly from measles pneumonia and/or neurologic complications. Case fatality rates are increased in children under age 5 and in children who are malnourished or those with immunocompromise. Seven to 10 years after wild measles infection, patients may develop subacute sclerosing panencephalitis (SSPE), a rare degenerative central nervous system disease. SSPE, seen more commonly in the prevaccine era, is an incurable disorder with convulsive seizures and behavioral/intellectual deterioration. SSPE has virtually disappeared in the United States since the widespread use of measles vaccine.

The World Health Organization (WHO) reports more than 400 deaths around the world each day associated with measles. It is critically important to recognize the potential lethality of measles complications in this era of antivaccine sentiment (WHO, n.d.). Society and the world economy have become increasingly global. Travel to and from countries where measles and other vaccine-preventable diseases remain endemic promotes the incidence of travel-related exposures. This is readily illustrated by the recent outbreak of more than 120 cases of measles originating from an index case at two southern California theme parks over the holidays in December 2014. The number of reported measles cases continues to increase annually, caused by the presence of nonimmune/ unvaccinated children and adults in this country. Infants who are too young to have received measles vaccine (routinely at 12 to 15 months) and those who are immunocompromised are especially at risk. Measles is highly contagious, requiring 90% or greater herd immunity to prevent spread. The PanAmerican Health Organization/World Health Organization, reporting more than 5,000 cases of imported measles in the past decade, recommends that levels of coverage with two doses of measles vaccine be maintained at 95% or greater to prevent the spread of imported cases (WHO, n.d.). The measles vaccine is highly effective, providing 95% effective protection with the first dose and 98% with the second dose.

C. Pertussis

Commonly known as whooping cough because of the whooping sound of inspiratory stridor associated with laryngospasm, pertussis is spread by human transmission, most commonly among the adult population. It is a bacterial illness commonly transmitted by adults in whom it is a relatively mild 6-week-long respiratory illness with annoying cough. Susceptible infants who have not been vaccinated are most vulnerable and at greatest risk of hospitalization and death caused by pertussis. Pertussis is readily preventable in all ages by immunization. California reported a pertussis epidemic in June 2014 with incidence more than 5 times greater than baseline levels. The last previous pertussis epidemic in California was in 2010 with over 9,000 cases reported, including 808 hospitalizations and 10 infant deaths. As of November 2014, California had reported 9,935 cases of pertussis (Winter, Glaser, Watt, & Harriman, 2014). Pregnant mothers should receive Tdap (tetanus/diphtheria/pertussis vaccine) with each pregnancy, preferably between 27 to 36 weeks gestation. If a mother did not receive her Tdap during pregnancy, she should receive it postpartum. If she has not previously been vaccinated for pertussis, she should complete the three-dose series at 4-week intervals.

D. Rubella

Before licensure of rubella vaccine, there were 40,000–50,000 cases of rubella annually in the United States. Rubella was historically called the "3-day measles" and generally thought to be a benign infectious disease with maculopapular rash, postauricular or sub occipital lymphadenopathy, and low-grade fever. Transient polyarthralgias are rare in children but common in adolescents and adults with rubella. Complications are more rare than with rubeola, with rubella encephalitis reported in 1 in 6,000 cases and thrombocytopenia reported in 1 in 3,000 cases. Worldwide rubella epidemics or pandemics occurred with fairly predictable frequency every 6 to 9 years until widespread use of the rubella vaccine. The vaccine was licensed in 1969 after the report of hundreds of cases of congenital rubella syndrome in the United States and throughout the world. Rubella "parties" were commonplace prior to vaccine implementation. Naively considering rubella a uniformly benign disease, mothers took their infants and toddlers to neighborhood gatherings where they could purposely be exposed and contract rubella, thus conveying natural immunity. Nonimmune pregnant mothers also contracted rubella, which is often subclinical in adults but can have devastating effects on the developing fetus. Although milder forms of the disease can be present with few clinical findings noted at birth, congenital defects occur in as many as 85% of infants if maternal infection occurs during the first trimester, 50% during the first 13 to 16 weeks, and 25% during the end of the second trimester of gestation. Congenital rubella syndrome birth defects include cataracts, congenital glaucoma, microphthalmia, cardiac anomalies (patent ductus arteriosus, peripheral pulmonary artery stenosis), sensorineural hearing loss, neurologic disorders including meningoencephalitis, and intellectual/developmental and behavioral disabilities.

E. Varicella

Commonly referred to as chickenpox, varicella is another usually benign infectious disease of childhood that consists of a generalized, pruritic, vesicular rash with 250 to 500 lesions distributed over the body in various stages of development and/or crusting, low-grade fever, and other systemic symptoms of viral exanthema. Less well appreciated are the complications of varicella, caused by the varicella-zoster virus (VZV). These include bacterial superinfection of skin lesions, pneumonia, encephalitis, acute cerebellar ataxia, thrombocytopenia, and less commonly glomerulonephritis, arthritis, and hepatitis. Reye syndrome can occur when salicylates are taken to alleviate fever associated with chickenpox. Severe progressive varicella with continuing eruption of lesion and high fever along with other complications can occur in immunocompromised children and adults. Children with atopic eczema are also at risk of secondary bacterial dermatitis and potential sepsis. Pneumonia is an uncommon complication of varicella in immunocompetent children, but it is the most common complication of varicella in adults. In children with HIV infections, recurrent varicella or disseminated herpes zoster can develop. VZV establishes latency in the dorsal root ganglia during primary varicella infection and/or breakthrough varicella, which may occasionally develop despite immunization. Reactivation of VZV results in shingles or herpes zoster, usually in the distribution of sensory dermatomes, and often accompanied by pain and/or pruritus. Postherpetic neuralgia may last for weeks or months, as persistent pain after resolution of the zoster rash.

Fetal infection after maternal varicella during the first or early second trimester of gestation may result in fetal death or varicella embryopathy. The latter is described as congenital varicella syndrome and is reported in approximately 1% to 2% of infants born to a mother who had varicella before 20 weeks of gestation. Also, varicella has a higher risk of fatality in infants born to mothers who develop varicella from 5 days before to 2 days after obstetric delivery, in whom there is decreased opportunity for transfer of VZV-specific maternal immunoglobulin (IgG) antibody.

F. Vaccination recommendations

The Advisory Committee on Immunization Practices (ACIP) annually develops and updates recommendations for the routine use of vaccines in children, adolescents, and adults. Chartered as a federal advisory committee, ACIP provides expert objective advice and guidance to the director of the Centers for Disease Control and Prevention on the use of vaccines and related agents for control of vaccine-preventable diseases in the civilian population of the United States. For children and adolescents, ACIP recommendations consider and generally incorporate recommendations from the American Academy of Pediatrics (AAP), American Academy of Family Physicians (AAFP), and the American College of Obstetricians and Gynecologists (ACOG). For vaccine use in adults, ACIP considers recommendations of AAFP, ACOG, the American College of Nurse Midwives (ACNM), and the American College of Physicians (ACP). Upon adoption of ACIP recommendations by the CDC director, these guidelines are published in the *Morbidity and Mortality Weekly Report* (MMWR), which is available online at ACIP.

Recommended U.S. Immunization Schedules and Catch-Up Schedules for Ages Birth Through 18 Years

Current immunization schedules for infants, children, and adolescents are available at http://www.cdc.gov/vaccines/acip and detailed immunization recommendations are at http://www.cdc.gov/vaccines/hcp/acip-recs/index.html. The CDC recommends use of combination vaccines, which are preferable to separate injections of the equivalent component vaccines. Any dose not administered at the recommended age should be administered at a subsequent visit, according to the CATCH-UP schedule (CDC, 2015a, 2015b).

I. Recommended pediatric vaccine schedule

A. Hepatitis B

Recommended preventive vaccinations should begin in the newborn with the initial dose of hepatitis B vaccine followed by a second dose between 6 and 8 weeks of age and a third dose between 6 and 18 months to complete the primary series.

B. Diphtheria and Tetanus Toxoids, and Acellular Pertussis (DTaP)

DTaP is recommended at 2, 4, 6, and 15 to 18 months with a booster fifth dose between 4 and 6 years of age. The DTaP vaccine is used for adolescents at age 11 to 12 years as the sixth dose of the series prior to middle school.

C. Rotavirus (RV)

Minimum age is 6 weeks for both RV vaccines. RV1 (Rotarix) is a two-dose series administered at 2 and 4 months of age. Alternatively, RV5 (RotaTeq) is administered as a three-dose series at 2, 4, and 6 months of age. The maximum age for the first dose of RV in the series is 14 weeks 6 days, and the maximum age for the final dose of RV is 8 months.

D. Haemophilus influenzae Type B (Hib)

Check CDC-ACIP schedule footnotes and vaccine package insert for specific product schedule: A two- or three-dose Hib vaccine primary series at 2, 4, and (6) months with a third or fourth booster dose at 12 or 15 months is recommended. Note: Multiple preparations of HIB are now available.

E. Pneumococcus, Pneumococcal Conjugate (PCV13)

PCV13 is a primary series of four doses with administration at 2, 4, 6, and 12 to 15 months. The pneumococcal polysaccharide vaccine (PCV23) may be recommended for children age 2 and older with certain high-risk conditions (including cyanotic congenital heart disease, chronic lung disease including asthma if treated with high-dose corticosteroids, diabetes mellitus, cerebrospinal fluid [CSF] leak, cochlear implants, sickle cell disease, other hemoglobinopathies, asplenia, HIV infection, chronic renal failure, immunosuppression, malignant neoplasms, leukemias, lymphomas, Hodgkin's disease, congenital immunodeficiency, and others). Check for guidance at http://www.cdc.gov/vaccines/hcp/acip for vaccine administration recommendations in high-risk children and youth age 6 through 18 years of age.

F. Inactivated Polio Virus (IPV)

Administer at 2, 4, and between 6 and 18 months plus a preschool dose at 4 to 6 years. Pediatric vaccines are routinely given at scheduled well-child health maintenance visits at 2, 4, and 6 to 18 months of age.

G. Influenza (IIV, LAIV)

Vaccination is recommended annually beginning at age 6 months. Children less than 2 years of age should be vaccinated with the inactivated influenza vaccine (IIV). After age 2, children may be vaccinated with either IIV or LAIV (live attenuated influenza vaccine). Note: LAIV should NOT be given to persons with previous severe allergic reactions to the product or another influenza vaccine, those receiving aspirin products, those with severe egg allergies, children age 2 through 4 with asthma and wheezing in the past 12 months, or persons who have taken influenza antiviral medications within the past 48 hours. See MMWR for other precautions and contraindications (Grohskopf et al., 2014).

H. Measles, Mumps, and Rubella (MMR)

Routine schedule is a two-dose series with one dose at 12–15 months and a booster dose between 4 and 6 years of age.

I. Measles, Mumps, Rubella, and Varicella (MMRV)

MMRV is indicated for simultaneous immunization against those respective diseases for children after 12 months through 12 years of age and is not indicated outside of this age group. Febrile seizures occur in 3 to 4 per 10,000 children ages 12 through 23 months receiving the first dose of MMR and varicella separately and in 7 to 9 per 10,000 receiving the first dose of MMRV. The MMRV vaccine schedule is the same as for the MMR. Single antigen measles vaccine is no longer available in the United States.

Children ages 6 to 11 months who are going to travel abroad prior to the recommended vaccine administration should have one dose of MMR vaccine administered before departure from the United States (www.cdc.gov/travel/yellowbook) (CDC, 2015c). Also, for children in this age group during a community-wide outbreak, a single dose of MMR is recommended. Seroconversion after MMR is lower for infants immunized before their first birthday, so these children will require initiation of their two-dose primary series beginning at 12 or 15 months of age. Similarly, if an infant aged 6–11 months is in a setting where disease risk is high, an initial dose can be administered with initiation of the primary series at 12 to 15 months, as long as the second dose is at least 4 weeks later. Note: Measles vaccine, if given within 72 hours of measles exposure, should provide protection or amelioration of symptoms and is the intervention of choice in outbreaks of measles in childcare centers and school settings. Intramuscular administration of immune globulin (IG) can be given within 6 days of exposure to a susceptible person, including susceptible household contacts, contacts younger than 12 months of age who have not yet been immunized, pregnant women, immunocompromised individuals, or others for whom measles vaccine is contraindicated. Children with egg allergy are at low risk of severe hypersensitivity reaction (anaphylaxis) to measles vaccines (MMR and MMRV). Skin testing of children for egg allergy is not reliable and nonpredictive of reactions to MMR vaccines. The measles vaccine is produced in chick embryo cell culture and does not contain significant amount of ovalbumin (egg white cross-reacting proteins). People with allergies to chickens or feathers are not at increased risk of allergic reaction to the vaccine. Measles (MMR and MMRV) vaccine is contraindicated for individuals who have severe hypersensitivity (anaphylaxis) to gelatin or neomycin. Read footnotes in ACIP vaccine schedules and guidelines for details (Wyckoff, 2015).

J. Varicella (VAR)

Varicella vaccine is to be administered as a two-dose series with first dose at 12–15 months and second dose at 4–6 years of age. Varicella vaccine is also available in a quadrivalent vaccine as MMRV. Note: In the event of household exposure or more than casual contact of an immunocompromised, nonimmune child or adult (including HIV infected) to an individual with contagious varicella, use of varicella-zoster immune globin (VZIG) may be indicated as soon as possible and no later than 10 days after exposure. In addition, patients with high-risk status (i.e., neonate whose mother had onset of varicella within 5 days before delivery or within 48 hours after delivery, hospitalized premature infants of birth weight 1,000 grams or less, hospitalized preterm infant more than 28 weeks of gestation whose mother lacks evidence of immunity, pregnant women without evidence of immunity) should be given VZIG if exposed to varicella. Oral acyclovir or valacyclovir is not recommended for routine use in otherwise healthy children with varicella, as administration within 24 hours of rash onset will result in only modest amelioration of symptoms. Consultation on an individual case basis with an infectious disease or public health expert is recommended for consideration of VZIG and IVIG use.

K. Hepatitis A (Hep A)

Routine two-dose series should be administered between 12 and 23 months of age with 6 to 18 months between doses. For catch-up immunization, a minimum interval of 6 months between the first and second dose is recommended.

L. Human Papillomavirus (HPV)

Administer a three-dose series of HPV vaccine beginning at 11 years of age in males and females, then at 1- to 2-month and 6-month intervals (females either HPV2, HPV4, or HPV9 and males HPV4 or HPV9). The vaccine series may be started at age 9. If not previously vaccinated, adolescents ages 13 through 18 should receive the three-dose series with a minimum of 4 weeks between the first and second doses and the third dose 16 weeks after the second dose or 24 weeks after the first dose. Note: Multiple preparations are available: HPV2/Cervarix for females only, minimum age 9 years; HPV4/Gardasil 4 for males or females; HPV9/Gardasil 9 for females or males aged 9–15.

M. Meningococcal Conjugate Vaccines

Minimum age 6 weeks for Hib-MenCY (MenHibrix), 9 months for MenACWY-D (Menactra), and 2 months for Men ACWY-CRM (Menveo). Routine vaccination is a single dose of Menactra or Menveo vaccine at age 11 through 12 plus a booster dose at age 16. Adolescents with human immunodeficiency virus (HIV) infection should receive a two-dose primary series with at least 8 weeks between doses. For children ages 2 months through 18 years with high-risk conditions, see footnotes at http://www.cdc.gov/vaccines/hcp/acip-recs/index.html.

II. Adult immunization recommendations

The annual ACIP Adult Immunization Schedule is approved by the CDC Advisory Committee on Immunization Practices, American Academy of Family Physicians, the American College of Obstetricians and Gynecologists, the American College of Nurse Midwives, and the American College of Physicians and published in January. Immunization schedules can be found at http://www.cdc.gov/vaccines/schedules/index.html.

ACIP and the CDC advise that all clinically significant postvaccination reactions be reported to the Vaccine Adverse Event Reporting System (VAERS) at www.vaers.hhs.gov or by telephone at 800-822-7967.

A. Pneumococcal Vaccine

The new recommendation for adult immunizations is the pneumococcal vaccination schedule for seniors. PCV13 (PREVNAR13), the pneumococcal conjugate vaccine, is now recommended for all adults age 65 and older, in addition to pneumococcal polysaccharide vaccine, PPSV23 (PNEUMOVAX 23), which has been recommended for seniors since 1997. All new ACIP recommendations have been evidence based since 2010. In 2014, the schedule included an evidence-based recommendation for PCV13

vaccination for all immunocompromised adults (age 19 or older) including those with functional or anatomic asplenia, cochlear implant, immunocompromising conditions, or CSF leaks. ACIP expanded routine PCV13 for all adults age 65 and older after reviewing the Community Acquired Pneumonia Immunization Trial in Adults of 85,000 seniors in the Netherlands (CAPiTA), which documented that older adults are also at increased risk for invasive pneumococcal disease. The order and timing of the two vaccines are complicated and important because polysaccharide and conjugate vaccines provoke immune responses in different ways. The two vaccines must not be given at the same visit. Seniors who have already received PPSV23 must wait at least a year before receiving PCV13. Clinicians are referred to the CDC vaccine schedule for extensive explanatory footnotes available at www.cdc.gov/vaccines/adult.

B. Influenza

All individuals age 6 months and older should receive an annual influenza vaccination. Individuals age 6 months and older, including pregnant women and individuals with hives-only egg allergy, can receive the inactivated influenza vaccine (IIV) appropriate for their age. Adults age 18 and older can receive the recombinant influenza vaccine (RIV) (FluBlok), which contains no egg protein. Healthy nonpregnant individuals age 2 to 48 years without high-risk medical conditions can receive the intranasally administered, live attenuated influenza vaccine (LAIV) (FluMist). Adults age 65 or older can receive the standard-dose influenza vaccine or the high-dose IIV (Fluzone High Dose) Currently available influenza vaccines are listed at http://www.cdc.gov/flu/fluvaxview/index.htm.

Precaution: Healthcare personnel who receive LAIV and care for severely immunocompromised individuals requiring care in a protected environment should avoid providing care to such individuals for 7 days after vaccination. IIV or RIV are the preferred influenza vaccination options for such healthcare personnel.

C. Tetanus, Diphtheria, Pertussis (Td/Tdap)

Adults with unknown or incomplete history of completing a three-dose primary series or those who have not been immunized should receive a three-dose series that includes one Tdap and two Td doses.

Note: Pregnant women should receive one dose of Tdap during each pregnancy (recommended during 27 to 36 weeks gestation) regardless of interval since prior Td or Tdap.

D. Varicella

Adults without evidence of immunity to varicella should receive two doses of single antigen varicella vaccine. Note: Varicella vaccine is contraindicated for individuals with immune-compromising conditions, excluding HIV unless severely immunocompromised. Clinicians are referred to the CDC-ACIP footnotes for indications on use of VZIG.

E. Human Papillomavirus (HPV, Gardasil 9)

Series of three doses may start as early as age 9 years. HPV can prevent most cases of cervical cancer if given before exposure to the virus. It also can prevent vaginal and vulvar cancer in females and genital warts and anal cancer, as well as oropharyngeal cancers in both males and females. HPV vaccination is recommended for all females ages 11 to 26 and for males ages 11 to 21. For males who have sex with men and for immunocompromised males, including those with HIV, HPV vaccination is recommended for ages 22–26.

F. Measles, Mumps, and Rubella

Most adults born prior to 1957 are considered immune to measles, but in view of recent outbreaks of measles and mumps, documentation of one or more doses of MMR or serologic evidence of immunity should be produced or vaccination is recommended. Rubella immunity should be established for all women of childbearing potential. If not immune and not pregnant, these women should be vaccinated with one dose of MMR. Note: MMR is contraindicated for individuals with immune-compromising conditions including HIV and for women who are pregnant.

G. Meningococcal Vaccine (MenACWY, Menactra, Menveo)

All adults with asplenia or persistent complement deficiencies should receive two doses of quadrivalent meningococcal conjugate vaccine. Refer to CDC-ACIP footnotes and recommendations for other high-risk individuals.

H. Hepatitis A (Havrix, Vaqta, Twinrix)

Two doses of an appropriate hepatitis A vaccine are recommended for all adults who are not immune. The single antigen vaccine formulation (Havrix) is administered in two doses 6 to 12 months apart or two doses with Vaqta at 6- to 18-month intervals. If the Twinrix vaccine (Hepatitis A and B) is used, administer three doses at 0, 1, and 6 months. Consult CDC footnotes on 2015 Adult Immunization Schedule.

I. Haemophilus influenzae B Vaccine (Hib)

Adults with functional or anatomic asplenia should receive a dose of Hib. Stem cell transplant recipients should receive three doses of Hib 6 to 12 months after transplant.

J. Zoster Vaccine (Zostavax, Merck)

One dose at age 60 or older is recommended by ACIP for prevention of herpes zoster (shingles) and complications including postherpetic neuralgia among older adults. Although the Food and Drug Administration (FDA) in 2011 approved the use of Zostavax for use in adults age 50 to 59, ACIP continues to recommend that the vaccine be routinely recommended for adults age 60 and older. Clinicians are referred to the CDC adult vaccine schedule: http://www.cdc.gov/vaccines/schedules/hcp/imz/adult.html

III. Immunization modalities

A. Intranasal Vaccine

Live attenuated influenza vaccine is the only vaccine licensed in the United States for intranasal administration and is for healthy, nonpregnant individuals 2 through 49 years of age. Administration of the vaccine requires the recipient to be upright in order to spray half of the sprayer contents (approximately 0.1 mL) into the first nostril. The dose–divider is then removed from the sprayer and the second half of the dose is sprayed into the second nostril. If the recipient sneezes after receiving the doses, administration should not be repeated.

B. Oral Vaccine

Oral polio vaccine (OPV) is not licensed for use in the United States. Rotavirus is available as an oral vaccine. Breastfeeding does not interfere with efficacy of either oral rotavirus or OPV. Vomiting within 10 minutes of receiving a dose of rotavirus vaccine is not an indication for repeat. (In countries where OPV is recommended, repeat dose administration is indicated.)

C. Parenteral Vaccines

Recommended routes of administration, sites, and aseptic technique are included in vaccine package inserts. Choice of site for intramuscular (IM) injectable vaccines is based on volume of the vaccine material and size of the muscle (usually anterolateral thigh for infants or deltoid muscle for older children and adults). The buttocks should not routinely be used for active immunizations, because of possibility of damaging the sciatic nerve and also the potential for decreased immunogenicity because of the subcutaneous fat layer over the gluteal area.

D. Informed Consent and Risk Versus Benefit

Standard consent forms and discussion of benefit versus risk of vaccines should be routinely included in encounters that include vaccination. Vaccine Information Statement (VIS) forms can be found at www.cdc.gov/vaccines/pubs/vis/default.htm. Anticipatory guidance on vaccines and providing schedules and handouts in advance are recommended.

Virtually no medical procedure is totally without risk. Informed discussion of anticipated risk and carefully addressing the questions of parents/patients are crucially important. Reactions to vaccines range from common discomfort at the injection site and low-grade fever to occasional fainting/syncope and rare untoward hypersensitivity reactions, which can be immediate or delayed. Checking for previous reactions to immunization components should be routinely done prior to any immunization, and having facilities, supplies, and trained staff available for treating immediate hypersensitivity reactions (anaphylaxis) wherever vaccines are administered is recommended. Observing patients, especially children, teens, and young adults, for 15 minutes after vaccination is recommended to monitor for syncope or other immediate side effects or adverse events.

IV. Active and passive immunizations

The administration of all or part of a modified form of a microorganism to produce the humoral or cellular responses to the immunization agent in the recipient constitutes active immunization. Modifications include purified antigens, genetically engineered antigens, or toxoids produced by those microorganisms. Active immunizations provoke an immune response that is similar to a natural infection but without the risk of the actual infection. The result is the development of protective antibodies in the actively immunized child or adult. Such vaccines may include infectious agents that are attenuated (i.e., weakened or modified), live, genetically engineered, or killed units of infectious agents. The CDC maintains a table of ingredients of licensed vaccines and is an excellent reference (CDC, 2015d; FDA, 2015).

The administration of an already formed antibody, such as immune globulin, constitutes passive immunization. Special circumstances indicate the need for passive immunization (i.e., when an individual is deficient in certain antibodies or the ability to produce antibodies, either from congenital or acquired immunodeficiencies or other lymphocyte defects). Another indication for passive immunization is for prophylactic use when a person is exposed to a high-risk disease and does not have time to produce adequate antibodies from active immunization. A third category is therapeutic indication, when a disease, such as botulism, tetanus, or other toxin-producing infection, is already present.

V. Herd immunity

The population of an immune herd is crucially important to prevent epidemic spread of vaccine-preventable infectious diseases. When the percentage of immunized or naturally immune individuals within a population declines, preventable infectious diseases that have not been eradicated again emerge among the unvaccinated/susceptible population. This has been demonstrated repeatedly with outbreaks of measles, mumps, rubella, pertussis, varicella, and other vaccine-preventable diseases. The percentage of protection required in the herd is related to the contagion rate of the individual disease.

VI. Adverse event reporting

The National Childhood Vaccine Injury Act (NCVIA) of 1986 mandates notification of all pediatric patients and parents about vaccine risks and benefits. Whether public or private funds are used to purchase vaccines, provision of a Vaccine Information Sheet is required with the administration of each vaccine covered under the National Vaccine Injury Compensation Program (VICP), preferably at least a day before the vaccination. Copies of the current VISs can be found online at www.cdc.gov/vaccines/pubs/vis/default.htm and the Immunization Action Coalition website www.immunize.org. Health professionals must read and comply with the recordkeeping requirements for VICP covered vaccines. Health professionals should be familiar with possible adverse reactions for all recommended vaccines and be prepared to provide any treatment indicated in the event of a rare severe hypersensitivity reaction, as well as to report to the federal monitoring entity Vaccine Adverse Events Reporting System (VAERS). Reporting forms and information are available at: http://vaers.hhs.gov or at 800-822-7967.

A. VAERS

VAERS is a passive monitoring system for vaccines licensed in the United States and is jointly administered by the CDC and the FDA. Submission of the report does not necessarily confirm a causal association of vaccine to the adverse event. Establishment of the Vaccine Safety Datalink Project (VSD) in 1990 supplements the passive monitoring surveillance of VAERS and provides continuous active monitoring of vaccine safety. More information on VSD is at www.cdc.gov/vaccinesafety/Activities/vsd.html.

B. Clinical Immunization Safety Assessment (CISA)

In 2001, the CDC established the CISA Network to develop research protocols for clinical evaluation of adverse events following immunization and to develop evidence-based guidelines for people at risk (including possible rare genetic and/or immunologic risk factors) for such adverse events (CDC, 2014b). Patients with rare and serious adverse events following immunization can be referred to CISA for inclusion in the CISA Vaccine Safety BioRepository for further safety studies. Current information is available at www.cdc.gov/vaccinesafety/Activities/CISA.html.

C. The Vaccine Injury Compensation Program (VICP)

The VICP was established in 1988 as an alternative to civil litigation when an individual was thought to have suffered injury or death as a result of administration of a covered vaccine. Although such events are uncommon, the list for possible injury or death is based on the Vaccine Injury Table and details can be found at www.hrsa.gov /vaccinecompensation/vaccinetable.html.

Information for parents or guardians about VICP is available through the Vaccine Information Statements (VISs) at http://www.cdc.gov/vaccines/hcp/vis/index .html. It is important for health professionals to discuss with parents the need for all vaccines with care and sensitivity, using the VISs readily available for download on the CDC website, www.cdc.gov/vaccines/pubs/vis/default.htm.

VII. Current concerns and vaccination rates

Immunizations have been so successful in preventing most of these diseases in the United States for more than a half century that many people, including parents, physicians, and nurses, have never seen a case of polio or possibly even measles, pertussis, or rubella. The unfortunate downside of such success is an increasing number of parents who choose to refuse immunizations for their children, assuming that their child will not be exposed or assuming that he or she will be protected by the immune status of his or her schoolmates. Apart from those few individuals for whom certain immunizations are contraindicated because of past severe allergic reactions or immunologic conditions, personal belief or religious exemptions can constitute grounds for parental refusal—differing from state to state to avoid mandatory compliance with adequate immunization status required for school entry at age 5. Parental belief exemptions have become law in several states. Such vaccine refusal has resulted in communities and states where immunization rates have fallen to far less than that required to have an immune "herd" or cohort of immunized individuals to protect those susceptible. This has led to several recent outbreaks of vaccine-preventable diseases, such as measles, mumps, and pertussis. The California Department of Health Services declared an epidemic of pertussis in July 2010 because of the excessively large and rapidly increasing number of cases reported. As of December 2014, approximately 10,000 cases of laboratory confirmed pertussis were reported for that year in California, mostly in children who had not been immunized (Winter et al., 2014). Several infants died of pertussis and others were seriously ill and hospitalized with the disease. The recent outbreaks of vaccine-preventable diseases have resulted in challenges to the personal belief and religious exemptions. In 2015, California repealed the state personal exemption and religious belief exemption and other states are considering similar action.

REFERENCES

Centers for Disease Control and Prevention. (2014a). *Measles cases and outbreaks*. Retrieved from http://www.cdc.gov/measles/cases -outbreaks.html.

Centers for Disease Control and Prevention. (2014b). *Vaccine safety*. Retrieved from http://www.cdc.gov/vaccinesafety/index.html.

Centers for Disease Control and Prevention. (2015a). *Birth–18 years & "catch-up" immunization schedules: United States, 2015*. Retrieved from www.cdc.gov/vaccines/schedules/hcp/child-adolescent.html.

Centers for Disease Control and Prevention. (2015b). *Immunization schedules*. Retrieved from http://www.cdc.gov/vaccines/schedules /index.html.

Centers for Disease Control and Prevention. (2015c). *Travelers' health: Yellow book homepage*. Retrieved from http://wwwnc.cdc.gov/travel /page/yellowbook-home.

Food and Drug Administration. (2015). *Complete list of vaccines licensed for immunization and distribution in the US*. Retrieved from http:// www.fda.gov/BiologicsBloodVaccines/Vaccines/ApprovedProducts /ucm093833.htm

Fryhofer, S. A. (2015). *ACIP adult vaccine schedule: What you need to know*. Retrieved from http://www.medscape.com/viewarticle/838658.

Grohskopf, L. A., Olsen, S. J., Sokolow, L. Z., Bresee, J. S., Cox, N. J., Broder, K. R., et al. (2014). Prevention and control of seasonal influenza with vaccines: Recommendations of the Advisory Committee on Immunization Practices (ACIP)—United States, 2014–15 influenza season. *MMWR Morb Mortal Wkly Rep, 63*(32), 691–697.

Kimberlin, D. W., Long, S. S., Brady, M. T., & Jackson, M. A. (Eds.). (2015). *Red book: 2015 report of the Committee on Infectious Disease* (30th ed.). Elk Grove Village, IL: American Academy of Pediatrics.

Pickering, L. K., Baker, C. J., & Kimberlin, D. W. (Eds.). (2012). *Red book: 2012 report of the committee on infectious diseases* (29th ed.). Elk Grove Village, IL: American Academy of Pediatrics

Winter, K., Glaser, C., Watt, J., & Harriman, K. (2014). Pertussis epidemic— California, 2014. *MMWR Morb Mortal Wkly Rep, 63*(48), 1129–1132.

World Health Organization. (n.d.). *Health topics: Vaccines*. Retrieved from http://www.who.int/topics/vaccines/en/.

Wyckoff, A.S. (2015). Red book online offers updated measles guidance. *AAP News*. Retrieved from http://aapnews.aappublications.org /content/early/2015/02/10/aapnews.20150211-1.full.pdf+html.

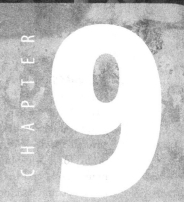

DEVELOPMENTAL ASSESSMENT: SCREENING FOR DEVELOPMENTAL DELAY AND AUTISM

Abbey Alkon

CHAPTER 9

I. Introduction

A. General background

The prevalence of children with developmental and behavioral problems is estimated to be 17% in the United States (Boyle et al., 2011). In the 2007 National Survey of Children's Health, over 25% of children younger than 5 years of age were at risk for developmental and behavioral problems or social delays but fewer than one in five received the recommended screening (U.S. Department of Health and Human Resources, Health Resources and Services Administration, & Maternal and Child Health Bureau, 2009). Screening instruments help identify children with possible developmental delays or disorders who require follow-up or referrals to undergo a comprehensive assessment.

In 2003, the President's New Freedom Commission on Mental Health included the goal for early mental health screening, assessment, and referral to services to be common practice and recommended that screening for mental disorders be included in primary health care and connected to treatment and support services. Title V of the Social Security Act and the Individuals with Disabilities Education Improvement Act (IDEA) of 2004 reaffirm the mandate for child health professionals to provide early identification of, and intervention for, children with developmental disabilities through community-based collaborative systems. The Early and Periodic Screening, Diagnostic, and Treatment (EPSDT) guidelines require that states provide regular health screenings and all medically necessary services to children and adolescents, including assessments of mental health development. The American Academy of Pediatrics (AAP) provides guidelines for screening for developmental and behavioral problems as part of primary care (AAP Council on Children with Disabilities, AAP Section on Developmental Behavioral Pediatrics, Bright Futures Steering Committee, & AAP Medical Home Initiatives for Children with Special Needs

Project Advisory Committee, 2006). A recent initiative by the U.S. Departments of Health and Human Services and Education, *Birth to 5: Watch Me Thrive!*, increases awareness about the importance of developmental and behavioral screening by providing a user guide on how to select and use these tools (U.S. Department of Health and Human Services & U.S. Department of Education, 2014).

Under the Affordable Care Act (ACA), screening for children less than 3 years of age and surveillance throughout childhood are covered under preventative services. The Current Procedural Terminology (CPT) code 96127 is used for an emotional and behavioral assessment and the CPT code 96110 is for a developmental assessment in primary care.

B. Primary care and screening

Primary care practices have failed to identify and refer 60–80% of children with developmental delays in a timely manner (Halfon et al., 2004). Only 57% of children 10 to 35 months old ever received a developmental screen. Although pediatric primary care practices are busy and primary care providers have a limited amount of time with children, children who are at risk for developing developmental and behavioral problems need to be identified early in life and referred for intervention services to prevent more serious problems later in life. The AAP developed a policy statement, "Identifying Infants and Young Children with Developmental Disorders: An Algorithm for Developmental Surveillance and Screening," which provides a strategy to incorporate ongoing developmental surveillance and screening of all children into primary care visits (AAP Council on Children with Disabilities et al., 2006).

C. Why screen?

Standardized screening tests are more accurate than clinical impressions and thus are recommended at targeted ages to augment developmental surveillance. Screening programs are provided to all children or those at risk for behavioral, developmental, and emotional problems. Children with positive screening tests may need to be referred for diagnostic testing because screening is not a diagnostic tool.

The goal of screening is to identify children who will benefit from early intervention services. Early intervention services for children with developmental problems have been shown to be extremely effective if children enter these programs at an early age (Glascoe, 2005a). Intervention programs can help children with behavior problems, autism, or developmental delays to reduce the likelihood of needing special education placement and increase the likelihood of future school success (Johnson & Myers, 2007).

D. Where?

Screening is most effective when embedded in a preventive services system in primary care, where screening is part of a preventive services schedule coordinated with other guidance and screening activities, and where concerns and observations always lead to a within-office guidance process even if a referral to an outside agency or service is made.

The AAP recommends that all children have a "medical home," defined as care that is accessible, continuous, comprehensive, family centered, coordinated, and compassionate (U.S. Department of Health and Human Services et al., 2009), but more than 4 out of 10 children do not have a medical home. Therefore, not all children are receiving the recommended screening in their primary care practices, and new, innovative screening programs need to be developed in primary care or community settings, such as public health departments or child care programs.

E. Prevalence of disorders

At least one in eight children has a developmental concern at some point during their childhood. Twelve to 17% of all children have:

- Speech or language delay
- Mental retardation
- Learning disability
- Hearing loss
- Emotional or behavioral concern
- Delay in growth or development

The prevalence of autism spectrum disorders is estimated at about 1 in 68. The prevalence differs for boys (1 in 42) compared to girls (1 in 189) (Autism and Developmental Disabilities Monitoring Network Surveillance Year 2010 Principal Investigators, 2014).

II. Developmental surveillance and screening algorithm

Figure 9-1a and **Figure 9-1b** provide a flowchart algorithm with numbers and headings with associated explanations about providing surveillance and screening as part of preventive primary care visits (AAP Council on Children with Disabilities et al., 2006).

A. Pediatric patient at preventive care visit (#1)

The AAP recommends surveillance to be included in every well-child visit and standardized screening to be included in well-child visits at 9, 18, 24, and 30 months of age. Developmental surveillance alone, without screening, captures only 30% of children with delays and disabilities before the age of 5 years (www.first5ecmh.org).

B. Developmental surveillance (#2)

1. Definition—Surveillance is the process of recognizing children who may be at risk of developmental delays. It is the process of gathering information about the family's well-being through report or observation, observing children's behavior, eliciting parents' concerns, and gathering data from medical history and current physical examination (Glascoe, 2005a).

2. The components of surveillance are:
   a. Eliciting and attending to the parents' concerns about their child's development
   b. Documenting and maintaining the child's developmental history
   c. Making informed and accurate observations of the child's development
   d. Identifying risk and protective factors for developmental delay
   e. Documenting the process and results of ongoing developmental surveillance and screening

C. Does surveillance demonstrate risk? (#3)

Any concerns raised by the parent or primary care provider during surveillance should be followed by the administration of a standardized screening tool. The screening should be done at a separate visit shortly after the initial surveillance visit.

D. Is this a 9-, 18-, or 30-month or prekindergerten visit? (#4)

A general developmental screen is recommended at the 9-, 18-, and 30-month and prekindergarten visits according to the current well-child guidelines *Bright Futures: Guidelines for Health Supervision for Infants, Children and Adolescents* (AAP, 2007). The AAP recommendations are based on recent research that credits standardized screening tools with capturing up to 80% of children with early developmental delays. Autism screening is recommended for all children before they are 24 months of age (Johnson & Myers, 2007; Robins, 2008).

E. Administer screening tool (#5)

1. Definition

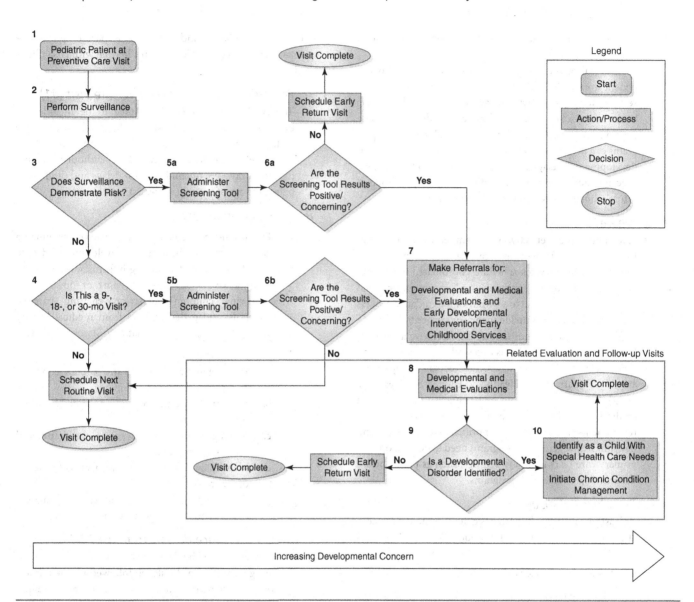

FIGURE 9-1A Developmental Surveillance and Screening Algorithm for Pediatric Primary Care
Reproduced with permission from *Pediatrics*, Vol. 118, Pages 407–408, Copyright © by the AAP.

a. Screening is the use of standardized tools to identify and refine a recognized risk (AAP Council on Children with Disabilities et al., 2006).

b. Assessments include gathering and synthesizing information across multiple domains, settings, and informants.

c. A list of selected screening tools is provided in **Table 9-1**.

F. Are the screening tool results positive? (#6)

Normal screening results provide an opportunity to focus on promoting health development. If the results of the screening test are positive, review the child's strengths and then review the child's areas of difficulty. Explain the results to the parents and refer the child for further evaluation.

G. Referrals and evaluation (#7 and #8)

1. Initial referrals may be needed to rule out hearing and visual impairments, and then referrals for specific diagnostic tests are needed.

2. Evaluation is defined as a complex process aimed at identifying specific developmental disorders that are affecting a child.

3. Referrals for developmental and medical evaluations and possibly referrals for early developmental intervention services are needed.

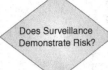

| Pediatric Patient at Preventive Care Visit | **1.** Developmental concerns should be included as one of several health topics addressed at each pediatric preventive care visit throughout the first 5 years of life. |

2. *Developmental surveillance* is a flexible, longitudinal, continuous, and cumulative process whereby knowledgeable healthcare professionals identify children who may have developmental problems. There are 5 components of developmental surveillance: eliciting and attending to the parents' concerns about their child's development, documenting and maintaining a developmental history, making accurate observations of the child, identifying the risk and protective factors, and maintaining an accurate record and documenting the process and findings.

Perform Surveillance

Does Surveillance Demonstrate Risk?

3. The concerns of both parents and child health professionals should be included in determining whether surveillance suggests the child may be at risk of developmental delay. If either parents or the child health professional express concern about the child's development, a developmental screening to address the concern specifically should be conducted.

4. All children should receive developmental screening using a standardized test. In the absence of established risk factors or parental or provider concerns, a general developmental screen is recommended at the 9-, 18-, and 30-month visits. Additionally, autism-specific screening is recommended for all children at the 18-month visit.

Is This a 9-, 18-, or 30-mo Visit?

Administer Screening Tool

5a and 5b. *Developmental screening* is the administration of a brief standardized tool aiding the identification of children at risk of a developmental disorder. Developmental screening that targets the area of concern is indicated whenever a problem is identified during developmental surveillance.

6a and 6b. When the results of the periodic screening tool are normal, the child health professional can inform the parents and continue with other aspects of the preventive visit. When a screening tool is administered as a result of concerns about development, an early return visit to provide additional developmental surveillance should be scheduled even if the screening tool results do not indicate a risk of delay.

Are the Screening Tool Results Positive/ Concerning?

Make Referrals for:

Developmental and Medical Evaluations and Early Developmental Intervention/Early Childhood Services

Developmental and Medical Evaluations

7–8. If screening results are concerning, the child should be scheduled for developmental and medical evaluations. *Developmental evaluation* is aimed at identifying the specific developmental disorder or disorders affecting the child. In addition to the developmental evaluation, a *medical diagnostic evaluation* to identify an underlying etiology should be undertaken. *Early developmental intervention/early childhood services* can be particularly valuable when a child is first identified to be at high risk of delayed development, because these programs often provide evaluation services and can offer other services to the child and family even before an evaluation is complete. Establishing an effective and efficient partnership with early childhood professionals is an important component of successful care coordination for children.

9. If a developmental disorder is identified, the child should be identified as a child with special healthcare needs and chronic condition management should be initiated (see No. 10 below). If a developmental disorder is not identified through medical and developmental evaluation, the child should be scheduled for an early return visit for further surveillance. More frequent visits, with particular attention paid to areas of concern, will allow the child to be promptly referred for further evaluation if any further evidence of delayed development or a specific disorder emerges.

Is a Developmental Disorder Identified?

Identify as a Child With Special Health Care Needs

Initiate Chronic Condition Management

10. When a child is discovered to have a significant developmental disorder, that child becomes a child with special healthcare needs, even if that child does not have a specific disease etiology identified. Such a child should be identified by the medical home for appropriate chronic condition management and regular monitoring and entered into the practice's children and youth with special healthcare needs registry.

FIGURE 9-1B Developmental Surveillance and Screening Algorithm for Pediatric Primary Care

Reproduced with permission from *Pediatrics*, Vol. 118, Pages 407–408, Copyright © by the AAP.

H. Is a developmental disorder identified? (#9)

1. If a developmental disorder is not identified, then the child should be scheduled for frequent surveillance to follow areas of concern.

2. If a developmental disorder is identified, the child should be identified as a child with special healthcare needs, a diagnosis is made, and referrals for early intervention services are needed.

TABLE 9-1 Developmental Screening Tools

Screening Instrument	Description	Age Range	No. of Items	Time (admin, scoring; minutes)	Psychometric Properties	Languages	Purchase/Obtainment Information	Key References
Multiple Developmental, Including Social-Emotional Screening Instruments								
Ages and Stages Questionnaires, Third Edition (ASQ-3)	Parent-completed questionnaire; series of 19 age-specific questionnaires screening communication, gross motor, fine motor, problem-solving, and personal adaptive skills; results in pass/fail score for domains	1–60 mo	30	10–15 adm, 2–3 score	Normed on 2008 children from diverse ethnic and socioeconomic backgrounds, including Spanish speaking; sensitivity: 0.70–0.90 (moderate to high); specificity: 0.76–0.91 (moderate to high)	English, Spanish, French, Korean	Brookes Publishing Co. http://www .brookespublishing .com/ Training at http:// www.agesandstages .com/	Squires & Bricker (2009)
Behavior Assessment System for Children, Second Edition (BASC-2)	Parent- or caregiver-completed questionnaire; assesses behavioral and emotional functioning; measures adaptive and problem behaviors in school, home, and community settings; includes Teacher Rating Scale (TRS), Parent Rating Scale (PRS), self-report of personality, student observation, developmental history.	2–21 y	TRS: 100–139 PRS: 134–160	10–20 adm	Normed based on current U.S. Census population characteristics. Internal consistency: acceptably high to strong results. Test-retest reliability, interrater reliability, and concurrent validity: moderate results.	English, Spanish	Pearson (PsychCorp) http://www .pearsonassessments .com/	Reynolds & Kamphaus (2004)
Brigance Screens II	Directly administered tool; series of 9 forms that screen articulation, expressive and receptive language, gross motor, fine motor, self-help, social-emotional, social skills and preacademic skills (when appropriate); for 0–23 mo, parent report	0–90 mo	8–10	10–15 adm	Normed on 1,156 children from 29 clinical sites in 21 states; sensitivity: 0.75–0.93 (moderate to high); specificity: 0.70–0.80 (moderate)	English, Spanish	Curriculum Associates http://www .curriculumassociates .com/	Glascoe (2002, 2005b)

Tool	Description	Age range		Administration time	Normative sample / sensitivity & specificity	Languages	Publisher	Reference
Child Development Inventories (CDI) Infant Development Inventory (IDI) Early Child Development Inventory (ECDI) Preschool Development Inventory (PDI)	Parent-completed questionnaire; measures social, self-help, motor, language, and general development skills; results in developmental quotients and age equivalents for different developmental domains; suitable for more in-depth evaluation	CDI: 15 mo–6 y IDI: 0–18 mo ECDI: 18–36 mo PDI: 36–60 mo	300	30–50 adm; IDI: 5–10 min., 5 min.	Normative sample included 568 children from south St Paul, MN, a primarily white, working class community; Doig et al. included 43 children from a high-risk follow-up program, which included 69% with high school education or less and 81% Medicaid; sensitivity: 0.80–1.0. (moderate to high); specificity: 0.94–0.96 (high); IDI: sensitivity 85%, specificity 77%	English, Spanish (IDI)	Pearson (PsychCorp) http://www.pearsonassessments.com/	Doig, Macias, Saylor, Craver, & Ingram (1999); Ireton (1992)
Denver II Developmental Screening Test	Directly administered tool; designed to screen expressive and receptive language, fine motor, gross motor, and personal-social skills; results in risk category (normal, questionable, abnormal)	0–6 y	125	10–20 adm	Normed on 2,096 term children in Colorado; not nationally representative; sensitivity: 0.56–0.83 (low to moderate); specificity: 0.43–0.80 (low to moderate)	English, Spanish	Denver Developmental Materials, Inc. http://www.denverii.com/	Glascoe, Byrne, Ashford, Johnson, Chang, & Strickland (1992); Frankenburg, Camp, & Van Natta (1971)
Parents' Evaluation of Developmental Status (PEDS)	Parent-completed form; designed to screen for developmental and behavioral problems needing further evaluation; single response form used for all ages; may be useful as a surveillance tool	0–8 y	10	5 to adm and 2 to score	Standardized with 771 children from diverse ethnic and socioeconomic backgrounds, including Spanish speaking; sensitivity: 0.74–0.79 (moderate); specificity: 0.70–0.80 (moderate)	English, Spanish, and 16 other languages	Ellsworth and Vandermeer Press, LLC http://pedstest.com/	Glascoe (2006)

(continues)

TABLE 9-1 Developmental Screening Tools (*Continued*)

Screening Instrument	Description	Age Range	No. of Items	Time (admin, scoring; minutes)	Psychometric Properties	Languages	Purchase/Obtainment Information	Key References
Socioemotional Screening Instruments								
Ages and Stages Questionnaire: Social-Emotional (ASQ-SE)	Parent/caregiver-completed questionnaire in 7 areas: screening self-regulation, compliance, communication, adaptive behaviors, autonomy, affect, and interaction with people	3–66 mo	30	10–15 adm, 1–3 score	Investigated with more than 3,000 questionnaires across the age intervals; reliability is 94%; validity is between 75% and 89%; sensitivity = 78%, specificity = 94%	English, Spanish	Brookes Publishing Co. http://www .brookespublishing .com/ Training at http:// www.agesandstages .com/	Squires, Bricker, & Twombley (2002)
Brief Infant/Toddler Social Emotional Assessment (BITSEA)	Parent or caregiver forms; brief comprehensive screening instrument to evaluate social and emotional behavior	12–36 mo	42	5–7 adm	Clinical groups in the normative sample (n = 600) included young children who had delayed language, were premature, and had other diagnosed disorders. Not geographically representative. Sensitivity = 80–85%, Specificity = 75–80%; Internal consistency for Problem = 0.83–0.89; for Competence = 0.66–0.75. Test-retest reliability, interrater reliability, internal consistency: acceptably high to strong results. Concurrent validity: moderate results.	English, Spanish, French, Hebrew, Dutch	Pearson (PsychCorp) http://www .pearsonassessments .com/	Briggs-Gowan, Carter, Irwin, Wachtel, & Cicchetti (2004)
Pediatric Symptom Checklist (PSC) Pediatric Symptom Checklist – Youth Report (PSC-Y)	Parent-or caregiver-completed questionnaire to identify emotional and behavioral problems. Identifies need for further evaluation.	4–16 years	35	10–15 minutes; Total score; clinical cutoff = 24 (4–5 year olds) and 28 (6–16 years old)	Normative sample of middle and low socioeconomic status. Test-retest reliability: high to strong; Internal consistency: high to strong; Predictive validity: moderate. Sensitivity: 80–95%; Specificity: 68–100%	English, Spanish, Japanese	www.dbpeds.org /pdf/psc.pdf	Jellinek, Murphy, Bishop, Pagano, Comer, & Kelleher (1999)

Measure	Description	Age range	Number of items	Administration/Cutoff	Norming/Psychometrics	Languages	Source	Citation
Preschool Pediatric Symptom Checklist (PPSC)	Parent-completed questionnaire. Based on PSC. Rating of 2 "very much," 1 "somewhat," 0 "not at all." Part of the comprehensive Survey of Well-being of Young Children (SWYC) instrument	18–60 mo	18	Cutoff scores = 9	Normed on 292 families from primary care and 354 families from referral clinics; Sensitivity: 79% to 85%; Specificity: 81% to 92%	English, Spanish	www.theswyc.org	Sheldrick, Henson, Merchant, Neger, Murphy, & Perrin (2012)
Preschool and Kindergarten Behavior Scales-Second Edition (PBKS-2)	Parent- or caregiver-completed questionnaire; social skills scale includes social cooperation, social interaction, and social independence; problem behavior scale includes externalizing problems and internalizing problems	36–60 mo	76	12 adm	Normative sample of 3,317 children ages 3 through 6. Ethnicity, socioeconomic status, and special education classification of sample are similar to characteristics of U.S. population, based on 2000 census. Internal consistency is 0.96–0.97. High concurrent validity. Interrater reliability: moderate results.	English, Spanish	Pro-Ed, Inc.; www.proedinc.com	Allin (2004)
Survey of Well-being of Young Children (SWYC); Includes Baby Pediatric Symptom Checklist (BPSC), Preschool Pediatric Symptom Checklist (PPSC), Parent's Observations of Social Interactions (POSI), The Developmental Milestones Checklist, and Family Risk Factors questions	Parent- or caregiver-completed questionnaire; cognitive, motor, language, social-emotional-behavioral functioning, autism, family factors	2–60 mo	54 total or 10-item age-specific forms	10–15 adm; Internet, tablet	Developed in Massachusetts with 864, 469 primary care & 395 specialty clinic & 308 in replication sample; Acceptable test-retest reliability and internal consistency; moderate construct validity, moderate sensitivity (55–100%) and specificity (63–96%).	English, Spanish, Burmese, Nepali, Portuguese	www.theswyc.org	Sheldrick & Perrin (2013)

(continues)

TABLE 9-1 Developmental Screening Tools *(Continued)*

Screening Instrument	Description	Age Range	No. of Items	Time (admin, scoring; minutes)	Psychometric Properties	Languages	Purchase/Obtainment Information	Key References
Vineland Social-Emotional Early Childhood Scales (SEEC)	Parent or caregiver interview by licensed professional; assesses interpersonal relationships, play and leisure time, and coping skills; the social-emotional composite assesses usual social-emotional functioning	0–71 mo	122	15–25 adm	Normative sample; nationally representative. Test–retest reliability and internal consistency; acceptably high to strong results; interrater reliability and concurrent validity: moderate results.	English	Pearson (PsychCorp) http://www .pearsonassessments .com/	Sparrow, Balla, & Cicchetti (1998)
Autism Screening Instruments								
Modified Checklist for Autism in Toddlers-Revised with Follow-up (M-CHAT-R/F)	Parent-completed questionnaire designed to identify children at risk of autism from the general population; responses are Pass or Fail	18–24 mo	23	5–10 adm; 2nd stage screen with interview questions	Standardization sample included 1,293 children screened, 58 evaluated, and 39 diagnosed with an autistic spectrum disorder; validated using Autism Diagnostic Interview-Revised, Autism Diagnostic Observation Schedule-Generic, Childhood Autism Rating Scale, Diagnostic and Statistical Manual of Mental Disorders-IV; sensitivity: 0.85–0.87 (moderate); specificity: 0.93–0.99 (high)	English, Spanish, French, Chinese, Japanese, and 23 other languages	m-chat.org	Robins et al. (2014)

I. Children with special healthcare needs: early intervention (#10)

1. Refer for early intervention services.

2. Coordination of services, monitoring progress and outcomes, and follow-up are needed.

III. Screening instruments

Table 9-1 lists a selected group of screening instruments that can be administered in a primary care office by the type of screening instrument, description of who completes the tool and why it is administered, age range, number of items, time for administration, psychometrics, languages available, how to purchase or obtain the tool, and primary references if available (AAP Council on Children with Disabilities et al., 2006; Glascoe, 2005a; Ringwalt, 2008; Sosna & Mastergeorge, 2005; Moodie et al., 2014). The tools were selected because they are designed to be administered to children less than 6 years of age, have a short administration time, have adequate reliability and validity, and are widely used in the primary care field. The cultural relevance or ability to generalize the results of the instrument's psychometrics to other cultural groups is reported in the psychometrics column. The key references are included in the reference list in this chapter.

A. General development, including socioemotional tools

1. Ages and Stages Questionnaires, Third Edition (Squires & Bricker, 2009)

2. Behavior Assessment System for Children, Second Edition (Reynolds & Kamphaus, 2004)

3. Brigance Screens II (Glascoe, 2002, 2005b)

4. Child Development Inventories (Doig, Macias, Saylor, Craver, & Ingram, 1999; Ireton, 1992)

5. Denver-II Developmental Screening Test* (Frankenburg, Camp, & Van Natta, 1971; Glascoe et al., 1992)

6. Parents' Evaluation of Developmental Status (Glascoe, 2006)

   *The Denver-II lacks adequate validation and over-refers or underdetects problems (Glascoe, 2005a).

B. Socioemotional screening tools

1. Ages and Stages Questionnaire: Social-Emotional (Squires, Bricker, & Twombly, 2002)

2. Brief Infant/Toddler Social Emotional Assessment (Briggs-Gowan, Carter, Irwin, Wachtel, & Cicchetti, 2004)

3. Pediatrics Symptom Checklist (Jellinek et al., 1999)

4. Preschool and Kindergarten Behavior Scales—Second Edition (Allin, 2004)

5. Survey of Well-being of Young Children (SWYC), Preschool Pediatric Symptom Checklist (Sheldrick et al., 2012), Baby Pediatric Symptom Checklist (BPSC)

6. Vineland Social-Emotional Early Childhood Scales (Sparrow, Balla, & Cicchetti, 1998)

C. Autism screening tools

1. Modified Checklist for Autism in Toddlers—Revised with Follow-Up (M-CHAT-R/F) (Robins et al., 2014)

2. Pervasive Developmental Disorders Screening Test (Siegel, 2004)

3. In combination with a standardized screening tool, the following Diagnostic and Statistical Manual IV criteria for autism spectrum disorders can be applied for children younger than 3 years of age (Johnson, 2008; Johnson & Myers, 2007):

   a. Impairment in social interaction
      i. Lack of spontaneous seeking to share enjoyment, interests, or achievements with other people (e.g., lack of pointing and showing)
      ii. Marked impairment in the use of multiple nonverbal behaviors, such as eye-to-eye gaze, facial expression, body postures, and gestures to regulate social interaction
      iii. Lack of social and emotional reciprocity

   b. Impairments in communication. Delay in or total lack of the development of spoken language (not accompanied by attempt to compensate using gestures or mime)

   c. Restricted repetitive and stereotyped patterns of behavior, interests, and activities

IV. Psychometrics (AAP Council on Children with Disabilities et al., 2006; Glascoe, 2005a; Ringwalt, 2008; Sosna & Mastergeorge, 2005)

A. Characteristics of accurate screening tests

1. Sensitivity
   a. Definition: the accuracy of the test in identifying children suspected to be at risk for a developmental problem. Sensitivity is also seen as the percentage of children with true problems correctly identified on a screening tool.

b. Example: if the screening tool has 70% sensitivity, it means that 70% of the children who receive a positive screening result truly have a developmental problem.

c. Standards: 70–80% sensitivity is considered moderate and 90% or higher is strong.

2. Specificity

a. Definition: the accuracy of a test in identifying children who are not delayed. Specificity is also seen as the percentage of children without true difficulties correctly identified by a negative result on a screening tool.

b. Example: if the test has 80% specificity, it means that 80% of the children screened who have a negative result have no developmental problem.

c. Standards: 80% or higher specificity is considered moderate to strong. This minimizes referrals for diagnostic tests for children with no developmental delays or problems.

3. Positive predictive value (PPV)

Definition: the percentage of children who have a positive screening test result and actually have the diagnosis of a developmental problem. The PPV tells the clinician what a positive test result means for the individual child. PPV is frequently used by clinicians.

a. Example: if four out of five children have positive screening test results and are found to have a developmental problem, then the PPV is 80%. Therefore, for the screening test there is an 80% chance that the child actually has a developmental problem.

b. Standards: there is no agreed-on standard for PPV. In reality, PPVs are rarely very high and can range between 30% and 50%.

4. Representative sample

Definition: the screening test should be standardized on a large nationally representative sample whose characteristics reflect those of the United States in terms of ethnicities and parents' level of education, income, and language spoken at home.

5. Reliability

Definition: the ability of a measure to produce consistent results. There are different types of reliability:

a. Test–retest reliability: the stability or consistency of results across different administrations.

b. Interrater reliability: the stability or consistency of results across different raters.

c. Internal consistency: the correlation across items on an instrument to show consistency or responses. Usually shown as the Cronbach's alpha coefficient.

6. Validity

Definition: the ability of a measure to discriminate between a child at a determined level of risk for delay and the rest of the population. There are many types of validity:

a. Concurrent validity: high correlation between the screening tool and a diagnostic measure with similar domains.

b. Discriminant validity: how well the screening tool distinguishes children with the problem or condition compared to those without the problem or condition.

c. Predictive validity: screening test results are compared to performance on diagnostic measures administered at a later time.

V. Conclusion

Regular surveillance and routine screening at recommended intervals help identify children at risk for behavioral, developmental, and emotional problems, refer them for diagnostics tests and early intervention services. Children develop at different paces and surveillance and screening tests can help differentiate normal, intermittent changes in behavior from persistent challenging behaviors. In addition, valid and reliable screening tests can help identify children whose development has changed or whose developmental milestones have regressed (e.g., autism). Early identification of developmental, behavioral, and emotional problems during childhood may help children succeed in school, develop social relationships, and contribute to society.

VI. Clinician resources

1. AAP National Center of Medical Home Initiatives for Children with Special Needs. Resources developed by the AAP and pilot projects implementing the AAP algorithm for developmental screening, including policies and protocols, screening algorithms, resources and tips on Medicaid billing, and parent resources; available at www.medicalhomeinfo.org.

2. AAP, Caring for Children with Autism Spectrum Disorders: A Resource Toolkit for Clinicians. Includes identification, surveillance and screening tools, referrals, fact sheets, and family handouts; available at aapnews.aappublications.org/content/34/4/30.2.full.pdf+html

3. AAP's Bright Futures provides health supervision guidelines and developmental, behavioral, and psychosocial screening and assessment tools used in primary care including questions to ask parents during the interview; available at https://brightfutures.aap.org/Pages/default.aspx.

4. Assuring Better Child Health and Development (ABCD Initiative). Research and resources promoting child health and development. Includes tools for clinicians and state resources; available at http://www.nashp.org/abcd-map/.

5. Center on the Social and Emotional Foundations for Early Learning; available at csefel.vanderbilt.edu/

6. Developmental Screening Toolkit for Primary Care Providers developed by the Maternal and Child Health Bureau and Children's Hospital Boston to implement validated screening instruments into their practice—includes information on screening tools, billing, and referral; available at www.developmentalscreening.org.

7. First Signs. Information for families on developmental screening and services; available at www.firstsigns.org/screening.

8. Ounce of Prevention Fund "Snapshots: Incorporating Comprehensive Developmental Screening into Programs and Services for Young Children"; available at www.ounceofprevention.org.

9. National Early Childhood Technical Assistance Center "Developmental Screening and Assessment Documents"; available at www.nactac.org.

10. The Commonwealth Fund. Research on innovations on child health and development, including the work of the ABCD initiative and screening in primary care settings; available at www.commonwealthfund.org.

11. Technical Assistance Center of Social Emotional Intervention; available at www.challengingbehavior.org/.

REFERENCES

Allin, J. D. (2004). Book review: Preschool and kindergarten behavior scales-second edition. *Journal of Psychoeducational Assessment, 22*(1), 81–86.

American Academy of Pediatrics. (2007). *Bright futures: Guidelines for health supervision of infants, children, and adolescents* (3rd ed.). Elk Grove, IL: American Academy of Pediatrics.

American Academy of Pediatrics Council on Children with Disabilities, AAP Section on Developmental Behavioral Pediatrics, Bright Futures Steering Committee, & AAP Medical Home Initiatives for Children with Special Needs Project Advisory Committee. (2006). Identifying infants and young children with developmental disorders in the medical home: An algorithm for developmental surveillance and screening. *Pediatrics, 118*(1), 405–420.

Autism and Developmental Disabilities Monitoring Network Surveillance Year 2010 Principal Investigators. (2014). Prevalence of autism spectrum disorder among children aged 8 years: Autism and developmental disability monitoring network, 11 sites, United States, 2010. *MMWR Surveillance Summaries, 63*(2): 1–24.

Boyle, C., Coulet, S., Schieve, L. A., Cohen, R. A., Blumberg, S. J., Yeargin-Allsopp, M., et al. (2011). Trends in the prevalence of developmental disabilities in US children, 1997-2008. *Pediatrics, 127*, 1034–1042.

Briggs-Gowan, M. J., Carter, A. S., Irwin, J. R., Wachtel, K., & Cicchetti, D. V. (2004). The brief infant-toddler social and emotional assessment: Screening for social-emotional problems and delays in competence. *Journal of Pediatric Psychology, 29*(2), 143–155.

Doig, K. B., Macias, M. M., Saylor, D. F., Craver, J. R., & Ingram, P. E. (1999). The child development inventory: A developmental outcome measure for the follow-up of the high risk infant. *Journal of Pediatrics, 135*, 358–362.

Frankenburg, W. K., Camp, B. W., & Van Natta, P. A. (1971). Validity of the Denver developmental screening test. *Child Development, 42*, 475–485.

Glascoe, F. P. (2002). The Brigance Infant-Toddler Screen (BITS): Standardization and validation. *Journal of Developmental and Behavioral Pediatrics, 23*, 145–150.

Glascoe, F. P. (2005a). Screening for developmental and behavioral problems. *Mental Retardation and Developmental Disabilities Research Reviews, 11*, 173–179.

Glascoe, F. P. (2005b). *Technical report for the Brigance screens.* North Billerica, MA: Curriculum Associates.

Glascoe, F. P. (2006). *Parents' evaluation of developmental status (PEDS).* Nashville, TN: Ellsworth & Vandermeer Press.

Glascoe, F. P., Byrne, K. E., Ashford, L. G., Johnson, K. L., Chang, B., & Strickland, B. (1992). Accuracy of the Denver-II in developmental screening. *Pediatrics, 89*, 1221–1225.

Halfon, N., Regalado, M., Sareen, H., Inkelas, M., Reuland, C. P., Glascoe, F. P., et al. (2004). Assessing development in the pediatric office. *Pediatrics, 113*(6), 1926–1933.

Ireton, H. (1992). *Child development inventory manual.* Minneapolis, MN: Behavior Science Systems.

Jellinek, M., Murphy, J., Little, M., Pagano, M., Comer, D., & Kelleher, K. (1999). Use of the Pediatric Symptom Checklist (PSC) to screen for psychosocial problems in pediatric primary care: A national feasibility study. *Archives of Pediatric and Adolescent Medicine, 153*(3), 254–260.

Johnson, C. P. (2008). Recognition of autism before age 2 years. *Pediatrics in Review, 29*(3), 86–95.

Johnson, C., & Myers, S. (2007). Identification and evaluation of children with autism spectrum disorders. *Pediatrics, 120*, 1183–1215.

Moodie, S., Daneri, P., Goldhagen, S, Halle, T., Green, K., & LaMonte, L (2014). Early childhood developmental screening: A compendium of measures for children ages birth to five. Washington, DC: Office of Planning, Research and Evaluation, Administration for Children and Families, U.S. Department of Health and Human Services.

Reynolds, C., & Kamphaus, R. (2004). *Behavior Assessment System for Children* (BASC-II, 2nd ed.). San Antonio, TX: Pearson (PsychCorp.).

Ringwalt, S. (2008). *Developmental screening and assessment instruments with an emphasis on social and emotional development for young children ages birth through five.* Chapel Hill, NC: The University of North Carolina, FPG Child Development Institute, and National Early Childhood Technical Assistance Center.

Robins, D. (2008). Screening for autism spectrum disorders in primary care settings. *Autism, 12*(5), 537–556.

Robins, D., Casagrande, K., Barton, M. L., Cehn, C. A., Dumont-Mathieu, T. M., & Fein, D. (2014). Validation of the Modified Checklist for Autism in Toddlers, Revised with Follow-Up (M-CHAT-R/F). *Pediatrics, 133*(1), 37–45.

Sheldrick, R., & Perrin, E.C. (2013). Evidence-based milestones for surveillance of cognitive, language, and motor development. *Academic Pediatrics, 13*(6), 577–586.

Sheldrick, R., Henson, B. S., Merchant, S., Neger, E. N., Murphy, J., & Perrin, E. C. (2012). The Preschool Pediatric Symptom Checklist (PPSC): Development and initial validation of a new social/emotional screening instrument. *Academic Pediatrics, 12*(5), 456–467.

Siegel, B. (2004). *Pervasive Developmental Disorders Screening Test-II (PDDST-II): Early childhood screener for autistic spectrum disorders.* San Antonio, TX: Harcourt Assessment.

Sosna, T., & Mastergeorge, A. (2005). *The infant, preschool, family, mental health initiative: Compendium of screening tools for early childhood social-emotional development.* Sacramento, CA: California Institute for Mental Health.

Sparrow, S. S., Balla, D. A., & Cicchetti, D. V. (1998). *Vineland Social-Emotional Early Childhood Scales.* Circle Pines, MN: American Guidance Services, Inc.

Squires, J., & Bricker, D. (2009). *Ages and Stages Questionnaires, Third Edition (ASQ-3).* Baltimore, MD: Paul H. Brookes Publishing.

Squires, J., Bricker, D., & Twombly, E. (2002). *Ages and Stages Questionnaires: Social-Emotional.* Baltimore, MD: Paul H. Brookes Publishing Co., Inc.

U.S. Department of Health and Human Services, Health Resources and Services Administration, & Maternal and Child Health Bureau. (2009). *The National Survey of Children's Health 2007.* Rockville, MD: U.S. Department of Health and Human Services.

U.S. Department of Health and Human Services and U.S Department of Education. (2014). *Birth to 5: Watch me thrive! A primary care provider's guide for developmental and behavioral screening.* Retrieved from www.hhs.gov/WatchMeThrive.

Weitzman, C., Wegner, L., & Section on Developmental and Behavioral Pediatrics, Committee on Psychosocial Aspects of Child and Family Health, Council on Early Childhood, Society for Developmental and Behavioral Pediatrics. (2015). Promoting optimal development: Screening for behavioral and emotional problems. *Pediatrics, 135*(2), 384–395.

CHILDHOOD ASTHMA

Nan Madden and Andrea Crosby Shah

C H A P T E R

10

I. Introduction and general background

A. Definition and overview

Asthma is a chronic lung disease causing narrowing of the airways. It is characterized by inflammation, broncho-constriction, and mucus production, causing variable and recurring symptoms (National Heart, Lung, and Blood Institute, National Asthma Education and Prevention Program, & National Institutes of Health [NHLBI/ NAEPP/NIH], 2007). Symptoms include coughing, wheezing, shortness of breath, and chest tightness. Airway obstruction is generally partially or fully reversible (NHLBI/NAEPP/).

B. Prevalence and incidence

Asthma onset often occurs during childhood (NHLBI/ NAEPP/NIH, 2007). Over 10 million children (14%) younger than age 18 in the United States have ever been diagnosed with asthma (Bloom, Jones, & Freeman, 2013). Non-Hispanic black children, children from low-income families, and children in fair or poor health are more likely to be diagnosed with asthma (Bloom et al., 2013).

II. Database (may include but is not limited to)

A. Subjective

1. Past health history
   a. Prematurity (particularly with known lung disease)
   b. Hospitalization for respiratory syncytial virus infection, pneumonia, or asthma
   c. Wheezing in first years of life
   d. Gastroesophageal reflux
   e. Diagnoses from the "atopic triad": allergic rhinitis, asthma, and atopic dermatitis (eczema).

The allergic component of asthma is much more prevalent and important in children.
   f. Frequency of emergency room (ER)/urgent care visits for asthma, in particular history of needing oral steroids
   g. Known allergies to medications, food, or environmental factors

2. Family history
   a. Asthma
   b. Allergic rhinitis
   c. Atopic dermatitis

3. Occupational and environmental history
   a. Maternal smoking during pregnancy
   b. Environmental exposure to tobacco smoke
   c. Environmental exposure to toxins (through parental occupation, neighborhood of residence, etc.)
   d. Home, school, or daycare exposure to environmental allergens (dust, animals, molds, etc.)

4. Review of systems
   a. Constitutional signs and symptoms: nighttime awakening, poor sleep patterns, chronic cough, other problems related to poor sleep, sedentary lifestyle, and avoidance of physical activity
   b. Pulmonary: wheezing, shortness of breath, nocturnal dry cough, exercise intolerance, and cough with exertion
   c. Allergy symptoms: itchy eyes and nose, sneezing, and dry itchy skin
   d. Growth and general nutritional status

5. Medications
   a. Past and current medications (some medications can trigger or worsen asthma symptoms, and it is also important to assess adherence and past medication failures)
   b. Actual use, as opposed to prescribed use, of medications
   c. Response of symptoms to past and current medications
   d. Spacer use, with or without mask

B. Objective

1. Physical examination findings
   a. Overall appearance: body habitus, level of distress, interaction with caregiver and provider
   b. Vital signs: particularly heart rate, respiratory rate, and oxygen saturation
   c. Skin: dry, erythematous patches and other symptoms of atopic dermatitis
   d. Allergy-related findings: "allergic shiners" (dark circles under eyes) and "allergic salute" (habitual upward wiping or rubbing of nose that can cause a crease across the nose)
   e. Ear, nose, and throat: boggy nasal turbinates, persistent ear effusions, and cobblestoning of posterior oropharynx from chronic postnasal drip
   f. In acute flare: general state of alarm and anxiety because of "air hunger"; posturing (leaning forward to increase air entry); grunting; and inability to speak in full sentences
   g. Pulmonary examination findings: most often normal when not in acute flare; however, many associated symptoms during flares
      i. Prolonged expiratory phase
      ii. Wheezing (expiratory more common than inspiratory)
      iii. Decreased air entry—when severe, may result in minimal to no wheezing, which is a warning sign
      iv. Use of accessory muscles (especially intercostal and supraclavicular)
      v. Cough (usually dry)
   h. Abdomen: increased use of accessory muscles to improve air entry

2. Supporting data from relevant diagnostic tests (not required for diagnosis and further detailed under the Plan section)
   a. Spirometry (pre- and postbronchodilator)
   b. Allergy testing
   c. Radiology: chest radiograph
   d. Laboratory measures: complete blood count and arterial blood gas

---

III. Assessment

A. Differential diagnosis (NHLBI/NAEPP/NIH, 2007)

1. Asthma
2. Allergic rhinitis
3. Sinusitis
4. Gastroesophageal reflux
5. Viral upper respiratory infection
6. Other causes of large airway obstruction
   a. Foreign body in trachea or bronchus
   b. Viral infection (e.g., croup)
   c. Vocal cord dysfunction
   d. Vascular rings or laryngeal webs
   e. Laryngotracheomalacia, tracheal stenosis, or bronchostenosis
   f. Enlarged lymph nodes or tumor
7. Other causes of small airway obstruction
   a. Bronchiolitis
   b. Cystic fibrosis
   c. Bronchopulmonary dysplasia
   d. Pulmonary edema (e.g., from congenital heart disease)
8. Habit cough or psychogenic cough

B. Classify severity or control (see Tables 10-1 and 10-2)

1. Classify **severity** if child *is not* currently on any controller medications, considering domains of both impairment and risk. Impairment refers to how the patient feels presently or in a typical week; risk refers to the likelihood that exacerbations will progress over time. A patient's severity level is defined by the most severe category. For example, if a patient has no symptoms during the day but wheezes every night, the severity level would be defined as severe persistent. Severity level is used to determine if a patient should be started on a daily controller medicine. Once the severity level is determined, pharmacotherapy may be initiated based on a stepwise approach. The higher steps correspond to more potent medications (**Table 10-3**). Asthma severity classifications are as follows:
   a. Intermittent
   b. Mild persistent
   c. Moderate persistent
   d. Severe persistent

2. Classify **control** if the child *is* currently on a controller medication, again considering domains of both impairment and risk. As with the severity domain, the control level is defined by the most severe category. Identifying a patient's control level helps determine if the patient's asthma medications should be stepped up or stepped down. For example, if a patient has been symptom free for at least 3 months, a step-down of the controller medication could be considered. On the other hand, if the patient's symptoms are not well controlled, the patient's controller medication should be stepped up at least one step and the patient should be reevaluated in 2 to 6 weeks. Asthma control levels are defined as follows:
   a. Well controlled
   b. Not well controlled
   c. Very poorly controlled

TABLE 10-1 Classifying Asthma Severity in Children 0–11 Years of Age

Impairment				
Symptoms	≤ 2 d/wk	> 2 d/wk but not daily	Daily	Throughout the day
Nighttime awakenings	0 ≤ 2×/mo	1–2×/mo 3–4×/mo	3–4×/mo >1×/wk but not nightly	>1×/wk Often 7×/wk
Short-acting β₂-agonist use for symptom control (not prevention of EIB)	≤ 2 d/wk	> 2 d/wk but not daily	Daily	Several times per day
Interference with normal activity	None	Minor limitation	Some limitation	Extremely limited
Lung function (ages 5–11)	Normal FEV_1 between exacerbations FEV_1 > 80% predicted FEV_1/FVC > 85%	FEV_1 > 80% predicted FEV_1/FVC > 80%	FEV_1 = 60–80% predicted FEV_1/FVC = 75–80%	FEV_1 < 60% predicted FEV_1/FVC < 75%

Risk				
Exacerbations requiring oral systemic corticosteroids	0–1/year	**Children 0–4 years:** ≥ 2 exacerbations in 6 mo requiring oral systemic corticosteroids, or ≥ 4 wheezing episodes/1 year lasting > 1 d and risk factors for persistent asthma **Children 5–11 years:** ≥ 2/year		
	Consider severity and interval since last exacerbation. Frequency and severity may fluctuate over time. Relative annual risk may be related to FEV_1. Exacerbations of any severity may occur in patients in any severity category.			

Recommended Step for Initiating Therapy (See Table 10-3 for recommended treatment steps)	Step 1	Step 2	Step 2	Step 3 and consider short course of oral systemic corticosteroids
	In 2–6 wk, depending on severity, evaluate level of asthma control that is achieved. If no clear benefit is observed in 4–6 wk, consider adjusting therapy or alternative diagnosis.			

Abbreviations: EIB = exercise-induced bronchospasm; FEV_1 = forced expiratory volume in the first second of expiration; FVC = forced vital capacity.

Reproduced from U.S. Department of Health and Human Services, National Institutes of Health, National Heart, Lung, and Blood Institute. (2008). *National Asthma Education and Prevention Program Expert Panel Report 3: Guidelines for the diagnosis and management of asthma—Summary Report 2007* (NIH Publication Number 08-5846, pp. 40–42). Bethesda, MD: Author.

TABLE 10-2 Assessing Asthma Control and Adjusting Therapy in Children 0–11 Years of Age

Impairment	Symptoms	≤2 d/wk but not more than once on each day	>2 d/wk or multiple times on <2 d/wk	Throughout the day
	Nighttime awakenings	≤1x/mo	>1x/mo ≥2x/mo	>1x/wk ≥2x/wk
	Interference with normal activity	None	Some limitation	Extremely limited
	Short-acting β₂-agonist use for symptom control (not prevention of EIB)	≤2 d/wk	>2 d/wk	Several times per day
	Lung function —FEV₁ (predicted) or peak flow personal best—FEV₁/FVC	N/A >80% >80%	N/A 60–80% 75–80%	N/A <60% <75%
Risk	Exacerbations requiring oral systemic corticosteroids	0–1x/year	2–3x/year ≥2x/year	>3x/year ≥2x/year
	Reduction in lung growth (ages 5–11)	Requires long-term follow-up		
	Treatment-related adverse effects	Medication side effects can vary in intensity from none to very troublesome and worrisome. The level of intensity does not correlate to specific levels of control but should be considered in the overall assessment of risk.		
Recommended Action for Treatment (see 10-3 for treatment steps) The stepwise approach is meant to assist, not replace, clinical decision making required to meet individual patient needs.		Maintain current step Regular follow-up every 1–6 mo Consider step-down if well controlled for at least 3 mo	Step up 1 step	Consider short course of oral systemic corticosteroids Step up 1–2 steps

Before step-up: Review adherence to medication, inhaler technique, and environmental control. If alternative treatment was used, discontinue it and use preferred treatment for that step. Reevaluate the level of asthma control in 2–6 wk to achieve control, every 1–6 mo to maintain control.
Children 0–4 years old: If no clear benefit is observed in 4–6 wk, consider alternative diagnosis or adjusting therapy.
Children 5–11 years old: Adjust therapy accordingly. For side effects, consider alternative treatment options.

Abbreviations: EIB = exercise-induced bronchospasm; FEV₁ = forced expiratory volume in the first second of expiration; FVC = forced vital capacity.

Reproduced from U.S. Department of Health and Human Services, National Institutes of Health, National Heart, Lung, and Blood Institute. (2008). *National Asthma Education and Prevention Program Expert Panel Report 3: Guidelines for the diagnosis and management of asthma—Summary Report 2007* (NIH Publication Number 08-5846, pp. 40–42). Bethesda, MD: Author.

IV. Goals of clinical management

A. *Few or no daytime asthma symptoms*

B. *No nighttime awakenings caused by asthma symptoms*

C. *Normal spirometry*

D. *Ability to do normal physical activity and sports*

E. *Child should not miss school and care provider should not need to miss work*

F. *Child is on the safest form and lowest dose of controller medication needed to achieve these goals*

V. Plan

A. *Diagnostic tests*

1. Spirometry
   a. Obtain a baseline in children ages 5 years and older, and repeat with changes in clinical status and/or major changes in medication regimen
   b. Forced expiratory volume in the first second of expiration (FEV_1), forced vital capacity (FVC) and forced expiratory flow, midexpiratory phase (FEF 25–75%) are most useful in children.
   c. May be difficult to obtain accurate results in children, but trends over time can be helpful even if values remain in normal range.
   d. Most often normal in children between asthma flares.
   e. The comparison of the results of spirometry performed before and after the administration of a bronchodilator demonstrates obstruction and assesses reversibility. An increase of greater than or equal to 12% in the FEV_1 and/or in the FEF 25–75% shows significant reversibility and is diagnostic for asthma.

2. Chest radiograph
   a. All young children (< 5) with a new diagnosis of asthma should have a baseline chest film. This is not to diagnose asthma but to evaluate for alternate diagnoses, such as structural abnormalities.
   b. May show hyperinflation, infiltrates, and bronchiolar cuffing.

3. Allergy testing
   a. Indicated in children with difficult to control asthma and those with suspected allergies, allergy symptoms, or severe eczema
   b. Tests for foods, airborne allergens, and known or possible triggers
   c. Testing to detect specific immunoglobulin E (IgE) sensitization can be done on children of any age, but it is more useful after the age of 2 years when meaningful positive reactions are more likely.
   d. Referral to a subspecialty clinic may be necessary for testing.
   e. Skin testing
      i. Results are immediate and generally considered more sensitive than in vitro testing.
      ii. Skin testing will not be accurate if antihistamine was taken recently.
   f. Specific IgE immunoassay (in vitro)
      i. Indicated if history of anaphylaxis to particular allergen or if severe atopic dermatitis makes it difficult to find clear skin on which to perform the prick tests.
      ii. More expensive and less sensitive than skin testing; however, not affected by recent doses of antihistamines.
      iii. Requires blood draw.

4. Laboratory measures
   a. Laboratory tests should not be routinely performed in the diagnosis or management of pediatric asthma patients. Consider only if results will help with differential diagnosis or meaningfully change management
   b. Complete blood count: eosinophilia may be supportive of allergic component to child's asthma.
   c. Blood gas: in acute asthma flare, can show retention of carbon dioxide, suggestive of impending respiratory failure. Should not be used alone to determine need for intubation

B. *Management*

1. Environmental controls
   a. Allergens: identify and minimize exposure to common allergens (dust mites, mold, animal dander, cockroaches, molds, and seasonal pollens).
      i. Carpeting: harbors dust mites, and children like to play on the floor. Should be removed or at least vacuumed frequently.
      ii. Stuffed animals: try to limit to one or two stuffed toys, wash them in hot water every 2 weeks, or freeze and then place in the dryer.
      iii. Allergen-proof mattress and pillow covers: for those with dust mite allergies.
      iv. All bed linen should be washed in hot water and dried in a dryer every week.

b. Irritants (smoke, perfumes, or fumes from cleaning solutions).

  i. Absolutely no one should smoke in the house or in a car with children, and those who choose to smoke outside should wear a smoking jacket that is never brought into the house.

  ii. Use environmentally safe cleaning products and clean when the child is out of the home.

2. Medication (see **Table 10-3**)

  a. Rescue medications are short-acting β-agonists (SABA) (albuterol HFA or levalbuterol HFA, also available in nebulized form). Give every 4 hours as needed for any signs of asthma, including coughing.

  b. Controller medication.

  i. Prescribe controller medications for any child with persistent asthma.

  ii. Inhaled corticosteroids (ICS) are first-line treatment because they offer the best and safest long-term control therapy (NHLBI/NAEPP/NIH, 2007).

  iii. Start with a low-to-medium dose depending on the child's risk and severity of symptoms.

  iv. Assess control after 4–6 weeks, and if well controlled, continue treatment for a total of 3 months. Step down to a lower dose if asthma remains under control. Goal is to find minimal effective dose.

  v. If after 4–6 weeks asthma is not well controlled, step up therapy and/or consider an alternative diagnosis.

  vi. Consider combining a long-acting β-agonist with the ICS for children who do not respond to a medium-dose ICS alone. Also consider the addition of a leukotriene receptor antagonist if the child has symptoms of exercise-induced bronchospasm or a strong allergic component to their asthma.

  c. Antihistamines.

  i. Medication to decrease allergy symptoms, such as itchy eyes, frequent sneezing, or a scratchy throat or mouth, should also be considered. Besides interfering with a child's normal life and academic achievements, untreated allergies can make the asthma symptoms worse by causing bronchial smooth muscle contractions that quickly narrow the airways (Mahr & Sneth, 2005; NHLBI/NAEPP/NIH, 2007).

  d. Oral systemic corticosteroids.

  i. Short-course steroid "pulse" doses: used to decrease airway inflammation during moderate or severe exacerbations or for patients who fail to respond promptly and completely to a SABA.

  ii. Oral prednisone or dexamethasone shown equally effective. Usually requires 3–10 days of therapy. No evidence that tapering "pulse" dose prevents relapse (NHLBI/NAEPP/NIH, 2007).

  iii. Daily long-term use of oral steroids is a treatment of last resort and is reserved for children with severe asthma who do not respond adequately to other controller medications.

TABLE 10-3 Stepwise Approach for Managing Asthma Long Term in Children 0–11 Years of Age: Preferred Medications*

SABA PRN	**Ages 0–4**				
	Low-dose ICS	Medium-dose ICS	Medium-dose ICS + LABA *or* montelukast	High-dose ICS + LABA *or* montelukast	High-dose ICS + LABA *or* montelukast + oral corticosteroids
	Ages 5–11				
	Low-dose ICS	Low-dose ICS + LABA or LTRA *or* medium-dose ICS	Medium-dose ICS + LABA	High-dose ICS + LABA	High-dose ICS + LABA + oral corticosteroids

Abbreviations: ICS = inhaled corticosteroids; LABA = long-acting β-agonists; LTRA = leukotriene receptor antagonist.

* See NHLBI/NAEPP/NIH (2007) guideline for full details of stepwise treatment, including alternative therapies.

e. Omalizumab (Xolair).

   i. A monoclonal IgE antibody, administered in subcutaneous injections.

   ii. Recommended for consideration for children older than 12 years of age who have severe allergic asthma, poorly controlled on other therapies (NHLBI/NAEPP/NIH, 2007).

   iii. Omalizumab's major potential side effect is anaphylaxis and is therefore administered in a specialist's office.

3. Treat comorbid conditions

a. Treatment of the following conditions that are frequently seen with asthma may improve asthma control: rhinitis, sinusitis, gastroesophageal reflux, obesity, depression, and allergic bronchopulmonary aspergillosis.

b. Vaccinate all asthmatic children over the age of 6 months with the inactivated form of the influenza vaccine. If the child has an egg allergy but has experienced only hives after ingesting egg, the vaccine should be administered by a healthcare provider who is familiar with the possible manifestations of egg allergy. In addition, the patient should be observed for at least 30 minutes after receiving each vaccine. If a child has had a severe reaction to ingesting eggs, such as respiratory distress, angioedema, or recurrent vomiting, the inactivated vaccine should be administered by a healthcare provider who is experienced in the recognition and management of severe allergic reactions. Available data are insufficient to determine the level of severity of asthma for which administration of the live attenuated influenza vaccine (LAIV) would be inadvisable. The influenza vaccine that is not egg based, trivalent recombinant influenza vaccine, RIV3/FluBloc, is not licensed for use in patients < 18 years old (Centers for Disease Control and Prevention, 2014).

c. When possible, young children should avoid contact with people who have viral respiratory infections, a common trigger and a major factor in the development, persistence, and possibly severity of asthma (NHLBI/NAEPP/NIH, 2007).

4. Encourage physical activity

If necessary, treat exercise-induced bronchospasm by use of a SABA 20 minutes before exercise. Increase or start a daily controller medication if exercise-induced symptoms persist or if symptoms occur during daily activities.

5. Consider allergy immunotherapy

Referral may be appropriate if the child has mild-to-moderate asthma, and there is a correlation between their asthma symptoms and their exposure to allergens.

6. Involve the family and child (if old enough) in all treatment decision making to encourage a partnership in the care and control of the child's asthma.

7. Follow-up

a. Patients with well-controlled asthma should be seen every 3–6 months by specialist or primary care provider, depending on the patient's past asthma history, the family's need for reinforcement and education, and social factors that might put the child at high risk.

b. At each follow-up visit, reassess asthma control, adjust medications as needed, and review medication technique.

8. Referral to specialist

a. Child is a severe asthmatic (multiple hospitalizations, history of intubation, poor control on typical controller medications).

b. Symptoms are not responding to appropriate treatment.

c. Child is candidate for immunotherapy or omalizumab therapy.

d. Allergy testing or spirometry is desired and cannot be performed by primary provider.

C. Patient and family education

1. Basic asthma education

a. Determine family's knowledge about asthma.

b. Show diagrams of the lungs and where they are located in the body to both the parent and child.

c. Explain that asthma is a chronic, inflammatory disease of the lungs. Although the child's asthma can be controlled and the child can lead a normal life, the asthma itself will not be cured. This is an important and difficult concept for some families and children to understand and accept.

2. Environmental controls

Allergy and trigger reduction or avoidance (see the Management section)

3. Medications

a. Explain the difference between rescue medication and controller medication. Lung diagrams showing normal lungs versus lungs affected by asthma and other diagrams showing the muscle-relaxing effect of bronchodilator versus the anti-inflammatory effects of controller medications can be very useful.

b. Review the use of their asthma action plan and identification of symptoms (see the Self-Management Resources and Tools section).

c. Demonstrate the proper use of spacer (with the appropriate-size mask for young children), inhalers, discus, and nebulizer.

d. Address, if necessary, the family's concerns about their child's use of ICS. Long-term studies have shown that children reach predicted adult height despite ongoing use of inhaled steroids (Guill, 2004). If needed, point out that the risks of inadequately treated asthma include death.

e. Teach methods of obtaining refills from a pharmacy.

4. Emergency care
   a. Recognition of severe asthma
   b. Use of medications for severe symptoms
   c. When to call the medical provider
   d. When to bring the child to the emergency room

5. Follow-up telephone calls or emails
   a. Answer questions.
   b. Review the action plan.
   c. Review knowledge of emergency care of the child.
   d. Remind the family of follow-up appointments.

6. Educational tools
   a. Videos are another useful tool in patient education. Some people are more likely to watch a video in the clinic or office than to read educational materials at home.
   b. Written material should be available to those who are interested with consideration of the family's literacy level.
   c. Computer programs, peer education, and other school-based programs can be effective educational tools for school-aged children and adolescents.

7. Barriers to learning
   a. Family: No parent wants to think that their child may have a chronic disease, so this can be very difficult emotionally for the parent to hear. Denial of the chronic nature of asthma is very common and frequently leads to nonadherence to medication routines and laxity in environmental controls. Fear of addiction to, or side effects from, medications is another common barrier.
   b. Patient: The child or teenager may also have difficulty accepting the diagnosis of asthma. After acknowledging this difficulty, naming famous athletes or celebrities who have controlled asthma might be reassuring.

8. Adherence
   a. Provide calendars with boxes for the parent or child to check when medicine has been given.
   b. Help the family or child coordinate the timing of taking their medication with another well-established habit, such as brushing teeth.
   c. Remind the family and child that adherence helps them achieve their desired outcomes and minimizes visits to the ED as well as the use of stronger medications.

9. Goal setting: it might help for a child or teenager to set a goal for improvement. For example, they might set a very concrete goal, such as being able to blow out all the candles on their next pulmonary function test or being able to sleep all night without symptoms by the next office or clinic visit.

VI. Resources

A. Self-management resources and tools

1. At home
   a. Asthma action plan. (See sample Action Plan, **Figure 46-2, in Chapter 46, Asthma in Adolescents and Adults.**)
      i. Complete a written asthma action plan, with a copy for any secondary home and for school or daycare.
      ii. To avoid confusion, keep the medication regimen as uncomplicated as the child's condition allows.
      iii. Provide a new plan every time medication is changed.
   b. Peak flow meter.
      i. Not recommended for all patients. Observation of the child's symptoms is often more useful, because of inconsistent use of peak flow meters.
      ii. Some motivated parents and patients find it helpful to monitor their child's asthma by using a peak flow meter twice a day. The purpose is to be able to detect or help recognize worsening symptoms by comparing the present reading with the child's best reading.

2. At child's school
   It is imperative that a school knows if a child has asthma, no matter how mild, and has an emergency care plan in place. Most schools require a written permission from the health provider and from the parent for the child to be able to use or receive his or her rescue medication in school. Ensuring that the school has

this permission should be part of the routine care of all children with asthma.

B. Asthma education resources

1. Allergy & Asthma Network Mothers of Asthmatics: www.breathville.org

2. American Academy of Allergy, Asthma and Immunology: www.aaaai.org

3. American Lung Association: www.lungusa.org

4. Centers for Disease Control and Prevention: www.cdc.gov/asthma

5. National Heart, Lung, and Blood Institute Information Center: www.nhlbi.nih.gov

6. National Jewish Medical and Research Center (Lung Line): www.nationaljewish.org

REFERENCES

Bloom, B., Jones, L. I., & Freeman, G. (2013). *Summary health statistics for U.S. children: National Health Interview Survey, 2012* (Vital Health Statistics, series 10, no. 258). Washington, DC: National Center for Health Statistics, Centers for Disease Control and Prevention.

Centers for Disease Control and Prevention (CDC). (2014, August 15). Recommendations of the Advisory Committee on Immunization Practices (ACIP) United States, 2014–2015 influenza season. *Morbidity and Mortality Weekly Report, 63*(32): 691–697. Retrieved from http://www.cdc.gov/mmwr/preview/mmwrhtml/mm6332a3.htm.

Guill, M. F. (2004). Asthma update: Clinical aspects and management. *Pediatrics in Review, 25*(10), 338–342.

Mahr, T. A., & Sneth, K. (2005). Update on allergic rhinitis. *Pediatrics in Review, 25*(8), 284–289.

National Asthma Education and Prevention Program, & National Heart, Lung, and Blood Institute. (2007). *Expert panel report 3: Guidelines for the diagnosis and management of asthma* (NIH publication no. 08-4051). Retrieved from http://www.nhlbi.nih.gov/health-pro/resources/lung/naci/asthma-info/asthma-guidelines.htm.

U.S. Department of Health and Human Services, National Institutes of Health, National Heart, Lung, and Blood Institute. (2007). *National Asthma Education and Prevention Program Expert Panel Report 3: Guidelines for the diagnosis and management of asthma—Summary Report 2007* (NIH Publication Number 08-5846). Bethesda, MD: Author.

ATOPIC DERMATITIS IN CHILDREN

Karen G. Duderstadt and Nan Madden

I. Introduction and general background

A. Definition and overview

Atopic dermatitis (AD) is classified as an eczematous eruption of the skin in childhood. The term "eczema" is often used interchangeably with AD. Eczema means "flaring up," which describes the acute symptom complex of erythema, scaling, vesicles, inflamed papules, plaques, and crusts seen with AD (Goodhue & Brady, 2009). The protective barrier of the skin is impaired and undergoes stages of dryness; pruritus; inflammation; and increased susceptibility to bacterial, viral, and fungal infections. AD is often the initial manifestation of atopic disease in children. Children with severe AD have a higher risk of developing other atopic diseases.

B. Prevalence and incidence

AD, or atopic eczema, is the most common skin disorder in young children and affects approximately 10–20% of the pediatric population. It is increasing in prevalence in the United States and there has been a twofold to threefold increase in the prevalence of AD in developing countries in the past 30 years (Leong, Boguniewicz, Howell, & Hamid, 2004). AD develops in 45% of affected children within the first 6 months of life, and in 60% of children by the first year of age. Allergic rhinitis develops in 50–80% of children with AD, and greater than 50% of children with AD develop asthma in adolescence or adulthood (Boguniewicz, 2005; Paller & Mancini, 2006). AD occurs more commonly in urban populations, in smaller family units with higher socioeconomic status, and in families with less exposure to infectious agents and antigenic triggers than in families living in rural settings.

C. Etiology

The exact etiology or immune mechanism of AD is unknown. Skin barrier dysfunction is now being recognized as having a key role in the development of AD. Defects in the outer layer of the skin, the stratum corneum, leads to a reduced ability of keratinocytes to maintain hydration and to restrict transepidermal water loss, which leads to extreme dryness of the skin, which produces itching and subsequently AD (Tollefson & Bruckner, 2014). An inadequate skin barrier might also allow for the entry of aeroallergens from the environment that could cause the elevated immunoglobulin E (IgE) levels, common in children with AD. Children with AD have elevated serum IgE levels. These antigens activate T lymphocytes, which leads to an increase in interleukins and peripheral eosinophilia. The mechanism of scratching or rubbing the skin releases cytokines from the epidermal cells and perpetuates the inflammation (Paller & Mancini, 2006). Children may have a genetic predisposition for this dysfunction of their skin barrier. About 75% of children with AD have a positive family history of the atopic disease indicating a genetic alteration as a causative factor.

II. Database (may include but is not limited to)

A. Subjective

1. History of the presenting illness and relevant past health history
   a. Feeding history: breastfed or formula fed
   b. When rash or lesions first appeared and on what areas of the body
   c. Has infant or child had periods without lesions or rash?
   d. Bathing routine? Soaps used? Emollients used?
   e. Sleep history? Quality of sleep and nighttime symptoms?
   f. Any known food or drug allergies?
   g. History of exposure to known allergens?
   h. What does the parent or child think about what makes the rash or lesions better or worse?

i. Factors that lead to flares include (National Institute of Arthritis and Musculoskeletal and Skin Diseases, 2009):
  i. Emotions: Especially anger, stress, and frustration
  ii. Bacterial skin infections (exotoxins of *Staphylococcus aureus* may act as superantigens and stimulate activation of T cells and macrophages) (Fitzpatrick & Wolff, 2005)
  iii. Climate: Low humidity (but sometimes high humidity if it causes excessive perspiration) and a dry year-round climate. Ideal humidity for the home is 45–55%.
  iv. Long or hot baths or showers
  v. Not using enough moisturizers after bath
  vi. Going from sweating to being chilled
j. History of other atopic skin disease, hives, or urticaria?
k. History of allergic rhinitis or asthma?
l. History of bacterial skin infections, herpes, fungal infections?
m. History of other chronic conditions or developmental delay?

2. Medication history
  a. Over-the-counter medications used, topical and oral
  b. Prescription medications used, topical and oral
  c. Frequency of medication use, daily or with flares
  d. In what areas are the medications applied?
  e. Complementary or alternative medications or therapies?
  f. Has child been on antibiotics in the past year?
3. Family history
  a. Any family history of allergies, AD, eczema, allergic rhinitis, or asthma?
  b. Siblings with atopic disease?
  c. Known food allergies in parent or sibling?
4. Environmental history
  a. Factors that trigger onset or exacerbation of AD are common but manifest differently in each individual (see **Figure 11-1**).
5. Social history
  a. Quality of life for children and families with AD. (Note: Quality of life is often diminished because of chronicity of condition, constant

FIGURE 11-1 *Common Triggering Factors*

TRIGGER	ASSOCIATED FINDINGS (may or may not include)
Food:	Food items include eggs, peanuts, cow's milk, fish, shellfish, soy, and wheat. Food preservatives and food color may trigger allergies but no testing mechanism exists for these substances.
Decreased humidity:	Cold seasons with reduced humidity often herald a flare-up for children with AD. Skin holds less moisture, dry skin becomes irritated, pruritus develops, and scratching begins.
Emotional stress:	Physical and emotional stress can precipitate flares of AD. It is not causative but worsens the condition.
Aeroallergens:	Most common trigger of aeroallergens: • Dust mites in household • Grass pollens • Animal dander • Molds
Temperature change and sweating:	Increased scratching and rubbing caused by sudden change in temperature are common in infants and children with AD. Sweating particularly causes scratching and flares of AD.

Data from Habif, T. P. (2010). Atopic dermatitis. In T. P. Habif (Ed.), *Clinical dermatology: A color guide to diagnosis and therapy* (5th ed.). Philadelphia, PA: Elsevier.

pruritus, and difficulty in identifying and avoiding triggers.)

6. Symptom history

a. Common constitutional signs and symptoms of AD include pruritus, sleep disturbance, nasal congestion, age-specific patterns, or distribution of skin involvement, sparing of diaper area in infants, and sparing of groin and axillae in older children and adolescents; occasionally, irritability in infants with moderate-to-severe disease.

b. Skin, hair, and nails

i. Dry skin (xerosis), erythema, occasional papules, vesicles, weeping lesions, and crusting

ii. Chronic skin changes include hyperpigmentation on lighter skin; hypopigmentation on darker skin; lichenification or leathery, thickened skin; and scarring from scratching

c. Lymphadenopathy

i. Enlarged lymph glands can be a common associated finding of children with AD, particularly in areas localized to exacerbations of AD or in children with associated bacterial, viral, or fungal infections.

d. Respiratory

i. Pulmonary findings of wheezing are common in children with atopic disease and asthma is a common associated condition.

B. Objective

1. Physical examination findings

a. AD presents differently at different ages. There are three distinct phases of clinical features: (1) infantile phase, (2) childhood phase, and (3) adult phase (see **Figure 11-2**).

b. Conditions and features often associated with AD in children and adolescents (see **Figure 11-3**).

c. Opportunistic infections are common in infants and children with AD (see **Figure 11-4**).

d. Additional physical examination findings of atopic disease:

i. General appearance: pallor, allergic shiners, allergic salute, and xerosis

ii. Head, eye, ear, nose, and throat: periorbital puffiness; tympanic membranes with effusion unilaterally or bilaterally; boggy nasal mucosa or erythematous turbinates with enlarged adenoids; and tonsilar hypertrophy, nonerythematous, nonexudative

iii. Neck: enlarged lymph nodes (cervical, occipital, postauricular)

iv. Chest: adventitious sounds such as wheezing

2. Supporting data from relevant diagnostic tests

a. Diagnosis of AD is most often a clinical diagnosis, and immunologic testing is reserved for moderate to severe disease (**Table 11-1**).

i. A low accuracy of food allergy tests has been reported in children with AD.

ii. Diagnostic testing for skin allergies should be reserved for children who are nonresponsive to traditional therapies or who may have gastrointestinal symptoms of AD.

b. At 6 months of age, 83% of children with severe AD show positive IgE sensitization to milk, eggs, and peanuts.

III. Assessment

A. Determine the diagnosis

Differential diagnoses (**Figure 11-5**)

B. Assess the severity of the disease

SCORAD is a clinical tool used by dermatologists to assess the extent and the severity of AD in children and to determine the effectiveness of the treatment regimen. The tool is available at http://dermnetnz.org/dermatitis/scorad.html

C. Assess the significance of the problem to the child and family

D. Assess the family functioning and ability to follow the treatment regimen

IV. Goals of clinical management

A. Improve quality of life for children with AD and their families

1. No nighttime awakening because of itching

2. No daytime discomfort or itching

3. No missed school because of AD

4. No missed workdays for the parents because of their child's symptoms

B. Prescribe medications that allow the minimum effective dose to prevent adverse reactions

C. Educate families so they understand and adhere to optimum skin care and medication regimens

FIGURE 11-2 *Phases of Atopic Dermatitis in Children*

PHASES	CLINICAL FEATURES (may or may not include)
Infantile phase	Begins from birth to 6 months of age: • May begin on cheeks and progress to scalp, arms, trunk, and legs; generalized dry skin (xerosis) including scalp • Progresses to lateral extensor surfaces of arms and legs • Pruritus and itch-scratch-itch cycle develops • Acute phase with intense itching causing irritability in infant; vesicle formation, oozing, and crusting with excoriated areas on the skin • Hallmark sign is diaper area and groin are usually spared of lesions • May resolve by 2 years of age but can continue into childhood; symptoms may become milder as the child ages and disappear at adolescence or may continue throughout life
Childhood phase	Begins around 2 years of age: • Involves wrists, hands, neck, ankles, popliteal and antecubital spaces, commonly on flexural surfaces • Lesions tend to be dry, papular, circumscribed, scaly patches • Pruritus is often severe Chronic manifestations include: • Lichenification, thickening of skin causing leathery appearance • Hyperpigmentation • Scratch marks Often worse during winter dryness or summer heat.
Adult phase	Begins at puberty or ~12 years of age: • Most commonly involves flexural skin folds; bends of elbows and knees; face; neck; upper arms; back; and dorsa of the hands, feet, fingers, and toes • May be a new occurrence or reoccurrence of chronic condition Often postinflammatory hyperpigmentation and hypopigmentation disappear in adolescence or young adulthood.

Data from Habif, T. P. (2010). Atopic dermatitis. In T. P. Habif (Ed.), *Clinical dermatology: A color guide to diagnosis and therapy* (5th ed.). Philadelphia, PA: Elsevier.

D. Control environmental factors that may adversely affect the child's skin

(Note: Food avoidance is no longer first-line management or mainstay of treatment for AD.)

E. Provide ongoing emotional and medical support for children and their families

V. Plan

A. Develop an optimum skin care routine with the family

New data have established that AD results from primary abnormalities of the skin barrier, suggesting the importance of skin-directed management of the disease

FIGURE 11-3 Conditions and Features Associated with Atopic Dermatitis

ASSOCIATED CONDITIONS (may or may not include)	CLINICAL FEATURES
Dennie line or Dennie-Morgan fold	Extra grooves or accentuated lines seen below lower eyelids bilaterally; may result from chronic edema of the eyelids and skin thickening
Allergic shiners	Dark discoloration below lower eyelids in lighter skin; slate-gray discoloration in individuals with darker skin; a result of vascular stasis
Allergic salute	Crease over the nasal bridge or exaggerated linear nasal crease caused by frequent rubbing of nose or nasal tip; most often associated with allergic rhinitis but common in atopic children
Pityriasis alba	Hypopigmented, slightly elevated plaques; occasionally with fine scaling, irregular borders; nonpruritic; occurring most often on the face of young children; also may appear on the upper arms and thighs; ~2–4 cm in diameter round-to-oval, often occur in summer or fall
Keratosis pilaris	Most predominant on the lateral aspects of the upper arms, buttocks, and thighs; appears in early childhood and persists into adulthood; papular with plugged hair follicles and surrounding inflammation; characterized by redness on lighter skin
Nummular eczema	Coin-shaped lesions or plaques ~1 cm or greater in diameter; erythematous and formed by confluent papules or occasionally vesicles
Ichthyosis vulgaris	Transmitted as an autosomal-dominant trait; can be associated with AD but a separate disease; may occur as early as 3 months of age, but most common onset in later childhood; characterized by large scales on extensor surfaces of extremities, particularly on lateral aspect of the lower legs in plate-like scales; flexural surfaces are spared

Data from Paller, A. S., & Mancini, A. J. (2011). Eczematous eruptions in childhood. In A. S. Paller & A. J. Mancini (Eds.), *Hurwitz clinical pediatric dermatology: A textbook of skin disorders of childhood and adolescence* (4th ed.). Philadelphia, PA: Elsevier ; Habif, T. P. (2010). Atopic dermatitis. In T. P. Habif (Ed.), *Clinical dermatology: A color guide to diagnosis and therapy* (5th ed.). Philadelphia, PA: Elsevier.

(Tollefson & Bruckner, 2014). Develop an optimum skin care routine with the family. Instruct the family to use the following "soak and seal" technique:

1. Daily bath with lukewarm water for about 10 to 15 minutes. Use a minimal amount of fragrance-free and dye-free gentle soap or cleanser that is formulated for sensitive skin, such as Cetaphil Cleanser, at the end of the bath. If the child is not too dirty, use soap or cleanser only on hands, feet, armpits, and genital area, not all over the body.

    a. If the child complains of burning when sitting in the bathtub, the addition of one cup of table salt may make the bath more tolerable (Paller & Mancini, 2011).

2. Gently pat away excess water, leaving skin slightly damp.

3. If rash is present, apply skin medication to the rash on body and face. Prescription medications should be applied to areas of the skin that are red, rough, or itchy, or where there is a rash when the skin is slightly damp. Apply in a thin layer and rub in well.

4. After drying, apply a generous amount of moisturizing cream or ointment to the entire body and face. This seals in the water from bathing and makes the skin less dry and itchy. Eucerin cream, Aquaphor™ ointment, and Cetaphil™ cream are effective products. Lotions are not recommended for adequate moisturizing in children with AD. Vaseline or petroleum jelly can be used as an inexpensive moisturizer and sealer, and it is a good occlusive preparation, although not a moisturizer. This application should be done within 3 minutes of exiting the bath before water loss in the

FIGURE 11-4 Secondary Opportunistic Skin Infections

OPPORTUNISTIC INFECTIONS	ASSOCIATED FINDINGS (may or may not include)
Staphylococcus aureus	Erythematous with pustular, exudative lesions and crusting; the most common opportunistic infection in AD and recovered in 93% of patients with AD lesions, 79% from nares of atopic children
Streptococcus pyogenes	A less common opportunistic infection in children with AD than *S. aureus*; skin findings as above
Herpes simplex	Vesicles often become umbilicated; eczema herpeticum, rapid development of vesiculopustular lesions over the sites of dermatitis, can occur in individuals with AD
Viral molluscum contagiosum	Small, dome-shaped papules often with central umbilication; commonly affect trunk, axillae, and antecubital and popliteal fossae in 25% of children with AD

Data from Habif, T. P. (2015). Atopic dermatitis. In T. P. Habif (Ed.), *Clinical dermatology: A color guide to diagnosis and therapy* (6th ed.). Philadelphia, PA: Elsevier.

TABLE 11-1 Common Laboratory Tests

Test	Definition	Clinical Implications	Comments
Skin prick test	Wheal response after skin prick with antigen	IgE-mediated food hypersensitivity	Often does not correlate with clinical manifestations in children with AD
Radioallergosorbent test	Circulating specific IgE	IgE-mediated food hypersensitivity	False-positive findings are common, particularly in older children

Data from Paller, A. S., & Mancini, A. J. (2011). Eczematous eruptions in childhood. In A. S. Paller & A. J. Mancini (Eds.), *Hurwitz clinical pediatric dermatology: A textbook of skin disorders of childhood and adolescence* (4th ed.). Philadelphia, PA: Elsevier.

skin occurs from evaporation. It can be repeated as needed to dry, itchy skin (Paller & Mancini, 2011). This bath routine should be continued even after the skin has improved and the prescription medication is no longer necessary.

5. When moisturizing products are not effective, some children may need a special preparation containing ammonium lactate or alpha-hydroxy acid lotion for maintenance care. These products have increased ability to hold water in the skin and the products may limit desquamation. However, they frequently cause burning of the affected skin and so should be used with caution with young children (Fitzpatrick & Wolff, 2005).

B. Avoid factors or allergic triggers that lead to flares

1. Irritants: things that may cause the skin to be red or itchy or to burn
   a. Wash all new clothes before wearing to remove chemicals. Double rinse the child's laundry so that the skin is not in contact with residual detergent in clothing.
   b. Do not use fabric softeners.
   c. Avoid clothes made of wool and artificial fibers. Dress the child in loose-fitting cotton clothes that allow air to pass freely to the skin.
   d. Avoid contact with harsh household cleaners. Use natural, environmentally safe products.

FIGURE 11-5 *Common Differential Diagnosis of Atopic Dermatitis*

CONDITION	ASSOCIATED FINDINGS (may or may not include)
Contact dermatitis	Irritant or allergic contact dermatitis is generally milder than AD; occurs on the cheeks and chin, extensor surfaces or diaper area of infants and young children; caused by harsh soaps, vigorous bathing, or saliva on cheek and chin area.
Seborrheic dermatitis	Greasy, yellow scales that involve the scalp, eyebrows, behind the ears, cheeks, and can spread to neck and chest area; generally nonpruritic. Often AD appears as seborrheic dermatitis subsides.
Psoriasis	Round, erythematous, well-marginated plaques; covered by grayish or silvery-white scales; ~1 cm or greater in diameter; commonly found on the scalp, elbows, knees, and lumbosacral area.
Scabies	Pruritic papules, nodules, vesiculopustules, and burrowing lesions; commonly occur on infants and young children; seen on trunk, between the fingers, wrists, ankles, axillae, waist, groin, palms of hands, and soles of feet; occasionally seen on the head of infants.

Data from Paller A. S., & Mancini, A. J. (2011). Eczematous eruptions in childhood. In A. S. Paller & A. J. Mancini (Eds.), *Hurwitz clinical pediatric dermatology: A textbook of skin disorders of childhood and adolescence* (4th ed.). Philadelphia, PA: Elsevier.

---

e. Wear long pants and long sleeves when playing around irritating substances, such as sand, dirt, and plants.

f. Eliminate the child's exposure to secondhand smoke because it can increase irritation and pruritus and may also increase the tendency for the development of asthma (Paller & Mancini, 2011).

g. Keep the child's fingernails short, smooth, and clean to help prevent skin irritation, infection, and damage caused by scratching. Explain to the family that when the child scratches the rash becomes worse and the skin becomes thicker.

2. Proved or suspected allergens

a. Consider food allergy only in children who have reacted immediately to a certain food and in infants and young children with moderate or severe uncontrolled AD, particularly with gastrointestinal symptoms or failure to thrive (National Institute for Health and Clinical Excellence [NICE], 2007). The National Institute of Allergy and Infection Disease (NIAID) guidelines state that allergy evaluation, specifically to milk, eggs, peanuts, wheat, and soy, should be considered in children less than 5 years with severe AD if the child has persistent AD despite optimal management. The guidelines state that food allergies can induce hives and itching, which may aggravate AD but do not cause AD. Egg allergy may be one exception. Up to half of infants with egg-specific IgE may have improvement in their AD when following an egg-free diet (Tollefson & Bruckner, 2014).

i. If cow's milk allergy is suspected, offer a 6- to 8-week trial of an extensively hydrolyzed protein formula as a substitute for cow's milk formula for bottle-fed infants younger than 6 months of age with moderate or severe AD. Refer to a dietary specialist if the baby needs to be on cow's milk-free diet for more than 8 weeks (Paller & Mancini, 2011).

ii. Inform breastfeeding mothers that it is not known whether altering a mother's diet is effective in reducing symptoms. However, if a food allergy is strongly suspected consider a trial of elimination of the more allergenic foods, such as cow's milk, soy, wheat, tree nuts, peanuts, fish, and egg, under dietary supervision.

b. Consider inhalant allergy in children with seasonal flares, associated asthma, and allergic rhinitis and in children older than 3 years of age with AD on the face. After 3 years of age, many children outgrow food allergies but become sensitive to airborne allergens, such as dust mites (Leong et al., 2004). Some children have shown improvement in symptoms when dust mites are controlled in their environment, especially in their bedroom:

    i.   Eliminate floor coverings and curtains

    ii.   Eliminate all upholstered furniture except the bed

    iii.   Cover box springs, mattress, and pillows in plastic zippered covers or obtain allergy-proof covers

    iv.   Eliminate clutter and limit the toys, especially stuffed animals

    v.   Wash all bedcovers and stuffed animals at least once a week in hot water

    vi.   Keep pets with fur or feathers out of the room because they attract dust

  c. Avoid only substances that are documented to cause an increase in symptoms. It is important not to deny children things unnecessarily, such as foods or outdoor activities.

  d. Most children with mild AD do not need diagnostic testing for skin allergies (NICE, 2007).

C. Treat symptoms when they occur

1. Topical corticosteroids are the therapeutic mainstay for AD. They not only suppress the inflammation and pruritus associated with AD, but they may also have an effect on bacterial colonization. Choosing which corticosteroid to prescribe depends on the severity and distribution of the lesions and the age of the child. Preparations are divided into seven groups based on relative potency, from very low preparations, such as hydrocortisone acetate, to very high preparations, such as clobetasol propionate. Ointment-based preparations are more potent, more occlusive, and less drying than chemically equivalent cream-based agents. The most effective, but least potent, should be used to prevent thinning of the skin. For children with mild-to-moderate disease, a group VII drug, such as hydrocortisone ointment 1% or 2.5%, is usually sufficient. When corticosteroids are prescribed, consider the following:

  a. Prescribe in adequate amounts to optimize control. Prescriptions that require frequent refills may lead to undertreatment or nonadherence.

  b. Prescribe for application only once or twice a day.

  c. Corticosteroids should be applied to areas of active lesions, not to clear skin for prophylaxis.

  d. Consider the possibility of secondary bacterial or viral infection if the regular application of corticosteroids has not controlled the AD within 2 weeks.

  e. Consider changing to a different topical corticosteroid of the same potency as an alternative to stepping up treatment if tachyphylaxis is suspected (NICE, 2007).

  f. Do not use potent topical corticosteroids on the face or neck.

  g. When inflammation is widespread, avoid high-potency corticosteroids because of the risk of systemic adverse effects.

  h. Refer to a specialist if potent corticosteroids are needed for children younger than 12 months of age.

  i. Explain to families that the benefits of topical corticosteroids outweigh the risks if applied correctly.

2. Topical calcineurin inhibitors are an option for treatment if the child's AD has not shown a satisfactory clinical response to adequate use of topical corticosteroids at the maximum strength and potency that is appropriate for the child's age and the area being treated (NICE, 2007). Both pimecrolimus cream 1% (Elidel) and tacrolimus ointment 0.03% and 0.1% (Protopic) are approved for treating AD in children 2 years of age and older.

  a. Pimecrolimus is efficacious in children with mild-to-moderate AD.

  b. Tacrolimus is appropriate for children with moderate-to-severe disease, and its effectiveness has been compared to midpotency topical steroids.

  c. Both medications are safe for use in the periorbital areas and on the head, neck, and intertriginous area (Paller & Mancini, 2011).

  d. A burning sensation may occur during the first few days of application in children with either medication, especially in children with more severe dermatitis.

  e. Use sun protection when using either medication.

3. Wet-wrap dressings reduce itching and inflammation by cooling the skin and improving penetration of topical corticosteroids for acute exacerbations. They also prevent excoriation from scratching. In the hospital, gauze is usually used for this procedure. At home, a method used for years at the National Jewish Medical and Research Center, Denver, Colorado, is a simpler approach. It uses wet clothing, such as long underwear and cotton socks, applied over an undiluted layer of topical corticosteroids with a dry layer of clothing on top.

  a. Use blankets to prevent chilling.

  b. Should not be used for more than 7–14 consecutive nights (NICE, 2007).

4. Antihistamines are thought to have little direct effect on pruritus. However, the tranquilizing and sedating effects of sedating antihistamines, such as hydroxyzine, diphenhydramine, and doxepin, may provide symptomatic relief if given at bedtime. Cetirizine may have limited value, but it is also somewhat sedating.

Nonsedating antihistamines are not effective in alleviating pruritus (Paller & Mancini, 2011).

    a. Ensure that the medication does not interfere with the child's functioning during the daytime.

    b. Topical antihistamines should be avoided because of possible local allergic reactions.

5. Phototherapy could be considered for severe AD or when other management options have failed. Refer to a pediatric specialty clinic where staff is experienced in dealing with children.

6. Systemic corticosteroids should be avoided except in rare instances (Fitzpatrick & Wolff, 2005). Although effective for most patients with AD, the rapid rebound after discontinuation and high risk of potential side effects make their use impractical in children.

7. Treating flares of symptoms is an important area of patient education. Flares can occur at any time and the family should be prepared to step up treatment when needed.

    a. Offer information on how to recognize flares.

    b. Give written instructions, such as an Eczema Action Plan, on how to manage flares by stepping up treatment and prescribe treatments accordingly.

    c. Treatment of flares should be started as soon as symptoms appear and should be continued for 48 hours after acute symptoms subside (NICE, 2007).

D. Treat complications

1. Bacterial superinfection with *S. aureus* is common in children with AD. First-generation cephalosporins, such as cephalexin, 25–50 mg/kg divided two or three times daily for 10 days, are commonly used, although in some communities it may be advisable to culture for methicillin-resistant *S. aureus* and then treat accordingly. The addition of one-quarter to one-eighth cup of chlorine bleach to a full tub of water, intermittent application of mupirocin ointment to the nares and hands of patients and caregivers daily for 3 weeks, and the use of a gentle antibacterial soap may decrease colonization (Paller & Mancini, 2011). Control of pruritus and prevention of excoriation with proper skin care and medications also helps prevent cutaneous infections.

2. Herpes simplex virus infection (eczema herpeticum) is a potentially life-threatening complication.

    a. Considered if the following is observed:

       i. Areas of rapidly worsening and painful dermatitis

       ii. Systemic symptoms, such as fever, lethargy, or distress

       iii. Clustered blisters with the appearance of early-stage cold sores

       iv. Punched-out erosions that are uniform in appearance and that may coalesce (NICE, 2007)

       v. Child's infected dermatitis fails to respond to antibiotic treatment and appropriate corticosteroids

    b. If suspected, treat immediately with systemic acyclovir and refer for same-day dermatologic advice.

    c. If there is involvement of the skin around the eyes, refer for a same-day consultation with an ophthalmologist and dermatologist.

VI. Self-management

A. Patient and family education and home management of bathing and medication regimens are the key factors in determining successful outcomes for children with AD. It is important to:

1. Involve the family in all treatment decisions. The family is likely to be more adherent with the treatment plans if they have been part of the decision-making process. Consider the family's cultural skincare and bathing practices when discussing options.

2. Explain that AD often improves with time, but not all children grow out of the condition; at times it becomes worse as the child gets older.

3. Educate families regarding the avoidance of environmental, behavioral, or emotional factors that may trigger symptoms. Referral to a public health nurse or community health worker for an environmental assessment in the home may be helpful.

4. Clearly explain the quantity of moisturizer to use on the child's skin. Applying an insufficient amount of moisturizer is a common problem.

B. Families need comprehensive written and verbal information in their native language regarding maintenance therapy, when and how to step treatment up and down, how to treat flares, and how to recognize complications. All procedures, even the application of ointments, should be demonstrated.

C. Discuss complementary therapies with the family and explain that their effectiveness and safety for AD has not been adequately assessed (NICE, 2007).

VII. Psychosocial and emotional support

A. *Considering the effect of AD on the quality of life of patients and their families, it is important to address possible psychosocial issues and to offer support:*

1. Parents may feel guilty about the child's condition and they may be exhausted from sleep deprivation and from caring for the child's needs.

2. School-age children may be teased by their peers about the appearance of their skin and may also fall behind in their schoolwork because of absences.

3. Adolescents may be particularly self-conscious about their appearance and may be leading isolated lives.

B. *Refer the family and child to a local support group or for counseling if needed.*

C. *AD education resources:*

1. National Eczema Association Support Network: www.nationaleczema.org/support

2. National Jewish Medical and Research Center: www.nationaljewish.org

3. National Institute for Health and Clinical Excellence "Understanding NICE Guidance—Information for Patients and Caregivers": www.nice.org.uk/CG57

4. National Eczema Society (UK): www.eczema.org

5. Changing Faces: www.changingfaces.org.uk

REFERENCES

Boguniewicz, M. (2005). Atopic dermatitis: Beyond the itch that rashes. *Immunology and Allergy Clinics of North America, 25,* 333–351.

Fitzpatrick, T., & Wolff, K. (2005). *Fitzpatrick's color atlas and synopsis of clinical dermatology* (5th ed.). New York, NY: McGraw-Hill.

Goodhue, J. G., & Brady, M. A. (2009). Atopic and rheumatic disorders. In C. E. Burns et al. (Eds.), *Pediatric primary care* (4th ed., pp. 553–583). St. Louis, MO: Saunders/Elsevier.

Habif, T. P. (2010). Atopic dermatitis. In T. P. Habif (Ed.), *Clinical dermatology: A color guide to diagnosis and therapy* (5th ed.). Philadelphia, PA: Elsevier.

Leong, D. Y. M., Boguniewicz, M., Howell, M. D., & Hamid, Q. A. (2004). New insight into atopic dermatitis. *Journal of Clinical Investigation, 113,* 651–657.

National Institute for Health and Clinical Excellence (NICE). (2007). *Atopic eczema in children* (NICE clinical guideline 57). London, UK: Author.

National Institute of Arthritis and Musculoskeletal and Skin Diseases Information Clearing House, National Institutes of Health. (2009). *Atopic dermatitis: Handout on health.* Bethesda, MD: Author. Full text available online: www.niams.nih.gov

Paller, A. S., & Mancini, A. J. (2011). Eczematous eruptions in childhood. In A. S. Paller & A. J. Mancini (Eds.), *Hurwitz clinical pediatric dermatology: A textbook of skin disorders of childhood and adolescence* (4th ed.). Philadelphia, PA: Elsevier.

Porth, C. M., & Matfin, G. (2009). *Pathophysiology: Concepts of altered health states* (8th ed.). Philadelphia, PA: Wolters Kluwer/Lippincott, Williams & Wilkins.

Tollefson, M. M., & Bruckner, A. L. (2014). Atopic dermatitis: Skin-directed management. *Pediatrics, 135*(6), 1735–1744.

ATTENTION-DEFICIT/ HYPERACTIVITY DISORDER IN CHILDREN AND ADOLESCENTS

CHAPTER **12**

Naomi Schapiro

I. Introduction and general background

Attention-deficit/hyperactivity disorder (ADHD) is one of the most common chronic conditions in childhood and the most common of the chronic neuropsychiatric conditions (Merikangas et al., 2010), with an estimated prevalence rate of 7.2% (Thomas, Sanders, Doust, Beller, & Glasziou, 2015). The major pediatric and child psychiatric organizations recognize the benefits and role of primary care providers in diagnosing and treating this condition in childhood and adolescence (Pliszka & American Academy of Child and Adolescent Psychiatry [AACAP] Work Group on Quality Issues, 2007; Subcommittee on Attention-Deficit/Hyperactivity Disorder et al., 2011). The advanced practice nurse (APN), working in either primary or specialty care, is well suited to detect, follow, refer, and manage children with ADHD (Vierhile, Robb, & Ryan-Krause, 2009).

II. Overview

A. Definitions

ADHD is defined by its features as a syndrome involving inattentiveness, hyperactivity, impulsivity or a combination (Feldman & Reiff, 2014). Diagnostic criteria for ADHD have been set historically by the *Diagnostic and Statistical Manual for Mental Disorders* (DSM). The current edition, DSM-V (American Psychiatric Association [APA], 2013, p. 61), describes the "essential feature" of ADHD as "a persistent pattern of inattention and/or hyperactivity-impulsivity that interferes with functioning or development." Under the current diagnostic criteria, the individual must have displayed some of these behaviors before age 12 years, and they must be present in at least two areas of the child's life, such as home and school. Changes from the DSM-IV-Text Revision (TR; APA, 2000) include a move of the upper limit for appearance of first symptoms from age 7 to age 12, a lowering of the number of required

symptoms in the categories described next for older adolescents and young adults, and added examples of core behaviors that are more applicable to adolescents and adults (APA, 2013). These changes were made in recognition of the developmental changes in behaviors across the lifespan and the difficulties adults might have in recalling childhood symptoms when presenting for diagnosis. Because current practice guidelines still follow the DSM-IV TR diagnostic criteria (Pliszka and AACAP Work Group on Quality Issues, 2007; Subcommittee on Attention-Deficit/Hyperactivity Disorder et al., 2011), it is important for the APN to be familiar with both sets of criteria. Fortunately, the core behaviors of ADHD remain the same across DSM versions (Dalsgaard, 2013).

To be diagnosed with ADHD under DSM-V criteria, the child or adolescent (under 17) must display at least six inattentive behaviors and/or at least six impulsive or hyperactive behaviors (APA, 2013). Adolescents and adults 17 and older must display at least five behaviors in either or both categories. Examples of inattentive behaviors include difficulty in performing tasks that require sustained attention, distractibility, difficulty in organizing sequential tasks, poor time management, forgetfulness, and appearing not to listen when spoken to directly. Examples of hyperactive or impulsive behaviors include fidgeting, leaving one's seat or running around in inappropriate settings or difficulty staying still in restaurants or meetings, difficulty taking turns, blurting out answers, taking over what others are doing and acting as if "driven by a motor" (APA, 2013, p. 60). In adolescents and young adults, hyperactive behaviors may be more subtle, and impulsivity may manifest as impaired decision making or impulsive driving errors (Adler, Mattingly, Montano & Newcorn, 2011).

Many of the symptoms and behaviors diagnostic of ADHD can be considered developmentally normal in younger children. Nevertheless, the current American Academy of Pediatrics (AAP) guidelines state that primary care clinicians can diagnose ADHD as young as 4 years of age, as long as the child is showing behavior that is out of range for developmentally appropriate peers and functional impairment in two domains (Subcommittee on Attention-Deficit/Hyperactivity Disorder et al., 2011).

B. Incidence and prevalence

According to the 2011 National Health Interview Survey (NHIS), 8.4% of U.S. children were reported by their parents to have been diagnosed with ADHD (Perou et al., 2013). Using part of the National Health and Nutrition Examination Survey sample, over 8% of children who were given a structured mental health diagnostic interview fit diagnostic criteria for ADHD (Merikangas et al., 2010). Only half of the children in this study with diagnosable mental health conditions had sought treatment with a mental health professional. A meta-analysis of 179 global prevalence studies over 36 years show a pooled prevalence rate of 7.2%, with somewhat increased rates using the DSM-IV and DSM-IV-TR criteria over earlier DSM versions (Thomas et al., 2015).

Prevalence studies of coexisting conditions in children with ADHD come from samples of children referred to psychiatric care, and so should not be interpreted as being representative of all children: 35% of children with ADHD in referral samples have oppositional defiant disorder, 26% have conduct disorder, 26% have anxiety, and 18% have depressive disorders (Stein & Perrin, 2003). A retrospective chart review of children from ages 5 to 10 diagnosed with ADHD found that African-American children, girls, and children of parents with lower educational levels were less likely to receive a comprehensive neurodevelopmental evaluation for coexisting conditions (Gipson, Lance, Albury, Gentner, & Leppert, 2015). There was no difference in polypharmacy or special education evaluation between those who did and did not receive this evaluation; however, authors expressed concern about potential differences in long-term outcomes. The APN should be alert to the possibility of coexisting conditions while taking a comprehensive history and performing a physical exam.

An estimated 60% to 80% of the behavioral problems of children with ADHD persist into adulthood (Sharma & Couture, 2014). In one 6-year follow-up study of adolescents with ADHD, Cheung and colleagues (2015) found that 79% of adolescents with ADHD still met diagnostic criteria for ADHD into adulthood, with hyperactivity and parent ratings in childhood predicting adult persistence, and low income and lower cognitive function in childhood predicting higher adult functional impairment. In an earlier 10-year longitudinal study, boys with ADHD who were treated with stimulants had lower rates of psychiatric disorders and academic failure than boys with ADHD who were not treated (Biederman, Monuteaux, Spencer, Wilens, & Faraone, 2009). These findings reinforce the importance of early diagnosis and effective treatment for children and adolescents with ADHD.

C. Theories of pathophysiology

Studies of heritability have found that 60% to 76% of the variance in ADHD could be explained by genetic factors, with multiple potential genetic contributions (Cortese, 2012). Genome-wide association studies have shown that heritability is polygenic, with a mixture of common and rare DNA variants (Faraone, 2014). Dopamine and adrenergic systems have been implicated in the core symptoms of ADHD, with alpha-2-adrenergic receptors responsible for inhibitory control of motor activity (Cortese, 2012). There may be involvement of serotonin and cholinergic systems, although animal studies are less consistent, and there is no animal model that completely replicates the core symptoms of ADHD. Current theories suggest structural abnormalities and delays in maturation in the prefrontal cortex, caudate, and cerebellum (Sharma & Couture, 2014). Functional brain studies reveal low activation in areas related to cognition, executive function, emotion and sensorimotor functions, and altered connectivity between regions (Cortese, 2012). Up to 45% of children with ADHD exhibit emotional dysregulation, with less sensitivity to positive stimuli than children without ADHD, problems regulating attention to emotional stimuli, and misperception of the emotions of others (Shaw, Stringaris, Nibb, & Leibenluft, 2014).

III. Database: History

A. Chief complaint: referrals from parents, teachers, and family members

Parents may initiate care if they have noticed disruptive or attention problems at home or at school and are also frequently encouraged by school personnel to have their child evaluated for ADHD. The initiating symptoms, and motivation for seeking a diagnosis or treatment, are an important part of the history. Because specific behaviors are both part of the diagnostic criteria and help guide the treatment plan, it is important to have parents and children be as specific as possible about the core behavioral symptoms and how they manifest in all the areas or domains of the child's life, particularly at home, at school, and with friends. Just as with a purely physical chief complaint, the APN can be guided in diagnosis by asking for the duration of the behaviors, specifically when they manifest (during which activities at home or which parts of the school day), any environmental characteristics or interventions that have made the behaviors better or worse, any associated problems, and any previous efforts by parents or teachers to manage the behaviors. For older adolescents and young adults, the functional impairment in school- and work-related settings may be the most salient part of the presenting complaint, and it may take skillful questioning to elicit the core behavioral symptoms that fit diagnostic criteria for ADHD and the age at which they began to manifest (Adler et al., 2011).

Sleep problems, including sleep apnea, may result in daytime fatigue and inattention. Seizure disorders, especially absence seizures, may masquerade as inattention (Subcommittee on Attention-Deficit/Hyperactivity Disorder, 2011). Allergy symptoms, and the medications used to treat them, can also be related to inattention (Selekman, 2010). The APN's documentation of patient history should include questions about sleep, snoring, and nighttime awakening and specific descriptions of inattentive behavior. Children with hearing impairments or learning disabilities, such as reading disorders and receptive language delays, and other psychiatric conditions, such as anxiety or depression, may also seem distractible and inattentive. History should include questions about any unusual movements or habits, such as tics or obsessive–compulsive behaviors, which may coexist with ADHD.

B. Screening for ADHD

The AAP states that primary care clinicians may use ADHD-specific screening scales to aid in the diagnosis of ADHD (Subcommittee on Attention-Deficit/ Hyperactivity Disorder, 2011). The screening questionnaire in the AAP ADHD Toolkit, the Vanderbilt questionnaire (Wolraich, Bard, Neas, Doffing, & Beck, 2013; Wolraich et al., 2003), is available without cost on several websites in English and Spanish (see **Table 12-1**). Broader questionnaires, such as the Achenbach Child Behavior Checklist, have not been found to be specific or sensitive enough for the diagnosis of ADHD in primary care settings (Subcommittee on Attention-Deficit/Hyperactivity Disorder, 2011) but may be used by psychiatric and mental health professionals as part of their assessment. Most clinical questionnaires for identifying ADHD include parent forms and teacher forms, and it is crucial to collect information directly from the child's teacher. Asking the parent to deliver and retrieve screening forms from the teacher saves the APN time and ensures that parents consent to the collection of this information.

C. Screening for coexisting psychiatric and behavioral issues

Screening questionnaires, such as the Vanderbilt or Conners forms, include questions whose positive answers raise the clinician's suspicion of coexisting oppositional, anxiety, or mood disorders. Children who are suffering the

TABLE 12-1 Screening Tools for ADHD (Partial List)

Name Contact Info	Cost	Individuals Screened	Languages	Additional Information
Vanderbilt Forms in *Caring for Children with ADHD: A Resource Toolkit for Clinicians*, 2nd ed. American Academy of Pediatrics http://www2.aap.org/pubserv/adhd2/1sted.html	$94.95	Parents Teachers	English Spanish	Screening forms Educational handouts Behavioral treatment guidelines
Vanderbilt Forms National Institute for Children's Health Quality (NICHQ) http://www.nichq.org/childrens-health/adhd /resources/vanderbilt-assessment-scales	No Cost	Parents Teachers	English	Screening forms (1st ed.) Educational handouts
Modified Vanderbilt Forms San Diego ADHD Project https://research.tufts-nemc.org/help4kids /forms.asp	No Cost	Parents Teachers	English Spanish	Screening forms Educational handouts Links to behavioral treatment guidelines
Conners Forms http://www.mhs.com/product.aspx?gr=cli&id =overview&prod=conners3	$269–$795, paper, online, software	Parents Teachers Youth (8–18)	English Spanish French	Screening—long & short forms
Barkley scales for children and adults http://www.guilford.com/search-products /ADHD	variable	Parents Teachers Adults	English	
CHADD list of screening resources http://www.help4adhd.org/en/treatment /scales	Links to rating scales listed here and others			

Partial list of screening forms. Additional forms described in Pliszka, S., & AACAP Work Group on Quality Issues. (2007). Practice parameter for the assessment and treatment of children and adolescents with attention-deficit/hyperactivity disorder. *Journal of the American Academy of Child & Adolescent Psychiatry, 46*, 894–921.

sequelae of family disruption, child abuse, or other traumas may exhibit distractibility, inattention, and fatigue from sleep problems related to anxiety or mood changes (Gerson & Rappaport, 2013; Selekman, 2010). Careful history-taking, including the use of additional screening questionnaires for depression, anxiety, and substance use (Levy & Kokotailo, 2011; Zuckerbrot, Cheung, Jensen, Stein, & Laraque, 2007), will aid in assessment of children with more complex behavioral and emotional symptoms. Unless the APN and collaborating clinicians within the practice are very experienced at diagnosing and managing mental health conditions in the primary care setting, children who may have coexisting conditions should be referred to mental health clinicians for diagnosis and co-management.

D. Screening for learning disabilities

If the child's functioning at school indicates the possibility of both learning disabilities and ADHD, both evaluations should proceed. Most health insurance plans, private or public, do not cover learning evaluations, which must be requested by the parent from an overburdened public school system. Although these evaluations are legally required for children who may need special education services, parents may need assistance from the APN in advocating for them (Selekman & Vessey, 2010). For children who do not improve in academic performance within 1 or 2 months of ADHD diagnosis and treatment, the AACAP recommends an evaluation at that point for learning disorders (Pliszka & AACAP Work Group on Quality Issues, 2007).

IV. Physical examination

A. Overview

The physical examination in ADHD should help the APN eliminate potential physical causes of inattention, hyperactivity, and disruptive behavior and any contraindications to medication that might be used to treat ADHD. There are no specific physical findings that confirm or rule out a diagnosis of ADHD.

B. Important to eliminate other potential physical causes of attention issues and disruptive behavior

The physical examination should include a thorough head, eye, ear, nose, and throat examination; a thorough cardiovascular evaluation; a thorough neurologic examination including documentation of any tics; and hearing and vision screening.

Many examiners look for signs of hyperthyroidism or hypothyroidism, anemia, or lead poisoning. These conditions typically present with more symptoms than just inattention or impulsivity (Pliszka & AACAP Work Group on

Quality Issues, 2007). Most children with ADHD have a normal physical examination (Pliszka & AACAP Work Group on Quality Issues, 2007), although some children may have "soft neurologic signs" (Gustafsson et al., 2009), demonstrating more clumsiness on tasks requiring cerebellar integration, such as rapid-finger or alternating hand tests, than most children of their age. A frankly abnormal neurologic examination should prompt a search for other diagnoses, additional testing, and referral.

Children with normal examinations do not need laboratory or other imaging tests (Pliszka & AACAP Work Group on Quality Issues, 2007). In particular, brain imaging studies, electroencephalograms, and continuous performance tests have not been found to be useful diagnostically, and the AAP recommends ordering laboratory tests for hematocrit, blood lead levels, and thyroid hormone only if concerns are raised from the history and physical exam (Subcommittee on Attention-Deficit/Hyperactivity Disorder, 2011). If the child also has symptoms of anxiety or mood disturbances, complete blood count, thyroid, lead, and metabolic panels may be indicated.

C. Monitor for possible cautions or contraindications to treatments

Concerns about possible cases of sudden death in children treated with stimulants for ADHD have prompted a call for screening all children with ADHD for cardiovascular disease before initiating treatment with medications (AAP & American Heart Association, 2008). This recommendation reinforces the need to take a history and perform a thorough physical examination to exclude cardiovascular disease (Subcommittee on Attention-Deficit/Hyperactivity Disorder, 2011). The joint statement recommends the clinician use judgment as to whether an electrocardiogram (ECG) should be done on any particular child before beginning medication to treat ADHD but does not recommend universal use of premedication ECGs. In a clarification, Vetter and colleagues (2008) recommended that all children with a family history of such conditions as hypertrophic cardiomyopathy, prolonged QT interval, and Wolff-Parkinson-White syndrome, which carry an increased risk for sudden cardiac death, be evaluated by a cardiologist before beginning stimulant medication.

When a range of medications is being considered, consulting mental health professionals may ask for chemistry panels that could reassure prescribers about kidney function (creatinine and blood urea nitrogen) and a lack of liver inflammation (aspartate aminotransferase and alanine aminotransferase).

D. Neuropsychiatric conditions and ADHD: tic disorders

Between 3% and 6% of all school-age children exhibit chronic vocal or motor tics, lasting over 1 year, and fewer than 1% have Tourette syndrome. However, up to 55% of this group has ADHD as a coexisting condition, and children with tics or Tourette syndrome should be evaluated for ADHD (Cohen, Leckman, & Bloch, 2013). Although most children with tics can suppress them for a time in public settings, they may show up on examination.

V. Assessment

A. History and examination that support a diagnosis of ADHD

No coexisting mental or behavioral health conditions are present. The child may be treated in a primary care setting or comanaged with mental health and learning professionals.

B. History and examination that support a diagnosis of ADHD and coexisting conditions

If additional coexisting conditions are suspected, consultation or referral to mental health and learning professionals for more definitive diagnosis is recommended, and the APN may comanage the conditions. Coexistence of anxiety, mood disorders, or tic disorders may complicate treatment, and children with a family history of bipolar disorder may react poorly to stimulant medications, even if they themselves do not have coexisting conditions.

C. History and examination that do not support a diagnosis of ADHD

Refer to psychiatric or mental health professionals or a neurologist, as indicated by the findings.

VI. Plan

Current practice guidelines recommend treating ADHD as a chronic condition, centered in the healthcare home, and recommend medication, psychosocial treatment, or both, depending on the age of the child (Pliszka & AACAP Work Group on Quality Issues, 2007; Subcommittee on Attention-Deficit/Hyperactivity Disorder, 2011). The AAP (2001) in particular recommends the choosing of three to six target behaviors that the parent and child would specifically like to improve. For school-age children and adolescents, the AAP and the AACAP have found that medication is the most effective treatment for core ADHD behaviors, with behavioral and educational interventions helpful in combination or instead, depending on severity of symptoms and family preference. For children from 4 to 6 years of age, the AAP recommends coordinated family and school behavioral interventions as first-line treatment. Current practice guidelines recommend treating ADHD as a chronic condition, centered in the healthcare home, and recommend medication or psychosocial

treatment, or both (Subcommittee on Attention-Deficit/Hyperactivity Disorder, 2011), with medication considered if behavioral treatments are insufficient.

A. Behavioral approaches (Subcommittee on Attention-Deficit/Hyperactivity Disorder, 2011)

1. Psychoeducation
   a. Long-term developmental implications of ADHD
   b. Effects on self-esteem and strategies for positive parenting
   c. Goals of treatment
   d. Bringing in school personnel as part of the team

2. Parent behavioral training to help parents work more effectively with their children, specifically using:
   a. Positive reinforcement (including point systems, token economy)
   b. Methods of negative reinforcement (e.g., cost response)
   c. Giving commands, shaping behavior effectively

B. Medication

1. Stimulant medications
   Although the exact mechanism of action is unclear, stimulant medications affect core symptoms of ADHD in up to 75% of children if tried systematically (Pliszka & AACAP Work Group on Quality Issues, 2007) and are still considered first-line treatment by most clinicians (see **Table 12-2**). All have potential side effects of appetite suppression, sleep disturbance (although this is also a core ADHD symptom), headaches, constipation, and irritability during the day as medication wears off. Stimulants can worsen anxiety or mania in children with anxiety or bipolar disorder or a family history of bipolar disorder. Although dextroamphetamine and mixed amphetamine salts are approved for children as young as 3, stimulants are not generally recommended for preschool-age children, because they seem to have increased adverse effects and may not be as effective as behavioral treatment in this age group. Extended-release medications can last anywhere from 6 to 12 hours, depending on the medication and absorption formulation. These medications obviate the need for midday dosing, may decrease irritability because the medication wears off more slowly, and may have less potential for abuse. They also offer coverage for after-school or after-work tasks, such as homework or driving (Adler et al., 2011; Pliszka & AACAP Work Group on Quality Issues, 2007; Taketomo, Hodding, & Kraus, 2014).
   a. Short-acting: rapid onset, duration of action 3–4 hours
      i. Advantages: dose clears system rapidly, effect rapid

TABLE 12-2 ADHD Medications: Food and Drug Administration (FDA) Approved

Class Medication	Duration	Examples	Advantages	Disadvantages	Dosing
Stimulants	Short-acting (3–6 hr)	Methylphenidate (chewable, liquid available) Dextroamphetamine Dexmethylphenidate	Quick onset Ease of making dosage adjustments without changing prescription	Must be dosed midday to last through school or work day. Higher abuse potential	Individualized, not mg/kg dosing, but starting dose adjusted to weight
	Medium-acting (4–8 hr)	Mixed amphetamine salts (sometimes listed as short acting, however effects may last through school day)	May last during school day, lower abuse potential.	Steady release during day, less effective for some children than bursts of medication	Individualized, not mg/kg dosing, but starting dose adjusted to weight
	Long-acting, variable forms of absorption/release (8–12 hr)	OROS methylphenidate Methylphenidate ER, SR Methylphenidate–LA* Methylphenidate CD* Methylphenidate patch Methylphenidate XR solution Dextroamphetamine XR Dexmethylphenidate XR* Mixed amphetamine salts XR* Lisdexamfetamine#	Last during entire school day, better coverage for driving, lower abuse potential	Cannot be crushed or altered, may effect sleep more	Dosing less flexible, conversion charts available from short-acting medications
Norepinephrine reuptake inhibitor	Long-acting, 24-hr effect, half-life 5–21 hr	Atomoxetine	24-hr coverage, low abuse potential, may be effective for depression	Extensive drug interactions, black box warnings re suicidality	Weight-based dosing for children < 70 kg
Alpha-2-agonist	Short- or long-acting (only extended-release FDA approved 2009), half-life 17 hr	Guanfacine Guanfacine ER	More effective for impulsivity, hyperactivity than for inattention	Rebound hypertension if withdrawn too quickly, some children c/o headache, somnolence; drug interactions	Start with 1 mg oral daily, may increase in increments of 1 mg/wk, weight-based suggested upper limits

* = capsule may be opened and sprinkled on applesauce

\# = capsule may be opened and dissolved in water

Data from Feldman, H. M., & Reiff, M. I. (2014). Clinical practice. Attention deficit-hyperactivity disorder in children and adolescents. *New England Journal of Medicine, 370,* 838–846; Pliszka, S., & AACAP Work Group on Quality Issues (2007). Practice parameter for the assessment and treatment of children and adolescents with attention-deficit/hyperactivity disorder. *Journal of the American Academy of Child and Adolescent Psychiatry, 46,* 894–921; Taketomo, C. K., Hodding, J. H., & Kraus, D. M. (2014). *Pediatric dosage handbook: 2014–2015* (21st ed.). Hudson, OH: Lexi-Comp.

ii. Disadvantages: given two or three times a day, including midday; issues of convenience (parent, school personnel), training, safety, and child's embarrassment; and more reports of irritability as medication wears off

b. Intermediate- and long-acting medication

i. Longer acting: 6–12 hours, no need for midday dose

ii. May start long acting directly, no need to start with short acting first, except in very young children

iii. May have slower onset, depending on formulation

iv. May have decreased abuse potential relative to short-acting medication

v. If slower, steady release, child may not "feel" that the medication is working as much as the short acting or medication released in several bursts, but literature shows equivalent effect

c. Absorption mechanisms available in long-acting medications (current available medications in parentheses accurate at time of publication)

i. Osmotically released oral therapy: shorter release and nonabsorbable plastic shell contains some medication for later release; later onset; longer effect than spheroidal oral drug absorption system (methylphenidate)

ii. Spheroidal oral drug absorption system: combination of immediate-release and longer release beads; capsules may be opened up and sprinkled on food (methylphenidate, dexmethylphenidate)

iii. Transdermal patch: releases medication over 9 hours; onset within 2 hours; duration 12 hours; applied on hip; site and patch changed daily (methylphenidate)

iv. Prodrug, converted slowly to active drug, in intestines and liver; slower onset and 10 hours of active effect; lower abuse potential (lisdexamfetamine to dexamphetamine)

2. Nonstimulant medication

a. Atomoxetine: affects norepinephrine receptors

i. Slow onset, effects may not be felt for several weeks

ii. 24-hour coverage, longest coverage

iii. More acceptable to child and adolescent if first medication, rather than switching from stimulant (patient may not "feel" that medication is taking effect)

iv. Rare reports of liver toxicity, cleared through CYP2D6 pathway, half-life up to 21 hours in individuals with less active CYP2D6

v. May increase effects of albuterol, sympathomimetic drugs in general

vi. Black box warnings of suicidality

b. α_2-Adrenergic agonists

i. More effective for impulsivity than for inattention

ii. Guanfacine approved for children 6 years and older in extended-release form only; clonidine used off label

iii. Clonidine patch available (off label) when steady dose reached; medication must be tapered off slowly

iv. Sometimes used for children with impulsive ADHD and tics (off label for tics and aggression)

v. Side effects: depression, headache, dizziness, fatigue, constipation, decreased appetite; rebound hypertension if discontinued suddenly; drug interactions

c. Tricyclic antidepressants (off label for ADHD): imipramine, nortriptyline, and desipramine

i. Not considered first line

ii. May be effective for ADHD combined with other conditions, such as anxiety, tics, or enuresis

iii. Many drug interactions (neuroleptics, selective serotonin reuptake inhibitors, H_2 blockers, combined hormonal contraceptives)

iv. Rate of metabolism may decrease after puberty

v. Side effects: anticholinergic; weight gain; cardiac arrhythmias (need premed ECG and repeat with increasing doses), dangerous in overdose

d. Bupropion

i. Off-label use for ADHD, Food and Drug Administration approved for depression, smoking cessation

ii. Not approved for children younger than 18 years

iii. Side effects: insomnia, fatigue, agitation, dry mouth, headaches, rash, and lower seizure threshold

iv. Contraindicated if history of seizures, traumatic head injury, or eating disorders

C. General considerations about medication

1. Contraindications for stimulants

a. Symptomatic cardiovascular disease (adults and children)

b. Glaucoma

c. Food and Drug Administration lists tics as a contraindication to stimulant medication; however, several studies of children with Tourette syndrome randomized to various treatment arms for ADHD showed no increase in tics with stimulant medicine

2. Tracking medication short-term effects

a. Encourage systematic follow-up of ADHD core symptoms: designation of core symptoms and follow-up with parent, child, and school about effects of medication

b. Initial dose should be increased weekly until core symptoms show improvement or side effects increase

   i. Clinician and family should expect some loss of appetite during the dosing period for stimulants, with normal appetite before dose and after wearing off; lack of this effect may indicate subtherapeutic dose

   ii. Carefully monitor side effects if child is on nonstimulant medication or if taking additional medications

   iii. Check in weekly with parent and child by telephone or in office when starting medication and increasing dose. Stimulants are Schedule II medications: no refills by telephone and new prescriptions must be written and picked up when continuing these medications.

   iv. Follow-up blood pressure, heart rate, and weight for stimulants; other medications as indicated (e.g., possible liver inflammation for atomoxetine)

c. Track adherence and diversion: especially an issue for adolescent and young adult patients taking shorter acting stimulant medication

d. Stimulant medication holidays

   i. Sometimes used or recommended on weekends and summer if core symptoms manageable outside of school; medication holidays are controversial

   ii. May increase side effects on restarting

   iii. May not be beneficial for adolescents, especially if they drive

3. Tracking medication long-term effects

a. Effects on academic and job performance and home and peer relationships

   i. Most documented benefits early in treatment (first 3 years) may be partly caused by more intensive management

   ii. May be more effective if started earlier in the course of ADHD

   iii. Interaction of ADHD and substance abuse is complex: in general, adolescents and adults with ADHD have higher rates of substance abuse compared to non-ADHD

peers; effective treatment with stimulants seems to lower this risk while treatment is maintained

b. Emergence or persistence of any mood-related symptoms

c. Growth (height, weight) and blood pressure

d. Diversion or substance use issues: in-depth psychosocial screen for adolescents

D. Follow-up and indications for referral

1. Lack of expected improvement

a. Most children respond to stimulants, but may require a switch in specific type, adjustments in dose, or addition or switch to a nonstimulant medication

b. Response to behavioral approaches

2. Coexisting learning, mood, or behavioral problems not improving or worsening

E. Parental/Patient Education

Encourage parental connection with other parents, peer support for children and youth, and community resources (see **Box 12-1**)

F. Long-term issues and transition to adulthood

1. Condition trajectory (Adler et al., 2011; Obioha & Adesman, 2014).

a. Initial presenting behavioral symptoms may diminish, functional impairments may improve or worsen

b. Increasing appearance of coexisting conditions (anxiety, mood, conduct, substance abuse); may be mitigated by appropriate medication and behavioral treatment in childhood and adolescence

c. Significantly increased risks of driving accidents, tickets, and impulsive errors, especially if not properly medicated

2. Long-term planning should begin with early adolescent and parent

a. Skill building to increase confidence, offer alternatives to risky behavior, and aid in career planning

   i. Reframing ADHD to highlight positive aspects of behavioral characteristics for appropriate careers

   ii. Jobs, chores to give youth a sense of accomplishment, instill work ethic

   iii. Focusing on strengths and interests

b. Advocating for educational accommodations as needed, involving the adolescent as a self-advocate (Selekman, 2010)

c. Shift to long-acting medication with decreased abuse potential and greater coverage for evening behaviors, especially driving

BOX 12-1 Resources

National Institute for Children's Health Quality (NICHQ)
Caring for Children with ADHD: A Resource Toolkit for Clinicians (first edition open access)
http://www.nichq.org/adhd_tools.html

American Academy of Pediatrics
Children's Health Topics—ADHD—with links to resource for parents (ADHD Toolkit second edition available for purchase)
http://www.healthychildren.org/English/health-issues/conditions/adhd/Pages/Attention-Deficit-Hyperactivity-Disorder.aspx

Implementing the Key Action Statements: An algorithm and explanation of care for the evaluation, diagnosis, treatment, and monitoring of ADHD in children and adolescents
http://pediatrics.aappublications.org/content/suppl/2011/10/11/peds.2011-2654.DC1/zpe611117822p.pdf

Developmental Behavioral Pediatrics Online
Materials related to screening and early identification of behavioral/mental health problems
http://www.dbpeds.org/

American Academy of Child and Adolescent Psychiatry
http://www.aacap.org/

Help4Kids with ADHD
Tufts University site with resources in Spanish and English, including San Diego ADHD Project Screening Packets in Spanish and English, parent and teacher educational forms
Last updated 2008
https://research.tufts-nemc.org/help4kids/default.asp

CHADD
Children and Adults with Attention Deficit Hyperactivity Disorder
http://www.chadd.org/

Adolescent Health Working Group
Behavioral Health: An Adolescent Provider Toolkit
Screening and treatment guidelines for providers, handouts for youth and parents, symptom and medication side effect tracking forms
http://www.ahwg.net/uploads/3/2/5/9/3259766/behavioral_health.pdf

3. Transition to adult systems of care
   a. Adult providers are often unfamiliar with ADHD, relative to pediatric providers
   b. Loss of insurance coverage and difficulty continuing stimulant medications through publicly funded or indigent mental health care
      i. May be greatly mitigated through 2010 healthcare reforms
      ii. Decreased access to care affects educational and job trajectories
      iii. Severities of coexisting conditions may increase and risk of substance abuse increases without access to effective care

REFERENCES

Adler, L. A., Mattingly, G. W., Montano, C. B., & Newcorn, J. H. (2011). Optimizing clinical outcomes across domains of life in adolescents and adults with ADHD. *Journal of Clinical Psychiatry, 72*, 1008–1014. doi: 10.4088/JCP.10063ah1

American Academy of Pediatrics. (2001). Clinical practice guideline: Treatment of the school-aged child with attention-deficit/hyperactivity disorder. *Pediatrics, 108*, 1033–1044.

American Academy of Pediatrics, & American Heart Association. (2008). American Academy of Pediatrics/American Heart Association clarification of statement on cardiovascular evaluation and monitoring of children and adolescents with heart disease receiving medications for ADHD: May 16, 2008. *Journal of Developmental Behavioral Pediatrics, 29*, 335.

American Psychiatric Association. (2000). *Diagnostic and statistical manual of mental disorders* (4th, Text Revision Ed.). Washington, DC: Author.

American Psychiatric Association. (2013). *Diagnostic and statistical manual of mental disorders* (5th ed.). Washington, DC: Author.

Biederman, J., Monuteaux, M. C., Spencer, T., Wilens, T. E., & Faraone, S. V. (2009). Do stimulants protect against psychiatric disorders in youth with ADHD? A 10-year follow-up study. *Pediatrics, 124*, 71–78.

Cheung, C. H., Rijdijk, F., McLoughlin, G., Faraone, S. V., Asherson, P., & Kuntsi, J. (2015). Childhood predictors of adolescent and young adult outcome in ADHD. *Journal of Psychiatric Research, 62*, 92–100. doi: 10.1016/j.jpsychires.2015.01.011

Cohen, S. C., Leckman, J. F., & Bloch, M. H. (2013). Clinical assessment of Tourette syndrome and tic disorders. *Neuroscience Biobehavioral Review, 37*, 997–1007. doi: 10.1016/j.neubiorev.2012.11.013

Cortese, S. (2012). The neurobiology and genetics of attention-deficit/hyperactivity disorder (ADHD): What every clinician should know. *European Journal of Paediatric Neurology, 16*, 422–433. doi: 10.1016/j.ejpn.2012.01.009

Dalsgaard, S. (2013). Attention-deficit/hyperactivity disorder (ADHD). *European Child Adolescent Psychiatry, 22*(Suppl. 1), S43–S48. doi: 10.1007/s00787-012-0360-z

Faraone, S. V. (2014). Advances in the genetics of attention-deficit/hyperactivity disorder. *Biological Psychiatry, 76*(8), 599–600. doi: 10.1016/j.biopsych.2014.07.016

Feldman, H. M., & Reiff, M. I. (2014). Clinical practice. Attention deficit-hyperactivity disorder in children and adolescents. *New England Journal of Medicine, 370*, 838–846. doi: 10.1056/NEJMcp1307215

Gerson, R., & Rappaport, N. (2013). Traumatic stress and posttraumatic stress disorder in youth: Recent research findings on clinical impact, assessment, and treatment. *Journal of Adolescent Health, 52,* 137–143. doi: 10.1016/j.jadohealth.2012.06.018

Gipson, T. T., Lance, E. I., Albury, R. A., Gentner, M. B., & Leppert, M. L. (2015). Disparities in identification of comorbid diagnoses in children with ADHD. *Clinical Pediatrics (Phila), 54,* 376–381. doi: 10.1177/0009922814553434

Gustafsson, P., Svedin, C. G., Ericsson, I., Linden, C., Karlsson, M. K., & Thernlund, G. (2009). Reliability and validity of the assessment of neurological soft-signs in children with and without attention-deficit-hyperactivity disorder. *Development Medicine and Child Neurology, 52,* 364–370.

Levy, S. J., & Kokotailo, P. K. (2011). Substance use screening, brief intervention, and referral to treatment for pediatricians. *Pediatrics, 128,* e1330–e1340. doi: 10.1542/peds.2011-1754

Merikangas, K. R., He, J. P., Brody, D., Fisher, P. W., Bourdon, K., & Koretz, D. S. (2010). Prevalence and treatment of mental disorders among US children in the 2001–2004 NHANES. *Pediatrics, 125,* 75–81.

Obioha, O., & Adesman, A. (2014). Pearls, perils, and pitfalls in the assessment and treatment of attention-deficit/hyperactivity disorder in adolescents. *Current Opinion in Pediatrics, 26,* 119–129. doi: 10.1097/mop.0000000000000053

Perou, R., Bitsko, R. H., Blumberg, S. J., Pastor, P., Ghandour, R. M., Gfroerer, J. C., et al. (2013). Mental health surveillance among children—United States, 2005–2011. *MMWR Surveillance Summaries, 62*(2), 1–35.

Pliszka, S., & AACAP Work Group on Quality Issues. (2007). Practice parameter for the assessment and treatment of children and adolescents with attention-deficit/hyperactivity disorder. *Journal of the American Academy of Child and Adolescent Psychiatry, 46,* 894–921.

Selekman, J. (2010). Attention-deficit/hyperactivity disorder. In P. J. Allen, J. A. Vessey, & N. A. Schapiro (Eds.), *Primary care of the child with a chronic condition* (5th ed., pp. 197–217). St. Louis, MO: Mosby Elsevier.

Selekman, J., & Vessey, J. A. (2010). School and the child with a chronic condition. In P. J. Allen, J. A. Vessey, & N. A. Schapiro (Eds.), *Primary care of the child with a chronic condition* (5th ed., pp. 42–59). St. Louis, MO: Mosby Elsevier.

Sharma, A., & Couture, J. (2014). A review of the pathophysiology, etiology, and treatment of attention-deficit hyperactivity disorder (ADHD). *Annals of Pharmacotherapy, 48*(2), 209–225. doi: 10.1177/1060028013510699

Shaw, P., Stringaris, A., Nigg, J., & Leibenluft, E. (2014). Emotion dysregulation in attention deficit hyperactivity disorder. *American Journal of Psychiatry, 171,* 276–293. doi: 10.1176/appi.ajp.2013.13070966

Stein, M. T., & Perrin, J. M. (2003). Diagnosis and treatment of ADHD in school-age children in primary care settings: A synopsis of the AAP practice guidelines. *Pediatrics in Review, 24,* 92–98.

Subcommittee on Attention-Deficit/Hyperactivity Disorder, Steering Committee on Quality Improvement and Management. (2011). ADHD: clinical practice guideline for the diagnosis, evaluation, and treatment of attention-deficit/hyperactivity disorder in children and adolescents. *Pediatrics, 128*(5), 1007–1022. doi: 10.1542/peds.2011-2654

Taketomo, C. K., Hodding, J. H., & Kraus, D. M. (2014). *Pediatric dosage handbook: 2014–2015* (21st ed.). Hudson, OH: Lexi-Comp.

Thomas, R., Sanders, S., Doust, J., Beller, E., & Glasziou, P. (2015). Prevalence of attention-deficit/hyperactivity disorder: A systematic review and meta-analysis. *Pediatrics.* doi: 10.1542/peds.2014-3482

Vetter, V. L., Elia, J., Erickson, C., Berger, S., Blum, N., Uzark, K., et. al. (2008). Cardiovascular monitoring of children and adolescents with heart disease receiving medications for attention deficit/hyperactivity disorder [corrected]: A scientific statement from the American Heart Association Council on Cardiovascular Disease in the Young Congenital Cardiac Defects Committee and the Council on Cardiovascular Nursing. *Circulation, 117,* 2407–2423.

Vierhile, A., Robb, A., & Ryan-Krause, P. (2009). Attention-deficit/hyperactivity disorder in children and adolescents: Closing diagnostic, communication, and treatment gaps. *Journal of Pediatric Health Care, 23*(Suppl. 1), S5–S23.

Wolraich, M. L., Bard, D. E., Neas, B., Doffing, M., & Beck, L. (2013). The psychometric properties of the Vanderbilt attention-deficit hyperactivity disorder diagnostic teacher rating scale in a community population. *Journal of Developmental Behavioral Pediatrics, 34,* 83–93. doi: 10.1097/DBP.0b013e31827d55c3

Wolraich, M. L., Lambert, W., Doffing, M. A., Bickman, L., Simmons, T., & Worley, K. (2003). Psychometric properties of the Vanderbilt ADHD diagnostic parent rating scale in a referred population. *Journal of Pediatric Psychology, 28,* 559–567.

Zuckerbrot, R. A., Cheung, A. H., Jensen, P. S., Stein, R. E., & Laraque, D. (2007). Guidelines for Adolescent Depression in Primary Care (GLAD-PC): I. Identification, assessment, and initial management. *Pediatrics, 120,* e1299–e1312.

CHILDHOOD DEPRESSION

Damon Michael Williams

CHAPTER 13

I. Introduction

A. General background

Clinical depression is a disease state with physical, emotional, and cognitive effects burdening children, adolescents, and adults. It is characterized by persistently low mood or loss of interest/pleasure (anhedonia) such that the patient's subjective quality of life is lessened. Functional impairment in school, work, home, and peer relationships is also often objectively observed, but this is not required for diagnosis. Subjective report of depressive symptoms by the patient suffices. This is an important distinction in evaluating the adolescent or child who, because of developmental misunderstanding or caregiver bias, may not be perceived as depressed or impaired. Alternatively, lack of emotional and intellectual insight by the child/adolescent may lead to a discrepancy between the caregiver's observation of depressive symptoms and the child/adolescent's ability to acknowledge or name these symptoms.

The clinician should keep in mind that the presenting symptomatology of the depressed child or adolescent may differ from that of the adult patient and that problematic behavior cannot be assumed to be developmentally normative or caused by depression. Popular wisdom suggests that adolescents go through expectable "phases" of depression or irritability (Arnett, 1999). Although this may be true to a minor degree (Hines & Paulson, 2006), the typically developing child or adolescent should not go through an extended period of depression, irritability, or rebelliousness as a part of normative development: any report by the parent, caretaker, or child of a prolonged period of irritability or oppositional behavior should trigger suspicion of depressive or other psychiatric illness and further inquiry. Additionally, a presenting recurrent or acute somatic complaint (stomachache, headache, etc.—especially in very young children), feeling "blah," appetite loss, appetite increase, weight fluctuation, or anxiety complaints may indicate the presence of depressive

illness (American Psychiatric Association [APA], 2013). In any of these cases, or in any case in which the clinician suspects or elicits the presence of depressive symptoms or other behavioral or mental health concerns, safety must be assessed as a priority. Suicidal ideation as well as bullying, sexual or physical abuse, and neglect should be chief among the safety concerns explored when a behavioral or mood change is the focus of the presenting complaint in the child or adolescent.

Mental health treatment and medication are not synonymous. It should be remembered that primary screening for and assessment of mood and behavioral disorders in the pediatric population is an *essential* component of the psychiatric assessment and treatment process and does not always necessitate prescription of psychotropic medication. *All* psychiatric treatment—pharmacologic and otherwise—including family and patient education, behavioral training, and play- or talk-based psychotherapies as well as specialty evaluation typically proceed from primary care screening and referral. The primary care provider is encouraged to appreciate the importance of their gatekeeping and educational function, regardless of comfort level in prescribing psychotropic medication in children. Additionally, it should be kept in mind that although reassurance and normalizing are necessary and useful practices, the primary care provider should not preference these activities above mood and behavioral assessment—especially in reference to safety, onset, duration, precipitants, severity, and extent of symptomatology. Screening instruments in the public domain—such as the PHQ-A (Patient Health Questionnaire for Adolescents)—can be invaluable in this regard, providing a quantifiable reference point for assessing symptomatology and treatment response over time.

Research suggests clinical depression is a relatively common occurrence in the pediatric population, with some estimates showing adolescents mirroring adult lifetime prevalence rates of 15–25% (March et al., 2004; Rao & Chen, 2009). Depression in younger children is not as prevalent but does occur. According to Cheung, Kozloff,

& Sacks (2013), it has been "reliably diagnosed in children as young as 3 years of age." Onset of depression in children (especially the very youngest children) rarely arises de novo because of purely internal biologic or psychologic factors as the young child's psyche is developmentally predicated upon the family environment, especially the relationship with the primary caregiver(s). Therefore, onset of depression in the very young child warrants assessment of abuse, neglect, trauma, child–caregiver fit, parental mental health, parenting styles, discipline approaches, parental/family conflict, and interactions with siblings.

Genetic, biologic, and environmental etiologic factors (Rao & Chen, 2009) are suggested as contributing to depression. Despite clear evidence of familial transmission of depression in the case of children and adolescents, it is unclear to what degree childhood depression is influenced by genetics, environment, or some combination thereof (Rao & Chen, 2009). In any case, it is believed that the single greatest risk factor for developing major depressive disorder (MDD) in childhood or adolescence is paternal or maternal loading for the disorder (Birmaher & Brent, 2007). Thus, the subjective and family history should include any history of depression in the family, especially the child's parents or siblings, any parental or family history of bipolar disorder, or alcohol or substance abuse.

B. Definition of clinical depression

In the clinical setting, diagnosis and assessment of the clinical syndromes of depression are defined and guided by the fifth edition of the *Diagnostic and Statistical Manual of Mental Disorders* (DSM) published by the APA (2013). DSM-V includes the following depressive syndromes, which have depressive features:

- Major Depressive Disorder (MDD)
- Persistent Depressive Disorder (includes DSM-IV diagnoses of Dysthymia & Chronic Major Depressive Disorder) (APA, 2013)
- Unspecified Depressive Disorder
- Bipolar Affective Disorder I and II (variously abbreviated as BAD or BPD)
- Cyclothymia
- Seasonal Affective Disorder
- Disruptive Mood Dysregulation Disorder
- Adjustment Disorder with Depressed Mood or Mixed Depression and Anxiety

Note: A review of the latter five diagnoses is beyond the scope of this chapter and the reader is referred to the 2013 DSM-V.

Presentation of depressive illness in the pediatric population shows remarkable similarity to the adult population. These symptoms can include sad, low, or disinterested mood; anhedonia; felt or observed decreased effectiveness at school; feelings of guilt; feelings of hopelessness; anorexia (literally "without appetite" as a symptom, versus anorexia nervosa, a diagnosable disorder) or hyperphagia (increased appetite); insomnia or hypersomnia; or fatigue (APA, 2013). However, the primary care clinician evaluating the child or adolescent for depressive illness should keep in mind that mood may show more as "irritability" (excessive anger or feeling mad) rather than sad and that the child may not report subjective change in appetite but instead show observable "failure to make expected weight gains" (APA, 2013, p. 163).

C. Major depressive disorder

MDD is the prototypical disease usually referred to when depression is spoken of generically. It is diagnosed based on the occurrence of one or more major depressive episodes (APA, 2013). A major depressive episode consists of 2 (or more) weeks of depressed mood/irritability or anhedonia and a minimum of four additional depressive symptoms (APA, 2013). The neurobiology underlying depression is not well understood, and continues to evolve. Current theories suggest more complicated and nuanced processes than the simplified vision of deficient serotonin or norepinephrine many were taught, though this remains the most credible explanation vis-à-vis the effects of antidepressants such as SSRIs (selective serotonin reuptake inhibitors) and SNRIs (serotonin norepinephrine reuptake inhibitors). Researchers have theorized depression from a strictly behavioral perspective as caused by a loss of environmental reward (positive reinforcement) leading to avoidance, withdrawal, and isolation via negative reinforcement (Dimidjian et al., 2011; Dobson et al., 2008).

In addition to depressed/irritable mood or anhedonia, depressive symptoms can include fatigue, psychomotor agitation or slowing, feelings of worthlessness or guilt, decreased ability to think or concentrate, indecisiveness, unintentional weight changes, and suicidal ideation (APA, 2013). The reader is referred to DSM-V directly for complete diagnostic criteria. Note that in the case of MDD and most other depressive syndromes, DSM-V qualifies most of these symptom criteria as "most of the day, nearly every day" or "nearly every day" (APA, 2013). According to DSM-V, in diagnosing any of the depressive syndromes, symptoms caused by a general medical condition or substance use or abuse must first be ruled out.

D. Persistent depressive disorder (dysthymia)

Persistent depressive disorder is similar in symptom profile to MDD but lacks its severity and demonstrates a course that is constant over a longer period of time without distinct episodes (APA, 2013). DSM-V criteria for persistent depressive disorder are not significantly different from the DSM-IV criteria for dysthymia. The major difference is that chronic major depressive disorder, which had been a distinct and separate diagnosis, was integrated into the single diagnosis of persistent depressive disorder along with dysthymia (APA, 2013).

The presence of MDD and comorbid dysthymia identified in a single individual is commonly known as "double depression." The clinician should keep in mind that 5–10% of children and adolescents have depressive symptoms that are not severe enough to warrant diagnosis of a depressive syndrome, such as MDD or dysthymia, but that are debilitating to some degree nonetheless (Birmaher & Brent, 2007); in some cases these depressive symptoms are attributable to an adjustment disorder caused by an acute stressor. Additionally, of those children and adolescents with diagnosable depressive syndromes, 40–90% have other psychiatric disorders (Birmaher & Brent, 2007). Thus, the clinician should observe for any potential signs of other comorbid psychiatric illness, such as attention-deficit/hyperactivity disorder, anxiety disorders, and autism spectrum disorder.

In terms of the diagnostic nomenclature used by DSM-V, a child with depressive symptoms that does not have enough signs and symptoms to meet criteria for MDD or dysthymia could be identified as having unspecified depressive disorder—formerly depressive disorder not otherwise specified (NOS) in DSM-IV-TR.

E. Bipolar spectrum

Clinical depression is also a significant component of the bipolar "spectrum" of illnesses, which include bipolar affective disorder I, bipolar affective disorder II, and cyclothymia. As would be suggested by the idea of a "spectrum," these three illnesses are differentiated from one another by severity and duration but all show similar cyclical episodic variations in mood reflecting elevated, expansive, energized mood symptoms (mania or hypomania) alternating or sometimes even intermixed with depressive symptoms. Patients experiencing a bipolar spectrum illness, like those with MDD, may also spend a period of time in a euthymic ("normal") mood state. Mania is differentiated from (less severe) hypomania by a greater duration (at least 1 week) and greater intensity of symptoms (more symptoms, need for hospitalization or presence of psychotic symptoms, among others) (APA, 2013). One might characterize the bipolar spectrum from most severe to least severe as follows: bipolar affective disorder I, bipolar affective disorder II, and cyclothymia.

The DSM-V, in an effort to address the controversy over the upswing in diagnosis of pediatric patients with bipolar disorder, also now includes a diagnosis called disruptive mood dysregulation disorder (APA, 2013). The differential between the two is best left to a specialist in mental health; suffice to say this diagnosis categorizes "children who present with chronic, persistent irritability relative to children who present with classic (i.e., episodic) bipolar disorder" (APA, 2013, p. 157).

Children and adults with bipolar illness often present in a depressed, rather than elevated state. In these cases, the clinician may mistakenly diagnose unipolar depression rather than bipolar depression if inquiry is not made about mood and behavior over the lifetime of the patient rather than the limited course of the current episode alone. In cases of undiagnosed bipolar disorder, psychotropic medications (especially antidepressants) may precipitate hypomanic or manic mood or behavior when administered—this is known as "activation" or an "activated mania." Thus, in the interest of "doing no harm," the clinician evaluating clinical depression in the child, adolescent, or adult must always entertain the possibility of a bipolar illness presenting in its depressed phase, especially if antidepressant medication is being considered. This evaluation can be assisted by asking about family history of mood lability or bipolar disorder and substance abuse, though the absence of these in the *family* history does not rule out bipolar disorder. Finally, in many cases of MDD, bipolar spectrum illness remains a "rule out" diagnosis; one should advise the patient and family about the possibility of activation when reviewing the risks and benefits of antidepressant medication.

II. Database (may include, but not limited to)

A. Subjective data

The primary care provider evaluating the child or adolescent is in an excellent position to assess for depression. The primary care provider usually has an established relationship with the child and family and some familiarity with the family dynamics and the child's developmental and other medical history, all essential components of a competent evaluation for pediatric depression. If this is not the case, the treating clinician should gather information from the child and parents about the family situation and the child's emotional, physical, and cognitive development and history since birth, including intrauterine conditions. Gathering these data may take several visits, especially with adolescents, as the clinician may choose to meet first with the family together and then on separate occasions with the child/adolescent alone and then the parents alone (or vice versa). Regardless of the number of visits, always prioritize the safety screening first. The safety screening will then provide the initial data to determine a referral course, if indicated. As the clinician lays out an initial plan for screening and assessment with the child and family, it is useful to clarify the parameters of confidentiality and what information will and will not be shared and how this will occur. Clarity around confidentiality is essential for maintaining rapport with the child and the caregivers throughout this process and may assist in data gathering.

Depending on age-appropriateness of the patient, the database review should include the following elements:

1. Cardiovascular, seizure, endocrine, and metabolic problems, and chronic conditions, such as diabetes, physical impairments, sleep-related disorders (including insomnia), pain, or other relevant medical conditions

2. Medications (prescribed and over-the-counter, including herbs and supplements)

3. Developmental data
   a. Temperamental or developmental difficulties
   b. Behavioral problems

4. Education
   a. Academic difficulties ("How is school going for you?" "What kind of grades are you getting?")
   b. Learning disabilities

5. Psychiatric history
   a. Self-injurious behavior, such as "cutting"
   b. Previous outpatient mental health treatment or inpatient psychiatric hospitalization
   c. Previous suicidal ideation (in the school-aged child this may be described as the desire to "disappear" or "not be here anymore")
   d. Previous suicide attempt (including type and lethality)
   e. Anxiety ("What worries you?" "Do you ever get so worried that you start to feel sweaty or like you can't breathe or are having an anxiety attack?")
   f. Hallucinations ("Besides my voice, do you hear anything or anyone else right now?" "Do you ever hear or see anything that other people cannot?" If the answer is affirmative: "Describe that for me" or "Tell me more about that.")
   g. Do you ever have trouble paying attention or getting assignments completed?
   h. Do your parents or teachers complain about you being "fidgety" or get on your case to hurry up? Do you do things without thinking that get you into trouble?

6. Substance use and abuse
   a. Cigarette, alcohol, marijuana, or other illicit or licit drug abuse. Often teens are more forthcoming when the clinician educates them regarding confidentiality and the fact that in most cases there is not an obligation to report such use to parents or law enforcement (reference your local laws, policies and other professional guidelines). Interview using the term "recreational drugs" and framing in terms of experimentation can also be useful.

7. Social and family history
   a. Peer relationships, including identifiable (namable) friends and peer support, and any peer bullying

   b. Romantic relationships or break-ups ("Are you dating anybody?" rather than "Do you have a girlfriend/boyfriend?")
   c. Sexual debut (e.g., "Have you ever had sex with anyone else?")
   d. Traumatic events ("Has anything really bad ever happened to you?" and "Has anything happened that you think about a lot or can't stop thinking about?")
   e. Sexual or physical abuse
   f. Family conflict (e.g., "How does your family get along?" "What's your relationship like with your parents?" "Is there any yelling or arguing in the household?")

B. Objective data

The mental status examination (MSE) is the psychiatric equivalent to the physical examination and it must be included in any evaluation of depressive conditions or other psychiatric illness. However, the MSE does not substitute for the physical examination, if indicated to rule out organic factors in a depressive presentation or identify other comorbid medical illness.

Generally speaking, the MSE begins with gross physical observations and progresses to description of the internal cognitive and emotional processes as observed by the clinician in the course of the interview, visit, or interaction, however brief. The MSE typically includes the following observations, adapted from Saddock and Saddock (2007):

1. General demeanor, response to clinician, and appearance (including remarkable identifiers) and grooming

2. Motor status: slowing, agitation, tremor, and hyperactivity

3. Speech: tone, volume, rate, rhythm, and production

4. Eye contact

5. Affect

6. Mood: the patient's direct report of how they feel in quotation marks (e.g., "sad," "tired," "bored," "none of your business," etc.)

7. Thought process: how organized, linear, cogent vs. disorganized, circumstantial/tangential, loose

8. Thought content: includes suicidal and homicidal ideation, perceptual changes, paranoia, intrusive thoughts/memories/worries or hallucinatory experience

9. Judgment

10. Insight

11. Some sources include impulsivity (important for safety assessment)

III. Assessment

DSM-V provides clear diagnostic criteria for each syndrome involving depressed mood and guidance on differential diagnosis. The primary care clinician is encouraged to refer to DSM-V for complete diagnostic criteria and procedures.

No assessment of depressive illness in the child or adolescent is complete without assessment of suicide risk and any self-injurious behaviors. Since 2000, suicide has remained the third leading cause of death among 10- to 14-year-olds and 15- to 19-year-olds in the United States (Gould, Greenberg, Velting, & Shaffer, 2003). Risk of suicide and lethality must be assessed on an individual basis. Keeping this in mind, the clinician must be aware that the following factors (*not* listed in order of importance) confer **higher risk for suicide attempt and completed suicide** and may warrant emergent referral to a psychiatric provider or hospital emergency room (Gould et al., 2003; Pelkonen & Marttunen, 2003):

- Male gender
- White race
- Substance abuse or dependence
- Posttraumatic stress disorder
- Panic attacks
- Prior suicide attempt or suicidal behavior
- Poor interpersonal problem-solving ability
- Aggressive–impulsive behavior
- Same-sex sexual orientation
- Family history of suicidal behavior
- Parental psychopathology, particularly depression and substance abuse
- Impaired parent–child relationship
- Family violence and arguments
- Precipitating incident or life stressors (e.g., interpersonal loss, legal problem, school change, being kicked out of school, disciplinary problems, or physical changes)
- Physical abuse
- Sexual abuse
- Difficulties in school
- Media coverage of suicide
- Nonintact family of origin
- Psychiatric disorder
- Presence of plan
- Intent to act on the plan
- Access to means to execute the plan

A comprehensive review of assessment, evaluation, and treatment of suicidal ideation in the child or adolescent is beyond the scope of this chapter. However, the reader is referred to the American Academy of Child and Adolescent Psychiatry (AACAP)'s Practice Parameter on the topic. Included in this parameter is a more thorough treatment of risk factors, safety planning, national resources on suicide for the family and clinician, and a comparative review of suicide screening instruments for the child and adolescent. It is available for free from the AACAP website; a link is provided in the "Resources" section.

IV. Plan

A. Diagnostics

Diagnostic laboratory tests are not used to establish or rule out a diagnosis of depression. However, a number of disease states can present with low energy, fatigue, loss of motivation, and other symptoms of depression. The following tests may be used to differentially assess an identifiable organic pathology (e.g., hypothyroidism or anemia) from a nonmedical depressive syndrome:

1. Thyroid-stimulating hormone (TSH), free T4
2. Complete blood count
3. Comprehensive metabolic panel
4. 25-OH-Vitamin D

Keep in mind that a patient may have a diagnosable depressive syndrome *along with* other pathology such as anemia, hypothyroidism, diabetes mellitus, or low vitamin D, which may exacerbate depressive symptoms and require concurrent treatment.

B. Treatment

1. Medications and the black box warning

   The Food and Drug Administration (FDA) issued a ruling in 2007 directing antidepressant manufacturers to include "black box" labeling identifying the possibility of increased suicidal ideation in children and adolescents up through age 24. The announcement of this black box warning was widely reported in the media. Since that time, there has been a marked drop in the prescription of first-line antidepressant treatment by primary care providers (Gibbons et al., 2007) and subsequent increase in completed suicides. The prudent clinician should continue circumspect prescribing and vigilant monitoring for increased suicidal ideation or behavior in the child or adolescent (through age 24) continuing on or initiated on antidepressant medication. However, considerable data continue to accumulate regarding the benefit of antidepressant treatment in children and adolescents and the importance of early intervention and potential negative sequelae associated with failure to prescribe (Gibbons et al., 2007; Hammad, Laughren, & Racoosin, 2006a, 2006b; March et al., 2004). With this in mind, the primary care provider who has identified a child or adolescent with uncomplicated unipolar depression is encouraged to consider the benefits and risks with the family of cautiously initiating first-line antidepressant treatment.

In addition to the very small but real potential risk of increased suicidal ideation and behavior, selective serotonin reuptake inhibitors (SSRIs), including escitalopram and fluoxetine, often have significant gastrointestinal, nervous system, and sexual side effects predominantly because of the effect on nontargeted serotonin receptors. Risk of various potential side effects (additional to suicidal ideation) must be reviewed with the child and their parents or guardians as part of the process for obtaining informed consent (**Table 13-1**). The medication guide in Table 13-1 may be helpful in assisting families through this process. For the most current version and other prescriber-directed medication advisories, see www.fda.gov. The process of initiating first-line antidepressant treatment for the child or adolescent with uncomplicated unipolar depression may be done in tandem with referral to a pediatric psychiatric specialist.

2. FDA-approved antidepressant agents

   Only two agents have FDA approval for use as antidepressants in children and adolescents: the SSRIs fluoxetine (Prozac™) and escitalopram (Lexapro™). **Table 13-2** summarizes data on these agents. Note that sertraline (Zoloft™) and fluvoxamine (Luvox™)—also SSRIs—do not have FDA approval for use in the pediatric age group for depressive disorders. They do, however, have FDA approval for treatment of obsessive–compulsive disorder in children and adolescents, the former for ages 6–17 years and the latter for ages 8–17 and have been used *off-label* for treatment of depressive disorders.

   After gaining appropriate consent, the clinician choosing to initiate antidepressant treatment in an uncomplicated case of major depressive disorder should begin with the lowest dose possible (often one-quarter to one-half the recommended adult dose depending on other factors) and titrate in very slow intervals, generally not sooner than every 3–4 weeks. However, face-to-face monitoring at more frequent intervals than those required to make a dosage change is recommended for children and adolescents receiving antidepressant medication. Vigilance is especially warranted when initiating, increasing, reducing, or otherwise changing dosage. The FDA recommends "at least weekly face-to-face contact with the prescriber during the first 4 weeks of treatment, then visits every other week for the next 4 weeks, then at 12 weeks, and as clinically indicated beyond 12 weeks" (Hughes et al., 2007, pp. 667–686), and this is now generally accepted as the standard of care. The provider should enlist parents in monitoring for adverse effects and, with proper consent, could consider educating the child's psychotherapist(s) and teachers to assist in monitoring.

   At a minimum, medication monitoring visits should include the following parameters:

   a. Patient's subjective response to the medication
   b. Objective evaluation of demeanor, energy, and affect
   c. Report of any adverse effects, including any changes in weight, sleep, behavior (activation), and sexual problems (adolescents). The clinician is referred to the manufacturer's literature for a comprehensive listing of drug side effects with frequency of occurrence.
   d. Dosing record and any difficulties with or obstacles to adherence, such as gastrointestinal complaints or sleep changes
   e. Suicidal ideation and self-harming behaviors
   f. Progress with psychiatric referral or response to psychotherapy or other nonpharmacologic treatments.

3. Psychotherapy and combined treatment

   Psychotherapy either alone or combined with pharmacotherapy is effective in treating pediatric depression. Specifically, cognitive behavioral therapy (CBT) shows the strongest evidence for improved outcome (March et al., 2004; Weisz, McCarty, & Valeri, 2006). Developed by Aaron Beck (and since elaborated by many other clinician-researchers), CBT uses behavioral interventions, structured exercises, and talk therapy to change negative thinking. In the depressed child, CBT is thought to exert a therapeutic effect because it leads to restructuring of the negatively distorted cognitions that engender and accompany depressive symptoms.

   The best data concerning CBT and depression in the pediatric population come from the Treatment for Adolescents with Depression Study (TADS). The TADS is a highly powered 13-site, national study funded by the National Institute of Mental Health that tested three conditions in randomized controlled trial design from spring through summer 2003 (March et al., 2004): fluoxetine alone, CBT alone, and fluoxetine plus CBT. The study was conducted with the adolescent population, so conclusions should be applied only to that population. Among the conclusions reached by the TADS team:

   - "despite calls to restrict access to medications, medical management of MDD with fluoxetine, including careful monitoring for adverse events, should be made widely available, not discouraged" (March et al., 2004, p. 819).
   - "given incremental improvement in outcome when CBT is combined with medication and,

TABLE 13-1 Revisions to Medication Guide

Read the Medication Guide that comes with your or your family member's antidepressant medicine. This Medication Guide is only about the risk of suicidal thoughts and actions with antidepressant medicines. **Talk to your, or your family member's, healthcare provider about:**

- All risks and benefits of treatment with antidepressant medicines
- All treatment choices for depression or other serious mental illness

What is the most important information I should know about antidepressant medicines, depression and other serious mental illness, and suicidal thoughts or actions?

1. **Antidepressant medicines may increase suicidal thoughts or actions in some children, teenagers, and young adults when the medicine is first started.**

2. **Depression and other serious mental illnesses are the most important causes of suicidal thoughts and actions. Some people may have a particularly high risk of having suicidal thoughts or actions.** These include people who have (or have a family history of) bipolar illness (also called manic-depressive illness) or suicidal thoughts or actions.

3. **How can I watch for and try to prevent suicidal thoughts and actions in a family member or myself?**
   - Pay close attention to any changes, especially sudden changes, in mood, behaviors, thoughts, or feelings. This is very important when an antidepressant medicine is first started or when the dose is changed.
   - Call the healthcare provider right away to report new or sudden changes in mood, behavior, thoughts, or feelings.
   - Keep all follow-up visits with the healthcare provider as scheduled. Call the healthcare provider between visits as needed, especially if you have concerns about symptoms.

Call a healthcare provider right away if you or your family member has any of the following symptoms, especially if they are new, worse, or worry you:

- Thoughts about suicide or dying
- Attempts to commit suicide
- New or worse depression
- New or worse anxiety
- Feeling very agitated or restless
- Panic attacks
- Trouble sleeping (insomnia)
- New or worse irritability
- Acting aggressive, being angry, or violent
- Acting on dangerous impulses
- An extreme increase in activity and talking (mania)
- Other unusual changes in behavior or mood

What else do I need to know about antidepressant medicines?

- **Never stop an antidepressant medicine without first talking to a healthcare provider.** Stopping an antidepressant medicine suddenly can cause other symptoms.
- **Antidepressants are medicines used to treat depression and other illnesses.** It is important to discuss all the risks of treating depression and also the risks of not treating it. Patients and their families or other caregivers should discuss all treatment choices with the healthcare provider, not just the use of antidepressants.
- **Antidepressant medicines have other side effects.** Talk to the healthcare provider about the side effects of the medicine prescribed for you or your family member.
- **Antidepressant medicines can interact with other medicines.** Know all of the medicines that you or your family member takes. Keep a list of all medicine to show the healthcare provider. Do not start new medicines without first checking with your healthcare provider.
- **Not all antidepressant medicines prescribed for children are FDA approved for use in children.** Talk to your child's healthcare provider for more information.

The U.S. Food and Drug Administration has approved this Medication Guide for all antidepressants.

Reproduced from U.S. Food and Drug Administration. *Medication guide: Antidepressant medicines, depression and other serious mental illnesses, and suicidal thoughts or actions.* Retrieved from http://www.fda.gov/downloads/drugs/drugsafety/informationbydrugclass/ucm100211.pdf.

TABLE 13-2 Antidepressant Medications with FDA Approval for Use in the Pediatric Population

Proprietary Name	Generic Name	Generic Available	FDA-Approved Pediatric Indication	Dosage
Prozac™	Fluoxetine hydrochloride	Yes	MDD, 8–18 years (also OCD, 7–17 years)	Initial: 10–20 mg/day, depending on weight (initial dose in OCD is 10 mg)
Lexapro™	Escitalopram	Yes	MDD, 12–17 years	Initial: 10 mg once daily Recommended: 10 mg once daily Maximum: 20 mg once daily

MDD = major depressive disorder; OCD = obsessive–compulsive disorder.

Data from U.S. Food and Drug Administration.

as importantly, increased protection from suicidality, CBT also should be readily available as part of comprehensive treatment for depressed adolescents" (March et al., 2004, p. 819).

In addition to CBT, family therapy and interpersonal therapy are often used in the treatment of pediatric depression (Weisz et al., 2006). The clinician should keep in mind that all therapeutic interventions must be chosen on the basis of the child's particular context, family situation, and unique presentation.

It should be noted that most of the research into psychotherapy treatment of pediatric depression has focused particularly on adolescents and only rarely on young school-age children. Although some CBT models have been adapted for use in younger children, generally speaking, for a chronologically preadolescent child (or developmentally young older child), play psychotherapies are going to be both more accessible and developmentally appropriate, though they may seem like a waste of time or simply esoteric to the parent or caregiver. CBT requires a certain level of cognitive, verbal, and social development on the part of the child. Very young or developmentally impaired persons do not and cannot process thoughts and feelings like some adolescents and adults. For these young children, expressing themselves with and through play is the developmental equivalent for the adult or older adolescent of talking through something using spoken words and conversation. Typically, a play psychotherapist will use the play itself to help the child explore feelings and thoughts by *acting them out* in the therapy room using toys, puppets, paint, drawing, and the like. The primary provider can facilitate a successful referral for evaluation or psychotherapy of the young child by helping to frame the caretaker's expectations of psychotherapy in a developmentally appropriate way.

C. Referral

Children and adolescents with depression and other psychiatric illness are optimally treated in the context of their families, school, and community within a developmental framework. Often the collateral contacts required for optimal assessment and treatment are not easily conducted within the confines of the 15-minute medical office visit. Thus, the primary care clinician should always feel free to consult with or refer to a pediatric psychiatric specialist. Referral or consultation should definitely be sought depending on severity, lethality, complexity, and comorbidity of the case. Cases in which emergent or urgent referral to a psychiatric colleague or hospital emergency room should be made include the following:

1. Suspected bipolar illness

2. Presence of suspected or identified suicidal ideation or suicide-related behavior or nonsuicidal self-harming behavior

3. Aggressive behavior

4. Comorbid or suspected psychiatric or medical illnesses

5. Comorbid or suspected substance abuse

6. Impaired parent–child functioning or other dysfunction in the family or support system

7. Significant family pathology or history of suicide in the family

8. Comorbid or suspected learning disability

9. Any case in which the treating clinician desires consultation or believes that the presenting problem exceeds his or her scope or knowledge base to provide competent care

V. Self-management resources

A. For providers

1. Information on antidepressant use in children, adolescents, and adults with advisories from the FDA available at http://www.fda.gov/Drugs/DrugSafety/InformationbyDrugClass/ucm096273.htm.

2. A toolkit for child and adolescent depression treatment in primary care, developed from consensus guidelines, available at www.glad-pc.org.

3. The general AACAP website also offers parameters for competent prescribing and evaluation in the child and adolescent population for licensed professionals available at http://www.aacap.org/AACAP/Resources_for_Primary_Care/Practice_Parameters_and_Resource_Centers/Practice_Parameters.aspx.

B. For patients and families

1. The general AACAP website also offers excellent educational material for families on a number of topics including medications available at http://www.aacap.org/AACAP/Families_and_Youth/Facts_for_Families/Facts_for_Families_Keyword.aspx.

2. Also from AACAP resources on the depression resource center available at http://www.aacap.org/AACAP/Families_and_Youth/Resource_Centers/Depression_Resource_Center/Home.aspx.

3. American Academy of Pediatrics resources on child health topics including depression and suicide available at https://healthychildren.org/English/health-issues/conditions/emotional-problems/Pages/default.aspx.

4. Information on depression in children and adolescents, available at http://www.nami.org/Content/NavigationMenu/Mental_Illnesses/Depression/Depression_in_Children_and_Adolescents.htm.

5. Child and adolescent mental health resources available at http://www.nimh.nih.gov/health/topics/child-and-adolescent-mental-health/index.shtml.

6. The National Center for Infants, Toddlers, and Families has excellent educationsal materials for parents and providers available at http://www.zerotothree.org/child-development/temperament-behavior/.

REFERENCES

American Psychiatric Association. (2013). *Diagnostic and statistical manual of mental disorders* (5th ed.). Washington, DC: Author.

Arnett, J. J. (1999). Adolescent storm and stress, reconsidered. *American Psychologist, 54*(5), 317–326.

Birmaher, B., & Brent, D. (2007). Practice parameter for the assessment and treatment of children and adolescents with depressive disorders. *Journal of the American Academy of Child & Adolescent Psychiatry, 46*(11), 1503–1526.

Cheung, A. H., Kozloff, N., & Sacks, D. (2013). Pediatric depression: An evidence-based update on treatment interventions. *Current Psychiatry Reports, 15*(8), 1–8.

Dimidjian, S., Barrera, M., Martell, C., Muñoz, R. F., & Lewinsohn, P. M. (2011). The origins and current status of behavioral activation treatments for depression. *Annual Review of Clinical Psychology, 7*, 1–38

Dobson, K. S., Hollon, S. D., Dimidjian, S., Schmaling, K. B., Kohlenberg, R. J., Gallop, R., et al. (2008). Randomized trial of behavioral activation, cognitive therapy, and antidepressant medication in the prevention of relapse and recurrence in major depression. *Journal of Consulting and Clinical Psychology, 76*(3), 468–477.

Food and Drug Administration. (2007). FDA proposes new warnings about suicidal thinking, behavior in young adults who take antidepressant medications. Retrieved from http://www.fda.gov/NewsEvents/Newsroom/PressAnnouncements/2007/ucm108905.htm.

Gibbons, R. D., Brown, C. H., Hur, K., Marcus, S. M., Bhaumik, D. K., Erkens, J. A., et al. (2007). Early evidence on the effects of regulators' suicidality warnings on SSRI prescriptions and suicide in children and adolescents. *American Journal of Psychiatry, 164*, 1356–1363.

Gould, M. S., Greenberg, T., Velting, D. M., & Shaffer, D. (2003). Youth suicide risk and preventive interventions: A review of the past 10 years. *Journal of the American Academy of Child & Adolescent Psychiatry, 42*(4), 386–405.

Hammad, T. A., Laughren, T. P., & Racoosin, J. A. (2006a). Suicidality in pediatric patients treated with antidepressant drugs. *Archives of General Psychiatry, 63*, 332–339.

Hammad, T. A., Laughren, T. P., & Racoosin, J. A. (2006b). Suicide rates in short-term randomized controlled trials of newer antidepressants. *Journal of Clinical Psychopharmacology, 26*(2), 203–207.

Hines, A. R., & Paulson, S. E. (2006). Parents' and teachers' perceptions of adolescent storm and stress: Relations with parenting and teaching styles. *Adolescence, 41*(164), 597–614.

Hughes, C. W., Emslie, G. J., Crismon, M. L., Posner, K., Birhamer, B., Ryan, N., et al. (2007). Texas children's medication algorithm project: Update from the Texas consensus panel on medication treatment of childhood major depressive disorder. *Journal of the American Academy of Child & Adolescent Psychiatry, 46*(6), 667–686.

March, J., Silva, S., Petrycki, S., Curry, J., Wells, K., Fairbank, J., et al. (2004). Fluoxetine, cognitive-behavioral therapy, and their combination for adolescents with depression. *JAMA, 292*, 807–820.

March, J. S., Silva, S., Petrycki, S., Curry, J., Wells, K., Fairbank, J., et al. (2007). Treatment for Adolescents with Depression Study (TADS): Long-term effectiveness and safety outcomes. *Archives of General Psychiatry, 64*(10), 1132–1144.

Pelkonen, M., & Marttunen, M. (2003). Child and adolescent suicide: Epidemiology, risk factors, and approaches to prevention. *Pediatric Drugs, 5*(4), 243–265.

Rao, U., & Chen, L. (2009). Characteristics, correlates, and outcomes of childhood and adolescent depressive disorders. *Dialogues in Clinical Neuroscience, 11*, 45–62.

Saddock, B. J., & Saddock, V. A. (2007). *Kaplan & Saddock's synopsis of psychiatry* (10th ed.). New York, NY: Lippincott, Williams & Wilkins.

Weisz, J. R., McCarty, C. A., & Valeri, S. M. (2006). Effects of psychotherapy for depression in children and adolescents: A meta-analysis. *Psychological Bulletin, 132*(1), 132–149.

FAILURE TO THRIVE DURING INFANCY

Annette Carley

CHAPTER 14

I. Introduction and general background

Growth failure in childhood, defined as inadequate sustained growth and/or weight gain compared to age-appropriate norms, must be appropriately identified and managed to optimize outcomes (Al Nofal & Schwenk, 2013). Weight is primarily affected when nutritional intake cannot support growth demands, although height and head circumference are affected by increasing malnutrition. Failure to thrive (FTT) is a sign of growth failure with multiple interacting causes, yet is itself poorly defined in the literature. Formerly labeled "organic" and "inorganic," FTT is now thought of in more useful terms based on its presumed etiology: (1) inadequate caloric intake, (2) inadequate caloric absorption or use, or (3) excess caloric consumption. Regardless of the etiology, growth failure and FTT may have long-term effects on cognitive and behavioral development and long-term growth (Al Nofal & Schwenk, 2013; Cole & Lanham, 2011; Jaffe, 2011; Stephens, Gentry, Michener, & Kendall, 2008).

A. FTT from all causes

1. Overview

   The most common cause of FTT worldwide is poverty and poor access to adequate nutrition (Block, Krebs, Committee on Child Abuse and Neglect, & Committee on Nutrition, 2005). It occurs across all populations, although the risk is increased in impoverished urban and rural populations (Gahagan, 2006; Rabinowitz, 2015).

   a. In developed countries, it is also commonly associated with poor caretaking skills, reflecting a disparity between infant interactive and growth needs and caretaker attentiveness.

   b. FTT may be the sole clinical finding suggesting neglect or abuse.

   c. FTT accounts for up to 5% of pediatric hospitalizations (Stephens et al., 2008; Rabinowitz, 2015) and is associated with 40–50% of nonorganic pediatric feeding disorders (Romano, Hartman, Privitera, Cardile, & Shamir, 2015).

2. Prevalence and incidence

   a. FTT is usually identified during the first 2 years of life; 80% are identified by 18 months of age (Cole & Lanham, 2011).

   b. It affects up to 5–10% of infants and children in primary care settings, although less than 10% can be attributed to a recognized disorder, such as cardiac disease or inborn errors of metabolism (Atalay & McCord, 2012; Block et al., 2005; Stephens et al., 2008).

   c. However, because there is a lack of consensus regarding criteria to establish the diagnosis, this likely affects the reported incidence.

B. FTT caused by inadequate caloric intake

1. Overview

   FTT may be the result of poorly sustained nutrient availability, infant inability to consume adequate foods, or ineffective feeding interactions leading to decreased intake (the most common cause of FTT).

   a. Improper formula preparation, limited formula or food availability, insufficient breastmilk production, or overuse of fruit juices at the expense of more nutrient-dense foods

   b. Motor feeding issues interfering with consuming adequate intake, such as inability to suck, chew, or swallow effectively

   c. Poor appetite

   d. Oral aversion

   e. Disturbed caregiver–infant interactions affecting feeding interest or success, including behavioral problems during the meal, caregiver inattention, or outright neglect (Gahagan, 2006; Stephens et al., 2008)

   f. One endocrinology clinic reported an association with family stress (34% of patients), ineffective feeding such as poor attention to cues or inadequate mealtime structure (28% of patients), and overreliance on a liquid diet such as excess juice (38% of patients) in their referred patients (Atalay & McCord, 2012).

C. FTT caused by inadequate caloric absorption or use

1. Overview

    A number of genetic, structural, or functional conditions may create ineffective nutrient absorption or use and must be recognized. Included among these conditions are:

    a. Celiac disease

    b. Cystic fibrosis

    c. Cow milk protein allergy

    d. Vitamin or mineral deficiencies

    e. Biliary atresia or hepatic dysfunction

    f. Short gut syndrome

    g. Genetic abnormalities, such as trisomy 13, 18, and 21

    h. Short-stature syndromes including Russell-Silver syndrome, Turner syndrome, Down syndrome, hypothyroidism, hypophosphatemic rickets, growth hormone deficiency, and fetal alcohol syndrome

    i. Metabolic disorders, such as glycogen storage disease and aminoacidopathies

    j. Chronic vomiting

    k. Gastroesophageal reflux

    l. Chronic renal disease (Gahagan, 2006; Jaffe, 2011; Stephens et al., 2008)

D. FTT caused by excess caloric consumption needs

1. Overview

    Increased metabolic demands may interfere with growth, which may occur with such conditions as:

    a. Chronic lung disease

    b. Congenital heart disease

    c. Chronic infection

    d. Hyperthyroidism

    e. Anemia

    f. Diabetes

    g. Renal tubular acidosis

    h. Fever

    i. Immunodeficiency

    j. Malignancy

    k. Intrauterine growth restriction (Cole & Lanham, 2011; Jaffe, 2011; Stephens et al., 2008)

II. Database (appropriate for the evaluation of FTT in developed countries) may include but is not limited to:

A. Subjective

1. History and review of systems

    A thorough history, the most critical element in establishing the diagnosis, uncovering causes, and posing a therapeutic plan (Block et al., 2005; Cole & Lanham, 2011; Gahagan, 2006; Jaffe, 2011; Rabinowitz, 2015), includes:

    a. Past health history

        i. Prenatal history, including gravida and parity of mother, maternal weight gain during pregnancy, pregnancy complications, prenatal care access

        ii. Intrauterine growth history (Jaffe, 2011)

        iii. Birth history, including gestational age, weight, type of delivery, infant Apgar scores, and delivery complications

        iv. Neonatal history; including weight at discharge; complications; congenital disorders; and oral instrumentation, such as intubation

        v. Early childhood history, including acute and chronic illness, hospitalizations, injuries, and developmental status

        vi. Current history, including presenting complaint onset and duration and associated symptoms

        vii. Elimination history, including voiding and frequency and character of stools

    b. Family history

        i. Age and health of parents, grandparents, and primary caretakers

        ii. Birth weight and height of parents and siblings

        iii. Congenital disorders; chronic illness; and mental health disorders, such as anxiety or depression

    c. Social and environmental history

        i. Marital status, education, and literacy of parents

        ii. Occupation and source of financial support and access to public assistance programs, such as the Special Supplemental Nutrition Program for Women, Infants, and Children (WIC) or food stamps

        iii. Type of housing and number of persons in household

        iv. Social or environmental concerns, such as unemployment, marital problems, abuse, and substance exposure

        v. Family and peer relationships, including physical and emotional closeness, communication, support, history of abuse or neglect, adaptive behaviors, positive social affect, and ability to ask for and receive support

vi. Parenting skills, including previous experience caring for children, attendance at parenting classes, ability to interpret infant cues, daily routines, play activity with child, caretaking routines related to behavior, crying, and elimination

vii. Disorganized or disruptive household environment, erratic family meals, and multiple caretakers

viii. Caretaker concerns about growth and development

d. Nutrition history

   i. Maternal nutrition before, during, and after pregnancy, including number of meals per day, type, and amount of food and fluid intake

   ii. Infant feeding history, including type of milk, volume and frequency of feedings, proper preparation of formula, strength of suck, burping, use of supplemental foods, and tolerance of food texture

   iii. Obtain minimum 24-hour dietary recall (Rabinowitz, 2015)

e. For breastfed infants: frequency of feeding, duration of feeding, perceived satiety, strength of suck, single or two breasts at feeding, and maternal breast fullness before feeding and emptying after feeding

f. For bottle-fed infants: frequency of feeding, duration of feeding, perceived satiety, strength of suck, and proper formula preparation

g. For infant transitioning to solid foods: time of introduction of solids and foods self-fed by infant

h. Review of systems and clinical findings may reveal

   i. Dysmorphic features suggesting a syndrome, such as low-set ears, hypertelorism, or long philtrum

   ii. Pallor

   iii. Hair loss

   iv. Thin or wasted appearance, loose folds of skin

   v. Irritability

   vi. Sleepiness or easy fatigue

   vii. Poor eye contact or social smile

   viii. Delayed vocalization

   ix. Delayed motor development, including late rolling, sitting, crawling, or walking (Lucile Packard Children's Hospital, 2009)

B. Objective

1. Physical examination findings

   a. Establish a growth trend, including measuring and plotting head circumference, weight, and length (height). For children less than 2 years of age, the WHO growth charts are recommended; beyond age 2 years, the CDC growth charts are recommended (Al Nofal & Schwenk, 2013).

      i. Weight-for-age ratio is not sufficient as the sole indicator of FTT because it does not accurately address infants who are genetically or constitutionally small or those born premature or small for gestational age (Joosten & Hulst, 2011).

      ii. Persistent weight below the third to fifth percentile on standardized curve, downward growth trend crossing two percentile lines, or change in weight-to-height ratio currently recommended in the determination of FTT (Joosten & Hulst, 2011).

      iii. Joosten and Hulst summarized multiple criteria to determine FTT and direct immediate nutritional management, based on age, weight, and/or height including:

         a. inadequate weight gain or growth for more than 1 month in a child less than age 2

         b. weight loss or failure of weight gain for more than 3 months in a child over age 2

         c. more than −1 standard deviation (SD) change in weight: age over 3 months in a child less than 1 year of age

         d. more than −1 SD change in weight: height over 3 months in a child over 1 year of age

         e. decrease in height gain of 0.5–1 SD per year in a child less than 4 years of age, or 0.25 SD per year in a child over age 4 years

         f. decrease in height gain of more than 2 cm compared with preceding year during early and middle puberty (Joosten & Hulst, 2011)

   b. Vital signs, including blood pressure

2. Observation and documentation of caregiver–child interactions

   a. Presence of eye contact, holding close to body, calling infant by name

   b. Observation during feeding

3. Supportive data from relevant diagnostic tests are rarely needed, although may be dictated by positive findings in the history (Stephens et al., 2008).

III. Assessment

A. Determine the diagnosis

Identify other causes of diminished growth, including those constitutionally small or genetically small.

B. Severity

Assess severity of the condition: severe malnutrition, dehydration, and suspected abuse are indications for hospitalization. Rarely hospitalization may be indicated for accurate observation of feeding interactions or to optimize investigation (Block et al., 2005; Cole & Lanham, 2011; Gahagan, 2006; Stephens et al., 2008).

C. Significance

Assess significance of the problem to caregiver and family.

D. Motivation and ability

Determine caregiver and family willingness and ability to follow through with the treatment plan.

IV. Goals of clinical management

A. Screening or diagnosing FTT

Choose a practical, cost-effective approach to screening and diagnosis.

B. Treatment

Select a treatment plan that achieves appropriate growth and growth velocity, provides necessary micronutrients and macronutrients, and is individualized for the caregiver and child as part of a therapeutic alliance

C. Patient adherence

Select an approach that maximizes caretaker compliance.

V. Plan

A. Screening

Elicit a thorough history and perform a thorough physical examination; assess growth and development at all well-child visits.

B. Diagnostic tests

Laboratory or radiographic tests are rarely necessary, because the diagnosis is generally apparent after review of history and physical examination findings (Cole & Lanham, 2011). In addition to routine childhood screening at 6–18 months for iron deficiency and lead poisoning, supportive testing suggested by positive findings may include:

1. Urinalysis and urine culture, urine pH
2. Complete blood count with smear
3. Stool pH, reducing substances, and ova and parasites or occult blood
4. Sweat chloride
5. Tuberculosis testing: skin (Mantoux tuberculin skin test) or blood (interferon-gamma release assays)
6. Radiographic studies, including skeletal survey and bone age (Al Nofal & Schwenk, 2013, 2010; Gahagan, 2006; Stephens et al., 2008).

C. Management

1. FTT is a chronic process, and management continues long term (Block et al., 2005).
2. Adequate growth is essential for survival, and interventions begin before completion of the diagnostic evaluation (Gahagan, 2006).
3. Most FTT cases can be managed on an outpatient basis, unless malnutrition is severe; hospitalization is indicated for evidence of severe dehydration, weight less than 70% of predicted weight-to-height, or suspected neglect or abuse (Block et al., 2005; Gahagan, 2006; Jaffe, 2011; Stephens et al., 2008).
4. A multidisciplinary approach is strongly encouraged, involving input from medicine, nursing, lactation specialists, pediatric nutritionist, physical therapy, behavioral psychology, and social services as part of a therapeutic alliance with the family (Cole & Lanham, 2011; Jaffe, 2011)
5. For breastfed infants, efforts should support breastfeeding where possible, including:
   a. Breast pumping using dual-pump
   b. Considering galactalogues to increase milk production
   c. Encouraging maternal nutrition, fluids, and rest
   d. Developing strategies to modify maternal and environmental stress and its negative impact on milk production
   e. Identifying sources of home and social support for breastfeeding
   f. If formula supplementation is deemed necessary to ensure sufficient nutrient intake, support the mother in efforts to resume or continue breastfeeding
6. For formula-fed infants, efforts to optimize intake include:
   a. Increasing the number of feeds per day, with a goal of 100–120 kcal/kg/d
   b. Demonstrating techniques to awaken a sleepy feeder
   c. Reviewing formula preparation with the caretaker
7. For infants consuming solid foods, encourage self-feeding while ensuring adequate intake of nutritious foods and nutritionally competent choices of finger foods. Discourage excess juice as this may interfere with more appropriate nutritional intake. Consider instructing parents to complement foods with calorie-dense supplements such as gravy, cream sauces, olive oil, or butter (Cole & Lanham, 2011; Gahagan, 2006).

8. Attention to optimizing interest by including appealing food textures, colors, or temperatures and rewarding desirable eating behaviors (Jaffe, 2011).

9. Catch-up growth should be promoted until previous growth percentiles have been attained. The refeeding plan is determined by the degree of malnutrition, with attention to potential risks from exceeding the child's absorptive capacity or creating refeeding syndrome. This condition is not well understood but may create electrolyte and fluid balance abnormalities that contribute to edema and impaired cardiac performance. The therapeutic nutrition plan must attend to careful monitoring of serum electrolytes, glucose, and acid-base balance as well as growth measures (Nutzenadel, 2011).

D. Client education

Offer ongoing caretaker support and education and reinforce consistent effective nutritional practices at all office visits by:

1. Providing a supportive environment for parents to discuss concerns or conflicts related to the infant or home setting

2. Role modeling infant feeding, holding, and stimulation

3. Discussing normal development and infant behavior

4. Reinforcing proper nutritional practices, such as discussing caloric needs to optimize growth, demonstrating proper formula preparation, proposing a regular feeding schedule with written instructions, and directly assessing a feeding interaction

5. Maintaining ongoing contact with the caregiver and family and modifying the nutritional plan accordingly

6. Referral to public health or home care nursing, as available in the community, for ongoing evaluation and support

E. Outcome

Most children with poor growth can demonstrate adequate improvement with intensive intervention. However, both cognitive and school outcomes of children with FTT are worse than their non-FTT counterparts, likely representing the cumulative effects of undernutrition and other environmental risks, such as inattention or lack of appropriate stimulation. These infants need ongoing developmental, behavioral, and growth monitoring to detect and manage long-term consequences of FTT (Gahagan, 2006).

VI. Resources

A. Patient–client education

The following resources provide online health library information for clients and professionals.

1. Children's National Medical Center, Washington, DC
http://childrensnational.org/choose-childrens/conditions-and-treatments/stomach-digestion-gi/poor-growth-failure-to-thrive

2. Johns Hopkins Children's Center, Baltimore, MD
http://www.hopkinschildrens.org/Failure-to-Thrive.aspx

3. Lucile Packard Children's Hospital, Palo Alto, CA
http://www.stanfordchildrens.org/en/topic/default?id=failure-to-thrive-90-P02297

4. University of California, San Francisco School of Medicine/Department of Pediatrics
http://pediatrics.ucsf.edu/blog/failure-thrive-rethinking-our-approach#.VawHpSpViko

5. Medscape eMedicine
http://emedicine.medscape.com/article/985007-overview

REFERENCES

Al Nofal, A., & Schwenk, W. F. (2013). Growth failure in children: A symptom or a disease? *Nutrition in Clinical Practice, 28*(6), 651–658.

Atalay, A., & McCord, M. (2012). Characteristics of failure to thrive in a referral population: Implications for treatment. *Clinical Pediatrics, 51*(3), 219–225. doi: 10.1177/000992281142100

Block, R. W., Krebs, N. F., & Committee on Child Abuse and Neglect, & Committee on Nutrition. (2005). Failure to thrive as a manifestation of child neglect. *Pediatrics, 116*(5), 1234–1237.

Cole, S. Z., & Lanham, J. S. (2011). Failure to thrive: An update. *American Family Physician, 83*(7), 829–834.

Gahagan, S. (2006). Failure to thrive: A consequence of undernutrition. *Pediatrics in Review, 27*(1), e1–e11.

Jaffe, A. C. (2011). Failure to thrive: Current clinical concepts. *Pediatrics in Review, 32*(3), 100–108. doi: 10.1542/pir.e2-3-100

Joosten, K. F. M., & Hulst, J. M. (2011). Malnutrition in pediatric hospital patients: Current issues. *Nutrition, 27*, 133–137. doi: 10.1016/j.nut.2010.06.001

Lucile Packard Children's Hospital. (2009). *Failure to thrive.* Retrieved from http://www.stanfordchildrens.org/en/topic/default?id=failure-to-thrive-90-P02297

Nutzenadel, W. (2011). Failure to thrive in childhood. *Deutsches Arzteblatt International, 108*(38), 642–649.

Rabinowitz, S. S. (2015). Nutritional considerations in failure to thrive. Retrieved from http://emedicine.medscape.com/article/985007-overview

Romano, C., Hartman, C., Privitera, C., Cardile, S., & Shamir, R. (2015). Current topics in the diagnosis and management of the pediatric non organic feeding disorders (NOFEDs). *Clinical Nutrition, 34*, 195–200. doi: 10.1016/j.clnu.2014.08.013

Stephens, M. B., Gentry, B. C., Michener, M. D., & Kendall, S. K. (2008). Clinical inquiries. What is the clinical workup for failure to thrive? *Journal of Family Practice, 57*(4), 264–266.

CHILD MALTREATMENT

CHAPTER 15

Naomi Schapiro

I. Introduction and general background

Child maltreatment encompasses physical, sexual, and emotional abuse and child neglect. Healthcare providers have legal, professional, and ethical responsibilities to assess children for maltreatment and to report suspected cases. Each of the 50 states, the District of Columbia, and territories such as Puerto Rico has its own definitions of child abuse and neglect, but all must conform to minimum federal standards set in the Child Abuse Prevention and Treatment Act: Any recent act or failure to act on the part of a parent or caretaker, which results in death, serious physical or emotional harm, sexual abuse, or exploitation, or an act or failure to act that presents an imminent risk of serious harm (Child Abuse Prevention and Treatment Act, 1998; Child Welfare Information Gateway, 2014). Advanced practice nurses (APNs) can consult the website https://www.childwelfare.gov /topics/systemwide/laws-policies/state/ for the specific definitions and reporting responsibilities in their own states.

The professional and ethical responsibilities to assess for, detect, and report child maltreatment are reinforced by a steadily accumulating body of literature on the myriad and long-lasting effects of these adverse events, including greater rates of depression and substance abuse, early onset of sexual activity, greater likelihood of becoming a teenage parent, and higher rates of type 2 diabetes mellitus and other adult chronic conditions (Herrenkohl, Hong, Klika, Herrenkohl, & Russo, 2013; Mersky, Topitzes, & Reynolds, 2013; Shonkoff & Garner, 2012). In 2013, 3.5 million reports were made to child protection agencies in the United States. From these reports, 678,932 children were deemed to be victims of child maltreatment, with a victimization rate of 9.1 per 1,000 children. An estimated 1,520 children died as a result of abuse or neglect, with a rate of 2.04 deaths for 100,000 children. Children who were less than 1 year old were most vulnerable to fatal maltreatment, at a rate of 18.09 per 100,000 infants (U.S. Department of Health and Human Services, 2015). However, these annual reporting rates understate the prevalence of child abuse and neglect in the pediatric population. Cumulative estimates from the National Child Abuse and Neglect Data System (NCANDS) are that 12.5% of all children will be reported and confirmed as maltreated during their childhood (Wildeman et al., 2014). A recent household survey of caregivers and older children found that 12% of children in the sample experienced some form of maltreatment just in the past year (Finkelhor, Vanderminden, Turner, Hamby, & Shattuck, 2014).

Assessing and responding to child maltreatment can be challenging for the APN, because the abuse or neglect may not be readily apparent and may not be the specific reason that the child is presenting for care. Epidemiologic risk factors for child maltreatment may be helpful in planning population-level interventions but are not as helpful in the clinical setting, where the APN should always keep maltreatment in mind as part of the differential diagnosis (Schapiro, 2008). Child abuse and neglect involve injuries to children or failure to protect them from harm; maltreatment assessments and reports are made to protect children, not to punish "bad" parents (Keeshin & Dubowitz, 2013). Keeping the child in mind helps the APN to sort through what is often a confusing and emotion-laden situation.

Child maltreatment has been associated in the literature with a variety of risk factors including poverty; income inequality; single parenthood; intimate partner violence; parental physical and mental illness; substance abuse; and child factors, such as disability, special healthcare needs, or temperamental mismatch with a parent (Eckenrode, Smith, McCarthy, & Dineen, 2014; IOM & NRC, 2014; Testa & Smith, 2009). Protective factors may include extended family cohesiveness; personal, financial, and community resources; religiosity; optimism on the part of the caregiver; and an engaging child (IOM & NRC, 2014). Just as it is important for the APN to explore the resources and coping strategies of all families who seem to have risk factors for maltreatment, it is also important to remember that child maltreatment can occur in families who do not have known risk factors. Research has shown that healthcare providers may underreport maltreatment in families they know well and assume to be socially and economically stable (Jones et al., 2008).

A. Physical abuse

1. Definition and overview

   Broadly, physical abuse is an inflicted (nonaccidental) injury to a child that results in physical impairment. Mechanisms of injury may include biting, burning, kicking, striking, shaking, grabbing, stabbing, dragging, throwing, strangling, or poisoning. Legal definitions of reportable physical abuse vary widely from state to state (Child Welfare Information Gateway, 2014).

2. Incidence and prevalence

   During 2013, 18% of victims of child maltreatment were physically abused. Physical abuse accounted for 46.8% of child fatalities, either alone or in combination with another type of maltreatment (U.S. Department of Health and Human Services, 2015). Lifetime prevalence estimates of severe physical abuse (not including hitting, slapping, or grabbing) from parental or self-reported surveys range from 5–35% (Gilbert, Widom et al., 2009). Widely differing definitions and overlap with nonabusive physical punishment make estimation of prevalence difficult.

B. Sexual abuse

1. Definition and overview

   Sexual abuse includes sexual contact between adults and children, including fondling, penetration, exposure to sexual activity or involvement in pornography, and unwanted sexual contact between minors. This contact may be carried out through violence, coercion, emotional manipulation, or the child's developmental inability to understand or consent to the activity (Child Welfare Information Gateway, 2013a). Sexual abuse includes commercial sexual exploitation of children (Greenbaum, 2014). In many states, consensual sexual activity of a minor with either an older minor or an adult may be reportable under sexual abuse laws (Assistant Secretary for Planning and Evaluation, n.d.).

2. Incidence and prevalence

   During 2013, 9% of child maltreatment victims were sexually abused (U.S. Department of Health and Human Services, 2015). Lifetime prevalence estimates range from 15–30% of girls and 5–15% of boys (Gilbert, Widom et al., 2009).

C. Psychologic or emotional abuse

1. Definition and overview

   Under federal standards, emotional abuse involves "a pattern of behavior that impairs a child's emotional development or sense of self-worth. This may include constant criticism, threats, or rejection, as well as withholding love, support, or guidance" (Child Welfare Information Gateway, 2013a, p. 4). Emotional abuse is difficult to substantiate unless the child exhibits severe psychologic sequelae. Such abuse is also a component of other forms of child maltreatment, which impedes reporting and tracking of emotional abuse in itself. In some states, witnessing domestic violence may be considered a form of child abuse, whereas in others committing intimate partner violence in the presence of a child may result in an enhanced sentence or a requirement to pay for counseling for the child (Child Welfare Information Gateway, 2013b).

2. Incidence and prevalence

   In 2013, 8.7% of child maltreatment victims were psychologically abused (U.S. Department of Health and Human Services, 2015). Prevalence studies over childhood in developed countries range from 4–9% of children (Gilbert, Widom et al., 2009).

D. Neglect

1. Definition and overview

   As the most commonly reported form of child maltreatment, neglect has been understudied, yet its long-term consequences may be just as devastating as other forms of abuse (Keeshin & Dubowitz, 2013). Broadly, neglect involves the failure of a parent or caregiver to provide for a child's basic physical and emotional needs (Child Welfare Information Gateway, 2014), including food, clothing, shelter, educational needs, medical care, supervision, and emotional care. Although neglect may involve one instance of a dangerous failure to supervise or provide care, it also may result from the accumulation of smaller lapses over time, making assessment a challenge. The standard for reporting neglect involves the APN's suspicion of actual or imminent harm to a child (Schapiro, 2008). States vary widely in their specific definitions of neglect, with some including or excluding drug use, homelessness, or parental refusal of health care for their child for personal or religious reasons. In some states, failure to educate is covered under truancy rather than child abuse law (Child Welfare Information Gateway, 2014). Child neglect has been associated with substance abuse, depression, and other caretaker stressors (IOM & NRC, 2014). Neglect has also been strongly associated with poverty, with increasing reports of neglect directly related to increasing unemployment, decreasing income, stricter limits on welfare payments, and decreased access to childcare and child health insurance, independent of parenting characteristics (IOM & NRC, 2014; Klevens, Barnett, Florence, & Moore, 2015.)

2. Incidence and prevalence

During 2013, 79.5% of child maltreatment victims in the United States were neglected, and 2.3% suffered from medical neglect (U.S. Department of Health and Human Services, 2015). Prevalence estimates range from 6–11.8% of children (Gilbert, Widom et al., 2009).

II. Database (may include but is not limited to)

A. Subjective

As with other sensitive subjects, history-taking about child maltreatment may be enhanced when written questionnaires on paper or computer are used in combination with direct questions by the practitioner (Gilbert, Kemp et al., 2009; Slep, Heyman, & Foran, 2015). Routinely asking questions about physical punishment or fighting, about forced or coerced sexual activity and inappropriate touching, and about general safety can send a message to the child and parent that these subjects are open topics of discussion during the visit, even if they do not answer them at first.

1. Chief complaint
   a. Injuries
      i. Detailed history of any new or old injuries: Is the injury consistent with the history?
      ii. History of similar injuries and general injury history.
      iii. Current or past history of delayed care for injuries.
      iv. History of seeking care for injuries at multiple facilities.
   b. Sudden changes in behavior
      Because children vary widely in temperament, and cultural influences may also affect their behavior in clinical settings, a sudden change in behavior is an important indicator of some kind of emotional trauma (including but not limited to child maltreatment): for example, the outgoing child who suddenly seems withdrawn, or the quiet child who suddenly seems driven by a motor.
   c. Sexual acting out
      Genital self-stimulation for pleasure, or masturbation, is a normal part of child development from toddlerhood through adolescence; children younger than school age may not have a well-developed sense of privacy and may masturbate in social settings considered inappropriate by adults. Sexual play between age mates, consisting of exploration of body parts and sexual

jokes, is developmentally normal and not in itself a sign of sexual abuse (Kellogg, 2010). In a media-saturated society in which sexual images are widely available, discerning age-appropriate from inappropriate sexual knowledge may be difficult. However, some activities should raise a suspicion of sexual abuse:
      i. Sexual play involving penetration or use of objects.
      ii. Sexual play that closely mimics adult sexual activity.
      iii. Sexual play between children with an age difference of 3 or more years or suspicion of emotional coercion.
   d. Personal and social history and activities of daily living
      i. How does the parent describe the child? Red flags include obvious lack of enjoyment of the child, labeling the child as bad, or inappropriate expectations for child's developmental stage.
      ii. Family routines and activities.
      iii. Methods of discipline used and their perceived effectiveness.
   e. Review of systems
      Recurrent headache, abdominal pain, or genitourinary discomfort may be related to somaticizing or actual recurrent injury. A thorough review of systems from both parent and child may be helpful in cases in which the history is confusing or inconsistent.

2. Situations that may heighten the risk of child maltreatment

   Children and families in these situations may need extra support, and should be asked how they are coping if they are experiencing any of the following situations (Dubowitz & Leventhal, 2014; Christian & Committee on Child Abuse, 2015; Saul et al., 2014):
   a. Sudden changes in family status
      Job loss, loss of health insurance, death, divorce, domestic violence, and parental illness, including mental health diagnoses and substance abuse, can all strain or overwhelm a parent's resources and ability to care for a child.
   b. Challenging stages in child development
      i. The inconsolable infant, the willful toddler, the school-age child with behavioral and learning difficulties, and normative developmental changes of adolescence can challenge all parents.
      ii. In some cases these typical challenges of parenting can exacerbate a stressed family system.

c. Children who are difficult to care for
This category encompasses a wide variety of conditions, from children with difficult temperaments to children with neuromuscular disabilities. Children who require a great deal of additional care or who are less able to give the parent positive reinforcement for that care may be at greater risk for maltreatment.

3. Special considerations for taking histories from children about suspected maltreatment
The APN should approach history-taking of injuries and physical complaints in a careful and systematic fashion. If children disclose abuse, the APN should avoid taking a comprehensive history of the disclosure, instead limiting questions to a brief review of who, what and when, gathering just enough information to report to Child Protective Services (CPS) or the police. The following are age-related considerations:

a. Toddlers and preschool-aged children
    i. Children under the age of 6 have limited vocabularies and a relatively undeveloped sense of time and sequence and are best interviewed by a trained expert in child maltreatment.
    ii. Well-meaning parents and healthcare professionals can inadvertently feed the child information and unwittingly distort the story.

b. School-age children
    i. School-age children have a developed sense of time and sequence. The challenge for the healthcare provider is to speak briefly with the school-age child without the parent present.
    ii. If history-taking is not possible, the APN with a reasonable suspicion of maltreatment should still file a CPS report.

c. Adolescents
    i. Adolescents may come in alone for care, and many clinics have established policies for taking written questionnaires and verbal histories from children over 12 without a parent in the room (see Chapter 7).
    ii. Each state has its own parameters for confidential services (Guttmacher Institute, 2015), and it is important to let the adolescent know which parts of the history are truly confidential and what the APN must report related to both sexual assault and consensual sexual activity between dissimilar-aged minors and between minors and adults (Assistant Secretary for Planning and Evaluation, n.d.; Child Welfare Information Gateway, 2014).

B. Objective

It is important to document any abnormal findings as thoroughly and accurately as possible, including measurement of injuries and drawings if appropriate. Photographic documentation may be useful if it conforms to local law enforcement standards for quality and chain of custody.

1. General overview of child's appearance and behavior
The demeanor and behavior of the child or adolescent in the clinic can provide the APN with valuable information. However, it is important to remember that the APN is seeing just a snapshot of the child in an artificial and sometimes stressful setting. Behavioral changes commonly seen in maltreated children may also occur after other adverse events of childhood, including death, incarceration, or divorce of a parent, or sudden death of a close friend (Fairbank & Fairbank, 2009; Naughton et al., 2013). Children may be overly compliant for their developmental age, may be withdrawn or attach readily to adults they do not know well, may exhibit hypervigilance, or may fail to seek comfort in the clinical setting from parents or caretakers (Child Welfare Information Gateway, 2013a).

2. Physical examination findings consistent with physical abuse
In some cases, an inflicted injury is obvious to the examiner. In other cases, it may be difficult to distinguish between inflicted and accidental injury or between injury and infection or a chronic medical condition. Yet timely identification of physical abuse can protect vulnerable children and may be able to prevent serious injury or fatalities, especially in infants and young children. Reviews of missed cases of physical abuse show that clinicians tend to miss "sentinel injuries" (Christian & Committee on Child Abuse, 2015, p. e1340) such as bruising, intraoral injuries including lingual and labial frena tears and fractures. Common errors include incomplete exams, failure to understand the significant of bruises in preambulatory children, failure to report discrepancies between the history and the physical findings, and failure to obtain imaging when recommended by protocols (Jackson et al., 2015). **Table 15-1** is a partial list of physical indicators of maltreatment and normal variants or medical conditions that may appear similar on exam.

a. Bruises are the most common injuries in physically abused children. Dating of bruises by appearance has been found to be unreliable (Grossman, Johnston, Vanezis, & Perrett, 2011). Bruising to the center of the face, ears, neck, back, buttocks, upper arms, and backs of the legs and any bruising in an infant that does not have a clear and plausible history raise suspicions of inflicted injury. Bruising over bony prominences is more consistent with accidental injury (Hornor, 2012).

TABLE 15-1 Physical Findings or Conditions That May Mimic Findings in Child Maltreatment

Findings	Inflicted Injury/Abuse	Normal Variant or Medical Condition
Circular crusted plaques with red margins	Burns from cigarettes or other hot circular-tipped objects	Impetigo Iatrogenic: wart removal
Bullae	Inflicted burns	Accidental burns Bullous impetigo
Marked erythema with or without vesicles or bullae	Immersion burns	Staphylococcal scalded skin syndrome Toxic epidermal necrolysis
Red or hyperpigmented handprint	Slapping	In sun-exposed areas: phytophotodermatitis
Ecchymoses	Inflicted injury from punching or slapping	Accidental injury Clotting or bleeding disorders, chronic or acute (e.g., hemophilia vs. idiopathic thrombocytopenic purpura) Infants: birthmarks (congenital dermal melanocytosis) Neonates: bruising from precipitous delivery Accidental impact to forehead with movement of ecchymoses during healing Allergic "shiners"
Swollen red eyelid or orbital area	Fresh inflicted injury	Periorbital cellulitis
Scratches on wrists, popliteal spaces, back	Scratching, restraining child	Self-inflicted secondary to atopic dermatitis or neuropsychiatric conditions
Fractures inconsistent with history or child's developmental level; multiple fractures at different stages of healing	Grabbing, twisting, throwing	Pathologic fractures related to osteogenesis imperfecta or other bone abnormalities
Mucopurulent vaginal discharge in prepubertal girl	*Neisseria gonorrhoeae* or *Chlamydia trachomatis* infection [Absence of discharge does not indicate lack of infection]	*Streptococcus pyogenes* or *Salmonella shigella* infection Intravaginal foreign body (e.g., toilet paper)
Clear, gray, or whitish vaginal discharge in early puberty	Nonspecific, or may indicate bacterial vaginosis, trichomoniasis	Physiologic leukorrhea common in Tanner stages 2 and 3
Anal fissure	Penetration (penis or foreign object)	Functional constipation
Weight loss or failure to thrive	Neglect	Metabolic, neuromuscular, or cardiac abnormalities, including malabsorption syndromes Depression Eating disorders

b. Burns may be inflicted or accidental. Accidental burns from hot objects, such as heaters or irons, may be difficult to distinguish from inflicted burns, because both have patterning. Splash burns, occurring for example when a toddler pulls a hot pot or cup off a surface, have typical and irregular formation, with the burn degree lessening as the liquid drips down the body. Immersion burns with a stocking or glove demarcation are more likely to be inflicted (Toon et al., 2011).

c. Fractures are common in children, and distinguishing inflicted from accidental fractures can be difficult. Spiral fractures and metaphyseal fractures can be the result of inflicted or accidental trauma, and some preambulatory infants in walkers have sustained accidental fractures. The following findings on physical or radiologic examination should raise suspicions of physical abuse:
   i. Fractures in a preambulatory infant.
   ii. Fractures in different stages of healing.

iii. Rib fractures, especially posterior, in the absence of documented accidental trauma.

iv. Bucket-handle or corner fractures (from shaking or squeezing).

d. Head trauma may be caused by shaking (coup contrecoup injuries), striking, or throwing an infant and is implicated in most cases of fatal physical abuse. Presentations may be acute or subtle, with children often misdiagnosed in emergency settings as suffering from a viral illness because of lethargy, vomiting, and poor feeding (Herman, Makoroff, & Corneli, 2011; Leventhal, Asnes, Pavlovic, & Moles, 2014). The following findings can be associated with abusive head trauma:

i. Altered mental status.

ii. Retinal hemorrhages (requires dilated examination by a pediatric ophthalmologist, and finding can be nonspecific).

iii. Skull fractures and possibly additional long bone or rib fractures.

iv. Intracranial hemorrhages (also may be present in coagulopathies and other medical conditions).

e. Thoracoabdominal trauma: squeezing or punching may result in rib fractures, trauma to underlying structures, or abdominal trauma. Children may not have surface bruising, and the examination can be confounded by other injuries or concurrent head injury. Imaging studies, including computed tomography, may be indicated (Hornor, 2012). Examination findings may include:

i. Decreased or absent bowel sounds.

ii. Guarding or abdominal muscle rigidity.

3. Physical examination findings consistent with sexual abuse

a. In examinations of sexually abused children, physical findings are rare (Jenny & Crawford-Jakubiak, 2013); over 90% of examinations of children who are evaluated for sexual abuse show no evidence of trauma or infection (Heger, Ticson, Velasquez, & Bernier, 2002; Jenny & Crawford-Jakubiak, 2013). Sexual abuse of prepubertal children most often consists of oral or digital contact. The elastic nature of genital and rectal tissues, added to delays in disclosure or examinations, contribute to the lack of findings (Adams, 2011). Some trauma to the genital area can occur accidentally, as with the asymmetric vulvar trauma consistent with straddle injuries. The APN who regularly examines the genital area of prepubertal girls during well-child examinations is more confident in distinguishing

normal from abnormal findings (Monasterio & Schapiro, 2014). However, apparently abnormal findings are often subtle, are difficult to determine without special magnification equipment (e.g., a colposcope), and can be caused by normal physiologic variations. Therefore, they should be confirmed by an expert in sexual abuse examinations.

b. The following are findings that are consistent with sexual abuse:

i. Vaginal trauma: trauma may occur anywhere in the vulvar area, the periurethral or perihymenal tissue, or in the perineum, from either forceful digital penetration, use of objects, or penile penetration. The following are consistent with sexual abuse (Adams, 2011):

a. Acute trauma or notches or transactions of inferior hymenal tissue (caution: normally occurring redundant hymenal folds may appear to be notched).

b. Thin or absent hymenal tissue.

ii. Anorectal trauma: penetration may cause fissures, and repeated penetration may lead to laxity of the sphincter. The most common cause of anal fissures is large hard stools, so fissures in themselves are nonspecific. Laxity of the anal sphincter should raise suspicions of abuse, but may also be related to neurologic conditions.

iii. Penile trauma: penile trauma is an uncommon finding in sexual abuse but may be associated with severe physical abuse.

iv. Sexually transmitted infections: most cases of vulvovaginitis in prepubertal children, including mucopurulent vaginal discharge, are caused by nonsexually transmitted infections, such as *Streptococcus pyogenes* and *Salmonella shigella*. Most cases of balanitis (inflammation of the foreskin) are also unrelated to sexual abuse. Gonorrhea and chlamydia are rare in sexually abused prepubertal children (0.7–3.7%) and are more common in sexually abused teenagers whose rates of infection (14%) are higher than teenagers who report only consensual activity with peers (Bechtel, 2010). Vertical transmission of gonorrhea, chlamydia, human papillomavirus, and herpes simplex virus is possible (Adams, 2011). Ulcers or verrucous papules in the genital area should be tested for herpes simplex virus and human papillomavirus typing.

4. Physical examination findings consistent with neglect
   a. Physical signs of neglect may include evidence of generally poor hygiene, inadequate clothing, and failure to grow and gain weight as expected during childhood. Most cases of failure to thrive have a variety of causes, including congenital heart disease, malabsorption syndromes, neuromuscular disorders, and a variety of interactional failures between parent or caregiver and child (Cole & Lanham, 2011; Harper, 2014). These interactional failures may be related to neglect or to a parent's appropriate anxieties about a medically fragile child who does not respond easily to the parent's customary caretaking strategies.
   b. A rare and puzzling form of child maltreatment, pediatric symptom falsification or medical child abuse, involves elements of physical abuse, psychologic abuse, and child endangerment (a type of neglect) (Flaherty & Macmillan, 2013; Mash, Frazier, Nowacki, Worley, & Goldfarb, 2011). Formerly known as Munchhausen syndrome by proxy, parents in this form of maltreatment induce or falsify symptoms of illness in their children, presenting them as victims of rare and serious medical conditions. The parent is typically a well-educated mother, often with training in a healthcare profession. Although uncommon, this form of maltreatment should be in the differential when children have repeated visits or hospitalizations for serious symptoms with negative diagnostic tests.

III. Assessment

Child maltreatment does not fit easily into a medical model or diagnostic algorithm in which one can "rule out" or "rule in" abuse or neglect. Many physical signs and behaviors associated with abuse are also associated with infections, serious chronic conditions, or variations of normal. Children and their caretakers, for a variety of reasons, may withhold elements of the history that could, alone or considered together with physical findings, aid in the determination or elimination of child maltreatment as a likely explanation for a given clinical picture.

However, the APN's legal responsibility usually hinges on a reasonable suspicion or concern, rather than a firm or even likely diagnosis (Child Welfare Information Gateway, 2014) (see **Table 15-2**). The following elements should be carefully assessed when the APN suspects child maltreatment:

A. Safety

1. Is further testing or examination warranted by experts in child physical or sexual abuse?
   a. Acute disclosure of sexual abuse or assault, especially involving penetration or exchange of body

TABLE 15-2 Child Maltreatment: Associated Factors That May Trigger an Independent Report

Adverse Conditions	Specific Reportable Behaviors	Variations from State to State
Domestic violence	Domestic violence committed in front of a child Physical injury to a child reportable under child abuse laws	Reportable in some states, but not others Adds to charges or sentencing of offender in some states Offender may have to pay for child's counseling
Substance abuse	Exposure of a child to substance abuse Manufacturing or using methamphetamine in front of a child Substance abuse affecting parenting ability Prenatal use of substances affecting a fetus Newborn testing positive for drugs of abuse	Specifically reportable in some states, but not others Providing substances to a child or failure to prevent access reportable in all states Some states have mandated follow-up for prenatally exposed newborns with evaluation by CPS before discharge
Poverty	Homelessness Failure to provide adequate food, clothing, shelter, health care	Homelessness reportable in some states, specifically excluded in others Inability to provide stable, adequate housing may be related to reporting in some states Some states have exemptions for personal or religious beliefs
Truancy	Failure to send child to school or provide home schooling, ensure child goes to school	Check individual state laws: in some states a violation of truancy laws; not under child protection laws

Data from U.S. Department of Health and Human Services, Child Welfare Information Gateway. (n.d.). State statutes search. Retrieved from https://www.childwelfare.gov/topics/systemwide/laws-policies/state/

fluids (within 72 hours, or in some states up to 108 hours): the child or adolescent should be transported to a specialized center for forensic examination, usually a designated emergency room or child advocacy center within or near the county where the abuse took place.

b. Equivocal examination, for example an apparently abnormal genital examination, which warrants a specialized examination with magnification.

c. Evaluation to determine if serious physical injuries are accidental or inflicted.

2. Is it safe for the child or adolescent to go home? Although CPS ultimately makes this decision, the APN's concerns will affect the urgency of reporting and referral.

   a. Do the suspected injuries or overall physical condition warrant hospitalization?

   b. Is there a disclosure or suspicion of sexual abuse in the home or physical abuse with imminent danger to the child?

   c. Can the caretaker with the child keep or transport the child safely?

      i. Willingness or ability to protect the child.

      ii. Safe transport (e.g., intoxicated caregiver who drove to the clinic with the child).

   d. Will the disclosure or reporting of maltreatment put the child or caretaker at risk in the home?

      i. Family reactions to disclosure.

      ii. For adolescents, potential harsh punishment for disclosing behaviors associated with extrafamilial abuse (e.g., going to a forbidden party).

3. Are there potential safety issues for the APN in reporting?

   a. Suspected offending parent or caretaker in the clinic.

   b. Reactions of nonoffending parent of child or adolescent.

B. Need to report

1. Does the situation warrant mandatory reporting in the state in which the APN is practicing?

   a. Consultation with other clinic providers.

   b. Consultation with local child abuse reporting hotline.

2. How urgent is the report (related to safety issues described previously)?

   a. Immediate.

      i. Immediate safety issues.

      ii. Legal issues: evidence collection or documentation.

b. End of the day (disclosures of past abuse, child and caretaker currently safe, sexual abuse outside of home beyond 72-hour period).

C. Are the child's and family's immediate needs being met?

1. When suspected maltreatment is part of the family's chief complaint

   a. Determine their expectations for outcome regarding housing safety (e.g., shelter versus arrest of suspected offender, which is not always immediate).

   b. Further testing desired by child and family that may or may not be indicated.

2. If suspected maltreatment is not the chief complaint of the child or caregiver

   a. It is important for APN not to lose sight of child and family priorities, which may be equally or more urgent than the investigation of maltreatment.

   b. If a report is necessary, a collaborative approach with the family and a respect for their priorities can help preserve provider-family relationships

IV. Plan

A. Diagnostic testing

1. Imaging: order in consultation with radiologist or child abuse specialist to determine occult, old, healing fractures. If inflicted fractures are suspected in children younger than 2 years, a full skeletal series should be ordered (Flaherty, Perez-Rossello, Levine, & Hennrikus, 2014; Hornor, 2012). Rib fractures, especially posterior, in children younger than 2, should prompt a head CT scan and ophthalmology consult to look for abusive head trauma (Hornor, 2012).

2. Laboratory testing

   a. If there is fresh disclosure of sexual assault or abuse within time period for forensic evidence, examination and laboratory testing should be ordered by a specialized sexual abuse forensic testing center.

   b. Bacterial or viral cultures as indicated for skin lesions or discharge in anogenital area and the oropharynx. Current guidelines recommend a NAAT (nucleic acid amplification test) from appropriate sites for gonorrhea, chlamydia, and *Trichomonas vaginalis* infections (Workowski & Bolan, 2015).

   c. Serologic testing as indicated (HIV, rapid plasma reagin, hepatitis panels).

B. Management

1. Treat injuries or infections as indicated.

   a. Prophylactic treatment of adolescents to prevent sexually transmitted infections in cases of sexual assault, including HIV prophylaxis if indicated (Workowski & Bolan, 2015).

   b. Current guidelines recommend prophylaxis for HIV only in prepubertal children, given low rates of infection and complications and importance of confirmed diagnosis; however, some parents and children may insist on treatment, which may be considered after all diagnostic testing has been done.

2. As indicated previously, refer any child or adolescent with sexual abuse or assault of less than 72 hours (or longer in some localities) to police and specialized child sexual abuse forensic team.

3. Make a child abuse report if maltreatment is suspected, following state and local procedures for verbal (telephone) and written reporting; usually both are required.

   a. Consider informing the parent about a report if it is safe for the provider, in order to maintain transparency and trust in the therapeutic relationship.

   b. Involve the adolescent in making a report.

      i. In most states, reporting is required by law, regardless of the adolescent's wishes; in some states, the provider has discretion and the adolescent can decline to report sexual abuse or assault if the suspected offender is not a parent or caretaker (Child Welfare Information Gateway, 2014).

      ii. Discuss APN legal responsibilities and adolescent decision making about disclosing versus withholding information.

4. Arrange follow-up care

   a. Counseling, if not arranged by law enforcement or CPS.

   b. For suspected neglect, follow-up supports for family.

      i. Practical and material (food banks, shelter assistance, transportation vouchers).

      ii. Health supervision and support: public health nursing and health education.

   c. Close clinic follow-up as indicated.

V. Resources

A. Patient education

Many states have excellent websites with parent and child educational material in multiple languages. The Child Welfare and Information Gateway at https://www.childwelfare.gov/ is an excellent site for parent and provider education, with some materials available in Spanish.

REFERENCES

Adams, J. A. (2011). Medical evaluation of suspected child sexual abuse: 2011 update. *Journal of Child Sexual Abuse, 20,* 588–605. doi: 10.1080/10538712.2011.606107

Assistant Secretary for Planning and Evaluation. (n.d.). Statutory rape: A guide to state laws and reporting requirements. Retrieved from http://aspe.hhs.gov/hsp/08/sr/statelaws/summary.shtml#_ftn9.

Bechtel, K. (2010). Sexual abuse and sexually transmitted infections in children and adolescents. *Current Opinions in Pediatrics, 22,* 94–99.

Child Abuse Prevention and Treatment Act (CAPTA). 42 U.S.C.A. § 5106g(2) (West Supp. 1998)

Child Welfare Information Gateway. (2014). *Definitions of child abuse and neglect: State statutes series.* Washington, DC: U.S. Department of Health and Human Services. Retrieved from https://www.childwelfare.gov/topics/systemwide/laws-policies/state/.

Child Welfare Information Gateway. (2013a). *What is child abuse and neglect? Recognizing the signs and symptoms.* Washington, DC: U.S. Department of Health and Human Services, Children's Bureau. Retrieved from https://www.childwelfare.gov/pubs/factsheets/whatiscan/.

Child Welfare Information Gateway. (2013b). *Child witnesses to domestic violence: Summary of state laws.* Retrieved from https://www.childwelfare.gov/topics/systemwide/laws-policies/statutes/witnessdv/.

Christian, C. W., & Committee on Child Abuse and Neglect. (2015). The evaluation of suspected child physical abuse. *Pediatrics, 135,* e1337-1354. doi: 10.1542/peds.2015-0356

Cole, S. Z., & Lanham, J. S. (2011). Failure to thrive: An update. *American Family Physician, 83,* 829–834.

Dubowitz, H., & Leventhal, J. M. (2014). The pediatrician and child maltreatment: Principles and pointers for practice. *Pediatric Clinics of North America, 61,* 865–871. doi: 10.1016/j.pcl.2014.06.001

Eckenrode, J., Smith, E. G., McCarthy, M. E., & Dineen, M. (2014). Income inequality and child maltreatment in the United States. *Pediatrics, 133,* 454–461. doi: 10.1542/peds.2013-1707

Fairbank, J. A., & Fairbank, D. W. (2009). Epidemiology of child traumatic stress. *Current Psychiatry Reports, 11,* 289–295.

Finkelhor, D., Vanderminden, J., Turner, H., Hamby, S., & Shattuck, A. (2014). Child maltreatment rates assessed in a national household survey of caregivers and youth. *Child Abuse & Neglect, 38,* 1421–1435. doi: 10.1016/j.chiabu.2014.05.005

Flaherty, E. G., & Macmillan, H. L. (2013). Caregiver-fabricated illness in a child: A manifestation of child maltreatment. *Pediatrics, 132,* 590–597. doi: 10.1542/peds.2013-2045

Flaherty, E. G., Perez-Rossello, J. M., Levine, M. A., & Hennrikus, W. L. (2014). Evaluating children with fractures for child physical abuse. *Pediatrics, 133,* e477–e489. doi: 10.1542/peds.2013-379

Gilbert, R., Kemp, A., Thoburn, J., Sidebotham, P., Radford, L., Glaser, D., et al. (2009). Recognizing and responding to child maltreatment. *Lancet, 373,* 167–180.

Gilbert, R., Widom, C. S., Browne, K., Fergusson, D., Webb, E., & Janson, S. (2009). Burden and consequences of child maltreatment in high-income countries. *Lancet, 373,* 68–81.

Greenbaum, V. J. (2014). Commercial sexual exploitation and sex trafficking of children in the United States. *Current Problems in Pediatric and Adolescent Health Care, 44,* 245–269. doi: 10.1016/j.cppeds.2014.07.001

Grossman, S. E., Johnston, A., Vanezis, P., & Perrett, D. (2011). Can we assess the age of bruises? An attempt to develop an objective technique. *Medicine Science & Law, 51,* 170–176.

Guttmacher Institute. (2015). *An overview of minors' consent law* (State Policies in Brief). Retrieved from http://www.guttmacher.org/statecenter/spibs/spib_OMCL.pdf.

Harper, N. S. (2014). Neglect: Failure to thrive and obesity. *Pediatric Clinics of North America, 61,* 937–957. doi: 10.1016/j.pcl.2014.06.006

Heger, A., Ticson, L., Velasquez, O., & Bernier, R. (2002). Children referred for possible sexual abuse: Medical findings in 2384 children. *Child Abuse & Neglect, 26,* 645–659.

Herman, B. E., Makoroff, K. L., & Corneli, H. M. (2011). Abusive head trauma. *Pediatric Emergency Care, 27,* 65–69. doi: 10.1097/PEC.0b013e31820349db

Herrenkohl, T. I., Hong, S., Klika, J. B., Herrenkohl, R. C., & Russo, M. J. (2013). Developmental impacts of child abuse and neglect related to adult mental health, substance use, and physical health. *Journal of Family Violence, 28.* doi: 10.1007/s10896-012-9474-9

Hornor, G. (2012). Medical evaluation for child physical abuse: What the PNP needs to know. *Journal of Pediatric Health Care, 26,* 163–170. doi: 10.1016/j.pedhc.2011.10.00

IOM (Institute of Medicine) & NRC (National Research Council) (2014). *New directions in child abuse and neglect research.* Retrieved from http://www.nap.edu/catalog/18331/new-directions-in-child-abuse-and-neglect-research.

Jackson, A. M., Deye, K. P., Halley, T., Hinds, T., Rosenthal, E., Shalaby-Rana, E., & Goldman, E. F. (2015). Curiosity and critical thinking: Identifying child abuse before it is too late. *Clinical Pediatrics (Phila), 54,* 54–61. doi: 10.1177/0009922814549314

Jenny, C., & Crawford-Jakubiak, J. E. (2013). The evaluation of children in the primary care setting when sexual abuse is suspected. *Pediatrics, 132,* e558–e567. doi: 10.1542/peds.2013-1741

Jones, R., Flaherty, E. G., Binns, H. J., Price, L. L., Slora, E., Abney, D., et al. (2008). Clinicians' description of factors influencing their reporting of suspected child abuse: Report of the child abuse reporting experience study research group. *Pediatrics, 122,* 259–266.

Keeshin, B. R., & Dubowitz, H. (2013). Childhood neglect: The role of the paediatrician. *Paediatric Child Health, 18,* e39–e43.

Kellogg, N. D. (2010). Sexual behaviors in children: Evaluation and management. *American Family Physician, 82,* 1233–1238.

Klevens, J., Barnett, S. B., Florence, C., & Moore, D. (2015). Exploring policies for the reduction of child physical abuse and neglect. *Child Abuse & Neglect, 40,* 1–11. doi: 10.1016/j.chiabu.2014.07.013

Leventhal, J. M., Asnes, A. G., Pavlovic, L., & Moles, R. L. (2014). Diagnosing abusive head trauma: The challenges faced by clinicians. *Pediatric Radiology, 44*(Suppl. 4), 537–542. doi: 10.1007/s00247-014-3074-1

Mash, C., Frazier, T., Nowacki, A., Worley, S., & Goldfarb, J. (2011). Development of a risk-stratification tool for medical child abuse in failure to thrive. *Pediatrics, 128,* e1467–e1473. doi: 10.1542/peds.2011-1080

Mersky, J. P., Topitzes, J., & Reynolds, A. J. (2013). Impacts of adverse childhood experiences on health, mental health, and substance use in early adulthood: A cohort study of an urban, minority sample in the U.S. *Child Abuse & Neglect.* doi: 10.1016/j.chiabu.2013.07.011

Monasterio, E. B., & Schapiro, N. A. (2014). Female genitalia. In K. G. Duderstadt (Ed.), *Pediatric physical examination: An illustrated handbook* (2d ed., pp. 242–258). St. Louis, MO: Mosby Elsevier.

Naughton, A. M., Maguire, S. A., Mann, M. K., Lumb, R. C., Tempest, V., Gracias, S., et al. (2013). Emotional, behavioral, and developmental features indicative of neglect or emotional abuse in preschool children: A systematic review. *JAMA Pediatrics, 167,* 769–775. doi: 10.1001/jamapediatrics.2013.192

Saul, J., Valle, L. A., Mercy, J. A., Turner, S., Kaufmann, R., & Popovic, T. (2014). CDC grand rounds: Creating a healthier future through prevention of child maltreatment. *Morbidity and Mortality Weekly Report (MMRR), 63*(12), 260–263.

Schapiro, N. A. (2008). Medical neglect of children: Reporting issues for nurse practitioners. *Journal for Nurse Practitioners, 4,* 531–534.

Shonkoff, J. P., & Garner, A. S. (2012). The lifelong effects of early childhood adversity and toxic stress. *Pediatrics, 129,* e232–e246. doi: peds.2011-2663 10.1542/peds.2011-2663

Slep, A. M., Heyman, R. E., & Foran, H. M. (2015). Child maltreatment in DSM-5 and ICD-11. *Family Process, 54,* 64–81. doi: 10.1111/famp.12131

Testa, M. F., & Smith, B. (2009). Prevention and drug treatment. *Future of the Child, 19,* 147–168.

Toon, M. H., Maybauer, D. M., Arceneaux, L. L., Fraser, J. F., Meyer, W., Runge, A., et al. (2011). Children with burn injuries—assessment of trauma, neglect, violence and abuse. *Journal of Injury & Violence Research, 3,* 98–110. doi: 10.5249/jivr.v3i2.91

U.S. Department of Health and Human Services. (2015). *Child maltreatment 2013.* Washington DC: Administration for Children and Families, Administration on Children, Youth and Families, Children's Bureau, U.S. Department of Health and Human Services. Retrieved from http://www.acf.hhs.gov/programs/cb/research-data-technology/statistics-research/child-maltreatment.

U.S. Department of Health and Human Services, Child Welfare Information Gateway. (n.d.). State statutes search. Retrieved from https://www.childwelfare.gov/topics/systemwide/laws-policies/state/.

Wildeman, C., Emanuel, N., Leventhal, J. M., Putnam-Hornstein, E., Waldfogel, J., & Lee, H. (2014). The prevalence of confirmed maltreatment among US children, 2004 to 2011. *JAMA Pediatrics, 168,* 706–713. doi: 10.1001/jamapediatrics.2014.410

Workowski, K. A., & Bolan, G. A. (2015). Sexually transmitted diseases treatment guidelines, 2015. *MMWR Recommendation Report, 64*(RR-03), 1–137.

CHILDHOOD OVERWEIGHT AND OBESITY

Victoria F. Keeton

I. Introduction and general background

Over 30% of children and adolescents between 2 and 19 years old in the United States are overweight or obese (body mass index [BMI] ≥ 85%), as defined by the Centers for Disease Control and Prevention (CDC) sex-specific BMI-for-age growth charts (Ogden, Carroll, Kit, & Flegal, 2014). Although the prevalence of childhood overweight has remained relatively stable in the United States over the last decade (Ogden, Carroll, Kit, & Flegal, 2012), there is still much work to be done to address this epidemic. Overweight and obesity in childhood have been linked to numerous serious health consequences, including increased risk for obesity in adulthood, as well as metabolic and cardiovascular disease (Daniels, 2009; de Onis et al., 2013; Friedemann et al., 2012; Harrington, Staiano, Broyles, Gupta, & Katzmarzyk, 2013).

Numerous changes in growth and development occur between infancy and adolescence. As such, it is important to consider the etiology and impact of overweight and obesity within a developmental context (National Association of Pediatric Nurse Associates & Practitioners, 2006).

A. Obesity in infancy

According to current statistics, approximately 8% of U.S. infants younger than 2 years of age have a high weight for recumbent length (≥ 95% on the CDC growth chart) (Ogden et al., 2014). Although the diagnosis of overweight or obesity is not generally used in this age group, there is increasing research to show that infants with high weight for length or rapid weight gain (Brisbois, Farmer, & McCargar, 2012; Koontz, Gunzler, Presley, & Catalano, 2014) may be at greater risk for remaining overweight in the future. Contributing factors to overweight in infancy include maternal overweight (via fetal metabolic programming) and overfeeding (Brisbois et al., 2012; Institute of Medicine [IOM], 2011). Preventive factors against overweight in infancy may include breastfeeding and delay of the introduction of solid foods to 4–6 months of age (Hunsberger et al., 2013; Moss & Yeaton, 2014; Oddy, 2012) .

B. Obesity in early childhood

Overweight and obesity in children between 2 and 5 years old are particularly concerning, and much attention is being paid to prevention in this age group. During this time, BMI generally reaches its minimum point before beginning to increase again (known as the "adiposity rebound") in early school age. This is a critical point for prevention of obesity, as there is evidence that an early adiposity rebound can be predictive of obesity later in life (Brisbois et al., 2012; Hughes, Sherriff, Ness, & Reilly, 2014). Increased intake of sugar-sweetened beverages (SSBs), nonnutritious snack foods, large portion sizes, lack of physical activity, and decreased sleep duration are all contributors to early childhood overweight (IOM, 2011).

C. Obesity in school-age children

Between 6 and 12 years of age, self-regulation becomes increasingly important, especially with regard to nutritional intake, as children with compromised abilities to self-regulate tend to have a higher BMI (Francis & Susman, 2009). In addition to the risk factors in early childhood described previously, children in this group are also beginning to consume more food outside of the home, which can include high rates of fast food or other "junk" foods. As children spend more time in school and after school programs, time spent in sedentary behaviors also increases (Tanaka, Reilly, & Huang, 2014), and opportunities for physical activity may be more difficult to find. Body awareness and teasing or bullying by peers may also surface during this period, which can negatively affect self-esteem and emotional health (Maggio et al., 2014; van Geel, Vedder, & Tanilon, 2014).

D. Obesity in adolescence

Some consider adolescence to be one of the most challenging periods with regard to overweight and obesity. Puberty brings physical and metabolic changes in the body that may exacerbate risk for negative sequelae such as insulin resistance (Jasik & Lustig, 2008; Pilia et al., 2009). Developmentally, teens are increasingly more independent from their parents, which often includes unsupervised decision making related to food and beverage choices. Excessive sedentary behavior and screen time are also a significant problem, when activities such as TV, social media, texting, and gaming become more common pastimes and sources of peer interaction (Li et al., 2013). Studies have shown that physical activity levels decrease significantly in early adolescence, especially among girls (Dumith, Gigante, Domingues, & Kohl, 2011). Body image may be more of a concern in this age group, and negative mental health consequences associated with being overweight are more prevalent (Maggio et al., 2014; Marmorstein, Iacono, & Legrand, 2014; National Association of Pediatric Nurse Associates & Practitioners, 2006).

E. Obesity in special populations

1. Children and adolescents with special healthcare needs (SHCN)

   Over the last decade there has been more awareness of the high prevalence of overweight in children with SHCN or developmental disabilities. Several factors may contribute to this issue (Bandini, Curtin, Hamad, Tybor, & Must, 2005; Murphy, Carbone, & American Academy of Pediatrics Council on Children with Disabilities, 2008; Reinehr, Dobe, Winkel, Schaefer, & Hoffmann, 2010; Rimmer & Rowland, 2008). Dietary restrictions or sensitive eating habits in some children with these conditions can provide challenges to caregivers' ability to consistently provide balanced and nutritious meals. Medications used to manage symptoms such as seizures or behavior concerns may cause weight gain. Children with physical impairments or significant cognitive deficits may have limited ability to participate in sufficient physical activity. The need for intense cognitive therapies, which are more often sedentary in nature, may also take precedence over physical activity.

2. Children and adolescents with mental health concerns

   Proper prevention and management of childhood overweight must include the integration of physical and behavioral health considerations. Children with mental health conditions such as depression may have unique risk factors for overweight as well as particular challenges in its prevention and management (Korczak, Lipman, Morrison, & Szatmari, 2013). Some psychotropic medications may exacerbate weight gain in an already overweight child (Cockerill, Biggs, Oesterle, & Croarkin, 2014; Mansoor et al., 2013). Especially when a mental health condition is exacerbated, a child's or teen's motivation and interest in physical activity may be negatively affected. The provider must also be aware of the potential for food and eating to be a significant source of coping for some patients. Conversely, the presence of overweight in a child may also contribute to the emergence or worsening of mental health conditions, especially if negative self-esteem or bullying is present (Geoffroy, Li, & Power, 2014; Rottenberg et al., 2014). General mental health assessment of the parents or guardian should be considered as well, as caregivers with impaired mental health may have a compromised ability to promote healthy behaviors in their children (National Association of Pediatric Nurse Associates & Practitioners, 2006).

II. Database

Figure 16-1 shows an algorithm for obesity risk assessment and recommended steps for prevention and treatment in all children (Barlow & Expert Committee, 2007). The following provides a comprehensive overview of pertinent assessment of the overweight child.

A. Subjective

1. Past medical/developmental history
   a. Investigate history of any physical illnesses that may contribute to weight gain and/or limitations in physical activity, as well as any related comorbid conditions and their management plans.
   b. Review current medications and note whether significant changes in weight occurred with their initiation or discontinuation.
   c. If the child is 5 years old or younger or has a significant developmental delay, review the developmental history and note any impact of current or previous delays on nutrition or mobility status.

2. Family history
   a. Take an accurate history of obesity, cardiovascular disease (including hypertension and/or hyperlipidemia), and diabetes in the immediate family, especially siblings, parents, and grandparents.
   b. Obtain a comprehensive family mental health history, including disordered eating and addiction.

3. Diet

   Request a detailed history of intake that includes type of food as well as serving size and overall quantity consumed per day or week. Consider having examples of cup sizes to help families accurately describe quantity of intake.
   a. Beverages
   b. Breakfast consumption
   c. Nonnutritious snack foods (sweets, chips, etc.)

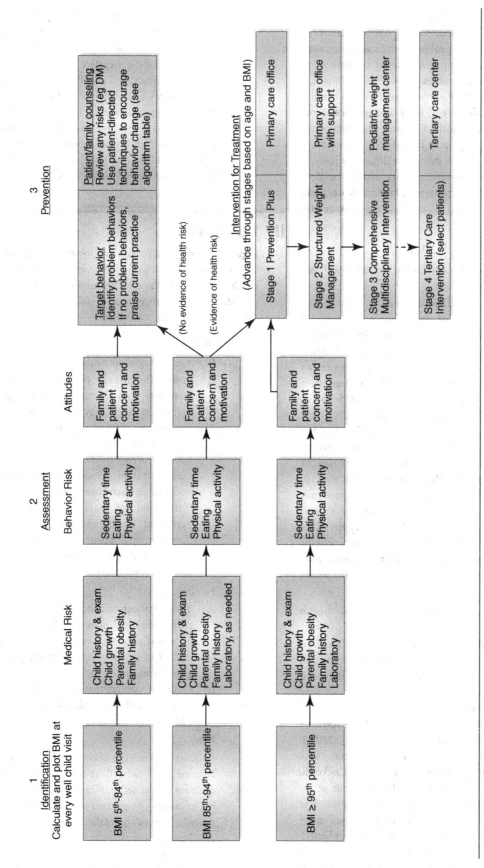

FIGURE 16-1 Assessment of Obesity Risk and Steps to Prevention and Treatment

Reproduced from Barlow, S. E., & Expert Committee. (2007). Expert committee recommendations regarding the prevention, assessment, and treatment of child and adolescent overweight and obesity: Summary report. *Pediatrics, 120*(Suppl. 4), S164–S192. doi:120/Supplement_4/S164

d. Intake of fast food or other food prepared outside the home

e. Fruit and vegetable consumption

f. Starches low in fiber (made from white flour or rice, corn, etc.)

4. Physical activity and sedentary behavior

a. Minutes per day spent engaged in moderate to vigorous physical activity (breathing hard, sweating, etc.), and type of physical activity

b. Minutes per day spent in screen-based activities (TV, computer, tablets, gaming, etc.)

c. Presence of a TV in the child's bedroom and frequency of eating in front of the TV

d. Quantity and quality of sleep

5. Emotional and social history

a. History of mental/behavioral health conditions and management

b. Screen for presence of active symptoms, for example, using a tool like the Pediatric Symptom Checklist (available at www.brightfutures.org)

c. Discuss family eating and activity patterns

6. Body image and self-identified concerns about weight

7. Previous strategies for losing/maintaining weight

8. Level of readiness, confidence, and motivation for lifestyle changes

9. Obesity-focused review of systems

a. General/constitutional: fatigue, unexplained weight gain/loss

b. Skin: presence of dark patches around neck, abdomen, or under arm area that can't be "scrubbed off"

c. Head, eyes, ears, nose, and throat (HEENT): snoring and/or gasping for air during sleep

d. Respiratory: shortness of breath, cough, or wheeze with exercise

e. Cardiac: history of elevated blood pressure

f. Gastrointestinal (GI): unexplained nausea or vomiting

g. Endocrine: irregular/absent menses, polydipsia, polyuria, polyphagia

h. Musculoskeletal: joint pain, especially in the hips

i. Psych/behavioral: moods, self-harm, suicidal ideation, stress, coping

B. Objective

1. Vital signs
   Measure blood pressure at every visit for children over 3 years of age. Be sure that the appropriate cuff size is used, and if using an electronic sphygmomanometer, confirm elevated results with a manual cuff. Calculate blood pressure percentile for sex, age, and height percentile using a National Heart, Lung,

and Blood Institute chart (National High Blood Pressure Education Program Working Group on High Blood Pressure in Children and Adolescents, 2004).

2. Anthropometric measurements
   Accurate weight and height should be measured at each visit. Calculate BMI, BMI percentile, and BMI z-score whenever possible.

3. Physical exam

a. General: observe overall appearance of health

b. Skin: inspect posterior neck, axilla, and lower abdomen for evidence of acanthosis nigricans

c. HEENT: inspect tonsils for hypertrophy

d. Neck: palpate thyroid in older children and adolescents

e. Chest: Auscultate breath and heart sounds

f. GI: palpate for masses and hepatosplenomegaly

g. Genitourinary: in males inspect for "buried penis"

h. Musculoskeletal: observe range of motion in all extremities; if pain in the hips, perform appropriate maneuvers to evaluate for acute slipped capital femoral epiphysis

i. Psych/behavioral: note affect and mood

4. Laboratory testing
   The primary goal of laboratory analysis in the obese child is to evaluate for comorbid conditions, based on the presence of risk factors and/or any current symptoms (Barlow & Expert Committee, 2007; Daniels, 2009). Elevated BMI can be a strong predictor of metabolic and cardiovascular disease risk (Daniels, 2009; de Onis et al., 2013; Friedemann et al., 2012; Harrington et al., 2013), and thus screening for these conditions should be considered.

When deciding whether to perform laboratory analysis, it is important to consider whether the results will in any way alter the treatment plan. If the answer is no, then the provider should consider whether there is true justification for the use of resources and subjecting the patient to the trauma of venipuncture. It is possible that abnormal lab results can be useful in patient/family education, regardless of whether they will affect the overall management plan. An example is a lab report that demonstrates mildly elevated lipids, which would most often be treated with lifestyle modification, but could still be a powerful visual indicator for the family that the child's condition has had a negative physical impact.

Consider risk-based screening for the following in children over 8–10 years of age and/or a child of any age with increased risk:

a. Diabetes: HgbA1c, fasting glucose (or if strong concerns about presence of hyperglycemia in clinic, perform a random fingerstick glucose)

b. Nonalcoholic fatty liver disease (NAFLD): Aspartate aminotransferase (AST), alanine aminotransferase (ALT)

c. Hyperlipidemia: Fasting lipid panel

d. Hypertension: Complete metabolic panel or renal panel

e. Hypovitaminosis D: 25-hydroxyvitamin D

5. Other diagnostics

Other diagnostic evaluation may be useful in the diagnosis of comorbid conditions, such as an ultrasound of the liver to confirm the diagnosis of NAFLD or a sleep study to confirm the diagnosis of obstructive sleep apnea or obesity hypoventilation syndrome. These conditions are generally comanaged with pediatric subspecialists, and thus it may be helpful to consult with such specialists prior to ordering additional studies to confirm what is needed.

III. Assessment

A. Classification using BMI percentile

BMI has been shown to be a reliable indicator of relative adiposity in children (Barlow & Expert Committee, 2007; Boeke et al., 2013) and as a noninvasive measure is commonly used in screening for overweight. In the United States, childhood overweight and obesity are classified in youth 2 to 20 years of age according to percentile of BMI as reflected on either the CDC or World Health Organization (WHO) age- and sex-specific growth charts. Current cutoff measures define a BMI percentile of 85–94% as overweight, whereas a BMI percentile of 95% or above is considered obese (Barlow & Expert Committee, 2007). Although BMI is not calculated in infants and young toddlers, a weight for recumbent length of 95% (CDC) or 97.7% (WHO) or above may be used as a foundation for overweight prevention counseling with families (National Association of Pediatric Nurse Associates & Practitioners, 2006; Ogden et al., 2014).

B. Rule out physiologic origin (endocrine, medication, etc.), particularly if weight gain is sudden over a brief period and/or not well explained by lifestyle or familial patterns

C. Identify comorbid illnesses or conditions, including mental health concerns

D. Motivation and confidence

Use motivational interviewing methods to determine the patient's and family's perception of the child's weight, as well as level of motivation and confidence in the ability to make lifestyle changes (National Association of Pediatric Nurse Associates & Practitioners, 2006; Rao, 2008).

IV. Plan

The foundation for the prevention or management of childhood overweight is lifestyle modification related to nutritional intake and physical activity, often by the entire family (Spear et al., 2007). The principal role of the primary care physician (PCP) is to provide the patient and family with sufficient education, counseling, and support to make and maintain these modifications (National Association of Pediatric Nurse Associates & Practitioners, 2006; Rao, 2008).

Table 16-1 illustrates a staged approach to treatment according to the child's age and BMI percentile (Barlow & Expert Committee, 2007). The following presents a complete plan for managing the child or adolescent with overweight in primary care. It is important to note that it may not be possible to cover everything in one visit, but rather the plan should include frequent follow-up to provide continuing education, review goal setting, and monitor progress. It is also possible that the following would not be carried out by the PCP alone but in collaboration with other professionals. Ideally, holistic and comprehensive care for the overweight patient will involve an interdisciplinary team of clinicians that may include a registered dietician, behavioral health provider, and/or pediatric specialists as indicated.

A. If secondary obesity, treat or refer for treatment of underlying cause.

B. Provide family-centered education.

1. Multifactorial etiology of obesity and associated health risks

2. Importance of healthy nutrition and physical activity routines for all members of the family

3. Need for support from all members involved in child/adolescent's daily life

4. Impact of weight and height changes on BMI for children who are still growing

5. Realistic expectations for weight or BMI changes over time

C. Encourage lifestyle modification where appropriate.

1. Nutrition counseling
   a. Use "My Plate" (**Figure 16-2**) to encourage a balanced distribution of nutrients and healthy portion sizes
   b. Encourage reduction/elimination of all SSBs
   c. Review healthy eating behaviors, such as eating meals at the table as a family and not eating in front of the TV
   d. Provide culturally tailored resources for grocery shopping and recipes for meals

TABLE 16-1 Staged Treatment of Obesity According to Age and BMI

BMI Percentile	Age of 2–5 y	Age of 6–11 y	Age of 12–18 y
5th-85th (normal)	Prevention stage	Prevention stage	Prevention stage
85th–94th (Overweight)[a]	Start at Prevention Plus stage. Advance to structured weight management stage after 3–6 mo if increasing BMI percentile and persistent medical condition or parental obesity, weight goal is weight maintenance until BMI of <85th percentile or slowing of weight gain, as indicated by downward deflection in BMI curve.	Start at Prevention Plus stage. Advance to structured weight management stage after 3–6 mo if increasing BMI percentile or persistent medical condition. Weight goal is weight maintenance until BMI of <85th percentile or slowing of weight gain, as indicated by downward deflection in BMI curve.	Start at Prevention Plus stage. Advance to structured weight management stage after 3–6 mo if increasing BMI percentile or persistent medical condition. Weight goal is weight maintenance until BMI of <85th percentile or slowing of weight gain, as indicated by downward deflection in BMI curve.
95th–98th	Start at Prevention Plus stage. Advance to structured weight management stage after 3–6 mo if not showing improvement. Weight goal is weight maintenance until BMI of <85th percentile, however, if weight loss occur with healthy, adequate-energy diet, it should not exceed 1 lb/mo, if greater loss is noted, monitor patient for causes of excessive weight loss.[b]	Start at Prevention Plus stage. Advance to structured weight management stage depending on response to treatment, age, degree of obesity, health risks, and motivation. Advance from structured weight management stage to comprehensive multidisciplinary intervention stage after 3–6 mo if not showing improvement. Weight goal is weight maintenance until BMI of <85th percentile or gradual weight loss of ~1 lb/mo if greater loss is noted, monitor patient for causes of excessive weight loss.[b]	Start at Prevention Plus or structured weight loss stage depending on age, degree of obesity, health risks, and motivation. Advance to more-intensive level of intervention depending on responses to treatment, age, health risks, and motivation. Weight goal is weight loss until BMI of <85th percentile, with no more than average of 2 lb/wk. If greater loss is noted, monitor patient for causes of excessive weight loss.[b]
≥99th	Start at Prevention Plus stage. Advance to structured weight management stage after 3–6 mo if not showing improvement. Advance from structured weight management stage to comprehensive multidisciplinary intervention stage after 3–6 mo if not showing improvement and comorbidity or family history indicates. Weight goal is gradual weight loss, not to exceed 1lb/mo. If greater loss occurs, monitor patient for causes of excessive weight loss.[b]	Start at Prevention Plus stage. Advance to structured weight management stage depending on responses to treatment, age, degree of obesity, health risks, and motivation. Advance from structured weight management stage to comprehensive multidisciplinary intervention stage after 3–6 mo if not showing improvement. After 3–6 mo with comorbidity present and patient not showing improvement. It may be appropriate for patient to receive evaluation in tertiary care center. Weight goal is weight loss not to exceed average of 2 lb/wk. If greater loss is noted, monitor patient for causes of excessive weight loss.[b]	Start at stage 1, 2 or 3 of treatment depending on age, degree of obesity, health risks, and motivation. Advance to more-intensive levels of intervention depending on responses to treatment age, health risks, and motivation of patient and family. Advance from comprehensive multidisciplinary intervention stage to tertiary care stage after 3–6 mo with comorbidity present and patient not showing improvement. Patients may warrant tertiary care evaluation to determine next level of treatment. Weight goal is weight loss not to exceed average of 2 lb/wk. If greater loss is noted, monitor patient for causes of excessive weight loss.[b]

In most circumstances, the general goal for all ages is for BMI to deflect downward until it is <85th percentile. Although long-term BMI monitoring is ideal, short-term (3<month) weight changes may be easier to measure. Resolution of comorbidities is also a goal.

[a] Children in this BMI category whose BMI has tracked in the same percentile over time and who have no medical risks may have a low risk for excess body fat Clinicians can continue obesity prevention strategies and not advance treatment stages.

[b] Because Youth Risk Behavior Surveillance Survey responses indicated that 15% of teens practice some unhealthy eating behaviors, all teens should be evaluated from these symptoms. Providers should be especially concerned if weight loss is >2 lb/week in this age group and should evaluate patients for excessive energy restrictions by the parent or children or unhealthy forms of weight loss (meal skipping, purging fasting, excessive exercise, and/or use of fixatives, diet pills, or weight loss supplements).

Reproduced from Barlow, S. E., & Expert Committee. (2007). Expert committee recommendations regarding the prevention, assessment, and treatment of child and adolescent overweight and obesity: Summary report. *Pediatrics, 120* (Suppl 4), S164-92. doi:120/Supplement_4/S164

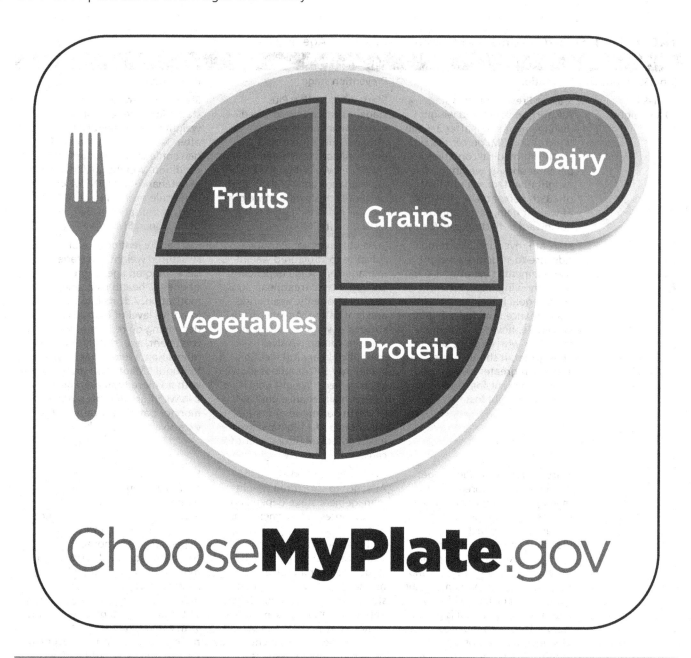

FIGURE 16-2 "My Plate" Guide for Making Healthy Eating Choices

Reproduced from the U.S. Department of Agriculture. Retrieved from http://www.choosemyplate.gov/print
-materials-ordering/graphic-resources.html

2. Exercise counseling
   a. Review recommendations for at least 60 minutes (cumulative) of moderate to vigorous activity and less than 2 hours of screen time daily
   b. Encourage turning off the TV during meals and removing the TV from the child's bedroom
   c. Discuss creative ways to find enjoyable physical activities for the family

   d. Provide resources for low-cost, safe local activity options
   e. For children with special needs, encourage participation in suitable physical activity whenever possible

3. Set SMART (Specific, Measurable, Achievable, Realistic, Timely) goals for nutrition and activity, to be followed up at next visit. Write them on a

prescription pad for the family to take home and post in a visible location.

D. Refer to specialty care as needed for management of comorbidities (otolaryngology, pulmonology, GI, endocrine, mental health, etc.).

E. Refer to tertiary obesity care if patient fails repeated attempts to control/lose weight. Tertiary interventions may include:

1. Medication management
   a. Metformin
      There is increasing evidence to suggest that the use of metformin may support weight loss in obese children with signs of insulin resistance (Adeyemo et al., 2014; Kendall et al., 2013; Yanovski et al., 2011).
   b. Sibutramine and Orlistat are the most commonly studied antiobesity medications used for adolescents and have shown modest results in supporting weight loss, with increased side effects noted with the use of Orlistat (Viner, Hsia, Tomsic, & Wong, 2010).

2. Bariatric surgery
   Adolescents who present with morbid obesity with either multiple comorbidities and/or the inability to lose weight via the methods described previously may progress to the need for surgical management. The types of surgery, course of recovery, and potential for complications vary from patient to patient but overall seem to be similar to that of adults (Levitsky, Misra, Boepple, & Hoppin, 2009).

F. The encouragement of weight maintenance versus weight loss depends on the age and BMI percentile of the child as follows (Barlow & Expert Committee, 2007; Spear et al., 2007):

1. Overweight (BMI 85–94%)
   Children of any age should be encouraged to maintain weight and/or slow weight gain until a BMI of < 85% is achieved

2. Obese (BMI 95–98%)
   a. Children under 12 should be encouraged to maintain weight or lose weight at a rate no greater than 1 lb per month.
   b. Adolescents 12 and older should be encouraged to lose weight at a rate no greater than 2 lbs per week.

3. Severely obese (BMI > 98%)
   a. Children under 6 years old should be encouraged to lose weight at a rate no greater than 1 lb per month.
   b. Children 6 years and older should be encouraged to lose weight at a rate no greater than 2 lbs per week.

G. Follow up with the patient at least every 3–6 months for weight/BMI monitoring and further support in lifestyle modification.

V. Helpful online resources

A. www.cdc.gov/obesity/childhood/
   CDC website that provides statistics and facts about obesity in the United States, tools for BMI measurement and tracking, and strategies for obesity prevention

B. http://ihcw.aap.org/
   Website for the American Academy of Pediatrics Institute for Healthy Childhood Weight, which includes information about programs and practice resources aimed toward obesity prevention and treatment

C. www.choosemyplate.gov
   U.S. Department of Agriculture-sponsored website that offers resources and tools for dietary assessment and nutrition education

D. www.letsmove.gov
   Official website of the "Let's Move" campaign launched by first lady Michelle Obama; provides information about nutrition, physical activity, and advocacy around obesity prevention initiatives in communities and schools

E. www.nchpad.org
   National Center on Health, Physical Activity and Disability website that provides information and resources to promote the health of people with disabilities through physical activity

F. www.chopchopmag.org
   Website and print magazine developed by the nonprofit organization, ChopChopKids, whose mission is to promote nutrition by teaching children and families to cook and eat together; offers a wide selection of easy recipes from a variety of cultural cuisines

REFERENCES

Adeyemo, M. A., McDuffie, J. R., Kozlosky, M., Krakoff, J., Calis, K. A., Brady, S. M., et al. (2014). Effects of metformin on energy intake and satiety in obese children. *Diabetes, Obesity & Metabolism, 17,* 363–370. doi:10.1111/dom.12426 [doi]

Bandini, L. G., Curtin, C., Hamad, C., Tybor, D. J., & Must, A. (2005). Prevalence of overweight in children with developmental disorders in the continuous national health and nutrition examination survey (NHANES) 1999–2002. *Journal of Pediatrics, 146*(6), 738–743. doi:10.1016/j.jpeds.2005.01.049

Barlow, S. E., & Expert Committee. (2007). Expert committee recommendations regarding the prevention, assessment, and treatment of child and adolescent overweight and obesity: Summary report. *Pediatrics, 120*(Suppl. 4), S164–S192. doi:120/Supplement_4/S164

Boeke, C. E., Oken, E., Kleinman, K. P., Rifas-Shiman, S. L., Taveras, E. M., & Gillman, M. W. (2013). Correlations among adiposity measures in school-aged children. *BMC Pediatrics*, 13(99). doi: 10.1186/1471-2431-13-99

Brisbois, T. D., Farmer, A. P., & McCargar, L. J. (2012). Early markers of adult obesity: A review. *Obesity Reviews: An Official Journal of the International Association for the Study of Obesity*, 13(4), 347–367. doi:10.1111/j.1467-789X.2011.00965.x

Cockerill, R. G., Biggs, B. K., Oesterle, T. S., & Croarkin, P. E. (2014). Antidepressant use and body mass index change in overweight adolescents: A historical cohort study. *Innovations in Clinical Neuroscience*, 11(11–12), 14–21.

Daniels, S. R. (2009). Complications of obesity in children and adolescents. *International Journal of Obesity*, 33(Suppl. 1), S60–S65. doi:10.1038/ijo.2009.20

de Onis, M., Martinez-Costa, C., Nunez, F., Nguefack-Tsague, G., Montal, A., & Brines, J. (2013). Association between WHO cut-offs for childhood overweight and obesity and cardiometabolic risk. *Public Health Nutrition*, 16(4), 625–630. doi:10.1017/S1368980012004776

Dumith, S., Gigante, D., Domingues, M. & Kohl, H. (2011). Physical activity change during adolescence: A systematic review and a pooled analysis. *International Journal of Epidemiology*, 40(3), 685–698.

Francis, L. A., & Susman, E. J. (2009). Self-regulation and rapid weight gain in children from age 3 to 12 years. *Archives of Pediatrics & Adolescent Medicine*, 163(4), 297–302. doi:10.1001/archpediatrics.2008.579

Friedemann, C., Heneghan, C., Mahtani, K., Thompson, M., Perera, R., & Ward, A. M. (2012). Cardiovascular disease risk in healthy children and its association with body mass index: Systematic review and meta-analysis. *BMJ (Clinical Research Ed.)*, 345, e4759. doi:10.1136/bmj.e4759

Geoffroy, M. C., Li, L., & Power, C. (2014). Depressive symptoms and body mass index: Co-morbidity and direction of association in a British birth cohort followed over 50 years. *Psychological Medicine*, 44(12), 2641–2652. doi:10.1017/S0033291714000142

Harrington, D. M., Staiano, A. E., Broyles, S. T., Gupta, A. K., & Katzmarzyk, P. T. (2013). BMI percentiles for the identification of abdominal obesity and metabolic risk in children and adolescents: Evidence in support of the CDC 95th percentile. *European Journal of Clinical Nutrition*, 67(2), 218–222. doi:10.1038/ejcn.2012.203

Hughes, A. R., Sherriff, A., Ness, A. R., & Reilly, J. J. (2014). Timing of adiposity rebound and adiposity in adolescence. *Pediatrics*, 134(5), e1354–e1361. doi:10.1542/peds.2014-1908

Hunsberger, M., Lanfer, A., Reeske, A., Veidebaum, T., Russo, P., Hadjigeorgiou, C., et al. (2013). Infant feeding practices and prevalence of obesity in eight European countries—the IDEFICS study. *Public Health Nutrition*, 16(2), 219–227. doi:10.1017/S1368980012003850

Institute of Medicine (IOM). (2011). *Early childhood obesity prevention policies*. Washington, DC: National Academies Press.

Jasik, C. B., & Lustig, R. H. (2008). Adolescent obesity and puberty: The "perfect storm." *Annals of the New York Academy of Sciences*, 1135, 265–279. doi:10.1196/annals.1429.009

Kendall, D., Vail, A., Amin, R., Barrett, T., Dimitri, P., Ivison, F., et al. (2013). Metformin in obese children and adolescents: The MOCA trial. *Journal of Clinical Endocrinology and Metabolism*, 98(1), 322–329. doi:10.1210/jc.2012-2710

Koontz, M. B., Gunzler, D. D., Presley, L., & Catalano, P. M. (2014). Longitudinal changes in infant body composition: Association with childhood obesity. *Pediatric Obesity*, 9(6), e141–e144. doi:10.1111/ijpo.253

Korczak, D. J., Lipman, E., Morrison, K., & Szatmari, P. (2013). Are children and adolescents with psychiatric illness at risk for increased future body weight? A systematic review. *Developmental Medicine and Child Neurology*, 55(11), 980–987. doi:10.1111/dmcn.12168

Levitsky, L. L., Misra, M., Boepple, P. A., & Hoppin, A. G. (2009). Adolescent obesity and bariatric surgery. *Current Opinion in Endocrinology, Diabetes, and Obesity*, 16(1), 37–44. doi:10.1097/MED.0b013e32832101ff

Li, J. S., Barnett, T. A., Goodman, E., Wasserman, R. C., Kemper, A. R., & American Heart Association Atherosclerosis, Hypertension and Obesity in the Young Committee of the Council on Cardiovascular Disease in the Young, Council on Epidemiology and Prevention, and Council on Nutrition, Physical Activity and Metabolism. (2013). Approaches to the prevention and management of childhood obesity: The role of social networks and the use of social media and related electronic technologies: A scientific statement from the American Heart Association. *Circulation*, 127(2), 260–267. doi:10.1161/CIR.0b013e3182756d8e

Maggio, A. B., Martin, X. E., Saunders Gasser, C., Gal-Duding, C., Beghetti, M., Farpour-Lambert, N. J., et al. (2014). Medical and non-medical complications among children and adolescents with excessive body weight. *BMC Pediatrics*, 14(232). doi:10.1186/1471-2431-14-232

Mansoor, B., Rengasamy, M., Hilton, R., Porta, G., He, J., Spirito, A., et al. (2013). The bidirectional relationship between body mass index and treatment outcome in adolescents with treatment-resistant depression. *Journal of Child and Adolescent Psychopharmacology*, 23(7), 458–467. doi:10.1089/cap.2012.0095

Marmorstein, N. R., Iacono, W. G., & Legrand, L. (2014). Obesity and depression in adolescence and beyond: Reciprocal risks. *International Journal of Obesity*, 38(7), 906–911. doi:10.1038/ijo.2014.19

Moss, B. G., & Yeaton, W. H. (2014). Early childhood healthy and obese weight status: Potentially protective benefits of breastfeeding and delaying solid foods. *Maternal and Child Health Journal*, 18(5), 1224–1232. doi:10.1007/s10995-013-1357-z

Murphy, N. A., Carbone, P. S., & American Academy of Pediatrics Council on Children With Disabilities. (2008). Promoting the participation of children with disabilities in sports, recreation, and physical activities. *Pediatrics*, 121(5), 1057–1061. doi:10.1542/peds.2008-0566

National Association of Pediatric Nurse Associates & Practitioners. (2006). NAPNAP healthy eating and activity together (HEAT) initiative. *Journal of Pediatric Health Care: Official Publication of National Association of Pediatric Nurse Associates & Practitioners*, 20(2 Suppl.), S3–S63.

National High Blood Pressure Education Program Working Group on High Blood Pressure in Children and Adolescents. (2004). The fourth report on the diagnosis, evaluation, and treatment of high blood pressure in children and adolescents. *Pediatrics*, 114(2 Suppl. 4th Report), 555–576. doi:114/2/S2/555

Oddy, W. H. (2012). Infant feeding and obesity risk in the child. *Breastfeeding Review: Professional Publication of the Nursing Mothers' Association of Australia*, 20(2), 7–12.

Ogden, C. L., Carroll, M. D., Kit, B. K., & Flegal, K. M. (2012). Prevalence of obesity and trends in body mass index among US children and adolescents, 1999–2010. *JAMA*, 307(5), 483–490. doi:10.1001/jama.2012.40

Ogden, C. L., Carroll, M. D., Kit, B. K., & Flegal, K. M. (2014). Prevalence of childhood and adult obesity in the United States, 2011–2012. *JAMA*, 311(8), 806–814. doi:10.1001/jama.2014.732

Pilia, S., Casini, M. R., Foschini, M. L., Minerba, L., Musiu, M. C., Marras, V., et al. (2009). The effect of puberty on insulin resistance in obese children. *Journal of Endocrinological Investigation*, 32(5), 401–405. doi:10.1007/BF03346475

Rao, G. (2008). Childhood obesity: Highlights of AMA expert committee recommendations. *American Family Physician, 78*(1), 56–63.

Reinehr, T., Dobe, M., Winkel, K., Schaefer, A., & Hoffmann, D. (2010). Obesity in disabled children and adolescents: An overlooked group of patients. *Deutsches Arzteblatt International, 107*(15), 268–275. doi:10.3238/arztebl.2010.0268

Rimmer, J. A., & Rowland, J. L. (2008). Physical activity for youth with disabilities: A critical need in an underserved population. *Developmental Neurorehabilitation, 11*(2), 141–148. doi:10.1080/17518420701688649

Rottenberg, J., Yaroslavsky, I., Carney, R. M., Freedland, K. E., George, C. J., Baji, I., et al. (2014). The association between major depressive disorder in childhood and risk factors for cardiovascular disease in adolescence. *Psychosomatic Medicine, 76*(2), 122–127. doi:10.1097/PSY.0000000000000028

Spear, B. A., Barlow, S. E., Ervin, C., Ludwig, D. S., Saelens, B. E., Schetzina, K. E., et al. (2007). Recommendations for treatment of child and adolescent overweight and obesity. *Pediatrics, 120*(Suppl. 4), S254–S288. doi:120/Supplement_4/S254

Tanaka, C., Reilly, J. J., & Huang, W. Y. (2014). Longitudinal changes in objectively measured sedentary behaviour and their relationship with adiposity in children and adolescents: Systematic review and evidence appraisal. *Obesity Reviews: An Official Journal of the International Association for the Study of Obesity, 15*(10), 791–803. doi:10.1111/obr.12195

van Geel, M., Vedder, P., & Tanilon, J. (2014). Are overweight and obese youths more often bullied by their peers? A meta-analysis on the relation between weight status and bullying. *International Journal of Obesity, 38*(10), 1263–1267. doi:10.1038/ijo.2014.117

Viner, R. M., Hsia, Y., Tomsic, T., & Wong, I. C. (2010). Efficacy and safety of anti-obesity drugs in children and adolescents: Systematic review and meta-analysis. *Obesity Reviews: An Official Journal of the International Association for the Study of Obesity, 11*(8), 593–602. doi:10.1111/j.1467-789X.2009.00651.x

Yanovski, J. A., Krakoff, J., Salaita, C. G., McDuffie, J. R., Kozlosky, M., Sebring, N. G., et al. (2011). Effects of metformin on body weight and body composition in obese insulin-resistant children: A randomized clinical trial. *Diabetes, 60*(2), 477–485. doi:10.2337/db10-1185

URINARY INCONTINENCE IN CHILDREN

Angel K. Chen

CHAPTER 17

I. Introduction and general background

Urinary incontinence by definition is the involuntary loss of urine (Neveus et al., 2006). The bladder is responsible for the storage and emptying of urine. During infancy, this occurs as reflexive behavior by the complex pathway controlled by an "integration of sympathetic, parasympathetic, and somatic innervation that involves the lower urinary tract, the micturation center in the sacral spinal cord, the midbrain, and the higher cortical centers" (Hinds, 2005, p. 79). The infant also may not empty to completion (Feldman & Bauer, 2006). The cortical inhibitory pathway develops between 1 and 3 years of age, which inhibits bladder contraction and allows for voluntary control of the external sphincter (Feldman & Bauer, 2006). By age 4, a child has learned to control and coordinate the voiding process and can become dry between urination. The detrusor muscle (bladder wall muscle) is relaxed during the filling stage while the bladder neck remains closed to achieve continence. Once the bladder is full, the external sphincter relaxes while the detrusor muscle contracts during voiding to allow for complete emptying of the bladder. An estimated bladder capacity in mL for a child over 2 years of age is now defined as **the child's age (in years) plus 1 × 30 mL** up until puberty (Austin et al., 2014). The normal range of voiding is between 3 and 7 times per day for children between the ages of 7 and 15 years (Austin et al., 2014). However, a wide range of conditions or dysfunctions may cause either continuous or intermittent urinary incontinence in children.

This chapter presents the latest standard terminology set forth by the International Children's Continence Society to standardize the language and avoid confusion among clinicians and researchers (Austin et al., 2014). Urinary incontinence is categorized as either continuous or intermittent. This chapter focuses on intermittent incontinence in children older than 5 years of age who are otherwise healthy and normal, both anatomically and neurologically. The assessment and management of both daytime and nighttime urinary incontinence (nocturnal enuresis) are discussed. There is also a brief review of the assessment and management of the common comorbid conditions associated with urinary incontinence including urinary tract infections (UTIs), stool retention, encopresis due to behavioral patterns (Feldman & Bauer, 2006; Franco, 2007a), and the psychological, social, and cultural impact on children with incontinence.

As a child learns to contract the external sphincter muscle, the muscle inhibits both detrusor contraction and stool motility, which can affect both systems. This is now referred to as bladder and bowel dysfunction (BBD), when both lower urinary tract dysfunction and bowel dysfunction coexist (Austin et al., 2014). Chronic contraction of the sphincter muscle promotes further stool retention and distention and/or incomplete emptying of the bladder, potentially leading to recurrent UTIs. In addition, a full rectum may exert pressure on the bladder, inducing bladder symptoms, such as sudden urgency or decreased bladder capacity, described as the "cross-talk" mechanism (Burgers et al., 2013; Franco, 2007a).

Possible early childhood risk factors, such as developmental delays in motor, communication, and social skills, or even difficult temperament may contribute to a higher chance of daytime incontinence and soiling (Joinson et al., 2008). Children with urinary incontinence have also been found to have social and psychological distress that must be addressed at the same time (Butler & Heron, 2008; Feldman & Bauer, 2006). Although correction of incontinence may not alter internalizing problems, such as anxiety or obsessive–compulsive disorders, it does normalize the incidence of externalizing problems, such as conduct disorders (Glassberg & Combs, 2009). Our society has little tolerance for bladder and bowel incontinence; thus children with such symptoms are at risk for further embarrassment and psychologic and emotional distress (Tobias, Mason, Lutkenhoff, Stoops, & Ferguson, 2008). Providers must handle both the initial workup and routine follow-up with much sensitivity and respect for the child's self-esteem.

A. Daytime (intermittent) incontinence

1. Definition and overview.

    Daytime urinary incontinence is the involuntary loss of urine while awake. It involves a wide array of clinical symptoms and causes, which differ in severity and reversibility. In addition, it may involve the maturation, functional, or behavioral process within the elimination cycle. Most commonly, children discover the power of controlling the external sphincter to postpone urination (by inhibiting the detrusor contraction) and thus eventually may reach a dyscoordination between the bladder and sphincter muscle control or have a delay in maturation of the bladder sphincter coordination (Franco, 2007a), both of which lead to daytime urinary leakage. Furthermore, after repeated dyscoordination, the child may also have a difficult time relaxing the external sphincter muscle enough to void to completion, thus increasing the risk of UTI and causing even more uninhibited contractions of the bladder (Austin & Ritchey, 2000).

    Some of the major causes of daytime incontinence include:

    a. Vaginal reflux and postvoid dribbling: involuntary leakage of urine immediately or within 10 minutes after voiding can be caused by urine trapped in the introitus during void or may occur with coughing, sneezing, or jumping; often due to voiding with adducted legs or presence of labial adhesions; may cause skin irritation.

    b. Voiding postponement: typically with classic postponing maneuvers ("potty dance," crossing legs fully, squatting with heel pressed into perineum, or penile grabbing) to externally contract the sphincter or compress urethra to temporarily relax the detrusor, postpone urination, or prevent urinary leakage, but followed by a sudden urge to void.

    c. Overactive bladder and urge incontinence: increased detrusor contractions that lead to pelvic floor contraction, can be diagnosed by urodynamics or accurate voiding diary; may or may not involve urinary frequency; high association with UTIs; associated with strong desire to void with tendency to perform classic postponing maneuvers (see item b.).

    d. Dysfunctional voiding: incomplete relaxation of external sphincter during voiding in an otherwise neurologically intact patient; may be verified by urodynamics or uroflow evaluation with staccato urinary flow pattern and prolonged voiding time potentially with incomplete emptying of the bladder (elevated postvoid residual [PVR]); associated with increased risk of UTI.

    e. Bladder and bowel dysfunction (BBD): combination of both bladder and bowel dysfunction, without identifiable neurologic abnormality and potentially affecting the upper urinary tract system if severe.

    f. Underactive bladder: low voiding frequency (three or less in 24-hour period) with need for intra-abdominal pressure (valsalva) to initiate, maintain, or complete voiding; caused by hypotonic detrusor muscle; large bladder volume with elevated PVR and increased risk for UTI.

    g. Giggle incontinence (enuresis risoria): a rare condition with complete involuntary emptying of bladder that occurs during or after laughter; bladder normal while not laughing; seen in girls.

    h. Stress incontinence: involuntary leakage of urine with physical exertion that increases abdominal pressure; on urodynamics the leakage is confirmed by lack of a detrusor muscle contraction.

    i. Extraordinary daytime urinary frequency or benign urinary frequency: frequent, small-volume voiding during the day only (> 1 time per hour with voided volume of < 50% estimated bladder capacity). Generally self-limiting.

2. Prevalence and incidence.

    Daytime urinary incontinence is generally considered a problem after 4 years of age (Feldman & Bauer, 2006). It may account for up to 40% of the visits in a pediatric urology clinic. In addition, dysfunctional voiding is associated with increased risk of UTIs, stool retention and encopresis, vesicoureteral reflux, and psychologic distress (Feldman & Bauer, 2006). Emotional stressors, such as sexual abuse, may sometimes trigger sudden dysfunctional voiding.

B. Nighttime (intermittent) incontinence— nocturnal enuresis

1. Definition and overview.

    a. Nighttime intermittent incontinence, also known as nocturnal enuresis, is the involuntary loss of urine in discrete episodes while asleep, occurring at least 2 nights per week (Butler, Heron, & The ALSPAC Study Team, 2006; Neveus et al., 2006; Austin et al., 2014). Enuresis is thought to be caused by a lack of arousal during nighttime with resultant bladder contractions and wetting, reduced nighttime bladder capacity, nighttime polyuria, bladder overactivity, or an elevated threshold for nighttime arousal (Butler et al., 2006; Neveus et al., 2010; Robson, 2009). To better understand nighttime incontinence, it is important to divide the children into subgroups based on symptoms or by onset of enuresis:

i.   Monosymptomatic enuresis: enuresis as the sole symptom, without any bladder dysfunction or other lower urinary tract symptoms; the etiology is unclear but possible cause is thought to be related to immaturity of the brainstem, with fluctuation or decreased production of serum arginine vasopressin, which leads to increased nocturnal urine production (Glassberg & Combs, 2009).

ii. Nonmonosymptomatic enuresis: enuresis along with additional daytime lower urinary tract symptoms (e.g., daytime incontinence, frequency, and urgency); the cause is thought to be overactive bladder or stool retention, or a combination of both (Franco, 2007a, 2007b).

iii. Primary enuresis: child has never been dry at night—can be for either monosymptomatic or nonmonosymptomatic enuresis.

iv. Secondary enuresis: child has had dry nights for at least 6 consecutive months but now with recurrence of enuresis; may have similar presentation as primary enuresis with the difference in degree of constipation and age of toilet training.

b.   Additional causes of enuresis may include genetic factors, maturational delay, upper airway obstruction (rare), psychologic factors, UTI, or decreased nighttime bladder capacity. Severe stool retention may also lead to decreased bladder capacity. Secondary nonmonosymptomatic enuresis requires further work-up for neurologic involvement especially if unresponsive to traditional treatments for enuresis or stool retention (Robson, 2009).

2.   Prevalence and incidence.

Approximately 15–25% of 5-year-olds have nocturnal enuresis despite cultural differences (Feldman & Bauer, 2006). A small percentage of this age group still wet two or more times per week (Robson, 2009). Recent studies have found more children with nonmonosymptomatic enuresis than monosymptomatic enuresis (Neveus et al., 2010; Robson, 2009), although the literature is mixed on actual prevalence. Children with nonmonosymptomatic enuresis tend to have higher rates of comorbidity, including both bladder and bowel dysfunction (Butler et al., 2006). In addition, they tend to have more severe symptoms including more wet episodes per night and more wet nights per week than those with monosymptomatic enuresis, because of persistent bladder overactivity throughout the night (Butler et al., 2006). The comorbid factors hinder the success of treatment

for enuresis if left unresolved. The spontaneous cure rate in children is about 15% per year, depending on their culture. Approximately 2–3% of older adolescents and 1–2% of adults continue to experience nocturnal enuresis. This occurs more in boys than girls (Bogan, 2005; Robson, 2009). Although most children do outgrow enuresis, studies have shown reduced self-esteem in children with even just once per month enuresis. By providing treatment, self-esteem improves regardless of actual success of treatment (Robson, 2009). Another study by Butler and Heron (2008) reveals that 9-year-old children view enuresis as extremely stressful life events, even more stressful than physical illnesses. Insurance companies may pay for bed alarm treatment for children over 7 years of age with monosymptomatic enuresis (Aetna, 2009), but daytime symptoms must be ruled out initially. The decision about when to start treatment depends on the child's degree of concern and motivation rather than the family's concerns and motivation (Robson, 2009).

II. Database (may include but is not limited to)

A. Subjective

1.   Detailed voiding and elimination history: most useful and most important (see **Table 17-1**).

a.   History provides critical information.

b.   Direct questions at both child and parent because the child knows best what occurs during the day; parents have been found to be unreliable in stating the voiding and elimination history alone.

2.   Past health history.

a.   Prenatal and birth history.

b.   Medical illnesses: significant congenital conditions especially of the genitourinary tract, heavy snoring.

c.   Surgical history: urologic or neurologic surgery.

d.   Obstetric and gynecological history: recent pregnancy.

e.   Growth and development: developmental milestones and any challenges or delays especially in neuromuscular area; attention-deficit/hyperactivity disorder; and school performance.

f.   Family history: renal or urologic diseases and history of enuresis.

g.   Diet: caffeine, soda, energy drinks, chocolate, or citrus intake (bladder irritants); fluid intake throughout the day and night; and fruit or fiber intake.

TABLE 17-1 Detailed Voiding and Elimination History from Child and Parent

Daily Activities & Related Symptoms	Information Gathering
Voiding habits	Potty training process (age, approach, and length of time)
	Number of voids throughout the day or at school (0–3 times)
	Postponing behavior ("potty dance")
	Urgency or frequency (number of times per hour; can sit through a movie?)
	Intermittent versus smooth urine stream
	Use of abdominal pressure to void (Valsalva)
	Nocturnal wetting or polyuria
Daytime incontinence	Frequency: number of times wet per day or per week
	Amount and severity: dampness versus soaking accidents
	• number of pads or liners used per day
	Pattern: morning versus afternoon
	• weekday versus weekend
	Sudden wetting versus wet along the way to the bathroom
	Amount of time between voiding and wetting (immediately, 10 min, or 2 hr)
	Aware of wetting and change clothes independently?
	Previous treatment and results
Nighttime incontinence	Frequency: number of nights per week
	Amount and frequency: wet before or after midnight
	• number of times per night (1 or > 1)
	• soak through pull-ups or diapers
	Previous treatment and results; compliance or appropriate use?
	Age when initial nighttime wetting resolved (if applicable)
	Family history of delayed resolution of nighttime wetting
	Responsible for changing wet sheets or clothing
History of urinary tract infection	Bladder versus kidney infection
	Fever or other symptoms at presentation
	Symptoms after treatment
	Previous work-up
	Total number of infections, dates, and treatment
Elimination habits	Frequency of stooling in toilet
	Size, shape, and consistency of stool; clog the toilet?
	Staining on underwear versus complete soiling
	Postponing of stooling (withholding behavior)
	Chronic abdominal pain
	Water, fruit, and fiber intake per day; evaluate timing of fluid intake
	Prior treatment and results
	Family history of constipation or infrequent stooling
Overall	Skin breakdown or rashes in perineum
	Awareness before or right after accident (urine or stool)?
	Which occurred first: urinary wetting or stool retention or soiling?
	Which is worse: daytime or nighttime wetting, or stool retention or soiling?
	Which is the child more motivated to correct?
	Which is the family more motivated to correct?
	Assess child's and family's readiness to address the issues

h. Personal–social–psychologic history: traumatic events or history of abuse, family and social support, reaction to accidents, recent major changes in the family; temperament in general.

3. Review of systems
   a. General: self-esteem, mood, attitude, patterns of behavior, fatigue, weight loss.
   b. Musculoskeletal and neurologic: gait and changes in lower extremity sensation or control.

B. Objective

1. Physical examination findings (see **Table 17-2**).

2. Supporting data from relevant diagnostic tests gathered from work-up and management plan (**Table 17-3**).

III. Assessment

A. Determine the diagnosis

1. Daytime (intermittent) urinary incontinence.

2. Nighttime (intermittent) urinary incontinence—nocturnal enuresis; monosymptomatic vs. nonmonosymptomatic; primary vs. secondary.

TABLE 17-2 Physical Examination

System	Details
General	Assess self-esteem, attitude, and mood
Abdomen	Abdominal tenderness or distention
	Abdominal masses
	• kidneys and bladder
	• stool masses
Genitourinary	Overall hygiene
	Dampness or stool staining on underwear
	Tanner stage
	Anatomic abnormality
	Signs of skin breakdown or skin excoriation
	Signs of infection
	Male: urine pooled under foreskin, balanitis, or meatal stenosis
	Female: urine in introitus or perineum, discharge, or labial adhesion
	Active urine leakage at baseline versus with straining
	Rectum
	• stool staining around rectum
	• rectal fissures
	• sphincter tone and sensation; anal wink
	If positive stool symptoms then consider digital rectal examination for assessment of rectal tone, presence of fecal or solid mass, or hemoccult testing
Spine	Sacral dimple, pit, or sinus tract
	Tuft of hair
	Hemangioma
	Subcutaneous lipoma
	Asymmetric gluteal crease
Neurologic	Gait
	Heel and toe walk
	Lower extremity muscle strength and tone
	Deep tendon reflexes
	Sensation in lower extremities

TABLE 17-3 Common Urologic Tests

Test	Definition	Clinical Implications	Comments
Urinalysis (UA)	Analysis of the urine by urine dipstick and, when available, evaluation under the microscope with spun urine	Specific gravity • < 1.000 may reveal concentrating defect • > 1.020 may reveal dehydration and insufficient fluid intake Positive glucose on dipstick: rule out diabetes mellitus Positive protein on dipstick: repeat and rule out renal disease Positive leukocytes or nitrites on dipstick: proceed with microscopic evaluation and culture and sensitivity to rule out UTI	UTIs must be ruled out as they may be the cause of or the result of the incontinence Can exacerbate bladder symptoms
Urine culture and sensitivity (urine C&S)	Cultured urine specimen to evaluate organism causing UTI and sensitivity to panel of antibiotics	Positive urine culture indicates UTI and requires treatment with antibiotics May follow with prophylactic antibiotics to prevent further infections until voiding dysfunction resolved	Method of obtaining specimen is important Use a catheterized specimen if not fully toilet trained to avoid contamination
Uroflowmetry (UF)	Noninvasive test measuring urinary flow rate, voiding pattern (degree of external sphincter relaxation), voiding volume, and time	Staccato flow (intermittent stream) indicates inability for sphincter to completely relax during voiding and may cause incomplete emptying in dysfunctional voiding Bell-shaped curve indicates proper sphincter relaxation during voiding Prolonged flow time with weak flow rate may indicate hypotonic bladder and detrusor contraction Best done with simultaneous pelvic floor electromyogram monitoring	Need to have at least half of estimated bladder capacity in the bladder to be effective Can be evaluated by listening and observing the urine flow if machine is not available
Bladder scan and PVR	Ultrasound of the bladder after voiding to determine residual urine within the bladder; noninvasive	Ideal goal of < 10% of expected bladder capacity Can detect bladder wall thickness (> 5 mm; caused by voiding dysfunction) and any masses within the bladder Useful as prognostic indicator Prevoid bladder volume is also helpful	
Renal bladder ultrasound (RBUS)	Ultrasound of the kidneys and bladder; noninvasive	Assess renal size and parenchyma and any evidence of hydronephrosis Assess bladder volume, bladder wall thickness, and any masses within the bladder May see rectal distention (indicate stool retention)	Normal renal bladder ultrasound can also be reassuring to both families and provider
Kidneys, ureter, bladder radiograph (KUB)	Plain film of kidneys, ureter, and bladder region	Assess degree of stool retention Assess for any spinal deformity	Complements clinical history and physical examination

(continues)

TABLE 17-3 Common Urologic Tests *(Continued)*

Test	Definition	Clinical Implications	Comments
Urodynamics (UDS)	Invasive study involving urethral catheter and filling of bladder for evaluation of bladder pressure, compliance, detrusor and uninhibited contractions, and bladder capacity Also evaluates pelvic floor muscle coordination and condition of bladder at time of urinary leakage (if any) Fluoroscopic urodynamics also is able to reveal VUR	Reserved for those without improvement or concern for neurogenic cause	Results may vary depending on how fast the bladder is filled and how cooperative is the patient
Spinal MRI	MRI of the spine to rule out tethered cord	Consider for those suspected of neurogenic bladder Should be MRI of entire spine	Children who require this work-up should also receive a full neurologic examination
Voiding cystourethrogram (VCUG)	Invasive fluoroscopic study with insertion of urinary catheter to fill the bladder and evaluate for signs of VUR; requires evaluation of voiding and PVR	Indicated if positive history of febrile UTI to rule out VUR Also reveals bladder volume, bladder trabeculation, sphincter relaxation during voiding, urethra, and PVR Includes scout film (kidneys, ureter, bladder radiograph); reveals spinal deformity and degree of stool retention Incomplete relaxation of external sphincter during urination is seen as "spinning top urethra" in girls	Consider fluoroscopic urodynamics rather than voiding cystourethrogram only if the child has a history of incontinence and pyelonephritis

Abbreviations: UTI, urinary tract infection; PVR, postvoid residual; VUR, vesicourethral reflux; MRI, magnetic resonance imaging.

3. Eliminate other conditions that may explain the patient's symptoms and presentation:
   a. UTIs
   b. Constipation or stool retention; bladder and bowel dysfunction
   c. Neurogenic bladder
   d. Diabetes insipidus or diabetes mellitus
   e. Ectopic ureter (typically continuous incontinence)

B. Severity
Assess the severity of the disease (mild, moderate, severe, or debilitating).

C. Significance
Assess the significance of the problem to the child and family.

D. Motivation and ability
1. Determine the child's motivation, willingness, and ability to follow an individualized treatment plan.
2. Provide individualized program and set realistic goals.
3. Provide frequent follow-up to monitor progress and sustain motivation.

IV. Goals of clinical management

A. Screening or diagnosing
1. Choose a cost-effective approach for screening or diagnosing daytime and nighttime urinary incontinence in children.

2. Eliminate other possible conditions causing urinary incontinence, which require referral to a specialty service.

B. Treatment

1. Improve the patient's bladder and bowel health, including skin integrity.

2. Properly treat conditions with minimal use of medication (both in dose and length of treatment).

3. Decrease the prevalence of UTIs.

4. Improve the quality of life for both patient and family.

5. Prevent psychological and emotional trauma caused by incontinence.

6. Foster a healthy and active lifestyle.

7. Empower the patient and family to manage bladder and bowel health.

C. Patient adherence

1. Select an approach that maximizes patient and family adherence, including positive reinforcement.

2. Provide close follow-up to maximize patient and family adherence.

V. Plan

A. Screening

1. Urinalysis or urine culture and sensitivities, if indicated, to rule out UTI and other abnormalities in the urine (Table 17-3).

2. Dysfunctional Voiding Scoring System (DVSS) Questionnaire—a 10-item questionnaire to quantify severity of symptoms (Farhat et al., 2000).

3. Additional psychological questionnaires may be used to determine behavioral comorbidities.

B. Diagnostic tests (Table 17-3)

1. Voiding or elimination diary as both a diagnostic tool and treatment via urotherapy—the timed voiding and elimination process (**Figure 17-1**).

2. Uroflowmetry (parents can watch child void and listen to urine flow for interruption or smooth flow); review past history and bladder scan (if available); evaluate patient's voiding pattern and PVR.

3. Renal bladder ultrasound if positive for UTI or severe wetting (see **Figures 17-2, 17-3**).

4. Abdominal plain film if there is stool retention or unclear history of constipation

5. Voiding cystourethrogram if positive history of febrile UTI; or video urodynamics study, which includes fluoroscopic voiding cystourethrogram in addition to the urodynamics study of the bladder (see Figures 17-2, 17-3).

6. Urodynamics study and spinal magnetic resonance imaging if suspicion of neurogenic bladder for both day and nighttime incontinence or no improvement with initial treatment regimen of nonmonosymptomatic enuresis.

C. Management including treatment, consultation, referral, and follow-up care (see **Tables 17-4, 17-5** and Figures 17-2, 17-3) (Burgers et al., 2013; Austin et al., 2014; Maternik, Krzeminska, & Zurowska, 2015)

1. Daytime incontinence.

   a. Bladder and bowel dysfunction: adhere to strict urotherapy, including education on normal bladder function, regular voiding and elimination habits and posture, fluid intake, prevention of stool retention, and instruction on the use of voiding and elimination diaries. Of note, not enough data exist regarding benefits of fiber or probiotics for them to be recommended routinely.

   b. Vaginal reflux and postvoid dribbling: sit on toilet with underwear all the way down by the ankles or sit backward on toilet to allow full abduction of legs during urination to prevent urine from backflowing into the vagina.

   c. Giggle incontinence and enuresis risoria: methylphenidate, 0.2–0.5 mg/kg orally daily for 2 months for trial.

      i. Children less than 10 years of age: short-acting (4-hr) form used midmorning

      ii. Children more than 10 years of age: intermediate-acting (8-hr) form used before school (Berry, Zderic, & Carr, 2009)

   d. Valsalva voiding habits should be referred to pediatric urology for consultation and work-up.

2. Nighttime incontinence.

   a. Nonmonosymptomatic: start with treatment for daytime incontinence and address any other comorbid factors (e.g., stooling) before achieving nighttime continence.

   b. Monosymptomatic primary nocturnal enuresis: following daytime urotherapy and ruling out of stool retention, choice of bed alarm or medication if appropriate.

   c. Secondary nonmonosymptomatic nocturnal enuresis: following daytime urotherapy and ruling out stool retention, if unresponsive, refer

FIGURE 17-1 Voiding and Elimination Diary

Date _____

	Mon	Tues	Wed	Thurs	Fri	Sat	Sun
When you wake up							
Mid AM recess							
Lunch							
Mid PM (before leaving school)							
Dinner							
Bedtime							
Poop							
Dry Days							
Dry Nights							

Date _____

	Mon	Tues	Wed	Thurs	Fri	Sat	Sun
When you wake up							
Mid AM recess							
Lunch							
Mid PM (before leaving school)							
Dinner							
Bedtime							
Poop							
Dry Days							
Dry Nights							

Date _____

	Mon	Tues	Wed	Thurs	Fri	Sat	Sun
When you wake up							
Mid AM recess							
Lunch							
Mid PM (before leaving school)							
Dinner							
Bedtime							
Poop							
Dry Days							
Dry Nights							

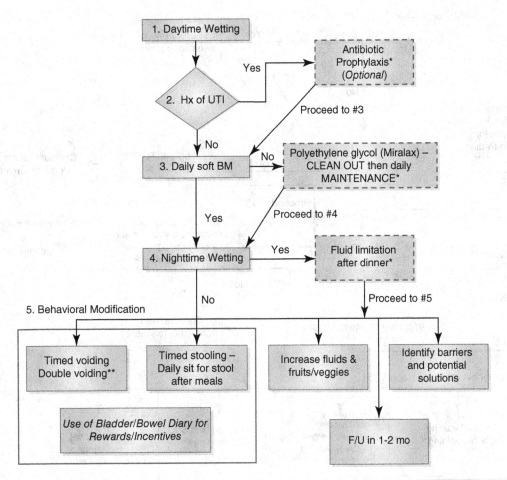

* Consider work-up and management accordingly; see Tables 17-3, 17-4, and 17-5. Stool retention must be addressed/resolved.
**Void every 1-2 hr; double void if elevated postvoid residual.

FIGURE 17-2 Algorithm for Diagnosis, Evaluation, and Treatment for Urinary Incontinence

to pediatric urology for full work-up possibly with renal bladder ultrasound, urodynamics, and/or spinal magnetic resonance imaging to rule out neurogenic bladder caused by possible tethered cord or other etiologies.

D. Client education

1. Information.
   Provide verbal and, preferably, written information regarding:
   a. Normal bladder and bowel functions, coordination of detrusor muscle with external sphincter muscle, and relationship between bladder and bowel functions.

b. The disease process, including but not limited to signs and symptoms and underlying etiologies. Emphasize that this condition is neither the child's nor parent's fault and that the healthcare provider will work together with family to resolve issues. Provide encouragement and motivation throughout the recovery process (average 3–6 months or as long as the length of dysfunction).

c. Diagnostic tests that include a discussion about preparation, cost, the actual procedures, and aftercare.

d. Management (rationale, action, use, side effects, associated risks, and cost of therapeutic

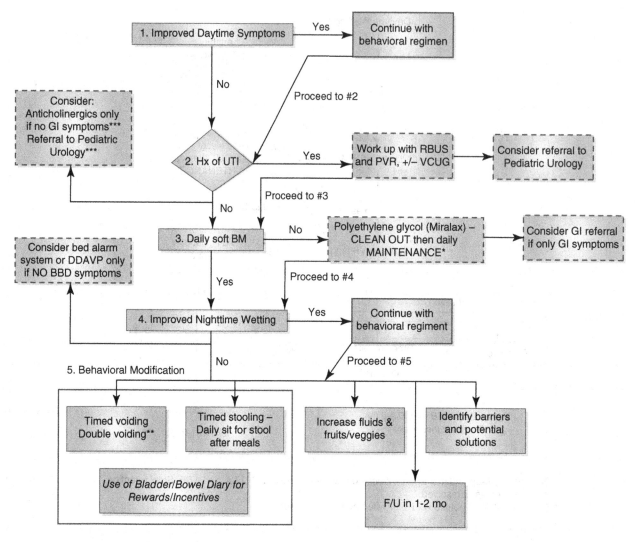

FIGURE 17-3 Algorithm for Follow-Up of Urinary Incontinence

interventions; and the need for adhering to long-term treatment plans).

2. Counseling.
   a. Recommended if symptoms have contributed to emotional distress or social isolation.
   b. If underlying issues contribute to the incontinence and encopresis, counseling or other psychotherapy may assist in addressing and correcting the issues.

VI. Resources

A. Provider resources

1. A number of validated tools are available to measure the psychologic and behavioral effects of incontinence, such as the Child Behavioral Check List (CBCL), or PinQ, a cross-cultural continence-specific pediatric quality-of-life measurement tool (Bower et al., 2006).

TABLE 17-4 Management of Daytime and Nighttime Urinary Incontinence*

Step	Recommendation	Comments
Step 1: Initial work-up or treatment	Antibiotic prophylaxis if needed (see **Table 17-5**)	If positive for recurrent urinary tract infection or incomplete emptying, consider daily low-dose prophylactic antibiotics at the same time as timed voiding and stooling May consider • trimethoprim-sulfamethoxazole • nitrofurantoin
	Timed voiding and double voiding	Initiate voiding every 1–2 hours during the day whether or not the child "feels the need"; approximately 6 times per day: first thing in the morning, midmorning recess, lunch, midafternoon before coming home, dinner, and bedtime. If elevated postvoid residual (> 10% estimated bladder capacity), perform double voiding by returning to void a few minutes after initial voiding; may consider antibiotic prophylaxis AVOID POSTPONING BEHAVIOR!
	Timed stooling	After a meal, typically dinner, sit on toilet for 10 minutes to attempt to have a bowel movement, and as needed Avoid rushing through the attempt Use of footstool to help with best posture in stooling
	Voiding and elimination diary (see Figure 17-1)	Document every voiding and elimination attempt each day, along with any dry days and nights May do a frequency–volume chart of shorter duration (i.e., 2-day diary) that includes fluid intake and volume voided Make note of size, shape, and consistency of stool
	Rewards system	Use the results on voiding–elimination diary to provide positive reinforcement Small treats, stickers, stamps, and privileges for voiding and elimination attempts rather than just for accident-free days and nights
	Dietary adjustments	Encourage fluids throughout the day (water best); avoid sodas and caffeinated beverages Increase fruit intake; natural best
	Stool retention and encopresis management (see Table 17-5)	If initial presentation with significant stool retention or encopresis, or on return with symptoms despite behavioral regimen, consider polyethylene glycol (Miralax) for cleanout and maintenance regimen May consider footstool to achieve best posture to relax external sphincter for stooling and voiding Refer to pediatric gastrointestinal service for further work-up if no improvement or gastrointestinal symptoms more severe than genitourinary symptoms Instruct families to expect 6–12 months of treatment, then wean therapy
	Fluid restriction (for nocturnal enuresis)	Avoid large amounts of fluids ingested at dinner and beyond Caution: children in afterschool sports activities require sufficient rehydration, thus significant fluid restriction may cause further dehydration Encourage fluid intake throughout the day
	Follow-up	Return to clinic in 1 month for close follow-up; best to maintain frequent contact especially if minor adjustments are necessary to behavior regimen
Step 2: Follow-up evaluation or treatment	Reevaluate	On return, review voiding–elimination diary and symptoms since last visit Repeat uroflowmetry and postvoid residual check (if available) If failed to comply with behavioral regimen, discuss barriers and possible ways to resolve barriers Continue with timed voiding, timed stooling, use of diary, and reward system

(continues)

TABLE 17-4 Management of Daytime and Nighttime Urinary Incontinence* *(Continued)*

Step	Recommendation	Comments
	Anticholinergic and antispasmodic medication (daytime incontinence or nonmonosymptomatic enuresis despite timed voiding) (see Table 17-5)	Use as adjunct to strict timed voiding for those with uninhibited bladder spasms and potentially increased functional bladder capacity
		May consider:
		• oxybutynin
		• tolterodine
		Second line of treatment for monosymptomatic enuresis or in conjunction with desmopressin acetate (DDAVP)
	Bed alarm system (monosymptomatic enuresis)	Consider for children greater than 6 years of age
		Choose loud sensor (sound/lights/vibration) to wake child up at the beginning of accident at night; not the same as setting an alarm at a specific time of the night
		Sensor is attached to underwear and is activated by the wetting of the underwear
		Child needs to get up (or to be woken up) at the time of alarm activation to void, then reattach alarm
		Should follow-up on results in 2–3 weeks; overall regimen for 2–3 months. If not effective, can consider pharmacologic regimen
		Pro: conditioning regimen; effective when used correctly in a motivated child and family (80%)
		Con: wakes up entire family with the loud sound; if soft then does not wake child up to void; relapse may occur after discontinuation
	Antidiuretic: desmopressin acetate (DDAVP) (monosymptomatic enuresis) (see Table 17-5)	First line of pharmacologic treatment for monosymptomatic enuresis
	Tricyclic antidepressant: imipramine (Tofranil) (see Table 17-5)	Third line of pharmacologic treatment for enuresis related to safety concerns
	Additional modalities: biofeedback	Consider biofeedback therapy to learn to relax sphincter and empty to completion; limited by child's ability to cooperate and follow directions (Franco, 2007b); "bladder stretching" exercises are not useful
	Other modalities (less evidence in the literature)	Alpha blocker therapy for overactive bladder
		Hypnosis
		Acupuncture
		Chiropractor
		Extracorporeal magnetic innervation therapy
		Botulinum A toxin for overactive bladder or sphincter dyssynergia
	Timed voiding and stooling regimen	Continue strict timed voiding and stooling along with medication trial
	Follow-up	Return in 1–2 months for follow-up and minor adjustments
		Continued support for patient and family
		Provide motivation in compliance with regimen
		Reminder regarding length of time required for full recovery
Step 3: Without improvement despite treatment compliance	Referral for further work-up	Pediatric gastroenterology if severe encopresis or stool retention
		Pediatric urology if recurrent urinary tract infection, persistent daytime or nighttime wetting, or suspicion of neurogenic bladder (require full work-up of renal bladder ultrasound, urodynamic study, spinal magnetic resonance imaging)
		Psychotherapy for emotional stressors to be assessed and treated

* Includes treatment, consultation, referral, and follow-up care.

TABLE 17-5 Common Urologic and Bowel Regimen Medication*

Category	Indication/Mechanism of Action	Name	Dosage	Side Effects	Comments
Anticholinergic	1. Treat daytime incontinence caused by bladder overactivity (uninhibited contractions) 2. Second line of treatment for monosymptomatic enuresis or in conjunction with desmopressin acetate (DDAVP)—must rule out constipation and daytime voiding dysfunction first	Oxybutynin	Daytime: 5 mg PO BID or TID dosing; or XL 10 mg PO daily Nighttime wetting: 5 mg PO QHS Immediate release, extended release, and transdermal forms available. Max dose 0.4 mg/kg	Dry mouth, constipation, occasional initial drowsiness; do not use in hot weather because of reduced perspiration, which leads to facial flushing; possible mood changes	Contraindication: incomplete emptying
		Tolterodine	2 mg PO QHS or 1 mg PO BID		
Antidiuretic	Synthetic antidiuretic hormone to reduce urine output at night Consider for children > 6 years of age 30% respond fully; 40% partial response May use only for sleepovers or camp	Desmopressin acetate (DDAVP)	Dose: 0.2-mg tablet 1–3 tablets PO QHS (1 hour before bedtime); may use higher dose then taper down	Risk of hyponatremia (rare) with mostly nasal spray formulation (longer half-life); limit fluids after dinner	Contraindication: excessive fluid intake in evening, (+) headache, nausea, or vomiting
Antidepressant	Mechanism unknown; used rarely; 50% response rate	Imipramine	0.5–1.5 mg/kg/d given 1–2 hours before bedtime OR 25–50 mg PO QHS (50 mg for children > 9 years of age)	Daytime sedation, anxiety, insomnia, dry mouth, nausea, and personality changes	Overdose can cause fatal cardiac arrhythmias, hypotension, respiratory distress, and convulsions

(continues)

TABLE 17-5 Common Urologic and Bowel Regimen Medication* *(Continued)*

Category	Indication/Mechanism of Action	Name	Dosage	Side Effects	Comments
Osmotic laxative	Induce catharsis by strong electrolyte and osmotic effect	Polyethylene glycol (Miralax)	Clean-out: 1.5 g/kg/d for 3 days (may split to BID dose) followed by daily maintenance dose and daily sit Maintenance: 2–11 years of age: 8.5 g (1/2 cap) in 4 oz. of water per day > 12 years of age: 17 g (1 cap) in 8 oz. of water per day; or 0.26–0.84 g/kg/d (titrate accordingly for daily soft stool)	Nausea, vomiting, cramps	If no stooling, return to cleanout procedure and then maintenance Parents will titrate depending on stool output, consistency, and staining
Antibiotic	Treatment of UTI; daily low-dose prophylaxis for prevention of UTIs	Trimethoprim (TMP)-sulfamethoxazole	UTI prophylaxis: 2 mg/kg/dose of TMP daily	Nausea, vomiting, Stevens-Johnson syndrome, rash	Contraindication: hypersensitivity to sulfa drug, trimethoprim, or components
		Nitrofurantoin	UTI prophylaxis: 1–2 mg/kg/d as single daily dose; maximum 100 mg/d	Nausea, vomiting, anorexia, Stevens-Johnson syndrome, rash	Avoid suspension; use capsule instead and sprinkle onto yogurt or ice cream Administer with food or milk

Abbreviation: UTI = urinary tract infection.

Data from Walia, R., Mahajan, L., & Steffen, R. (2009). Recent advances in chronic constipation. *Current Opinion in Pediatrics, 21,* 661–666.

B. Patient and client education websites

1. www.Kidshealth.org

   Part of Nemours Foundation's Center for Children's Health Media, Kidhealth.org is a website dedicated to providing health and safety information and helpful tips, in both English and Spanish. Content is designed to specifically address parents, kids, and teenagers. Search "bedwetting" to retrieve helpful information.

2. www.Healthychildren.org

   Sponsored by American Academy of Pediatrics. Contains health topics ranging from regular development to conditions such as enuresis and constipation.

3. www.i-c-c-s.org

   International Children's Continence Society official website. Includes resources for providers and patients on bladder and bowel dysfunction.

4. www.Bedwettingstore.com

   Offers both resources and products to help manage daytime and nighttime urinary incontinence.

REFERENCES

Aetna, Inc. (2009). *Clinical policy bulletin: Nocturnal enuresis treatments.* Retrieved from http://www.aetna.com/cpb/medical/data/400_499/0431.html.

Austin, P. F., & Ritchey, M. L. (2000). Dysfunctional voiding. *Pediatrics in Review, 21*(10), 336–341.

Austin, P. F., Bauer, S. B., Bower, W., Chase, J., Franco, I., Hoebeke, P., et al. (2014) The standardization of terminology of lower urinary tract function in children and adolescents: Update report from the Standardization Committee of the International Children's Continence Society. *Journal of Urology, 191,* 1863–1865.

Berry, A. K., Zderic, S., & Carr, M. (2009). Methylphenidate for giggle incontinence. *Journal of Urology, 182*(Suppl. 4), 2028–2032.

Bogan, P. A. (2005). Nocturnal enuresis. In L. Baskin & B. Kogan (Eds.), *Handbook of Pediatric Urology* (2nd ed., pp. 92–97). Philadelphia, PA: Lippincott Williams & Wilkins.

Bower, W. F., Sit, F. K., Bluyssen, N., et al. (2006). PinQ: A valid, reliable and reproducible quality-of-life measure in children with bladder dysfunction. *Journal of Pediatric Urology, 2*(3), 185–189.

Burgers, R. E., Mugie, S. M., Chase, J., Cooper, C. S., von Gontard, A., Rittig, C. S., et al. (2013). Management of functional constipation in children with lower urinary tract symptoms: Report from the Standardization Committee of the International Children's Continence Society. *Journal of Urology, 190,* 29–36.

Butler, R., & Heron, J. (2008). An exploration of children's views of bedwetting at 9 years. *Child Care, Health and Development, 34*(1), 65–70.

Butler, R., Heron, J., & The ALSPAC Study Team. (2006). Exploring the differences between mono- and polysymptomatic nocturnal enuresis. *Scandinavian Journal of Urology and Nephrology, 40*(4), 313–319.

Farhat, W., Bagli, D. J., Capolicchio, G., O'Reilly, S., Merguerian, P. A., Khoury, A., et al. (2000). The dysfunctional voiding scoring system: Quantitative standardization of dysfunctional voiding symptoms in children. *Journal of Urology, 164*(3), 1011–1015.

Feldman, A. S., & Bauer, S. B. (2006). Diagnosis and management of dysfunctional voiding. *Current Opinion in Pediatrics, 18*(2), 139–147.

Franco, I. (2007a). Overactive bladder in children. Part 1: Pathophysiology. *Journal of Urology, 178*(3), 761–768.

Franco, I. (2007b). Overactive bladder in children. Part 2: Management. *Journal of Urology, 178*(3), 769–774.

Glassberg, K. I., & Combs, A. J. (2009). Nonneurogenic voiding disorders: What's new? *Current Opinions in Urology, 19,* 412–418.

Hinds, A. (2005). Daytime urinary incontinence (in the otherwise healthy child). In L. Baskin & B. Kogan (Eds.), *Handbook of Pediatric Urology* (2nd ed., pp. 79–91). Philadelphia, PA: Lippincott Williams & Wilkins.

Joinson, C., Heron, J., von Gontard, A., Butler, U., Golding, J., & Emond, A. (2008). Early childhood risk factors associated with daytime wetting and soiling in school-age children. *Journal of Pediatric Psychology, 33*(7), 739–750.

Maternik, M., Krzeminska, K., & Zurowska, A. (2015). The management of childhood urinary incontinence. *Pediatric Nephrology, 30*(1), 41–50.

Neveus, T., Eggert, P., Evans, J., Macedo, A., Rittig, S., Tekgül, S., et al. (2010). Evaluation of and treatment for monosymptomatic enuresis: A standardization document from the International Children's Continence Society. *Journal of Urology, 183*(2), 441–447.

Neveus, T., von Gontard, A., Hoebeke, P., Hjälmås, K., Bauer, S., Bower, W., et al. (2006). The standardization of terminology of lower urinary tract function in children and adolescents: Report from the Standardization Committee of the International Children's Continence Society. *Journal of Urology, 176*(1), 314–324.

Robson, W. L. (2009). Clinical practice. Evaluation and management of enuresis. *New England Journal of Medicine, 360*(14), 1429–1436.

Steers, W. D. (1997). Physiology and pharmacology of the bladder and urethra. In P. C. Walsh, A. B. Retol, E. D. Vaughan, A. J. Wein (Eds.), *Campbell's urology* (7th ed., pp. 870–916). Philadelphia: WB Saunders.

Tobias, N., Mason, D., Lutkenhoff, M., Stoops, M., & Ferguson, D. (2008). Management principles of organic causes of childhood constipation. *Journal of Pediatric Health Care, 22*(1), 12–23.

Walia, R., Mahajan, L., & Steffen, R. (2009). Recent advances in chronic constipation. *Current Opinion in Pediatrics, 21,* 661–666.

ABNORMAL UTERINE BLEENING

CHAPTER 18

Pilar Bernal de Pheils

I. Introduction and general background

Abnormal uterine bleeding (AUB) is one of the most common presenting healthcare complaints of women. Most commonly the origin of genital bleeding is from the uterus; however, other genital track bleeding etiologies are discussed in this chapter as the evaluation is very similar. AUB is responsible for 25% of all gynecological surgical procedures in the United States (Jain & Santoro, 2005). Menorrhagia (heavy or prolonged menstrual bleeding) alone has been noted as the primary cause for 12% of referrals to gynecological specialty practices (Mohan, Page, & Higham, 2007). Changes in the menstrual cycle accounted for 19.1% of the 20.1 million visits to healthcare providers for gynecological conditions observed in a 2-year study (Nicholson, Ellison, Grason, & Powe, 2001).

Menstruation, ovulation, and the coordinated sequence of endocrine signals that distinguish the menstrual cycle are the foundation for the regularity, predictability, and consistency of menstrual bleeding (Fritz & Speroff, 2011). Although an extensive review of the endocrinology of the menstrual cycle is beyond the scope of this chapter, an overview of the normal menstrual cycle provides important background and context for understanding AUB.

There are essentially three phases to a normal menstrual cycle: (1) the follicular phase, (2) ovulation, and (3) the luteal phase, all of which are managed by the hypothalamic–pituitary–ovarian (HPO) axis, a complicated system of feedback between the hypothalamus, the pituitary, and the ovary (Fritz & Speroff, 2011). During the follicular phase, increasing levels of follicle-stimulating hormone cause the development and maturation of the dominant ovarian follicle, which in turn leads to increased production of estrogen and the proliferation of the endometrium. Increasing levels of estrogen also stimulate a surge of luteinizing hormone and ovulation occurs in response. After ovulation, the corpus luteum, which develops from the dominant ovarian follicle, continues to produce estrogen and also begins to produce progesterone. As this

luteal phase progresses, the corpus luteum continues to enlarge, producing greater levels of progesterone and estrogen, and the endometrium becomes more organized in preparation for implantation. If conception does not occur, the corpus luteum regresses spontaneously on a predictable and stable timetable. With this regression, estrogen and progesterone levels drop rapidly and menstruation begins again. According to Fritz and Speroff (2011), "The sequence of events is so controlling that most ovulatory women have a pattern, volume, and duration of menstrual flow they recognize as their own and come to expect, very often accompanied by an equally consistent and predictable pattern of premenstrual molimina (bloating, breast tenderness, and mood swings)" (p. 593).

New terminology is being adapted to define clinical presentations of abnormal uterine bleeding (Munro, Critchley, & Fraser, 2012). Definitions such as menorrhagia and metrorrhagia have been replaced by heavy or prolonged menstrual bleeding for the former and irregular bleeding for the latter (see **Table 18-1** for a description of new terminology as well as the characteristic of the normal limits of the menstrual cycle/bleeding).

Etiologies of AUB have been recently classified as related or unrelated to uterine structural abnormalities, categorized with the acronym PALM-COEIN (Munro et al., 2011). Structural abnormalities (PALM) are polyps, adenomyosis, leiomyoma, and malignancy/hyperplasia; and nonstructural abnormalities (COEIN) are coagulopathy, ovulatory dysfunction, endometrial, iatrogenic, and not otherwise classified (see **Table 18-2**).

Abnormal uterine bleeding can manifest as acute or chronic. Acute refers to "an episode of bleeding in a woman of reproductive age, who is not pregnant, that, in the opinion of the provider is of sufficient quantity to require immediate intervention to prevent further blood loss" (Munro, Critchley, & Fraser, 2012, p. 3). A woman's perception of menstrual blood loss may differ significantly from the measured amount of blood loss (Hallberg, Högdahl, Nilsson, & Rybo, 1966); as such, a better description that addresses women's concerns is that from the National Institute for Health and Health Care

TABLE 18-1 Clinical Presentations of Abnormal Uterine Bleeding

Clinical presentation	Descriptive terms—New terminology: International Federation of Gynecology and Obstetrics (FIGO) (Munro, Critchley, & Fraser, 2012)	Descriptive terms—Old terminology	Frequency of menses Normal limits (5th to 95th percentiles)
Frequency of menses	Normal		Normal 24–38 days
	Frequent	Polymenorrhea	< 21–24 days
	Infrequent	Oligomenorrhea	> 38 days
	Absent	Amenorrhea	No menses × 3 regular cycles or < 9 cycles × year
Regularity of menses, cycle-to-cycle variation over 12 months (timing)	Regular	Regular	(2–20 days, FIGO) (±5 days)
	Irregular	Metrorrhagia	Variation > 20 days acyclical
Duration of flow	Prolonged	Menorrhagia	> 8.0 days
	Normal		4.5–8 days
	Shortened	Hypomenorrhea	< 4.5 (2 days)
Volume of monthly blood loss	Heavy	Menorrhagia	> 80 cc
	Normal	Normal	5–80 cc
	Light	Hypomenorrhea	< 5 cc

Data from Munro, M G, Critchley, H O, & Fraser, I S. (2012). *American journal of obstetrics and gynecology, 207*(4), 259–265.

Excellence Clinical Guideline, which defines heavy menstrual bleeding as "excessive menstrual blood loss which interferes with the woman's physical, emotional, social and material quality of life, and which can occur alone, or in combination with other symptoms" (National Collaborating Centre for Women's and Children's Health, 2007, p. 35).

Acute uterine bleeding can present without prior occurrences or within the context of chronic abnormal uterine bleeding. Chronic AUB is defined as being present for most of the last 6 months and not needing urgent attention (Munro, Critchley, & Fraser, 2012).

Some episodes of AUB can occur during the women's reproductive years as a result of alterations in the menstrual cycle (frequently seen in perimenopause) or can be superimposed over a regular menstrual cycle. Other less common sites of bleeding are the vagina and vulva or, rarely, the fallopian tubes or ovaries.

When abnormal bleeding occurs before menarche or after menopause, malignancy is a primary concern. Pregnancy should always be considered in women with AUB who are in the reproductive years, as bleeding in early pregnancy can lead to severe health consequences like a ruptured ectopic pregnancy. The reader is referred to an obstetric book for a discussion of the work-up and management of abnormal bleeding in a pregnant patient.

This chapter addresses both acute and chronic AUB in hemodynamically stable patients.

A. PALM (structural) etiologies: Polyps, adenomyosis, leiomyomas, malignancy

1. Definition and overview:
   a. **Polyps** are focal outgrowths of the endometrium, found in the endometrial cavity or in the cervical canal; often seen in association with uterine bleeding in premenopausal and postmenopausal women. Polyps are often asymptomatic and most frequently benign. Bleeding from polyps is uncommon and most likely will present as intermenstrual bleeding.
   b. **Adenomyosis** is a benign condition in which the endometrium invades the myometrium, producing a diffusely enlarged uterus. It causes heavy bleeding and dysmenorrhea, although it may also be asymptomatic. Definite diagnosis is made via uterine pathology after hysterectomy.
   c. **Leiomyomas** are benign tumors originating mainly from myometrium (smooth muscles of the uterus). They are also called myomas and fibroids. Depending on their location in the uterus, they may be subserous (originating at the serosal surface of the uterus), intramural (developing from within the uterine wall), or submucosal (originating from the myometrial cells just underneath the endometrium and may

TABLE 18-2 Abnormal Uterine Bleeding Etiologies Outside of Pregnancy

Classification	Likely Etiology

PALM (structural-organic and pelvic tract pathology)	• Polyps, AUB-P
	Can be found in the cervix or the endometrium.
	• Adenomyosis: AUB-A, benign lesion in the endometrium
	• Leiomyomata: AUB-L$_{SM}$ for submucosal myoma or AUB-L$_O$ for myomas in other layers of the muscle. This distinction is important as the submucosal leiomyomas are the most likely to contribute to the origin of AUB (Munro et al., 2011).
	• Malignancy: is preceded by endometrial hyperplasia, which also causes abnormal bleeding.
	  ☐ Other malignant etiologies to consider are:
	    – Premalignant lesions: cervical dysplasia
	    – Malignant lesions: cervical squamous cell carcinoma, endometrial adenocarcinoma, estrogen- or testosterone-producing ovarian tumors, leiomyosarcoma

COEIN (nonstructural-systemic pathology)	• **Coagulation disorders:**
	Encompasses a spectrum of systemic disorders of hemostasis, most commonly von Willebrand disease. Other conditions to consider are idiopathic thrombocytopenia purpura, coagulation factor deficiencies and other thrombophilias, dysfibrogenemias, disorders like leukemia that produce platelet deficiency, severe sepsis, hypersplenism, severe hepatic or renal disease, and rarely HIV-related thrombocytopenia
	• **Ovulatory dysfunction:** may be due to endocrinopathies (thyroid dysfunction, polycystic ovary syndrome, obesity) and ovulatory disorders that frequently occur at either end of the reproductive age: adolescence and the menopause transition
	  ☐ Other endocrine disorders can produce abnormal uterine bleeding; however, one is more likely to see amenorrhea or oligomenorrhea with:
	    – Hypothalamic dysfunction—habit changes, stress, anxiety, eating disorders, excessive weight loss, aggressive exercise, organic disease
	    – Pituitary diseases—hyperprolactinemia, acromegaly, pituitary adenoma; adrenal diseases—Cushing syndrome, Addison disease, tumors, congenital adrenal hyperplasia
	• **Endometrial:** local endometrial disorders due to homeostasis problems, which are difficult to diagnose (previously called idiopathic AUB), or secondary to local inflammation or infection, most commonly seen with subclinical infection with *Chlamydia trachomatis*. In such cases, bleeding is superimposed on a normal menstrual cycle.
	If no infection is identified, consider as a diagnosis of exclusion.
	  ☐ Other pelvic tract etiology of abnormal bleeding may include:
	    – Infections: salpingitis, cervicitis, endometritis, myometritis, pelvic inflammatory disease, tubo-ovarian abscess
	    – Vulvovaginal trauma: foreign body, abrasions, lacerations, sexual abuse or assault
	Iatrogenic (see under pharmacologic).

| Pharmacologic (the "I" for iatrogenic in the COEIN etiologies) | • Combined estrogen–progestin contraceptives (unscheduled breakthrough bleeding)
• Progestin-only contraceptives (prolonged and spotting, but many develop amenorrhea)
• Intrauterine devices: Nonhormonal (most likely heavy menstrual bleeding, may have spotting); levonorgestrel IUD (most likely spotting, absent bleeding in up to 40% of women at 2 years of use).
• Hormonal therapy: unscheduled postmenopausal bleeding with hormonal treatment
  ☐ Medications interfering with coagulation
    - Anticoagulants
    - Aspirin and other prostaglandin synthetase inhibitors
  ☐ Medications causing dopamine receptor blockade (see Chapter 19)
  ☐ Others
    - Anabolic steroid use
    - Chemotherapeutic medications
    - Herbal and other supplements: ginseng, ginkgo biloba, garlic, ginger, soy
    - Tamoxifen
    - Thyroid replacement hormone |
| Not yet classified | Conditions not demonstrated conclusively to contribute to AUB or others not yet identified by current diagnostic assays |

Data from American College of Obstetrics and Gynecology (ACOG). (2013). Committee opinion no. 557: Management of acute abnormal uterine bleeding in nonpregnant reproductive-aged women. *Obstetrics and Gynecology, 121*(4), 891–896; Munro, M. G., Critchley, H. O., Broder, M. S., et al. (2011). FIGO classification system (PALM-COEIN) for causes of abnormal uterine bleeding in nongravid women of reproductive age. *International Journal of Gynecology and Obstetrics, 113*(1), 3–13.

protrude in different degrees into the uterine cavity).

Leiomyomas may be asymptomatic, although chronic pelvic pain and heavy and prolonged menstrual bleeding is the most common presentation (Khan, Shehmar, & Gupta, 2014). Submucosal leiomyomas are thought to cause AUB although bleeding can be significant regardless of location and size (Doherty, Mutlu, Sinclair, & Taylor, 2014). On physical exam, the uterus can be enlarged and irregular. Growth of leiomyomas is associated with exposure to circulating estrogen; thus, these lesions can grow rapidly in the premenopausal years. Growth of leiomyomas is greater earlier in pregnancy, but early elevation of hormones alone does not sufficiently explain this rapid growth (Benaglia et al., 2014).

d. **Malignancy** and endometrial hyperplasia must be considered in nearly all women of reproductive age when presenting with abnormal vaginal bleeding (AVB) or AUB. Endometrial hyperplasia is the result of endometrial gland proliferation by unopposed chronic estrogen stimulation. It is classified as simple or complex, and both can be seen with or without atypia. Atypical endometrial hyperplasia can progress to adenocarcinoma if left untreated (Fritz & Speroff, 2011; Horn, Meinel, Handzel, & Einenkel, 2007).

2. Prevalence and incidence

Polyps are detected in an estimated 20–40% of women with abnormal uterine bleeding (Lasmar et al., 2008) but are not always the source of bleeding. During the reproductive years, uterine leiomyomas are the most common solid pelvic tumor. They are rarely observed before menarche and significantly decrease in size in the postmenopausal years. The prevalence of these lesions can be up to 70% in Caucasians and 80% in women of African ancestry (Day Baird, Dunson, Hill, Cousins, & Schectman, 2003). Prevalence of adenomyosis varies widely, ranging from 5% to 70% (Dueholm, 2006). Endometrial cancer (EC) is the most common malignancy of the female genital tract in the Western world with an estimated incidence of 39,080 annual new cases in the United States (Jemal, 2007).

B. COEIN etiologies (nonstructural anomalies): coagulopathy, ovulatory, endometrial, iatrogenic, not yet classified

1. Definition and overview

   a. **Coagulopathy** encompasses a variety of systemic disorders of hemostasis that include clotting defects, thrombocytopenia, or platelet/ fibrin function defects. The most common coagulopathy is von Willebrand disease, which is classified as mild, moderate, or severe. Diagnosis occurs usually at menarche, although clinical symptoms can present at any age, with heavy menstrual bleeding being one of the most significant morbidities (ACOG, 2013b; Ng, Motto, & Di Paola, 2015).

   b. **Ovulatory disorders** commonly present with changes in frequency and flow of menses (see Table 18-1). Previously called dysfunctional uterine bleeding, the new term is ovulatory dysfunction. Menstrual bleeding is considered abnormal if it persists for longer than 7 days (prolonged or menorrhagia) or less than 2 days (light or hypomenorrhea); occurs more often than every 21 days (frequent or polymenorrhea); or exceeds a total blood loss of 80 mL (heavy or menorrhagia) (see Table 18-2). Women with anovulatory cycles undergo disrupted and unpredictable patterns of hormonal production that result in irregular and variable menstrual bleeding. These women are essentially in a continuous follicular phase because there is no stimulus for ovulation or subsequent luteal phase development. As a result, the endometrium is continually exposed to estrogen, with resulting proliferation. Ultimately, without the organizing support of progesterone produced during the luteal phase, focal areas of the structurally fragile endometrium begin to break down, leading to a pattern of heavy (menorrhagia) and/or irregular heavy menstrual bleeding (menometrorrhagia) (Fritz & Speroff, 2011).

   c. **Endometrial** etiologies of AUB present as heavy menstrual bleeding in the context of regular predictable menstrual cycles when no other etiology is identified, previously called idiopathic menorrhagia. It is primarily a disorder of the endometrium either due to problems of homeostasis, which currently are difficult to diagnose, or may be secondary to endometrial inflammation or infection (Munro et al., 2011).

   d. **Iatrogenic** etiologies include anticoagulants (such as warfarin and heparin), anticonvulsants, or certain antibiotics (e.g., rifampin and griseofulvin) or medications that influence ovulation, like hormonal medications (estrogens, progestins, or androgens). Because of enhanced hepatic metabolism, cigarette smoking can increase the incidence of breakthrough bleeding in women on hormonal combined contraceptive (Rosenberg, Waugh, & Stevens, 1996).

Systemic medications that interfere with dopamine metabolism resulting in inhibition of prolactin released (e.g., tricyclic antidepressants and phenothiazines) may lead to absent or infrequent menses. See Chapter 19, "Amenorrhea and Polycystic Ovary Syndrome," for a list of medications causing amenorrhea and oligomenorrhea. Hormonal contraceptive agents result in regular withdrawal bleeding when provided in a cyclical manner, although it can be normal for bleeding not to occur in some cycles. Unscheduled bleeding (also called breakthrough bleeding) may be related to missed, delayed, or improper use of hormonal contraceptive methods. Women using progestin-only contraceptives such as levonorgestrel IUS (intrauterine system), the progestin-only pill, or the implant may have unscheduled bleeding. Women on the copper intrauterine device (IUD) may have increased menstrual flow after insertion.

   e. **Not yet classified** etiologies are those conditions that have not been demonstrated conclusively to contribute to AUB or other disorders that have not yet been identified by current diagnostic assays.

2. Prevalence and incidence:

As many as 20% of women with AUB have an underlying coagulation disorder (AGOG, 2013a); a large majority of these women have a variant of von Willebrand disease (VWD). This condition is the most common coagulation disorder in American women (ACOG, 2013b).

Anovulation results in sustained high levels of estrogen, which manifest with heavy and/or irregular bleeding. Examples of this phenomenon are polycystic ovary syndrome (PCOS), obesity, postmenarchal adolescents, and women in their perimenopausal period (Fritz & Speroff, 2011). Anovulation occurs most often at the extremes of reproductive life: soon after menarche due to immaturity of the hypothalamic–pituitary axis and in the years before menopause due to declining ovarian function. AUB is more frequent in the first 18 months postmenarche, particularly in obese teens, whereas AUB in perimenopausal women is a result of intermittent anovulation (ACOG, 2013c). In both scenarios, bleeding patterns are noncyclic and the flow may be heavy or light, with few if any moliminal symptoms (Fritz & Speroff, 2011). After all the underlying problems resulting in AUB are evaluated and addressed, medical treatment to reestablish cycle regularity and provide endometrial protection should be instituted (ACOG, 2013c).

II. Database (may include but is not limited to)

A. Subjective

1. Past medical history (Fritz & Speroff, 2011)

   a. Obstetric history

     i. History of postpartum hemorrhage

     ii. History of pregnancy complicated by leiomyoma

     iii. Recent history of pregnancy ending in miscarriage or abortion

   b. Gynecological history

     i. Gynecological disorders and surgeries including evaluation, findings, and treatment

     ii. Previous episodes of AUB including workup and treatments

     iii. Pap smear history including last Pap smear

     iv. Sexually transmitted infections or upper reproductive tract infection (i.e., pelvic inflammatory disease, tubo-ovarian abscess) Note dates and treatments.

     v. Menstrual cycle history

       a. Age at menarche

       b. Last normal menstrual period

       c. Previous normal menstrual periods (preferably the previous three menses): usual cycle duration, flow, interval length, molimina symptoms (breast tenderness, bloating, mood changes, and dysmenorrhea, which suggest ovulatory cycles)

       d. Date of onset of change in menses: rapid or gradual change

       e. Amount of flow: number of pads or tampons used and degree of saturation. Numerous studies to clarify amounts of blood lost have not been successful or practical, and evaluation ultimately depends on the woman's perception of her blood loss (Hallberg et al., 1996).

       f. Presence of intermenstrual bleeding, premenstrual or postmenstrual bleeding, and postcoital bleeding

     vi. Contraception history: methods, complications, and adverse outcomes

     vii. Future fertility concerns

     viii. Sexual history: number of lifetime sexual partners, and sexual practices

   c. Medical history: medical illnesses (see Table 18-2); general medical health; complete history of any and all medical problems including evaluation and treatments, ongoing and previous

d. Medication history: medications, vitamins, and supplements (see Table 18-2)

e. Trauma: sexual assault or sexual abuse

f. Exposure history: radiation (e.g., breast cancer, thyroid cancer, pelvic malignancies and associated treatments)

2. Family history

a. Gynecological problems: Family history of excessive menstrual blood loss; uterine, breast, and ovarian malignancies, endometriosis, leiomyomata, and diethylstilbestrol exposure

b. Medical diseases: endocrine dysfunction, blood clotting disorders

3. Occupational hazards: e.g., pelvic trauma (motor vehicle accident) or straddle injuries

4. Personal and social history

a. Education, occupation, social and family support systems, situational life stress, social and personal anxiety level, and cultural influences

b. Habits: tobacco

c. Nutrition: dietary history (weight loss or gain)

d. Impact of AVB/AUB on lifestyle (sexual practices, deterrence of exercise, work time loss)

5. Review of systems

a. Constitutional signs: fatigue, weight gain or loss, weakness, malaise, hot or cold sensitivity, appetite change, headaches, obesity, and edema. Suspect hemodynamic instability when patient reports shortness of breath, dizziness, and/or loss of consciousness

b. Skin, hair, and nails: hair loss or unwanted hair growth, petechiae, bruising, jaundice, acne, acanthosis nigricans, and sweating

c. Cardiac: palpitations

d. Abdomen: nausea and bloating

e. Genitourinary: pelvic pain, dyspareunia, dysmenorrhea, hot flashes, night sweats, vaginal dryness, vaginal discharge. Precipitating factors associated with abnormal bleeding (i.e., coitus, trauma, douching, diaphragm use, and the presence of a pessary)

f. Hematologic: suspect bleeding disorder (particularly VWD) when the patient reports heavy menstrual bleeding since menarche; one of the following conditions: excessive blood loss with dental work, postpartum hemorrhage, or surgery-related bleeding; or two or more of the following conditions: epistaxis one to two times per month, frequent gum bleeding, or family history of bleeding symptoms (ACOG, 2013b)

B. Objective (physical examination)

A complete physical examination and assessment of the following systems is essential in the evaluation of a woman complaining of AUB. The following is appropriate for both AUB of structural and nonstructural etiologies.

1. Vital signs (VS): orthostatic VS, temperature, body mass index

2. General: body habitus, posture, stature, motor activity, gait, mood, affect, dress, grooming, and personal hygiene

3. Hair: texture, hirsutism, pattern of loss if present (axillary, pubic, and scalp hair)

4. Eyes and ears: stare, lid lag, exophthalmos, and visual field abnormalities

5. Neck: thyroid nodules or enlargement and lymph nodes

6. Skin: pallor, jaundice, petechiae, ecchymosis, hematomas, palmar erythema, spider hemangiomata, rough or velvety, striae, acanthosis nigricans, acne, color of nail beds

7. Extremities: edema, perfusion, and wasting

8. Cardiovascular: tachycardia and murmurs

9. Lungs: hypoxia and accessory muscle use

10. Abdomen: striae, ascites, hepatomegaly, splenomegaly, tenderness, inguinal nodes, uterine height if palpable

11. Genital/anal

a. External genitalia: pubic hair distribution and developmental stage, clitoromegaly, lesions, edema, cysts, bruising, trauma, urethral prolapse, and atrophy

b. Vagina: traumatic lesions, bruising, erythema, type of discharge, foreign bodies, prolapse, and atrophy

c. Cervix: polyps, eversion, ectopy, lesions, inflammation, erythema, mucopurulent discharge, cervical motion tenderness, atrophy

d. Uterus: enlargement, contour, mobility, shape, consistency, tenderness, and masses

e. Adnexae: masses and tenderness

f. Anus/rectum: masses and bleeding

C. Assessment

1. Determine the appropriate diagnosis.

a. Establish if acute or chronic.

b. Assess for conditions that may underlie AUB—PALM (structural) or COEIN (nonstructural) etiologies (see Table 18-2).

c. Rule out complications of pregnancy in reproductive-age women.

d. Rule out malignancies as indicated.

2. Assess severity of AUB and associated conditions.

3. Assess significance of AUB to the patient and to family and significant others.

4. Evaluate the ability of the patient to adhere to a treatment plan and follow-up.

D. Goals of clinical management

1. Choose a cost-effective approach for screening and evaluating AVB/AUB.

2. Develop a treatment plan that addresses AUB and associated conditions and returns the patient to stability and optimal health in a safe and effective manner.

3. Work with patient to ensure that the plan enables adherence to treatment and follow-up and that is designed to reduce long-term complications AUB such as anemia and endometrial hyperplasia.

E. Plan

1. Diagnostic tests

   As a general rule, the patient's age, reproductive status, and data from the history and physical examination guide decision making regarding the appropriate diagnostic tests. Diagnostic testing is generally organized into three categories: (1) diagnostic tools, (2) initial testing, and (3) secondary or specialty-based testing.

   a. Diagnostic tools.

      i. For patients presenting with a history of irregular cycles, menstrual calendars can be very helpful to establish bleeding patterns. Several online sites are available but may include product advertisements and potentially biased information (e.g., www.MyMonthlyCycles.com). Number of pads or tampons and degree of saturation are of limited use in evaluation of blood loss (Hallberg et al., 1996).

   b. Initial testing (**Table 18-3a**).

   c. Secondary and specialty-based testing (**Table 18-3b**). These tests are often done by or in consultation with gynecology and women's health specialists.

2. Treatment and management

   Therapeutic management of AUB depends on the acuity, chronicity, and etiology of the disorder along with the goals of the woman, including her desire for pregnancy and the long-term consequences of any underlying medical conditions.

   a. Acute hemorrhagic bleeding

      Patients with acute hemorrhagic bleeding who are hemodynamically unstable (signs of hypovolemia, including orthostatic changes on physical examination) or who have a positive pregnancy test, warrant urgent referral to gynecology. Clinical evaluation and management of such patients are beyond the scope of this discussion.

   b. Acute heavy bleeding in the hemodynamically stable woman

      i. Hormonal management (combined oral contraceptives and progestins) is in most cases sufficient (ACOG, 2013a). For non-pregnant women of reproductive age, the goal of initial therapy is to stabilize the endometrial lining, prevent recurrence, and establish regular, orderly, and synchronous bleeding patterns. Hormonal therapies are equally effective in most cases for the management of acute heavy menstrual bleeding. The following regimens have been studied and found to be effective (Munro, Mainor, Basu, Brisinger, & Barreda, 2006):

         a. 35 ethinyl estradiol/1 mg norethindrone combined oral contraceptive (COC) taken by mouth daily three times a day for 7 days followed by 35 ethinyl estradiol/1 mg norethindrone daily for the next 3 weeks.

         b. Medroxyprogesterone acetate (MPA) 20 mg taken by mouth 3 times daily for 7 days followed by MPA 20 mg daily for 3 weeks.

            Compliance was higher in MPA than COC group. All of the MPA group and 95% of COC group avoided emergency surgical procedures. Eighty-eight percent of the COC group and 76% of MPA group achieved cessation of bleeding. The median time to bleeding cessation was 3 days for both groups. Compliance was higher in the MPA than in the COC group. (Munro et al., 2006).

         c. A third alternative treatment can also be considered: MPA 20 mg taken by mouth 3 times daily for 3 days plus depo medroxyprogesterone acetate (DMPA) 150 mg intramuscular, once. All patients stopped bleeding within 5 days, with a mean time to bleeding cessation of 2.6 days, with infrequent side effects and high patient satisfaction (Ammerman & Nelson, 2013).

            If desired, the patient may continue with COC to prevent anovulatory bleeding; otherwise the women will experience regular COC withdrawal.

TABLE 18-3A Essential Initial Testing in the Investigation of Abnormal Uterine Bleeding

Test	Definition	Clinical Implications	Comments
Urine pregnancy test (urine hCG)	Measures the beta subunit of human chorionic gonadotropin hormone (B-hCG). Urine hCG is a qualitative measurement of B-hCG and gives negative or positive results.	A positive urine pregnancy test (qualitative) warrants ordering a pelvic sonogram. If intrauterine sac is not visible, a quantitative serum B-hCG should be ordered and guide referral to an obstetrics specialty clinic (Fritz & Speroff, 2011; Levine, 2006)	Urine pregnancy test should be ordered in all sexually active women in their reproductive years, even those who have had a tubal ligation (ACOG, 2013a)
Complete blood count (CBC) with platelets	To assess the presence of significant anemia and bleeding disorders	Excessive vaginal bleeding can lead to iron deficiency anemia. CBC and platelet count are some of the initial tests in the investigation of von Willebrand disease.	Because the prevalence of blood dyscrasias (particularly von Willebrand diseases) in adolescents can be quite high (5–20%), and may present with heavy menstrual bleeding at menarche, routine screening for coagulation disorders is appropriate (ACOG, 2013b).
Highly sensitive thyroid-stimulating hormone (TSH)	Measurement of thyroid-stimulating hormone: an anterior pituitary hormone that stimulates growth and function of thyroid cells	An elevated TSH is diagnostic of primary hypothyroidism; a low TSH indicates hyperthyroidism (both can be implicated in AUB)	Thyroid disease is common in women. See Chapter 69 for more information on diagnostic testing and treatment.
Pap smear	To screen for cervical cancer	Early cervical cancer is frequently asymptomatic. Late cervical cancer may manifest as irregular, heavy, or postcoital bleeding (Monk & Tewari, 2007).	Endocervical and ectocervical sampling required for accuracy. See Chapter 20 for more discussion.
Testing for *Neisseria gonorrhoeae* (GC) and *Chlamydia trachomatis* (CT)	Gold standard method to test for *GC* and *CT* is nucleic acid amplification test (NAAT)	Cervicitis, caused by *GC* or *CT*, can cause postcoital or intermenstrual bleeding	As indicated for sexually active women. It can be collected in the endocervix or in the vagina. First-catch urine (no clean catch) can also be submitted to NAAT testing.
Wet mount of vaginal secretions with normal saline and potassium hydroxide	Evaluate for vaginal infections: trichomoniasis, bacterial vaginosis, and vulvovaginal candidiasis	Severe trichomoniasis, vulvovaginal candida, bacterial vaginosis, and may present with postcoital bleeding	Useful only if the woman is not bleeding heavily and vaginitis is suspected

Transvaginal ultrasonography of the pelvis (TVS)	Ultrasound imaging (most important, transvaginal) plays a pivotal role in the evaluation of AUB	a. Indicated to rule out anatomical lesions (endometrial polyps, leiomyomas, or adenomyosis), women with regular cycles but heavy menstrual bleeding or long duration or intermenstrual bleeding (Dueholm, 2006; Valentin, 2014), and when medical management has failed (Fritz & Speroff, 2011). b. To measure the thickness of the endometrial lining in the postmenopausal woman. If the lining is 4 mm or less, endometrial cancer is very unlikely (Giannella et al., 2014). c. In the evaluation of AUB in pregnancy. d. In the evaluation of adnexal and ovarian masses.	Leiomyomas are very common beginning in the third decade of life, and heavy menstrual bleeding is the most common symptom of leiomyoma (most commonly of submucosal origin), thus altering the endometrial lining. However, most leiomyomas are not the major cause of abnormal uterine bleeding, and the evaluation of abnormal uterine bleeding should not necessarily cease with this finding. In the case of asymptomatic leiomyomas, treatment is not mandatory (Bignardi, Van den Bosch, & Condous, 2009; Fritz & Speroff, 2011). For women on cyclic hormone therapy, do TVS after the progestin withdrawal bleed (Bignardi et al., 2009).
Endometrial biopsy (EMB)	Office sampling of the endometrium with low-pressure cannula (e.g., Pipelle), evaluates for the presence of endometrial hyperplasia and cancer	All women > 35 years of age with suspected anovulatory bleeding should be evaluated for endometrial hyperplasia and cancer (after excluding pregnancy). Endometrial cancer is more common in older women. However abnormal endometrial histology in premenopausal woman with irregular bleeding is relatively high—14%; or at any age if the duration of unopposed estrogen is significant (Fritz & Speroff, 2011). EMB is indicated in obese women who have prolonged bleeding. EMB is also indicated in postmenopausal women who are not on hormone therapy or in those who have been on hormone therapy for 6 months or more with unpredicted and unscheduled bleeding episodes (Fritz & Speroff, 2011).	Incidence of endometrial carcinoma in women ages 40–54 years is 17.8%, increasing to 34.2% at ages 55–64. Obesity, high blood pressure, and diabetes mellitus may increase the risk of endometrial cancer (http://seer.cancer.gov/statfacts/).

TABLE 18-3B Second-Line Testing in the Investigation of AUB, Including Tests Where Consultation or Referral Is Suggested

Test	Definition	Clinical Implications	Comments
Coagulation panel: prothrombin time, partial thromboplastin time, bleeding time	Second-line testing when coagulation disorder is suspected	Abnormal coagulation panel tests indicate coagulopathies	Abnormalities warrant a referral to hematology (ACOG, 2013b)
Ristocetin cofactor assay	Measures the ability of a patient's plasma to agglutinate in the presence of the antibiotic Ristocetin. Related to the concentration and functional activity of the von Willebrand factor	Evaluation for von Willebrand disease is appropriate in adolescents, women with a worrisome family history, and in the case of unexplained menorrhagia.	These tests should be ordered and interpreted in conjunction with hematology (ACOG, 2013b).
Magnetic resonance imaging (MRI)	MRI is a noninvasive imaging technology	Should be reserved for those women in whom adenomyosis diagnosis by TVS is inconclusive (Dueholm, 2006). MRI can help evaluate masses, adenomyosis, and the presence of endometrial polyps	MRI has a greater cost than TVS. Consult with physician.
Saline infusion sonography (sonohysterography)	Visualizes the contours of the uterine cavity	Indicated when polyps are not clearly identified with TVS	Safe and highly sensitive. Specific imaging used for the diagnosis of endometrial polyps (Radwan, Radwan, Kozarzewski, Polac, & Wilczyński, 2014).
Hysteroscopy	A small lighted scope is inserted via cervix into the uterus to visualize the endometrial cavity. Also allows for instrumentation as described in next column. Usually performed by gynecologist.	Direct visualization of the endometrium allows for: • Assessment of intrauterine adhesions • Assessment and removal of submucosal fibroids or endometrial polyps • Removal of embedded intrauterine devices (IUDs) • Assessment and biopsy of any lesions for pathologic evaluation (Farquhar, Ekeroma, Furness, & Arroll, 2003; Bignardi et al., 2009)	This instrumentation can be performed in the office setting by MD specialist to remove small endometrial lesions.
Biopsy		Indicated for suspicious vulvar, vaginal, or cervical lesion.	
Dilatation and curettage (D&C)		Indicated for severe acute bleeding events where hypovolemia is present or where suspicion of malignancy is high. It is valuable for the removal of endometrial polyps and for histologic diagnosis when endometrial sampling has been unsuccessful or inadequate.	This instrumentation can be performed in the office setting by gynecology specialist, often in conjunction with hysteroscopy. D&C can also be a curative treatment for AUB.

High-dose estrogen therapy and COC are both contraindicated in any woman at risk of or with a personal or family history of thromboembolic events.

c. Chronic bleeding

While the acute bleeding is being controlled, the clinician should initiate a diagnostic investigation to determine the underlying etiology. Table 18-3a will promptly assist the clinician in evaluation and long-term management of AUB. If pregnancy is desired, the clinician should promptly consult or refer the woman to an infertility specialist as AUB etiologies and their management may prevent or complicate pregnancy. Otherwise, some of the PALM etiologies (structural: adenomyosis and leiomyomas) and intractable heavy bleeding may ultimately be treated with surgery; however, pharmacologic management can be attempted as the initial treatment and, if successful, as a long-term treatment.

Management of chronic bleeding is addressed in three sections:

i. Common long-term pharmacology therapies for the management of heavy menstrual bleeding (addressing medical therapies for AUB in patients diagnosed with adenomyosis, leiomyomas, coagulation disorders, and idiopathic endometrial conditions): after includes progestin IUS, combined hormonal contraceptives, depo-medroxyprogesterone acetate, nonsteroidal anti-inflammatory drugs (NSAIDs), and gonadotropin-releasing hormone agonists.

a. Levonorgestrel-releasing IUD (Mirena®). LNG20-IUS has been observed to reduce heavy menstrual bleeding by 75–95% after 3 to 12 months of use (Doherty et al., 2014; Lethaby, Irvine, & Cameron, 2003). LNG20-IUS is very cost effective compared to hysterectomies for the management of heavy menstrual blood loss (Edlund, 2011; Ganz et al., 2013). In women with a maximum 12-week-size uterus without cavity distortion, LNG-IUS is a safe and effective treatment option for heavy menstrual bleeding characteristic of leiomyomas (Doherty et al., 2014). This IUD has been shown to work well in larger uteruses with cavity distortion; however, placement by an experienced clinician under sonogram guidance is advised. Limited data suggest that the LNG-IUS is equally effective in women with adenomyosis (Bitzer, Heikinheimo, Fraser, Calaf-Alsina, & Fraser, 2015).

b. Combined oral contraceptives (COC): COC may reduce heavy menstrual flow by promoting the development of an atrophic endometrium and can increase levels of factor VIII and von Willebrand factor, combating potential underlying coagulopathies (ACOG, 2013c). Oral contraceptive pills will not improve symptoms related to fibroid size. However, they are inexpensive and may be used as first-line therapy in patients with fibroids and heavy menstrual bleeding (Doherty et al., 2014). Daily cyclic use (withdrawal every 28 days), sequential withdrawal (every 90 days), or continuous use may be considered as treatment strategies and is particularly helpful for patients with anemia. Sequential withdrawal and continuous use require careful counseling to improve adherence.

c. Progestin-only treatment of leiomyomas with depo-medroxyprogesterone acetate (DMPA) may improve bleeding parameters and increase hemoglobin with a modest reduction in leiomyoma volume (Doherty et al., 2014).

d. NSAIDS have been observed to reduce heavy menstrual flow in several studies, possibly by reducing prostaglandin levels in the endometrium by enzyme (cyclo-oxygenase) inhibition (Lethaby, Augood, Duckitt, & Farquhar, 2007; Fritz & Speroff, 2011). Efficacy of NSAIDs in women with leiomyomas with heavy bleeding is limited (Bitzer et al., 2015). NSAIDS do not appear to reduce blood loss in women with myomas but can help to decrease painful menses. Counseling regarding the potential for gastrointestinal side effects should be provided. Options include:

i. Ibuprofen: 600 mg orally three times a day for the first 3 days of menses, or longer as needed.

ii. Naproxen sodium: 500 mg at onset and followed 3 to 5 hours later. Then 250 to 500 mg twice a day for the first 3 days. May continue throughout the menstrual cycle.

   iii. Mefenamic acid: 500 mg by mouth 3 times daily for the first 3 days of menses or for the duration of the cycle, as needed.

e. Gonadotropin-releasing hormone agonists, such as depo leuprolide (Lupron®), 3.75 mg intramuscularly monthly or 11.25 mg every 90 days, or nafarelin, 0.2–0.4 mg intranasally twice a day, can be useful for short-term management of heavy menstrual bleeding, particularly in the setting of leiomyoma or adenomyosis, as they reduce fibroid and uterine volume (Doherty et al., 2014). However, this therapy is limited to short-term use because of its expense and unpleasant side effects (menopausal vasomotor symptoms and bone loss), which resolve after discontinuation of therapy. Therefore, these medications are most often used as a preoperative adjunctive therapy for women intending conservative (myomectomy or endometrial ablation) or definitive (hysterectomy) surgery for abnormal bleeding and should be done in close collaboration with a gynecologist.

For perimenopausal women, the methods listed previously are all appropriate.

ii. Therapeutic management of ovulatory dysfunction and the management of simple endometrial hyperplasia without atypia. The goals for management of ovulatory dysfunction are to eliminate acute bleeding and its complications, to prevent future episodes, and to reduce the patient's lifetime risk of complications arising from long-term anovulation (endometrial hyperplasia and cancer). Treatment should induce or reestablish regular patterns of menstrual bleeding (ACOG, 2013c). Adherence issues may complicate treatment, because heavy bleeding may continue for several cycles after one of the treatment strategies for acute presentation has been initiated. Counseling the patient regarding treatment approaches and long-term goals improves adherence.

Treatment options include hormonal medications with and without contraceptive effects.

a. Combined estrogen and progestin contraceptive options include:

   i. Low-dose, monophasic COC, the contraceptive vaginal ring, or transdermal contraceptive patch: this treatment is contraindicated for women over 35 who smoke, women with evidence of vascular disease, or those with a personal or family history of thromboembolic events (ACOG, 2013c).

b. Progestin-only medications include:

   i. Levonorgestrel 20 IUS. Treatment of endometrial hyperplasia is generally more effective than with systemic progesterone treatments, and should be offered as a first line treatment (Abu Hashim, Ghayaty, & El Rakhawy, 2015). Management should be done in consultation with MD, and close follow-up is advisable (Bitzer et al., 2015).

   ii. Subdermal implant releasing etonogestrel 68 mg over a 3-year period (Nexplanon®). Indicated for women with ovulatory dysfunction. Not studied for the management of endometrial hyperplasia.

   iii. Depo-MPA (Depo-Provera®), 150 mg intramuscularly every 12 weeks. Indicated for women with ovulatory dysfunction.

c. Progestins without contraceptive activity

   i. Medroxyprogesterone acetate (MPA), 10 mg by mouth daily for the first 10–14 days of each month for three to six cycles, with careful follow-up. Alternatively, continuing monthly cyclic MPA induces regular withdrawal and reduces the likelihood for long-term complications of anovulation. However, it does not provide pregnancy protection (Fritz & Speroff, 2011).

   ii. Norethindrone acetate, 5–10 mg orally once to three times a day for the first 10–14 days of each month.

   iii. Micronized progesterone, 200 mg orally twice a day for the first

10–14 days of each month (Hickey, Higham, & Fraser, 2009).

iii. Surgical options managed by the gynecologist. Complex endometrial hyperplasia, hyperplasia with atypia, or cancer is managed by the gynecologist and is beyond the scope of this chapter.

a. Polyps: best managed with removal, most likely with hysteroscopy.

b. Leiomyoma: myomectomy; uterine fibroid: embolization or hysterectomy.

c. D&C is most commonly considered in the acute care setting.

d. Conservative management with endometrial ablation can be done with hysteroscopic guidance or with newer "blind" techniques. In all cases the goal is to prevent further menorrhagia by eliminating the endometrium. Not indicated for women who desire further childbearing, who are menopausal, or who are at high risk of endometrial cancer. Because endometrial ablation can be done in the office or an outpatient surgical unit, it is less costly than hysterectomy, involves less risk of surgical complications, and requires less recovery time. It is appropriate for women with conditions that make them poor candidates for major surgery (Fritz & Speroff, 2011; Lethaby, Hickey, Garry, & Penninx, 2009).

e. Hysterectomy remains the definitive treatment for menorrhagia and all abnormal bleeding patterns. It is appropriate for cases where treatment has failed or has been too noxious to tolerate, and where childbearing is no longer desired.

iv. Postmenopausal bleeding
Both endometrial biopsy and D&C provide information regarding the state of the endometrium, including evaluation for the presence of endometrial carcinoma. The pathologic examination of the sample identifies the presence of hyperplasia, atypia, polyps, and other endometrial lesions. The presence of atypia is of particular importance in determining an appropriate treatment plan (Fritz & Speroff, 2011).

An initial transvaginal ultrasound (TVUS) finding of an endometrial lining less than or equal to 4 mm may reduce the need for endometrial sampling in some cases, but EMB together with TVUS establishes the most precise diagnosis (Farquhar et al., 2003). If atypia is not present, cyclic or daily progestin therapy with MPA or norethindrone acetate every month for 3 months may be considered, followed by resampling. Close follow-up is strongly recommended and evaluation should be accelerated if abnormal bleeding patterns recur. The presence of atypia mandates specialty consultation for further evaluation, and hysterectomy is generally recommended. For postmenopausal women on hormone therapy, EMB findings can guide dose adjustments once endometrial pathology has been excluded.

F. **Additional considerations and follow-up**

1. All patients should be evaluated for anemia and treated as needed. Specialty referral should be instituted for:

a. Patients with suspected coagulation disorders

b. When medical treatment fails or AUB is persistent or recurrent

2. Patients with acute bleeding require follow-up soon after initiation of therapy to evaluate for further bleeding or to evaluate for success of treatment.

a. The schedule of follow-up care varies depending on the etiology (PALM or COEIN) and treatment of AUB and associated conditions.

b. Assessment at regular intervals should be established as warranted (i.e., 3–6 months, or as needed).

c. For leiomyomas, evaluation for symptoms and growth may be done every year, although TVUS may not be required if symptoms remain unchanged.

G. **Client education**

1. Information: ACOG provides many educational pamphlets available online: http://www.acog.org /Resources-And-Publications/Patient-Education-FAQs-List

2. Counseling: detailed explanation of the etiologies of AUB, essential diagnostic tests, and treatment plans is imperative for patient understanding and adherence. Patient involvement in the decision-making process, inclusion of family members when desired, and consideration of cultural issues are essential for promoting adherence. The clinician should:

a. Discuss medication side effects, risks versus benefits, and expected outcomes (e.g., withdrawal bleeding after progestin therapy).

b. Discuss all treatment options (medical versus surgical) and initiate referrals to specialists or surgeons.

c. Consider associated issues, such as weight management, interference with exercise, stress management, and management of chronic disorders. Referral for psychologic support may be necessary.

3. Self-management resources and tools

a. The most important tool for the patient is the menstrual calendar. Selected resources include:

i. American Society for Reproductive Medicine (http://www.asrm.org/)

ii. *Harvard Women's Health Watch* is a monthly publication providing information regarding issues in women's health written by the researchers and clinicians at Harvard Medical School (www.harvardwomenshealthwatch.org/)

REFERENCES

Abu Hashim, H., Ghayaty, E., & El Rakhawy, M. (2015). Levonorgestrel-releasing intrauterine system vs oral progestins for non-atypical endometrial hyperplasia: A systematic review and metaanalysis of randomized trials. *American Journal of Obstetrics and Gynecology.* Epub ahead of print.

American College of Obstetricians and Gynecologists (ACOG). (2013a). Committee opinion no. 557: Management of acute abnormal uterine bleeding in nonpregnant reproductive-aged women. *Obstetrics and Gynecology, 121*(4), 891–896.

American College of Obstetricians and Gynecologists (ACOG). (2013b). Committee Opinion No. 580: von Willebrand disease in women. *Obstetrics and Gynecology, 122*(6), 1368–1373.

American College of Obstetricians and Gynecologists (ACOG). (2013c). Practice bulletin no. 136: management of abnormal uterine bleeding associated with ovulatory dysfunction. *Obstetrics and Gynecology, 122*(1), 176–185.

Ammerman, S. R., & Nelson, A. L. (2013). A new progestogen-only medical therapy for outpatient management of acute, abnormal uterine bleeding: A pilot study. *American Journal of Obstetrics and Gynecology, 208*(6), 499–500.

Benaglia, L., Cardellicchio, L., Filippi, F., Paffoni, A., Vercellini, P., Somigliana, E., et al. (2014). The rapid growth of fibroids during early pregnancy. *PLoS ONE, 9*(1), e85933.

Bignardi, T., Van den Bosch, T., & Condous, G. (2009). Abnormal uterine bleeding and post-menopausal bleeding in the acute gynaecology unit. *Best Practice and Research Clinical Obstetrics and Gynecology, 23,* 595–607.

Bitzer, J., Heikinheimo, O., Nelson, A. L., Calaf-Alsina, J., & Fraser I. S. (2015). Medical management of heavy menstrual bleeding: A comprehensive review of the literature. *Obstetrical & Gynecological Survey, 70*(2), 115–130.

Day Baird, D., Dunson, D. B., Hill, M. C., Cousins, D., & Schectman, J. M. (2003). High cumulative incidence of uterine leiomyoma in black and white women: Ultrasound evidence. *American Journal of Obstetrics & Gynecology, 188*(1), 100–107.

Doherty, L., Mutlu, L., Sinclair, D., & Taylor, H. (2014). Uterine fibroids: clinical manifestations and contemporary management. *Reproductive Sciences, 21*(9), 1067–1092.

Dueholm, M. (2006). Transvaginal ultrasound for diagnosis of adenomyosis: A review. *Best Practice Research Clinical Obstetrics & Gynecology, 20*(4), 569–582.

Edlund, M. (2011). Nonhormonal treatments for heavy menstrual bleeding. *Journal of Women's Health, 20,* 1645–1653.

Farquhar, C., Ekeroma, A., Furness, S., & Arroll, B. (2003). A systematic review of transvaginal ultrasonography, sonohysterography and hysteroscopy for the investigation of abnormal uterine bleeding in premenopausal women. *Acta Obstetricia et Gynecologica Scandinavica, 82,* 493–504.

Fritz, M. A., & Speroff, L. (2011). Abnormal uterine bleeding. In *Clinical gynecologic endocrinology and infertility* (8th ed., pp. 591–620). Philadelphia, PA: Wolters Kluwer/Lippincott Williams & Wilkins.

Ganz, M. L., Shah, D., Gidwani, R., Filonenko, A., Su, W., Pocoski, J., et al. (2013). The cost-effectiveness of the levonorgestrel-releasing intrauterine system for the treatment of idiopathic heavy menstrual bleeding in the United States. *Value in Health, 16*(2), 325–333.

Giannella, L., Mfuta, K., Setti, T., Cerami, L. B., Bergamini, E., et al. (2014). A risk-scoring model for the prediction of endometrial cancer among symptomatic postmenopausal women with endometrial thickness > 4 mm. *BioMed Research International.* dx.doi.org/10.1155/2014/130569

Hallberg, L., Högdahl, A. M., Nilsson, L., & Rybo, G. (1966). Menstrual blood loss—a population study. Variation at different ages and attempts to define normality. *Acta Obstetricia et Gynecologica Scandinavica, 45*(3), 320–351.

Hickey, M., Higham, J. M., & Fraser, I. (2009). Progestogens versus oestrogens and progestogens for irregular uterine bleeding associated with anovulation (review). *Cochrane Database System Review, 4,* CD001895.

Horn, L., Meinel, A., Handzel, R., & Einenkel, J. (2007). Histopathology of endometrial hyperplasia and endometrial carcinoma: An update. *Annals of Diagnostic Pathology, 11*(4), 297–311.

Jain, A., & Santoro, N. (2005). Endocrine mechanisms and management of abnormal bleeding due to perimenopausal changes. *Clinical Obstetrics and Gynecology, 48*(2), 295–311.

Jemal A., Siegel, R., Ward, E., Murray, T., Xu, J., & Thun, M. J. (2007). Cancer statistics, 2007. *CA: A Cancer Journal for Clinicians, 57,* 43–66.

Khan, A. T., Shehmar, M., & Gupta, J. K. (2014). Uterine fibroids: Current perspectives. *International Journal of Women's Health, 6,* 95–114.

Lasmar, R. B., Dias, R., Barrozo, P. R., Oliveira, M. A., Coutinho, E. S., & da Rosa, D. B. (2008). Prevalence of hysteroscopic findings and histologic diagnoses in patients with abnormal uterine bleeding. *Fertility & Sterility, 89,* 1803–1807.

Lethaby, A., Augood, C., Duckitt, K., & Farquhar, C. (2007). Nonsteroidal anti-inflammatory drugs for heavy menstrual bleeding (review). *Cochrane Database of Systematic Reviews, 4,* CD000400.

Lethaby, A., Hickey, M., Garry, R., & Penninx, J. (2009). Endometrial resection/ablation techniques for heavy menstrual bleeding. *Cochrane Database Systematic Reviews,* CD001501.

Lethaby, A., Irvine, G., & Cameron, I. (2003). Cyclical progestogens for heavy menstrual bleeding (review). *Cochrane Database of Systematic Reviews,* CD001016.

Levine, S. (2006). Dysfunctional uterine bleeding in adolescents. *Journal of Pediatric Adolescent Gynecology, 19,* 49–51.

Mohan, S., Page, L. M., & Higham, J. M. (2007). Diagnosis of abnormal uterine bleeding. *Best Practice & Research in Clinical Obstetrics and Gynecology, 21*(6), 891–903.

Monk, B. J., & Tewari, K. S. (2007). Invasive cervical cancer. In P. J. Di Saia & W. T. Creasman (Eds.), *Clinical gynecologic oncology* (7th ed., pp. 55–124). Philadelphia, PA: Mosby.

Munro, M. G., Critchley, H. O., & Fraser, I. S. (2012). The FIGO systems for nomenclature and classification of causes of abnormal uterine bleeding in the reproductive years: Who needs them? *American Journal of Obstetrics and Gynecology, 207*(4), 259–265.

Munro, M. G., Critchley, H. O., Broder, M. S., Fraser, I. S., & FIGO Working Group on Menstrual Disorders. (2011). FIGO classification system (PALM-COEIN) for causes of abnormal uterine bleeding in nongravid women of reproductive age. *International Journal of Gynecology and Obstetrics, 113*(1), 3–13.

Munro, M. G., Mainor, N., Basu, R., Brisinger, M., & Barreda, L. (2006). Oral medroxyprogesterone acetate and combination oral contraceptives for acute uterine bleeding: A randomized controlled trial. *Obstetrics & Gynecology, 108*, 924–929.

National Collaborating Centre for Women's and Children's Health. Heavy menstrual bleeding (NICE Clinical Guidelines, No. 44).

London: RCOG Press, Retrieved from http://www.ncbi.nlm.nih.gov/books/NBK56536/.

Ng, C., Motto, D. G., & Di Paola, J. (2015). Diagnostic approach to von Willebrand disease. *Blood, 125*(13), 2029–2037.

Nicholson, W. K., Ellison, S. A., Grason, H., & Powe, N. R. (2001). Patterns of ambulatory care use for gynecologic conditions: A national study. *American Journal of Obstetrics and Gynecology, 184*(4), 523–530.

Radwan, P., Radwan, M., Kozarzewski, M., Polac, I., & Wilczyński, J. (2014). Evaluation of sonohysterography in detecting endometrial polyps—241 cases followed with office hysteroscopies combined with histopathological examination. *Wideochirurgia i Inne Techniki Maloinwazyjne, 9*(3), 344–350.

Rosenberg, M. J., Waugh, M. S., & Stevens, C. M. (1996). Smoking and cycle control among oral contraceptive users. *American Journal of Obstetrics & Gynecology, 174*(2), 628–632.

Valentin, L. (2014). Imaging techniques in the management of abnormal vaginal bleeding in non-pregnant women before and after menopause. Best practice & research. *Clinical Obstetrics & Gynecology, 28*(5), 637–654.

AMENORRHEA AND POLYCYSTIC OVARY SYNDROME

Pilar Bernal de Pheils

CHAPTER 19

I. Introduction and general background

Amenorrhea is classified as primary or secondary. Primary amenorrhea is defined as the lack of initiation of menses by age 13 with concomitant lack of growth of secondary sexual characteristics, such as breast development. If growth of secondary sexual characteristics is present, this diagnosis may be delayed until age 15, or within 5 years of breast development, if this happens before age 10 (Practice Committee of the American Society for Reproductive Medicine, 2008). Secondary amenorrhea is defined as menstrual cessation after three previous regular menstrual cycles or irregular menses (oligomenorrhea) or less than nine menstrual cycles per year (Practice Committee of the American Society for Reproductive Medicine, 2008).

Distinguishing primary and secondary amenorrhea is important because the former encompasses a more extensive differential diagnosis that includes genetic or anatomic abnormalities. As the most likely diagnosis is constitutional delay, early categorization may lead to an unnecessary work-up (Fritz & Speroff, 2011).

Amenorrhea may result from disturbances at the level of the hypothalamus, pituitary, ovaries, uterus, or outflow tract or may result from chronic illness or other endocrine abnormalities. Polycystic ovarian syndrome (PCOS) is one of the most common causes of amenorrhea, with disturbances that involve the hypothalamic–pituitary–ovarian (HPO) axis. Amenorrhea is physiologic during pregnancy, menopause, and in the postpartum period in lactating women. It can also be iatrogenic caused by hormonal contraception, exogenous androgens, or medications blocking dopamine receptors.

A. Hypothalamic amenorrhea

1. Definition and overview

   Hypothalamic amenorrhea is often used interchangeably with functional hypothalamic amenorrhea (FHA), the most common cause of amenorrhea in this category. In FHA, there is a decrease in gonadotropin-releasing hormone pulsatile secretion causing absent midcycle surges in luteinizing hormone secretion, failure to ovulate, and low serum estradiol concentrations. Low estrogen levels place the woman at risk for osteopenia and osteoporosis. Factors contributing to FHA include nutritional deficiencies, such as marked weight loss, malnutrition, eating disorders (anorexia and bulimia), excessive exercise, and severe physical or emotional stress. In many women with FHA, no obvious precipitating factor is evident.

   Untreated primary hypothyroidism can lead to hypothalamic amenorrhea (primary or secondary) by decreasing the hypothalamic content of dopamine and increasing prolactin levels with or without resulting galactorrhea (Khawaja et al., 2006). Dopaminergic drugs (e.g., phenothiazines, antipsychotics, and antiemetic-gastrointestinal agents) may also be responsible for hypothalamic amenorrhea. Menses usually return to normal after discontinuation of medications. Rarely, hypothalamic amenorrhea may be associated with congenital GnRH deficiency, called Kallmann syndrome, if there is associated anosmia or hyposmia (Fritz & Speroff, 2011).

2. Prevalence and incidence

   Prevalence of adult-onset hypothalamic amenorrhea is 35%, representing 20% of primary amenorrhea cases (Reindollar, Byrd, & McDonough, 1981; Reindollar, Novak, Tho, & McDonough, 1986). The "female athlete triad" is defined as amenorrhea, disordered eating, and osteoporosis or osteopenia. This syndrome is especially common in amenorrhea associated with ballet dancing. It is also prevalent in high school (Hoch et al., 2009) and college athletes (Beals & Hill, 2006).

B. Amenorrhea associated with pituitary dysfunction

1. Definition and overview

   Prolactin-secreting tumors are responsible for most cases of amenorrhea attributed to the pituitary gland. Increased prolactin levels lead to anovulation and low ovarian estradiol levels, causing the same problems as seen in FHA. Hyperprolactinemia can cause galactorrhea. Most prolactinomas are small (< 10 mm in diameter), called microadenomas, and maintain normal pituitary function. Macroadenomas are 10 mm or larger and can exert mass effects causing headaches and vision changes. Prolactin-secreting tumors can occur in the premenarchal female and present as primary amenorrhea.

Pituitary functional tumors should be suspected when patients have acromegaly caused by excessive secretion of growth hormone, Cushing's disease caused by excessive secretion of adrenocorticotropic hormone, or secondary hyperthyroidism caused by a thyroid-stimulating hormone secreting tumor. These tumors are rare but potential causes of amenorrhea. Most of these tumors are associated with headaches and visual changes (bitemporal hemianopsia/blurred vision) (Fritz & Speroff, 2011).

Hyperprolactinemia can also be caused by decreased clearance of dopamine in patients with chronic renal or liver impairment. Other causes of pituitary amenorrhea are Sheehan syndrome (severe postpartum hemorrhage causing acute infarction and necrosis of the pituitary gland) and empty sella syndrome. Hyperprolactinemia may be functional (idiopathic), found in about one-third of women (Fritz & Speroff, 2011).

2. Prevalence and incidence
Prolactin-secreting pituitary tumor (prolactinoma) is responsible for almost 20% of cases of secondary amenorrhea and is the most common pituitary etiology of amenorrhea (Reindollar et al., 1986). Pituitary disease is less common in primary amenorrhea, accounting for 5% of cases (Reindollar et al., 1981).

C. Amenorrhea originating from disorders of the ovaries

1. Definition and overview
   a. Polycystic ovarian syndrome (PCOS) (discussed later as a separate category).
   b. Primary ovarian insufficiency (POI), also known as premature ovarian failure, is defined as menopause before the age of 40. The average age of menopause is 51 with a range from 47–55. Ovarian insufficiency is more accepted as this condition may have periods of follicular development, ovulation, and menstrual bleeding followed by periods of hypoestrogenemia and anovulation. Causes of POI include autoimmune disorders, such as hypothyroidism, diabetes, and adrenal insufficiency; karyotypic abnormalities (Turner syndrome and mosaicism);

fragile X premutations; and idiopathic causes. Radiation therapy and chemotherapy can also cause ovarian failure.
   c. Gonadal dysgenesis (karyotypic abnormalities as described previously) can present with primary or secondary amenorrhea.

2. Prevalence and incidence
Premature ovarian insufficiency develops in approximately 1% of women before age 40 (Fritz & Speroff, 2011). Chromosomal abnormalities and gonadal dysgenesis are more common causes of primary amenorrhea than secondary amenorrhea (Fritz & Speroff, 2011; Reindollar et al., 1981).

D. Amenorrhea originating from disorders of the outflow tract or uterus

1. Definition and overview
End-organ abnormalities are rare in secondary amenorrhea. If present, the etiology is usually caused by Asherman syndrome, manifested clinically by very scant menstrual bleeding or amenorrhea. In almost all cases, there is a history of uterine manipulation, such as a dilatation and curettage, other surgical procedures resulting in uterine scarring, or miscarriage.

Congenital anomalies can lead to anatomic alterations in the genital tract, causing primary amenorrhea. These abnormalities include congenital developmental anomalies (imperforate hymen, vaginal septum, or cervical atresia) and müllerian agenesis (absence of the uterus and upper vagina). Ovaries are present as are secondary sex characteristics.

Androgen insensitivity is another etiology of primary amenorrhea. These patients are phenotypic females with some breast development, minimal axillary and pubic hair, external genitalia, blind vaginal canal, and absent uterus; however, they are genotypic males with testes, XY karyotype, and unresponsive androgen receptors but normal to high range of male testosterone levels.

2. Prevalence and incidence
Prevalence of Asherman syndrome is unknown because it is difficult to define the denominator (Berman, 2008). Müllerian abnormalities and complete androgen sensitivity are, with gonadal dysgenesis described previously, the most common causes of primary amenorrhea; androgen insensitivity is rare (Fritz & Speroff, 2011).

E. PCOS

1. Definition and overview
PCOS is one of the most common causes of anovulation. It is a syndrome, not a disease, reflecting multiple potential etiologies with variable clinical expression.

Hallmarks of the syndrome are chronic anovulation, insulin resistance, and hyperandrogenism. Women with PCOS are frequently overweight (Vrbikova & Hainer, 2009). Regardless of obesity, insulin resistance is present, which poses risks for long-term metabolic sequelae and cardiovascular disease. Up to 30% of patients with PCOS also have metabolic syndrome (American College of Obstetricians and Gynecologists [ACOG], 2009). Depression, anxiety, and obstructive sleep apnea are seen more frequently in women with PCOS, independent of obesity (Jedel et al., 2010; Tasali, Van Cauter, & Ehrmann, 2008; Vrbikova & Hainer, 2009). Endometrial cancer may also be increased in women with PCOS because anovulation, central obesity, and diabetes are all risk factors for this cancer.

The 2003 Rotterdam ESHRE/ASRM-Sponsored PCOS Consensus Workshop Group (2004) redefined the diagnosis of PCOS as the presentation of two of the following three criteria (ACOG, 2004b): (1) oligo-ovulation or anovulation (irregular cycles), (2) clinical or biochemical markers of hyperandrogenism, and (3) polycystic ovaries on ultrasonography and exclusion of other etiologies. The Androgen Society considers hyperandrogenism as essential to this diagnosis (ACOG, 2009).

PCOS remains a diagnosis of exclusion and can be diagnosed clinically meeting the criteria just described, including clinical or biochemical markers of hyperandrogenism. Other conditions to be ruled out are hypothyroidism, hyperprolactinemia, ovarian or adrenal tumors, late-onset adrenal hyperplasia, and Cushing syndrome. Women with PCOS are at risk for infertility. If they become pregnant, they are at an increased risk for gestational diabetes and hypertension (Altieri et al., 2010).

2. Prevalence and incidence
PCOS is frequently undiagnosed in the community. Prevalence varies from a high of 17.8 ± 2.8% to a low of 10.2 ± 2.2% (March et al., 2010; Rotterdam ESHRE/ASRM-Sponsored PCOS Consensus Workshop Group, 2004).

II. Database (may include but is not limited to)

A. Subjective

1. Amenorrhea
   a. Past health history
      i. Medical illnesses (**Table 19-1**)
      ii. Obstetric and gynecological: recent history of severe postpartum hemorrhage or oophorectomy (should also ask about miscarriages and postpartum course). Recent history of dilatation and curettage
      iii. Exposure history: radiation or chemotherapy directed to the pelvic organs
      iv. Medication history: dopamine adrenergic drugs or hormonal contraceptives (particularly progestin-only contraceptives and psychiatric medication) (Table 19-1)
   b. Family history
      i. Delayed or absent puberty
      ii. POI
      iii. Fragile X syndrome, developmental or intellectual disabilities
      iv. Congenital abnormalities (e.g., Turner syndrome)
      v. Autoimmune disorders
   c. Occupational and environmental history
      i. Work-related exposures: radiation
   d. Personal and social history
      i. Severe stress, malnutrition, crash dieting, excessive exercise
   e. Review of systems
      i. Constitutional symptoms: hot flushes or night sweats
      ii. Skin, hair, and nails: lanugo (anorexia)
      iii. Nose: anosmia (Kallmann syndrome)
      iv. Eyes: blurred vision if pituitary tumor (may be a late symptom in patients with macroadenomas)
      v. Breast: galactorrhea (hyperprolactinemia)
      vi. Genitourinary: oligomenorrhea (may precede amenorrhea), vaginal dryness if hypoestrogenic state, cyclical pelvic pain in primary amenorrhea (imperforated hymen, transverse septum, cervical atresia)
      vii. Endocrine: hot or cold sensitivity (suspect thyroid disease); fatigue, polydipsia, polyphagia (pituitary disease)
      viii. Neurologic: headaches (may be a late symptom in patients with macroadenomas and other pituitary lesions) particularly associated with blurred vision; change in personality, report of marked mood changes (infiltrative pituitary lesions)

2. PCOS
   a. Ethnicity
   Consider congenital adrenal hyperplasia in women of Ashkenazi Jewish descent, Hispanics, Yugoslavs, Native American Inuits, Alaskans, or Italians (ACOG, 2009).

TABLE 19-1 Amenorrhea and PCOS: Important Etiologies

Classification	Etiology
Hypothalamic amenorrhea	Functional hypothalamic amenorrhea (common etiology for primary or secondary amenorrhea)
	• Anorexia
	• Stress
	• Rapid weight loss
	• Excessive exercise
	• Idiopathic
	Most likely presenting with primary amenorrhea
	• Gonadotropin-releasing hormone deficiency, Kallmann syndrome if associated with anosmia
	Infiltrative lesions of the hypothalamus
Amenorrhea associated with pituitary dysfunction	Physiologic: breastfeeding
	Pathologic (pituitary):
	• Pituitary adenomas: functional prolactin-secreting hormone (most common)
	Other nonfunctional adenomas
	• Adrenocorticotropic hormone–secreting tumor causing Cushing syndrome
	• Thyroid-stimulating hormone–secreting tumor causing hyperthyroidism
	○ Somatotroph adenomas secreting growth hormone and causing acromegaly
	• Other masses (cyst, tuberculosis, sarcoidosis, fat deposits)
	• Renal failure
	• Cirrhosis
	• Sheehan syndrome
	• Empty sella syndrome
	• Drugs
Amenorrhea originating from disorders of the ovaries	Physiologic: menopause, constitutional delay
	Pathologic:
	• Polycystic ovary syndrome (caused by internal–external sources)—most likely explanation of secondary amenorrhea
	• Premature ovarian failure (common): supply of oocytes is depleted before age 40; consider autoimmune disorders, karyotype abnormalities
	Other conditions:
	Local disturbance of ovarian conditions:
	• History of infection (tuberculosis, mumps)
	• History of radiation therapy or cytotoxic drugs
	• Problems in gonadal development that can present either with primary or secondary amenorrhea
	• Turner syndrome
	• Mosaicism

(continues)

TABLE 19-1 Amenorrhea and PCOS: Important Etiologies *(Continued)*

Classification	Etiology
Amenorrhea originating from disorders of the outflow tract	Abnormalities in the first compartment are rare in secondary amenorrhea
	If present, is caused by destruction of the endometrium, from dilatation and curettage or other surgery or miscarriage resulting in uterine scarring (Asherman syndrome)
	Congenital anomalies can lead to anatomic alterations in the genital tract mostly causing primary amenorrhea
	• Imperforate hymen, transverse vaginal septum, or cervical atresia
	• Müllerian agenesis (ovaries are present because they are not müllerian structures)
	• Complete androgen insensitivity (testicular feminization)
Pharmacologic	Medications causing dopamine receptor blockade:
	• Tranquilizers (phenothiazine derivatives)
	• Antipsychotics (risperidone)
	• Antidepressants (desipramine, monoamine oxidase)
	• Antihypertensive (methyldopa, reserpine, verapamil)
	• Narcotics: opiates and heroin
	• Gastrointestinal medications: metoclopramide (Reglan), cimetidine, domperidone
	• Hormonal contraceptives (high-dose progestin)
	• Danazol (androgen-like medication for endometriosis treatment)
Polycystic ovary syndrome	Unknown etiology. It is a syndrome, not a disease, reflecting multiple potential etiologies with variable clinical expression comprised of anovulation, hyperandrogenism, and insulin resistance

b. Past health history
   i. Medical illnesses: metabolic syndrome may be present concomitantly or be the result of PCOS
   ii. Obstetric and gynecological history: menstrual irregularities and infertility or pregnancy complications (gestational diabetes and pregnancy-induced hypertension), obstructive sleep apnea.
   iii. Mental illness: depression or anxiety
c. Family history
   i. PCOS or other endocrinopathies
d. Personal and social history
e. Review of systems
   i. Constitutional signs and symptoms: fatigue
   ii. Skin and hair: acne, oily skin, acanthosis nigricans (neck, axilla, under breast, or groin), hirsutism, and androgenic alopecia
   iii. Genitourinary: irregular menses or amenorrhea, cyclical pelvic pain in primary amenorrhea (anatomical defects cause accumulation of blood behind the obstruction)
   iv. Neurologic: depressive symptoms

B. Objective

1. Physical examination findings (**Table 19-2**). Patient may also have a benign examination.

2. Supporting data from relevant diagnostic tests (**Tables 19-3A–19-3C**).

III. Assessment

A. Diagnosis

Diagnosis of amenorrhea is determined by its onset (primary or secondary); significant findings from the history, physical examination; and diagnostic tests (see Tables 19-3A–19-3C). Most common etiologies encountered in primary care are as follows:

1. Primary amenorrhea caused mainly by constitutional delay

2. Primary or secondary amenorrhea caused by:
   a. Hypothalamic etiology, most likely functional hypothalamic.
   b. Pituitary etiology, most likely hyperprolactinemia or prolactinoma
   c. Ovarian disorders, most likely premature ovarian failure (POF) in secondary amenorrhea or ovarian dysgenesis in primary amenorrhea (Turner syndrome and mosaicism).
   d. Disorders of the outflow tract, most likely Asherman syndrome in secondary amenorrhea

(precipitated by an insult to the endometrium) or müllerian agenesis or complete androgen insensitivity in primary amenorrhea
   e. PCOS

3. Other conditions that may explain the patient's amenorrhea or oligomenorrhea and need to be ruled out in the investigation of PCOS are:
   a. Thyroid disease (most likely primary hypothyroidism)
   b. Hyperprolactinemia
   c. Late-onset adrenal hyperplasia

IV. Goals of clinical management

Select a treatment plan that helps the patient restore normalcy of her menstrual cycle and fertility, if she desires, and reduces risk from hypoestrogenic state or unopposed estrogen stimulation of the endometrium.

V. Plan

A. Diagnostic tests

Tables 19-3A–19-3C provide descriptions of relevant diagnostic studies.

1. All women late for their menses or with oligomenorrhea should have a urine pregnancy test to rule out pregnancy.

2. Laboratory testing: prolactin, TSH, and FSH (Table 19-3A).

3. Some clinicians perform a progesterone withdrawal test in the initial evaluation of amenorrhea to determine endogenous estrogen status; others do not advocate for this test arguing poor sensitivity and specificity (ACOG, 2004a; Fritz & Speroff, 2011).

4. Diagnostic work-up in the adolescent with primary amenorrhea is based on the presence of breast development; secondary sexual characteristics; and the presence of the uterus and an intact outflow tract, likely determined with an ultrasound. If all are present and FSH is normal, the work-up should focus on the etiology of secondary amenorrhea. If there is no breast development and the FSH level is elevated, the probable diagnosis is gonadal dysgenesis. A karyotype should then be ordered. If the uterus or outflow tract is not present and the FSH values are normal, then the diagnostic test should be directed to diagnose müllerian agenesis or androgen insensitivity syndrome. In the latter, circulating testosterone is in the male range and a karyotype confirms the presence of a Y chromosome.

TABLE 19-2 Physical Examination Findings and Likely Etiologies in Amenorrhea and PCOS*

Organ or System	Examination Findings	Likely Etiologies
Vitals	Increased blood pressure	High blood pressure may be present in pituitary diseases (e.g., Cushing disease); karyotype abnormalities (e.g., Turner syndrome); or associated with PCOS
Anthropometric measurements Body mass index	< 18.5 kg/m²—underweight or 25.0–29.9 kg/m²—overweight and > 30 kg/m²—obesity	Underweight may be present in functional hypothalamic amenorrhea (e.g., anorexia) Overweight or obesity may be present in PCOS Waist circumference > 80 cm (31½ in) is predictive of PCOS (Chen, Xu, & Zhang, 2014) or waist–hip ratio > 0.85 (Fritz & Speroff, 2011).
Height	Short stature: less than 60 inches—152.40 cm (Fritz & Speroff, 2011)	Consistent with Turner syndrome
General appearance	Mood/affect (depression, anxiety) Change in personality, marked mood changes	Depression associated with PCOS Rare hypothalamic lesions
Hair	Excess terminal (thick, pigmented) body hair in a male distribution, as seen in upper lip, sideburn area, chin, chest, inner thighs, lower back, lower abdomen, and buttocks	PCOS Androgen-secreting tumor
	Thinning of hair	Thyroid disease
	Absent axillary and pubic hair	Androgen insensitivity
	Lanugo	Anorexia
Eyes	Visual field defects	Pituitary tumor
	Stare, lid lag, exophthalmos	Hypothyroidism
Neck	Thyroid enlargement	Thyroid disease
	Webbed neck	Turner syndrome
Breast	Secretions and galactorrhea expressed from multiple ducts	Occurs in 80% of patients with hyperprolactinemia
	Undeveloped breast in primary amenorrhea	Primary amenorrhea likely caused by karyotype abnormalities
Pelvic examination	Scant/absent hair on mons pubis	Androgen insensitivity
	Vulvar or vaginal atrophy	Hypoestrogenic state as in premature ovarian failure
	Clitoromegaly	Virilizing effect as in androgen tumor
	Imperforate hymen, transverse vaginal septum Cervical atresia	Congenital developmental abnormalities (primary amenorrhea)
	Vaginal pouch (blind or absent vagina), no uterus	Müllerian agenesis (primary amenorrhea)
	Enlarged ovaries	May be palpable if PCOS

Abbreviation: PCOS = polycystic ovary syndrome.

* Directed to organs and systems based on subjective information; examination may be benign.

5. Second-line diagnostic tests in the investigation of amenorrhea include tests where consultation and referral are suggested (Table 19-3B).

6. Magnetic resonance imaging (MRI) or computerized tomography scanning (not as sensitive but less expensive) for the evaluation of a pituitary tumor in the setting of hyperprolactinemia, galactorrhea, or headaches and vision field changes.

7. Karyotype, including fragile X testing, in any woman younger than 30 years of age diagnosed with POF (Fritz & Speroff, 2011), or for women presenting with primary amenorrhea with no uterus on ultrasound.

TABLE 19-3A Essential Testing in the Investigation of Amenorrhea

Test	Definition	Clinical Implications	Comments
Urine pregnancy test	Measures the beta subunit of human chorionic gonadotropin hormone (HCG)	Pregnancy is the most common cause of amenorrhea. This diagnosis must be ruled out in sexually active women before embarking on any additional work-up.	Pregnancy detection by urine HCG relative to the expected first day of menses: • Two days before (79%) • Seven days after (97%) • Eleven days after (100%) (Wilcox, Baird, Dunson, McChesney, & Weinberg, 2001)
Prolactin	Prolactin is produced by the lactotrophs of the anterior pituitary. Serum prolactin elevation causes amenorrhea by inhibiting pulsatile gonadotropin-releasing hormone secretion. This inhibits FSH and LH secretion resulting in anovulation and low ovarian estrogen production. Normal prolactin varies from 15 to 20 mcg.	Prolactin levels measured > 50 ng/mL (or galactorrhea, or visual disturbances) deserve consultation to order a magnetic resonance imaging (MRI) to rule out pituitary tumors or lesions (some practitioners would say 100 ng/mL). Prolactin < 100 mcg may be caused by dopamine agonist drugs, polycystic ovary syndrome, hypothyroidism, or functional (idiopathic); or may be caused by a microadenoma. Prolactin > 150 most likely indicates a prolactinoma (Casanueva et al., 2006)	Prolactin is best drawn fasting, early in the morning. Pregnancy, stress, intercourse, breast stimulation, and meals can increase levels. Prolactin may be mildly elevated in patients with polycystic ovary syndrome (Casanueva et al., 2006) or with long-standing hypothyroidism (Fritz & Speroff, 2011). If prolactin elevations are mild, repeat on a different day (Casanueva et al., 2006). Drugs are a common cause of elevated prolactin, primarily psychotropic medications.
Highly sensitive thyroid-stimulating hormone (TSH)	Measurement of TSH: anterior pituitary hormone that stimulates growth and function of thyroid cells	An elevated TSH accompanying prolactin levels < 100 ng/mL is diagnostic of primary hypothyroidism (Fritz & Speroff, 2011).	Very few patients with amenorrhea or galactorrhea may have subclinical hypothyroidism that is not clinically apparent (Fritz & Speroff, 2011).
Follicle-stimulating hormone (FSH)	Measures the amount of follicle-stimulating hormone produced by the anterior pituitary	FSH ≥ 30 IU/L (found persistently) points to premature ovarian failure or insufficiency or gonadal dysgenesis in primary amenorrhea (with absent breast development in the latter case) a. Normal or low FSH concentrations indicate anovulation likely caused by hypothalamic or pituitary etiology in secondary amenorrhea, or polycystic ovary syndrome	Intermittent follicular development and normalization of FSH values may occur in premature ovarian failure
Progesterone challenge test	Useful in evaluating the status of estrogen production. Administer progestins for 3–10 days. Bleeding is expected 2–7 days after discontinuation of the progestin (may bleed as late as 15 days later if ovulation triggered). Oral progestins available: Provera, 10 mg daily for 5–10 days, or micronized progesterone, 200 mcg at bedtime for 3–5 days	Progesterone challenge test is negative in patients who do not bleed after progestin withdrawal, which indicates lack of estrogen or end-organ problems (Asherman syndrome). Progesterone challenge test is positive in patients who bleed 2–7 days after progestin withdrawal. This indicates that estrogen is being produced by the ovaries. If a progesterone challenge test is negative, you can give combined oral contraceptives to ensure that Asherman syndrome is not present.	Some clinicians advocate for the progesterone challenge test to help in the interpretation of FSH values, and to assist in therapy decision making; need for estrogen therapy for prevention of bone loss (Fritz & Speroff, 2011). Other clinicians do not advocate for the progesterone challenge test due to high rates of false-positive and false-negative results.

TABLE 19-3B Second-Line Testing in the Investigation of Amenorrhea, Including Tests Where Consultation or Referral Is Suggested

Test	Definition	Clinical Implications	Comments
Abdominal–pelvic ultrasound	Ultrasound imaging to evaluate internal organs if unable to perform a pelvic examination, particularly in the case of primary amenorrhea.	Absent uterus, vaginal septum, or congenital absence of the vagina.	May be useful to confirm the presence of a uterus and ovaries. Absent uterus and vagina is likely caused by müllerian agenesis or androgen insensitivity in primary amenorrhea. If absent uterus, then karyotype and renal ultrasound indicated. Abnormalities of the urinary tract frequently accompany müllerian anomalies. Referral to a specialist is indicated.
MRI of the sella turcica to evaluate for prolactinomas (prolactin-secreting tumors) or other rare pituitary–hypothalamic tumors	The goal of imaging is to evaluate the possibility of a hypothalamic or pituitary lesion.	In the case of a prolactinoma, the image allows determination of a microadenoma or a macroadenoma ($\leq$ 1 or > 1 cm, respectively). Abnormal imaging (or hyperprolactinemia) requires referral to a specialist.	All women with high serum prolactin values ($\geq$ 50 mcg/L; some practitioners would say > 100 mcg/L) should have imaging of the sella turcica (MRI). MRI is also indicated if galactorrhea, headaches, or visual field disturbances are present in the evaluation of amenorrhea. MRI is indicated for delayed puberty and hypogonadism.
Karyotype evaluation	To evaluate for abnormal XY chromosomes in any woman diagnosed with premature ovarian failure, if younger than 30 years of age, or in women older than 30 years with short stature or family history of early menopause (Fritz & Speroff, 2011).	Mosaicism with a Y chromosome requires excision of gonads. Malignant tumor formation is highly possible with the presence of any testicular component within the gonad.	Most gonadal tumors appear before 20 years of age. A significant number of cases appear between ages 20 and 30. None have been found above age 30 (Fritz & Speroff, 2011).
Fragile X premutations	To evaluate fragile X syndrome premutation carriers who are at risk for having a fragile X syndrome (Fritz & Speroff, 2011)	Premutation of fragile X syndrome can result in premature ovarian failure (POF) or POI. Indicated when diagnosis of POF/POI is made.	The mechanism by which a premutation causes ovarian failure is not known.
Antiadrenal and anti thyroid antibodies, fasting blood sugar (FBS), and electrolytes	To evaluate autoimmune disorders involved in POF/POI.	Abnormal values for these tests are indicated in the work-up for autoimmune disorders causing POF/POI.	Autoimmune abnormalities (AA) are common in women with POF. Addison's disease has the strongest association with POF (Fritz & Speroff, 2011).
Saline-infusion hysterography or hysterosalpingogram	Imaging procedure allows for confirmation of Asherman syndrome.	Presence of intrauterine synechiae.	Hysteroscopy is used for the final diagnosis and treatment. Hysteroscopic lysis of adhesions is the main method of treatment.

Abbreviations: MRI, magnetic resonance imaging; mcg, micrograms; ng, nanograms; IU, international units.

TABLE 19-3C Additional Tests in the Investigation of Polycystic Ovary Syndrome*

Test	Definition	Clinical Implications	Comments
Total and free testosterone	Serum testosterone provides the best estimate of androgen production. Total testosterone is more widely available and better standardized than free testosterone (free testosterone is the best estimate of bioavailable testosterone).	Testosterone values may be normal in women with PCOS. Testosterone in the male range is seen in women with androgen insensitivity. Total testosterone may be elevated (> 60 ng/dL), but is not required for the diagnosis of PCOS. Testosterone twice the upper limit is most likely caused by androgen-producing tumors.	If testosterone levels are normal in a woman with high suspicion of PCOs, consider repeating testosterone and order sex hormone binding globulin (SHBG) in a specialized center. Low SHBG indicates PCOS (Conway et al., 2014). Be aware that local laboratory values for free testosterone vary greatly and the sensitivity and reliability are poor (ACOG, 2009).
Dehydroepiandrosterone sulfate	A direct measurement of adrenal androgen activity. This test may be ordered to rule out androgen-secreting tumor.	Upper limit of normal is 350 ng/dL. It may vary by laboratory. It may also be mildly elevated in PCOS.	It is most useful in the evaluation of rapid virilization, not as useful in common hirsutism (ACOG, 2009).
17-Hydroxy-progesterone	Serum blood test that evaluates adult-onset adrenal hyperplasia (caused by 21-hydroxylase deficiency).	Fasting, in the follicular phase: < 200 ng/dL excludes adult-onset adrenal hyperplasia	Limit test to high-risk women with hirsutism (Fritz & Speroff, 2011).
Pelvic ultrasound	To evaluate for presence of polycystic ovaries, perform sonogram ideally on days 3–5 of the menstrual cycle.	Polycystic ovaries are present when 12 or more follicles are seen in one of the ovaries. Recent studies raised the number to ≥ 19 in one of the ovaries (Conway et al., 2014). <ul><li>Follicles measure 2–9 mm in diameter</li><li>Increase in ovarian volume > 10 mL</li></ul>	The appearance of polycystic ovaries is nonspecific. It can also be seen in women with normal hormonal function or with other androgen excess disorders. Hence it is not recommended solely for the evaluation of PCOS. If done, patients should not be on oral contraceptives because these medications can change the ovarian morphology.

Abbreviation: PCOS = polycystic ovary syndrome; ng = nanograms.

* PCOS is a diagnosis of exclusion. If initial testing for the investigation of amenorrhea and oligomenorrhea is unrevealing, other conditions are advised to rule out other hyperandrogenic conditions.

8. Saline infusion hysterography or hysterosalpingogram, for the confirmation of intrauterine synechiae present in Asherman syndrome. Initial investigation of Asherman syndrome, in the setting of secondary amenorrhea and history of instrumentation, is performed by "priming" the uterus with 1 month of any low-dose combined oral contraceptive. Lack of withdrawal bleeding is highly suspicious of Asherman syndrome (Fritz & Speroff, 2011).

9. Abdominal and pelvic ultrasound to confirm the presence of the uterus.

10. There are no specific tests for the diagnosis of PCOS.

Conditions that can mimic PCOS must first be excluded.

11. Women diagnosed with PCOS should have testing for the investigation of insulin resistance and metabolic abnormalities, including 2-hour oral glucose tolerance test and fasting lipids. Hemoglobin A1C can be used if unable or unwilling to do the 2-hour glucose tolerance test (GTT) (Legro et al., 2013). In addition they should be screened for mood disorders and obstructive sleep apnea (Legro et al., 2013)

12. Additional testing to consider may be found in Table 19-3C.

B. Management

Therapeutic management of amenorrhea depends on the etiology, the goals of the woman including her desire for pregnancy, and the long-term consequences of her condition.

1. Hypothalamic amenorrhea
   a. Address the underlying condition and issues related to hypothalamic amenorrhea (e.g., eating disorders or excessive exercise) that may negatively affect ovulation and normal menstrual cycle. Cognitive behavioral therapy, designed to identify maladaptive attitudes toward eating and weight, and problem-solving strategies and coping skills to improve healthy eating behaviors have demonstrated improvement of hypothalamic function (Berga et al., 2003).
   b. Begin oral replacement with estrogen to prevent osteoporosis. Any low-dose oral contraceptive method provides the necessary estrogen replacement in a woman during the reproductive years, in addition to providing contraception. OCPs are preferable to estrogen alone as these women need the higher doses of estrogens.
   c. Supplement with calcium and vitamin D to strengthen bone health.
   d. Refer to reproductive endocrinology if pregnancy is desired. Some women may respond to clomiphene citrate; most require gonadotropin-releasing hormone.

2. Amenorrhea associated with pituitary dysfunction
   a. In hyperprolactinemia with pituitary macroadenomas, the treatment goal is to establish normal estrogen secretion, menstrual function, and tumor reduction. Therapy is indicated for all patients with macroadenoma and in most patients with microadenomas, particularly if there are bothersome symptoms and desired fertility and for the prevention of osteoporosis (Casanueva et al., 2006). Women with macroadenomas may need transsphenoidal surgery or radiation therapy (Casanueva et al. , 2006). Women desiring fertility may need induction of ovulation, although in many cases pharmacologic management of hyperprolactinemia establishes ovulatory cycles.
   b. Dopamine agonists, such as bromocriptine and cabergoline, are the drugs of choice for women with hyperprolactinemia and prolactinomas. These medications decrease the size of the prolactinomas, restore menstrual function and prolactin levels to normal, and ameliorate galactorrhea. Cabergoline is better tolerated, is more convenient, and has been demonstrated to be more effective in reduction of prolactin levels when used up to 2 years (Dekkers et al., 2010). Bromocriptine, however, has been used for many more years and is less expensive.
      i. If cost is an issue start with bromocriptine tablets, 2.5 mg at bedtime or half a pill twice a day, increasing levels weekly to the lowest possible that maintains normal prolactin levels, generally twice or occasionally three times a day dosing (Fritz & Speroff, 2011).
      ii. Side effects of bromocriptine are nausea, constipation, faintness caused by orthostatic hypotension, headache, and nasal stuffiness. Side effects can be minimized by taking the pill at bedtime along with a snack, by increasing the dose slowly as described previously, or by administering the 2.5-mg tablet high into the vagina at bedtime avoiding the first pass through the liver and achieving therapeutic results at lower doses (Fritz & Speroff, 2011).
      iii. Cabergoline can be started at a dose of 0.5 mg, one-half to one tablet administered once or twice weekly. The dose is increased monthly until prolactin levels normalize. The lowest dose to normalize prolactin should be attempted as well as medication discontinuation when prolactin levels have been normal for 2 years or more to prevent valvular heart disease, which can occur with doses > 3 mg daily (Fritz & Speroff, 2011). Doses over 3 mg per week are rarely necessary (Casanueva et al., 2006).
      iv. In a considerable proportion of patients, discontinuation of dopamine agonist medication results in resumption of symptoms, the tumor, and hyperprolactinemia.
   c. Dopaminergic treatment may reestablish ovulation, even before the first normal menstruation. The woman needs contraception if she wants to prevent pregnancy (Casanueva et al., 2006).
   d. Very few patients with microadenomas progress to larger tumors. Amenorrheic women with microadenomas do not need to be treated with dopamine agonists unless they want to become pregnant or they have bothersome galactorrhea. However, they need to be treated with estrogen and should have annual evaluations of serum prolactin. Request an MRI when prolactin rises significantly (or symptoms of tumor expansion ensue (Casanueva et al., 2006). Estrogen should be provided with progestins. Any low-dose oral hormonal contraception can be recommended (Fritz & Speroff, 2011).

e. Calcium and vitamin D supplementation is advised in the amenorrheic patient for the prevention of osteoporosis.

f. Correct hypothyroidism.

g. Address hyperprolactinemia induced by medications. Review the patient medication profile for drugs that cause hyperprolactinemia and amenorrhea, such as dopamine agonist drugs and estrogen or danazol. Withdrawal of the drug for 72 hours, if able to do this safely, helps elucidate if the drug is responsible for hyperprolactinemia. MRI should be considered if this alternative is not feasible, particularly in patients with neurologic symptoms to rule out a pituitary lesion (Casanueva et al., 2006).

3. Ovarian disorders

a. Primary amenorrhea: refer patients diagnosed with Turner syndrome or mosaicism to a physician. Patients with Turner syndrome need a multidisciplinary approach for management including the approach for primary or secondary amenorrhea. It is critical to review with the woman in a sensitive manner the consequences of POF and the need for early estrogen to induce pubertal development in the case of primary amenorrhea and to protect bone health during the adult life (Bondy, 2007).

b. Secondary amenorrhea caused by POF

i. Order a karyotype if woman is 30 years old or younger. Refer if the karyotype is abnormal. Malignant tumor formation within the gonad is associated in mosaicism with a Y chromosome. Removal of the gonadal areas is required (Fritz & Speroff, 2011).

ii. In women younger than 35 consider an evaluation of autoimmune disorders.

iii. Advise all women with POF to establish standard hormonal therapy with estrogen. Advised at least until age 50 to prevent osteoporosis (Kalantaridou & Nelson, 2000; Ostberg et al., 2007). Progestin should be added to estrogen to protect the endometrium if there is an intact uterus. Hormonal treatment also reduces menopausal symptoms.

iv. Women with POF commonly experience unpredictable and intermittent ovarian function (Rebar & Connolly, 1990). For women who wish to avoid pregnancy, offer any low-dose combined oral contraception instead of hormonal therapy because the estrogen doses in the hormonal therapy are not high enough to prevent pregnancy.

The possibility of vasomotor symptoms during the cyclical hormone-free pill interval should be addressed.

v. Refer women who desire pregnancy to an infertility specialist. Women with POF are candidates for ovum donation or adoption. Although rare, these women may become pregnant spontaneously (Check & Katsoff, 2006).

4. Disorders of the outflow tract

a. Primary amenorrhea

i. Refer patients suspected of or diagnosed with androgen insensitivity to a specialist. Patients with this condition need removal of gonads to prevent the development of gonadal neoplasia. Gonadectomy is usually delayed until puberty in patients with complete androgen insensitivity syndrome. These patients have a normal pubertal growth spurt and feminize at the time of expected puberty; tumors do not usually develop until after this time. These patients require psychological counseling given that they have female phenotype and male karyotype (Fritz & Speroff, 2011).

ii. Refer patients diagnosed with müllerian abnormalities or agenesis to a specialist. Surgery is needed if there is vaginal outlet obstruction to allow passage of menstrual blood. Creation of a neovagina for patients with müllerian agenesis is usually delayed until the woman is emotionally mature and ready to participate in the postoperative care required to maintain vaginal patency (Fritz & Speroff, 2011).

b. Secondary amenorrhea: refer patients to a specialist if Asherman syndrome is suspected. Final diagnosis is made with hysteroscopy performed by lysis of adhesions during the diagnostic procedure (Fritz & Speroff, 2011).

5. PCOS

Treatment goals should be directed to control menstrual irregularities, management of hyperandrogenic manifestations (acne and hirsutism), infertility issues, and the long-term consequences of hyperinsulinemia.

a. Advise weight loss (via caloric restricted diet) and regular exercise. Although the best treatment approach in obese PCOS patients remains to be defined, weight loss is the first-choice recommendation for the treatment of the clinical manifestations of PCOS, such as menstrual cycle irregularities, infertility, and hirsutism (Conway et al., 2014; Vrbikova & Hainer, 2009). A 5% weight loss has shown improvement in ovulatory cycles (ACOG, 2009). Bariatric surgery is now recommended for morbidly obese women (central obesity), as it may restore the HPO axis function, prevent or even reverse the metabolic syndrome and its consequences, and improve pregnancy outcomes (Conway et al., 2014).

b. Pharmacologic treatment for menstrual irregularities and hyperandrogenic manifestations include:

   i. If no contraindication for combined hormonal contraception use any low-dose oral contraceptives in order to decrease bioavailable testosterone levels (ACOG, 2009; Sheehan, 2004). Contraceptive patch and vaginal ring are also alternatives (Legro et al., 2013). Cyclic progestin is a good choice for menstrual regulation if contraception is not needed (200 mg daily micronized progestin or10 mg medroxyprogesterone acetate 10–14 days/month if contraception is not needed for menstrual regulation) (Conway et al., 2014).

   ii. Metformin, although not approved by the Food and Drug Administration for PCOS management, is widely used for its anti-insulinic effects. It is recommended as a second-line treatment for the prevention of diabetes when lifestyle modifications have not been successful (Legro et al., 2013). The dose suggested to treat women with PCOS is 1,500–2,000 mg per day given in divided doses (De Leo et al., 2009). Metformin is preferred over other classes of anti-insulinic drugs because the medication tends to decrease weight (ACOG, 2009). Metformin has limited effect in treating hirsutism, acne, and infertility and has a higher incidence of gastrointestinal side effects (Johnson, 2014).

   iii. Discuss contraception in women who do not desire pregnancy and are taking metformin because ovulation rates can improve with metformin.

c. Management of hirsutism can be additionally accomplished by:

   i. Oral contraceptives: although the Food and Drug Administration has not approved them for the management of hirsutism, observational and nonrandomized studies have shown some benefit (ACOG, 2009). OCPs help with hirsutism by increasing SHBG and reducing free testosterone.

   ii. Antiandrogen medications: consult with a specialist for the prescription of these medications (ACOG, 2009). For spironolactone the usual dosage is 25–100 mg, twice a day. It may take up to 6 months to observe full clinical effect. One-fifth of women on this medication may experience metrorrhagia if the dose is in the upper limit (Helfer, Miller, & Rose, 1988). Use cautiously in women with renal impairment because of hyperkalemia. Rarely, exposure has resulted in ambiguous genitalia in male infants. Offer mechanical hair removal (laser treatment). Eflornithine is a topical option.

d. Screen and treat to reduce risk of cardiovascular disease and diabetes.

   i. Adolescents and women with PCOS should be screened for impaired glucose tolerance every 3–5 years, or earlier if clinical suspicion of diabetes with a 2-hour glucose level using a 75-g oral glucose load (Legro et al., 2013; Salley et al., 2007)

   ii. Screen women for cardiovascular risk factors: smoking, obesity (central), hypertension, dyslipidemia, diabetes, obstructive sleep apnea, family history of early cardiovascular disease

e. Medical therapy for women with PCOS desiring pregnancy: the antiestrogen clomiphene citrate remains the drug of choice for ovulation induction. Recent data suggest that an aromatase inhibitor is more effective, particularly when BMI > 30 (Franik, Kremer, Nelen, & Farquhar, 2014). Discussion of ovulation induction is beyond the scope of this chapter.

C. Client education

1. Information: provide verbal and, preferably, written information regarding:

   a. Risk-reduction strategies and screening for osteoporosis in women with hypothalamic and pituitary amenorrhea and for metabolic syndrome and endometrial hyperplasia in women with PCOS.

   b. The disease process: signs and symptoms and underlying etiologies.

   c. Diagnostic tests: preparation, cost, the procedures, and aftercare.

   d. Medication management: rationale, action, use, side effects, associated risks, cost of therapeutic interventions, and the need for adhering to long-term treatment plans.

2. Counseling
    Women interested in becoming pregnant should be counseled on possible therapeutic options and possible referral to reproductive endocrinology specialists.

VI. Self-management resources and tools

A. Patient and client education

The Mayo Clinic website also has excellent patient information at www.mayoclinic.org. Resources are found under "Patient Care & Health Information"; click on "Diseases and Conditions" and search for "amenorrhea."

B. Community support groups

Women with POF can consult the Premature Ovarian Failure Support group at www.posupport.org, created by the nonprofit organization The International Premature Ovarian Failure Support Group, Alexandria, VA (email: info@pofsupport.org; telephone: 703-913-4787).

REFERENCES

Altieri, P., Gambineri, A., Prontera, O., Cionci, G., Franchina, M., & Pasquali, R. (2010). Maternal polycystic ovary syndrome may be associated with adverse pregnancy outcomes. *European Journal of Obstetrics, Gynecology and Reproductive Biology, 149*(1), 31–36.

American College of Obstetrics and Gynecology. (2004a). Current evaluation of amenorrhea. *Fertility and Sterility, 82*(Suppl. 1), 266–272.

American College of Obstetrics and Gynecology. (2004b). Revised 2003 consensus on diagnostic criteria and long-term health risks related to polycystic ovary syndrome. *Fertility and Sterility, 81*(1), 19–25.

American College of Obstetricians and Gynecologists. (2009). ACOG Practice Bulletin No. 108: Polycystic ovary syndrome. *Obstetrics and Gynecology, 114*(4), 936–949.

Beals, K. A., & Hill, A. K. (2006). The prevalence of disordered eating, menstrual dysfunction, and low bone mineral density among US collegiate athletes. *International Journal of Sport Nutrition and Exercise Metabolism, 16*(1), 1–23.

Berga, S. L., Marcus, M. D., Loucks, T. L., Hlastala, S., Ringham, R., & Krohn, M. A. (2003). Recovery of ovarian activity in women with functional hypothalamic amenorrhea who were treated with cognitive behavior therapy. *Fertility and Sterility, 80*(4), 976–981.

Berman, J. M. (2008). Intrauterine adhesions. *Seminars in Reproductive Medicine, 26*(4), 349–355.

Bondy, C. A. (2007). Care of girls and women with Turner syndrome: A guideline of the Turner Syndrome Study Group. *Journal of Clinical Endocrinology and Metabolism, 92*(1), 10–25.

Casanueva, F., Molitch, M. E., Schlechte, J. A., Abs, R., Bonert, V., Bronstein, M. D., et al. (2006). Guidelines of the Pituitary Society for the diagnosis and management of prolactinomas. *Clinical Endocrinology, 65*(2), 265–273.

Check, J. H., & Katsoff, B. (2006). Successful pregnancy with spontaneous ovulation in a woman with apparent premature ovarian failure who failed to conceive despite four transfers of embryos derived from donated oocytes. *Clinical and Experimental Obstetrics & Gynecology, 33*(1), 13–15.

Chen, L., Xu, W.M., Zhang, D. (2014). The association of abdominal obesity, insulin resistance, and oxidative stress in adipose tissue in women with polycystic ovary syndrome. *Fertility & Sterility, 102*(4), 1167–1174.

Conway, G., Dewailly, D., Diamanti-Kandarakis, E., Escobar-Morreale, H. F., Franks, S., Gambineri, A., et al. (2014). The polycystic ovary syndrome: A position statement from the European Society of Endocrinology. *European Journal of Endocrinology, 171*(4), P1–P29.

De Leo, V., Musacchio, M. C., Palermo, V., Di Sabatino, A., Morgante, G., & Petraglia, F. (2009). Polycystic ovary syndrome and metabolic comorbidities: Therapeutic options. *Drugs Today, 45*(10), 763–775.

Dekkers, O. M., Lagro, J., Burman, P., Jørgensen, J. O., Romijn, J. A., & Pereira, A. M. (2010). Recurrence of hyperprolactinemia after withdrawal of dopamine agonists: Systematic review and meta-analysis. *Journal of Clinical Endocrinology and Metabolism, 95*(1), 43–51.

Franik, S., Kremer, J. A. M., Nelen, W. L. D. M., & Farquhar, C. (2014) Aromatase inhibitors for subfertile women with polycystic ovary syndrome. *Cochrane Database of Systematic Reviews, 2*.

Fritz, M. A., & Speroff, L. (2011). *Clinical gynecologic endocrinology and infertility* (8th ed.). Philadelphia, PA: Lippincott Williams & Wilkins.

Helfer, E. L., Miller, J. L., & Rose, L. I. (1988). Side-effects of spironolactone therapy in the hirsute woman. *Journal of Clinical Endocrinology and Metabolism, 66*(1), 208–211.

Hoch, A. Z., Pajewski, N. M., Moraski, L., Carrera, G. F., Wilson, C. R., Hoffmann, R. G., et al. (2009). Prevalence of the female athlete triad in high school athletes and sedentary students. *Clinical Journal of Sport Medicine, 19*(5), 421–428.

Jedel, E., Waern, M., Gustafson, D., Landén, M., Eriksson, E., Holm, G., et al. (2010). Anxiety and depression symptoms in women with polycystic ovary syndrome compared with controls matched for body mass index. *Human Reproduction, 25*(2), 450–456.

Johnson, N. P. (2014). Metformin use in women with polycystic ovary syndrome. *Annals of Translational Medicine, 2*(6), 56. doi:10.3978/j.issn.2305-5839.2014.04.15.

Kalantaridou, S. N., & Nelson, L. M. (2000). Premature ovarian failure is not premature menopause. *Annals of the New York Academy of Sciences, 900*, 393–402.

Khawaja, N. M., Taher, B. M., Barham, M. E., Naser, A. A., Hadidy, A. M., Ahmad, A. T., et al. (2006). Pituitary enlargement in patients with primary hypothyroidism. *Endocrine Practice, 12*(1), 29–34.

Legro, R. S., Arslanian, S. A., Ehrmann, D. A., Hoeger, K. M., Murad, M. H., Pasquali, R., et al. (2013). Diagnosis and treatment of polycystic ovary syndrome: An Endocrine Society clinical practice guideline. *Journal of Clinical Endocrinology and Metabolism, 98*(12), 4565–4592.

March, W. A., Moore, V. M., Willson, K. J., Phillips, D. I., Norman, R. J., & Davies, M. J. (2010). The prevalence of polycystic ovary syndrome in a community sample assessed under contrasting diagnostic criteria. *Human Reproduction, 25*(2), 544–551.

Ostberg, J. E., Storry, C., Donald, A. E., Attar, M. J., Halcox, J. P., & Conway, G. S. (2007). A dose-response study of hormone replacement in young hypogonadal women: Effects on intima media thickness and metabolism. *Clinical Endocrinology, 66*(4), 557–564.

Practice Committee of the American Society for Reproductive Medicine. (2008). Current evaluation of amenorrhea. *Fertility and Sterility, 90*(5), S219–S225.

Rebar, R. W., & Connolly, H. V. (1990). Clinical features of young women with hypergonadotropic amenorrhea. *Fertility and Sterility, 53*(5), 804–810.

Reindollar, R. H., Byrd, J. R., & McDonough, P. G. (1981). Delayed sexual development: A study of 252 patients. *American Journal of Obstetrics and Gynecology, 140*(4), 371–380.

Reindollar, R. H., Novak, M., Tho, S. P., & McDonough, P. G. (1986). Adult-onset amenorrhea: A study of 262 patients. *American Journal of Obstetrics and Gynecology, 155*(3), 531–543.

Rotterdam ESHRE/ASRM-Sponsored PCOS Consensus Workshop Group (2004). Revised 2003 consensus on diagnostic criteria and long-term health risks related to polycystic ovary syndrome. *Fertility and Sterility, 81*(1), 19–25.

Salley, K. E., Wickham, E. P., Cheang, K. I., Essah, P. A., Karjane, N. W., & Nestler, J. E. (2007). Glucose intolerance in polycystic ovary syndrome—a position statement of the Androgen Excess Society. *Journal of Clinical Endocrinology and Metabolism, 92*(12), 4546–4556.

Sheehan, M. T. (2004). Polycystic ovarian syndrome: Diagnosis and management. *Clinical Medicine & Research, 2*(1), 13–27.

Tasali, E., Van Cauter, E., & Ehrmann, D. A. (2008). Polycystic ovary syndrome and obstructive sleep apnea. *Sleep Medicine clinics, 3*(1), 37–46.

Vrbikova, J., & Hainer, V. (2009). Obesity and polycystic ovary syndrome. *Obesity Facts, 2*(1), 26–35.

Wilcox, A. J., Baird, D. D., Dunson, D., McChesney, R., & Weinberg, C. R. (2001). Natural limits of pregnancy testing in relation to the expected menstrual period. *JAMA, 286*(14), 1759–1761.

SCREENING FOR INTRAEPITHELIAL NEOPLASIA AND CANCER OF THE LOWER GENITAL TRACT

Mary M. Rubin and Lynn Hanson

I. Introduction and general background

A. Abnormal cytology

1. Intraepithelial neoplasia (IN), often referred to as dysplasia, is an abnormal precancerous change in cells as they mature. This abnormality can be found in multicentric areas of the lower genital tract, such as the cervix (CIN), vagina (VAIN), vulva (VIN), anus (AIN), and perianal epithelium (PAIN). The natural history of the disease is unpredictable. Mediated by the immune system, the abnormality can regress, persist at the same level, or progress to malignancy.

2. The etiology of the condition is multifactorial, but the dominant agent is human papillomavirus (HPV). Over 100 different HPV types exist, but 14 types are considered oncogenic (Markowitz et al., 2014). Worldwide, types 16 and 18 are responsible for 70% of cervical cancers (Li, Franceschi, Howell-Jones, Snijders, & Clifford, 2010). HPV is necessary for malignant cellular transformation, but other cofactors, such as age of first intercourse, number of sexual partners, other sexually transmitted infections (STIs), smoking, diet, stress, and host immunologic status all play a role (Winer et al., 2003). Persistence of high-risk HPV types is also required for progression to high-grade lesions (Kosiol et al., 2008; Kjaer, Frederiksen, Munk, & Iftner, 2010). The virus is for the most part sexually transmitted and is responsible for other noncancerous conditions, such as genital warts (condyloma acuminata).

B. Screening guidelines

1. Guidelines for the use of cytology for cervical cancer screening (Pap tests) have undergone major revision (American College of Obstetrics and Gynecology [ACOG], 2012; Saslow et al., 2012; U.S. Preventive Services Task Force [USPSTF], 2012).

    The Pap test remains an important modality in determining the health of a woman's cervix, whether it is obtained by using the conventional Pap test or the liquid-based test. It screens for both glandular and squamous cell abnormalities. The use of HPV testing in combination with cervical cytology was approved for screening women 30 years of age or older and as a reflex test in younger women who have atypical cells of undetermined significance reported on their results. Reflex testing involves testing the cervical sample for the presence of high-risk HPV types. It is not necessary to test for low-risk types because they lack the potential for oncogenic transformation. HPV testing should not be used in women younger than 21 years. In April 2014, the Food and Drug Administration (FDA) approved Roche Diagnostics' cobas® HPV test as a primary screening test for cervical cancer. This action received unanimous support from an FDA advisory committee (Huh et al., 2015).

2. According to all three guidelines—ACOG (2012), American Cancer Society (Saslow et al., 2012), and USPSTF (2012), the recommendations for initiation, frequency, and cessation of cervical screening are:

    a. Begin Pap test screening at age 21 and continue every 3 years through age 29.

    b. Women age 30 and older may continue to be screened with cytology alone every 3 years or with HPV testing plus cytology every 5 years.

    c. Discontinuation of cervical cancer screening can be at age 65 in women who have had three or more consecutive negative cytology test results or two consecutive negative cytology plus HPV tests within 10 years before cessation of screening, with the most recent test performed within 5 years. Women with a history of CIN 2 or greater should continue routine screening for at least 20 years after diagnosis, even if that extends beyond age 65.

d. Women who have undergone a total hysterectomy for benign conditions and have not had prior CIN 2 (moderate dysplasia) or CIN 3 (severe dysplasia or carcinoma in situ) may discontinue Pap smear screening.

According to the American Cancer Society guidelines, the following conditions may increase a patient's risk for CIN and may necessitate more frequent Pap test screening. A specific interval of time is not stated for these special circumstances and should be a decision made between clinician and patient.

i. Women who have human immunodeficiency virus (HIV)

ii. Women with other immunosuppressive conditions (e.g., organ transplantation)

iii. Women who were exposed to diethylstilbestrol (DES) in utero

iv. Women previously treated for CIN 2, CIN 3, or cancer

3. With the introduction of the quadrivalent and bivalent HPV vaccines, screening guidelines for the vaccinated population may be modified in the future. At the present time the recommendation is to adhere to the current guidelines (Markowitz et al., 2014). In addition, at the end of 2014, the FDA approved the use of the 9-valent vaccine that protects against not only the four types included in the quadrivalent HPV vaccine (6, 11, 16, 18), available since 2006, but five other types known to cause HPV-associated cancers (31, 33, 45, 52, and 58). The combination of these genotypes in this vaccine is designed to protect against 90% of HPV-associated cancers as well as most external genital warts (FDA, 2014).

C. Pap smear classifications

The Bethesda System Pap test classification remains the preferred method for reporting cytology results in the United States (**Table 20-1**). This system has been used since 1988 for reporting cytologic evaluation for the cervix, vagina, and anus and has had only minor revisions since 2004, the latest being in June 2015 (Nayar & Wilbur, 2015; Solomon & Nayar, 2004). The

TABLE 20-1 2014 Revised Bethesda System Terminology for the Pap Test

Specimen Criteria	Comments
Type	Note the type of Pap test (conventional, liquid-based or other)
Adequacy (satisfactory for evaluation)	Note presence or absence of endocervical transformation zone component and any other indicators, e.g., blood partially obscuring specimen, inflammation, etc.)
Inadequacy (unsatisfactory for evaluation)	Specify reasons for rejection/not processing Specify reasons for a processed specimen yet is unsatisfactory for an epithelial abnormality evaluation
General categorization (optional)	*Negative for intraepithelial lesion or malignancy* *Other*: see Interpretation/Results (e.g., Endometrial cells are noted in a woman older than 45 years) *Epithelial cell abnormality*: see Interpretation/Results (stipulate "squamous" or "glandular," if relevant)
Interpretation (negative for intraepithelial lesion or malignancy and non-neoplastic findings)	*Negative for Intraepithelial Lesion or Malignancy*: no cellular evidence of neoplasia. (Result(s) is/are noted in the General Categorization and/or in the Interpretation/Result section of the report.) *Non-neoplastic findings (optional to report)* Nonneoplastic cellular variants • Atrophy • Keratotic changes • Pregnancy-associated • Squamous metaplasia • Tubal metaplasia Associated reactive cellular changes • Inflammation • Intrauterine devices Glandular cells changes following a hysterectomy

TABLE 20-1 2014 Revised Bethesda System Terminology for the Pap Test *(Continued)*

Specimen Criteria	Comments
	Non-neoplastic findings: Organisms • *Trichomonas vaginalis* • Fungal organisms consistent with *Candida* sp. • Shift in vaginal flora suggestive of bacterial vaginosis • Bacteria consistent with *Actinomyces* sp. • Cellular changes consistent with herpes simplex virus *Other:* Endometrial cells are noted in a woman older than 45 years (Note if "negative for squamous intraepithelial lesion").

Interpretation (cell abnormalities)	*Epithelial cell abnormalities*
	(Result(s) is/are noted in the General Categorization and/or in the Interpretation/Result section of the report.)
	• Squamous cell
	  ○ Atypical squamous cells of undetermined significance (ASC-US)
	  ○ Cannot exclude HSIL (ASC-H) L
	  ○ Low-grade squamous intraepithelial lesion (LSIL) encompassing: human papillomavirus/mild dysplasia/CIN 1
	  ○ High-grade squamous intraepithelial lesion (HSIL) encompassing moderate and severe dysplasia, CIN 2, and CIN 3/CIS with features suspicious for invasion (if invasion is suspected).
	  ○ Squamous cell carcinoma
	• Glandular cell
	  ○ Atypical
	    - Endocervical cells, endometrial cells and/or glandular cells (NOS or specify in comments)
	  ○ Atypical
	    - Endocervical and/or glandular cells, favor neoplastic
	  ○ Endocervical adenocarcinoma in situ
	  ○ Adenocarcinoma
	    - Endocervical
	    - Endometrial
	    - Extrauterine
	    - Not otherwise specified (NOS)
	
	Other malignant neoplasm

Adapted from Nayar R, Wilbur DC (Eds.) The Bethesda system for reporting cervical cytology. Definitions, criteria, and explanatory notes (3rd edition). New York, NY. Springer; 2015.

report encompasses the components of the specimen type, a statement of adequacy, a general categorization, the use of automated review or ancillary testing, and the interpretation of results. The following nomenclature is used for categorizing cytologic dysplasia or abnormality:

1. Atypical squamous cells of undetermined significance (ASC-US): refers to those samples where the cells are either equivocal or nondiagnostic for either benign conditions or squamous intraepithelial neoplasia.

2. Atypical squamous cells of undetermined significance cannot rule out high grade (ASC-H): refers to the presence of cells that are not clearly high grade but it cannot be ruled out.

3. Low-grade squamous intraepithelial lesion (LSIL): refers to any combination of HPV (cells characteristic of HPV), mild dysplasia, or CIN 1.

4. High-grade squamous intraepithelial lesion (HSIL): refers to the presence of moderate to severe dysplasia, carcinoma in situ, or intraepithelial neoplasia grades 2 or 3 (CIN 2 or 3).

5. Squamous cell cancer or suspicious for squamous cell cancer

6. Atypical glandular cells of undetermined significance (AGC): refers to endocervical or endometrial cell abnormalities or glandular cells not otherwise specified for site. The range of abnormality can be reactivity (e.g., from an intrauterine device string), adenocarcinoma in situ, or adenocarcinoma (Saslow et al., 2012). The presence of AGC necessitates referral for colposcopy not just a repeat Pap test.

D. Management of abnormal cytology

1. Triaging of each category of abnormal cytology is outlined in the algorithms developed at the 2012 consensus conference sponsored by the American Society for Colposcopy and Cervical Pathology (ASCCP). The evidence-based guidelines, including the most recent version, were developed by participants representing all disciplines involved in caring for patients with abnormal cytology (**Figures 20-1** through **20-12**) (Massad et al., 2013).

2. Evaluation techniques: Throughout the algorithms (Figures 20-1 through 20-12), choices can be made as to repeating the Pap smear in a specified interval of time, performing HPV DNA testing, or proceeding to colposcopic evaluation. The high incidence of low-grade squamous intraepithelial lesion with a small proportion of those cases progressing to high-grade squamous intraepithelial lesion has led to a conservative approach to managing adolescent and young women with abnormal cytology (Moscicki & Cox, 2010).

   a. Repeat Pap smear evaluation confirms the persistence or regression of abnormal cells over time.

   b. HPV DNA testing provides an opportunity to categorize HPV into low-risk and high-risk types. Type-specific HPV testing is also available once the presence of high-risk HPV has been confirmed. Data show that the persistence of high-risk HPV is a risk factor for progression to high-grade intraepithelial neoplasia.

   c. Colposcopic evaluation with directed biopsy allows the clinician to visually assess the lower genital tract under high-power magnification and evaluate lesions according to color, borders,

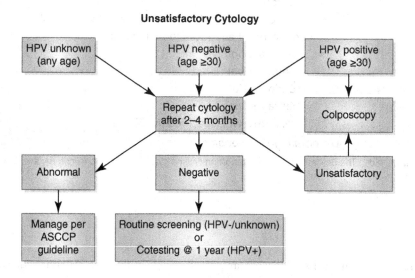

FIGURE 20-1 Unsatisfactory Cytology

Reprinted from the *Journal of Lower Genital Tract Disease*, Volume 17, Number 5, with the permission of ASCCP © American Society for Colposcopy and Cervical Pathology 2013. No copies of the algorithms may be made without the prior consent of ASCCP.

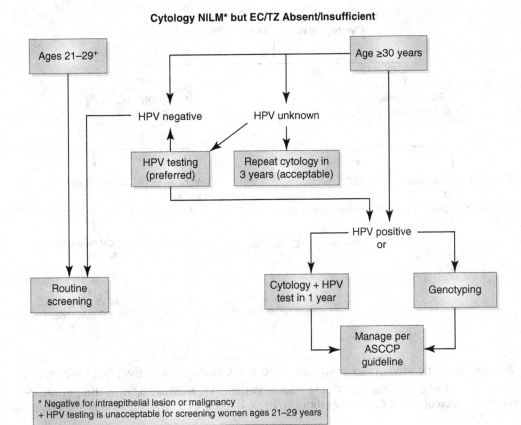

FIGURE 20-2 Cytology NILM but EC/TZ Absent/Insufficient
Reprinted from the *Journal of Lower Genital Tract Disease*, Volume 17, Number 5, with the permission of ASCCP ©
American Society for Colposcopy and Cervical Pathology 2013. No copies of the algorithms may be made without the
prior consent of ASCCP.

vessels, and surface. Colposcopically directed biopsies are obtained to determine the pathologic diagnosis of the lesions and guide the treatment and management strategies (Apgar, Brotzman, & Rubin, 2008; Mayeaux & Cox, 2012). The vulva and vagina should be included in the comprehensive evaluation of an abnormal Pap test because the cells from those areas can play a role in the abnormal reading. However, vulvar cytology is not considered effective for evaluating the keratinized epithelium in that site. Biopsy will facilitate obtaining an accurate diagnosis for vulvar lesions.

d. Endocervical sampling with a curette or a cytobrush is sometimes included in the colposcopic evaluation to further evaluate the endocervical canal. This occurs when glandular abnormality

is present or the colposcopic evaluation is unsatisfactory (the junction of the cervical squamous and columnar epithelium is not visualized on the surface of the cervix).

e. Endometrial sampling should also be included when atypical glandular cells are present and the woman is older than 35 years or at risk for endometrial cancer. In the 2014 Bethesda Update, benign-appearing endometrial cells should be reported in women ≥ 45 years, noting that endometrial evaluation be done only in postmenopausal women. *Atypical* endometrial cells should always be evaluated with endometrial biopsy regardless of age.

The following figures illustrate the triage and follow-up of abnormal cytology readings. They are meant to be a guide and not a comprehensive review. For greater detail regarding the evidence-based rationale

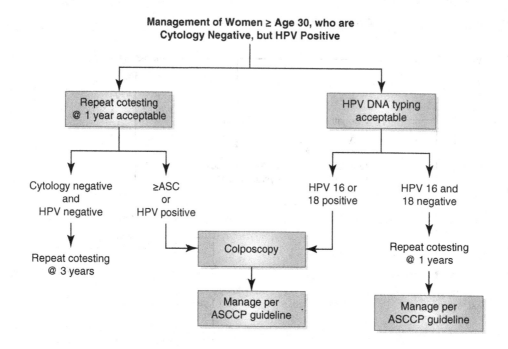

FIGURE 20-3 Management of Women ≥ Age 30, Who Are Cytology Negative, but HPV Positive

Reprinted from the *Journal of Lower Genital Tract Disease*, Volume 17, Number 5, with the permission of ASCCP © American Society for Colposcopy and Cervical Pathology 2013. No copies of the algorithms may be made without the prior consent of ASCCP.

for the choices, consult the consensus guidelines for cervical cancer screening from the ASCCP (Massad et al., 2013).

II. Database (may include but is not limited to)

A. Subjective

1. Past health history
   a. Medical illnesses: immune disorders including HIV, systemic lupus erythematosus, organ transplant, or blood dyscrasias.
   b. Medication history: medications that affect immune response (e.g., prednisone), hormone therapy, or anticoagulant or aspirin therapy.
   c. Allergy history: iodine
   d. Surgical history: hysterectomy and excisional or ablative treatment.
   e. Obstetric and gynecological history: parity, current or recent pregnancy, desire for future pregnancy, history of intraepithelial neoplasia, condylomata, abnormal cytology or positive HPV testing, menstrual history, history of STIs, history of DES exposure, HPV vaccination.

2. Family history: gynecological cancers

3. Personal and social history: age at onset of sexual activity; number of sexual partners; birth control method and condom use; sexual preference; and tobacco, alcohol, and drug use.

4. Review of systems
   a. General health.
   b. Psychosocial: ability to understand disease and relation to sexual activity, depression, anxiety, and guilt or shame.
   c. Reproductive: presence of pruritus; vulvar, vaginal, or anal pain; dyspareunia; abnormal bleeding; abnormal anogenital growths; and vaginal discharge or odor.

B. Objective

1. External: gross inspection of vulvar and perianal skin, noting presence of condylomata, ulcers, pigmented lesions, leukoplakia, microtears, inflammation,

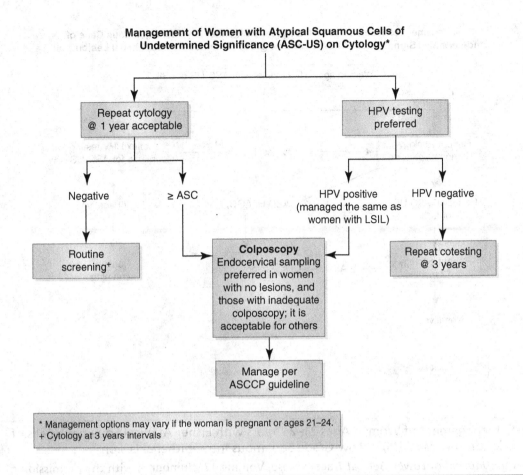

Management of Women with Atypical Squamous Cells of Undetermined Significance (ASC-US) on Cytology*

- Repeat cytology @ 1 year acceptable
  - Negative → Routine screening+
  - ≥ ASC → Colposcopy
- HPV testing preferred
  - HPV positive (managed the same as women with LSIL) → Colposcopy
  - HPV negative → Repeat cotesting @ 3 years

Colposcopy
Endocervical sampling preferred in women with no lesions, and those with inadequate colposcopy; it is acceptable for others

→ Manage per ASCCP guideline

* Management options may vary if the woman is pregnant or ages 21–24.
+ Cytology at 3 years intervals

FIGURE 20-4 Management of Women with Atypical Squamous Cells of Undetermined Significance (ASC-US) on Cytology

Reprinted from the *Journal of Lower Genital Tract Disease*, Volume 17, Number 5, with the permission of ASCCP © American Society for Colposcopy and Cervical Pathology 2013. No copies of the algorithms may be made without the prior consent of ASCCP.

atrophy, raised lesions; colposcopic inspection noting acetowhite epithelium with or without vessel patterns, such as punctation, mosaic, or atypical vessels; and Lugol's nonstaining lesions (avoid if allergic to iodine).

2. Speculum examination: gross inspection of cervix and vagina noting discharge, inflammation, atrophy, leukoplakia, ulcers, and raised lesions; colposcopic examination noting location of squamocolumnar junction, acetowhite epithelium with or without vessel patterns, and Lugol's nonstaining lesions (Mayeaux & Cox, 2012).

3. Supporting data from relevant diagnostic tests, including wet smear and potassium hydroxide (KOH), cytology and histology, and HPV testing, urine or swab.

III. Assessment

A. Determine the diagnosis
Genital warts, AIN, VIN, VAIN, CIN, AIS, invasive cancer, or other lesions

B. Determine the severity and location
1. Low-grade: mild dysplasia (intraepithelial neoplasia grade 1)

2. High-grade: moderate (intraepithelial neoplasia grade 2) and severe or carcinoma in situ (intraepithelial neoplasia grade 3). The conclusions from the Lower Anogenital Squamous Terminology (LAST) consensus conference for cervical histopathology

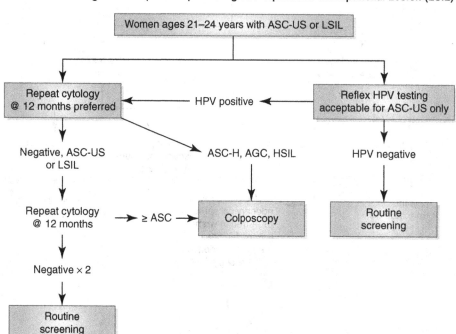

FIGURE 20-5 Management of Women Ages 21–24 Years with Either Atypical Squamous Cells of Undetermined Significance (ASC-US) or Low-Grade Squamous Intraepithelial Lesion

Reprinted from the *Journal of Lower Genital Tract Disease*, Volume 17, Number 5, with the permission of ASCCP © American Society for Colposcopy and Cervical Pathology 2013. No copies of the algorithms may be made without the prior consent of ASCCP.

and its implications for management of high-grade squamous intraepithelial lesions of the cervix have been adopted. Revised terminology for high-grade now combines CIN 2 and CIN 3 and does not try to differentiate between the two (Waxman et al., 2012). The current ASCCP 2013 guidelines do not yet reflect combining CIN 2 and 3 into one high-grade category, thus allowing young women with CIN 2 to be managed expectantly (see **Figure 20-9**). Management of young women with biopsy confirmed CIN 2, 3.

3. Unifocal versus multifocal, exocervical, endocervical, vaginal, or vulvar.

C. *Significance*

Assess the significance of the diagnosis to the patient and partner(s)

D. *Motivation and ability*

Determine the patient's willingness and ability to follow the treatment plan.

IV. Goals of clinical management

The choice of treatment is influenced by a number of factors, including the patient's preference; age; parity; the location, extent, and degree of abnormality; cost of treatment; the limitations of the healthcare facility to provide certain treatments; the patient's desire for future fertility; the patient's ability to understand and follow the treatment protocol; and probability of patient follow-up. The dose and duration of treatment should be determined by referring to product guidelines.

A. *Screening for the purpose of diagnosing or preventing cervical, vaginal, and vulvar cancer*

Anal and perianal intraepithelial neoplasia are also a growing concern but are not covered in this chapter. Choose a cost-effective available approach for diagnosing precancerous and cancerous lesions. More information regarding the evolving science for screening of the anal canal with digital exam, cytology evaluation, or high-resolution anoscopy (HRA) can be found in a recent review by Moscicki et al., 2015.

Management of Women with Low-grade Squamous Intraepithelial Lesions (LSIL)*‡

| LSIL with negative HPV test among women ≥ 30 with cotesting | LSIL with no HPV test | LSIL with positive HPV test among women ≥ 30 with cotesting |

Preferred

Acceptable

Repeat cotesting @ 1 year

Colposcopy

Cytology negative and HPV negative

≥ ASC or HPV positive

Non-pregnant and no lesion identified	Endocervical sampling "**preferred**"
Inadequate colposcopic examination	Endocervical sampling "**preferred**"
Adequate colposcopy and lesion identified	Endocervical sampling "**acceptable**"

Repeat cotesting @ 3 years

No CIN2, 3

CIN2, 3

Manage per ASCCP guideline

Manage per ASCCP guideline

* Management options may vary if the woman is pregnant or ages 21–24 years
‡ Manage women ages 25–29 as having LSIL with no HPV test

FIGURE 20-6 Management of Women with Low-Grade Squamous Intraepithelial Lesions

Reprinted from *The Journal of Lower Genital Tract Disease*, Volume 17, Number 5, with the permission of ASCCP © American Society for Colposcopy and Cervical Pathology 2013. No copies of the algorithms may be made without the prior consent of ASCCP.

B. Treatment

Select a treatment plan that reduces symptoms and prevents progression. See under management (treatment of CIN) for more detail.

C. Patient adherence

Select an approach that maximizes patient adherence.

V. Plan

A. Screening

Screening for cervical, vaginal, and vulvar cancer is influenced by the age of the patient, the presence of immunosuppressive diseases or medications, history of DES exposure, and history of CIN 2+ or positive HPV tests (Reed & Fenton, 2013; Rubin, 2007).

B. Diagnostic tests

May include the following: cervical cytology, HPV DNA testing, anal cytology, biopsy, endocervical curettage, cervical cultures for gonorrhea and *Chlamydia*, wet smear and KOH, and urine human chorionic gonadotropin.

C. Management

1. May include treatment of vaginitis, STIs, vaginal atrophy, and dermatosis if symptomatic.

2. Treatment of genital warts: trichloroacetic acid 0.5%, imiquimod (Aldara®) 5% cream, 5-fluorouracil (Efudex®) 3–5%, and sinecatechin (Veregen®); cryotherapy with liquid nitrogen or cryoprobe; surgical excision; laser therapy; or interferon alfa-2b (Intron®) or observation.

3. Treatment of VIN 2, 3: wide local excision, laser therapy, skinning vulvectomy, imiquimod (Aldara®) 5%, 5-fluorouracil 2–5%, cryotherapy, or observation (Riberio, Figueiredo, Paula, & Borrego, 2012). VIN 1 is no longer categorized as intraepithelial neoplasia that requires treatment. Refer to the International Society for the Study of Vulvovaginal Disease (http://issvd.org/) for more detail (Reyes & Cooper, 2014).

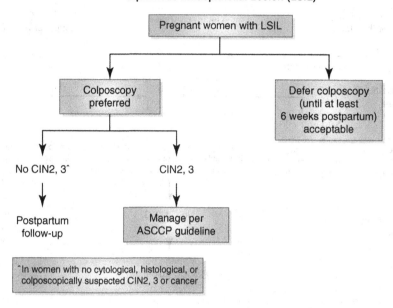

FIGURE 20-7 Management of Pregnant Women with Low-Grade Squamous Intraepithelial Lesion

Reprinted from the *Journal of Lower Genital Tract Disease*, Volume 17, Number 5, with the permission of ASCCP © American Society for Colposcopy and Cervical Pathology 2013. No copies of the algorithms may be made without the prior consent of ASCCP.

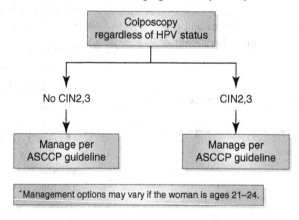

FIGURE 20-8 Management of Women with Atypical Squamous Cells: Cannot Exclude High-Grade SIL (ASC-H)

Reprinted from *The Journal of Lower Genital Tract Disease*, Volume 17, Number 5, with the permission of ASCCP © American Society for Colposcopy and Cervical Pathology 2013. No copies of the algorithms may be made without the prior consent of ASCCP.

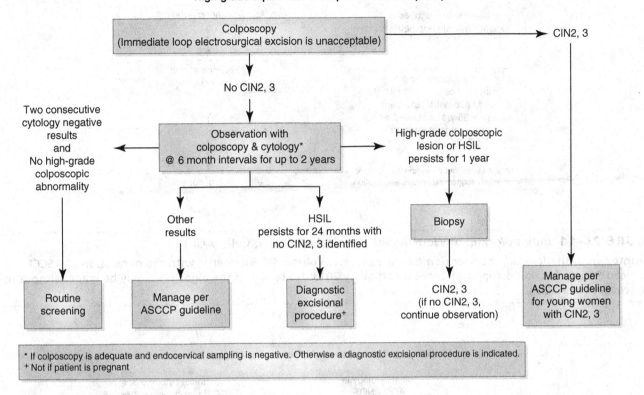

FIGURE 20-9 Management of Women Ages 21–24 Years with Atypical Squamous Cells, Cannot Rule Out High-Grade SIL (ASC-H) and High-Grade Squamous Intraepithelial Lesion (HSIL)

Reprinted from the *Journal of Lower Genital Tract Disease*, Volume 17, Number 5, with the permission of ASCCP © American Society for Colposcopy and Cervical Pathology 2013. No copies of the algorithms may be made without the prior consent of ASCCP.

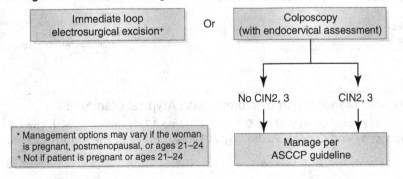

FIGURE 20-10 Management of Women with High-Grade Squamous Intraepithelial Lesions

Reprinted from the *Journal of Lower Genital Tract Disease*, Volume 17, Number 5, with the permission of ASCCP © American Society for Colposcopy and Cervical Pathology 2013. No copies of the algorithms may be made without the prior consent of ASCCP.

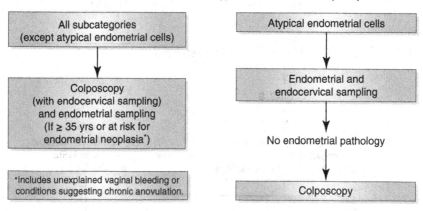

FIGURE 20-11 Initial Workup of Women with Atypical Glandular Cells (AGC)

Reprinted from the *Journal of Lower Genital Tract Disease*, Volume 17, Number 5, with the permission of ASCCP © American Society for Colposcopy and Cervical Pathology 2013. No copies of the algorithms may be made without the prior consent of ASCCP.

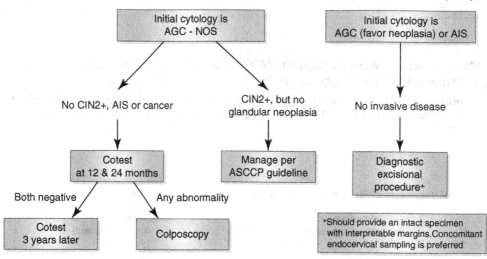

FIGURE 20-12 Subsequent Management of Women with Atypical Glandular Cells

Reprinted from the *Journal of Lower Genital Tract Disease*, Volume 17, Number 5, with the permission of ASCCP © American Society for Colposcopy and Cervical Pathology 2013. No copies of the algorithms may be made without the prior consent of ASCCP.

4. Treatment of VAIN: 5-fluorouracil 2–5%, laser therapy, surgical or electrosurgical excision, or observation.

5. Treatment of CIN: follow ASCCP Management Guidelines (**Figures 20-13** through **20-18**). These algorithms allow for appropriate management once colposcopic evaluation has been completed. Treatments include cryotherapy, laser vaporization or excision, loop electrosurgical excision procedure (LEEP), and cold knife cone biopsy. The choice of procedure and whether to use excision or ablation depend on many factors including experience of the provider, availability of equipment, size of the transformation zone and lesions, satisfactory colposcopic examination, insurance coverage, and desires of the patient, especially future fertility (Arbyn et al., 2008; Massad et al., 2013).

D. Client education

1. Concerns and feelings
   a. Discuss the emotional impact of HPV-associated disease on the patient's self-esteem, body image, and feelings of trust and safety with her sexual partner.
      i. Most women will be exposed to HPV at some time during their lifetime.
      ii. Partners are usually unaware of their exposure to the virus and their ability to transmit it to their partner. Evaluation of male partner is not usually recommended due to lack of available testing. Males have a very low risk of HPV-related cancer. Female partners should be advised to consult their clinician if recent Pap or HPV testing has not been done.
   b. Discuss concerns about cancer and fertility (Rubin & Tripsas, 2010).
      i. Cancer is preventable with early detection. It typically takes 10–20 years for HPV infection to develop into cancer. Intraepithelial neoplasia is treatable. However, HPV infection may persist after treatment. Follow-up is important.

c. After surgical excision treatment there is an increased risk of preterm labor. Young patients who desire more pregnancies should discuss ablation treatments such as cryotherapy or laser vaporization as an alternative to excision.

2. Information
   a. Discuss smoking cessation, healthy diet and lifestyle, safer sex, and HPV in pregnancy.
      i. Smoking is a known cofactor in the development of genital and oral cancers.
      ii. Diets high in fruits and vegetables may be beneficial in boosting the immune response.
      iii. Condom use reduces but does not eliminate transmission of HPV. Reducing the number of sexual partners can reduce the risk of HPV acquisition and transmission.
      iv. HPV transmission to the fetus is low. Patient may safely deliver vaginally.
   b. Discuss the relationship between HPV and cancer, and the need for ongoing follow-up (refer to ASCCP guidelines).
   c. Discuss diagnostic tests including colposcopy, biopsy, and endocervical curettage.
   d. Discuss treatments and side effects.
      i. All treatment methods are associated with some bleeding and discharge. Cryotherapy is also followed by heavy watery discharge for 2–4 weeks. Pelvic rest and avoidance of strenuous activity are recommended for that time after all treatments.
   e. Discuss HPV vaccination benefits and limitations.

3. Resources and tools
   a. http://www.asccp.org
   b. http://www.cdc.gov/std/hpv/
   c. www.cervicalcancerfacts.com
   d. http://www.cancer.org
   e. http://www.analcancerinfo.ucsf.edu

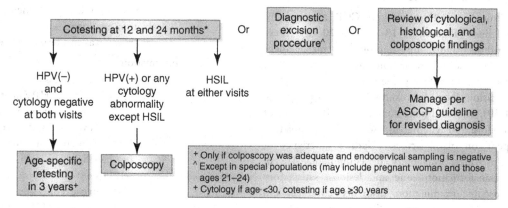

FIGURE 20-13 Management of Women with No Lesion or Biopsy Confirmed Cervical Intraepithelial Neoplasia–Grade 1 (CIN1) Preceded by ASC-H or HSIL Cytology

Reprinted from the *Journal of Lower Genital Tract Disease*, Volume 17, Number 5, with the permission of ASCCP © American Society for Colposcopy and Cervical Pathology 2013. No copies of the algorithms may be made without the prior consent of ASCCP.

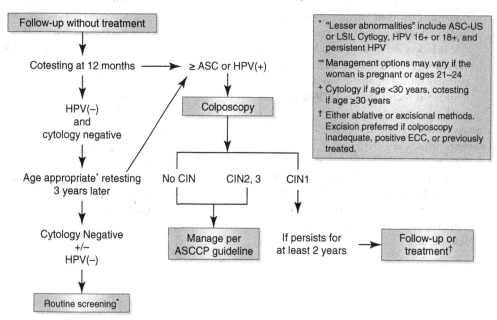

FIGURE 20-14 Management of Women with No Lesion or Biopsy-Confirmed Cervical Intraepithelial Neoplasia–Grade 1 Preceded by Lesser Abnormalities

Reprinted from the *Journal of Lower Genital Tract Disease*, Volume 17, Number 5, with the permission of ASCCP © American Society for Colposcopy and Cervical Pathology 2013. No copies of the algorithms may be made without the prior consent of ASCCP.

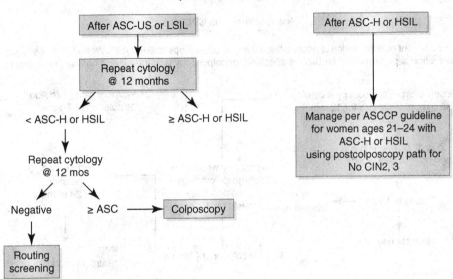

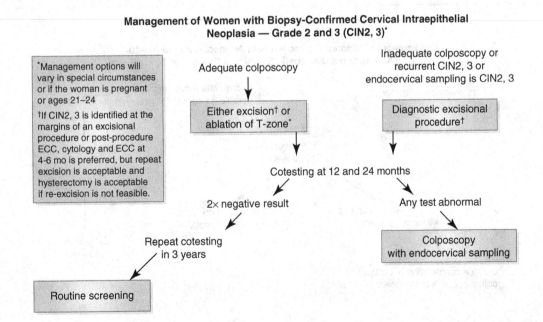

FIGURE 20-15 Management of Women Ages 21–24 with No Lesion or Biopsy-Confirmed Cervical Intraepithelial Neoplasia–Grade 1

Reprinted from the *Journal of Lower Genital Tract Disease*, Volume 17, Number 5, with the permission of ASCCP © American Society for Colposcopy and Cervical Pathology 2013. No copies of the algorithms may be made without the prior consent of ASCCP.

FIGURE 20-16 Management of Women with No Lesion or Biopsy-Confirmed Cervical Intraepithelial Neoplasia–Grades 2 and 3 (CIN2, 3)

Reprinted from the *Journal of Lower Genital Tract Disease*, Volume 17, Number 5, with the permission of ASCCP © American Society for Colposcopy and Cervical Pathology 2013. No copies of the algorithms may be made without the prior consent of ASCCP.

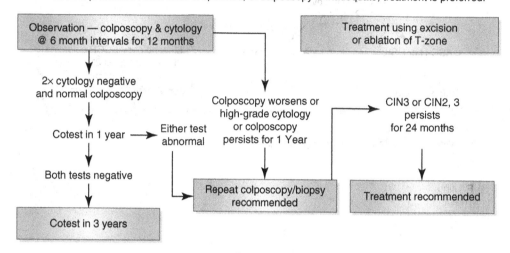

FIGURE 20-17 Management of Young Women with Biopsy-Confirmed Cervical Intraepithelial Neoplasia–Grades 2 and 3 in Special Circumstances

Reprinted from the *Journal of Lower Genital Tract Disease*, Volume 17, Number 5, with the permission of ASCCP © American Society for Colposcopy and Cervical Pathology 2013. No copies of the algorithms may be made without the prior consent of ASCCP.

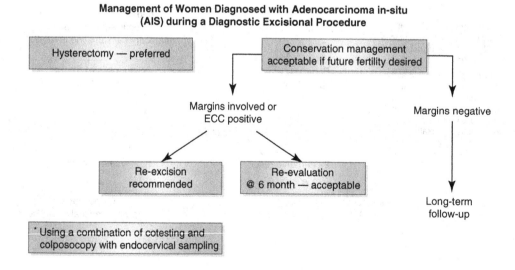

FIGURE 20-18 Management of Women Diagnosed with Adenocarcinoma In Situ (AIS) During a Diagnostic Excisional Procedure

Reprinted from the *Journal of Lower Genital Tract Disease*, Volume 17, Number 5, with the permission of ASCCP © American Society for Colposcopy and Cervical Pathology 2013. No copies of the algorithms may be made without the prior consent of ASCCP.

REFERENCES

American College of Obstetricians and Gynecologists. (2012). ACOG practice bulletin No 131: Screening for cervical cancer. *Obstetrics and Gynecology, 120*(5), 1222–1238.

Apgar, B., Brotzman, G., & Rubin, M. (2008). Principles and technique of the colposcopic exam. In B. Apgar, G. Brotzman, & M. Spitzer (Eds.). *Colposcopy principles and practice: An integrated textbook and atlas* (2nd ed., pp. 101–125). Philadelphia, PA: W.B. Saunders.

Arbyn, M., Kyrgiou, M., Simoens, C., Raifu, A. O., Koliopoulos, G., Martin-Hirsch, P., et al. (2008). Perinatal mortality and other severe adverse pregnancy outcomes associated with treatment of cervical intraepithelial neoplasia: Meta-analysis. *British Medical Journal, 337*, a1284.

Food and Drug Administration. (2014, December 10). FDA approves Gardasil 9 for prevention of certain cancers caused by five additional types of HPV. FDA News Release. Retrieved from http://www.fda.gov/NewsEvents/Newsroom/PressAnnouncements/ucm426485.htm.

Huh, W. K., Ault, K. A., Chelmow, D., Davey, D., Goulart, R., Garcia, F., et al. (2015). Use of primary high-risk human papillomavirus testing for cervical cancer screening: Interim clinical guidance. *Gynecologic Oncology, 136*, 178–182.

Kjær, S., Frederiksen, E., Munk, C., & Iftner, T. (2010). Long-term absolute risk of cervical intraepithelial neoplasia grade 3 or worse following human papillomavirus infection. *JNCI: Journal of the National Cancer Institute, 102*(1), 1478–1488.

Kosiol, J., Lindsay, L., Pimenta, J., Poole, C., Jenkins, D., & Smith, J. (2008). Persistence of human papillomavirus infection and cervical neoplasia: A systematic review and meta analysis. *American Journal of Epidemiology, 168*(2), 123–137.

Li, N., Franceschi, S., Howell-Jones, R., Snijders, P. J., & Clifford, G. M. (2011). Human papillomavirus type distribution in 30,848 invasive cervical cancers worldwide: Variation by geographical region, histological type and year of publication. *International Journal of Cancer, 128*(4), 927–935. doi: 10.1002/ijc.25396.

Markowitz, L., Dunne, E., Saraiya, M., Chesson, H., Curtis, C., Gee, J., et al. (2014). Human papillomavirus vaccination: Recommendations of the Advisory Committee on Immunization Practices (ACIP). *MMWR Recommendations and Reports, 63*(RR05), 1–30.

Massad, S., Einstein, M., Huh, W., Katki, M., Kinney, W., Schiffman, M., et al. (2013). 2012 updated consensus guidelines for the management of abnormal cervical cancer screening tests and cancer precursors. American Society for Colposcopy and Cervical Pathology. *Journal of Lower Genital Tract Disease, 17*(5), S1Y–S27.

Mayeaux, E. J., & Cox, J. T. (Eds.). (2012). *Modern colposcopy textbook and atlas* (3rd ed.). Philadelphia, PA: Wolters Kluwer/Lippincott William & Wilkins.

Moscicki, A. B., & Cox, J. T. (2010). Practice improvement in cervical screening and management (PICSM): Symposium on management of cervical abnormalities in adolescents and young women. *Journal of Lower Genital Tract Disease 14*, 73Y80.

Moscicki, A. B., Darragh, T., Berry-Lawhorn, M. J., Roberts, J., Kjhan, M., Boardman, L., et al. (2015). Screening for anal cancer in women. *Journal of Lower Genital Tract Disease, 19*(3, Suppl. 2), 27–42.

Nayar, R., & Wilbur, D. (2015). The Pap test and Bethesda 2014: "The reports of my demise have been greatly exaggerated" (after a quotation from Mark Twain). *Journal of Lower Genital Tract Disease, 19*(3), 175–184.

Reed, C., & Fenton, S. (2013). Exposure to diethylstilbestrol during sensitive life stages: A legacy of heritable health effects. *Birth Defects Research Part C: Embryo Today, 99*(2), 10.1002/bdrc.21035.

Reyes, M., & Cooper, K. (2014). An update on vulvar intraepithelial neoplasia: terminology and a practical approach to diagnosis. *Journal of Clinical Pathology, 67*(4), 290–294. doi: 10.1136/jclinpath-2013-202117. Epub 2014 Jan 7.

Ribeiro, F., Figueiredo, A., Paula, T., Borrego, F. (2012). Vulvar intraepithelial: evaluation of treatment modalities. *Journal of Lower Genital Tract Disease, 16*(3), 313–317.

Rubin, M. (2007). Antenatal exposure to DES: Lessons learned . . . concerns for the future. *Obstetrical and Gynecological Survey, 62*(8), 1–7.

Rubin, M., & Tripsas, C. (2010). Uncertainty, coping strategies and adaptation in women with human papillomavirus (HPV) on Papanicolaou smears. *Journal of Lower Genital Tract Disease, 14*(3), 81–89.

Saslow, D., Solomon, D., Lawson, H., Killackey, M., Kulasingam, S., Cain, J., et al. (2012). American Cancer Society, American Society for Colposcopy and Cervical Pathology, and American Society for Clinical Pathology Screening Guidelines for the Prevention and Early Detection of Cervical Cancer. *Journal of Lower Genital Tract Disease, 16*(3), 1–29.

Solomon, D., & Nayar, R. (2004.) *The Bethesda system for reporting cervical cytology: Definitions, criteria, and explanatory notes.* New York: Springer.

U.S. Preventive Services Task Force. (2012). Cervical cancer: Screening. Retrieved from http://www.uspreventiveservicestaskforce.org/Page/Document/UpdateSummaryFinal/cervical-cancer-screening.

Waxman, A. G., Chelmow, D., Darragh, T. M., Lawson, H., & Moscicki, A. (2012). Revised terminology for cervical histopathology and its implications for management of high-grade squamous intraepithelial lesions of the cervix. *Obstetrics and Gynecology, 120*(6), 1465–1471.

Winer, R., Lee, S., Hughes, J., Adam, D., Kiviat, N., & Koutsky, L. (2003). Genital human papillomavirus infection: Incidence and risk factors in a cohort of female university students. *American Journal of Epidemiology, 157*(3), 218–226.

FEMALE AND MALE STERILIZATION

Janis Luft

CHAPTER 21

I. Introduction and general background

Approximately 37% of reproductive age couples who desire contraception use sterilization, making this the most commonly used form of contraception in the United States (Bartz & Greenberg, 2008).

Female sterilization describes a number of surgical procedures intended to physically prevent sperm from uniting with and fertilizing an egg. Although sterilization surgeries can include the removal of the uterus (hysterectomy), the term "female sterilization" in this chapter describes the more typically performed, less invasive procedures for disrupting fallopian tubal patency. Tubal ligation, either by excision of a portion of the tube, electrosurgical dessication, or tubal occlusion through the use of surgical clips or rings is generally performed via laparoscopy. Tubal occlusion using fallopian inserts (Essure®) can be done hysteroscopically through the cervix, thus avoiding surgical incision. All of these procedures effectively end a woman's fertility. About 700,000 women choose some form of sterilization procedures annually. Vasectomy is the male form of sterilization. Approximately half a million men a year choose this permanent form of contraception. A vasectomy is a minor surgical procedure that is performed under local anesthesia. One or two small punctures or incisions are made in the scrotum and the vas deferens is ligated, cauterized, or occluded, thus preventing sperm from admixing with semen.

A. Tubal ligation

1. Definition and overview
   a. Sterilization is a permanent form of contraception that is highly effective. Recent evaluation of data collected by the U.S. Collaborative Review of Sterilization (CREST), which followed more than 10,000 women with surgical sterilization for up to 14 years, reported a 5-year failure rate of 13/10,000 procedures. These data do not

include operative sterilization using the Filshie clip or hysteroscopic sterilization (Gariepy, Creinin, Smith, & Xu, 2014).
   b. Laparoscopy can be performed under general, regional, or local anesthesia with sedation. Fallopian tubes can be ligated, dessicated with electrosurgery, or clamped.
   c. Minilaparotomy involves a small abdominal incision and requires general anesthesia. Salpingectomy (removal of the fallopian tubes) or any of the previously mentioned procedures can be performed using minilaparotomy.

2. Benefits
   a. Both surgeries provide immediate and permanent contraception.
   b. Highly effective but failure rates have been shown to be dependent on the age of the woman and the method used (Creinin & Zite, 2014).
   c. Extremely safe with rare operative complications.
   d. Covered benefit of Medi-Cal, Medicaid programs, and the Affordable Care Act.
   e. Large case control studies have demonstrated a 39% reduction in the risk of ovarian cancer in women who have had surgical sterilization (Rice, Hankinson, & Tworoger, 2014).

3. Risks and disadvantages
   a. There are no absolute contraindications to these procedures, but people with certain health conditions, such as obesity, pelvic adhesions, diabetes, or severe cardiac or lung disease, may not be ideal surgical candidates.
   b. General anesthesia may be required.
   c. A 30-day waiting period post counseling and post consenting is required by federal Medicaid guidelines.
   d. There is an increased risk of ectopic pregnancy if the method fails.

e. This method affords no protection against sexually transmitted infections (STIs).

f. Possibility of regret exists.

B. Transcervical tubal occlusion

1. Definition and overview

Currently, Essure® is the only system of transcervical sterilization available in the United States approved by the Food and Drug Administration. The procedure is done via hysteroscopy and involves placing micro-inserts into the horns of the uterus, causing scarring and occlusion of the fallopian tubes. This is done using local anesthesia only, requires no incision, and thus can be done in an outpatient setting. This method requires an appropriately trained clinician. Accurate insertion of the devices can fail in as many as one in seven placements. Verification of tubal occlusion requires hysterosalpingography (HSG) 3 months after placement of the occluding devices.

Essure® microinsert is a tiny coil that consists of a stainless steel inner coil, a nickel titanium outer coil, and polyethelene fibers. After placement, there is a delay in efficacy until tubal fibrosis occurs (typically 3 months) during which alternate contraception must be used.

2. Benefits

a. Hysteroscopy precludes the need for a surgical incision. There is less risk of infection and faster recovery time. It may be a better choice for women who are not ideal candidates for even minimally invasive pelvic surgery.

b. There is no need for general or regional anesthesia. Generally, only paracervical block or mild oral or intravenous sedation is used, and thus it can be done in an outpatient setting.

c. Initial studies found the method to be highly effective, but failure rates may be underestimated and are probably lower than with surgical sterilization. Effectiveness can be dependent on the experience of the provider and the compliance of the patient during the 3-month interval until tubal occlusion can be verified (Gariepy et al., 2014).

d. It is covered by Medi-Cal, most Medicaid programs, and the Affordable Care Act.

3. Risks and disadvantages

a. There is a delay in the efficacy of these methods of 3 months or more to allow for sufficient tubal fibrosis to take place. A hysterosalpingogram is required to ensure that the tubes are occluded. Other methods of contraception (but not an intrauterine device) must be used in the 3-month interim between the procedure and until tubal fibrosis can be demonstrated.

b. The provider must be trained in the use and placement of these devices. Rates of successful bilateral coil placement can range from 76% to 96%.

c. Certain uterine malformations (e.g., bicornuate uterus) may preclude proper placement of the devices.

d. Women must be at least 6 weeks postpartum.

e. A 30-day waiting period post counseling and post consenting is required by federal Medicaid guidelines.

f. This method affords no protection against STIs.

g. Possibility of regret exists.

C. Vasectomy

1. Definition and overview

Vasectomy is male sterilization accomplished by severing the vas deferens, thus preventing sperm from entering the ejaculate. Vasectomies can be done either by making a small incision in the scrotum using a scalpel to access and sever the vas or by using the no-scalpel technique. No incision is made. Rather, the vas is grasped with specialized ring forceps externally and a small puncture is made using dissecting forceps to externalize the vas for cutting. The benefits of this procedure include less bleeding, a smaller hole in the skin, and fewer complications. Both techniques are equally effective (Sharlip et al., 2012).

2. Benefits

a. Provides permanent contraception with low failure rates, ranging from 0% to 0.5% when used perfectly

b. Requires local anesthesia and can be done in the outpatient setting.

c. Cost effective. Covered by Medi-Cal and some Medicaid programs but not the Affordable Care Act.

d. Not partner dependent.

3. Risks and disadvantages

a. It can take up to 3–6 months to achieve complete aspermia. Effective contraception must be used until ejaculate tests negative for the presence of sperm. Most vasectomy "failures" occur within the first 3 months after the procedure.

b. There is postprocedure pain and swelling.

c. A 30-day waiting period post counseling and post consenting is required by federal Medicaid guidelines.

d. This method affords no protection against STI.

e. Possible regret exists. Although vasectomy reversal is often possible, success rates for pregnancy vary from 40% to 90% and can be dependent on the length of time since the original procedure, type of procedure, and the skill of the provider performing the reversal (Sharlip et al., 2012).

II. Database (may include but is not limited to)

A. Subjective

1. Gynecological, urologic, medical, and psychosocial history
   a. Patient desires permanent sterilization.
   b. Patient has considered and declined other contraceptive options.
   c. There are no medical contraindications to the procedure that would incur high surgical risk.

B. Objective

1. Complete gynecological and urologic examination; negative pregnancy test for women.
2. Absence of psychiatric or mental disability.
   a. For guidance on the issues of mental competency and ability to give informed consent for sterilization see http://www.acog.org/Resources-And-Publications/Committee-Opinions/Committee-on-Ethics/Sterilization-of-Women-Including-Those-With-Mental-Disabilities

III. Assessment

A. Patient is a candidate for sterilization

1. According to federal guidelines, candidate must be at least 21 years of age.
2. Mentally competent.
3. Women not currently pregnant.
4. No medical contraindications to procedure.

B. Understands and accepts the permanent nature of the procedure and is prepared to end childbearing

IV. Plan

A. Client education

1. Information and counseling
   a. Before undergoing sterilization, patients must be sure that they no longer want to bear children and will not want to bear children in the future, even if life circumstances change. Information must also be provided about the many effective contraceptive choices available.
   b. Discuss risks, benefits, discomforts, and recovery times associated with various procedures.
   c. Review follow-up testing as appropriate. Discuss plan for and provide interim contraception as needed.

2. Consenting
   a. In California, clinicians are required to provide a copy of the sterilization booklet published by the Department of Health Services. In other states, check the state department of health for similar requirements.
   b. Obtain informed consent. Federal Medicaid guidelines require written consent signed at least 30 days and no more than 180 days before the planned procedure for patients receiving public funding. A copy must be placed in the medical record and a copy provided to the patient.
   c. Assure the patient of his or her right to revoke consent at any time.

V. Self-management resources

A. The American Congress of Obstetricians and Gynecologists: Sterilization for men and women: http://www.acog.org/-/media/For-Patients/faq011.pdf?dmc=1&ts=20150920T1518453944

B. Planned Parenthood, Sterilization for women (tubal ligation): http://www.plannedparenthood.org/learn/birth-control/sterilization-women

C. Planned Parenthood, Vasectomy: http://www.plannedparenthood.org/learn/birth-control/vasectomy

REFERENCES

American College of Obstetricians and Gynecologists. (2007). *Sterilization of women, including those with mental disabilities* (ACOG Committee Opinion Number 371). Washington, DC: Author.

Bartz, D., & Greenberg J. A. (2008). Sterilization in the United States. *Reviews in Obstetrics and Gynecology, 1*(1), 23–32.

Creinin, M. D., & Zite, N. (2014). Female tubal sterilization: The time has come to routinely consider removal. *Obstetrics and Gynecology, 124*(3), 596–599.

Daniels, K., Daugherty, J., & Jones, J. (2014). *Current contraceptive status among women aged 15–44: United States, 2011–2013* (NCHS Data Brief, no.173). Hyattsville, MD: National Center for Health Statistics, Centers for Disease Control and Prevention.

Gariepy, A. M., Creinin, M. D., Smith, K. J., & Xu, X. (2014). Probability of pregnancy after sterilization: A comparison of hysteroscopic versus laparoscopic sterilization. *Contraception, 90*, 174–181.

Pollack, A. E., Thomas, L. J., & Barone, M. A. (2008). Female and male sterilization. In R. A. Hatcher, J. Trussell, A. E. Nelson, W. Cates, F. Stewart, & D. Kowal (Eds.). (2009). *Contraceptive technology* (19th rev. ed., pp. 362–401). New York, NY: Ardent Media.

Rice, M. S., Hankinson, S. E., & Tworoger, S. S. (2014). Tubal ligation, hysterectomy, unilateral oophorectomy, and risk of ovarian cancer in the Nurses' Health Studies. *Fertility and Sterility, 102*(1), 192–198.

Sharlip, I. D., Honig, S., Labrecque, M., Marmar, J. L., Ross L. S., Sandlow, J. L., et al. (2012). Vasectomy: American Urologic Association Guideline. Retrieved from www.auanet.org/education/guidelines/vasectomy.cfm.

Shih, G., Zhang, Y., Bukowski, K., & Chen, A. (2014). Bringing men to the table: Sterilization can be for him or for her. *Clinical Obstetrics and Gynecology, 57*(4), 731–740.

HORMONAL CONTRACEPTION

Lynn Hanson

CHAPTER 22

I. Introduction and general background

Hormonal contraception is used extensively and successfully throughout the world for family planning. When used properly, it is highly effective and safe. The most common form of hormonal contraception is the combined oral contraceptive (COC) pill. Other forms include the progestin-only pill (POP; Minipill), transdermal contraceptive patch, vaginal contraceptive ring, medroxyprogesterone acetate (Depo-Provera®) injection, etonogestrel implant (Implanon®, Nexplanon®), and levonorgestrel intrauterine system (LNG-IUS) (Mirena®, Skyla). Levonorgestrel alone or in a COC pill is used as the emergency contraception pill (ECP). (This should not be used as a regular method of contraception. Ulipristal acetate, an antiprogestin, is the newest option for emergency contraception, and the most effective.) All of these methods except for Ulipristal contain a form of progestin alone or in combination with an estrogen. The mechanism of contraception is primarily supplied by the progestin, through thickening of the cervical mucus, change in fallopian tube motility, inhibition of ovulation, and prevention of sperm capacitation, and in some cases endometrial atrophy. The addition of estrogen can further inhibit ovulation, and may alter the endometrial lining to prevent implantation. Estrogen helps to prevent breakthrough bleeding and maintain normal cycle patterns (Nelson, Contraceptive Technology, 2011).

Many factors must be weighed in determining if hormonal contraception is appropriate for a patient. Certain medical conditions present contraindications or relative contraindications to hormone use (see U.S. Medical Eligibility Criteria, **Table 22-1**). Patient compliance and tolerance of side effects are mandatory. Efficacy may be of primary importance to a woman where pregnancy is contraindicated for medical or personal reasons. Time to return of fertility may be important. Cost may be prohibitive for some patients. High-risk sexual behavior should also be considered, because many patients are less likely to use condoms when using hormonal

contraception, placing them at higher risk for sexually transmitted infections (STIs). Comfort with and ease of use of the method must also be considered. Age is an important factor, especially with adolescents, who continue to have high unintended pregnancy rates.

The Centers for Disease Control and Prevention have published recommendations for *Providing Quality Family Planning Services* (Gavin et al., 2014), with a focus on improved counseling through a client-centered approach that asks about reproductive life plan; respecting age, sexual preference, race, ethnicity, disability, and language limitations. A five-step counseling approach with a focus on interactive communication that establishes and maintains rapport is recommended. A special section addresses the needs of adolescents with regard to long-acting reversible contraception (LARC) and recommends the discussion of hormonal implants and intrauterine contraception as a safe and highly effective method for adolescent clients. For all patients, LARC provides the best contraceptive efficacy by avoiding less than optimal patient compliance.

A. Combined hormonal contraception

Combined hormonal contraception (CHC) includes methods that contain both estrogen and a progestin. These include the COC pill, transdermal patch, and vaginal ring. Combined injectable contraceptives are not currently available in the United States. CHC has many advantages beyond prevention of pregnancy. Dysmenorrhea and menorrhagia are often significantly reduced, and menstrual cycle regularity is improved. Symptoms and severity of endometriosis may be reduced, potentially preserving fertility. Premenstrual syndrome and migraine headaches are often improved but may also be increased. Many women benefit from a reduction in incidence of ovarian cyst-related problems when using estrogen-containing methods. Symptoms related to polycystic ovary syndrome, such as acne and hirsutism, often improve. Lighter menstrual cycles contribute to lower incidence of iron deficiency anemia. CHC is associated

TABLE 22-1 Summary Chart of U.S. Medical Eligibility Criteria for Contraceptive Use

Key:
1. No restriction (method can be used)
2. Advantages generally outweigh theoretical or proven risks
3. Theoretical or proven risks usually outweigh the advantages
4. Unacceptable health risk (method not to be used)

Updated June 2012. This summary sheet only contains a subset of the recommendations from the US MEC. For complete guidance, see: http://www.cdc.gov/reproductivehealth/unintendedpregnancy/USMEC.htm

Most contraceptive methods do not protect against sexually transmitted infections (STIs). Consistent and correct use of the male latex condom reduces the risk of STIs and HIV.

Condition	Sub-condition	Combined pill, patch, ring		Progestin-only pill		Injection		Implant		LNG-IUD		Copper-IUD	
		I	C	I	C	I	C	I	C	I	C	I	C
Age		Menarche to <40=1 ≥40=2		Menarche to <18=1 18–45=1 >45=1		Menarche to <18=2 18–45=1 >45=2		Menarche to <18=1 18–45=1 >45=1		Menarche to <20=2 ≥20=1		Menarche to <20=2 ≥20=1	
Anatomic abnormalities	a) Distorted uterine cavity									4		4	
	b) Other abnormalities									2		2	
Anemias	a) Thalassemia	1		1		1		1		1		2	
	b) Sickle cell disease‡	2		1		1		1		1		2	
	c) Iron-deficiency anemia	1		1		1		1		1		2	
Benign ovarian tumors	(including cysts)	1		1		1		1		1		1	
Breast disease	a) Undiagnosed mass	2*		2*		2*		2*		2		1	
	b) Benign breast disease	1		1		1		1		1		1	
	c) Family history of cancer	1		1		1		1		1		1	
	d) Breast cancer‡												
	i) current	4		4		4		4		4		1	
	ii) past and no evidence of current disease for 5 years	3		3		3		3		3		1	
Breastfeeding (see also Postpartum)	a) < 1 month postpartum	3*		2*		2*		2*					
	b) 1 month or more postpartum	2*		1*		1*		1*					
Cervical cancer	Awaiting treatment	2		1		2		2		4	2	4	2
Cervical ectropion		1		1		1		1		1		1	
Cervical intraepithelial neoplasia		2		1		2		2		2		1	
Cirrhosis	a) Mild (compensated)	1		1		1		1		1		1	
	b) Severe‡ (decompensated)	4		3		3		3		3		1	

(continues)

TABLE 22-1 Summary Chart of U.S. Medical Eligibility Criteria for Contraceptive Use *(Continued)*

Key:
1. No restriction (method can be used)
2. Advantages generally outweigh theoretical or proven risks
3. Theoretical or proven risks usually outweigh the advantages
4. Unacceptable health risk (method not to be used)

Updated June 2012. This summary sheet only contains a subset of the recommendations from the US MEC. For complete guidance, see: http://www.cdc.gov/reproductivehealth/unintendedpregnancy/USMEC.htm

Most contraceptive methods do not protect against sexually transmitted infections (STIs). Consistent and correct use of the male latex condom reduces the risk of STIs and HIV.

Condition	Sub-condition	Combined pill, patch, ring I	C	Progestin-only pill I	C	Injection I	C	Implant I	C	LNG-IUD I	C	Copper-IUD I	C
Deep venous thrombosis (DVT)/Pulmonary embolism (PE)	a) History of DVT/PE, not on anticoagulant therapy												
	i) higher risk for recurrent DVT/PE	4		2		2		2		2		1	
	ii) lower risk for recurrent DVT/PE	3		2		2		2		2		1	
	b) Acute DVT/PE	4		2		2		2		2		2	
	c) DVT/PE and established on anticoagulant therapy for at least 3 months												
	i) higher risk for recurrent DVT/PE	4*		2		2		2		2		2	
	ii) lower risk for recurrent DVT/PE	3*		2		2		2		2		2	
	d) Family history (first-degree relatives)	2		1		1		1		1		1	
	e) Major surgery												
	(i) with prolonged immobilization	4		2		2		2		2		1	
	(ii) without prolonged immobilization	2		1		1		1		1		1	
	f) Minor surgery without immobilization	1		1		1		1		1		1	
Depressive disorders		1*		1*		1*		1*		1*		1*	
Diabetes mellitus (DM)	a) History of gestational DM only	1		1		1		1		1		1	
	b) Non-vascular disease												
	(i) non-insulin dependent	2		2		2		2		2		1	
	(ii) insulin dependent‡	2		2		2		2		2		1	
	c) Nephropathy/ retinopathy/ neuropathy‡	3/4*		2		3		2		2		1	
	d) Other vascular disease or diabetes of > 20 years' duration‡	3/4*		2		3		2		2		1	
Endometrial cancer‡		1		1		1		1		4	2	4	2
Endometrial hyperplasia		1		1		1		1		1		1	
Endometriosis		1		1		1		1		1		2	
Epilepsy‡	(see also Drug Interactions)	1*		1*		1*		1*		1		1	

TABLE 22-1 Summary Chart of U.S. Medical Eligibility Criteria for Contraceptive Use *(Continued)*

Key:
1. No restriction (method can be used)
2. Advantages generally outweigh theoretical or proven risks
3. Theoretical or proven risks usually outweigh the advantages
4. Unacceptable health risk (method not to be used)

Updated June 2012. This summary sheet only contains a subset of the recommendations from the US MEC. For complete guidance, see: http://www.cdc.gov/reproductivehealth/unintendedpregnancy/USMEC.htm

Most contraceptive methods do not protect against sexually transmitted infections (STIs). Consistent and correct use of the male latex condom reduces the risk of STIs and HIV.

Condition	Sub-condition	Combined pill, patch, ring I	C	Progestin-only pill I	C	Injection I	C	Implant I	C	LNG-IUD I	C	Copper-IUD I	C
Gallbladder disease	a) Symptomatic												
	(i) treated by cholecystectomy	2		2		2		2		2		1	
	(ii) medically treated	3		2		2		2		2		1	
	(iii) current	3		2		2		2		2		1	
	b) Asymptomatic	2		2		2		2		2		1	
Gestational trophoblastic disease	a) Decreasing or undetectable ß-hCG levels	1		1		1		1		3		3	
	b) Persistently elevated ß-hCG levels or malignant disease‡	1		1		1		1		4		4	
Headaches	a) Non-migrainous	1*	2*	1*	1*	1*	1*	1*	1*	1*	1*	1*	
	b) Migraine												
	i) without aura, age < 35	2*	3*	1*	2*	2*	2*	2*	2*	2*	2*	1*	
	ii) without aura, age ≥ 35	3*	4*	1*	2*	2*	2*	2*	2*	2*	2*	1*	
	iii) with aura, any age	4*	4*	2*	3*	2*	3*	2*	3*	2*	3*	1*	
History of bariatric surgery‡	a) Restrictive procedures	1		1		1		1		1		1	
	b) Malabsorptive procedures	COCs: 3 P/R: 1		3		1		1		1		1	
History of cholestasis	a) Pregnancy-related	2		1		1		1		1		1	
	b) Past COC-related	3		2		2		2		2		1	
History of high blood pressure during pregnancy		2		1		1		1		1		1	
History of pelvic surgery		1		1		1		1		1		1	
HIV	High risk	1		1		1*		1		2	2	2	2
	HIV infected (see also Drug Interactions)‡	1*		1*		1*		1*		2	2	2	2
	AIDS (see also Drug Interactions)‡	1*		1*		1*		1*		3	2*	3	2*
	Clinically well on therapy	If on treatment, see Drug Interactions								2	2	2	2
Hyperlipidemias		2/3*		2*		2*		2*		2*		1*	

(continues)

TABLE 22-1 Summary Chart of U.S. Medical Eligibility Criteria for Contraceptive Use *(Continued)*

Key:
1. No restriction (method can be used)
2. Advantages generally outweigh theoretical or proven risks
3. Theoretical or proven risks usually outweigh the advantages
4. Unacceptable health risk (method not to be used)

Updated June 2012. This summary sheet only contains a subset of the recommendations from the US MEC. For complete guidance, see: http://www.cdc.gov/reproductivehealth/unintendedpregnancy/USMEC.htm

Most contraceptive methods do not protect against sexually transmitted infections (STIs). Consistent and correct use of the male latex condom reduces the risk of STIs and HIV.

Condition	Sub-condition	Combined pill, patch, ring		Progestin-only pill		Injection		Implant		LNG-IUD		Copper-IUD	
		I	C	I	C	I	C	I	C	I	C	I	C
Hypertension	a) Adequately controlled hypertension	3*		1*		2*		1*		1		1	
	b) Elevated blood pressure levels (properly taken measurements)												
	(i) systolic 140–159 or diastolic 90–99	3		1		2		1		1		1	
	(ii) systolic ≥ 160 or diastolic ≥ 100‡	4		2		3		2		2		1	
	c) Vascular disease	4		2		3		2		2		1	
Inflammatory bowel disease	(Ulcerative colitis, Crohn's disease)	2/3*		2		2		1		1		1	
Ischemic heart disease‡	Current and history of	4		2	3	3		2	3	2	3	1	
Liver tumors	a) Benign												
	i) Focal nodular hyperplasia	2		2		2		2		2		1	
	ii) Hepatocellular adenoma‡	4		3		3		3		3		1	
	b) Malignant‡	4		3		3		3		3		1	
Malaria		1		1		1		1		1		1	
Multiple risk factors for arterial cardiovascular disease	(such as older age, smoking, diabetes, and hypertension)	3/4*		2*		3*		2*		2		1	
Obesity	a) ≥ 30 kg/m² body mass index (BMI)	2		1		1		1		1		1	
	b) Menarche to < 18 years and ≥ 30 kg/m² BMI	2		1		2		1		1		1	
Ovarian cancer‡		1		1		1		1		1		1	
Parity	a) Nulliparous	1		1		1		1		2		2	
	b) Parous	1		1		1		1		1		1	
Past ectopic pregnancy		1		2		1		1		1		1	
Pelvic inflammatory disease	a) Past (assuming no current risk factors of STIs)												
	(i) with subsequent pregnancy	1		1		1		1		1	1	1	1
	(ii) without subsequent pregnancy	1		1		1		1		2	2	2	2
	b) Current	1		1		1		1		4	2*	4	2*

TABLE 22-1 Summary Chart of U.S. Medical Eligibility Criteria for Contraceptive Use *(Continued)*

Key:
1. No restriction (method can be used)
2. Advantages generally outweigh theoretical or proven risks
3. Theoretical or proven risks usually outweigh the advantages
4. Unacceptable health risk (method not to be used)

Updated June 2012. This summary sheet only contains a subset of the recommendations from the US MEC. For complete guidance, see: http://www.cdc.gov/reproductivehealth/unintendedpregnancy/USMEC.htm

Most contraceptive methods do not protect against sexually transmitted infections (STIs). Consistent and correct use of the male latex condom reduces the risk of STIs and HIV.

Condition	Sub-condition	Combined pill, patch, ring I	C	Progestin-only pill I	C	Injection I	C	Implant I	C	LNG-IUD I	C	Copper-IUD I	C
Peripartum cardiomyopathy‡	a) Normal or mildly impaired cardiac function												
	(i) < 6 months	4		1		1		1		2		2	
	(ii) ≥ 6 months	3		1		1		1		2		2	
	b) Moderately or severely impaired cardiac function	4		2		2		2		2		2	
Postabortion	a) First trimester	1*		1*		1*		1*		1*		1*	
	b) Second trimester	1*		1*		1*		1*		2		2	
	c) Immediately post-septic abortion	1*		1*		1*		1*		4		4	
Postpartum (see also Breastfeeding)	a) < 21 days	4		1		1		1					
	b) 21 days to 42 days												
	(i) with other risk factors for VTE	3*		1		1		1					
	(ii) without other risk factors for VTE	2		1		1		1					
	c) > 42 days	1		1		1		1					
Postpartum (in breastfeeding or non-breastfeeding women, including post-cesarean section)	a) < 10 minutes after delivery of the placenta									2		1	
	b) 10 minutes after delivery of the placenta to < 4 weeks									2		2	
	c) ≥ 4 weeks									1		1	
	d) Puerperal sepsis									4		4	
Pregnancy		NA*		NA*		NA*		NA*		4*		4*	
Rheumatoid arthritis	a) On immunosuppressive therapy	2		1		2/3*		1		2	1	2	1
	b) Not on immunosuppressive therapy	2		1		2		1		1		1	
Schistosomiasis	a) Uncomplicated	1		1		1		1		1		1	
	b) Fibrosis of the liver‡	1		1		1		1		1		1	
Severe dysmenorrhea		1		1		1		1		1		2	

(continues)

TABLE 22-1 Summary Chart of U.S. Medical Eligibility Criteria for Contraceptive Use *(Continued)*

Key:
1. No restriction (method can be used)
2. Advantages generally outweigh theoretical or proven risks
3. Theoretical or proven risks usually outweigh the advantages
4. Unacceptable health risk (method not to be used)

Updated June 2012. This summary sheet only contains a subset of the recommendations from the US MEC. For complete guidance, see: http://www.cdc.gov/reproductivehealth/unintendedpregnancy/USMEC.htm

Most contraceptive methods do not protect against sexually transmitted infections (STIs). Consistent and correct use of the male latex condom reduces the risk of STIs and HIV.

Condition	Sub-condition	Combined pill, patch, ring I	C	Progestin-only pill I	C	Injection I	C	Implant I	C	LNG-IUD I	C	Copper-IUD I	C
Sexually transmitted infections (STIs)	a) Current purulent cervicitis or chlamydial infection or gonorrhea	1		1		1		1		4	2*	4	2*
	b) Other STIs (excluding HIV and hepatitis)	1		1		1		1		2	2	2	2
	c) Vaginitis (including trichomonas vaginalis and bacterial vaginosis)	1		1		1		1		2	2	2	2
	d) Increased risk of STIs	1		1		1		1		2/3*	2	2/3*	2
Smoking	a) Age < 35	2		1		1		1		1		1	
	b) Age ≥ 35, < 15 cigarettes/day	3		1		1		1		1		1	
	c) Age ≥ 35, ≥ 15 cigarettes/day	4		1		1		1		1		1	
Solid organ transplantation‡	a) Complicated	4		2		2		2		3	2	3	2
	b) Uncomplicated	2*		2		2		2		2		2	
Stroke‡	History of cerebrovascular accident	4		2	3	3		2	3	2		1	
Superficial venous thrombosis	a) Varicose veins	1		1		1		1		1		1	
	b) Superficial thrombophlebitis	2		1		1		1		1		1	
Systemic lupus erythematosus‡	a) Positive (or unknown) antiphospholipid antibodies	4		3	3	3		3		3		1	1
	b) Severe thrombocytopenia	2		2		3	2	2		2*		3*	2*
	c) Immunosuppressive treatment	2		2		2	2	2		2		2	1
	d) None of the above	2		2		2	2	2		2		1	1
Thrombogenic mutations‡		4*		2*		2*		2*		2*		1*	
Thyroid disorders	Simple goiter/ hyperthyroid/ hypothyroid	1		1		1		1		1		1	
Tuberculosis‡ (see also Drug Interactions)	a) Non-pelvic	1*		1*		1*		1*		1		1	
	b) Pelvic	1*		1*		1*		1*		4	3	4	3
Unexplained vaginal bleeding	(suspicious for serious condition) before evaluation	2*		2*		3*		3*		4*	2*	4*	2*
Uterine fibroids		1		1		1		1		2		2	

TABLE 22-1 Summary Chart of U.S. Medical Eligibility Criteria for Contraceptive Use *(Continued)*

Key:
1. No restriction (method can be used)
2. Advantages generally outweigh theoretical or proven risks
3. Theoretical or proven risks usually outweigh the advantages
4. Unacceptable health risk (method not to be used)

Updated June 2012. This summary sheet only contains a subset of the recommendations from the US MEC. For complete guidance, see: http://www.cdc.gov/reproductivehealth/unintendedpregnancy/USMEC.htm

Most contraceptive methods do not protect against sexually transmitted infections (STIs). Consistent and correct use of the male latex condom reduces the risk of STIs and HIV.

Condition	Sub-condition	Combined pill, patch, ring		Progestin-only pill		Injection		Implant		LNG-IUD		Copper-IUD	
		I	C	I	C	I	C	I	C	I	C	I	C
Valvular heart disease	a) Uncomplicated	2		1		1		1		1		1	
	b) Complicated‡	4		1		1		1		1		1	
Vaginal bleeding patterns	a) Irregular pattern without heavy bleeding	1		2		2		2		1	1	1	
	b) Heavy or prolonged bleeding	1*		2*		2*		2*		1*	2*	2*	
Viral hepatitis	a) Acute or flare	3/4*	2	1		1		1		1		1	
	b) Carrier/Chronic	1	1	1		1		1		1		1	
Drug Interactions													
Antiretroviral therapy	a) Nucleoside reverse transcriptase inhibitors	1*		1		1		1		2/3*	2*	2/3*	2*
	b) Non-nucleoside reverse transcriptase inhibitors	2*		2*		1		2*		2/3*	2*	2/3*	2*
	c) Ritonavir-boosted protease inhibitors	3*		3*		1		2*		2/3*	2*	2/3*	2*
Anticonvulsant therapy	a) Certain anticonvulsants (phenytoin, carbamazepine, barbiturates, primidone, topiramate, oxcarbazepine)	3*		3*		1		2*		1		1	
	b) Lamotrigine	3*		1		1		1		1		1	
Antimicrobial therapy	a) Broad spectrum antibiotics	1		1		1		1		1		1	
	b) Antifungals	1		1		1		1		1		1	
	c) Antiparasitics	1		1		1		1		1		1	
	d) Rifampicin or rifabutin therapy	3*		3*		1		2*		1		1	

I = initiation of contraceptive method; C = continuation of contraceptive method; NA = not applicable

* Please see the complete guidance for a clarification to this classification: www.cdc.gov/reproductivehealth/unintendedpregnancy/USMEC.htm

‡ Condition that exposes a woman to increased risk as a result of unintended pregnancy.

This table includes criteria for the copper intrauterine device (IUD) as well as the hormonal methods. Please see the chapter on nonhormonal contraceptive methods for a discussion of the copper IUD.

Reproduced from Centers for Disease Control and Prevention. (Updated June 2012). *Summary chart of U.S. medical eligibility criteria for contraceptive use*. Retrieved from http://www.cdc.gov/reproductivehealth/UnintendedPregnancy/USMEC.htm.

with a decrease in ectopic pregnancy, pelvic inflammatory disease (PID), and benign breast disease. In perimenopausal women, use of estrogen-containing methods may reduce hot flashes, vaginal dryness, and bone loss. Finally, ovarian, endometrial, and colorectal cancer risk is reduced in users of CHC.

Much data has been collected about the safety of the COC pill, and although less is available about the safety of the patch and ring, they seem to have a similar profile. The World Health Organization (WHO) 2015 Medical Eligibility Criteria provide detailed information on hormonal contraceptive safety and is available on the WHO website (http://apps.who.int/iris/bitstream/10665/181468/1/9789241549158_eng.pdf?ua=1). The U.S. Medical Eligibility Criteria modify these recommendations to include situations specific to the U.S. population, and are listed in this chapter in Table 22-1.

1. COC pill

   COC pills have been in use for more than 50 years. When used correctly, the failure rate is 0.3% in perfect use and 8% in typical use (Trussell and Guthrie, Contraceptive Technology, 2011). There are many different combinations of estrogen- and progestin-containing pills marketed today (for a complete up-to-date list, see Comparison of Hormonal Contraceptive Methods, **Appendix 22-1**). Most contain ethinyl estradiol, whereas a few of the higher estrogen pills contain mestranol (although 50 mcg is equivalent to only 35 mcg of ethinyl estradiol). Ethinyl estradiol doses range from 20 to 50 mcg, although doses above 35 mcg are rarely used. A new COC pill containing the natural estrogen estradiol is now available under the name Natazia®. This COC contains the progestin dienogest and has been shown to be effective for heavy menstrual bleeding as well as contraception. It has a quadriphasic (four-phase) regimen that necessitates unique "missed pill" instructions (Nelson, 2012). Eight other synthetic progestins are in use in the United States, ranging in dosage from 0.1 to 1 mg. The combination of estrogen and progestin determine the efficacy and characteristics of the COC pill.

   All COC pills have four biologic activities: (1) endometrial activity (defined as the percentage of breakthrough bleeding in the third cycle of use); (2) estrogenic activity; (3) progestational activity; and (4) androgenic activity (Dickey, 2010). The side effects experienced by many pill users relate to these activities and may be reduced by switching to COC pills with different biologic profiles. For instance, breast swelling and tenderness, nausea, mood changes, and fluid retention resulting in weight gain or headaches are related to the estrogen effect and may be relieved by switching to a pill with greater progestational activity. COC pills with greater progestational activity may cause weight gain from appetite stimulation, increased varicosities, increased vaginal discharge including moniliasis, and mood changes. Pills with high androgenic activity can cause acne, hirsutism, and increased libido. Appendix 22-1 lists the hormonal contraceptive options available at the time of publication, with comments describing characteristics of each category. Two excellent pocket guides for quick reference for COC pill selection are *Managing Contraceptive Pill Patients* (Dickey, 2010) and *A Pocket Guide to Managing Contraception* (Zieman et al., 2010–2012).

Additionally, different COC pill combinations have varying effects on high-density lipoprotein and low-density lipoprotein cholesterol, thus affecting the potential for serious complications, such as venous thrombosis (VTE) and cardiovascular disease (CVD). This effect is mainly related to the dose of estrogen and only slightly to the type of progestin (Nelson, Contraceptive Technology, 2011). This should be considered when choosing COCs for users with other risk factors for VTE and CVD (e.g., older age, smoking, diabetes, hypertension, obesity, and family history of VTE or CVD).

After COC pills are initiated, patients must be counseled about the symptoms of serious or potentially serious side effects, and the possible need for immediate discontinuation. These include:

- Loss or distortion of vision (retinal artery thrombosis)
- Severe chest pain (myocardial infarction)
- Hemoptysis (pulmonary embolism)
- Severe unilateral leg pain, swelling, and redness (VTE, thrombosis)
- Severe persistent headaches, unilateral numbness, weakness or tingling, and slurring of speech (stroke)
- Abdominal pain (thrombosis, myocardial infarction, pulmonary embolism, and gallbladder or liver disease)
- Headaches: Patients who develop migraine headaches with aura after starting COC pills should be switched to a progestin-only method.

COC pills may be monophasic, with each pill containing the same dose, or multiphasic, with pill weeks containing varying doses of estrogen and progestin. Most COC pills have 21 active pills and 7 inactive or "placebo" pills, allowing for regular menstrual cycling. Several newer formulations extend the active pill days to reduce menstrual flow and related problems. Some have 24 days of active pills and 3 days of placebos. The shortened pill-free interval improves pill efficacy and lessens withdrawal bleeding (Endrikat et al., 2001; Spona et al., 1996). Others have 84 days of active pills, followed by 7 days of placebos. One COC pill formulation is continuous with no placebo days. Extended COC pill use is ideal for women who suffer from menstrual-related (catamenial) problems or who have conditions, such as endometriosis, that are suppressed by COC pill use. There is no medical necessity for withdrawal bleeding (Miller & Notter, 2001).

Women may experience breakthrough bleeding with extended COC pill use and should be counseled that this is not harmful. COC pills offer advantages and disadvantages. COC pills are often preferred by women who feel most comfortable with an oral as opposed to transdermal or vaginal delivery system. However, failure rates are often higher, because timely and consistent dosing requires discipline and motivation. Because of the variety of pill types, more options are available for managing side effects. Most COC pills are now sold generically, thus reducing the cost. A woman may choose to start COC pills in one of three ways:

a. Quick start allows her to take her first pill on the day she receives the prescription, increasing compliance and reducing the risk of subsequent pregnancy. A pregnancy test should be performed at the time of her visit, and if indicated, emergency contraception should be given, followed by initiation of the first COC pill no later than the next day. She should use a backup method for the first 7 days and return for a urine pregnancy test in 2–3 weeks if pregnancy before starting the COC pill is a possibility.

b. First day start is another option. The user begins her COC pill on the first day of her menses. This approach reduces the risk of ovarian follicle development in the first cycle, thus reducing the risk of pregnancy.

c. Sunday start requires the user to start her first pill on the Sunday after her menstrual cycle begins. Many women find it is easier to remember to start a new pill cycle on a Sunday and enjoy the lower likelihood of bleeding on the weekend. However, this approach has the disadvantage of possible ovarian follicle formation, so a backup method should be used for the first 7 days.

2. Transdermal patch

The transdermal patch currently marketed under the name Ortho Evra® is scheduled to be discontinued, but a new generic version, Tulane, is now available. It contains norelgestromin and ethinyl estradiol in a three-layered adhesive polyester patch. The hormonal dose is absorbed through the skin, thus bypassing the liver and gastrointestinal system. A new patch is applied once a week for 3 weeks, followed by a patch-free week, during which withdrawal bleeding will likely occur. The transdermal patch is equivalent to COC pills in efficacy in women who weigh less than 198 pounds (Zieman et al., 2002). Additionally, ease of use improves compliance, although pregnancy rates for women over 90 kg (198 pounds) are slightly higher. Care must be taken to ensure that the patch is completely adhered, because partial or complete separation from the skin has occurred. Although fewer long-term data are available for the patch, it seems to provide similar advantages, risks, and side effects as the COC pill. Serum levels of ethinyl estradiol are higher in patch users by 60% compared to users of a 35-mcg pill, but epidemiological data are inconsistent as to whether this increases the risk of VTE (Nanda, Contraceptive Technology, 2011). Some users of the patch have experienced localized reactions, including rash and skin irritation at the site of application. Women with dermatologic conditions may not be candidates for patch use. The same options for starting COC pills are available for patch users; backup methods should be used for quick start and Sunday start options. Management of missed or late patches depends on the week of use; manufacturer instructions should be given to the user.

3. Vaginal contraceptive ring

The vaginal contraceptive ring (NuvaRing®) is a soft, flexible ring made of ethylene vinyl acetate that releases ethinyl estradiol and etonogestrel (a metabolite of desogestrel) in a low and steady dose. It is worn in the vagina for 3 weeks, and removed for 1 week to allow for withdrawal bleeding. The hormones are absorbed transvaginally, and like the patch, bypass the liver and gastrointestinal system. Circulating levels of hormone are lower than in the transdermal patch or COC pill and do not fluctuate throughout the day. Cycle control is often better than with the COC pill, and there are relatively few side effects (Bjarnadottir, Tuppurainen, & Killick, 2002).

Efficacy is comparable to the transdermal patch and COC pill, but similar to patch use, compliance is improved. Users are subject to the same advantages, risks, and side effects as with the other combined hormonal methods; however, some users also experience vaginal discomfort and discharge. The ring may inadvertently be removed with intercourse, so care should be taken to check for its presence postcoitus.

When initiating ring use, it is recommended that the first ring be inserted any time within the first 5 days of onset of menses, with backup contraception for the first 7 days.

A 1-year vaginal ring containing the progestin Nestorone® and ethinyl estradiol has completed trials and is being prepared for the approval process. A 3-month Nestorone®-only ring is currently in use in some countries and is designed for breastfeeding women.

B. Progestin-only contraception

Progestin-only contraception is an option for women who cannot take estrogen because of medical contraindications or estrogen-related side effects. Progestin can be taken orally (POP), by injection (medroxyprogesterone acetate), by implant (Implanon®, Nexplanon), or through an intra-uterine system (LNG-IUS; Mirena® and Skyla). Each has its advantages, risks, and potential side effects. The only absolute contraindication to progestin use is current or recent breast cancer, although additional absolute contraindications exist for LNG-IUS (Table 22-1). Relative contraindications to progestin and its delivery systems and conditions that may require monitoring are also listed in Table 22-1 (U.S. Medical Eligibility Criteria guidelines).

1. POP (Progestin-Only Pill)

   The POPs contain norethindrone or norgestrel, and no estrogen. The POP has a perfect use failure rate of 0.3%, and a typical use failure rate of 8%, and requires diligent pill-taking (pill should be taken within 3 hours of same time every day). It is often prescribed during lactation. The main action of the POP is to thicken the cervical mucus; ovulation may or may not be inhibited. Therefore, ovarian cysts are more likely to occur with the POP than with the COC pill (Tayob, Adams, Jacobs, & Guillebaud, 1985). Without the cycle-regulating effect of estrogen, irregular bleeding (breakthrough bleeding, amenorrhea, or shortened cycles) can occur. There are no placebo pills; active pills are taken every day. If POPs are started within 5 days of the first day of menses, backup contraception is not necessary. If started at other times in the cycle, a pregnancy test should be performed and a backup method used for 2 days. POPs are in general more expensive than COC pills and less effective in controlling medical conditions, such as dysmenorrhea, acne, and hirsutism. POPs protect against uterine and ovarian cancer, PID, and benign breast disease.

2. Injectable progestin (Depo-Provera®)

   Depo-Provera® (depo medroxyprogesterone acetate), 150 mg, is given by intramuscular injection every 11–13 weeks. A subcutaneous dose of 104 mg is also available for self-administration (Depo-subQ Provera). Medroxyprogesterone acetate is highly efficacious, with a failure rate of 0.3–3%. It is discreet and convenient and can be used by women with contraindications to estrogen. Medroxyprogesterone acetate suppresses the follicle-stimulating hormone and luteinizing hormone surge, resulting in ovulation suppression. Additionally, it thickens the cervical mucus, thins the endometrium, and slows tubal motility. Disadvantages include irregular or heavy bleeding; amenorrhea; weight gain; depression; unfavorable lipid changes in some women; and decrease in bone density, which is largely reversible (Kaunitz, Arias, & McClung, 2008). Users should be encouraged to take calcium supplements and exercise regularly. Additionally, there can be a delay in return of fertility averaging 10 months from last injection. Medroxyprogesterone acetate is contraindicated in women with breast cancer and should be used with caution in women with CVD and risk factors for CVD, liver disease, and vaginal bleeding without explanation. Advantages include convenience; high efficacy; possible decreased menorrhagia and dysmenorrhea; and a reduction in PID, endometrial cancer, fibroids, sickle cell anemia crises, and seizures. Medroxyprogesterone acetate should be initiated any time during the first 7 days of onset of menstruation or at any time if the candidate is not pregnant. A backup method should be used for 7 days if injection occurs outside of the first 7 days of the cycle.

3. Implants (Implanon®, Nexplanon)

   Implanon® and Nexplanon are single implants containing etonogestrel in an ethylene vinyl acetate capsule. The implant is inserted under the skin of the nondominant upper arm by a trained clinician (training can be obtained through a company-sponsored training session). Nexplanon is the next-generation implant; it is identical to Implanon® with the exception of having a preloaded applicator and the addition of radio-opaque barium sulphate. The implant is the most effective form of birth control, with a 0.05% failure rate, exceeding tubal ligation efficacy. It is effective for at least 3 years; efficacy is not dependent on user compliance. Its mechanism of action is to thicken the cervical mucus, suppress ovulation, and cause atrophy of the endometrium. It is discrete and can be easily removed at any time with a single incision. Among the advantages of the implant are reduction in menstrual flow and cramping, rapid return of fertility, and high acceptability and continuation. Disadvantages include irregular bleeding, amenorrhea, pain or infection at implant site postinsertion, and possible weight gain (in clinical studies, mean weight gain in implant users was 2.8 pounds after 1 year and 3.7 pounds after 3 years). Implants can be inserted at any time in the cycle, if pregnancy has been ruled out. If inserted within the first 7 days of onset of menses, no additional contraception is needed; otherwise, backup should be used for 7 days. Fertility is restored within 3–6 weeks of removal in 94% of women. Initially cost is high, but if spread out over 3 years of use, it can be less expensive than many other hormonal options.

4. Levonorgestrel intrauterine system (LNG-IUS)

LNG-IUS (Mirena®, Skyla®) is an intrauterine system containing levonorgestrel in a capsule molded to a polyethylene T-shaped device. Mirena® releases 20 mcg of levonorgestrel a day for 5 years, and Skyla® releases 14 mcg a day for 3 years. The progestin is released directly into the uterine cavity, with only a small amount of systemic absorption. The amount of plasma concentration is lower than for implants and POPs, but the contraceptive effect remains high. Skyla® is smaller in diameter than Mirena® and has a narrower inserter, making it easier to insert in nulliparous women and better tolerated by teens and perimenopausal women with smaller uterine cavities. LNG-IUS is more than 99% effective in pregnancy prevention. Two strings are attached to the base, extending through the cervix into the vagina. The strings allow users to check for the presence of the device and facilitate removal. A total of 2–10% are expelled in the first year of use, often without the awareness of the user (it is important to teach the patient to check for her strings regularly). Mechanism of action is through thickening of the cervical mucus, inhibition of sperm capacitation, suppression of the endometrium, and in some cases suppression of ovulation. It is discrete and well tolerated.

Noncontraceptive benefits include decrease in menstrual flow and pain and in risk of endometrial cancer. LNG-IUS has been used in the treatment of women with menorrhagia, endometriosis, adenomyosis, and fibroids, and Mirena® is approved by the Food and Drug Administration (FDA) for the treatment of menorrhagia. Disadvantages include pain with and after insertion, especially in nulliparous women; infection postinsertion (0.1%); perforation of uterus at the time of insertion (less than 0.1%); spontaneous expulsion; irregular spotting and bleeding (usually limited to first 6 months); amenorrhea; ovarian cyst problems; and rare side effects, such as headaches, acne, mood changes, and back and abdominal cramping. The cumulative risk for PID for users of LNG-IUS is 0.8% over a 5-year period and

is higher in women younger than age 25 (Anderson, Odlind, & Rybo, 1994).

Cervical cultures for chlamydia and gonorrhea should be performed before insertion in high-risk women, and women should be counseled to use condoms with new or high-risk partners. The insertion process requires clinician training. It can be inserted immediately after abortion or delivery, and if inserted within the first 7 days of menstrual onset, no backup method is needed. It can be inserted at other times in the menstrual cycle if pregnancy is ruled out. Backup contraception should be used for 7 days. Cost of the LNG-IUS is high, but if it is used for 5 years the overall cost is lower than other hormonal methods.

C. ECP

ECP provides the only postcoital method of contraception (other than the highly effective insertion of a copper-releasing intrauterine device within 5 days of unprotected intercourse). Thus, it is an excellent option after unplanned intercourse, rape, or contraceptive failure (condom breakage, missed COC pills or POPs, delay of more than 14 days in getting medroxyprogesterone acetate injection, delay of 2 or more days in starting a new ring or patch cycle). Prepackaged ECPs containing progestin only (Plan B One-Step, Next Choice, and other generic equivalents) contain 1.5 mg of levonorgestrel taken once. Ulipristal acetate, a progesterone receptor modulator, is packaged in a 30 mg tablet know as Ella. A third option, CHC pills containing ethinyl estradiol and norgestrel or levonorgestrel, can also be used in two doses taken 12 hours apart (Yuzpe method).

ECPs have varying actions depending on the phase of the cycle in which they are taken. They may disrupt normal follicular maturation; interfere with corpus luteal function; or alter the endometrium, cervical mucus, and tubal transport. The first dose should be taken immediately or within 120 hours of unprotected intercourse. Ulipristal is the most effective ECP and is more effective through the fifth day postcoitus than the other ECPs. It may also be more effective in overweight women. Progestin-alone ECPs reduce the risk of pregnancy by 52–100% depending on how soon after coitus they are taken, Ulipristal reduces the risk by an additional 42% up to 72 hours, and 65% in the first 24 hours. Combined estrogen and progesterone pills are less effective than eitherprogestin-only pills or Ulipristal. Efficacy is dependent on what phase in the woman's cycle she takes the ECP and how many hours have elapsed since intercourse. Side effects include headache, nausea, and abdominal pain. If a woman vomits within 3 hours of taking ECP she should repeat the dose. ECP may cause early or later menstrual flow. If no bleeding occurs within 3 weeks of taking the dose, a pregnancy test should be performed.

ECP should not be used as a primary birth control method, because it is less effective than other methods. However, all patients using CHC methods, POP, medroxyprogesterone acetate, and nonhormonal contraceptives should be advised to obtain ECP as a backup method ahead of need. Pharmacies provide progestin-only ECP to all women without a prescription regardless of age. Ulipristal acetate requires a prescription.

II. Database (may include but is not limited to)

A. Subjective

1. Combined hormonal contraceptive (CHC)
   a. Medical illnesses
   b. Family history (especially deep VTE, pulmonary embolism, breast and ovarian cancer)
   c. Personal and social history
   d. Age
   e. Parity and desire for future fertility
   f. Breastfeeding, postpartum
   g. Postabortion
   h. Smoking
   i. Sexual history: recent history of unprotected intercourse, current risk for sexually transmitted disease
   j. Previous contraceptive use: satisfaction, compliance, problems
   k. Preference for and comfort with different hormone delivery systems
   l. Tolerance of side effects: weight change, breast tenderness, bleeding irregularities, melasma and chloasma, nausea, headaches, libido changes, mood swings, vaginal discharge (vaginal contraceptive ring)
   m. Financial constraints
   n. Current medication use
   o. Menstrual history: age of menarche, character of menses, date of last menstrual period

2. Progestin-only contraception
   a. Medical illness
   b. Family illness
   c. Personal and social history
   d. Age
   e. Parity and desire for future fertility
   f. Breastfeeding, postpartum
   g. Postabortion
   h. Smoking
   i. Sexual history: recent history of unprotected intercourse, current risk for sexually transmitted disease
   j. Previous contraceptive use and satisfaction, compliance, problems
   k. Preference for and comfort with different hormonal delivery systems (e.g., not fearful of needles and willing to return for repeat injections) (medroxyprogesterone acetate)
   l. Willingness to undergo a minor procedure (LNG-IUS, implants)
   m. Tolerance of side effects: menstrual cycle disturbances, weight gain (medroxyprogesterone acetate), breast tenderness, mood changes, and possible local inflammation and infection (implants)
   n. Financial constraints
   o. Current medications
   p. Menstrual history: age of menarche, character of menses, and date of last menstrual period
   q. Noncontraceptive benefits: scant or no menses (less anemia), decreased menstrual problems, decreased risk of endometrial and ovarian cancer, decreased risk of PID and fibroids, decreased pain from endometriosis, and fewer seizures and sickle cell crises (medroxyprogesterone acetate)

3. ECP
   a. Age
   b. Date of last menstrual period
   c. Time of unprotected intercourse
   d. Medical conditions
   e. Contraceptive methods used and nature of failure or misuse
   f. Occurrence of rape

B. Objective (note: the only essential and mandatory components of the exam are blood pressure for combined hormonal contraception and bimanual examination and cervical inspection for IUS insertion. All other components are optional and should be directed by the patient's history)

1. CHC
   a. Blood pressure and weight
   b. Breast examination
   c. Speculum and pelvic examination (not required unless symptomatic)
   d. Pap smear and testing for sexually transmitted diseases as indicated
   e. Assessment for skin conditions (patch use)
   f. Pregnancy test

2. Progestin-only contraception
   a. Blood pressure and weight
   b. Breast examination

c. Speculum examination with Pap smear and cultures for gonorrhea and chlamydia (LNG-IUS), assess for cervical stenosis (LNG-IUS)

d. Pelvic examination (required for LNG-IUS and if symptomatic)

e. Pregnancy test

3. ECP

4. Pregnancy test

III. Assessment

A. CHC

1. No medical contraindications to estrogen or progestin

2. Nonsmoker (if older than age 35)

3. Not breastfeeding

4. Noncontraceptive benefits: decreased acne and hirsutism; less endometrial and ovarian cancer; decreased benign breast disease; improved cycle control; suppression of endometriosis; less gonorrheal PID; improvement in premenstrual syndrome and perimenopausal symptoms; decreased anemia; fewer ovarian cyst problems; possible reduction in such diseases as polycystic ovary syndrome, rheumatoid arthritis, uterine fibroids, seizure and asthma episodes, colorectal cancer, and osteoporosis; possible improvement of lipid profile

5. Normotensive

6. No breast masses

7. No lifestyle barriers: need for discretion, difficulty remembering to use method, difficulty with storage or access, need for protection against sexually transmitted infections, financial constraints, desire for rapid return to fertility (delayed in some COC users)

8. No skin rashes (patch)

9. No physical or psychologic limitations with vaginal insertion or removal (ring)

10. Willing to tolerate side effects

B. Progestin-only contraception

1. No medical contraindications to progestin or vehicle for progestin

2. Noncontraceptive benefits: reduction in menstrual flow and pain, migraine headaches, and ovarian cyst formation (implants)

3. Appropriate when estrogen contraindicated (smoker, hypertension, lactation, or migraine headache)

4. No breast masses

5. No lifestyle barriers: need for discretion (POP), difficulty remembering to use method (POP), difficulty with storage or access, need for protection against sexually transmitted infections, financial constraints, desire for rapid return to fertility (medroxyprogesterone acetate), and intolerance of irregular bleeding

6. Obesity (medroxyprogesterone acetate and transdermal patch)

7. High efficacy desired (medroxyprogesterone acetate, implants, and LNG-IUS)

8. No PID, chlamydia, gonorrhea, or cervical or uterine anomalies (LNG-IUS)

9. Willing to tolerate discomfort of delivery (implants and medroxyprogesterone acetate)

10. Willing to tolerate side effects

C. ECP

1. Within window of effective use (120 hours from unprotected intercourse)

2. Willing to tolerate side effects

IV. Goals of clinical management

A. Screen for contraindications to contraceptive method

B. Management and patient adherence

1. Select appropriate contraceptive method; discuss risks, benefits, and costs.

2. Provide counseling and tools to increase compliance. Discuss smoking cessation and prevention of sexually transmitted infections with all methods of contraception.

V. Plan

A. Screening and diagnostic tests

In addition to Pap smear and sexually transmitted infection testing, may include mammogram, pelvic ultrasound (rule out fibroids or other anomalies), lipid testing (if family history of premature CVD), fasting blood sugar (if family history of diabetes), Leiden factor V.

B. Management and patient adherence

1. COC pills

a. Choose any low-dose (≤ 35 mcg) pill. If patient has polycystic ovary syndrome, hirsutism, or acne, choose pill with low androgenic activity. Choose monophasic pill if cycle suppression planned.

b. Select starting option (first day, quick start, Sunday start) based on patient desire, compliance, and willingness to use backup.

c. Select cycling pattern based on patient desire and medical indications (endometriosis, dysmenorrhea, and menstrual migraines).

d. May choose prepackaged extended cycle pills or skip placebo pills.

e. Discuss possible side effects and option for changing pill type, breakthrough bleeding, and lack of withdrawal bleeding.

f. Review warning signs (ACHES):
   i. Abdominal pain
   ii. Chest pain
   iii. Headaches
   iv. Eye problems
   v. Severe leg pain

g. Discuss compliance (take at same time every day), tips for remembering pills (e.g., set alarm, put near toothbrush), what to do if pill missed, when to use backup.

h. Recommend ECP be purchased in advance as backup method.

i. Discuss interactions with medications (certain antiretroviral therapy, certain anticonvulsant therapy, rifampicin, St. John's Wort may interfere with efficacy; most antibiotics do not lower effectiveness).

2. Transdermal patch

a. Select starting option (same as for COC pills).

b. Discuss patch placement.
   i. Place on clean, dry, skin of lower abdomen, buttock, upper arm, or upper back without rash or abrasion; rotate sites
   ii. Avoid use of body lotions and oils; can be worn in shower and bath, during exercise and swimming

c. Discuss compliance including daily patch inspection, tips for remembering patch removal and replacement dates, what to do if dates missed (patch effective for 2 extra days), when to use backup.

d. Discuss side effects, warning signs (ACHES).

e. Provide prescription for replacement patch if patch dislodged.

f. Recommend ECP be purchased in advance as backup method.

g. Dispose of used patch in product package to avoid environmental contamination.

3. Vaginal contraceptive ring

a. Instruct to insert first ring within first 5 days of onset of menses or at any time if not pregnant (use backup for 7 days).

b. When possible, have patient insert and remove ring at time of examination to demonstrate comfort and ease of insertion.

c. Ring is usually worn during intercourse but can be removed before intercourse if replaced within 3 hours. If worn with intercourse, check for presence in vagina postcoitus.

d. Dispose of used ring in product package.

e. Discuss side effects and warning signs (ACHES).

f. Discuss compliance, tips for remembering insertion and removal dates, what to do if dates missed (ring offers 1 extra week of efficacy), and backup.

g. Recommend ECP be purchased in advance as backup method.

4. POP

a. Begin first pill at any time during the first 5 days of menses, or begin at any time if not pregnant (use backup for 2 days).

b. Discuss compliance, tips for remembering to take pills, what to do if pill missed or late by 3 or more hours (use backup for at least 48 hours).

c. Manage side effects: for amenorrhea, rule out pregnancy, then reassure. For irregular bleeding, rule out underlying pathology, then reassure. Explain that bleeding is likely to improve within 3 months. For heavy bleeding, nonsteroidal anti-inflammatory medications (NSAIDs) for 3-day course may be beneficial.

d. Discuss interactions with medications (see COC pills).

e. Recommend ECP be purchased in advance as backup method.

5. Injectable progestin (medroxyprogesterone acetate)

a. Provide first injection within 7 days of onset of menses (no backup method needed) or at any time if not pregnant (use backup for 7 days).

b. Inject 150 mg intramuscularly deeply into deltoid or gluteus maximus.

c. Schedule subsequent injections every 11–12 weeks. If more than 13 weeks from previous injection, test for pregnancy. Assess for weight gain and depression.

d. Review potential side effects: weight gain, depression, severe headaches, heavy bleeding, and amenorrhea.

e. Manage bleeding problems. For heavy bleeding, rule out underlying pathology, then may provide NSAIDs (800 mg ibuprofen every 8 hours for 3 days) or conjugated estrogen (2.5, 1.25, or 0.625 mg one to four times a day for 4–6 days), or COC pills for 1–2 months. For spotting or breakthrough bleeding, rule out underlying pathology, reassure, or treat as for heavy bleeding. For amenorrhea, test for pregnancy if indicated and reassure.

f. Discuss delayed return to fertility of up to 1.5 years.

g. Discuss bone health, recommend 1,000–1,200 mg of calcium daily and 1,000 IU of vitamin D$_3$ daily, discuss weight-bearing exercise.

h. Recommend ECP be purchased in advance as back up method.

6. Implants

a. Implants should be inserted by a trained practitioner according to manufacturer guidelines. It may be inserted within 7 days of onset of menses (no backup method needed) or at any time in the cycle if not pregnant (backup should be used for 7 days).

b. Discuss possible side effects: irregular bleeding and infection or abscess at insertion site.

c. Manage side effects: for amenorrhea, perform pregnancy test, then reassure. For spotting or breakthrough bleeding, rule out underlying pathology, then treat as for medroxyprogesterone acetate. For arm pain and swelling, rule out infection, then treat with icepacks and NSAIDs. For infection without abscess, treat with oral antibiotics, and recheck in 24–48 hours. For abscess, treat with antibiotics, drain pus, and remove implant.

d. Remove implant according to manufacturer guidelines after 3 years or as desired by patient. Discuss rapid return to fertility with patient.

7. LNG-IUS

a. Insertion of LNG-IUS should be performed by a trained clinician, according to manufacturer guidelines. The system can be inserted within the first 7 days of onset of menses; no backup method is needed. It may be inserted at other times if pregnancy is excluded; use backup for 7 days.

b. Cervical dilation may be necessary, either with graduated dilators, or misoprostol, 200-µg tablet placed in the vagina or buccal cavity 1–2 hours before insertion. Patients can be premedicated with ibuprofen or with a paracervical block.

c. Patients should be observed postinsertion for adverse events, including signs of perforation and vasovagal reaction.

d. Advise NSAIDs for postinsertion pain.

e. Patients may be scheduled for a follow-up visit in 2 months to assess for presence of strings and for side effects; return sooner if problems.

f. Discuss side effects, including menstrual changes and warning signs of expulsion and infection. Teach patient how to check for strings.

g. Discuss signs of PID, including prolonged heavy bleeding, unusual discharge, pelvic pain, fever and chills, and dyspareunia. If PID is diagnosed, treat with antibiotics.

8. ECP

a. All women who are using COC pills and POPs, rings, and patch should be advised to have ECP available.

b. Advise patients to purchase ECP in advance.

c. Provide ECP to all patients if unprotected intercourse has occurred within 120 hours; review directions for taking ECP.

d. Discuss possible side effects (nausea and vomiting with COC pills; may prescribe antiemetic to take 1 hour before first dose).

e. Discuss possible changes in menstrual cycle post-ECP (early or delayed menses). Recommend pregnancy test if no menses in 3 weeks.

f. Report rape; provide or refer for trauma services.

g. Discuss prevention of sexually transmitted disease, offer testing.

h. Advise no teratogenic effect if pregnancy occurs.

i. Advise no prolonged contraceptive effect after ECP dose, may begin new cycle of CHC or POC immediately.

j. Discuss contraceptive compliance, reason for contraceptive failure if indicated.

REFERENCES

Anderson, K., Odlind, V., & Rybo, G. (1994). Levonorgestrel-releasing and copper releasing (Nova-T) intrauterine devices during five years of use: A randomized comparative trial. *Contraception, 49,* 56–72.

Bjarnadottir, R. I., Tuppurainen, M., & Killick, S. R. (2002). Comparison of cycle control with a combined contraceptive vaginal ring and oral levonorgestrel/ethinyl estradiol. *American Journal of Obstetrics and Gynecology, 186,* 389–395.

Centers for Disease Control and Prevention. (2012). Update to U.S. medical eligibility criteria for contraceptive use. *Morbidity and Mortality Weekly Report (MMWR), 61*(24), 449–452.

Dickey, R. P. (2010). *Managing contraceptive pill patients* (14th ed.). New Orleans, LA: EMIS Medical Publishers.

Endrikat, J., Cronin, M., Gerlinger, C., Ruebig, A., Schmidt, W., & Düsterberg, B. (2001). Open, multicenter comparison of efficacy, cycle control, and tolerability of a 23-day oral contraceptive regimen with 20 microg ethinyl estradiol and 150 microg desogestrel. *Contraception, 64*(3), 201–207.

Gavin, L., Moskosky, S., Carter, M., Curtis, K., Glass, E., Godfrey, E. et al. (2014). Providing quality family planning services: Recommendations of CDC and the U.S. Office of Population Affairs recommendations and reports. *Morbidity and Mortality Weekly Report, 63*(RRO4), 1–29.

Hatcher, R. A., Trussell, J., Nelson, A. L., Cates, W., Jr., Kowal, D., & Policar, M. S. (2011). *Contraceptive technology* (20th rev. ed.). New York, NY: Ardent Media, Inc..

Kaunitz, A. M., Arias, R., & McClung, M. (2008). Bone density recovery after depot medroxyprogesterone acetate injectable contraception use. *Contraception, 77,* 67–76.

Miller, L., & Notter, K. M. (2001). Menstrual reduction with extended use of combination oral contraceptive pills: Randomized controlled trial. *Obstetrics and Gynecology, 98*(5, Pt. 1), 771–778.

Nelson, A. L. (2012). New developments in oral contraception: Clinical utility of estradiol valerate/dienogest (Natazia) for contraception and treatment of heavy menstrual bleeding: Patient considerations. *Open Access Journal of Contraception, 2012:3,* 49–63.

Pharmacist's Letter/Prescriber's Letter. (2013). *Comparison of oral contraceptives and non-oral alternatives.* Stockton, CA: Therapeutic Research Center.

Spona, J., Elstein, M., Feichtinger, W., Sullivan, H., Lüdicke, F., Müller, U., et al. (1996). Shorter pill-free interval in combined oral contraceptives decreases follicular development. *Contraception, 54*(2), 71–77.

Tayob, Y., Adams, J., Jacobs, H. S., & Guillebaud, J. (1985). Ultrasound demonstration of increased frequency of functional cysts in women using progestogen-only oral contraception. *British Journal of Obstetrics and Gynaecology, 92,* 1003–1009.

World Health Organization, Department of Reproductive Health and Research. (2015). *Medical eligibility criteria for contraceptive use* (5th ed.). Geneva: Author.

Zieman, M., Guillebaud, J., Weisberg, E., Shangold, G. A., Fisher, A. C., & Creasy, G. W. (2002). Contraceptive efficacy and cycle control with the Ortho Evra/Evra transdermal system: The analysis of pooled data. *Fertility and Sterility, 77*(Suppl. 2), S13–S18.

Zieman, M., Hatcher, R. A., Cwiak, C., Darney, P. D., Creinin, M. D., & Stosur, H. R. (2010–2012). *A pocket guide to managing contraception.* Tiger, GA: Bridging the Gap Foundation.

APPENDIX 22–1: COMPARISON OF HORMONAL CONTRACEPTIVE METHODS

TABLE 22-2 Comparison of Oral Contraceptives

Products	Manufacturer	Estrogen	Progestin	Comments
LOW-DOSE MONOPHASIC PILLS				
Aviane-28 Falmina Lessina Lutera Orsythia Sronyx	Teva Novast Teva Actavis Qualitest Actavis	EE 20 mcg	Levonorgestrel 0.1 mg	Low estrogen; low progestin; low androgen. Low estrogen dose may cause more spotting and less margin of error for missed pills. Good choice to minimize risk of estrogen side effects like nausea, breast tenderness, etc.
Gildess Fe 1/20 Junel 1/20 Junel Fe 1/20 Loestrin-21 1/20 Loestrin Fe 1/20 Microgestin 1/20 Microgestin Fe 1/20	Qualitest Teva Teva Warner Chilcott Warner Chilcott Actavis Actavis	EE 20 mcg	Norethindrone 1 mg	Low estrogen; high progestin; medium androgen. Low estrogen dose may cause more spotting and less margin of error for missed pills. Good choice to minimize risk of estrogen side effects like nausea, breast tenderness, etc.
Generess Fe Chewable	Actavis	EE 25 mcg	Norethindrone 0.8 mg	High progestin, low estrogen, high androgen. Good choice to minimize estrogen side effects like nausea, breast tenderness, etc.
Altavera Kurvelo Levora Marlissa Nordette-28 Portia-28	Sandoz Lupin Actavis Glenmark Duramed/Teva Teva	EE 30 mcg	Levonorgestrel 0.15 mg	Low estrogen; medium progestin; medium/high androgen. Good choice to minimize estrogen side effects like nausea, breast tenderness, etc. Good choice to minimize spotting and/or breakthrough bleeding.
Cryselle-28 Elinest Low-Ogestrel-21 Low-Ogestrel-28 Lo/Ovral-28	Teva Novast Actavis Actavis Wyeth	EE 30 mcg	Norgestrel 0.3 mg	Low estrogen; medium progestin; medium/high androgen. Good choice to minimize estrogen side effects like nausea, breast tenderness, etc. and to minimize spotting and/or breakthrough bleeding.
Gildess Fe 1.5/30 Junel 1.5/30 Junel Fe 1.5/30 Loestrin 1.5/30-21 Loestrin Fe 1.5/30 Microgestin 1.5/30 Microgestin Fe 1.5/30	Qualitest Teva Teva Warner Chilcott Warner Chilcott Actavis Actavis	EE 30 mcg	Norethindrone acetate 1.5 mg	Low estrogen; high progestin; high androgen. Good choice to minimize estrogen side effects like nausea, breast tenderness, etc.

(continues)

TABLE 22-2 Comparison of Oral Contraceptives *(Continued)*

Products	Manufacturer	Estrogen	Progestin	Comments
Apri Desogen Emoquette Ortho-Cept Reclipsen Solia	Teva Organon Qualitest Ortho Actavis Prasco	EE 30 mcg	Desogestrel 0.15 mg	Low estrogen; high progestin; low androgen. Increased risk of DVT with desogestrel over other progestins (controversial data). Good choice to minimize spotting and/or breakthrough bleeding and to minimize androgenic effects. Has favorable lipid profile.
Levonorgestrel/ ethinyl estradiol Ocella Safyral Syeda Zarah Yasmin	Lupin Teva Bayer Sandoz Activis Bayer	EE 30 mcg	Drospirenone 3 mg	Low estrogen; progestin potency unclear; antiandrogenic and antimineralocorticoid activity. Does not appear to cause cyclic fluid retention. May be good choice for women with premenstrual syndrome, premenstrual dysphoric disorder, acne, hirsutism, or PCOS. Can increase potassium: avoid in renal/hepatic dysfunction or renal insufficiency. Check potassium during first cycle if another potassium-sparing drug (NSAID, ACE inhibitor, angiotensin receptor blocker, potassium-sparing diuretic, aldosterone antagonist) is given. Safyral contains folate.
Kelnor 1/35 Zovia 1/35	Teva Actavis	EE 35 mcg	Ethynodiol diacetate 1 mg	Medium estrogen; high progestin; low androgen. Good choice to minimize androgenic effects.
Mono-Linyah Ortho-Cyclen-28 MonoNessa Norgestimate/ ethinyl estradiol Previfem Sprintec	Novast Ortho Actavis Glenmark Qualitest Teva	EE 35 mcg	Norgestimate 0.25 mg	Medium estrogen; low progestin; low androgen. Good choice to minimize spotting and/or breakthrough bleeding and to minimize androgenic effects. Has favorable lipid profile.
Necon 1/50 Norinyl 1+50	Actavis Actavis	Mestranol 50 mcg	Norethindrone 1 mg	Medium estrogen; medium progestin; medium androgen.
Ovcon-35 Balziva Briellyn Femcon Fe chewable Gildagia Philith Zenchent Zeosa chewable	Warner Chilcott Teva Glenmark Warner Chilcott Qualitest Novast Actavis Teva	EE 35 mcg	Norethindrone 0.4 mg; total of 8.4 mg/cycle	Medium estrogen; low progestin; low androgen. Good choice to minimize androgenic effects. Has favorable lipid profile.

TABLE 22-2 Comparison of Oral Contraceptives *(Continued)*

Products	Manufacturer	Estrogen	Progestin	Comments
Brevicon-28 *Modicon-28* *Necon 0.5/35* *Nortrel 0.5/35* *Wera*	Actavis Ortho Actavis Teva Novast	EE 35 mcg	Norethindrone 0.5 mg; total of 10.5 mg/cycle	Medium estrogen; low progestin; low androgen. Good choice to minimize androgenic effects. Has favorable lipid profile.
Alyacen 1/35 *Cyclofem 1/35* *Dasetta 1/35* *Necon 1/35-28* *Norinyl 1+35-28* *Nortrel 1/35-28* *Ortho-Novum 1/35-28*	Glenmark Qualitest Novast Actavis Actavis Teva Ortho	EE 35 mcg	Norethindrone 1 mg; total of 21 mg/cycle	Medium estrogen; medium/high progestin; medium androgen.

HIGH-DOSE MONOPHASIC PILLS

Products	Manufacturer	Estrogen	Progestin	Comments
Ovcon-50	Warner Chilcott	EE 50 mcg	Norethindrone 1 mg	High estrogen; medium progestin; medium androgen.
Ogestrel 0.5/50-28	Actavis	EE 50 mcg	Norgestrel 0.5 mg	High estrogen; high progestin; high androgen.
Zovia 1/50-28	Actavis	EE 50 mcg	Ethynodiol diacetate 1 mg	High estrogen; high progestin; medium/high androgen.

BIPHASIC PILLS

Products	Manufacturer	Estrogen	Progestin	Comments
Azurette *Mircette* *Kariva* *Viorele*	Actavis Teva Teva Glenmark	EE 20 mcg × 21 days, placebo × 2 days, 10 mcg × 5 days	Desogestrel 0.15 mg × 21 days	Low estrogen; high progestin; low androgen. Shorter hormone-free interval may help menstrual migraine, dysmenorrhea, PMS. Increased risk of deep vein thrombosis (DVT) with desogestrel over other progestins.
Necon 10/11	Actavis	EE 35 mcg	Norethindrone 0.5 mg × 10 days, 1 mg × 11 days	High estrogen; medium progestin; low/medium androgen. Poor cycle control compared with levonorgestrel triphasic pill.

TRIPHASIC PILLS

Products	Manufacturer	Estrogen	Progestin	Comments
Estrostep Fe *Tilia* *Tilia Fe* *Tri-Legest Fe*	Warner Chilcott Actavis Actavis Teva	EE 20 mcg × 5 days, 30 mcg × 7 days, 35 mcg × 9 days	Norethindrone 1 mg × 21 days	Low estrogen; high progestin; medium androgen. FDA-labeled for acne. Good choice to minimize estrogen side effects like nausea, breast tenderness, etc. and to minimize spotting and/or breakthrough bleeding.
Norgestimate/ ethinyl estradiol *Ortho Tri-Cyclen Lo* *Tri-Lo Sprintec*	Lupin Ortho Actavis	EE 25 mcg × 21 days	Norgestimate 0.18 mg × 7 days, 0.215 mg × 7 days, 0.25 mg × 7 days	Low estrogen; low progestin; low androgen. Good choice to minimize spotting, breakthrough bleeding, and androgenic effects. Has favorable lipid profile.

(continues)

TABLE 22-2 Comparison of Oral Contraceptives *(Continued)*

Products	Manufacturer	Estrogen	Progestin	Comments
Caziant Cesia Cyclessa Velivet	Actavis Prasco Schering-Plough Teva	EE 25 mcg × 21 days	Desogestrel 0.1 mg × 7 days, 0.125 mg × 7 days, 0.15 mg × 7 days	Low estrogen; high progestin; low androgen. First triphasic pill with desogestrel. Increased risk of DVT with desogestrel over other progestins. Better cycle control and less weight gain than *Ortho-Novum 7/7/7*.
Enpresse Levonest Myzilra Trivora	Teva Novast Qualitest Actavis	EE 30 mcg × 6 days, 40 mcg × 5 days, 30 mcg × 10 days	Levonorgestrel 0.05 mg × 6 days, 0.075 mg × 5 days, 0.125 mg × 10 days. Total of 1.925 mg/cycle.	Medium estrogen; low progestin; low/medium androgen. Better cycle control than with norethindrone biphasic pill (*Ortho-Novum 10/11*).
Ortho Tri-Cyclen Tri-Estarylla Tri-Linyah TriNessa Tri-Previfem Tri-Sprintec	Ortho Sandoz Novast Actavis Qualitest Teva	EE 35 mcg × 21 days	Norgestimate 0.18 mg × 7 days, 0.215 mg × 7 days, 0.25 mg × 7 days	Medium estrogen; low progestin; low androgen. FDA-labeled for treatment of acne.
Aranelle Leena Tri-Norinyl	Teva Actavis Actavis	EE 35 mcg × 21 days	Norethindrone 0.5 mg × 7 days, 1 mg × 9 days, 0.5 mg x 5 days. Total of 15 mg/ cycle.	Medium estrogen; medium progestin; low/medium androgen.
Alyacen 7/7/7 Cyclafem 7/7/7 Dasetta 7/7/7 Ortho-Novum 7/7/7 Nortrel 7/7/7 Necon 7/7/7	Glenmark Qualitest Novatest Ortho Teva Actavis	EE 35 mcg × 21 days	Norethindrone 0.5 mg × 7 days, 0.75 mg × 7 days, 1 mg x 7 days. Total of 15.75 mg/cycle.	Medium estrogen; medium progestin; low/medium androgen.
FOUR-PHASIC				
Natazia	Bayer	Estradiol valerate 3 mg x 2 days, then 2 mg x 22 days, then 1 mg x 2 days, then 2-day pill-free interval	Dienogest none x 2 days, then 2 mg x 5 days, then 3 mg x 17 days, then none x 4 days	Strong endometrial effect, low androgen effect. Four-phase regimen with minimal effect on lipid profile, fewer metabolic changes. Good choice for heavy menstruation.
EXTENDED-CYCLE PILLS				
Lo Loestrin Fe	Warner Chilcott	EE 10 mcg x 26 days	Norethindrone 1 mg x 24 days	High progestin, ultra-low estrogen, medium androgen. Good choice for women with endometriosis, perimenopause, migraine with higher dose estrogen (without aura), smoker < 35 years old.

TABLE 22-2 Comparison of Oral Contraceptives *(Continued)*

Products	Manufacturer	Estrogen	Progestin	Comments
Loestrin-24 Fe	Warner Chilcott	EE 20 mcg × 24 days	Norethindrone 1 mg × 24 days	Low estrogen; high progestin; medium androgen. Low estrogen dose may cause more spotting and less margin of error for missed pills. Good choice to minimize risk of estrogen side effects like nausea, breast tenderness, etc. 24/4-day cycle combination may be helpful for women wanting to stay on a 28-day cycle, but minimize duration of withdrawal bleeding and menstrual-related symptoms.
Amethia Lo *Ethinyl estradiol/ levonorgestel* *LoSeasonique*	Actavis Lupin Teva	EE 20 mcg × 84 days, 10 mcg × 7 days	Levonorgestrel 0.1 mg × 84 days	A low dose version of *Seasonique*.
Introvale *Jolessa* *Levonorgestrel/ ethinyl estradiol* *Quasense* *Seasonale*	Sandoz Teva Lupin Actavis Teva	EE 30 mcg × 84 days	Levonorgestrel 0.15 mg × 84 days	84-day active pills then 7-day pill-free interval. More intermenstrual bleeding and/ or spotting than with 28-day cycle; total days of bleeding and/or spotting similar. May allow women to experience menstruation-related symptoms less frequently.
Amethia *Seasonique*	Actavis Teva	EE 30 mcg × 84 days, 10 mcg × 7 days	Levonorgestrel 0.15 mg × 84 days	84-day active pills then 7-day low-dose estrogen instead of placebo pills. Extended cycle and lack of hormone-free interval may help menorrhagia, dysmenorrhea, menstrual migraine, and PMS.
Beyaz *Gianvi* *Loryna* *Vestura* *Yaz*	Bayer Teva Sandoz Actavis Bayer	EE 20 mcg × 24 days	Drospirenone 3 mg × 24 days	FDA-approved for premenstrual dysphoric disorder and moderate acne. Follows 24/4-day cycle and contains ingredients of *Yasmin*, but with lower estrogen dose (20 mcg EE compared to 30 mcg EE in *Yasmin*). Also see *Yasmin* comments. Beyaz contains folate.
CONTINUOUS-CYCLE PILLS				
Amethyst	Actavis	EE 20 mcg	Levonorgestrel 90 mcg	Active pill taken every day (NO pill-free interval). Breakthrough bleeding/spotting common initially and decreases with continued use. May allow women to experience menstruation-related symptoms less frequently.

(continues)

TABLE 22-2 Comparison of Oral Contraceptives *(Continued)*

Products	Manufacturer	Estrogen	Progestin	Comments
PROGESTIN-ONLY PILLS—"Mini-pill"				
Camila *Errin* *Heather* *Jolivette* *Micronor* *Nor-QD* *Nora-BE*	Teva Teva Glenmark Actavis Ortho Actavis Actavis	Not applicable	Norethindrone 0.35 mg	Irregular menses, but overall blood loss reduced. Preferred over COCs in women who are breastfeeding.
EMERGENCY CONTRACEPTION				
Levonorgestrel *Ella* *Plan B* *Next Choice*	Perrigo Rand D Actavis Teva Actavis	Not applicable Ella: Not applicable	Levonorgestrel 0.75 mg tablets × 2 Ella: Ulipristal 30 mg tablet (progesterone receptor modulator)	For prevention of pregnancy for women who present within 72 hours of unprotected intercourse or contraceptive failure. Traditional FDA-approved regimen consists of two tablets with the first tablet taken as soon as possible within 72 hours and the second tablet taken 12 hours later. Alternatively, taking both tablets at once is equally effective and is recommended by some experts. *Plan B* can be considered for a woman who presents within 5 days of unprotected or inadequately protected sexual intercourse; however, it is more effective the earlier it is taken. *Plan B* is about 89% effective if used within 3 days after sex. Ella: Most effective ECP, may be more effective in overweight women, requires prescription
Next Choice One Dose *Plan B One-Step*	Actavis Teva	Not applicable	Levonorgestrel 1.5 mg tablet	One tablet for prevention of pregnancy for women who present within 72 hours of unprotected intercourse or contraceptive failure. Similar efficacy and adverse effects as *Plan B*.

Data from Therapuetic Research Center. (2013). Pharmacist's Letter / Prescriber's Letter.

TABLE 22-3 Hormonal Alternatives to Oral Contraception

Brand Name	Manufacturer	Estrogen	Progestin	Failure Rate	Comments
Depo-Provera® CI Medroxyprogesterone Acetate Injection	Pfizer Sicor	None	Medroxyprogesterone acetate 150 mg	0.3%	Intramuscular injection once every 3 months. Long duration of action may be inappropriate for some women. Noncontraceptive benefits in women with sickle cell disease. May decrease risk of seizures in women with epilepsy. May decrease bone mineral density.
Depo-SubQ Provera 104	Pfizer	None	Medroxyprogesterone acetate 104 mg	N/A	Subcutaneous injection once every 3 months. FDA approved for use as a contraceptive in December 2004 and for management of pain associated with endometriosis in March 2005. Efficacy similar to *Depo-Provera®* and medroxyprogesterone injections, but at lower doses. Long-term adverse effects similar to *Depo-Provera*.
Nexplanon®	Schering-Plough	None	Etonogestrel (release rate varies over time)	N/A	Implantable (subdermal) rod. Provides contraception for up to 3 years. Failure rate = < 1 pregnancy per 100 women using *Implanon* for 1 year. Effectiveness rate in very overweight women unknown.
Mirena®	Bayer	None	Levonorgestrel 20 mcg/day for 5 years	0.1%	Intrauterine device (IUD). In October 2009, approved to treat heavy menstrual bleeding in women who use IUDs for contraception.
Skyla (IUS)	Bayer	None	Levonorgestrel 14 mcg/day (after first 24 days of insertion) for up to 3 years		Smaller in diameter, narrower inserter, easier to insert in nulliparous women, better tolerated in teens and perimenopausal women.

(continues)

TABLE 22-3 Hormonal Alternatives to Oral Contraception *(Continued)*

Brand Name	Manufacturer	Estrogen	Progestin	Failure Rate	Comments
NuvaRing®	Schering-Plough	Ethinyl estradiol 15 mcg/day	Etonogestrel (active form of desogestrel) 0.12 mg/day	0.3%	Vaginal ring that is left in for 3 weeks and removed for 1 week. May have higher incidence of vaginal discharge than pills.
Ortho Evra®	Ortho	Ethinyl estradiol 35 mcg/day (Release rate extrapolated from Canadian product monograph, which shows identical pharmacokinetic data for *Evra* [Canada] and *Ortho Evra®* [U.S.])	Norelgestromin (active form of norgestimate) 200 mcg/day (Release rate extrapolated from Canadian product monograph, which shows identical pharmacokinetic data for *Evra* [Canada] and *Ortho Evra®* [U.S.])	0.3%	Transdermal patch applied weekly (for 3 weeks, then week 4 is patch free). Application site reactions. Cycle control poor in 20% of women in first cycle. More breast discomfort in first two cycles than with combined oral contraceptive. Body weight > 90 kg may increase risk of unintended pregnancy. Has been used continuously with nine active patches in a row followed by 7-day patch-free interval. Compliance may improve compared with combined oral contraceptive.

Data from Therapuetic Research Center. (2013). Pharmacist's Letter / Prescriber's Letter.

MENOPAUSE TRANSITION

CHAPTER 23

Priscilla Abercrombie

I. Introduction and general background

Menopause is the result of the natural decline in the hormones produced in the ovaries. As hormone levels decrease, a number of symptoms may emerge, although their presentation and severity varies greatly from woman to woman. Menopause is a retrospective diagnosis made after complete cessation of the menstrual period for 12 consecutive months (Speroff & Fritz, 2005). The average age of menopause is 51.4 years old. Women who smoke reach menopause 1.74 years earlier than nonsmokers (McKinlay, Bifano, & McKinlay, 1985). The Stages of Reproductive Aging Workshop (STRAW) +10 (Harlow et al., 2012) is an updated version of the original STRAW criteria developed to more precisely describe the reproductive aging process in women (Soules et al., 2001). Menopause usually occurs between the mid-40s and the mid-50s. The menopause transition is not only marked by physiologic changes; there are also important developmental changes that occur at this time of life. During this transition, women face such issues as the meaning of midlife and aging, role and purpose in life, and changes in interpersonal relationships (children, spouse, and parents) (Deeks, 2002). The experience of the menopause transition is influenced by sociocultural background. Women with a negative attitude toward menopause seem to report more symptoms (Forshaw & Hunter, 2010). This chapter addresses the management of the major symptoms experienced by women during the menopause transition.

A. Types of menopause

1. Surgical menopause occurs when both ovaries are surgically removed (bilateral oophorectomy).

2. Medical menopause can be induced by the use of certain drugs, such as gonadotropin-releasing hormone antagonists, or treatments, such as chemotherapy or radiation therapy.

3. Premature ovarian insufficiency is the loss of ovarian function before the age of 40 years (Davies &

Cartwright, 2012). Previously, the condition was referred to as premature ovarian failure.

B. Symptoms

1. Vasomotor changes

   a. Definition and overview: Symptoms range from flushing or warmth in the face and upper body to sweating and chills lasting about 1–5 minutes (Kronenberg, 1990). Hot flashes can lead to severe sleep disturbances in some women. Hot flashes typically begin when cycles become irregular. Unfortunately, emerging research suggests that women with hot flashes may have an increased risk for cardiovascular disease especially if they have other risk factors (Thurston et al., 2011).

   b. Etiology: Hot flashes stem from declining levels of estradiol affecting the hypothalamic temperature regulating center. This results in altered thermoregulation, although the exact mechanism is unknown. In addition, genetic polymorphisms may play a role in how estradiol is synthesized and metabolized, thus affecting vasomotor symptoms (Rebbeck et al., 2010).

   c. Prevalence and incidence: Sixty to eighty percent of women will have vasomotor symptoms at some point during the menopause transition (Gold et al., 2007). African-American women are more likely to report bothersome vasomotor symptoms and Asian women are least likely to report them (Thurston et al., 2008). They commonly occur up to 5 years after the last menstrual period but about one-third of women have them for up to 10 years (Freeman, Sammel, & Sanders, 2014).

2. Genitourinary syndrome of menopause (GSM)

   a. Etiology and definition: Decreasing estrogen levels lead to a decrease in the production of vaginal lubrication and loss of vaginal elasticity and thickness of the epithelium (Speroff &

Fritz, 2005). GSM is a new term endorsed by the North American Menopause Society and International Society for the Study of Women's Sexual Health to describe changes in the genital tract associated with a decrease in sex hormones. It includes symptoms of vaginal dryness, burning, and irritation; lack of lubrication, discomfort, impaired function or pain during intercourse; and urinary urgency, dysuria and recurrent urinary tract infections (Portman, Gass, & Vulvovaginal Atrophy Terminology Consensus Conference Panel, 2014).

b. Prevalence and incidence: In a cohort study involving over 1,000 women, 50% experienced problematic vaginal dryness and 40% of the sexually active women had dyspareunia (Huang et al., 2010). In a large online survey of women with vulvovaginal symptoms 55% experienced dryness, 44% had dyspareunia, and 37% reported irritation (Kingsberg, Wysocki, Magnus, & Krychman, 2013). Vulvovaginal atrophy symptoms affected enjoyment of sex in 59% of participants.

3. Mood and cognition

Women are at increased risk for depressive symptoms and depressive disorders during perimenopause (Bromberger & Kravitz, 2011). Women who experience vasomotor symptoms and insomnia are more at risk for depression (Gyllstrom, Schreiner, & Harlow, 2007). Women with a history of depression especially during reproductive events may be more vulnerable to relapse during perimenopause.

a. Difficulty thinking, forgetfulness, and other cognitive disturbances are frequently reported during the menopause transition.

b. Estrogens not only act as hormones but as neurosteroids and neuromodulators that influence cognition (Luine, 2014). The Women's Health Initiative (WHI) Memory study concluded that hormone therapy (HT) did not improve cognitive function (Rapp et al., 2003) and increased the risk for dementia in women 65 years and older (Shumaker et al., 2003).

c. The "critical period hypothesis" suggests that in order for estrogens to exert positive benefits on the brain they should be given early in the menopause transition (Luine, 2014). There is some evidence that giving only short-term HT during perimenopause may have long-term benefits.

d. Estradiol has differing effects on the brain than conjugated equine estrogen used in the WHI studies. There is some evidence that estrogen may reduce the risk of Alzheimer's disease, a devastating disease that largely affects women

(Morrison, Brinton, Schmidt, & Gore, 2006). More research is needed to determine whether estrogen may be beneficial when initiated after surgical menopause or early in the menopause transition to prevent cognitive decline.

4. Sexual functioning

The most common sexual complaints during menopause are vaginal dryness and painful sex, low desire, and poor orgasm and satisfaction (Nappi & Lachowsky, 2009). Population-based studies show a decline in many aspects of sexual functioning in conjunction with a decline in estradiol levels, not androgen levels (Dinnerstein, 2003). In one Australian study, scores indicating sexual dysfunction rose from 42% to 88% during perimenopause. Sexual function in midlife women is a complex issue that is affected not only by hormonal changes but also by many other factors, such as premorbid sexual functioning, personality, educational level, stress, physical and psychological health status, partner health status, and the woman's feelings toward her partner. The level of distress experienced as a result of the sexual problems should also be assessed. Sexual dysfunction can be categorized into disorders of desire, arousal, orgasm, or pain.

a. Hypoactive sexual desire disorder is a lack of desire for sexual activity and lack of responsiveness to sexual stimulation. Decreased sexual desire is a relatively common problem for women. About 24–43% of women complain of low sexual desire. It can become particularly problematic for women during life transitions, such as pregnancy, postpartum, and menopause.

b. Sexual aversion disorder: intermittent or persistent avoidance of sexual contact with a partner because of fear or loathing of such an experience.

c. Sexual arousal disorder: intermittent or persistent inability to attain or maintain adequate sexual excitement. Sexual thoughts that typically produce somatic changes, such as vaginal lubrication or swelling, are absent.

d. Orgasmic disorder: intermittent or persistent difficult or inability to attain orgasm after sufficient stimulation and arousal.

e. Sexual pain disorder: dyspareunia, vaginismus, noncoital sexual pain.

5. Sleep disturbance

During the menopause transition, many women suffer from poor sleep and it can have a severe impact on quality of life.

a. The prevalence of sleep disturbance is higher in perimenopausal, postmenopausal, and surgical menopausal women than in premenopausal women (Xu & Lang, 2014).

b. Severity of insomnia is associated with frequency of moderate to severe hot flashes (Ensrud et al., 2009).

c. HT has been shown to improve perceived sleep quality and sleeping problems better than placebo (Joffe, Massler, & Sharkey, 2010).

d. Sleep disturbance is associated with anxiety and depression, aging, primary sleep disorders, medical conditions, and medications.

e. Psychosocial and behavioral factors also contribute to sleep issues, making it difficult to treat. A multimodal approach to treatment is preferred.

C. Menstrual cycle disturbances

Disturbances in the menstrual cycle are a hallmark of the menopausal transition. Fluctuations in hormone levels lead to variations in cycle length and menstrual flow. Periods of amenorrhea caused by anovulatory cycles can be followed by heavy and prolonged menstrual bleeding. Menstrual cycle length eventually increases especially in the year preceding cessation of menses. During the perimenopause transition follicle-stimulating hormone (FSH) and estradiol levels rise (Speroff & Fritz, 2005), whereas luteinizing hormone (LH) levels remain normal. Although FSH levels can be high, ovarian follicular development is unpredictable; thus the use of contraceptive methods is encouraged to prevent unwanted pregnancy. In the postmenopause, FSH and LH levels remain high and estrogen is low. Dysfunctional uterine bleeding may occur because of hormonal fluctuations. Abnormal menstrual bleeding may be a symptom of endometrial hyperplasia or cancer, and further evaluation with endometrial biopsy may be warranted.

1. Menorrhagia is excessive or prolonged bleeding. Gynecological conditions, such as fibroids, endometrial polyps, adenomyosis, and anovulation, contribute to menorrhagia.

2. Menometrorrhagia is irregular or frequent excessive bleeding.

3. Intermenstrual bleeding is bleeding that occurs between menstrual periods. It may be a symptom of endometrial hyperplasia or cancer.

4. Persistent abnormal vaginal bleeding, suspected ovulation resulting in unopposed estrogen, and any postmenopausal bleeding should be investigated further.

II. **Database** (may include but is not limited to)

A. Subjective: menopause transition

1. Past medical history: cardiovascular disease, stroke, venous thromboembolism (VTE), hypertension, hyperlipidemia, thyroid disease, depression or anxiety, liver disease, obesity, prolactinoma, and anorexia.

2. Surgical history: hysterectomy with bilateral oophorectomy.

3. Gynecological history

a. Obstetric history: pregnancies, deliveries, abortions, and postpartum issues

b. Contraception and family planning: current and past use, experience with hormonal contraception

c. Urinary: recurrent cystitis, interstitial cystitis, overactive bladder, and urinary incontinence

d. Gynecological: vulvar disease, vulvar pain disorders, abnormal uterine or vaginal bleeding, cervical cancer screening, uterine fibroids, endometriosis, and ovarian cysts

e. Anatomic issues: organ prolapse, stenosis, scarring, cervical mass and Asherman syndrome

4. Sexually transmitted infections

5. Cancer: gynecological and breast malignancies; history of treatment with surgery, radiation, chemotherapy, and/or drugs

6. Sexual history

a. Sexual experience or inexperience

b. Sexual orientation and gender identity

c. Baseline and current receptivity to sex play

d. Assess current pattern and explore if pattern has changed

e. Discuss disparity between patient and partner's desire

f. Assess nonpartner initiated sexual expression (masturbation, erotic dreams, and sexual thoughts)

g. Assess sexual trauma history

7. Exposure history: environmental exposures that affect hormone production.

8. Medication history: medications that affect hormone production (antipsychotics, contraceptives, gonadotropin-releasing hormone antagonists, and so forth) platelet function, liver or kidney function, or sexual function.

9. Family history: age of menopause, breast and ovarian cancer, and osteoporosis.

10. Occupational and environmental history: workplace stress.

11. Personal social history: religious or cultural considerations, current or past relationship issues, and perception of menopause.

12. Review of systems.

a. Constitutional signs and symptoms: fatigue, mood, and hot flashes

b. Genitourinary: heavy menses or amenorrhea, intermenstrual bleeding, dysuria, urinary incontinence, dyspareunia, vaginal dryness, decreased sexual arousal or orgasm, and postcoital bleeding

c. Musculoskeletal: joint stiffness or pain, myalgias

d. Neurologic: lethargy, depressed mood, moodiness, decreased libido, and poor short-term memory

B. Objective

1. Physical examination findings

   a. Vasomotor changes: may witness flushing

   b. Urogenital atrophy (Castelo-Branco, Cancelo, Villero, Nohales, & Julia, 2005).

      i. Visual inspection changes seen in vaginal epithelium is the most common diagnostic indicator

      ii. Vaginal pH greater than 4.5

      iii. Pale dry vaginal tissues with decreased rugae

      iv. Shrinkage of labia minora, check for lesions, inflammation, and friability

      v. Inspect for urethral caruncle, prolapse, or polyps

      vi. Tightening of introitus secondary to atrophic changes or other vulvar conditions

   c. Thinning of pubic hair

   d. Cystocele or rectocele and/or genital prolapse

   e. Menstrual cycle disturbances: menstrual flooding at time of examination, intermenstrual spotting on examination, cervical mass or stenosis, uterine fibroids, and ovarian cysts and adnexal mass

   f. Mood and cognition: inappropriate affect, depressed or anxious affect, crying, and poor cognition during interview

   g. Cotton swab Q-tip test to assess for vulvodynia

   h. Assess pelvic floor muscles to rule out pelvic floor muscle dysfunction

   i. Vulvar lesions

III. Assessment

A. Determine the diagnosis

Menopause transition is diagnosed based on chronologic age, menstrual cycle history, and menopausal symptoms

B. Other conditions to consider based on symptoms and examination findings

1. Vasomotor symptoms

   a. Cardiovascular disease

   b. Hyperthyroidism

   c. Pheochromocytoma

   d. Cancer

   e. Effect of medications

2. Urogenital atrophy

   a. Urinary incontinence

   b. Urinary tract infection

   c. Vulvar disease

   d. Atrophic vaginitis

3. Menstrual cycle disturbances

   a. Causes of secondary amenorrhea: hyperprolactinemia or prolactinoma, pregnancy, hypothalamic dysfunction, thyroid disease, and Asherman syndrome (see Chapter 19 on amenorrhea).

   b. Abnormal vaginal bleeding: endometrial hyperplasia and unopposed estrogen, endometrial or cervical cancer, endometrial polyps, adenomyosis, pregnancy, thyroid disease, and spontaneous abortion (SAB) (see Chapter 18 on abnormal uterine bleeding).

4. Mood and cognition

   a. Depression and anxiety disorders

   b. Dementia and Alzheimer's disease

   c. Sleep disorders

5. Sexual dysfunction

   a. Anxiety and depression disorders and relationship issues

   b. Vulvar disease, vulvar pain disorder, and pelvic floor muscle dysfunction, vaginal atrophy

   c. Sexual trauma history

C. Severity

Assess the severity of the symptoms and transition

1. The menopausal rating scale can be found at http://www.menopause-rating-scale.info/

2. See the review of instruments to measure quality of life during the menopause transition (Shin & Shin, 2012).

D. Significance

Assess the significance of the transition to the patient and significant others

IV. Goals of clinical management

A. Alleviate symptoms of the menopause transition that affect quality of life

B. Rule out abnormalities

C. Prevent major causes of morbidity and mortality

1. Osteoporosis

2. Cardiovascular disease and stroke

3. Cancer: lung, breast, and colorectal

V. Plan

A. Screening

1. Consult guidelines on healthcare maintenance of the adult for age-appropriate physical exam and screening test recommendations.

B. Diagnostic testing based on symptoms

1. For abnormal bleeding: endometrial biopsy, pelvic ultrasound, complete blood count, and thyroid-stimulating hormone (see Chapter 18 on abnormal uterine bleeding for a more in-depth discussion).

2. For amenorrhea: pregnancy test, prolactin, thyroid-stimulating hormone, and FSH (see Chapter 19 on amenorrhea for more in-depth discussion).

3. For mood and cognition symptoms: screen for depression, anxiety, and dementia.

4. For sexual dysfunction symptoms: consider baseline free testosterone level, lipid profile, and liver enzyme levels, especially important before initiating testosterone therapy.

C. Management

1. Hormone therapy (Note: as with prescribing any drug be aware of drug interactions, contraindications for use, and side effects)

   The results of two large clinical trials, the Women's Health Initiative and the Heart and Estrogen/Progestin Replacement Study in 2002, greatly influenced HT prescribing practices. In 2013 the Global Consensus Statement on Menopausal Hormone Therapy was released (de Villiers et al., 2013). This consensus statement was created by an international panel and is endorsed by many professional organizations including the Endocrine Society, American Menopause Society, and the American Society for Reproductive Medicine. Key points include:

   - Menopause hormone therapy (MHT) is the most effective treatment for vasomotor symptoms and the benefits outweigh the risks before age 60 or within 10 years of menopause.
   - MHT is effective for the prevention of osteoporosis-related fractures before age 60 or within 10 years of menopause.
   - Estrogen-alone MHT may decrease the risk of coronary heart disease (CHD) and all-cause mortality in women younger than 60 or within 10 years of menopause.
   - The addition of a progestogen has not shown a benefit for CHD.
   - Vaginal estrogen should be used for women with vaginal dryness or related dyspareunia.
   - Estrogen can be used alone in women post hysterectomy; otherwise, it should be used with a progestogen to protect against increased risk of endometrial cancer.
   - MHT is an individual decision based on quality of life, health priorities, and risk factors such as age, time since menopause, risk for venous thromboembolism, stroke, ischemic heart disease, and breast cancer.
   - Oral MHT increases the risk of venous thromboembolism and ischemic stroke.
   - The increased risk of breast cancer with MHT is small. It is primarily associated with the progestogen and the duration of use. The risk decreases once treatment stops.
   - The dose and duration of MHT should be individualized based on goals and safety issues.
   - The use of custom compounded bioidentical hormone therapy is not recommended.
   - Safety data do not support the use of MHT in breast cancer survivors.

   a. Benefits: HT is the most effective treatment for vasomotor symptoms and is recommended for women who are experiencing moderate to severe hot flashes. It is also beneficial for the symptoms of genitourinary syndrome. It may improve overall quality of life. The "timing hypothesis" suggests that there may be some cardiovascular disease (CVD) protection when estrogen is started near the onset of menopause (Grodstein, Manson, & Stampfer, 2006).

   b. Contraindications (Al-Safi & Santoro, 2014):
      i. History of breast or endometrial cancer, cardiac disease
      ii. Thromboembolic disease, uncontrolled hypertension
      iii. Acute liver disease
      iv. Active gallbladder disease
      v. Migraine headache with aura
      vi. Undiagnosed vaginal bleeding

   c. Risks: there is an increased risk of ischemic stroke, VTE, and breast cancer with HT. The "gap theory" suggests that the risk of breast cancer may be highest when HT is started near menopause (Bhupathiraju & Manson, 2014). Women should not take HT to prevent CVD or to treat heart disease.

d. Estrogen therapy: there are multiple types of estrogen available in many doses and formulations including pills, creams, lotions, and patches. Transdermal administration of estrogen has been associated with a decreased risk of deep vein thrombosis, stroke, and MI in observational studies (North American Menopause Society, 2012). It may also be more advantageous in the setting of hypertension, gallbladder disease, and diabetes but more research is needed. Start at the lowest effective dose for the shortest duration possible. For examples of preparations and starting doses, see **Table 23-1**. Of note, vaginal preparations are for the treatment of vaginal symptoms and do not require progesterone for endometrial protection.

e. Progestogen therapy: women with an intact uterus should receive progestogen in addition to estrogen to prevent endometrial hyperplasia. Progestins seem to attenuate the beneficial effects of estrogen on lipids. Oral micronized progesterone may be more advantageous because it appears to have little or no effect on lipids (Writing Group for the PEPI Trial, 1995). Note: Progestogens may worsen depression. For examples of preparations and starting doses, see **Table 23-2**.

f. Combination therapies: See **Table 23-3.**

g. Dosing considerations: advantages, disadvantages, and the patient's preferences should be taken into account when prescribing HT. Options are:
   i. Daily administration of both estrogen and progestogen.
   ii. Intermittent progestogen with daily estrogen. The progestogen could be given on days 1–14 each month. At this time there are inadequate data to support the use of long-cycle regimens, such as a progestogen, every 3 months, vaginal administration of progesterone, or ultralow-dose estrogen without progestogen (North American Menopause Society [NAMS], 2012).

h. Discontinuing therapy: There is a 50% risk of symptoms recurring after HT is discontinued (NAMS, 2008). Recurrence of vasomotor symptoms is similar whether tapered or if cessation is abrupt.

i. Bioidentical HT: bioidentical hormones are thought to more closely mimic the hormones normally found in the female body. There are three different types of estrogen produced in the body: (a) E_2 or estradiol is produced primarily during the reproductive years, (b) E_1 or estrone is produced primarily after menopause, and (c) E_3 or estriol is produced primarily during pregnancy. Each form of estrogen works differently throughout the body. It is thought that estriol may be protective against

TABLE 23-1 Estrogen Therapy

Oral preparations	Starting dose and frequency
estradiol	0.5 mg per day
ethinyl estradiol	2.5 mcg per day
conjugated estrogen	0.3–0.45 mg per day
Transdermal preparation	**Starting dose and frequency**
estradiol patch	0.025–0.0375 mg changed once or twice weekly depending on product
Intramuscular preparations	**Starting dose and frequency**
estradiol cypionate	1–5 mg every 3–4 weeks
estradiol valerate	10–20 mg every 4 weeks
Topical preparations	**Starting dose and frequency**
estradiol: gel 0.06% pump	0.75 mg/1.25 g per day
estradiol: 0.06% spray emulsion	1.53 mg/spray per day
Vaginal preparations	**Starting dose and frequency**
estradiol 0.01%	1 g one to three times per week after daily use of 2 g for 1–2 weeks
conjugated estrogen	0.25–2 g one to three times per week after daily use for 2 weeks
estradiol tablet	10 mcg/tab twice weekly after daily use for 2 weeks
estradiol ring	2 mg ring every 3 months

TABLE 23-2 Progestogen Therapy

Oral preparations for cyclic use	Starting dose
medroxyprogesterone acetate	5–10 mg
norethindrone acetate	2.5–5 mg
micronized progesterone	100–200 mg
Intrauterine system for long-term use	
levonorgestrel-releasing intrauterine system*	

*A levonorgestrel-releasing intrauterine system appears to offer adequate endometrial protection according to a meta-analysis, but further study is warranted (Somboonporn, Panna, Temtanakitpaisan, Kaewrudee, & Soontrapa, 2011)

TABLE 23-3 Combination Therapies

Progesterone and Estrogen Combinations	Starting dose and frequency
estradiol/levonorgestrel transdermal patch	0.045/0.015 mg once weekly
estradiol/norethindrone acetate transdermal patch	0.05/0.14 mg. twice weekly
conjugated estrogen/ medroxyprogesterone oral preparation	0.3/1.5, 0.45/1.5, 0.625/2.5, 0.625/5 mg per day
Estrogen and Aldosterone Antagonist	**Starting dose and frequency**
estradiol/drospirenone oral preparation	0.5/0.5 mg per day
Estrogen and Selective Estrogen Receptor Modulator	**Starting dose and frequency**
conjugated estrogen/ bazedoxifene oral preparation	0.45/20 mg per day

breast cancer but it has not been well studied. Progesterone is the progestogen naturally found in the body. Counseling women about bioidentical hormone therapy can be challenging because terms such as compounded and bioidentical are often times confused. An evidence-based guide for counseling women about bioidentical hormone therapy can be found in the *Journal of the American Board of Family Medicine* (Sood, Shuster, Smith, Vincent, & Jatoi, 2011).

i. There is mounting evidence that estradiol and micronized progesterone may have some beneficial effects over other synthetic hormones (Holtorf, 2009; Moskowitz, 2006). There is evidence from animal models and observational studies that micronized progesterone may pose less risk for breast cancer than medroxyprogesterone acetate (Gadducci, Biglia, Cosio, Sismondi, & Genazzani, 2009). One of the side effects of the breakdown of oral progesterone is sedation; therefore, it can be very helpful for women with insomnia when it is given before bed. Unfortunately, the bioavailability of progesterone is low when given orally (< 2%); thus, it may not offer adequate endometrial protection (Stanczyk, Hapgood, Winer, & Mishell, 2013). When given per vagina it probably affords better

endometrial protection (Miles et al., 1994) though this needs to be studied further.

ii. There are Food and Drug Administration (FDA)-approved bioidentical hormones available by prescription. Estradiol comes in many different forms including pills, patches, creams, lotions, and vaginal products. Oral micronized progesterone is also available.

iii. Compounded hormones are non-FDA approved prescription hormones that are prepared by a compounding pharmacist. By compounding the hormones, pharmacists are able to provide a wide range of types of hormones, dosages, and formulations that are not available from pharmaceutical companies. In 2008, the FDA sent warning letters to seven compounding pharmacies for making false claims about the safety and effectiveness of bioidentical hormonal replacement therapy.

iv. There is no evidence that salivary or blood hormone testing should be used to adjust hormone levels (Boothby & Doering, 2008). NAMS has made a statement against the use of compounded hormones and salivary testing (NAMS, 2012).

2. Nonhormonal drug (Note: as with prescribing any drug, be aware of drug interactions, contraindications for use, and side effects.)

These drugs include selective serotonin reuptake inhibitors (SSRIs), serotonin-norepinephrine reuptake inhibitors, clonidine, and gabapentin. These drugs are less effective than HT but are a good alternative for women who are not candidates for HT. Most of these drugs have been studied in women with breast cancer, not women experiencing naturally occurring menopause, and were found to be safe for use.

a. SSRIs: paroxetine, citalopram, escitalopram, venlafaxine, and desvenlafaxine are all effective in reducing the number and severity of hot flashes (Handley & Williams, 2014). Fluoxetine and sertraline appear to be less effective. Side effects of selective serotonin reuptake inhibitors include dry mouth, insomnia, sedation, decreased appetite, constipation, and decreased libido. Severe withdrawal syndrome if discontinued abruptly.

i. Paroxetine: 10–25 mg daily. The FDA-approved drug for menopause is Brisdelle 7.5 mg.

ii. Venlafaxine: 37.5 or 75 mg daily. May cause heavy uterine bleeding, galactorrhea, or mastodynia.

b. Gabapentin: 900 mg daily. Side effects include somnolence, fatigue, dizziness, and palpitations. May be especially helpful in women with poor sleep and night sweats.

c. Clonidine: 0.025–0.075 mg twice daily. Side effects include drowsiness, dry mouth, constipation, insomnia, postural hypotension, and reaction to skin patch. Discontinue slowly to reduce dose to avoid rebound hypertension, headaches, and agitation.

d. Only paroxetine is FDA approved for the treatment of hot flashes.

3. Alternative treatments (Note: as with prescribing any drugs, be aware of drug interactions, contraindications for use, and side effects of any herbal supplements.)

a. Phytoestrogens (red clover, soy isoflavones, etc.): according to a Cochrane review there is no conclusive evidence that they decrease vasomotor symptoms (Lethaby et al., 2013). In contrast, a meta-analysis found an improvement in hot flushes but not the Kupperman Index when compared to placebo (Chen, Lin, & Liu, 2014). No serious side effects were noted.

b. Black cohosh: A Cochrane review of the evidence for the use of black cohosh (*Cimicifuga racemosa*) was insufficient to support its use for the treatment of menopausal symptoms though other reviewers of the scientific literature found benefit and challenge the Cochrane conclusions (Beer et al., 2013).

   i. Study doses ranged from 20 to 80 mg twice daily.

   ii. Mechanism of action is unknown but unlikely hormonal. A systematic review of the clinical evidence for the safety of black cohosh found that clinical studies suggest that it is safe, although case reports including liver toxicity have been reported (Borrelli & Ernst, 2008). The U.S. Pharmacopeia also reviewed the case reports and concluded that dietary supplements containing black cohosh should have a cautionary statement on the label: One should discontinue use and consult a healthcare practitioner if there is a liver disorder or if symptoms of liver trouble develop, such as abdominal pain, dark urine, or jaundice (Mahady et al., 2008). Baseline and periodic evaluations of liver enzymes when prescribing black cohosh may be prudent.

c. A meta-analysis found that acupuncture reduced hot flash frequency and severity and improved menopause-related symptoms and quality of life (Chiu, Pan, Shyu, Han, & Tsai, 2014).

d. Maca (*Lepidium meyenii*) has been found to have some positive effects on menopausal symptoms but the quality of studies has been poor and there is little safety data (Lee, Shin, Yang, Lim, & Ernst, 2011). Typical doses in studies were 2–3.5 grams. A review of its use for sexual function also showed mixed results (Shin, Lee, Yang, Lim, & Ernst, 2010).

e. Other herbs: Maritime pine bark (Pycnogenol®) and flaxseed show some promise in the treatment of vasomotor symptoms but more research is needed (Depypere & Comhaire, 2014).

4. Multiple lifestyle strategies are suggested but there has been little research done to support their efficacy.

a. Regulation of core body temperature

b. Regular exercise

c. Relaxation techniques

d. Paced breathing

e. Weight loss

f. Smoking cessation

5. Urogenital atrophy

a. Vaginal dryness or dyspareunia related to atrophy

   i. Vaginal estrogen

      a. Low-dose vaginal tablets, rings, and creams are equally effective (see Table 23-1).

      b. Less systemic and endometrial effects with low-dose vaginal estradiol tablets and estriol-containing formulations. Low-dose vaginal estrogen therapy does not generally require a progestogen (NAMS, 2012).

      c. May be of some benefit for women with urge incontinence (NAMS, 2010).

      d. May reduce the risk of recurrent urinary tract infection (Perrotta, Aznar, Mejia, Albert, & Ng, 2008).

      e. Estriol is a weaker estrogen that is well absorbed from vaginal mucosa and improves vaginal atrophy (Griesser, Skonietzki, Fischer, Fielder, & Suesskind, 2012) but must be ordered from a compounding pharmacist in the United States. It is usually given as 1 mg/g nightly for 2 weeks then twice weekly.

   ii. Estrogen receptor agonist/antagonist: ospemifene is a selective estrogen receptor modulator (SERM) that has been FDA approved for the treatment of dyspareunia related to vaginal atrophy. Side effects include hot flashes.

    iii. Vaginal moisturizers
       a. Lubricants for sexual intercourse
    iv. Maintain sexual activity: women who are sexually active have less vaginal atrophy
    v. There is mounting evidence that DHEA suppositories improve vaginal atrophy, sexual pain, and sexual desire. It is usually given as 12.5 mg ovule (Archer, 2015).

6. Urinary frequency, urgency, or incontinence (see Chapter 25 on urinary incontinence in women).
    a. These symptoms may not be related to estrogen deficiency and often are not relieved with the administration of estrogen alone.
    b. Refer for urogynecology assessment.

7. Mood and cognition
    a. Depression
      i. HT may be particularly useful in treating new onset of depression during the menopausal transition. HT may play a role in alleviating depressive symptoms during the menopause transition either alone or in combination with antidepressants (Toffol, Heikinheimo, & Partonen, 2014). Progestogens may counteract the beneficial effects of estrogen on mood.
      ii. Psychotherapy referral
      iii. Antidepressants
      iv. Regular physical activity and optimum nutrition avoiding stimulants and sugar
    b. Cognition: consider referral for neuropsychiatric assessment, physical activity, cognitive stimulation through games, languages, new activities, etc.

8. Sexual dysfunction: See Al-Azzawi et al. (2010) for a review of therapeutic options for postmenopausal women with sexual dysfunction. Hypoactive sexual desire disorder (HSDD) is a complex condition that is poorly understood among women. Consider hormone therapy. HT (estrogen alone or with a progestogen) given during the perimenopause or early postmenopause has been associated with a mild to moderate improvement in sexual function, particularly pain (Nastri et al., 2013). For decreased desire:
    a. Treat contributing psychological (e.g., depression or relationship issues) or underlying medical conditions.
    b. Change or discontinue medication contributing to decreased desire.
    c. Refer to a sex therapist or sexologist.
    d. Testosterone deficiency may be considered one of the underlying causes of HSDD.
      i. A review of clinical trials has demonstrated that transdermal testosterone improves sexual function and activity among postmenopausal women (Davis & Braunstein, 2012).

Specifically, the addition of an androgen to estrogen therapy has demonstrated a significant positive incremental effect on sexual functioning in women (Somboonporn et al., 2005).

    ii. The use of testosterone in women with disorders of sexual desire is controversial. The role of testosterone therapy in postmenopausal women: position statement of The North American Menopause Society (2005) states that postmenopausal women who are distressed by decreased sexual desire and have no other known cause (physical or psychological) are candidates for testosterone therapy.
    iii. Side effects: decreased high-density lipoprotein and increased low-density lipoprotein, acne, and hirsutism (Elraiyah et al., 2014). In addition, there is a potential for clitoral enlargement, voice deepening, weight gain, menstrual irregularities, and possibly an increased risk of breast cancer. There are inadequate long-term safety data for the use of testosterone.
    iv. Benefits: increased clitoral sensitivity, vaginal lubrication, and libido
    v. Contraindications: history of breast or uterine cancer, liver disease, and cardiovascular disease
    vi. Consider initiating therapy if below normal or low normal free testosterone. Transdermal use preferred. Counsel regarding risks and benefits of therapy. The use of testosterone in women is off label; there are no FDA-approved products for women. The use of products designed for men may lead to supraphysiologic levels of testosterone in women.
    vii. Testosterone 0.5–2 mg/g cream compounded: apply 2–3 times per week to lower abdomen, mons pubis, inner thigh, or buttocks. Results seen in 6–12 weeks, may first experience erotic dreams. Reevaluation at 3 months: monitor testosterone levels before and after therapy for supraphysiologic levels, lipid profile, and liver enzymes; monitor symptoms and side effects. Goal: free testosterone levels in upper normal range. Continued therapy: taper to lowest effective dose, monitor lipids and liver enzymes at 3 months then one to two times per year.

e. Discuss sexual issues when a new medication is prescribed, presurgery and postsurgery for bilateral oophorectomy

f. Consider lifestyle issues: boredom with sexual routine (give permission for experimentation); stress (importance of relaxation); and children (privacy and relationship time)

g. Directed resexualization: take 20 minutes three times a week for erotic literature; exercises that increase blood flow to genitals, such as biking; masturbation; and be aware of sexual cues

h. Herbal alternatives include American ginseng (*Panax quinquefolius*), damiana (*Turnera aphrodisiaca*), maca (*Lepidium meyenii*), and wild oats milky seed (*Avena sativa*). Although there is a long history of traditional use of herbs for decreased sexual desire, there is little research evidence to support their use.

9. Disorders of arousal

a. Over-the-counter products include L-arginine (oral), Zestra

b. Enhance stimulation and eliminate routine: use erotic materials, masturbation, encourage communication during sex; use vibrators, varying positions, times of day or places, and make a date for sex

10. Sexual pain disorder

a. Provide distraction techniques (helps with anxiety, increasing relaxation): erotic or nonerotic fantasy, Kegel exercises with sex, background music, or videos or television

b. Encourage noncoital behaviors: sensual massage, sensate-focus exercises, oral or noncoital stimulation with or without orgasm

D. Client education

1. Concerns and feelings: discuss menopause transition as a normal physiologic and developmental process that affects each woman uniquely.

2. Information: provide verbal and preferably written information regarding the menopause transition, diagnostic tests, and management strategies

3. Nutrition

a. Seven to nine servings of fresh fruits and vegetables

b. Plentiful use of grains and beans for 25–30 g of fiber daily

c. Healthy fats: monounsaturated (olive oil, canola oil, avocados, and so forth) and polyunsaturated fats and omega-3 fatty acids (flaxseed, fish, walnuts, and so forth)

d. Protein primarily from fish, poultry, and beans

e. Calcium from dark green vegetables and nonfat dairy to meet the need of 1,200 mg/day

f. Avoid exposure to plastics, pesticides, and other potential endocrine disruptors. See University of California San Francisco (2015) for more information.

4. Physical activity

a. Weight-bearing exercise for bone strength: walking, dancing, and jump rope

b. 30 minutes of aerobic exercise at least 5 days per week

c. Flexibility training, such as yoga, to decrease falls two to three times per week

d. Strength training to improve muscle mass two to three times per week

5. Spiritual life

a. Participate in activities that bring purpose and meaning to life

b. Take time for reflection

i. Journaling

ii. Women's group

iii. Walks in nature

iv. Religious activities: prayer, meditation, and ritual

v. Reflective questioning:

- What keeps you going? What sustains you?
- Where do you find meaning and purpose in life?
- Where do you find joy?
- What or whom do you turn to when you get down?

VI. Self-management resources and tools

A. *North American Menopause Society: http://www.menopause.org/Consumers.aspx*

B. *American College of Obstetricians and Gynecologists: http://www.acog.org/Patients*

C. *Association of Reproductive Health Professionals: http://www.arhp.org/topics/menopause*

VII. Clinical practice guidelines

A. *American Association of Clinical Endocrinologists: https://www.aace.com/publications/guidelines*

B. NAMS: http://www.menopause
.org/for-women/-i-menopro-i-mobile-app.
They have a mobile application called MenoPro
for health professionals and consumers. In
addition, see the NAMS clinical guidelines
(Shifren et al., 2014).

C. Obstetrics and Gynaecology of Canada
Guidelines: Managing Menopause (Reid et al.,
2014).

REFERENCES

Al-Azzawi, F., Bitzer, J., Brandenburg, U., Castelo-Branco, C., Graziottin, A., Kenemans, P., et al. (2010). Therapeutic options for postmenopausal female sexual dysfunction. *Climacteric, 13*(2), 103–120.

Al-Safi, Z. A., & Santoro, N. (2014). Menopausal hormone therapy and menopausal symptoms. *Fertility and Sterility, 101*(4), 905–915.

Archer, D. (2015). Dehydroepiandrosterone intra-vaginal administration for the management of postmenopausal vulvovaginal atrophy. *Journal of Steroid Biochemistry and Molecular Biology, 145*, 139–143.

Beer, A. M., Osmers, R., Schnitker, J., Bai, W., Mueck, A. O., & Meden, H. (2013). Efficacy of black cohosh (cimicifuga racemosa) medicines for treatment of menopausal symptoms - comments on major statements of the Cochrane Collaboration report 2012 "Black Cohosh (*Cimicifuga* spp.) for Menopausal Symptoms (Review)." *Gynecological Endocrinology: The Official Journal of the International Society of Gynecological Endocrinology, 29*(12), 1022–1025.

Berlin Center of Epidemiology and Health Research (2008). MRS—the Menopause Rating Scale. Retrieved from http://www.menopause-rating-scale.info/about.htm.

Bhupathiraju, S. N., & Manson, J. E. (2014). Menopausal hormone therapy and chronic disease risk in the Women's Health Initiative: Is timing everything? *Endocrine Practice: Official Journal of the American College of Endocrinology and the American Association of Clinical Endocrinologists, 20*(11), 1201–1213.

Boothby, L. A., & Doering, P. L. (2008). Bioidentical hormone therapy: A panacea that lacks supportive evidence. *Current Opinion in Obstetrics and Gynecology, 20*(4), 400–407.

Borrelli, F., & Ernst, E. (2008). Black cohosh (*Cimicifuga racemosa*): A systematic review of adverse events. *American Journal of Obstetrics and Gynecology, 199*(5), 455–466.

Bromberger, J. T., & Kravitz, H. M. (2011). Mood and menopause: Findings from the Study of Women's Health Across the Nation (SWAN) over 10 years. *Obstetrics and Gynecology Clinics of North America, 38*(3), 609–625.

Castelo-Branco, C., Cancelo, M., Villero, J., Nohales, F., & Julia, M. (2005). Management of post-menopausal vaginal atrophy and atrophic vaginitis. *Maturitas, 52S*, 546–552.

Chen, M. N., Lin, C. C., & Liu, C. F. (2014). Efficacy of phytoestrogens for menopausal symptoms: A meta-analysis and systematic review. *Climacteric: The Journal of the International Menopause Society, 18*(2), 260–269.

Chiu, H. Y., Pan, C. H., Shyu, Y. K., Han, B. C., & Tsai, P. S. (2014). Effects of acupuncture on menopause-related symptoms and quality of life in women on natural menopause: A meta-analysis of randomized controlled trials. *Menopause (New York, N.Y.), 22*(2), 234–244.

Davies, M. C., & Cartwright, B. (2012). What is the best management strategy for a 20-year-old woman with premature ovarian failure? *Clinical Endocrinology, 77*(2), 182–186.

Davis, S. R., & Braunstein, G. D. (2012). Efficacy and safety of testosterone in the management of hypoactive sexual desire disorder in postmenopausal women. *Journal of Sexual Medicine, 9*(4), 1134–1148.

de Villiers, T. J., Gass, M. L., Haines, C. J., Hall, J. E., Lobo, R. A., Pierroz, D. D., et al. (2013). Global consensus statement on menopausal hormone therapy. *Climacteric: The Journal of the International Menopause Society, 16*(2), 203–204.

Deeks, A. (2002). Is this menopause? Women in midlife—psychosocial issues. *Australian Family Physician, 33*(11), 889–893.

Depypere, H. T., & Comhaire, F. H. (2014). Herbal preparations for the menopause: Beyond isoflavones and black cohosh. *Maturitas, 77*(2), 191–194.

Dinnerstein, L., Alexander, J., & Kotz, K. (2003). The menopause and sexual functioning: A review of population-based studies. *Annual Review of Sex Research, 14*, 64–82.

Elraiyah, T., Sonbol, M. B., Wang, Z., Khairalseed, T., Asi, N., Undavalli, C., et al. (2014). Clinical review: The benefits and harms of systemic testosterone therapy in postmenopausal women with normal adrenal function: A systematic review and meta-analysis. *The Journal of Clinical Endocrinology and Metabolism, 99*(10), 3543–3550.

Ensrud, K. E., Stone, K. L., Blackwell, T. L., Sawaya, G. F., Tagliaferri, M., Diem, S. J., et al. (2009). Frequency and severity of hot flashes and sleep disturbance in postmenopausal women with hot flashes. *Menopause (New York, N.Y.), 16*(2), 286–292.

Forshaw, M., & Hunter, M. (2010). The impact of attitudes towards the menopause on women's symptom experience: A systematic review. *Maturitas, 65*, 28–36.

Freeman, E. W., Sammel, M. D., & Sanders, R. J. (2014). Risk of long-term hot flashes after natural menopause: Evidence from the Penn Ovarian Aging Study cohort. *Menopause (New York, N.Y.), 21*(9), 924–932.

Gadducci, A., Biglia, N., Cosio, S., Sismondi, P., & Genazzani, A. R. (2009). Progestagen component in combined hormone replacement therapy in postmenopausal women and breast cancer risk: A debated clinical issue. *Gynecological Endocrinology: The Official Journal of the International Society of Gynecological Endocrinology, 25*(12), 807–815.

Gold, E. B., Lasley, B., Crawford, S. L., McConnell, D., Joffe, H., & Greendale, G. A. (2007). Relation of daily urinary hormone patterns to vasomotor symptoms in a racially/ethnically diverse sample of midlife women: Study of Women's Health Across the Nation. *Reproductive Sciences (Thousand Oaks, Calif.), 14*(8), 786–797.

Griesser, H., Skonietzki, S., Fischer, T., Fielder, K., & Suesskind, M. (2012). Low dose estriol pessaries for the treatment of vaginal atrophy: A double-blind placebo-controlled trial investigating the efficacy of pessaries containing 0.2mg and 0.03mg estriol. *Maturitas, 71*(4), 360–368.

Grodstein, F., Manson, J. E., & Stampfer, M. J. (2006). Hormone therapy and coronary heart disease: The role of time since menopause and age at hormone initiation. *Journal of Women's Health (2002), 15*(1), 35–44.

Gyllstrom, M. E., Schreiner, P. J., & Harlow, B. L. (2007). Perimenopause and depression: Strength of association, causal mechanisms and treatment recommendations. *Best Practice & Research Clinical Obstetrics & Gynaecology, 21*(2), 275–292.

Handley, A. P., & Williams, M. (2014). The efficacy and tolerability of SSRI/SNRIs in the treatment of vasomotor symptoms in menopausal women: A systematic review. *Journal of the American Association of Nurse Practitioners, 27*(1), 54–61.

Harlow, S. D., Gass, M., Hall, J. E., Lobo, R., Maki, P., Rebar, R. W., et al. (2012). Executive summary of the stages of reproductive aging workshop + 10: Addressing the unfinished agenda of staging reproductive aging. *Fertility and Sterility, 97*(4), 843–851.

Holtorf, K. (2009). The bioidentical hormone debate: Are bioidentical hormones (estradiol, estriol, and progesterone) safer or more efficacious than commonly used synthetic versions in hormone replacement therapy? *Postgraduate Medicine, 121*(1), 73–85.

Huang, A., Moore, E. E., Boyko, E. J., Scholes, D., Lin, F., Vittinghoff, E., et al. (2010). Vaginal symptoms in postmenopausal women: Self reported severity, natural history, and risk factors. *Menopause, 17*(1), 121–126.

Joffe, H., Massler, A., & Sharkey, K. M. (2010). Evaluation and management of sleep disturbance during the menopause transition. *Seminars in Reproductive Medicine, 28*(5), 404–421.

Kingsberg, S. A., Wysocki, S., Magnus, L., & Krychman, M. L. (2013). Vulvar and vaginal atrophy in postmenopausal women: Findings from the REVIVE (REal women's VIews of treatment options for menopausal vaginal ChangEs) survey. *Journal of Sexual Medicine, 10*(7), 1790–1799.

Kronenberg, F. (1990). Hot flashes: Epidemiology and physiology. *Annals of the New York Academy of Sciences, 592*, 52–86; discussion 123–133.

Lee, M. S., Shin, B. C., Yang, E. J., Lim, H. J., & Ernst, E. (2011). Maca (lepidium meyenii) for treatment of menopausal symptoms: A systematic review. *Maturitas, 70*(3), 227–233.

Lethaby, A., Marjoribanks, J., Kronenberg, F., Roberts, H., Eden, J., & Brown, J. (2013). Phytoestrogens for menopausal vasomotor symptoms. *Cochrane Database of Systematic Reviews, 12*, CD001395.

Luine, V. N. (2014). Estradiol and cognitive function: Past, present and future. *Hormones and Behavior, 66*(4), 602–618.

Mahady, G. B., Dog, T. L., Barrett, M. L., Chavez, M. L., Gardiner, P., Ko, R., et al. (2008). United States Pharmacopeia review of the black cohosh case reports of hepatotoxicity. *Menopause, 15*(4), 628–638.

McKinlay, S. M., Bifano, N. L., & McKinlay, J. B. (1985). Smoking and age at menopause in women. *Annals of Internal Medicine, 103*(3), 350–356.

Miles, R. A., Paulson, R. J., Lobo, R. A., Press, M. F., Dahmoush, L., & Sauer, M. V. (1994). Pharmacokinetics and endometrial tissue levels of progesterone after administration by intramuscular and vaginal routes: A comparative study. *Fertility and Sterility, 62*(3), 485–490.

Morrison, J. H., Brinton, R. D., Schmidt, P. J., & Gore, A. C. (2006). Estrogen, menopause, and the aging brain: How basic neuroscience can inform hormone therapy in women. *Journal of Neuroscience: The Official Journal of the Society for Neuroscience, 26*(41), 10332–10348.

Moskowitz, D. (2006). A comprehensive review of the safety and efficacy of bioidentical hormones for the management of menopause and related health risks. *Alternative Medicine Review, 11*(3), 208–223.

Nappi, R. E., & Lachowsky, M. (2009). Menopause and sexuality: Prevalence of symptoms and impact on quality of life. *Maturitas, 63*(2), 138–141.

Nastri, C. O., Lara, L. A., Ferriani, R. A., Rosa-E-Silva, A. C., Figueiredo, J. B., & Martins, W. P. (2013). Hormone therapy for sexual function in perimenopausal and postmenopausal women. *Cochrane Database of Systematic Reviews, 6*, CD009672.

North American Menopause Society. (2005). The role of testosterone therapy in postmenopausal women: Position statement of the North American Menopause Society. *Menopause, 12*(5), 496–511; quiz 649.

North American Menopause Society. (2008). Estrogen and progestogen use in postmenopausal women: July 2008 position statement of The North American Menopause Society. *Menopause, 15*(4 Pt 1), 584–602.

North American Menopause Society. (2012). The 2012 hormone therapy position statement of: The North American Menopause Society. *Menopause (New York, N.Y.), 19*(3), 257–271.

Perrotta, C., Aznar, M., Mejia, R., et al. (2008). Oestrogens for preventing recurrent urinary tract infection in postmenopausal women. *The Cochrane Database of Systematic Reviews, (2)*, CD005131-.

Portman, D. J., Gass, M. L., & Vulvovaginal Atrophy Terminology Consensus Conference Panel. (2014). Genitourinary syndrome of menopause: New terminology for vulvovaginal atrophy from the International Society for the Study of Women's Sexual Health and the North American Menopause Society. *Menopause (New York, N.Y.), 21*(10), 1063–1068.

Rapp, S. R., Espeland, M. A., Shumaker, S. A., Henderson, V. W., Brunner, R. L., Manson, J. E., et al. (2003). Effect of estrogen plus progestin on global cognitive function in postmenopausal women: The Women's Health Initiative Memory Study: A randomized controlled trial. *JAMA, 289*(20), 2663–2672.

Rebbeck, T. R., Su, H. I., Sammel, M. D., Lin, H., Tran, T. V., Gracia, C. R., et al. (2010). Effect of hormone metabolism genotypes on steroid hormone levels and menopausal symptoms in a prospective population-based cohort of women experiencing the menopausal transition. *Menopause (New York, N.Y.), 17*(5), 1026–1034.

Reid, R., Abramson, B. L., Blake, J., Desindes, S., Dodin, S., Johnston, S., et al. (2014). Managing menopause. *Journal of Obstetrics and Gynaecology Canada: JOGC = Journal d'Obstetrique et Gynecologie du Canada: JOGC, 36*(9), 830–833.

Shifren, J., Gass, M., & NAMS Recommendations for Clinical Care of Midlife Women Working Group 2014. The North American Menopause Society recommendations for clinical care of midlife women. *Menopause, 21*(10), 1038–1062.

Shin, B. C., Lee, M. S., Yang, E. J., Lim, H. S., & Ernst, E. (2010). Maca (L. meyenii) for improving sexual function: A systematic review. *BMC Complementary and Alternative Medicine, 10*, 44-6882-10-44.

Shin, H., & Shin, H. S. (2012). Measurement of quality of life in menopausal women: A systematic review. *Western Journal of Nursing Research, 34*(4), 475–503.

Shumaker, S. A., Legault, C., Rapp, S. R., Thal, L., Wallace, R. B., Ockene, J. K., et al. (2003). Estrogen plus progestin and the incidence of dementia and mild cognitive impairment in postmenopausal women: The Women's Health Initiative Memory Study: A randomized controlled trial. *JAMA, 289*(20), 2651–2662.

Somboonporn, W., Davis, S., Seif, M., & Bell, R. (2005). Testosterone for peri- and postmenopausal women. *Cochrane Database of Systematic Reviews, 19*(4), CD004509.

Somboonporn, W., Panna, S., Temtanakitpaisan, T., Kaewrudee, S., & Soontrapa, S. (2011). Effects of the levonorgestrel-releasing intrauterine system plus estrogen therapy in perimenopausal and postmenopausal women: Systematic review and meta-analysis. *Menopause (New York, N.Y.), 18*(10), 1060–1066.

Sood, R., Shuster, L., Smith, R., Vincent, A., & Jatoi, A. (2011). Counseling postmenopausal women about bioidentical hormones: Ten discussion points for practicing physicians. *Journal of the American Board of Family Medicine, 24*(2), 202–210.

Soules, M. R., Sherman, S., Parrott, E., Rebar, R., Santoro, N., Utian, W., et al. (2001). Executive summary: Stages of reproductive aging workshop (STRAW). *Climacteric: The Journal of the International Menopause Society, 4*(4), 267–272.

Speroff, L., & Fritz, M. (2005). Menopause and perimenopause transition. In L. Speroff & M. Fritz, *Clinical gynecologic endocrinology and infertility* (7th ed., pp. 621–688). Philadelphia, PA: Lippincott Williams & Wilkins.

Stanczyk, F. Z., Hapgood, J. P., Winer, S., & Mishell, D. R., Jr. (2013). Progestogens used in postmenopausal hormone therapy: Differences in their pharmacological properties, intracellular actions, and clinical effects. *Endocrine Reviews, 34*(2), 171–208.

Thurston, R. C., Bromberger, J. T., Joffe, H., Avis, N. E., Hess, R., Crandall, C. J., et al. (2008). Beyond frequency: Who is most bothered by vasomotor symptoms? *Menopause (New York, N.Y.), 15*(5), 841–847.

Thurston, R. C., Sutton-Tyrrell, K., Everson-Rose, S. A., Hess, R., Powell, L. H., & Matthews, K. A. (2011). Hot flashes and carotid intima media thickness among midlife women. *Menopause (New York, N.Y.), 18*(4), 352–358.

Toffol, E., Heikinheimo, O., & Partonen, T. (2014). Hormone therapy and mood in perimenopausal and postmenopausal women: A narrative review. *Menopause (New York, N.Y.), 22*(5), 564–578.

University of California San Francisco, Program on Reproductive Health and the Environment (2015). Information for families. Retrieved from http://www.prhe.ucsf.edu/prhe/toxicmatters.html.

The Writing Group for the PEPI Trial. (1995). Effects of estrogen or estrogen/progestin regimens on heart disease risk factors in postmenopausal women. The Postmenopausal Estrogen/Progestin Interentions (PEPI) Trial. *JAMA, 273*(3), 199–208.

Xu, Q., & Lang, C. P. (2014). Examining the relationship between subjective sleep disturbance and menopause: A systematic review and meta-analysis. *Menopause (New York, N.Y.), 21*(12), 1301–1318.

NONHORMONAL CONTRACEPTION

Kimberley Chastain

CHAPTER 24

I. Introduction and general background

Nonhormonal contraception is a form of family planning used by couples during coitus or postcoitally to prevent pregnancy without the use of exogenous hormones. It includes barrier methods that can be used by either the male or female partner and placed before genital contact; spermicides, placed inside the vagina moments or minutes before genital contact; the ParaGard® intrauterine contraceptive (IUC), placed inside a woman's uterus by her provider in advance or in some cases up to 5 days after unprotected intercourse as emergency contraception (EC); and natural family planning (NFP) methods, which are learned behaviors and include fertility awareness methods (FAM) and the lactational amenorrhea method (LAM).

Nonhormonal contraception can be an appropriate option for most women, although most of the methods, excluding the IUC and strict NFP, have effectiveness rates that are lower than those containing hormones. Still, many women or couples prefer to use nonhormonal methods for a variety of reasons including but not limited to contraindication to hormones, reduced side effect profile, past experience, religious beliefs, and personal values. Advantages of nonhormonal contraception include few or no side effects for most methods, low long-term cost, no clinic visit required for several of the methods, and in all cases near immediate effectiveness and an immediate return to fertility once the method is stopped. With all of the methods discussed in this chapter, a patient should also be offered the EC pill or a prescription as a backup in case of user or method failure. The EC pill is discussed in a separate chapter.

Choosing a method of family planning is a multifaceted process. Patients need current, factual information about all methods of contraception and must be allowed to participate fully in the decision-making process. Efficacy rate is an important component in choosing a contraceptive method. In this chapter, efficacy rates are reported rather than failure rates. Terms used to identify these rates are "perfect use" and "typical use." Perfect use (reported as a percentage) refers to the number of women out of 100 who prevent pregnancy in 1 year with correct and consistent use of the method. Typical use refers to the percentage of women out of 100 who do not use the method consistently or correctly each time and over 1 year still avoid pregnancy (Trussell, 2008).

A. Barrier methods

A barrier method of contraception is one that is designed to physically prohibit sperm from entering the vagina or the uterus during intercourse. The current barrier methods available in the United States include the male condom, the female condom, the diaphragm, the FemCap, and the sponge. Effectiveness rates increase when combined with a spermicidal agent, such as nonoxynol-9, discussed in a later section.

1. Male condom

   The condom is a barrier method of contraception designed to prevent sperm from entering the vagina. Made of latex, polyurethane, or lambskin, male condoms come in a variety of textures, colors, and sizes, and with or without spermicide and with or without lubrication, each intended to improve user acceptance of the method. Additionally, they are available with or without reservoir tips, designed to help prevent spillage of the ejaculate; therefore, reservoir tips are usually recommended. Male condoms are placed on a man's erect penis before genital contact with a partner. Condom use instructions should be carefully followed because correct placement and removal are essential to avoid pregnancy. Perfect use efficacy rate for the male condom is 98%, whereas typical use rate is 85% (Trussell, 2008).

   One of the major advantages of using either latex or polyurethane male condoms for contraception is that they also help prevent sexually transmitted infections (STIs) including HIV (NIAID, 2011). However, although lambskin condoms protect equally as well against pregnancy as other condoms, they do not protect against most STIs or HIV. Other advantages to condoms include cost (male condoms are relatively inexpensive compared with other methods), the ability to offer men a role in contraception, the lack of physical examination or prescription requirement, ready availability over the counter, and a low side effect profile. Additionally, they can be used simultaneously with every other available birth control method except the female condom. Disadvantages include possible allergies or sensitivities to latex, reduction in sexual spontaneity, need for cooperation by the partner, and the possibility for breakage or slipping off, resulting in method failure.

2. Female condom

Currently, there is only one female condom approved by the Food and Drug Administration (FDA) for use in the United States. Formerly known as the "Reality," the second-generation female condom is called the FC2®, and is produced by the Female Health Company. Made of synthetic nitrile, the FC2® has a flexible inner ring that facilitates insertion into the vagina, with a second outer ring designed to hold it in place and cover part of the vulva. Perfect use of the female condom confers a 95% efficacy rate, compared with 79% with typical use in the first year (Trussell, 2008).

Advantages to using the female condom include the fact that it is relatively inexpensive (although more expensive than the male condom) and is available over the counter without an examination or prescription. Additionally, it reduces the risk of STIs including HIV in laboratory testing (French et al., 2003), giving women an opportunity to actively play a role in preventing HIV and STI transmission during intercourse. Disadvantages are that it can be somewhat awkward to place correctly and can become dislodged easily. Of note is that the female condom should not be used simultaneously with a male condom, because they can stick to one another, causing one or both to slip off or tear.

3. Contraceptive sponge

The contraceptive sponge was first introduced to the U.S. market as the Today® Sponge in 1983. However, after multiple production stops and starts, it was reintroduced most recently in May 2009 by Mayer Laboratories. The polyurethane sponge acts as a physical barrier to sperm by trapping them within the sponge before they can enter the cervix. Additionally, the sponge contains the spermicide nonoxynol-9 for added protection. Before insertion, the sponge must be moistened with water to activate the spermicide. It is then placed deep inside the vagina, with the concave side toward the cervix, up to 24 hours before intercourse. The sponge must be left in place a minimum of 6 hours after intercourse to ensure that all sperm are immobilized. The sponge should not be left in the vagina longer than 30 hours because of the risk of toxic shock syndrome. Perfect use efficacy rates for the contraceptive sponge are 91% for nulliparous women and 80% for parous women, whereas typical use yields efficacy of 84% for nulliparous and 68% for parous women (Trussell, 2008).

Advantages to using the sponge are that it is readily available over the counter and does not require a prescription or examination. Disadvantages include risk of sensitivity or allergy to nonoxynol-9 and the fact that it must be moistened with water before insertion, requiring advance preparation. The only absolute contraindications to use are current cervical cancer or women at high risk for HIV (WHO, 2009) because of the nonoxynol-9 component (see the section on spermicides).

4. Diaphragm

The diaphragm is one of the first female-worn barrier methods to be used in the United States. The diaphragm is a physical barrier made of silicone in the shape of a dome surrounded by a flexible "spring" rim, designed to be placed deep inside the vagina blocking the cervix entirely. Diaphragms are available in several different rim styles and diameters ranging from 55 to 95 mm. Because of the wide range of female anatomic differences, the diaphragm style and size must be fit for the patient during a pelvic examination by a trained provider. To use the diaphragm, a woman should check for integrity before insertion. A dime-sized amount of spermicidal jelly or cream is placed in the cup side of the dome and extra spermicide is placed around the rim. Pinching the diaphragm in half, the user places it deep inside her vagina making sure to completely cover the entire cervix, requiring both education and practice. The diaphragm must be kept in the vagina for at least 6 but no more than 24 hours after intercourse. Spermicide must be reinserted vaginally with every new act of intercourse while the diaphragm is in place. Perfect use effectiveness rate for the diaphragm is 94%, whereas typical use is 84% (Trussell, 2008).

Advantages to the diaphragm are that it is nonlatex, it can be placed well in advance of sexual intercourse (≤ 24 hours), it is discrete, and it is relatively inexpensive considering that each one lasts up to 2 years, with the only additional cost being extra spermicide. Additionally, it has been observed that the diaphragm may reduce the risk of human papillomavirus transmission (by blocking the cervix) and therefore lower the risk of cervical dysplasia (Cates & Raymond, 2007). Disadvantages are that it is available by prescription only and must be fit in the clinic by a provider.

It should normally be replaced every 2 years, but refitting is required after any full-term pregnancy, second-trimester abortion, or a weight gain or loss of 20% or more. Although not contraindicated, diaphragms should be used with caution in women with a history of repeated urinary tract infections. Absolute contraindications include women with current cervical cancer and those women at high risk for HIV (WHO, 2009) because of the necessary spermicide use. In 2014, Janssen, the manufacturer of OrthoFlex diaphragms, discontinued their manufacture due to low usage. Only Omniflex diaphragms are currently available in the United States, and providers can order these directly for their patients through their customer service department, as pharmacies typically do not stock them.

5. FemCap

    Because former contraceptive cervical caps, such as the Prentif and Lea's Shield®, have gone by the wayside, the FemCap is currently the only cap available on the U.S. market. Approved by the FDA in March 2003, the current version is a small silicone device shaped similarly to a sailor's cap, designed to cover the cervix and be held in place by the muscular walls of the vagina. The major difference between the current and original FemCap device introduced in 1999 is that it now includes a strap for easier removal. The FemCap comes in three diameter sizes: small (22 mm) for nulligravida women, medium (26 mm) for women with prior pregnancies that resulted in only abortion or cesarean delivery, and large (30 mm) for parous women with a history of vaginal delivery. Although not required, fit is best determined by a provider to check sizing in the clinic because of differences in female anatomy regardless of parity.

    FemCap must be used along with a spermicidal jelly, placed both in the "bowl" of the cap and around its "brim." It is then placed by the user with its concave side directly over her cervix up to 40 hours before intercourse and ideally at least 15 minutes before any female sexual arousal. Effectiveness data for the first generation FemCap showed a failure rate of 14% among nulliparous women and 29% among women who have had a vaginal delivery (FemCap, 2015). Like the diaphragm and sponge, the FemCap must be left in place at least 6 hours after intercourse; however, it can be left in place for a full 48 hours if necessary.

    Advantages of the FemCap are that it is nonlatex, is discrete, and can be placed well ahead of sexual intercourse. Disadvantages are that it requires a prescription, sizing and fit are best done by an experienced provider, and it must be replaced every year or after any new pregnancy. The only absolute contraindications to use of the FemCap are current cervical cancer or women at high risk for HIV (WHO, 2009) because of the use of a spermicide. Patients must be given a prescription for the FemCap, which they can use to order it online through www.femcap.com.

B. Spermicides

Contraceptive spermicides are formulations of a gel, foam, cream, suppository, or film base that have an added surface-active chemical to kill sperm. The only currently approved spermicidal chemical in the United States is nonoxynol-9. If a spermicidal formulation is correctly inserted into the vagina before intercourse, the efficacy rate for perfect use is 85%, whereas typical use is 71% (Trussell, 2008). Following package instructions is essential because of the fact that each formulation may require different amounts of time to dissolve or disperse to be effective. Spermicidal formulations require reinsertion after 1 hour and after each act of intercourse. They are commonly used with barrier methods, such as male and female condoms; come already imbedded in the sponge; and are recommended as standard practice with diaphragms and the FemCap to achieve full efficacy rates.

Advantages of spermicides are that no examination or prescription is required, they are readily available over the counter, they are relatively inexpensive, they provide lubrication during sex, and they increase efficacy of other methods. Disadvantages are that they can be somewhat messy, suppositories or film may require up to 15 minutes to dissolve, and some people experience allergies or irritation with use.

Additionally, studies have shown that there is a possible increased risk of genital ulceration or epithelial disruption from the use of nonoxynol-9, which could actually facilitate STI transmission including HIV, especially in frequent users (considered more than two times per day) (WHO, 2002). For women who are at low risk for STIs, spermicides remain a good contraception option.

C. Copper T 380-A intrauterine contraceptive (ParaGard ®)

1. IUC as long-acting reversible contraceptive

    Approved by the FDA in 1984, the Copper T 380-A, also known as the ParaGard®, is an IUC made of polyethylene shaped like a "T," wrapped in fine copper wire. Placed inside a woman's uterine cavity through the cervix by a trained provider, the IUC is considered a long-acting reversible contraceptive (LARC) and is highly effective at preventing pregnancy. Two monofilament threads (strings) are attached to the base of the device, extending through the cervix into the vaginal cavity. The strings are provided to facilitate removal but are also a convenient way for the patient to check for the presence of her IUC monthly by feeling for them with her finger. Because there is nothing for the patient to do after receiving the IUC to activate it, perfect use and typical use efficacy rates are similar at 99.4% and 99.2%, respectively (Trussell, 2008). This difference results from a perfect user checking her "strings" regularly at home and being more aware of spontaneous expulsion than a typical user. The ParaGard® works primarily by preventing sperm from fertilizing an egg by increasing copper ions, enzymes, prostaglandins, and macrophages in uterine fluid, both altering transport and affecting the sperm and egg, ultimately preventing fertilization (Grimes, 2007).

There is renewed interest in intrauterine contraception in the United States (Hubacher, Finer, & Espey, 2011). Although IUCs that were on the market before the 1980s had a design flaw that caused an increased prevalence of pelvic infection, current studies of today's IUCs show no increased incidence or only a slight increased incidence of infection in the first 30 days after and related to insertion. Additionally, IUCs decrease the risk of ectopic pregnancy and are safe in nulliparous women (Grimes, 2007).

An ideal candidate for the IUC is any woman looking for a highly effective, long-term, reversible method and who is able to tolerate minor discomfort with insertion. Absolute contraindications to the use of the ParaGard® according to the WHO (category 4) include current untreated chlamydia or gonorrhea; current pelvic inflammatory disease (or infection within the last 3 months); known cervical cancer that has yet to be treated; known endometrial cancer; known pelvic tuberculosis; persistent gestational trophoblastic disease; endometritis or septic abortion in the past 3 months; physical distortion of the uterine cavity, such as fibroids that would prevent proper placement; and undiagnosed suspicious, abnormal vaginal bleeding (WHO, 2009). Allergy to copper or history of Wilson disease is also a contraindication.

Advantages of the IUC include high effectiveness, reversibility, and relatively low long-term cost. Although initial cost may seem high, if used for at least 2 years, the ParaGard® is the most cost-effective contraceptive on the U.S. market (Trussell et al., 1995). Currently, the ParaGard® IUC is approved for use up to 10 years, at which time it can be removed and replaced immediately by another, if desired. Insertion can be done at any time during a woman's menstrual cycle (including the postpartum period) as long as pregnancy is reliably excluded. It has been shown to be highly safe and effective when inserted immediately post aspiration abortion (Goodman et al., 2008). Another advantage of the IUC is that there is nothing for the patient to remember at home other than checking her strings. Disadvantages include an increase in menstrual bleeding and cramping in the first several cycles, rare insertion risks including perforation and infection, and possible spontaneous expulsion.

2. IUC as EC

First reported in 1976, the ParaGard® IUC is the most highly effective method of postcoital EC available today. When placed within 5 days of unprotected intercourse, the ParaGard® has an efficacy rate of over 99% compared with only 75–89% for the EC pills (Trussell et al., 1995). It is recommended as an appropriate method of EC for all women who meet the standard criteria for ParaGard® IUC insertion and have none of the contraindications as listed in the previous section (American College of Obstetricians and Gynecologists, 2005).

Once an existing pregnancy has been ruled out by a good history and a high-sensitivity urine pregnancy test, the patient may have the ParaGard® IUC placed immediately by a trained provider in the same normal manner. Aside from the fact that it is highly effective as an EC, a great advantage to this method is that it is excellent for women who also desire long-term contraception, because it can confer up to another 12 years of protection. Disadvantages are the same as listed for ParaGard® as a LARC method.

D. Natural family planning (NFP)

NFP methods are for the most part behavioral methods of contraception requiring body awareness, self-control, education, and commitment. Methods include FAM and the LAM. Coitus interruptus (or withdrawal) and abstinence can also be considered methods of NFP, and both can be incorporated into the other methods, although neither is discussed in this chapter.

1. Fertility awareness method (FAM)

FAM is the practice of detecting and interpreting a woman's fertile ovulation period and avoiding all intercourse during that time. Two ways of identifying this fertile window are through either calendar-based or symptom-based methods. Simple periodic abstinence based on misinformation or guesswork without formal instruction regarding "safe" times yields an overall typical use rate of only about 75% (Trussell, 2008). However, actual FAMs depend on careful instruction, understanding, and strict adherence. If a specific method is adhered to correctly, perfect use rates have been shown to be very successful.

Calendar methods involve keeping track of the menstrual cycle and include the calendar rhythm method, with a 91% perfect use rate, and the standard days method, with a 95% perfect use rate. The calendar rhythm method involves tracking menstrual cycles for 6–12 months and using a simple mathematical formula to calculate fertile days, whereas the standard days method uses a tool called CycleBeads® for keeping track of fertile days and is ideal for low-literacy patients (Trussell, 2008). It is now also available online and as a smartphone app. These methods along with the basal body temperature method, for which there are no reliable data for effectiveness rate, have been largely replaced in favor of newer methods that use other physical signs of fertility, such as cervical secretions (Pallone & Bergus, 2009). The "2-day method" and the "ovulation method" confer a 96% and 97% effectiveness, respectively (Trussell, 2008), whereas the "symptothermal method," using a combination of basal body temperature and cervical mucus, has a perfect use rate of 98% (Trussell, 2008).

Teaching these methods can take considerably more time than teaching other methods of contraception, with an estimated 4–6 hours for a woman to learn the necessary skills (Jennings, Arevalo, & Kowal, 2007). Therefore, it is important that referrals to specialized instructors be provided if none are available in the clinical setting, or that literate couples be encouraged to read at least one or two books on the method of choice before beginning.

Advantages of FAMs are that there are no health risks or side effects, they can be acceptable for couples with religious concerns about other contraceptive methods, they can increase body awareness, and they are either free or very low cost. Additionally, some of the methods can be used in reverse for couples wanting to plan a pregnancy. Disadvantages are primarily that learning a method takes time and effort and using it requires considerable commitment and self-control. Additionally, many of the methods cannot be reliably used by women with irregular cycles or a vaginal infection, those who have recently reached menarche, those approaching menopause, those in the immediate postpartum period or while breastfeeding, or women who have recently discontinued hormonal contraceptive. Finally, there is no protection against STIs with FAM.

2. Lactational amenorrhea method (LAM)

LAM is a very effective method of NFP but is limited to the 6 months postpartum period for women meeting specific criteria. A woman must have had no return to menses since giving birth; be breastfeeding almost exclusively, with less than 10% of infant calories from supplements; feed at least every 4 hours during the day and at least every 6 hours at night; and not be "pumping" for an effectiveness rate of 98% to be achieved. However, if she pumps even part of her milk, the rate is reduced to 95% (Pallone & Bergus, 2009).

II. Database (may include but is not limited to)

A. Subjective

1. Barrier methods
   a. Medical illnesses: current cervical cancer (FemCap) and history of urinary tract infections (diaphragm)
   b. Personal and social history
      i. Gravida and para (FemCap and sponge)
      ii. Allergies: (male and female) latex, nonoxynol-9 (condoms, FemCap, diaphragm, sponge, and spermicide)
      iii. Sexual history: recent history of unprotected intercourse and current risk of STI
      iv. Previous contraceptive use and satisfaction, compliance, or problems
      v. Preference for and comfort with method
      vi. Tolerance of side effects: potential allergy or sensitivity to latex or nonoxynol-9
      vii. Financial constraints

2. Spermicides
   a. Personal and social history
      i. Allergies: (male and female) nonoxynol-9
      ii. Sexual history: current risk of STI
      iii. Previous contraceptive use and satisfaction, compliance, or problems
      iv. Preference for and comfort with method
      v. Tolerance of side effects: potential skin irritation or ulceration

3. Cu T380-A IUC
   a. Medical illnesses (cervical or endometrial cancer, history of Wilson disease, pelvic tuberculosis, pelvic inflammatory disease, endometritis or septic abortion in past 3 months, or persistent gestational trophoblastic disease)
   b. Personal and social history
      i. Allergies (to copper)
      ii. Postpartum (first 48 hours best, or wait 4 weeks after delivery for insertion)
      iii. Postabortion (immediate insertion appropriate)
      iv. Sexual history: recent history of unprotected intercourse (last 5 days for EC) and current risk for STI
      v. Previous contraceptive use and satisfaction, compliance, or problems
      vi. Preference for and comfort with method (i.e., can tolerate insertion process including minor pain or discomfort)

vii. Tolerance of side effects: possible increased bleeding or menstrual cramping in first several cycles

viii. Financial constraints

4. NFP

  a. Medical illnesses

  b. Personal and social history

    i. Postpartum

    ii. Breastfeeding

    iii. Sexual history: current risk for STI

    iv. Previous contraceptive use and satisfaction and compliance problems

    v. Preference for, comfort with, and expressed ability to learn and strictly adhere to chosen FAM or LAM

  c. Menstrual history and problems: length and regularity of cycles, recent menarche, or approaching menopause

  d. Current and recent medications (i.e., hormonal contraceptives)

B. Objective

1. Barrier methods

  a. Screening or testing for STIs as indicated

  b. Speculum examination with screening Pap if not up to date to rule out cervical cancer

  c. Pelvic examination and sizing for diaphragm; fitting for FemCap

2. Spermicides

  Screening and testing for STIs as indicated

3. Cu T 380-A IUC as LARC or EC

  a. Pregnancy test

  b. Screening for STIs

  c. Speculum examination with Pap if not up to date to rule out cervical cancer

  d. Pelvic examination to determine size, shape of uterus, and position of fundus; "sounding" to measure length of uterine cavity (minimum 6 cm required)

4. NFP

  Screening and testing for STIs as indicated

III. Assessment

A. Needs

Determine the current and future childbearing plans of the patient.

B. Significance

Determine the significance of an unplanned pregnancy to the patient.

C. Motivation and ability

Determine the patient's willingness and ability to correctly and consistently use the method of choice.

D. Meets criteria

No contraindications to the method of choice.

IV. Goals of clinical management

A. Desired outcomes met

1. Patient provided with methods that support his or her family planning needs; pregnancy prevention, planning, and spacing as desired

2. Screening, diagnosis, and treatment of any STIs or other infections

B. Patient adherence

Select an approach that maximizes patient adherence and satisfaction.

V. Plan

A. Screening for all methods

1. STI, human papilloma virus, and Pap screening as indicated. Major authorities including the United States Preventative Services Task Force recommend chlamydia and gonorrhea screening for all sexually active women 25 years of age and younger and men and women in geographically high-risk areas (Meyers et al., 2008). Additionally, screening for HIV and syphilis is recommended for all men and women engaging in high-risk sexual behavior (U.S. Department of Health and Human Services, 2014).

B. Management (includes treatment, consultation, referral, and follow-up care)

1. Barrier methods

  a. Provide method of choice in office or by prescription

  b. Follow-up for resizing of diaphragm after weight gain or loss of 20 pounds or more, or after vaginal childbirth

  c. Follow-up for refitting of new FemCap after any pregnancy beyond first trimester

2. Spermicides

  a. Provide in office or direct patient to convenient locations for purchase

  b. Have patient return to clinic for evaluation if vaginal or penile ulceration noted to rule out pathology

  c. Provide EC pills or a prescription

3. Cu T 380-A IUC
   a. Insert IUC at office visit per protocols
   b. Follow-up with clinic visit in 2 to 3 months after insertion to check for expulsion and trim strings if desired by patient
   c. Return to clinic for evaluation if experiencing extended, heavy menses or amenorrhea
4. NFP
   a. Refer to well-trained individuals for instruction if not experienced or comfortable with teaching methods
   b. Encourage follow-up to reinforce learning
   c. Support and encourage breastfeeding moms who choose LAM and refer to lactation specialist if necessary
   d. Provide EC pills or prescription

C. Client education

1. Information: provide verbal and written information regarding
   a. Risk reduction and screening
   b. Action, use, side effects, associated risks, and importance of adherence
2. Counseling
   a. Encourage full client participation in the contraceptive selection process; ideally meet with both patient and partner
   b. Discuss benefits and risks of all available methods
   c. Discuss possible outcomes and choices if user or method failure occurs
   d. Discuss risk factors for STIs
   e. Document discussion on patient records

VI. Self-management resources and tools

A. Patient and client education

Both of these sites have excellent patient information and interactive tools that allow the user to filter and search through different options to find the right method for them.

1. Planned Parenthood Federation of America website at www.plannedparenthood.org has full-color pictures and detailed information about all available contraception. They also have an interactive tool called "My Method" that can be reached directly: https://www.plannedparenthood.org/all-access/my-method.

2. The Association of Reproductive Health Professionals (ARHP) site at www.arhp.org has patient information and an interactive tool at http://www.arhp.org/methodmatch.

REFERENCES

American College of Obstetricians and Gynecologists. (2005). ACOG practice bulletin no. 59. *Obstetrics & Gynecology, 105*, 223–232.

Cates, W., & Raymond, E. (2007). Vaginal barriers and spermicides. In R. A. Hatcher, J. Trussell, A. L. Nelson, W. Cates, F. H. Stewart, & D. Kowal (Eds.), *Contraceptive technology* (19th ed., pp. 317–335). New York, NY: PDR Network, LLC.

FemCap. (2015). *Natural birth control for health-conscious women*. Retrieved from http://www.femcap.com/

French, P. P., Latka, M., Gollub, E. L., Rogers, C., Hoover, D. R., & Stein, Z. A. (2003). Use-effectiveness of the female versus male condom in preventing sexually transmitted disease in women. *Sexually Transmitted Disease, 30*, 433–439.

Goodman, S., Hendlish, C., Benedict, M., Reeves, M., Pera-Floyd, A., & Foster-Rosales, S. (2008). Increasing intrauterine contraception use by reducing barriers to post-abortal and interval insertion. *Contraception, 78*(2), 136–142.

Grimes, D. (2007). Intrauterine devices (IUDs). In R. A. Hatcher, J. Trussell, A. L. Nelson, W. Cates, F. H. Stewart, & D. Kowal (Eds.), *Contraceptive technology* (19th ed., pp. 117–143). New York, NY: PDR Network, LLC.

Hubacher, D., Finer, L. B.,& Espey, E. (2011). Renewed interest in intra-uterine contraception in the United States: Evidence and explanation. *Contraception, 83*(4), 291–294.

Jennings, V., Arevalo, M., & Kowal, D. (2007). Vaginal barriers and spermicides. In R. A. Hatcher, J. Trussell, A. L. Nelson, W. Cates, F. H. Stewart, & D. Kowal (Eds.), *Contraceptive technology* (19th ed., pp. 317–335). New York, NY: PDR Network, LLC.

Meyers, D., Wolff, T., Gregory, K. Marion, L., Moyer, V., Nelson, H., & USPSTF. (2008). *USPSTF recommendations for STI screening*. Originally published in *American Family Physician, 77*, 819–824. Rockville, MD: Agency for Healthcare Research and Quality.

National Institute of Allergy and Infectious Disease. Workshop Summary: Scientific Evidence on Condom Effectiveness for Sexually Transmitted Disease (STD) Prevention, July 20, 2011.

Pallone, S., & Bergus, G. (2009). Natural family planning. *Journal of the American Board of Family Medicine, 22*, 147–157.

Trussell, J. (2008). Contraceptive efficacy. In R. A. Hatcher, J. Trussell, A. L. Nelson, W. Cates, F. H. Stewart, & D. Kowal (Eds.), *Contraceptive technology* (19th ed., pp. 747–826). New York, NY: PDR Network, LLC.

Trussell, J., & Ellerston, C. (1995). Efficacy of emergency contraception. *Fertility Control Review, 4*, 8–11.

Trussell, J., Leveque, J. A., Koenig, J. D., London, R., Borden, S., Henneberry, J., & Wysocki, S. (1995). The economic value of contraception: A comparison of 15 methods. *American Journal of Public Health, 85*, 494–503.

U.S. Department of Health and Human Services. (2014). The guide to clinical preventive services. Retrieved from http://www.ahrq.gov/clinic/pocketgd1011/gcp10s1.htm.

World Health Organization. (2002). *Nonoxynol-9 ineffective in preventing HIV infection*. Retrieved from http://www.who.int/mediacentre/news/releases/who55/en/index.html

World Health Organization. (2009). *Medical eligibility criteria for contraceptive use* (4th ed.). Geneva, Switzerland: Department of Reproductive Health and Research. Retrieved from http://www.who.int/reproductivehealth/publications/family_planning/MEC-5/en/.

URINARY INCONTINENCE IN WOMEN

Janis Luft

CHAPTER 25

I. Introduction and general background

Involuntary loss of urine, or urinary incontinence (UI), affects more than 13 million American women, including 25% of reproductive age women, 44–57% of middle-age and postmenopausal women, and 75% of those aged 75 and older (Anger, Saigal, Litwin, & Urologic Diseases of America Project, 2006; Melville, Katon, Delaney, & Newton, 2005; Qaseem et al. for the Clinical Guidelines Committee of the American College of Physicians, 2014). The condition is associated with a profound adverse impact on quality of life and a higher risk of falls, fractures, nursing home admissions, and social isolation. Each year, consumers spend more than $30 billion on incontinence, including $20 billion in out-of-pocket costs for incontinence management. Yet, UI among adult women is a frequently unrecognized and undertreated problem.

A. Types of UI

UI classification is based on clinical presentation and severity. The primary circumstances leading to leakage of urine determine the type of incontinence. Most patients seen in the ambulatory care setting with UI present with stress, urge, or mixed UI (**Table 25-1**).

1. Stress UI

   Stress UI (SUI) is defined as the involuntary loss of urine as a result of physical stress or increased abdominal pressure from coughing, sneezing, straining, or exercise.

2. Urge incontinence and overactive bladder

   a. Urge incontinence (UUI) describes the loss of urine associated with a strong urge or need to void. Urinary frequency and nocturia are a frequent part of the clinical presentation of this condition. Some patients report nocturnal enuresis.

   b. Women with overactive bladder (OAB) can be characterized as having wet or dry OAB. Wet OAB includes episodes of UUI. Women with dry OAB experience frequency, urgency, or nocturia but manage to avoid accidents with various behavioral strategies (e.g., limiting fluids, voiding often, and avoiding dietary bladder irritants).

3. Mixed incontinence

   Women with mixed incontinence have symptoms of both stress and urge incontinence, although one or the other condition may predominate.

4. Overflow incontinence

   Bladder outlet obstruction or hypocontractility of the detrusor muscle can cause incomplete bladder emptying. An abnormally full bladder can overspill resulting in overflow incontinence. This is a less common bladder dysfunction in women.

TABLE 25-1 Differential Diagnosis of Urinary Incontinence in Women

Type	Presentation	Timing	Volume
Stress	Leakage associated with greater abdominal pressure from coughing, sneezing, straining, or exercise	Immediate	Small to moderate
Urge	Leakage occurs with a strong urge or need to void	Delayed	Drops to large
Mixed	Combination of stress and urge incontinence; one or the other may predominate	Varies	Varies

5. Functional incontinence

Functional incontinence is defined as urine loss that occurs because of factors exogenous to the lower urinary tract, such as diminished cognition or limited ambulation.

6. Reflex incontinence or neurogenic bladder

Reflex incontinence, also known as neurogenic bladder, is incontinence associated with neurologic dysfunction (e.g., multiple sclerosis or spinal cord injury). This can occur without warning or sensory awareness.

B. Prevalence

The prevalence of UI types varies according to age and underlying health status. Stress incontinence is more common in younger, ambulatory women, whereas urge and mixed incontinence increase with age and other health conditions. The proportion of women with UI varies widely (from 2% to 55%) depending on the definitions researchers used and the populations they surveyed. Researchers in the United States followed 64,000 women for at least 2 years in the Nurses' Health Study. The 2-year incidence of UI was 13.7%, but the 2-year remission rate (i.e., the percentage of women who reported leaking at least once a month at baseline and no leaking on follow-up) was 13.9% (Townsend et al., 2007). This surprising result underscores the dynamic nature of UI as a clinical condition.

C. Risk factors

1. Nonmodifiable: age, race or ethnicity, and possibly genetics.

2. Potentially modifiable: pregnancy, vaginal delivery, other obstetric events, and hysterectomy.

3. Modifiable or preventable: obesity, diabetes, smoking, chronic cough, and constipation.

II. Initial evaluation

Initial evaluation of UI begins with a thorough medical, surgical, obstetric, and gynecological history and a complete list of the patient's medications. Clinicians can use a three-part screening tool to determine the type of incontinence (**Table 25-2**). These questions reliably correlate with clinical findings.

TABLE 25-2 Initial Screening for Urinary Incontinence

1. **During the last 3 months, have you leaked urine (even a small amount)?**
   ☐ Yes   ☐ No

2. **During the last 3 months, did you leak urine (*check all that apply*):**
   ☐ When you were performing some physical activity, such as coughing, sneezing, lifting, or exercise?
   ☐ When you had the urge or the feeling that you needed to empty your bladder, but you could not get to the toilet fast enough?
   ☐ Without physical activity and without a sense of urgency?

3. **During the last 3 months, did you leak urine most often (*check only one*):**
   ☐ When you were performing some physical activity, such as coughing, sneezing, lifting, or exercise?
   ☐ When you had the urge or the feeling that you needed to empty your bladder, but you could not get to the toilet fast enough?
   ☐ Without physical activity and without a sense of urgency?
   ☐ About equally as often with physical activity as with a sense of urgency?

Type of Urinary Incontinence Is Based on Responses to Question 3	
Responses to Question 3	**Type of Incontinence**
a. Most often with physical activity	Stress only or stress predominant
b. Most often with the urge to empty the bladder	Urge only or urge predominant
c. Without physical activity or a sense of urgency	Other cause only or other cause predominant
d. About equally with physical activity and a sense of urgency	Mixed

Reproduced from Brown, J. S., Bradley, C. S., Subak, L. L., Richter, H. E., Kraus, S. R., Brubaker, L., et al. (2006). The sensitivity and specificity of a simple test to distinguish between urge and stress urinary incontinence. *Annals of Internal Medicine*, *144*, 715–723. Reprinted with permission.

TABLE 25-3 Urinary Diary*

Time	Urinate in Toilet	Leaking Accident	Reason for Accident	Fluid Intake	
				Type	Amount
6 A.M.					
7 A.M.					
8 A.M.					
9 A.M.					
10 A.M.					
11 A.M.					
12 NOON					
1 P.M.					
2 P.M.					
3 P.M.					
4 P.M.					
5 P.M.					

NOTES

INSTRUCTIONS

1. In the first column, mark an (x) every time you urinate into the toilet.

2. In the second column, mark an (x) every time you accidentally leaked urine.

3. If an accident occurred, indicate the reason or circumstances surrounding the accident, for example, "coughed, bent over, sudden urge."

4. Under "Fluid Intake" describe the type (coffee, tea, juice, etc.) and amount (a cup, 1 quart, etc).

5. Circle the time when you went to bed and when you got up in the morning.

6. Record number and type of pads used.

7. Under "Notes" write any additional information you would like to include. For example, type and dose of medication you may be on for your urinary incontinence.

*Actual diary contains 24 rows labeled for each hour.

A. Subjective

1. Urinary symptoms
   a. Timing, frequency, severity, and precipitants of incontinence episodes
   b. Number of daytime and nighttime urinations
   c. Urinary diary (**Table 25-3**)

2. Amount and nature of fluid intake

3. Bowel habits (e.g., constipation, diarrhea, or straining)

B. Objective

1. Although not a prerequisite to diagnosis and the initiation of nonsurgical treatment for UI, the following may provide data that aid in individualization of treatment or assist in the management of UI refractory to treatment
   a. Assess for genital atrophy

   b. Directed pelvic examination to assess for uterine prolapse or other pathology, such as a pelvic mass

2. Simple neurologic examination: mental status and sensory and motor function of the perineum and lower extremities

III. Assessment

A. Determine the diagnosis

The screening tool found in Table 25-2 can be used to determine the initial diagnosis of UI type (Table 25-1).

B. Severity

Assess the severity of the condition.

1. Number and types of pads or hygienic products used

2. Psychological distress and depression associated with the condition (e.g., limitation to travel, time with family, social isolation, fear of odor or accidents, restriction of exercise)

3. Disruption of sleep

C. Significance

Assess the significance of the problem to the patient and significant others.

D. Motivation and ability

1. Determine the patient's goals for treatment (e.g., reduction in incontinent episodes vs. complete dryness, less daytime urination, or less nocturia).

2. Determine the patient's preferences for treatment (e.g., behavioral modification, medication, combination of these, or other treatment options).

3. Determine the patient's willingness and ability to follow the treatment plan.

IV. Goals of clinical management

A. Screening or diagnosing UI

Choose a cost-effective approach for screening or diagnosing UI that is compatible with the patient's goals and preferences.

B. Treatment

Select a treatment plan that achieves the patient's objectives for bladder control in a safe and effective manner.

C. Patient adherence

Select an approach that maximizes patient adherence.

V. Plan

A. Screening

Although an extremely common chronic condition in women, UI is underreported by patients and unaddressed by many clinicians (Brown et al., 1999). Primary or women's healthcare providers can effectively screen patients by simply asking about issues of bladder control or using the simple questionnaire provided in Table 25-2.

B. Diagnostic tests (Table 25-2)

1. Incontinence Questionnaire

2. A urinary diary that the patient keeps for 1–3 days (Table 25-3)

3. A dipstick urinalysis to rule out underlying infection

4. Postvoid residual urine to rule out overflow incontinence. This can be done by catheterizing or bladder ultrasonography within 15 minutes of urination.

5. Urodynamic testing measures detrusor function, bladder capacity and compliance, and sensation to void. Although such testing may be useful in evaluating patients with complex symptoms or voiding dysfunction, it is not necessary for all patients with incontinence before proceeding to treatment based on clinical presentation.

C. Management (includes treatment, consultation, referral, and follow-up care)

1. Nonpharmacologic management

   a. Bladder training helps patients reestablish voluntary bladder control. Patients learn how to void on a set schedule, beginning with about 30–60 minutes between voids and then slowly increasing the interval to 3 or 4 hours (**Table 25-4**)

   b. Relaxation and urge suppression techniques effectively suppress the strong urge to void that is associated with urge UI (**Table 25-5**).

   c. Pelvic floor muscle exercises or Kegel exercises strengthen the muscles of the pelvic floor and improve urethral pressure and inhibit involuntary detrusor contractions (Table 25-5).

   d. Biofeedback uses electromyography or manometry to help patients learn pelvic floor muscle exercises through directed instructions as they receive feedback in the form of dynamic graphs or tones that reinforces their actions. This modality can help women isolate pelvic muscles and improve the efficacy of pelvic floor muscle exercises.

   e. Weight loss has been shown to improve continence symptoms (Subak et al., 2005; Subak et al., 2009). Weight loss as little as 3–5% has been shown to reduce weekly incontinence episodes by 50–60%.

   f. Diet modification can be helpful. Some patients find that reduction or elimination of "bladder triggers," such as caffeine, alcohol, spicy foods, and concentrated citrus, can improve urinary urgency and frequency. Overhydration and underhydration should be discouraged. Fluid intake sufficient to maintain "lemon juice" colored urine is ideal.

2. Pharmacologic treatment options

   A growing number of medications are available to treat UUI, urgency, frequency, and nocturia (**Table 25-6**). Generally, these agents, which inhibit

TABLE 25-4 Bladder Retraining

Bladder retraining is a behavioral treatment for urinary incontinence that uses scheduled toileting to help you relearn normal bladder function. The purpose of bladder retraining is to

   a.   increase the amount of time between emptying your bladder.

   b.   increase the amount of fluids your bladder can hold.

   c.   diminish the sense of urgency and/or leakage associated with your problem.

Keeping the diary of your bladder activity is very important. This helps us to determine the correct starting interval for you and to monitor your progress throughout your program.

INSTRUCTIONS

1. Empty your bladder as soon as you get up in the morning. This begins your retraining schedule.

2. Go to the bathroom every _____

   Wait the full amount of time before you urinate again *AND* when it is your scheduled time, be sure to empty your bladder even if you feel no urge to urinate. Follow the schedule during waking hours ONLY. During the night time go to the bathroom only if you awaken and find it necessary.

3. A helpful hint: When the urge to urinate is felt before the next designated time, use the "urge suppression" technique described on the pink handout, or try relaxation techniques like deep breathing. Focus on relaxing all other muscles. If possible, sit down until the sensation passes. If the urge is suppressed, adhere to the schedule. If you cannot suppress the urge, wait 5 minutes then slowly make your way to the bathroom; then reestablish the schedule. Repeat this process each time an urge is felt.

4. When you have accomplished this goal, gradually increase the time between emptying your bladder by 15-minute intervals. Try to increase your interval each week, but you will be the best judge of how quickly you can advance to the next step. The time between each urination is increased until you reach a 3- to 4-hour voiding interval.

5. It should take between 6 and 12 weeks to accomplish your goal. Don't be discouraged by setbacks. You may find you have good days and bad days. As you continue bladder retraining you will start to notice more and more good days, so keep practicing.

6. You will hasten your success by doing your pelvic muscle exercises faithfully every day. Your diaries will help you see your progress and identify your problem times.

7. If you need more help, medication or other treatments are available and may be useful.

the bladder's contractile activity, have an anticholinergic and/or antimuscarinic effect. Although they provide excellent symptom relief and reduce weekly incontinent episodes by 15–60%, they may also cause bothersome side effects, such as dry mouth, constipation, drowsiness, and blurred vision (Nygaard & Heit, 2004). Sustained-release medications may cause fewer side effects.

A newer type of overactive bladder medication is now available. Mirabegron (Myrebetriq®) is the only FDA-approved β3-adrenergic receptor agonist. It acts to relax the smooth muscle that surrounds the bladder and helps to increase the bladder's ability to store urine.

A review of studies evaluating the use of vaginal estrogen in postmenopausal women for the treatment of genitourinary symptoms, including UUI and SUI concluded that such vaginal estrogen creams, tablets, and rings can be safe and a helpful adjunct to treatment (Rahn et al., 2014).

Medical treatment of SUI has been largely unsuccessful. There are no pharmaceutical agents for the treatment of SUI on the U.S. market. Treatment of incontinence with oral or transdermal estrogen is not recommended. Two large randomized controlled trials (the Women's Health Initiative and the Heart and Estrogen Replacement Study) demonstrated an increase in the prevalence of UI with the use of both estrogen-only and combined hormone-replacement therapy on stress, urge, and mixed UI (40–50% over a 4-year period and 20–60% at 12 months) (Grady et al., 2001; Hendrix et al., 2005).

TABLE 25-5 Urge Suppression

Urge incontinence is the loss of urine when you have a strong desire to urinate and are unable to reach a bathroom in time. The urge is a signal that it is time to urinate. Your goal is to maintain bladder control until you reach a toilet. A normally functioning bladder can wait until the appropriate opportunity to empty; an unstable bladder cannot.

For a person with urge incontinence, *rushing* to the bathroom when you have a strong urge to urinate is the worst thing you can do. Rushing actually causes bladder irritability to increase and interferes with your ability to concentrate on controlling your bladder. When urgency strikes, you should use the "urge suppression" technique to maintain control.

1. Stop all movement immediately and stand still. Sit down if possible. Remaining still increases your ability to stay in control.

2. Squeeze your pelvic floor muscles quickly and tightly several times. Do not relax the muscles fully between these very quick squeezes. Squeezing your pelvic floor muscles this way signals the bladder to relax and increases your feeling of being in control.

3. Take a deep breath and relax. Shrug your shoulders and let them go limp. Release the tension in the rest of your body.

4. Concentrate on suppressing the urge feeling. Some women find distraction an effective technique.

5. When the strong urgency subsides, walk *slowly and calmly* to the bathroom. If the urge begins to build again, repeat these steps. You can also try contracting your muscles as you walk to the bathroom.

Remember: going to the bathroom is not an emergency!

TABLE 25-6 Medications for Overactive Bladder

Short-acting oral anticholinergics/ muscarinic receptor antagonists	Oxybutynin (Ditropan®), 5 mg	0.50–1 tablet two to four times a day
	Tolterodine (Detrol®), 1 and 2 mg	1 tablet twice daily (start with 2 mg and decrease to 1 mg if severe side effects)
	Trospium chloride (Sanctura®), 20 mg	1 tablet twice daily on an empty stomach
Extended-release oral anticholinergics/MRAs	Oxybutynin ER (Ditropan XL®), 5–15 mg	1 tablet daily
	Tolterodine ER (Detrol LA®), 2 and 4 mg	1 capsule daily (start with 4 mg and decrease to 2 mg if severe side effects)
	Darifenacin (Enablex®), 7.5 and 15 mg	1 tablet daily
	Solifenacin (VesiCare®), 5 and 10 mg	1 tablet daily
	Fesoterodine (Toviaz®), 4 and 8 mg	1 tablet daily
Transdermal anticholinergics/MRAs	Oxybutynin transdermal patch (Oxytrol®), 3.9 mg/day (OTC—no Rx needed)	1 patch on dry skin (hip, abdomen, or buttocks) every 3–4 days
	Oxybutynin transdermal gel 10% (Gelnique®), 100 mg/g	1 sachet daily to dry, intact skin on the abdomen, upper arms or shoulders, or thighs
Nonanticholinergic medications	Mirabegron (Myrbetriq®) 25 and 50 mg	1 tablet daily

Notes for anticholinergic/muscarinic receptor antagonist (MRA) medications

Contraindications: Narrow-angle glaucoma or severe liver or kidney disease.

Side effects: Dry mouth and constipation are the most common. Adjust dose to balance drug effectiveness versus side effects.

Alternative: Imipramine, 10 mg, at bedtime and adjust as often as weekly. Adjust per the patient's urinary diary and symptoms to a maximum of 100 mg at bedtime. Use with caution in the elderly because of hypotension or cognitive impairment.

Notes for Mirabegron

This is a β3-adrenergic receptor agonist. Monitor changes in blood pressure after initiation of medication.

3. Treatment requiring referral to a continence specialty practice

   a. Pessaries: well-fit incontinence ring or incontinence dish pessaries can relieve the symptoms of S UI. The pessary compresses the urethra against the upper posterior portion of the symphysis pubis and elevates the bladder neck. This causes an increase in outflow resistance and corrects the angle between the bladder and the urethra.

   b. Electrical stimulation

      i. Vaginal or rectal electrical stimulation uses an internal sensor to deliver electrical currents at preset frequencies. Higher frequency causes involuntary levator ani contractions that improve pelvic floor tone and assist in learning to contract these muscles at will. Lower frequencies are used to blockade the sacral nerve plexus, reducing detrusor irritability.

      ii. Percutaneous tibial nerve stimulation is used to treat OAB. A fine-needle electrode is inserted into the lower, inner aspect of the leg, slightly cephalad to the medial malleolus. The goal is to send stimulation through the tibial nerve. The needle electrode is connected to an external pulse generator that delivers an adjustable electrical pulse that travels to the sacral plexus via the tibial nerve. The treatment protocol requires once-a-week treatments for 12 weeks, roughly 30 minutes per session.

   c. Percutaneous tibial nerve stimulation
   Patient Instructions:
   Percutaneous tibial nerve stimulation (PTNS) is a minimally invasive treatment for overactive bladder symptoms. Although many options are available for the treatment of OAB, including behavioral modification, pelvic floor muscle rehabilitation (PFMR), and medication, not all patients have success with these. PTNS works by gentle electrical stimulation of the nerves of the sacral nerve plexus to modify the bladder's activity, sometimes referred to as neuromodulation. The tibial nerve, located in the lower leg, can be accessed with a sensor placed through the skin, the impulses then travel along the tibial nerve and to the sacral nerve plexus.

   After your clinician determines that you may benefit from PTNS, you return for an initial evaluation with our nurse practitioner who specializes in urinary incontinence. A small needle electrode is inserted adjacent to the tibial nerve in your lower leg and connected to the battery-powered stimulator. These gentle impulses travel up the tibial nerve to the sacral nerve plexus to modify the bladder's activity. Each treatment lasts about 30 minutes. An initial series of 12 treatments are scheduled, each about a week apart. The entire procedure is carried out in the comfort of our office, and following the initial series of treatments you are evaluated by your doctor to assess your response to treatment.

   d. Surgical treatments

      i. Multiple surgical options are available to treat stress incontinence. The most common sling procedure is the midurethral synthetic sling, in which the surgeon places a narrow piece of polypropylene mesh under the midurethra; this can be done by either a retropubic (passed behind the pubic bone through the anterior abdominal wall) or transobturator (passed through the obturator foramen) approach.

      ii. Patients whose stress incontinence results from intrinsic sphincter deficiency may benefit from urethral bulking agents, such as Coaptite® and Macroplastique®, which are injected transurethrally as an outpatient surgery (Ghoniem & Boctor, 2014).

      iii. Sacral nerve stimulation, also called sacral nerve neuromodulation (InterStim®) therapy, is a reversible treatment for people with UUI caused by OAB who do not respond to behavioral treatments or medication. InterStim® is a surgically implanted neurostimulation system that sends mild electrical pulses to the S3 sacral nerve root, a nerve that influences bladder control.

      iv. Botox® (botulinum toxin A) injection into the detrusor muscle is an option for neurogenic or idiopathic UUI unresponsive to conservative measures. Botox® is injected into numerous sites in the bladder wall using a cystoscope. The toxin works by inactivating proteins involved in neurotransmitter release from nerve terminals. As neurotransmitter levels decrease, underlying muscle spasm may be diminished or ablated. The Food and Drug Administration approved Botox® for the treatment of OAB in June 2013.

      v. Bladder augmentation is infrequently used and reserved for people with UUI who do not benefit from bladder retraining or medication. This procedure increases the capacity of a small, hyperactive, or nonresilient bladder by adding bowel segments or by reducing the muscle-squeezing ability of the bladder.

D. Client education

1. Information

    Provide verbal and, preferably, written information regarding:

    a. Prevalence, morbidity, cost, and available treatments for UI.

    b. Modifiable risk factors for UI, such as obesity, diabetes, and smoking.

    c. Management rationale, action, use, side effects, associated risks, and cost of therapeutic interventions; and the need for adhering to long-term treatment plans.

2. Counseling

    a. Weight loss counseling and advice as needed.

    b. Management of diabetic glucose levels.

    c. Avoidance of constipation.

    d. Decision making regarding elective pelvic surgery.

VI. Self-management resources and tools

A. Patient and client education

1. National Institute for Diabetes, Digestive and Kidney Diseases (NIDDK)

    The NIDDK is a division of the National Institutes of Health. According to their website, "the NIDDK conducts and supports research on many chronic and costly diseases affecting the public health. Several diseases studied by the NIDDK are among the leading causes of disability and death in the Nation; all affect seriously the quality of life of those suffering from them." Both patient and provider literature is available on their website (www2.niddk.nih.gov).

2. UCSF Women's Continence Center website (http://coe.ucsf.edu/wcc/)

    The UCSF Women's Continence Center website provides information about women's UI, pelvic floor prolapse, and treatment options. Downloadable diaries and handouts are available for public use.

B. Community support groups

1. National Association for Continence (NAFC)

    Founded in 1982, the NAFC was originally known as Help for Incontinent People. Today, the renamed National Association for Continence is the largest private consumer organization dedicated to educating and advocating for people with bladder and pelvic floor dysfunction. The NAFC provides educational resources, healthcare referrals, public education, and personal support for those with incontinence (www.nafc.org or 1-800-BLADDER).

2. The Simon Foundation for Continence

    The mission statement of the Simon Foundation is that of "bringing the topic of incontinence out into the open, removing the stigma surrounding incontinence, and providing help and hope for people with incontinence, their families, and the health professionals who provide their care." The organization provides public education materials (www.simonfoundation.org).

REFERENCES

Anger, J. T., Saigal, C.S., Litwin, M.S., & Urologic Diseases of America Project. (2006). The prevalence of urinary incontinence among community dwelling adult women: Results from the National Health and Nutrition Examination Survey. *Journal of Urology, 175*(2), 601–604.

Brown, J. S., Bradley, C. S., Subak, L. L., Richter, H. E., Kraus, S. R., Brubaker, L., et al. (2006). The sensitivity and specificity of a simple test to distinguish between urge and stress urinary incontinence. *Annals of Internal Medicine, 144*, 715–723.

Brown, J., Grady, D., Ouslander, J. G., Herzog, A. R., Varner, R. E., & Posner, S. F. (1999). Prevalence of urinary incontinence and associated risk factors in postmenopausal women. Heart & Estrogen/Progestin Replacement Study (HERS) Research Group. *Obstetrics & Gynecology, 94*(1), 66–70.

Ghoniem, G., & Boctor, N. (2014). Update on urethral bulking agents for female stress urinary incontinence due to intrinsic sphincter deficiency. *Journal of Urology and Research, 1*(2), 1009.

Grady, D., Brown, J. S., Vittinghoff, E., Applegate, W., Varner, E., Snyder, T., & HERS Research Group. (2001). Postmenopausal hormones and incontinence: The Heart and Estrogen/Progestin Replacement Study. *Obstetrics & Gynecology, 97*(1), 116–120.

Hannestad, Y. S., Rortveit, G., Sandvik, H., & Hunskaar, S. (2000). A community-based epidemiological survey of female urinary incontinence: The Norwegian EPINCONT study. Epidemiology of Incontinence in the County of Nord-Trøndelag. *Journal of Clinical Epidemiology, 53*(11), 1150–1157.

Hendrix, S., Cochrane, B., Nygaard, I., Handa, V., Barnabei, V., Iglesia, C., et al. (2005). Effect of estrogen with and without progestin on urinary incontinence. *Journal of the American Medical Association, 293*(8), 935–948.

Melville, J. L., Katon, W., Delaney, K., & Newton, K. (2005). Urinary incontinence in U.S. women: A population-based study. *Archives of Internal Medicine, 165*, 537–542.

Nygaard, I., & Heit, M. (2004). Stress urinary incontinence. *Obstetrics & Gynecology, 104*, 607–620.

Qaseem, A., Dallas, P., Forciea, M., Starkey, M., Denber, T. & Shekelle, P. for the Clinical Guidelines Committee of the American College of Physicians. (2014). Nonsurgical management of urinary incontinence in women: A clinical practice guideline from the American College of Physicians. *Annals of Internal Medicine, 161*(6), 429–440.

Rahn, D., Carberry C., Sanses, T., Mamik, M., Ward, R., Meriwether, K., et al. for the Society of Gynecologic Surgeons Systemic Review Group. (2014). Vaginal estrogen for genitourinary syndrome of menopause: A systematic review. *Obstetrics & Gynecology, 124*(6), 1147–1156.

Subak. L. L., Whitcomb, E., Shen, H., Saxton, J., Vittinghoff, E., & Brown, J. S. (2005). Weight loss: A novel and effective treatment for urinary incontinence. *Journal of Urology, 174*(1), 190–195.

Subak, L., Wing, R., West, D., Franklin, F., Vittinghoff, E., Creasman, J., et al. for the PRIDE Investigators. (2009). Weight loss to treat urinary incontinence in overweight and obese women. *New England Journal of Medicine, 360*(5), 481–490.

Townsend, M., Danforth, K., Lifford, K., Rosner, B., Curhan, G.. Resnick, N., et al. (2007). Incidence and remission of urinary incontinence in middle-aged women. *American Journal of Obstetrics & Gynecology, 197*(2), 167.e1–e5.

THE INITIAL PRENATAL VISIT

CHAPTER 26

Rebekah Kaplan

I. Definition and background

Pregnancy is a time of great physical and emotional changes in a woman's life. Careful, regular monitoring during pregnancy can reassure the mother-to-be and detect variations from a normal pregnancy.

Ideally prenatal care begins before conception. The basic components of prenatal care include early and continuing risk assessment, health promotion and education, and medical and psychosocial interventions and follow-up. Not only is pregnancy a time when most women are unusually open to making positive lifestyle changes, but prenatal care offers the clinician an opportunity to develop a relationship with women over the duration of the pregnancy.

Current evidence does not show that the standard model of individual prenatal care visits improves birth outcomes including the rates of low-birth-weight infants or preterm delivery. However, the various components of prenatal care may allow practitioners to identify risks for a woman and her family in many aspects of her life and initiate appropriate interventions (Fiscella, 1995; Lu et al., 2003; Vintzileos, Ananth, Smulian, Scorza, & Knuppel, 2002). The guiding principles prenatal care should include:

- Nonintervention: the reproductive cycle is a normal and essentially healthy process.
- Consideration of the patient as a member of the health-care team.
- Provision of education appropriate to age, culture, and needs including anticipatory guidance and nutrition.
- Promotion of self-esteem and empowerment.
- Individualization of care: respecting cultural background, sexual orientation, and patient priorities (Walker, McCully, & Vest, 2001).

The initial prenatal visit includes a health and psychosocial history and physical exam with a special focus on establishing a due date and identifying women and/or fetuses at risk for complications. Additional data are gathered through routine laboratory tests and additional ultrasound or diagnostic studies as indicated by findings of history, physical and/or gestational age.

II. Database (may include, but is not limited to)

A. Subjective

1. History of the current pregnancy
   a. Pregnancy symptoms: e.g., nausea, vomiting, fatigue, sore breasts, headache, and fetal movement
   b. Problems: e.g., vaginal bleeding, excessive vomiting
   c. Feelings about pregnancy: e.g., unplanned but wanted, anxious, happy

2. Information for dating of pregnancy (**Box 26-1**)
   a. Past menstrual history: menarche, cycle interval, length and amount of flow
   b. First day of last normal menstrual period: sureness of date, length of flow, previous menstrual period if last period abnormal and any factors that potentially interfere with duration of cycle or ovulation (e.g., hormonal contraceptives)
   c. Dates and results of home pregnancy testing
   d. Information related to conception—dates of intercourse, use of ovulation predictor, use of reproductive technology
   e. Symptoms of pregnancy including onset and evolution, and fetal movement if present
   f. Previous ultrasound if done

3. Obstetric history
   a. Total number of pregnancies including ectopic, abortions (spontaneous and therapeutic) and number of term, preterm, and living children
   b. Deliveries: date, mode of delivery (vaginal birth, cesarean, vacuum or forceps assisted and indication if operative birth), gestational age, gender, birth weight, length of labor,

Box 26-1 Establishing a Due Date

Dating the pregnancy is an essential part of the first prenatal visit. The practitioner must take into consideration all the information for dating the pregnancy and establish a best estimate of the delivery date (EDD). For most women a sure and "normal" last menstrual period (LMP) is the most useful method. Calculate the EDD based on LMP by using a gestational wheel, one of many apps, or Naegle's rule (LMP + 7 days – 3 months, based on 28-day cycle). Use an ultrasound EDD if first-trimester ultrasound dates differ by more than 5–7 days or second-trimester dates differ by more than 10 days.

Accuracy of Dating

- In vitro fertilization ± 1 day
- Ovulation indication ± 3 days
- Single intercourse record/insemination ± 3 days
- Basal body temperature record ± 4 days
- Ultrasound 6–9 weeks (crown-rump length) ± 5 days
- Ultrasound 9–14 weeks (crown-rump length) ± 7 days
- "Regular" and certain LMP with 28-day cycle ± 10–14 days
- Second-trimester ultrasound 10–14 days
- Third-trimester ultrasound 14–28 days
- First-trimester physical examination ± 2 weeks
- Second-trimester physical examination ± 4 weeks
- Third-trimester physical examination ± 6 weeks

Data from Hunter, L. A. (2009). Issues in pregnancy dating: Revisiting the evidence. *Journal of Midwifery & Women's Health, 54*(3), 184–190; ACOG. (2014). Committee Opinion No 611: Method for Estimating Due Date. *Obstetrics and Gynecology, 124*(4), 863.

anesthesia, pregnancy weight gain, spontaneous or induced labor

c. Pregnancy complications such as preterm labor, gestational diabetes, preeclampsia, gestational hypertension, cholestasis, small or large for gestational age newborn

d. Delivery complications such as: shoulder dystocia, postpartum hemorrhage, third- or fourth-degree laceration

e. Postpartum complications such as blood transfusion, infection, wound issues, depression, or mastitis

f. Neonatal or newborn complications such as prolonged hospitalization including diagnosis, jaundice, congenital anomalies

4. Gynecological history

a. Sexually transmitted infections including HIV and genital herpes simplex virus of patient or partner

b. Fibroids or reproductive tract malformations

c. Gynecological surgery, particularly uterine

d. Abnormal Pap smears and related loop electro-surgical excision procedure or cone procedures

e. Vulvovaginal disorders or vaginismus

5. Medical history

a. Present medications: prescriptions, over the counter, supplements

b. Significant illnesses: asthma, diabetes, hypertension, frequent urinary tract infections, cardiovascular, thyroid, hepatitis, anemia, tuberculosis, seizures, psychiatric illnesses

c. Allergies: medications, latex, foods, environmental

d. Surgeries, hospitalizations, blood transfusions

6. Family history

a. Significant illnesses with genetic risk: diabetes, hypertension, renal disease, cardiovascular disease, blood disorders, multiple gestation.

b. Significant illnesses with risk for fetal outcomes: congenital or chromosomal abnormalities, cystic fibrosis, intellectual disability, substance dependence.

7. Social history

a. Country of origin (recent immigrant)

b. Current living situation

c. Supports

d. Financial stability, healthcare coverage

e. Food access

f. Occupation and work safety (exposure to hazards: chemical, biologic, or physical)

g. Intimate partner violence

h. History of violence or sexual abuse

i. Substance use (cigarettes, alcohol, narcotics, current and past use)

j. HIV risk factors

k. Educational history (reading level, years of schooling, how they learn best)

8. Nutritional history

a. Prepregnancy weight and body mass index (BMI)

b. Weight gain or loss

c. Current diet: restrictions (vegetarian or lactose intolerant), adequate protein, calcium, grains, fruits and vegetables

B. Objective

1. Baseline data: height, weight, basal metabolic index, and blood pressure
2. Complete physical examination: for many women pregnancy is their only contact with medical care, hence an opportunity for overall health assessment.
   a. Head, ears, eyes, nose, and throat, teeth
   b. Skin, neck, and thyroid
   c. Breasts, heart, chest, and lungs
   d. Abdomen: including uterine size or fundal height and fetal heart tones (after 10 weeks)
   e. Neurologic: deep tendon reflexes, extremities
   f. Pelvic examination
      i. External genitalia
      ii. Vagina: discharge
      iii. Cervix: polyps, dilation of os, length, consistency, and position
      iv. Uterus: size, position, and symmetry
      v. Adnexa: difficult to palpate after 12 weeks
      vi. Rectum: note hemorrhoids

III. Assessment

A. Estimated gestational age and date of delivery: Size (S)/Dates (D) relationship (S = D, S < D, or S > D)

B. Creation of a "problem list" that will guide future care based on issues/risk factors identified from history and physical examination or existing laboratory data—could include:

1. Unknown LMP
2. Prior cesarean delivery
3. BMI: 41
4. Rh-negative blood type

C. Role assessment: need for consultation or collaborative management (see Chapter 30 for guidelines for medical consultation and referral during pregnancy)

IV. Goals of clinical management

A. Establish a date of delivery

B. Identify medical, nutritional, and psychosocial problems and risk factors and a plan of care for each problem

C. Anticipatory guidance related to pregnancy, birth, parenting, and medical care

D. Individualize care to meet both the family and medical needs and maximize maternal and fetal well-being

V. Plan

A. Discuss and order diagnostic and laboratory screening (see **Boxes 26-2** and **26-3**)

B. Discuss and recommend therapeutic interventions and medications

1. Prenatal vitamins
2. Other vitamins or supplementation as indicated by history or nutritional assessment may include:
   a. Iron, 325 mg daily if anemic (hemoglobin < 10, hematocrit < 32) (Graves & Barger, 2001; Grieger & Clifton, 2014)
   b. Calcium if dietary intake less than 1,200 mg daily (Grieger & Clifton, 2014; Hofmeyr, Lawrie, Atallah, & Duley, 2014)
   c. Vitamin D_3 (Harvey et al., 2014; Wei, Qi, Luo, & Fraser, 2013)
   d. Fish oil: omega-3 fatty acids (Mozurkewich & Klemens, 2012)
3. Prescriptions (assess safety in pregnancy): clinicians need to be mindful of the U.S. Food and Drug Administration risk category for drugs during pregnancy when prescribing medications for the pregnant woman (**Box 26-4**).
4. Vaccines:
   a. Influenza vaccine recommended for all pregnant women (seasonal).
   b. Tetanus/diphtheria/pertussis (Tdap) recommended for all pregnant women with each pregnancy, between 27–36 weeks, gestation.
   c. Hepatitis A and B if at risk (Bridges, Woods, & Coyne-Beasley, 2013).

C. Patient education includes (**Figure 26-1**):

1. Prenatal care and compliance
2. Common discomforts
3. Physiologic and emotional changes
4. Fetal growth and development
5. Options for prenatal screening and diagnosis offered, reviewed, and discussed
6. Nutrition and exercise

Box 26-2 Laboratory Data

Initial screening "routine"

- Complete blood count with platelets and mean corpuscular volume (MCV)
- Maternal blood type with antibody screen
- Hepatitis B surface antigen
- Rubella immunity
- Syphilis serology
- HIV antibody with consent
- Urine culture with sensitivities
- Pap smear if due

Initial screening "risk based" based on population served or individual risk may include:

- Hepatitis C antibody
- Varicella antibody if immunity is unknown
- Purified protein derivative (PPD tuberculosis skin test)
- Toxoplasmosis (IgG, IgM)
- Early glucose load test
- Hemoglobin A1c
- Tay-Sachs carrier status
- Cystic fibrosis
- Hemoglobin electrophoresis
- Wet mount
- Gonorrhea and chlamydia
- Thyroid function tests

Box 26-3 Timing of Elective Genetic Diagnostic and Screening Tests Offered to Women Before 20 Weeks

This may vary by location and what is available
Screening tests:

- First-trimester blood screen (10 weeks–13 weeks and 6 days)
- Nuchal translucency screening ultrasound (11 weeks and 2 days–14 weeks and 2 days weeks)
- Second-trimester or quadruple marker blood screen (15–20 weeks)
- Noninvasive prenatal testing/cell-free DNA blood test (after 10 weeks)
- Fetal survey/screening ultrasound (18–20 weeks, routine in many practices)

Diagnostic tests

- Chorionic villus sampling (10–14 weeks)
- Amniocentesis (15–20 weeks)

Box 26-4 Food and Drug Administration (FDA) Prescription Drug Safety Categories

A. No risk of harm to the fetus

B. No risk seen in animals, but no controlled studies in women; probably little risk

C. Animal studies may show some risk to fetus; studies in women unavailable. Give only if benefit outweighs risk

D. Positive evidence of human fetal risk, but benefits may be acceptable in life-threatening situation (D)

E. Known fetal abnormalities

7. Over-the-counter medications

8. Substance use and abuse

9. Food safety (e.g., listeria, mercury, and pasteurization)

10. Teratogens

11. Workplace safety and exposure

12. Safer sex

13. Danger signs (specific to gestational age)

14. Community resources

15. Sexuality during pregnancy

D. Consultation and referrals (could include)

1. Genetic counseling for advanced maternal age; family history of genetic disorder, developmental delays, and cardiovascular defects; as indicated by ethnic background, multiple miscarriages, consanguinity, and exposure to potential teratogens (**Box 26-5**)

2. Ancillary services: social worker, nutritionist, health educator, prenatal classes, psychiatry as needed or desired

3. Community resources (e.g., Women, Infants, Children nutritional program, public health nurse, smoking cessation, community-based organizations, support groups)

4. Medical consultation and referral

E. Follow-up

1. Patient should return per the return visit schedule guideline. This should be flexible, individualized, and depend on parity and risk (**Box 26-6**).

FIGURE 26-1 OB Provider Education Flow Sheet

First and Second Trimester

❑ Centering Offered ❑ Accepted ❑ Declined Why? _____

❑ Orientation to clinic/service ❑ Dental referral

Common Discomforts:

Back pain _____ N/V _____

Constipation _____ Dizziness _____

HA _____ Round ligament pain _____

SOB _____ Urinary frequency _____

Other: _____

Food and drug safety _____ Fetal growth and development _____

Dating/sonogram _____ Fetal movement _____

Exercises (back care, stretching, yoga, keeping fit) _____

Additional Education:

_____

_____

Method of infant feeding: ❑ breast ❑ bottle ❑ both

Breastfeeding:

❑ Received Breastfeeding class info

Breastfeeding experience _____ ❑ Benefits of breastfeeding _____

❑ Exclusive Breastfeeding 6 mo _____

Method of contraception _____ ❑ Consent signed ❑ Attended TL class

S/sx Preterm Labor (UCs, VB, LOF or ROM, pelvic pressure) _____

Danger signs (fever, VB, severe abd pain, dysuria) _____

Danger signs: preeclampsia (H/A, scotoma, RUQ or epigastric pain) _____

Third Trimester

❑ Gave childbirth class info ❑ Attended childbirth class ❑ Tdap vaccination

Danger signs: general (VB, ROM, severe abdominal pain, decreased FM, fever) _____

Labor and Delivery

Birth plan ❑ Relaxation techniques ❑ Pain control options ❑ _____

Fetal monitoring methods ❑ _____ ❑ Signs/Symptoms labor (UCs, bloody show, ROM)

Early labor comfort measures ❑ Support people in labor _____

(continues)

FIGURE 26-1 *OB Provider Education Flow Sheet* (Continued)

Breastfeeding:

❑ Attended breastfeeding class ❑ Early initiation of breastfeeding ❑ Skin to skin/rooming in

❑ Infant feeding cues _____ ❑ Latch _____ ❑ Colostrum/milk production _____

❑ Breastfeeding and returning to work _____ ❑ Breastfeeding resources _____

Baby Care:

❑ Experience with baby care _____ ❑ Help with baby at home _____

❑ Sibling rivalry ❑ Preparing for baby at home ❑ Calming your baby ❑ Car seat

Additional Education:

_____

_____

❑ Fetal movement _____ ❑ Kick counts _____

Developed by San Francisco General Hospital Nurse-Midwifery Service

---

Box 26-5 *Medical Conditions Requiring Transfer of Care to High-Risk Clinic*

(These may differ in different settings)

Maternal Conditions

- Chronic hypertension diagnosed before pregnancy
- Active or uncontrolled seizure disorder
- Severe asthma (hospitalization or requiring systemic steroids during pregnancy)
- Cardiac disease (except asymptomatic mitral valve prolapse)
- Pulmonary hypertension
- Platelet count less than 100,000
- Deep vein thrombosis
- Sickle cell disease
- Lupus, scleroderma, or any connective tissue disease
- Cancer
- Active tuberculosis
- Active viral hepatitis
- HIV positive
- Hyperthyroidism
- Diabetes: type 1 and type 2
- Multiple gestation

Box 26-6 *Visit Schedule Guidelines*

Frequency of prenatal visits

- 1–28 weeks—every 4 weeks
- 28–36 weeks—every 2–3 weeks
- 36+ weeks—every week

Reduced visit schedule

One visit during each gestational age or age range (approximately eight visits)

- 6–8 weeks
- 14–16 weeks
- 24–28 weeks
- 32 weeks
- 36 weeks
- Weekly from 38 weeks

2. Patient should return to a physician if she is assessed to be high risk per guidelines or for consultation around a specific problem (see Chapter 30 on guidelines for medical consultation during pregnancy).

VI. Internet resources

A. American College of Nurse-Midwives Consumer Education website:

There is information regarding pregnancy, labor and birth, parenting, and women's health including easy to use patient education handouts (some in Spanish) from the "Share with Women Series" (http://www.mymidwife.org/).

B. March of Dimes:

Information is available for providers and patients in both written and audio–video formats in English and Spanish on pregnancy, birth, and newborn development and care (http://www.marchofdimes.com/).

C. National Women's Health Information Center:

This is a U.S. Department of Health and Human Services women's health information website. There are numerous fact sheets on all aspects of women's health including pregnancy in both Spanish and English (http://www.womenshealth.gov).

D. Childbirth Connection:

This organization promotes evidenced-based maternity care and helps women and providers to make informed decisions. There are numerous patient education, pregnancy, and childbirth resources (http://www.childbirthconnection.org/).

E. American College of Obstetricians and Gynecologists:

There are limited numbers of patient education handouts available by provider request (http://www.acog.org/).

REFERENCES

American College of Obstetricians and Gynecologists. (2014). Committee opinion No. 611: Method for estimating due date. *Obstetrics and Gynecology, 124*(4), 863–866.

Bridges, C. B., Woods, L., & Coyne Beasley, T. (2013). Advisory Committee on Immunization Practices (ACIP) recommended immunization schedule for adults aged 19 years and older—United States, 2013. *MMWR. Surveillance Summaries, 62*(Suppl. 1), 9–19.

Dowswell, T., Carroli, G., Duley, L., Gates, S., Gülmezoglu, A. M., Khan-Neelofur, D., et al. (2010). Alternative versus standard packages of antenatal care for low-risk pregnancy. *Cochrane Database of Systematic Reviews, 10*, CD000934.

Fiscella, K. (1995). Does prenatal care improve birth outcomes? A critical review. *Obstetrics & Gynecology, 85*(3), 468–479.

Graves, B. W., & Barger, M. K. (2001). A conservative approach to iron supplementation during pregnancy. *Journal of Midwifery and Women's Health, 45*(3), 163–166; 159–163 (for N282A).

Grieger, J. A., & Clifton, V. L. (2014). A review of the impact of dietary intakes in human pregnancy on infant birthweight. *Nutrients, 7*(1), 153–178.

Harvey, N. C., Holroyd, C., Ntani, G, Javid, K., Cooper, P., Moon, R., et al. (2014). Vitamin D supplementation in pregnancy: A systematic review. *Health Technology Assessment, 18*(45), 1–190.

Hofmeyr, G. J., Lawrie, T. A., Atallah, A. N., & Dully, L. (2014). Calcium supplementation during pregnancy for preventing hypertensive disorders and related problems. *Cochrane Database of Systematic Reviews, 6*, CD001059.

Hunter, L. A. (2009). Issues in pregnancy dating: Revisiting the evidence. *Journal of Midwifery & Women's Health, 54*(3), 184–190.

Lu, M. C., Tache, V., Alexander, G. R., Kotelchuck, M., & Halfon, N. (2003). Preventing low birth weight: Is prenatal care the answer? *Journal of Maternal-Fetal & Neonatal Medicine, 13*(6), 362–380.

Mozurkewich, E. L., & Klemens, C. (2012). Omega-3 fatty acids and pregnancy: Current implications for practice. *Current Opinion in Obstetrics & Gynecology, 24*(2), 72–77.

Vintzileos, A., Ananth, C. V., Smulian, J. C., Scorza, W. E., & Knuppel, R. A. (2002). The impact of prenatal care on neonatal deaths in the presence and absence of antenatal high-risk conditions. *American Journal of Obstetrics and Gynecology, 186*(5), 1011–1016.

Walker, D. S., McCully, L., & Vest, V. (2001). Evidence-based pre-natal care visits: When less is more. *Journal of Midwifery and Women's Health, 46*(3), 146–151.

Wei, S. Q., Qi, H. P., Luo, Z. C., & Fraser, W. D. (2013). Maternal vitamin D status and adverse pregnancy outcomes: A systematic review and meta-analysis. *Journal of Maternal, Fetal, and Neonatal Medicine, 26*, 889–899.

PRENATAL GENETIC SCREENING AND DIAGNOSIS

Deborah Anderson

CHAPTER 27

I. Introduction and general background

Recent scientific advances in human genetics, combined with new prenatal screening and diagnostic technologies, have resulted in a proliferation of genetic testing options and a concomitant change in the landscape of prenatal genetic testing. All pregnant women now have the option of numerous genetic screening and diagnostic tests.

Traditionally, genetic tests such as hemoglobin electrophoresis for hemoglobinopathies, cystic fibrosis carrier screening, and first and second-trimester serologic screening with fetal ultrasound to determine risk for aneuploidy and selected structural defects are routinely offered to all pregnant women (Minkoff & Berkowitz, 2014). When patients test positive for these screening tests, or have genetic risk factors such as a family history of inherited disorders, advanced maternal age, a history of offspring with anomalies, or an ethnicity-based risk for autosomal recessive disorders, they are referred for genetic counseling and possible genetic diagnostic testing.

The recent introduction and acceptance of new technologies such as noninvasive prenatal testing (NIPT) for fetal aneuploidy (also known as cell-free fetal DNA) and expanded carrier gene panels offer benefits such as early genetic screening, improved specificity and sensitivity for aneuploidy, and capacity to identify genetic carrier status for over 100 recessive diseases. The limitations of these tests underlie current debate about how and when to best incorporate these new tests into established prenatal genetic testing algorithms (Han & Platt, 2014; Langlois, Benn, & Wilkins-Haug, 2015; Wienke, Brown, Farmer, & Strange, 2014). Nevertheless, incorporation of these tests is already beginning to alter testing paradigms. In 2014, for example, Larion, Warsof, and Romary reported that an increased use of NIPT was associated with a decrease in chronic villus sampling and amniocentesis procedures.

As more and more screening and diagnostic tools become available, genetic counselors with requisite knowledge about the multitude of optional genetic tests are key to providing patients with information about all screening and diagnostic options. Included in counseling are the benefits, limitations, and risks of prenatal genetic testing, individualized genetic information, options, and assistance with interpretation and understanding of test results.

A. Prenatal genetic screening for trisomies 21, 18, 13; neural tube defects (NTD); abdominal wall defects; and Smith-Lemli-Opitz syndrome (SLOS)

Several optional first and second trimester screening strategies are available to assess risk for trisomy 21 (Down syndrome), trisomy 18 (Edward syndrome), open neural tube defects (NTD), abdominal wall defects, and Smith-Lemli-Opitz syndrome (SLOS). The tests use serum biochemical markers and fetal ultrasound to refine and improve risk assessment beyond standard population-based risk assessments. Combining these first- and second-trimester screening strategies to assess risk, rather than using them as single-method testing, improves accuracy and detection rates for Down syndrome and trisomy 18 (California Department of Public Health, 2014). See **Table 27-1** for detection rates and timing of these genetic screening strategies.

1. Combined first-trimester screening: first-trimester maternal serum and fetal nuchal translucency (NT)

   Combined first-trimester screening is performed in two steps and determines risk for trisomies 21 and 18. Maternal serum testing for pregnancy-associated plasma protein A (PAPP-A) and human chorionic gonadotropin (hCG) is obtained; the serum analyte values are combined with ultrasound examination of fetal NT to determine risk.

   Nuchal translucency refers to a measurement of a clearly demarcated fluid-filled space behind the fetal neck that is present in all fetuses. Skill at obtaining NT measurement requires training for a standardized method of measurement; therefore, this screening tool may not be available in all communities. NT measurement alone has a detection rate for

TABLE 27-1 Selected Prenatal Screening Strategies, Detection Rates, and Timing of Screening

Timing of Screening (Laboratory dependent)	Screening Strategy	Detection Rate	Clinical Application
First-trimester serum: 10–13 weeks 6 days	**First-trimester serum**		There are no risk assessments for the first trimester as a stand-alone test. (May vary with screening program.) The test combines with the NT and/or the quad marker.
First-trimester serum: 10–13 weeks 6 days Nuchal translucency: 11 weeks 2 days–14 weeks 2 days	**Combined first-trimester screen** (Combines maternal serum testing results and NT results)	Trisomy 21: 85% Trisomy 18: 60%	Test performed in two steps. If results are positive, first-trimester screening allows for the option of early diagnostic testing and decision making regarding the course of the pregnancy.
> 10 weeks	**Noninvasive prenatal testing or cell-free fetal DNA testing** (Maternal serum)	Trisomy 21: 99% Trisomy 18: 99% Trisomy 13: 92%	Offered to women at high risk for aneuploidy
15–20 weeks (Optimal time 16–18 weeks)	**Quadruple or quad marker screen** (Maternal serum)	Trisomy 21: 80% Trisomy 18: 67% Anencephaly: 97% Open spina bifida: 80% Abdominal wall defects: 85% Smith-Lemli-Opitz: 60%	Can be used alone or combined with first-trimester serum or combined first-trimester screen. Detection rates for trisomy 21 and 18 are improved when combined. May be used in women with late entry to prenatal care.
First-trimester serum: 10–13 weeks 6 days Second-trimester serum: 15–20 weeks	**Serum integrated screen** (Combines first-trimester maternal serum with quad marker)	Trisomy 21: 85% Trisomy 18: 79% Anencephaly: 97% Open spina bifida: 80% Abdominal wall defects: 85% Smith-Lemli-Opitz: 60%	Test is performed in two steps.
First-trimester serum: 10–13 weeks 6 days Nuchal translucency: 11 weeks 2 days–14 weeks 2 days Second-trimester serum: 15–20 weeks	**Sequential integrated screen** (Combines first-trimester serum and NT with quad marker test results)	Trisomy 21: 90% Trisomy 18: 81% Anencephaly: 97% Open spina bifida: 80% Abdominal wall defects: 85% Smith-Lemli-Opitz: 60%	Test is performed in three steps.

Data from California Department of Public Health Prenatal Screening Program. (2014).

trisomy 21 of 64–70% with a 5% false-positive rate (California Department of Public Health, 2014). Detection rates improve and can modify risk assessment when combined with first-trimester serum testing and the quadruple marker serum screen. An increased NT measurement (> 3 mm) is associated with fetal chromosomal abnormalities and cardiac defects. NT measurement of 3.5 mm or greater is associated with fetal structural anomalies, such as congenital hydrocephalus; agenesis, hypoplasia, and dysplasia of the lung; atresia and stenosis of the small intestine; osteodystrophies; genetic disorders such as Noonan syndrome; and diaphragm anomalies (Baer et al., 2014). As such, women with an NT greater than or equal to 3 mm should be offered genetic counseling and diagnosis, targeted ultrasound, and fetal echocardiogram.

2. Quadruple (quad) marker serum examination
The quad marker estimates the risk for trisomies 21 and 18, open NTD, abdominal wall defect, and

SLOS. Four biochemical markers are assessed: alpha fetoprotein (AFP), human chorionic gonadotropin (hCG), unconjugated estriol (uE3), and dimeric inhibin-A (DIA).

It can be used alone, combined with first-trimester serum, or combined with first-trimester screen to improve detection rates.

3. Serum integrated screening: first- and second-trimester serum testing

Serum integrated screening combines first-trimester blood test results with quad marker blood test results. This test may be useful when NT measurements cannot be obtained because of timing, patient wishes, or where NT programs are not available.

4. Sequential integrated screening: first- and second-trimester serum testing, and NT

Sequential integrated screening combines three tests: first- and second-trimester serum screening, and NT. It provides higher detection rates for aneuploidy when compared to combined first-trimester screen or serum integrated screening.

5. Noninvasive prenatal testing (NIPT) or cell-free fetal DNA testing

Noninvasive prenatal testing screens for trisomy 21 (Down syndrome), trisomy 18 (Edward syndrome), trisomy 13 (Patau syndrome), and some sex chromosome abnormalities have been available for clinical use since 2011. NIPT can also determine fetal Rhesus status and fetal sex. The test analyzes maternal serum cell-free fetal DNA fragments circulating in maternal plasma and has been shown to be highly sensitive and specific, with a > 99.1% detection rate for Down syndrome and a low false-positive rate (< 1%) (Bianchi et al., 2013; Gil et al., 2015; Norton et al., 2012). The American College of Obstetricians and Gynecologists (ACOG Committee on Genetics, 2012) currently recommends offering NIPT to women who are at high risk for aneuploidy: women with maternal age of 35 years or older at delivery, fetal ultrasonographic findings indicating an increased risk of aneuploidy, history of

a prior pregnancy with a trisomy, positive test result for aneuploidy (including first-trimester, sequential, integrated screen, or quadruple screen), and parental balanced robertsonian translocation. The California Prenatal Screening Program recommends offering the option of NIPT or chorionic villus sampling (CVS) when the first-trimester combined screening (first-trimester serum and NT) is positive for trisomy 21 or 18.

B. Carrier screening for recessive conditions

Carrier screening is available to individuals and couples who are at risk of conceiving children affected by recessive diseases. Currently, all pregnant women are routinely screened for hemoglobinopathies (hemoglobin electrophoresis and mean corpuscular volume [MCV]) and are offered carrier screening for cystic fibrosis (ACOG Committee on Genetics, 2011). The American College of Medical Genetics and Genomics (ACMG) recommends the option of general population screening for spinal muscular atrophy, as well, although this is unsupported by ACOG (ACOG Committee on Genetics, 2009). Additionally, parents with personal or family histories of inherited disorders such as Tay-Sachs disease, Canavan disease, familial dysautonomia, fragile-X syndrome, sickle cell anemia, α-thalassemia, β-thalassemia, and cystic fibrosis are offered carrier testing along with genetic counseling.

In the absence of family history, ethnicity-based carrier screening is offered to women who are at risk of targeted genetic diseases that are found to have increased prevalence in certain ethnic groups. **Table 27-2** lists ACOG recommendations (ACOG Committee on Genetics, 2005, 2009, 2010, 2011; ACOG Committee on Obstetrics, 2007) for genetic diseases for which carrier screening is recommended and the patient populations that carry an increased risk for these disorders. Limitations of ethnicity-based carrier screening include difficulty assigning a specific ethnicity in individuals with mixed racial ancestry, patient preferences against use of racial and ethnic categorization in medicine, and noninclusion of groups with lower risks for the diseases. Recent research demonstrated

TABLE 27-2 Ethnicity-Based Recommendation for Carrier Screening

Ethnic Group/Geographic Ancestry	Disease
All ethnicities	Cystic fibrosis
Cajun, French-Canadian	Tay-Sachs disease
Ashkenazi Jewish	Tay-Sachs, Canavan disease, familial dysautonomia
African, African-American	Sickle cell anemia
Southeast Asian, Mediterranean	Alpha- or beta-thalassemia

that ethnicity-based approaches to genetic screening are not aligned with the current distribution of carrier frequencies of severe genetic disease and suggested that new carrier screening guidelines are needed (Lazarin et al., 2013).

Recent advances in genetic technology now make it possible to screen for hundreds of causal mutations for genetic disease (Lazarin et al., 2013). Expanded prenatal carrier screening panels are currently available to the public and medical providers through commercial laboratories. Evidence-based guidelines are not yet available to guide practitioners about how to best incorporate expanded prenatal carrier screening panels into current screening algorithms. When consumers request expanded prenatal carrier panels from commercial laboratories, formal genetic counseling prior to and after the test will provide patients with support and information for understanding the test's benefits, limitations, and interpretation. Current controversies related to expanded carrier screening include questions about which diseases to include in the prenatal carrier screening panel and implications of the test results in reproductive decision making. The American College of Medical Genetics and Genomics (Grody et al., 2013) position statement on prenatal/preconception expanded carrier screening provides criteria to laboratories for the selection of appropriate tests to be included in prenatal carrier screening panels.

II. Database

A. Subjective

1. All women regardless of age should have the option for genetic screening or diagnostic testing (ACOG Committee on Obstetrics, 2007). Advanced maternal age (35 years old) alone is no longer used as a determining factor for who is offered prenatal screening or diagnostic testing.

2. Last menstrual period. If unsure or unreliable, order an ultrasound to determine gestational age. Screening tests for aneuploidy and neural tube defects are sensitive to gestational age.

3. Ethnicity

4. Genetic, obstetric, and family history. Identify any genetic risk factors such as chromosome abnormalities, inherited genetic disorders, unexplained mental retardation or developmental delay, primary ovarian insufficiency of unknown etiology, autism, or congenital malformation.

5. Determine whether the patient desires prenatal testing. Factors to be considered if women choose to have or decline testing include

    a. Gestational age at entry into prenatal care
    b. Ethnicity-based risk factors
    c. Personal, family, genetic, and obstetric history
    d. Number of fetuses
    e. NT availability
    f. Test sensitivity and limitations
    g. Desire for testing
    h. Risks of diagnostic procedures
    i. Options for early termination
    j. Insurance coverage

B. Objective

1. Establish expected date of delivery (EDD). Because first and second-trimester testing is sensitive to gestational age, ultrasound dating of pregnancy reduces rates of false-positive and false-negative results caused by incorrect dating. If the expected date of delivery is changed (≥ 10 days difference) after submission of screening tests, the laboratory must be informed of the new EDD for reinterpretation of test results.

2. Routine laboratory: complete blood count (CBC) with mean corpuscular volume and hemoglobin electrophoresis to screen for hemoglobinopathies and cystic fibrosis carrier testing if desired by the patient.

3. Routine ultrasound to assess fetal anatomy at approximately 18–20 weeks' gestation

4. Weight

III. Assessment

Patient desires/declines prenatal genetic screening tests (specify test) or carrier testing.

IV. Goals for clinical management

A. Identify infants with specific genetic and/or neural tube disorders previous to birth in requesting families.

B. Establish inherited and/or historical risk for genetic disorders.

C. Establish patient desires for genetic screening using principals of informed consent and shared decision making.

D. Allow for identification of increased risk for neural tube defects and genetic disorders and give families the option of diagnostic screening.

V. Plan

A. Counseling regarding tests and results

1. All patients are offered first and second-trimester serologic screening, NT ultrasound examination, and cystic fibrosis carrier status testing. The option of NIPT and expanded carrier screening will vary with practice site.

2. If personal, family, or obstetric history are positive for genetic risk factors such as aneuploidy, inherited genetic disorder, offspring with birth defects, or consanguinity, offer referral to a genetic counselor or a perinatal specialist for counseling and possible prenatal diagnosis.

3. Provide information regarding screening tests in a nondirective, sensitive, and nonjudgmental manner. Include information about the difference between risk assessment and diagnosis, the limitations of the screening tests, the rates and meaning of false positives and negatives, and the difference between carrier traits and diseases. Offer unbiased support for their decisions (Sheets et al., 2011).

4. Document acceptance or refusal of genetic screening tests. Some state-run programs require a standardized signed accept/decline form for first-trimester serum screen, NT, or quad marker.

5. When reviewing combined first-trimester, quad marker, or sequential integrated screen results with women, it is preferred to communicate the numerical risk assessment of the final analysis rather than a "positive" or "negative" result. Numerical risk of a genetic condition can be communicated in both ratio and percentages and may include the chances of having or not having the genetic condition. For example, "There is a 1:50 chance of Down syndrome, which means there is a 49:50 chance that there is not Down syndrome. That equates to a 2% chance of Down syndrome or a 98% chance there is not Down syndrome." It may also be useful to compare their screening risk to their age-related risk.

B. Laboratory

1. See Table 27-1 for timing of genetic screening tests. Timing of the first-trimester serum screen, NT, and quad marker testing is limited by gestational age.

2. Fill out the appropriate laboratory forms including the best dating parameter, current weight, number of fetuses, race, diabetes, and tobacco use. Additional data are used to adjust interpretation of test results.

C. Consultation and referral

If the risk is screen positive, or if the risk is higher than the procedure-related risk of loss from diagnostic testing, refer to a genetic counselor for further counseling regarding interpretation of results, recommendations for follow-up examinations, possible confirmatory diagnostic testing, and supportive counseling.

I. Prenatal genetic diagnosis: Introduction and general background

Invasive prenatal diagnosis allows for the identification of multiple genetic disorders and provides parents with the information necessary to help make well-informed reproductive decisions. Although all women have the option of prenatal diagnosis, it is most often performed in women who have known risk factors for heritable genetic diseases or in women whose prenatal screening tests return positive. Chorionic villus sampling and amniocentesis permit a multitude of genetic diagnoses to be made in early pregnancy; preimplantation genetic diagnosis provides genetic diagnosis in an embryo obtained through in vitro fertilization prior to implantation.

A patient's decision to choose prenatal genetic diagnosis includes consideration of the anticipated risk that the fetus will have an abnormality, gestational age of the fetus, previous obstetric history, risk of pregnancy loss from an invasive procedure, feelings about having a child with a chromosomal abnormality, desire for a definitive diagnosis, and beliefs about termination.

A. Chorionic villus sampling

Under ultrasound guidance, a small sample of the placenta is obtained through a transcervical or transabdominal route.

1. Timing of test: 10–14 weeks of gestation

2. Benefits
   a. CVS tests for aneuploidy. If there is an indication, it can also test for biochemical abnormalities, single gene conditions, and collagen abnormalities. Microarray analysis can be performed to test for microdeletions and duplications.
   b. Because CVS is generally performed in the first trimester, it allows for early diagnosis and decision making about reproductive choices.
   c. Results are usually available 1–2 weeks after the procedure.

3. Risks
   a. Risk rates approach or may be the same as amniocentesis (see amniocentesis).
   b. Amniotic fluid leak or infection, vaginal bleeding, or cell culture failure.
   c. Mosaicism that may or may not be confined to the placenta. When mosaicism is detected on CVS, amniocentesis is recommended.

B. Amniocentesis

Under ultrasound guidance a small amount of amniotic fluid is aspirated via a transabdominal puncture of the uterus and amnion.

1. Timing of test: 15–20 weeks' gestation

2. Benefits

   a. Amniocentesis tests for aneuploidy and neural tube defects. If indicated, it can test for fetal blood type and selected inherited diseases. Microarray analysis can be performed to test for microdeletions and duplications.

   b. Results are usually available 1–2 weeks after the procedure.

   c. Cytogenetic diagnostic accuracy is greater than 99%.

3. Risks

   a. Procedure-related loss is 1 in 300–500, depending on provider (ACOG Committee on Obstetrics, 2007).

   b. Amniotic fluid leakage or rupture, transient vaginal spotting, chorioamnionitis, rare needle injury to fetus, and failure of amniotic fluid cell culture.

C. Preimplantation genetic diagnosis

Preimplantation genetic diagnosis is performed on cells removed from preimplantation embryos conceived through in vitro fertilization. Single gene or chromosomal abnormalities can be identified in the embryo, allowing for transfer of only unaffected embryos back to the uterus.

1. Benefits

   a. Tests for aneuploidy, single gene disorders, and chromosomal abnormalities, such as deletions and translocations (ACOG, 2014).

   b. Allows for very early reproductive decision making, prior to the establishment of pregnancy.

2. Risks

   a. Requires in vitro fertilization with its associated risks and expense.

   b. False-positive and -negative test results leading to misdiagnosis. Confirmatory CVS or amniocentesis is recommended for pregnancies conceived after prenatal diagnosis.

   c. May decrease the chance of pregnancy depending on type of testing.

II. Database

A. Subjective

1. Identify genetic indications for prenatal diagnosis.

   a. Chromosomal abnormality in previous offspring, parent, or close relative

   b. Structural anomalies identified by ultrasound examination

   c. History of previous fetus or child with any chromosome abnormality

   d. Parental carrier of chromosome translocation or chromosome inversion

   e. Parental aneuploidy or mosaicism for aneuploidy

   f. Abnormal prenatal screening test results

   g. Parents are carriers of mendelian conditions, such as cystic fibrosis, hemophilia, muscular dystrophy, Tay-Sachs disease, inborn errors of metabolism, or hemoglobinopathies

   h. All women regardless of age should have the option for genetic screening or diagnostic testing.

B. Objective

1. Gestational age

2. Results of prenatal screening tests for aneuploidy, ultrasound evaluations, and carrier screening status of parents

3. Rh status, hemoglobin electrophoresis, MCV

III. Assessment

Patient desires/declines CVS, amniocentesis, or preimplantation genetic diagnosis

IV. Goals for Clinical Management

A. Establish patient desires for genetic testing using principles of informed consent and shared decision making.

B. Identify infants with specific genetic defects and neural tube disorders previous to birth in requesting families.

C. Give families information in order to prepare for an affected child or allow for pregnancy termination.

V. Plan

A. Diagnosis

1. Refer patient for preimplantation genetic diagnosis, CVS, or amniocentesis during appropriate testing window.

B. Education and Counseling

1. Review the risks and benefits of procedures; include comparisons to screening tests.

2. Provide genetic counseling prior to testing; patients should return to their genetic counselors for reporting and interpretation of test results.

3. A positive diagnosis result is delivered to the patient by a knowledgeable healthcare provider. Provide accurate and balanced information as soon as possible, in the patient's preferred language, and in a private setting. Use neutral language, in a sensitive and caring manner while avoiding value judgments (Sheets et al., 2011); offer in-person follow-up.

4. Consider referral to social workers, parent support networks, clergy, and therapeutic counselors for further support and information.

C. Medication

1. Rh-negative nonsensitized women need Rh (D) immune globulin (Rhogam) administration after CVS or amniocentesis.

REFERENCES

ACOG Committee on Genetics. (2005). ACOG committee opinion. Number 318, October 2005. Screening for Tay-Sachs disease. *Obstetrics and Gynecology, 106*(4), 893–894.

ACOG Committee on Genetics. (2009). ACOG committee opinion no. 442: Preconception and prenatal carrier screening for genetic diseases in individuals of Eastern European Jewish descent. *Obstetrics and Gynecology, 114*(4), 950–953.

ACOG Committee on Genetics. (2010). ACOG committee opinion no. 469: Carrier screening for fragile X syndrome. *Obstetrics and Gynecology, 116*(4), 1008–1010.

ACOG Committee on Genetics. (2011). ACOG committee opinion no. 486: Update on carrier screening for cystic fibrosis. *Obstetrics and Gynecology, 117*(4), 1028–1031.

ACOG Committee on Genetics. (2012). Noninvasive prenatal testing for fetal aneuploidy. Committee opinion no. 545: Noninvasive prenatal testing for fetal aneuploidy. *Obstetrics and Gynecology, 120*(6), 1532–1534.

ACOG Committee on Obstetrics. (2007). ACOG practice bulletin no. 78: Hemoglobinopathies in pregnancy. *Obstetrics and Gynecology, 109*(1), 229–237.

American College of Obstetricians and Gynecologists. (2014). ACOG technology assessment no. 11: Genetics and molecular diagnostic testing. *Obstetrics and Gynecology, 123*(2, Pt. 1), 394–413.

Baer, R. J., Norton, M., Shaw. G., Flessel, M. C., Goldman, S., Currier, R. J., et al. (2014). Risk of selected structural abnormalities in infants after increased nuchal translucency measurement. *American Journal of Obstetrics and Gynecology, 211*(6), 675–719.

Bianchi, D. W., Prosen, T., Platt, L. D., Goldberg, J. D., Abuhamad, A. Z., Rava, R. P., et al. (2013). Massively parallel sequencing of maternal plasma DNA in 113 cases of fetal nuchal cystic hygroma). *Obstetrics and Gynecology, 121*(5), 1057–1062.

California Department of Public Health. (2014). California Prenatal Screening Program. Retrieved from www.cdph.ca.gov/pns.

Gil, M M, Quezada, M S, Revello, R, Akolekar, R. & Nicolaides, K.H. (2015). Analysis of cell-free DNA in maternal blood in screening for fetal aneuploidies: Updated meta-analysis. *Ultrasound in Obstetrics & Gynecology, 45*(3), 249-66.

Grody, W., Thompson, B., Gregg, A., Bean, L. H., Monaghan, K. G., Schneider, A., et al. (2013). ACMG position statement on prenatal/preconception expanded carrier screening. *Genetic Medicine, 15*(6), 482–483.

Han, C. S., & Platt, L. D. (2014). Noninvasive prenatal testing: Need for informed enthusiasm. *American Journal of Obstetrics and Gynecology, 211*(6), 577–580.

Langlois, S., Benn, P., & Wilkins-Haug, L. (2015). Current controversies in prenatal diagnosis 4: Pre-conception expanded carrier screening should replace all current prenatal screening for specific single gene disorders. *Prenatal Diagnosis, 35*(1), 23–28.

Larion, S., Warsof, S. L., & Romary, L. (2014). Uptake of noninvasive prenatal testing at a large academic referral center. *American Journal of Obstetrics and Gynecology. 211*(6), 651–657.

Lazarin, G. A., Haque, I. S., Nazareth, S., Iori, K., Patterson, A. S., Jacobson, J. L., et al. (2013). An empirical estimate of carrier frequencies for 400+ causal mendelian variants: Results from an ethnically diverse clinical sample of 23,453 individuals. *Genetics in Medicine, 15*(3), 178–186.

Minkoff, H., & Berkowitz, R. (2014). The case for universal prenatal genetic counseling. *Obstetrics and Gynecology, 123*(6), 1335–1338.

Norton, M. E., Brar, H., Weiss, J., Karimi, A., Laurent, L. C., Caughey, A. B., et al. (2012). Non-invasive chromosomal evaluation (NICE) study: Results of a multicenter prospective cohort study for detection of fetal trisomy 21 and trisomy 18. *American Journal of Obstetrics and Gynecology, 207*(2), 137–138.

Sheets, K., Crissman, B., Feist, C., Sell, S. L., Johnson, L. R., Donahue, K. C., et al. (2011). Practice guidelines for communicating a prenatal or postnatal diagnosis of down syndrome: Recommendations of the national society of genetic counselors. journal of genetic counseling. *Journal of Genetic Counseling, 20*(5), 432–441.

Wienke, S., Brown, K., Farmer, M., & Strange, C. (2014). Expanded carrier screening panels-does bigger mean better? *Journal of Community Genetics, 5*(2), 191–198.

CHAPTER 28

THE RETURN PRENATAL VISIT

Rebekah Kaplan and Margaret Hutchison

I. Definition and background

The purpose of return prenatal visits is to evaluate the pregnancy through ongoing health, nutritional, and psychosocial assessments. Referrals within the healthcare system and assistance with movement toward positive health behavior changes are also integral parts of the prenatal care process. The frequency and content of prenatal visits can be tailored to the specific needs of each client (medical risk factors, psychosocial needs, and parity).

The format of care delivery may also vary depending on the site. Although most prenatal care in the United States is still structured around one-to-one visits with a medical care provider, there is increasing use of group-based prenatal care models, most notably CenteringPregnancy. For sites using CenteringPregnancy, care is moved out of the examination room and into a group space, and cohorts of 8–12 women go through pregnancy together. Each of the 10 Centering sessions includes three components: Women receive medical assessment, health education with interactive learning, and social support within the group space. Randomized controlled trial research has shown that women who participate in CenteringPregnancy, when compared with women in one-to-one care, are less likely to have a premature birth, more likely to be satisfied with care, and feel more prepared for labor and childbirth (Ickovics et al., 2007). Numerous other studies support these findings and suggest other positive health outcomes associated with CenteringPregnancy (Baldwin, 2006; Tilden, Hersh, Emeis, Weinstein, & Caughey, 2014).

For more information on the CenteringPregnancy model, go to www.centeringhealthcare.org/.

Table 28-1 provides a summary of the Essential Elements of CenteringPregnancy.

II. Database

A. Subjective

1. Gestational age
2. Estimated delivery date: review dating
3. Problems or concerns since her last visit (e.g., uterine activity, change in vaginal discharge, or psychosocial issues)
4. Follow-up on problems from previous visit (e.g., nausea, back pain, fetal position, psychosocial issues)
5. Follow-up on problems from "problem list" (e.g., Was medication taken for urinary tract infection? Is housing issue resolved?)
6. Danger signs (e.g., signs of spontaneous abortion, preterm labor, urinary tract infection, preeclampsia, or intimate partner violence) (**Table 28-2**)
7. History and health screening review (current pregnancy, obstetric, medical, family, psychosocial-including depression and violence, and nutrition). The Family Violence Prevention Fund recommends screening for intimate partner violence and abuse at each prenatal visit (**Table 28-3**).
8. Consults: Results and management plans (physician, social worker, public health nurse, and so forth)

B. Objective

1. Vital signs and urine
   a. Weight
   b. Blood pressure
   c. Urinalysis: if indicated to screen for preeclampsia or urinary tract infection (evidence does not support routine urine screening in low-risk women [Alto, 2005; Siddique, Lantos, VanderWeele, & Lauderdale, 2012])
2. Laboratory data
   a. Results for current problems (e.g., urine dip or wet mount)
   b. Are laboratory values up to date? (e.g., chest radiograph after a positive purified protein derivative, third-trimester testing for group B streptococcus) (**Table 28-4**)

TABLE 28-1 CenteringPregnancy®: Essential Elements

The following are what are considered to be the "Essential Elements" of CenteringPregnancy, with a brief description of the significance of each element. These function as the guiding precepts that make prenatal care conducted in a group setting "centering."

1. Health assessment occurs within the group space.
   Normalizes pregnancy and prenatal care

2. Participants are involved in self-care activities.
   Promotes sense of self-efficacy

3. A facilitative leadership style is used.
   Promotes sense of self-efficacy, supports community building

4. The group is conducted in a circle.
   Supports open, nonhierarchic communications

5. Each session has an overall plan.
   There is an agenda for each session

6. Attention is given to the core content, although emphasis may vary.
   The facilitative leadership model supports flexibility in discussion content, as dictated by the needs of the group

7. There is stability of group leadership.
   Group leaders (a provider/nonprovider team) become trusted members of the group

8. Group conduct honors the contributions of each member.
   Creating a safe group environment supports group cohesion and learning

9. The composition of the group is stable but not rigid.
   Supports community -building and development of trust among participants

10. Group size is optimal to promote the process.
    8–12 pregnant participants are recommended; supports optimal engagement by of participants, sustainable use of staff

11. Involvement of family support people is optional.
    Support people included as determined by site

12. Opportunity for socializing within the group is provided.
    Supports community building

13. There is ongoing evaluation of outcomes.
    Given challenges inherent in prenatal care system redesign, supports sustainability

Modified from materials developed by the Centering Healthcare Institute (used with permission).

3. Physical examination
   a. General appearance (e.g., new striae or signs of depression)
   b. Abdominal examination
      i. Fundal height: measure by landmarks before 22–24 weeks, then with measuring tape (from the superior border of the symphysis pubis to the fundus)
      ii. Leopold's maneuvers (position and presentation) after 32–36 weeks
      iii. Estimated fetal weight after 36 weeks
   c. Fetal heart rate
      i. Doppler 9–12 weeks
      ii. Fetoscope 18–20 weeks
      iii. Ultrasound after 6–7 weeks (if indicated)
   d. Other physical examination as indicated by client problems or concerns (e.g., costovertebral angle tenderness or vaginal discharge)

TABLE 28-2 Signs of Pregnancy Complications

First Trimester
- Vaginal bleeding
- Fever, chills, dysuria
- Persistent nausea and vomiting

Second and Third Trimesters
- Vaginal bleeding
- Fever, chills, dysuria, flank pain
- Uterine cramping or contractions
- Leaking of amniotic fluid
- Decreased fetal movement
- Severe headache without relief from analgesics
- Visual changes (blurry vision or seeing spots)
- Pelvic pressure
- Continuous pruritus without rash (with affected palms and soles)

III. Assessment

A. *Gestational age/fetal size:*

1. Establish due date using best criteria if not previously done (**Table 26-5**)

2. Identify any size and date discrepancy

TABLE 28-3 Abuse Assessment Screen

1. Have you ever been emotionally or physically abused by your partner or someone important to you?

   ❏ YES ❏ NO

2. Within the last year, have you been hit, slapped, kicked, or otherwise physically hurt by someone?

   ❏ YES ❏ NO

   If YES, by whom? _____

   Total number of times: _____

3. Since you've been pregnant, were you hit, slapped, kicked, or otherwise physically hurt by someone?

   ❏ YES ❏ NO

   If YES, by whom? _____

   Total number of times: _____

Adapted from Centers for Disease Control and Prevention. (2007). *Intimate partner violence and sexual violence victimization assessment instruments.* Retrieved from http://www.cdc.gov/violenceprevention /pdf/ipv/ipvandsvscreening.pdf

TABLE 28-4 Timing of Testing/Procedures for Women Without Significant Medical Risk Factors

Initial visit (see Chapter 26, Obstetric Health Maintenance and Promotion: The Initial Prenatal Visit)
8–20 weeks
- $10–13^6$ weeks: offer first-trimester serum genetic screening test
- $11^2–14^2$ weeks: offer ultrasound for nuchal translucency
- 15–20 weeks: offer second-trimester serum genetic screening test

Diagnostic/screening testing and vaccines as indicated
- 10+ weeks: noninvasive prenatal testing (cell-free DNA)
- 10–14 weeks: chorionic villi sampling
- 15–20 weeks: amniocentesis
- 18–20 weeks: fetal survey screening ultrasound
- 26–28 weeks: complete blood count, 1-hour glucose load test, antibody screen if rhesus factor negative; if indicated, venereal disease reference laboratory, HIV
- 27-36 weeks: Tdap vaccine (American College of Obstetricians and Gynecologists [ACOG], 2013b)
- 32–36 weeks: if indicated, repeat sexually transmitted infection testing
- 35–37 weeks: group B *Streptococcus* (GBS) culture

TABLE 28-5 When to Redate a Pregnancy by Ultrasound Findings

Gestational Age Range (Based on LMP)	Method of Measurement	Discrepancy Between Ultrasound Dating and LMP Dating That Supports Redating
≤ 8 6/7 wk	CRL	More than 5 days
9 0/7 to 13 6/7 wk	CRL	More than 7 days
14 0/7 to 15 6/7	BPD, HC, AC, FL	More than 7 days
16 0/7 wk to 21 6/7 wk	BPD, HC, AC, FL	More than 10 days
22 0/7 wk to 27 6/7 wk	BPD, HC, AC, FL	More than 14 days
28 0/7 wk and beyond	BPD, HC, AC, FL	More than 21 days

Abbreviations: AC, abdominal circumference; BPD, biparietal diameter; CRL, crown–rump length; FL, femur length; HC, head circumference; LMP, last menstrual period.

Reproduced from ACOG. (2014). ACOG committee opinion No 611: Method for estimating due date. *Obstetrics and Gynecology, 124*(4), 863–866.

B. *Differential diagnosis:*

1. Establish for identified abnormal physical examination or laboratory findings (e.g., anemia, preterm labor, or urinary tract infection)

C. *Determine appropriateness of weight gain and nutritional status (Tables 28-6 and 28-7)*

D. *Determine prenatal educational needs*

E. *Identify psychosocial issues (e.g., food insecurity, violence, immigration problems, housing, or social isolation)*

F. *Role assessment: identify the need for consultation or collaborative management with other health team members*

IV. Goals of clinical management

A. *Identify medical, nutritional, and psychosocial problems and risk factors and develop a plan of care for each problem*

B. *Anticipatory guidance related to pregnancy, birth, parenting, and medical care*

C. *Individualize care to meet both the family and medical needs and maximize maternal and fetal well-being*

TABLE 28-6 Recommended Pattern of Weight Gain for Pregnancy

First trimester 1.1–4.4 lb
Rates for second and third trimesters by body mass index (BMI)
• Underweight—BMI less than 18.5: 1 lb/wk (1–1.3): TWG 28–40 lbs
• Normal weight—BMI 18.5–24.9: 1 lb/wk (0.8–1): TWG 25–35 lbs
• Overweight—BMI 25–29.9: 0.6 lb/wk (0.5–0.7): TWG 15–25 lbs
• Obese (all classes)—BMI 30 or greater: 0.5 lb/wk (0.4–0.6): TWG 11–20 lbs

Abbreviation: TWG, total weight gain.

Data from Institute of Medicine. (2009). *Report brief. Weight gain during pregnancy: Reexamining the guidelines.* Washington, DC: National Academies Press; ACOG. (2013a). ACOG committee opinion no. 548: Weight gain during pregnancy. *Obstetrics and Gynecology, 121*(1), 210–212.

TABLE 28-7 Daily Dietary Needs for Normal-Weight Women

Second and third trimesters: Approximately 300 additional calories a day (e.g., 8 oz 1% milk, one hardboiled egg, and one apple)
• Protein: 60 g (teenagers, 75–80 g)
• Grains: 6 oz
• Vegetables: 2.5 cups
• Fruit: 2 cups
• Calcium: 1,000 mg

V. Plan (Figure 28-1)

A. *Laboratory*

1. Laboratory or diagnostic testing (Table 28-4)

2. Other laboratory tests needed related to physical examination findings (e.g., urine culture, chlamydia test, or anemia work-up)

3. Follow-up on any previous abnormal laboratory studies

B. *Medication*

1. Refill prenatal vitamins as necessary

2. Supplementation: calcium, fish oil, vitamin D_3, and iron if deficient

3. Treatment of specific problems (e.g., urinary tract infection or vaginitis)

C. *Education and counseling*

1. Client concerns

2. Current laboratory data

3. Weight gain and diet

4. Teaching appropriate to gestational age and client needs (Figures 28-1 and 26-1)

5. Danger signs of pregnancy (e.g., spontaneous abortion, preterm labor, and preeclampsia)

6. Emotional preparation for motherhood

7. Exercise, stress management, and behavior modification

D. *Refer for consultation or antepartum fetal evaluation*

1. Refer any clients as indicated for physician consultation or transfer of care (see Chapter 30 on guidelines for medical consultation and referral

FIGURE 28-1 *Prenatal Care Flow Sheet*

8–14 Weeks	15–20 Weeks	20–28 Weeks
LABS/TESTS	**LABS/TESTS/VACCINES**	**LABS/TESTS**
Sono/dating	Quadruple marker screen	CBC, glucose load test
Blood type, Rh, antibody screen complete blood count (CBC), Hgb electrophoresis	Sono fetal survey (18–20 weeks)	(26–28 weeks)
Rapid plasma reagin (RPR), rubella, varicella (by hx or titers), HIV, purified protein derivative (PPD), hepatitis B surface antigen	Flu vaccine (Oct–May)	HIV, RPR (if indicated)
Urine culture + sensitivity (C+S), urine dip screening		
Pap (if due), GC/Chlamydia		
First-trimester diagnostic screen		
Nuchal translucency		
SELECTIVE TESTING	**SELECTIVE TESTING**	**SELECTIVE TESTING**
Early glucose load test, fasting glucose and/or hemoglobin A1C	Amniocentesis	3-hour glucose tolerance test
Hepatitis C	Early glucose load test or hemoglobin A1c	Antibody screen
Urine toxicology screen	Urine toxicology screen	Rhogam at 28 weeks (or with any vaginal bleeding) in Rh-negative woman
Chorionic villus sampling, noninvasive DNA testing	Chest x-ray (if + PPD)	
Cystic fibrosis, Ashkenazi screening	Urine C+S	
Genetic screening based on family medical history/ethnicity	Hepatitis B vaccine (high-risk behaviors)	
Refusal of blood products consent	Level 2 ultrasound, fetal echo	
EDUCATION	**EDUCATION**	**EDUCATION**
Orientation to clinic/service	Breastfeeding (BF) benefits	Signs/symptoms preterm labor (PTL)
Prenatal Classes referral	Exclusive breast milk 6 months	Contraception
Danger signs	BF class referral	Danger signs
Common discomforts	Fetal movement and quickening	Fetal movement
Nutrition, weight gain, and exercise	Exercise in pregnancy	Vaginal birth after cesarean/trial of labor (VBAC/TOL) discussion
Genetic testing options	Common discomforts	Postpartum tubal ligation (PPTL) class referral (PPTL papers can be signed after 17 weeks)
OTC/Rx med use	Danger signs	
Drug, tobacco, and alcohol use		Breastfeeding benefits
Dental services information		Exercise in pregnancy
		Attended breastfeeding class
		Attended Prenatal Classes

(continues)

FIGURE 28-1 *Prenatal Care Flow Sheet* (Continued)

28–32 Weeks

LABS/TESTS/VACCINES

Optional/Indicated

Antenatal testing

Kick counts

Tdap (recommended between 27–36 weeks)

EDUCATION

Contraception

Birth control method _____

Consent signed ❑

Attended PPTL class ❑

VBAC/TOL consent ❑

Signs and symptoms of PTL

Other danger signs

Newborn procedures

Referral to birth prep class ❑

32–37 Weeks

LABS/TESTS/VACCINES

GBS (35–37 weeks)

Tdap

Optional/Indicated

Antenatal testing

Disability

EDUCATION

Early initiation of breastfeeding

Skin to skin and rooming in

Latch, infant feeding cues

BF and returning to work

Colostrum and milk production

BF resources

Circumcision

Danger signs

Signs and symptoms labor

Infant car seat and baby supplies

Choosing a pediatric provider

Last chance for PPTL papers

37–41 Weeks

LABS/TESTS

Optional/Indicated

Antenatal testing: NST/AFI

(after 41 weeks)

EDUCATION

Labor comfort measures

Pain management options

Signs and symptoms labor

Managing early labor at home

Fetal monitoring options

Birth plan

Danger signs

Going past due date

(induction 41–42 weeks)

Attended labor prep class

Pain control preference

_____

Support system

_____

Pediatric provider

_____

Courtesy of Community Health Network of San Francisco, Department of Public Health.

during pregnancy) or for genetics, nutrition, or social services.

2. Initiate and refer for fetal evaluation and antenatal testing if indicated (**Table 28-8**)

E. *Update problem list*

1. Add or resolve any outstanding problems or concerns

F. *Follow-up visit*

1. This should be flexible and individualized based on client needs, parity, and risk following a standard or reduced visit schedule reviewed in Chapter 26, Obstetric Health Maintenance and Promotion: The Initial Prenatal Visit.

2. Postterm pregnancy (see **Table 28-9**)

TABLE 28-8 Antepartum Fetal Evaluation

Conditions posing risk for fetal compromise include, but are not limited to:

- Postterm pregnancy; hypertensive disease; fetal growth restriction; diabetes; previous unexplained stillbirth; decreased fetal movement; abnormal analytes on serum genetic screening tests; increased serum human chorionic gonadotropin; cholestasis of pregnancy; twins with discordant growth; BMI greater than or equal to 40; preterm premature rupture of membranes; oligohydramnios; unexplained severe polyhydramnios; rhesus factor isoimmunization; active substance abuse; lupus; gastroschisis; and medical problems (e.g., cardiac disease, hyperthyroidism)

Management

- Review of dating criteria
- Leopold's for good estimation of fetal weight

Initiation of testing

- Begin testing at the gestational age at which the provider is willing to intervene to save the life of the fetus balanced with the age at which one would expect to detect abnormal testing (generally 34–36 weeks)

Methods of testing

- Fetal movement assessments (kick counts)
- Nonstress test
- Amniotic fluid index
- Vibroacoustic stimulation
- Biophysical profile
- Contraction stress test

First line:

No consistent evidence suggests that formal kick counts decrease incidence of intrauterine fetal demise, although the method is widely used in practice for higher-risk pregnancies (Darby-Stewart, Strickland, & Jamieson, 2009).

Second line:

Modified biophysical profile: nonstress test plus amniotic fluid index.

If modified biophysical profile is not reassuring, consult for biophysical profile, Doppler flow studies, and induction of labor after a contraction stress test.

TABLE 28-9 Postterm Pregnancy

Definitions

- Term delivery is considered between 37–42 weeks.
- Early Term: 37 wks + 0 days to 38 wks + 6 days
- Full Term: 39 wks + 0 days to 40 wks + 6 days
- Late Term: 41 wks + 0 days to 41 wks + 6 days
- Postterm: 42 wks +

Management

- Examine cervix; Bishop's score greater than 5 is favorable for induction of labor
- Consider sweeping membranes at 38–41 weeks
- Consider alternative methods of induction

Education

- Counsel risks and benefits of induction versus expectant management

Follow-up

- Biweekly antenatal testing (nonstress test [NST], amniotic fluid index [AFI]) by 41 weeks, gestation
- Kick counts should be initiated at 40–41 weeks
- Offer induction of labor between 41–42 weeks

Data from ACOG. (2013c). ACOG committee opinion no. 579: Definition of term pregnancy. *Obstetrics and Gynecology, 122*(5), 1139–1140.

REFERENCES

Alto, W. A. (2005). No need for glycosuria/proteinuria screen in pregnant women. *Journal of Family Practice, 54*(11), 978–983.

American College of Obstetricians and Gynecologists. (2013a). ACOG committee opinion no. 548: Weight gain during pregnancy. *Obstetrics and Gynecology, 121*(1), 210–212.

American College of Obstetricians and Gynecologists. (2013b). ACOG committee opinion no. 566: Update on immunization and pregnancy: tetanus, diphtheria, and pertussis vaccination. *Obstetrics and Gynecology, 121*(6), 1411–1414.

American College of Obstetricians and Gynecologists. (2013c). ACOG committee opinion no. 579: Definition of term pregnancy. *Obstetrics and Gynecology, 122*(5), 1139–1140.

American College of Obstetricians and Gynecologists. (2014). ACOG committee opinion no. 611: Method for estimating due date. *Obstetrics and Gynecology, 124*(4), 863–866.

Baldwin, K. A. (2006). Comparison of selected outcomes of centering pregnancy versus traditional prenatal care. *Journal of Midwifery & Women's Health, 51*(4), 266–272.

Centers for Disease Control and Prevention. (2007). *Intimate partner violence and sexual violence victimization assessment instruments.* Retrieved from http://www.cdc.gov/violenceprevention/pdf/ipv/ipvandsvscreening.pdf.

Darby-Stewart, A. L., Strickland, C. & Jamieson, B. (2009). Do abnormal fetal kick counts predict intrauterine death in average-risk pregnancies? *Journal of Family Practice, 58*(4), 220a–220c.

Ickovics, J. R., Kershaw, T. S., Westdahl, C., Magriples, U., Massey, Z., Reynolds, H., et al. (2007). Group prenatal care and perinatal outcomes: A randomized controlled trial. *Obstetrics & Gynecology, 110*(2, Pt. 1), 330–339.

Institute of Medicine. (2009). *Report brief. Weight gain during pregnancy: Reexamining the guidelines.* Washington, DC: National Academies Press.

Siddique, J., Lantos, J. D., VanderWeele, T. J., & Lauderdale, D. S. (2012). Screening tests during prenatal care: Does practice follow the evidence? *Maternal and Child Health Journal, 16*(1), 51–59.

Tilden, E. L., Hersh, S. R., Emeis, C. L., Weinstein, S. R., & Caughey, A. B. (2014). Group prenatal care: Review of outcomes and recommendations for model implementation. *Obstetrical and Gynecological Survey, 69*(1), 46–55.

THE POSTPARTUM VISIT

CHAPTER 29

Jenna Shaw-Battista and Holly Cost

I. Introduction and general background

The postpartum period is a time of tremendous physical and emotional change for new mothers. Although childbearing women experience the most profound adaptations during this 6–8 week period, their partners, older children, extended family, and community may also experience significant transitions (Declerq, Sakala, Corry, Applebaum, & Herrlich, 2013). The goals of family-centered postpartum care include skilled support for optimal health during the transition with the prevention, identification, management, and resolution of abnormal physical, psychologic, and psychosocial adaptations. Postpartum visits include monitoring and education related to parturition complications with short-term or lifelong health implications. They serve as a transition from obstetric to primary health care with opportunities to initiate or resume routine screening and health maintenance activities.

There is little research on optimal postpartum care, and no evidence to support some routine counseling and recommendations often made by healthcare providers in the postpartum period, e.g., stair climbing and lifting restrictions (Minig et al., 2006). However, accurate health education and promotion activities may be particularly effective in the postpartum period because many new mothers have knowledge deficits (Declerq et al., 2013) and most are highly motivated to make lifestyle and other changes to improve their health and that of their growing family. The postpartum period is also a key time for interventions because perinatal care is often the entry point into health care for marginalized populations whose healthcare access and use may decrease between pregnancies (DiBari, Yu, Chao, & Lu, 2014) and who experience disparate adverse perinatal outcomes with lifelong implications for survivors. Postpartum education may include self- and infant care, symptoms that require immediate evaluation, and recommendations for primary care and health promoting activities such as exercise, healthful nutrition, breastfeeding, immunizations, sleep hygiene, child safety, contraception, and sexually transmitted infection prevention.

New mothers commonly appreciate opportunities to discuss their experience of childbirth and early parenting, although there are few data to guide the format or content of these conversations. Women may desire to review clinical details and ask questions to "fill in the blanks" in their childbirth memories (Rowan, Bick, & Bastos 2007). They may not have anticipated the intensity of the experience and benefit from reassurance that their coping behaviors and choices were respected. Postpartum care providers can prioritize sensitive and effective therapeutic communications because vulnerability, changes in self-perception, uncertainty, and disequilibrium are common during the postpartum role transition (Association of Women's Health, Obstetric and Neonatal Nurses [AWHONN], 2006). Ideally, women are provided an opportunity for a postpartum visit conducted by the provider who attended their labor and birth after visits in pregnancy, to extend or facilitate new continuity of care, exchange of information, and feedback (Barimani, Oxelmark, Johansson & Highland; Sandall, Soltani, Gates, Shennan, & Devane, 2015).

This chapter uses the SOAP (subjective, objective, assessment, and plan) note format to outline essential elements of postpartum care, which should be customized for individual women. The timing, number, and content of postpartum visits vary (Haran, van Driel, Mitchell, & Brodribb, 2014). Women are typically followed daily during their inpatient postpartum stay and scheduled for outpatient follow-up one or more times 1–8 weeks later (Declerq et al., 2013; Haran et al., 2014), per individual risk factors and recommendations by the American Academy of Pediatrics (AAP) and the American College of Obstetricians and Gynecologists (ACOG) (2012). The timing of the standard 6-week postpartum visit may be based on tradition as much as research, as well as the understanding that uterine involution is typically complete then (Speroff & Mishell, 2008).

Six weeks may be too late to detect or prevent some postpartum complications or to provide optimal contraceptive counseling because many women resume sexual intercourse before this time (Jackson & Glasier, 2011; Speroff & Mishell, 2008). Women may be examined earlier or more frequently, or visits may be supplemented with telephone encounters (Lavender,

Richens, Milan, Smyth, & Dowswell, 2013), to follow-up on birth complications, when significant risk factors for adverse postpartum conditions are present or for other reasons such as breastfeeding difficulties, management of chronic or perinatal health conditions, or optimal timing of birth control initiation. For example, women who gave birth by cesarean section may be evaluated 1–2 weeks postpartum with targeted assessments for postoperative complications including trauma, excessive blood loss, anemia, thrombophlebitis, oliguria, and infection, e.g., surgical wound infections that most commonly present 3–8 days postpartum (AWHONN, 2006). A 1–2 week postpartum visit may also be helpful to evaluate mother–infant bonding, mood, risks for discontinuing breastfeeding, and family support and integration (Yonemoto, Dowswell, Nagai, & Mori, 2013).

Appointment reminders or incentives may increase postpartum visit attendance and prove particularly useful in the care of high-risk populations, e.g., women with a history of mood disorders or adolescent mothers (Stevens-Simon, O'Connor, & Bassford, 1994). Perinatal outcomes may also be improved in vulnerable and high-risk populations with home visits, phone calls, web-based programs, and referrals to postpartum education, fitness classes, and peer support groups, among other interventions (Teychenne & York, 2013; Thomson, Dykes, Hurley, & Hoddinott, 2012). Counseling, social support facilitation, reinforcement of healthful coping strategies, and discussion of role transition and self-perception alterations may help to reestablish psychologic equilibrium (MacArthur et al., 2003; Ruchat & Mottola, 2012), particularly for women who experienced unanticipated obstetrical procedures, emergencies or trauma related to pregnancy and childbirth (Andersen, Melvaer, Videbech, Lamont, & Joergensen, 2012; Gamble & Creedy, 2009; Shaw, Levitt, Wong, & Kaczorowski, 2006). Women who experienced perinatal loss, had an infant removed from their custody by child protective services, placed their infant with an adoptive family, or served as a surrogate mother may require unique or additional supports during their postpartum transition. In addition to considerations of women's health status and risk factors, the time elapsed since childbirth informs the type of screening, intervention, education, and referrals provided in postpartum visits.

II. Database (may include but is not limited to)

Data may be gleaned from postpartum patient interviews and review of medical records when available.

A. Subjective data

1. History of medical conditions, antenatal, intrapartum, or postpartum complications requiring follow-up, including:
   a. Mental health conditions including mood and anxiety disorders
   b. Endocrine disorders (e.g., thyroid disorder and preexisting or gestational, type 1, or type 2 diabetes mellitus)
   c. Hypertension (e.g., chronic or gestational hypertension or preeclampsia–eclampsia)
   d. Infectious processes such as sexually transmitted infections, latent tuberculosis, or chronic hepatitis infection
   e. Body mass index (BMI) outside the normal range
   f. Tobacco exposure, either first or second hand
   g. Substance use disorders
   h. Intimate partner or family violence
   i. Psychosocial stressors including housing and food insecurity
   j. Any other primary care issues that may need to be addressed

2. Description of the woman's intrapartum experience, including:
   a. Date and type of birth and hospital postpartum course with information about any clinical variants or complications including perineal lacerations
   b. Her understanding and feelings about her labor and the birth of her infant; note and explore any traumatic feelings expressed about her experience, which may be most likely after obstetrical emergencies and unplanned cesarean or forceps-assisted vaginal birth (Andersen et al., 2012; Gamble & Creedy, 2009; Rowlands & Redshaw, 2012).

3. General health, well-being, and psychological status should be assessed screening for:
   a. Report of feeling generally unwell or specific symptoms, which may indicate primary health concerns or parturition complications including mood disorders (Cerimele et al., 2013).
   b. Self-care:
      i. What is the woman doing to care for herself?
      ii. Does she have the opportunity to get exercise and leave the house?
      iii. Can she nap/sleep when the baby sleeps?
      iv. If she sustained a perineal laceration, is she using sitz baths at home? How often?
   c. Adjustment, capabilities, and satisfaction with parenting
   d. Perinatal mood disorders, the most common postpartum complication
      i. Women with depression and/or anxiety frequently present with physical symptoms in primary care oriented visits during the first 12 months postpartum, which should prompt careful screening for risk factors and psychologic symptoms (Cerimele et al., 2013).

ii. Risk factors: History of depression or anxiety, perinatal loss, complications of pregnancy, hyperemesis, multiple gestation, major life events unrelated to pregnancy and childbirth, lack of support or resources, and social stigma, e.g., single or adolescent motherhood (Tharp & Farley, 2013).

iii. Symptoms: Inability to cope with demands of new role, disorganized daily routine, poor sleep hygiene, excessive fatigue that interferes with self- or infant care, depression or mania, anhedonia, frequent crying, insomnia, anxiety, hypervigilance, or thoughts of harming self or infant (Cerimele et al., 2013).

e. Postpartum psychosis, a medical emergency characterized by disorganized behavior, visual or auditory hallucination, and delusions (Tharp & Farley, 2013).

f. Posttraumatic stress disorder, which may recur due to childbirth-related stressors among women with a prior diagnosis or present for the first time as a consequence of trauma experienced during pregnancy and childbirth. Risk factors for new postpartum onset of posttraumatic stress disorder include subjective report of distress during labor, obstetrical emergencies, and unplanned mode of delivery (Andersen et al., 2012; Gamble & Creedy, 2009; Rowlands & Redshaw, 2012).

g. Substance use or abuse, which frequently co-occurs with perinatal mood disorders and intimate partner violence (AWHONN, 2006).

4. How is her infant?

a. Any health or growth issues?

b. Does the infant have pediatric care?

c. Is the infant in a safe sleeping environment at home and/or in other care situations

d. Using a car seat?

e. Ask about methods being used to soothe the infant—skin to skin, swaddling, movement, sounds

5. Infant feeding

a. If infant is nursing, determine if breastfeeding is exclusive or if there is formula supplementation.

i. If supplementation, how much and why?

ii. How is nursing going—any questions or concerns? Does the woman have support for nursing from her partner/family/friends?

iii. Does she feel her milk supply is adequate?

iv. How long does she plan to nurse? Does she plan to return to work, and if so, when? Will she have support for pumping and milk storage at work?

v. Does she have information about milk collection and storage? Does she need a breast pump?

b. If formula feeding, does she have information on how to properly make and store formula and how to properly clean bottles and nipples?

6. Nutrition status, including

a. Daily nutritional intake including adequacy of protein, calcium sources, and fruits and vegetables

b. Does she require additional support or education to obtain diet appropriate for lactation, iron deficiency, or other common postpartum circumstances?

c. Other nutritional risk factors such as BMI outside of the normal range, gestational diabetes, or eating disorders that would benefit from ongoing nutritional support

d. Any use of vitamins, minerals, herbs, or other supplements

e. Adequate water intake

7. Medications with dosage and indication, if any

8. Sexual health, including

a. Altered self-perception

b. Libido and satisfaction

c. Resumption of sexual activity and need for contraception

9. Family, social, and community integration and support

a. Bonding with infant

b. What types of physical and emotional support and daily help does she have?

c. Housing and economic status: Does she have what she needs to care for self and infant?

d. Any plans to start or return to work outside the home, with impact on infant care and feeding and self-care

e. Relationship conflict or interpersonal violence

f. Partner adjustment

g. Sibling, grandparent, extended family, and social support network adjustment

h. Cultural or religious practices in the postpartum period (Dennis et al., 2007)

10. Review of systems (screen for)

a. Breasts

i. Breast or nipple pain

ii. Masses or erythema noted

iii. Concerns about insufficient breast milk or infant feeding

b. Abdomen

i. Abdominal or uterine pain or cramping that has increased since delivery or is unrelieved with pain medication

    ii. Report of pain, redness, odor, or discharge at the site of a cesarean incision

  c. Pelvis, genitals, and lochia

    i. Pelvic pain, particularly over the symphysis pubis or coccyx, which may result from injury during childbirth

    ii. Vaginal, vulvar, or perineal pain that has increased since delivery or is unrelieved by pain medication, with or without edema

    iii. Abnormal, excessive or prolonged bleeding (e.g., fills pad in < 1–2 hours, large recurrent clots, lochia serosa or alba that reverts to lochia rubra, or lochia that persists beyond 6 weeks postpartum)

    iv. Foul-smelling lochia

    v. Resumption of menses

  d. Elimination

    i. Urinary, fecal, or flatus incontinence

    ii. Urinary retention

    iii. Dysuria

    iv. History of intrapartum or postpartum bladder catheterization, or other risk factors for urinary tract infection

    v. Constipation

  e. Extremities

    i. Calf pain, heat, or redness

    ii. Edema that increases or persists beyond 7 days postpartum, particularly if unilateral

B. Objective data

1. General well-being and psychologic status: Observe affect, eye contact, and appearance

2. Family integration: Observe interactions between mother, child, and family members present

3. Weight and vital signs

4. Head and neck

  a. Thyroid gland: palpate for size and nodularity

  b. Lymph nodes: palpate for size and tenderness

5. Breasts

  a. Observe size, color, and symmetry

  b. Palpate for tenderness, masses, and warmth

  c. Examine the nipples for cracks, fissures, bleeding, lesions, and compression stripes

  d. If possible, observe infant position and latch during breastfeeding

6. Abdomen

  a. Inspect and palpate for masses, tenderness, uterine involution, hernias, diastasis recti, and muscle tone

  b. Check surgical site for closure, pain, masses, exudate, and erythema if applicable, e.g., cesarean or postpartum tubal ligation

7. Pelvis, genitals, and lochia

  a. Palpate over symphysis pubis and coccyx if report of pain

  b. External genitalia and perineum

    i. Inspect for symmetry, excoriation, and varicosities

    ii. Assess any lacerations for approximation, exudate, and healing

    iii. Visualize the amount and appearance of lochia

    iv. Assess for leakage of urine

  c. Pelvic examination as indicated

    i. Vagina: assess for uterine prolapse, cystocele, or rectocele; check the strength of pelvic musculature during a Kegel exercise

    ii. Uterus: assess position, size, and tenderness

    iii. Cervix: assess os appearance and closure

  d. Rectal exam: Assess for hemorrhoids, fissures, fistulas, masses, and sphincter tone

8. Extremities

  a. Assess for calf pain, heat, or redness on inspection and palpation

  b. Assess for edema that increases or persists beyond 7 days postpartum or is unilateral

III. Assessment

Assessment should incorporate subjective and objective data and address the woman's physical, emotional, and social postpartum adaptation along with any complications noted.

IV. Goals for clinical management

The goals of family-centered postpartum care include skilled support for optimal health during the transition with the prevention, identification, management, and resolution of abnormal physical, psychologic, and psychosocial adaptations.

A. Identify women at risk for postpartum complications including mood disorders and individualize care to promote health and minimize harm.

B. Assess postpartum adjustment and support families during the postpartum transition period; provide care and referrals as needed.

C. Screen for dangers to the mother, baby, and family.

D. Breastfeeding support: Provide lactation care, anticipatory guidance, and nutritional counseling.

E. *Family planning: Provide families access to desired contraception and encourage a healthy pregnancy interval.*

F. *Identify and address health education, maintenance, and primary care needs; provide or refer as indicated by availability of services.*

V. Plan

A. Diagnostics

1. Laboratory testing as indicated by history or examination, for example
   a. Urine dipstick to assess for protein or nitrites if hypertensive or symptomatic for urinary tract infection
   b. Urine culture and sensitivity to rule out urinary tract infection
   c. Complete blood count to assess for infectious processes or anemia
   d. Wet mount to assess for vaginitis or infection
   e. Sexually transmitted infection testing
   f. Postpartum screening for women with diagnosis of gestational diabetes in pregnancy, e.g., a 2-hour, 75 gram oral glucose tolerance test performed 6–12 weeks after delivery (Leuridan et al., 2015).

2. Women's health screening as indicated
   a. Pap smear
   b. Occult fecal blood
   c. Mammography if not breastfeeding
   d. Screening tests indicated by age or health history, such as hemoglobin or lipid profile (results confounded by breastfeeding)

B. Treatment and follow-up

1. Visit schedule and providers
   a. Daily inpatient postpartum visits by a maternity or primary care provider is standard, with outpatient follow-up one or more times, 1–8 weeks later (Haran et al., 2014)
   b. Early or repeated outpatient visits or telephone consultations may be indicated for women who experienced obstetrical complications or have adverse health conditions or other risk factors for postpartum complications (Lavender et al., 2013).
   c. Visits should be conducted by competent and qualified providers, ideally with access to medical records if continuity of care is not feasible or desired by the patient. Visits may be performed by interprofessional team members such as physicians, registered nurses, lactation consultants, nutritionists, social workers, therapists, psychologists or psychiatrists, and health educators in addition to, or instead of, nurse practitioners and nurse-midwives (MacArthur et al., 2003).

2. Medications and therapeutics
   a. Continue daily prenatal vitamins or multivitamin during lactation if diet is lacking in whole foods, variety and balance (AAP & ACOG, 2012).
   b. Other medications as warranted by subjective and objective data (e.g., stool softener, analgesics, antibiotics).
   c. Consider recommending or supplying vaginal lubricant due to vaginal dryness commonly reported during lactation.
   d. Vaccinations such as influenza and Tdap (if not given during pregnancy); measles, mumps, rubella; varicella; or hepatitis A and B vaccines, with reminders and follow-up appointments as required for series.
   e. Contraception initiation will depend on lactation, desired method, and timing of resumption of sexual activity. Contraceptive methods and return to fertility are included in antepartum teaching to ensure informed consent and develop a postpartum implementation plan in advance.
      i. Estrogen-containing hormonal contraception is not generally recommended until 6 weeks postpartum, because of the increased risk of venous thromboembolism secondary to the resolving hypercoaguable state of pregnancy (Speroff & Mishell, 2008). In addition, there are some concerns about estrogen affecting milk supply, although research findings are inconclusive (Tepper, Phillips, Kapp, Gaffield, & Curtis, 2015).
      ii. If women have difficulty accessing care or managing their fertility, access to long-acting reversible contraceptives such as intrauterine devices or hormonal implants may be provided in the immediate postpartum period to avoid the risk of unintended pregnancy (Speroff & Mishell, 2008). An immediate postpartum intrauterine contraceptive may be placed under ultrasound guidance following delivery of the placenta. Although expulsion rates are higher following placement immediately versus 4–8 weeks postpartum, pregnancy prevention is effective when the device is retained.

iii. Women may benefit from a prescription for emergency contraception in case of contraceptive failure.

f. Therapeutics for postpartum conditions or complications, including

i. Discomfort from genital edema and perineal laceration is often treated with application of witch hazel, topical analgesia, local cooling with ice or gel packs (Minassian & Jazayeri, 2002; Moore & James, 1989), and/or hydrotherapy sitz baths, which are thought to promote healing as well as comfort despite limited supportive data (Aderhold & Perry, 1991; East, Begg, Henshall, Marchant, & Wallace, 2012). Complementary therapies commonly used for these purposes despite little to no evidence base include topical castor oil and herbal perineal packs.

ii. Compression stockings and hydrotherapy may be considered for symptomatic varicosities.

iii. A pelvic brace or binder may reduce discomfort from pelvic girdle pain or symphysis pubis mobility and separation. In severe cases, a walker or cane may be indicated.

C. Patient education

1. Answer questions and address concerns of the postpartum woman and her family, which often include

a. Clarifying questions about the labor and birth experience, and any impact of complications or procedures on future health or childbearing (Declercq et al., 2013)

b. Recovery after cesarean birth (AWHONN, 2006; Tharp & Farley, 2013)

i. Postoperative self-care and pain management

ii. Alternate infant feeding positions per maternal comfort, e.g., football hold (infant is not on incision) or side-lying (abdominal muscles are not engaged through feeding)

iii. Possible discomforts from surgery or anesthesia, e.g., edema and constipation

iv. Surgical complications such as excessive blood loss, thrombophlebitis, oliguria, and infection of the surgical wound, uterus, or urinary tract

v. The choice between vaginal birth after cesarean and elective repeat cesarean birth in future pregnancies is multifactorial and can be deferred in the postpartum period with referral to informational resources and future obstetrical care providers if applicable. In most cases, women with one or two prior cesareans may be counseled to consider vaginal birth after cesarean (ACOG, 2010).

c. Return to normal daily activities, exercise, and work.

d. Infant care including feeding, soothing, pediatric visits, immunizations, circumcision, and safety measures such as sleeping arrangements and car seats

e. Women experience many postpartum physical changes (Cheng & Li, 2008) that may be unexpected or concerning and prompt questions about normal versus abnormal symptoms, e.g., average versus excessive bleeding (soaking a large menstrual pad in 1 hour or less), breast pain from engorgement (bilateral) versus mastitis (usually signaled by unilateral mass with fever), etc.

f. Sexual health and dysfunction, which are critical topics but frequently omitted from postpartum visits (Declerq et al., 2013)

i. Sexual practices, libido, arousal, and orgasm

ii. Dyspareunia, frequently related to genital laceration and insufficient lubrication related to postpartum hormonal changes and breastfeeding

iii. Postpartum and other changes in psychologic aspects of sexuality including self-perception and partner relationships

g. Return of fertility and menses

h. Contraception

i. Optimal pregnancy interval: although conclusive data are lacking, women may be advised that maternal and neonatal outcomes are improved when pregnancies are 18–60 months apart (Conde-Agudelo, Rosas-Bermúdez, & Kafury-Goeta, 2007)

2. Counseling about nutrition and exercise is essential in the postpartum period, may have lifelong impact on all family members (Ruchat & Mottola, 2012), and may include:

a. Basic principles of optimal nutrition and hydration

b. Encouragement to achieve and maintain a normal body mass index to reduce immediate and long-term health risks (Amorim, Linne, & Lourenco, 2013)

c. Advice that regular exercise may improve health and prevent or reduce depressive symptomatology (Teychenne & York, 2013)

d. Continue daily 400–800 mcg folate throughout childbearing years for the prevention of neural tube defects in case of unintended pregnancy; dosage is adjusted according to maternal risk factors up to 4–5 mg per day (Gomes, Lopes, & Pinto, 2015)

e. Nutritional supplementation specific to the postpartum period
   i. Fluid and fiber to support bowel function
   ii. Iron supplementation following postpartum hemorrhage or anemia diagnosis
   iii. Routine supplementation is not indicated in the absence of nutritional deficiencies, in which case a multivitamin including calcium and vitamins B and D may be helpful (AAP & ACOG, 2012)
   iv. Essential fatty acids intake may minimize incidence and severity of postpartum depression in women and optimize brain development in breastfed infants (Genuis & Schwalfenberg, 2006; Wojcicki & Heyman, 2011)

f. Nutrition during breastfeeding (AAP & ACOG, 2012)
   i. Minimal daily caloric intake required for milk production in the average woman is 1,800, with 500 calories typically used for this purpose each day
   ii. Weight loss of 2 pounds per month does not typically affect lactation
   iii. Although common, routine vitamin supplementation is not indicated during lactation if a woman's diet is wholesome, balanced, and varied, in the absence of identified deficiencies

3. Additional health maintenance counseling should include
   a. Signs and symptoms that require immediate evaluation
   b. Resumption of routine gynecological and primary care
   c. Self-knowledge and examination (e.g., breasts and skin)
   d. Kegel exercises for pelvic muscle tone, continence, and sexual health
   e. If urinary or fecal incontinence is present, advise this is not uncommon and is reported by 10–50% and up to 25% of postpartum women respectively (Handa et al., 2007). Pelvic floor muscle training, pessary fitting, and surgical intervention may be discussed if Kegel exercises do not result in improved symptoms within 1–2 months postpartum (Dumoulin & Hay-Smith, 2010).

D. Consultation and referral as indicated

1. Conditions that warrant medical consultation or referral may include, and are not limited to (Tharp & Farley, 2013):
   a. Endometritis
   b. Infection or dehiscence of surgical site or perineal laceration site
   c. Excessive or prolonged vaginal bleeding
   d. Breast abscess
   e. Postpartum thyroiditis
   f. Chronic medical conditions requiring follow-up, if outside of the advanced practice nurse's scope of practice
   g. Intimate partner violence
   h. Poor maternal adaptation
   i. Postpartum depression, anxiety, mania, or psychosis
   j. Substance abuse treatment
   k. Suspected child abuse or neglect (notify pediatrician and child protective services)
   l. Housing, food, and financial assistance programs

2. Local and web-based resources
   a. Public health programs, visiting nurses associations, lactation consultants, nutritionists, breastfeeding and birth trauma support groups, therapists, social workers, psychologists, psychiatrists, and postpartum doulas may have services for the evaluation, monitoring, and treatment of select maternal physical and psychosocial problems and infant or breastfeeding concerns.
   b. Women can be encouraged to seek support groups and other services for new parents, particularly if they lack family and social support, experienced childbirth-related trauma, or have special circumstances such as multiples or perinatal loss. Online forums may be a useful adjunctive or primary source of meaningful support if local resources are limited, particularly for women with unusual diagnoses or infants with rare conditions that are not addressed by programs in the community.

3. Primary care: Women and their families need a medical home for ongoing health maintenance. This might be a nurse practitioner or midwife-led practice setting, a community clinic, or other primary care location. Postpartum clients may be guided to access ongoing healthcare elsewhere if they will not remain in your practice beyond the postpartum period.

Midwives and nurse practitioners are uniquely situated to have a profound effect on the health of women and their families. The relationships we establish with our clients in the antepartum period, as we assist them to have the safest and healthiest pregnancies possible, provides the platform for further growth in the postpartum period. We can have an ongoing positive impact on the lives of our clients and their families, ideally resulting in intergenerational health promotion and improved public health.

REFERENCES

Aderhold, K. J., & Perry, L. (1991). Jet hydrotherapy for labor and postpartum pain relief. *MCN, the American Journal of Maternal Child Nursing, 16*(2), 97–99.

American Academy of Pediatrics & American College of Obstetricians and Gynecologists. (2012). *Guidelines for perinatal care* (7th ed.). Washington, DC: American College of Obstetricians and Gynecologists.

American College of Obstetricians and Gynecologists. (2010). ACOG practice bulletin no. 115: Vaginal birth after previous cesarean delivery. *Obstetrics & Gynecology, 116,* 450.

Amorim, A. R., Linne, Y. M., & Lourenco, P. M. (2013). Diet or exercise, or both, for weight reduction in women after childbirth. *Cochrane Database of Systematic Reviews, 7,* CD005627

Andersen, L. B., Melvaer, L. B., Videbech, P., Lamont, R. F., & Joergensen, J. S. (2012). Risk factors for developing post-traumatic stress disorder following childbirth: A systematic review. *Acta Obstetricia et Gynecologica Scandinavica, 91*(11), 1261–1272.

Association of Women's Health, Obstetric and Neonatal Nurses, (2006). *The compendium of postpartum care* (2nd ed.). Washington, DC: Author.

Barimani, M., Oxelmark, L., Johansson, S., & Highland, I. (2015). Support and continuity during the first 2 weeks postpartum. *Scandinavian Journal of Caring Sciences, 29*(3), 409–17.

Cerimele, J., Vanderlip, E., Croicu, C., Melville, J., Russo, J., Reed, S., et al. (2013). Presenting symptoms of women with depression in an obstetrics and gynecology setting. *Obstetrics & Gynecology, 122*(2), 313–318.

Cheng, C.-Y., & Li, Q. (2008). Integrative review of research on general health status and prevalence of common physical health conditions of women after childbirth. *Women's Health Issues, 18*(4), 267–280.

Conde-Agudelo, A., Rosas-Bermúdez, A., & Kafury-Goeta, A. C. (2007). Effects of birth spacing on maternal health: A systematic review. *American Journal of Obstetrics and Gynecology, 96*(4), 297–308.

Declercq, E. R., Sakala, C., Corry, M. P., Applebaum, S., & Herrlich, A. (2013). *Listening to mothers III: New mothers speak out.* New York: Childbirth Connection.

Dennis, C. L., Fung, K., Grigoriadis. S., Robinson, G. E., Romans, S., & Ross, L. (2007). Traditional postpartum practices and rituals: A qualitative systematic review. *Women's Health, 3*(4), 487–502.

DiBari, J. N., Yu, S. M., Chao, S. M., & Lu, M. C. (2014). Use of postpartum care: Predictors and barriers. *Journal of Pregnancy, 2014,* 530769.

Dumoulin, C., & Hay-Smith, J. (2010). Pelvic floor muscle training versus no treatment, or inactive control treatments, for urinary incontinence in women. *Cochrane Database of Systematic Reviews, 1,* CD005654.

East, C. E., Begg, L., Henshall, N. E., Marchant, P., & Wallace, K. (2012). Local cooling for relieving pain from perineal trauma sustained during childbirth. *Cochrane Database of Systematic Reviews, 5,* CD006304.

Gamble, J., & Creedy, D. K. (2009). A counseling model for postpartum women after distressing birth experiences. *Midwifery, 25*(2), e21–e30.

Genuis, S. J., & Schwalfenberg, G. K. (2006). Time for an oil check: The role of essential omega-3 fatty acids and maternal and pediatric health. *Journal of Perinatology, 26,* 59–65.

Gomes, S., Lopes, C., & Pinto, E. (2015). Folate and folic acid in the periconceptional period: Recommendations from official health organizations in thirty-six countries worldwide and WHO. *Public Health Nutrition,* 1–14.

Haran, C., van Driel, M., Mitchell, B. L., & Brodribb, W. E. (2014). Clinical guidelines for postpartum women and infants in primary care: A systematic review. *BMC Pregnancy and Childbirth, 14,* 51.

Jackson, E., & Glasier, A. (2011). Return of ovulation and menses in postpartum nonlactating women: A systematic review. *Obstetrics & Gynecology, 117*(3), 657–662.

Lavender, T., Richens, Y., Milan, S., Smyth, R., & Dowswell, T. (2013, July 18). Telephone support for women during pregnancy and the first six weeks postpartum. *Cochrane Database of Systematic Reviews, 7,* CD009338.

Leuridan, L., Wens, J., Devlieger, R., Verhaeghe, J., Mathieu, C., & Benhalima, K. (2015). Glucose intolerance in early postpartum in women with gestational diabetes: Who is at increased risk? *Primary Care Diabetes, 9*(4), 244–252.

MacArthur, C., Winter, H. R., Bick, D. E., Lilford, R. J., Lancashire, R. J., Knowles, H., et al. (2003). Redesigning postnatal care: A randomised controlled trial of protocol-based midwifery-led care focused on individual women's physical and psychological health needs. *Health Technology Assessment, 7*(37), 1–98.

Minassian, V., & Jazayeri, A. (2002). Randomized trial of lidocaine ointment versus placebo for the treatment of postpartum perineal pain. *Obstetrics & Gynecology, 100*(6), 1239–1243.

Minig, L., Trimble, E. L., Sarsotti, C., Sebastiani, M. M., & Spong, C. Y. (2009). Building the evidence base for postoperative and postpartum advice. *Obstetrics & Gynecology, 114*(4):892–900.

Moore, W., & James, D. K. (1989). A random trial of three topical analgesic agents in the treatment of episiotomy pain following instrumental vaginal delivery. *Journal of Obstetrics & Gynaecology, 10*(1), 35–39.

Rowan, C., Bick, D., & Bastos, M. H. (2007). Postnatal debriefing interventions to prevent maternal mental health problems after birth: Exploring the gap between the evidence and UK policy and practice. *Worldviews on Evidence-Based Nursing, 4*(2), 97–105.

Rowlands, I. J., & Redshaw, M. (2012). Mode of birth and women's psychological and physical wellbeing in the postnatal period. *BMC Pregnancy and Childbirth, 12,* 138.

Ruchat, S. M., & Mottola, M. F. (2012). Preventing long-term risk of obesity for two generations: Prenatal physical activity is part of the puzzle. *Journal of Pregnancy, 2012,* Article ID 470247. doi:10.1155/2012/470247.

Sandall, J., Soltani, H., Gates, S., Shennan, A., & Devane, D. (2015). Midwife-led continuity models versus other models of care for childbearing women. *Cochrane Database of Systematic Reviews, 9,* CD004667.

Shaw, E., Levitt, C., Wong, S., & Kaczorowski, J. (2006). Systematic review of the literature on postpartum care: Effectiveness of postpartum support to improve maternal parenting, mental health, quality of life, and physical health. *Birth, 33*(3), 210–220.

Speroff, L., & Mishell, D. (2008). The postpartum visit: It's time for a change in order to optimally initiate contraception. *Contraception, 78*(2), 90–98.

Stevens-Simon, C., O'Connor, P., & Bassford, K. (1994). Incentives enhance postpartum compliance among adolescent prenatal patients. *Journal of Adolescent Health, 15*(5), 396–399.

Tepper, N. K., Phillips, S. J., Kapp, N., Gaffield, M. E., & Curtis, K. M. (2015, May 19). Combined hormonal contraceptive use among breastfeeding women: An updated systematic review. *Contraception.* doi: 10.1016/j.contraception.2015.05.006

Teychenne, M., & York, R. (2013). Physical activity, sedentary behavior, and postnatal depressive symptoms: A review. *American Journal of Preventive Medicine, 45*(2), 217–227.

Tharp, N., & Farley, C. (2013). *Clinical practice guidelines for midwifery and women's health* (4th ed.). Sudbury, MA: Jones & Bartlett Publishing.

Thomson, G., Dykes, F., Hurley, M. A., & Hoddinott, P. (2012). Incentives as connectors: Insights into a breastfeeding incentive intervention in a disadvantaged are of North-West England. *BMC Pregnancy and Childbirth, 12,* 22.

Wojcicki, J. M., & Heyman, M. B. (2011). Maternal omega-3 fatty acid supplementation and risk for perinatal maternal depression. *Journal of Maternal, Fetal and Neonatal Medicine, 24*(5), 680–686.

Yonemoto, N., Dowswell, T., Nagai, S., & Mori, R. (2013, July 23). Schedules for home visits in the early postpartum period. *Cochrane Database of Systematic Reviews, 7,* CD009326.

GUIDELINES FOR MEDICAL CONSULTATION, INTERPRO-FESSIONAL COLLABORATION, AND TRANSFER OF CARE DURING PREGNANCY AND CHILDBIRTH

Jenna Shaw-Battista

I. Introduction and general background

Pregnant women are frequently dichotomized as being at "low" or "high" risk for suboptimal perinatal outcomes despite a continuum of medical and obstetric risk. There is little disagreement as to what constitutes a normal pregnancy or physiologic childbirth in a healthy parturient, and nurse practitioners and nurse-midwives routinely provide independent care for these low-risk women (American College of Nurse-Midwives, Midwives Alliance of North America, & National Association of Certified Professional Midwives, 2012). At the other end of the spectrum are women for whom exclusive physician care and referral to perinatology or neonatology services is immediately indicated due to high-risk medical conditions or unstable and severe complications of pregnancy and parturition. In the middle are women with one or more moderate risk factors, for whom informed consent for care and decisions about consultation and referral to medical providers are unclear due to lack of relevant data from robust studies to guide clinical management including the selection of healthcare provider type (Chauhan, Hendrix, Berghella, & Siddiqui, 2010; Wright et al., 2011).

Gray areas in clinical decision making necessitate partnership with women to develop care plans guided by their values, culture, and preferences for providers and care practices. Individual clinicians' past experience, skill set, values, and scope of practice also influence clinical decisions including consultations, collaborations, and referral. Additional influential factors include state and federal regulatory language, institutional policies and interprofessional practice protocols, research findings, community standards, healthcare ethics, and financial considerations (Avery, 2000; Bailey, Jones, & Way, 2006; Porter, Crozier, Sinclair, & Kernohan, 2007). Within this complex context, nurse practitioners and nurse-midwives frequently collaborate with physician colleagues to care for pregnant women with perinatal risk factors for adverse outcomes and high-risk conditions including selected disorders of the endocrine, cardiovascular, hematologic, neurologic, musculoskeletal, pulmonary, gastrointestinal, and renal systems; and specific psychiatric diagnoses, infectious diseases, malignancies, and abnormal diagnostic testing (Office of Technology Assessment, 1986).

A. Perinatal risk factors and complications include, but are not limited to:

1. History of pregnancy or childbirth complications
   a. Gestational diabetes, hypertensive disorder, or other pregnancy complication
   b. Habitual abortion (< 12–20 weeks gestation), stillbirth (≥ 20 weeks gestation) or death of a newborn or infant in the first year of life
   c. Large or small for gestational age infant
   d. Preterm delivery
   e. Dystocia, maternal or neonatal birth injury, postpartum hemorrhage, or other complication of parturition
   f. Previous cesarean section or other uterine surgery

2. Variants and complications of current pregnancy and parturition
   a. Prenatal diagnosis of minor or major fetal anomaly
   b. Multiple gestation
   c. Nonvertex fetal presentation at term or fetal malpresentation incompatible with vaginal birth
   d. Prolonged pregnancy (41–42 weeks gestation) or postterm pregnancy (≥ 42 weeks gestation)
   e. Preterm labor or ruptured membranes before term (20–36 weeks gestation)
   f. Prolonged premature rupture of membranes at term
   g. Polyhydramnios or oligohydramnios
   h. Abnormal placentation (e.g., previa or accreta)
   i. Unexplained vaginal bleeding
   j. Rhesus factor sensitization or other IgG antibody sensitization
   k. Hypertensive disorders (essential or gestational hypertension, or preeclampsia–eclampsia)

l. Hemolysis, elevated liver enzymes, and low platelets syndrome

m. Idiopathic thrombocytopenic purpura

n. Cholestasis of pregnancy

o. Preexisting or gestational diabetes mellitus

p. Selected anemias or hemoglobinopathies(e.g., thalassemias and hemoglobin less than 10 g/dL, not responsive to iron therapy)

q. Sickle cell crisis

3. Selected maternal infections with potential fetal sequelae (e.g., human immunodeficiency virus, cytomegalovirus, parvovirus, rubella, syphilis, toxoplasmosis, primary herpes infection, or presence of genital lesions at term)

4. Additional maternal illnesses (e.g., unstable new or chronic health conditions, severe asthma requiring hospitalization during pregnancy, autoimmune disorders, cardiac disease other than asymptomatic mitral valve prolapse, renal disease or recurrent urinary tract infections, or thyroid disorders)

5. Psychosocial risk factors (e.g., psychiatric diagnoses, substance abuse, interpersonal violence, social deprivation, poverty, and homelessness)

B. *Intrapartum and postpartum complications and procedures for which medical consultation, comanagement, or referral is recommended include:*

1. Preterm labor and delivery

2. Induction or augmentation of labor

3. Abnormal fetal surveillance and variant fetal heart rate tracings (category II and III)

4. Amnioinfusion

5. Prolapsed cord

6. Chorioamnionitis or other maternal infection

7. Prodromal or protracted labor, or arrest of labor or fetal descent

8. Anticipated or actual shoulder dystocia

9. Indications for, and occurrence of, operative vaginal delivery or cesarean section

10. Severe perineal laceration (third or fourth degree) or cervical laceration

11. Prolonged third stage of labor (> 30 minutes), with or without postpartum hemorrhage (> 500–1000 mL)

12. Unstable genitourinary hematoma

13. New maternal disease or exacerbation of chronic illness

14. Child abuse or neglect, suspected or observed (notify pediatrician and child protective services)

15. Neonatal health conditions, anticipated or observed

Figure 30-1 contains an algorithm for medical consultation and referral during pregnancy. Interprofessional practices benefit from applied algorithms in the form of clinical guidelines and written policies regarding methods and types of consultation and referral in their practice settings. These and other formal and informal strategies to encourage interprofessional communication and standardize collaborations may facilitate mutual understanding of varied scopes of practice and improve care team efficacy and job satisfaction along with patient outcomes (Bailey et al., 2006; Brooten et al., 2005; Hutchison et al., 2011; Kennedy, Grant, Shaw-Battista, Walton, & Sandall, 2010; Shaw-Battista, Fineberg, Skubic, Wooley, & Tilton, 2011; Zwarenstein, Goldman, & Reeves, 2009).

Interprofessional guidelines for maternity care frequently describe consultation and comanagement of women with specific medical, obstetric, and neonatal risk factors. Varied levels of consultation may be delineated, with or without direct physical assessment and documentation of collaborative management plans required of the medical consultant for specific diagnoses. When pregnant women experience complications that require ongoing medical or obstetric management, comanagement or transfer of care to a physician rather than consultation may be indicated. High-risk patients may return to the nurse practitioner or nurse-midwife caseload for pregnancy or childbirth care if their condition stabilizes and collaborative or independent advance practice nursing care becomes feasible and mutually agreeable.

For many childbearing women, risk status and maternity care provider type are determined by the severity rather than presence of a specific condition. For example, nurse practitioners and nurse-midwives may independently or collaboratively care for women with gestational diabetes who can maintain euglycemia with diet and exercise or oral hypoglycemic agents, but comanage care with obstetrician colleagues if insulin becomes necessary or transfer care to physicians if blood sugars are poorly controlled regardless of treatment type (Avery, 2000; Jacobson et al., 2005; Nicholson et al., 2009). Similarly, collaborative practice guidelines may suggest transfer to physician care when women have severe hypertensive disorders of pregnancy or require pharmacological treatment (e.g., antihypertensive medications or magnesium sulfate for seizure prophylaxis), but endorse independent advance practice nursing care or interprofessional comanagement of women with mild or stable gestational hypertension or preeclampsia (e.g., no pharmacological treatment is required, or the physician provides medication management while the nurse practitioner or nurse-midwife continues other aspects of maternity care) (Chummun, 2009). These details, and other specifics of clinical protocols and collaborative

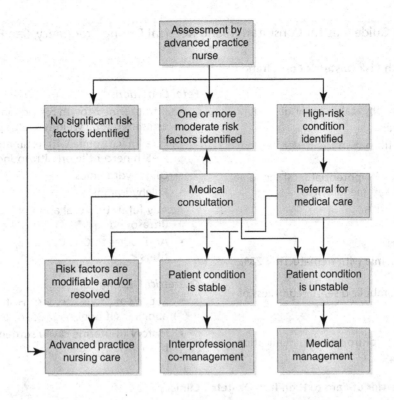

FIGURE 30-1 Algorithm for Medical Consultation and Referral During Pregnancy

practice agreements, necessarily differ among practice sites. Variation also occurs over time as interprofessional practices evolve in response to changes in clinical team members, patient populations, and supportive data (Bailey et al., 2006; Zwarenstein et al., 2009). **Table 30-1** contains a sample policy for community health center obstetric providers and high-risk obstetric physician consultation and transfer of care during pregnancy.

Regardless of the indication for collaborative care, comanagement must include ongoing communication among providers to ensure patient safety (Bailey et al., 2006; Brooten et al., 2005; Zwarenstein et al., 2009). The structure of interprofessional communication varies among sites but typically includes periodic conversations about specific patients to achieve consensus about management plans via electronic medical record, telephone, secure email, or in person. Interprofessional practices may use regularly scheduled meetings to discuss their high-risk prenatal caseload. This formalizes the comanagement process and ensures timely review of women's evolving health status to facilitate optimal outcomes. These interprofessional communications about risk assessment and plans of care should be documented prominently in the medical record in addition to routine charting following clinical encounters and any written consultant reports. Patients should be kept apprised

of changing assessments, participate in formulating and revising care plans, and receive information about healthcare providers' responsibilities and relationships when consultation, comanagement or transfer of care occurs.

In addition to formal interprofessional relationships, effective communications, and shared clinical guidelines, optimal perinatal outcomes are fostered through collegial interactions that are characterized by mutual respect, professionalism, and trust (American College of Nurse-Midwives & American College of Obstetricians and Gynecologists, 2014). Shared goals related to high-quality patient-centered care, healthcare education, research, and public health may also strengthen interprofessional practice relations (Avery, Montgomery, & Brandl-Salutz, 2012; Hutchison et al., 2011; King, Laros, & Parer, 2012; Shaw-Battista et al., 2011). Interprofessional clinical practices that include nurse practitioners and nurse-midwives contribute to public health by increasing access to safe and effective maternity care with comprehensive physiological and psychosocial support services, facilitation of normal childbirth, and decreased use of unnecessary costly obstetric interventions among childbearing women across the spectrum of health and perinatal risk (Cragin & Kennedy, 2006; Priddis, Schmied, Sneddon, & Dahlen, 2014). To this end, public health policies and clinical organizations should

TABLE 30-1 Sample Guidelines for Consultation and Referral During Pregnancy, San Francisco General Hospital

Conditions Requiring High-Risk Obstetric Consultation

Maternal Conditions

- Pelvic mass noted by physical exam or ultrasound
- Uterine malformations
- Patients with large fibroids in the lower uterine segment
- Maternal infections with potential fetal sequelae, e.g., toxoplasmosis, cytomegalovirus
- Recurrent pyelonephritis
- Nephrolithiasis
- Persistent proteinuria
- Persistent severe anemia with hematocrit < 28% despite iron therapy
- History of thromboembolic disease regardless of etiology
- Hypothyroidism
- Seizure disorder well controlled with medication
- Body mass index ≥ 45

Fetal Conditions

- Intrauterine growth restriction with ultrasound-estimated fetal weight ≤ 10th percentile
- Fetal macrosomia with estimated fetal weight ≥ 95th percentile on ultrasound
- Oligohydramnios
- Polyhydramnios
- Any fetal structural abnormality detected by ultrasound
- Antibodies to C, c, D, Kell, E, e, or Duffy with titers < 1:8

Obstetrical History

- Recurrent pregnancy loss: History of ≥ 3 spontaneous abortions if under age 35, or ≥ 2 if over age 35
- History of uterine cavity surgery other than cesarean birth

Conditions Requiring Transfer of Care to High-Risk Obstetric Clinic

Maternal Conditions

- Chronic hypertension diagnosed before pregnancy
- Hypertension in pregnancy requiring medication
- Active or uncontrolled seizure disorder
- Severe asthma with hospitalization for asthma during pregnancy
- Cardiac disease (except asymptomatic mitral valve prolapse)
- Pulmonary hypertension
- Platelet count less than 100,000
- Deep vein thrombosis
- Sickle cell disease
- Lupus/scleroderma/any connective tissue disease
- Cancer
- Active tuberculosis
- Active viral hepatitis
- HIV positive
- Hyperthyroidism
- Diabetes: type 1, type 2, or poorly controlled gestational diabetes requiring medication
- Hyperemesis gravidarum with hospital admission, until resolved
- Paraplegia or quadriplegia

Fetal Conditions

- Complete placenta previa or partial previa in the third trimester
- Chronic placental abruption diagnosed by hospital admission
- Presence of antibodies to C, c, D, Kell, E, e, or Duffy, with antibody titers ≥ 1:8
- Multiple gestation

Obstetrical History

- Incompetent cervix, or history suggestive thereof, i.e., painless cervical dilatation < 24 weeks gestation

Other Conditions

- Transfer of care is recommended for the following conditions. However, in some cases, the benefits of continued client engaged in prenatal care at their original site may outweigh the benefits of services available in high-risk clinic.
- Active drug or alcohol use
- Mental illness characterized by the use of psychotropic medication, history of suicide attempts, violence, trauma, or hospitalization for psychiatric problems, with a probability of recurrence

support nurse and midwife-led care, and interprofessional team-based care, as alternatives to conventional physician-led maternity care service models (Campbell, 2007; Hoope-Bender et al., 2014; Sakala & Corry, 2008; Sandall, Soltani, Gates, Shennan, & Devane, 2013).

REFERENCES

American College of Nurse-Midwives & American College of Obstetricians and Gynecologists. (2014). *Joint statement of practice relations between obstetrician-gynecologists and certified nurse-midwives/certified midwives.* Washington, DC: American College of Nurse-Midwives.

American College of Nurse-Midwives, Midwives Alliance of North America, & National Association of Certified Professional Midwives. (2012). *Supporting health and normal physiologic childbirth: A consensus statement by ACNM, MANA and NACPM.* Washington, DC: American College of Nurse-Midwives.

Avery, M. D. (2000). Diabetes in pregnancy: The midwifery role in management. *Journal of Midwifery & Women's Health, 45*(6), 472–480.

Avery, M. D., Montgomery, O., & Brandl-Salutz, E. (2012). Essential components of successful collaborative maternity care models: The ACOG-ACNM project. *Obstetrics and Gynecology Clinics of North America, 39*(3), 423–434.

Bailey, P., Jones, L., & Way, D. (2006). Family physician/nurse practitioner: Stories of collaboration. *Journal of Advanced Nursing, 53*(4), 381–391.

Brooten, D., Youngblut, J., Blais, K., Donahue, D., Cruz, I., & Lightbourne, M. (2005). APN-physician collaboration in caring for women with high-risk pregnancies. *Journal of Nursing Scholarship, 37*(2), 178–184.

Campbell, K. P. (Ed.). (2007). *Investing in maternal and child health: An employer's toolkit.* Washington, DC: Center for Prevention and Health Services, National Business Group on Health.

Chauhan, S. P., Hendrix, N. W., Berghella, V., & Siddiqui, D. (2010). Comparison of two national guidelines in obstetrics: American versus royal college of obstetricians and gynecologists. *American Journal of Perinatology, 27*(10), 763–770.

Chummun, H. (2009). Hypertension: A contemporary approach to nursing care. *British Journal of Nursing, 18*(13), 784–789.

Cragin, L., & Kennedy, H. P. (2006). Linking obstetric and midwifery practice with optimal outcomes. *Journal of Obstetric, Gynecologic, and Neonatal Nursing, 35*(6), 779–785.

Hoope-Bender, P. T., de Bernis, L., Campbell, J., Downe, S., Fauveau, V., Fogstad, H., et al. (2014). Improvement of maternal and newborn health through midwifery, *The Lancet, 384*(9949), 1226–1235.

Hutchison, M., Ennis, L., Shaw-Battista, J., Delgado, A., Myer, K., & Cragin, L. (2011). Great minds don't think alike: Collaborative maternity care at San Francisco General Hospital. *Obstetrics & Gynecology, 118*(3), 678–682.

Jacobson, G. F., Ramos, G. A., Ching, J. Y., Kirby, R. S., Ferrara, A., & Field, D. R. (2005). Comparison of glyburide and insulin for the management of gestational diabetes in a large managed care organization. *American Journal of Obstetrics and Gynecology, 193*(1), 118–124.

Kennedy, H. P., Grant, J., Shaw-Battista, J., Walton, C., & Sandall, J. (2010). Normalizing birth: A study of childbirth in two NHS hospitals. *Journal of Midwifery and Women's Health, 55*(3), 262–269.

King, T. L., Laros, R. K., & Parer, J. T. (2012). Interprofessional collaborative practice in obstetrics and midwifery. *Obstetrics and Gynecology Clinics of North America, 39*(3), 411–422.

Nicholson, W., Bolen, S., Witkop, C. T., Neale, D., Wilson, L., & Bass, E. (2009). Benefits and risks of oral diabetes agents compared with insulin in women with gestational diabetes: A systematic review. *Obstetrics and Gynecology, 113*(1), 193–205.

Office of Technology Assessment. (1986). *Health technology case study 37. Nurse practitioners, physician assistants, and certified nurse-midwives: A policy analysis.* Washington, DC: Congress of the United States.

Porter, S., Crozier, K., Sinclair, M., & Kernohan, W. G. (2007). New midwifery? A qualitative analysis of midwives' decision-making strategies. *Journal of Advanced Nursing, 60*(5), 525-34.

Priddis, H. S., Schmied, V., Sneddon, A. & Dahlen, H. G. (2014, July 18). "A patchwork of services"—Caring for women who sustain severe perineal trauma in New South Wales—from the perspective of women and midwives. *BMC Pregnancy and Childbirth, 18*(14), 236.

Sakala, C., & Corry, M. P. (2008). *Evidence based maternity care: What it is and what it can achieve.* New York, NY: The Milbank Memorial Fund.

Sandall, J., Soltani, H., Gates, S., Shennan, A., & Devane, D. (2013). Midwife-led continuity models versus other models of care for childbearing women. *Cochrane Database of Systematic Reviews, 8*, CD004667.

Shaw-Battista, J., Fineberg, A., Skubic, B., Wooley, D., & Tilton, Z. (2011). Collaborative maternity care: A successful model of public health and private practice partnership. *Obstetrics & Gynecology, 118*(3), 663–672.

Wright, J. D., Pawar, N., Gonzalez, J. S., Lewin, S. N., Burke, W. M., Simpson, L. L., et al. (2011). Scientific evidence underlying the American College of Obstetricians and Gynecologists' practice bulletins. *Obstetrics and Gynecology, 118*(3), 505–512.

Zwarenstein, M., Goldman, J., & Reeves, S. (2009). Interprofessional collaboration: Effects of practice-based interventions on professional practice and healthcare outcomes. *Cochrane Database of Systematic Reviews, 3*, CD000072.

BIRTH CHOICES FOR WOMEN WITH A PREVIOUS CESAREAN DELIVERY

Rebekah Kaplan

CHAPTER

31

I. Introduction and general background

Because currently almost a third of births in the United States are by cesarean section, increasing numbers of women are faced with the choice of whether to have a repeat cesarean or a trial of labor (TOL) and attempt a vaginal birth after a cesarean (VBAC). Cesarean delivery rates in the United States have risen by almost 60% from a rate of 21% in 1996 to a record high of 32.9% in 2009. In the last few years the rate has fallen slightly to 32.7% in 2013 and 32.2% in 2014 (Hamilton et al., 2015).

For most of the 20th century, women who had a primary cesarean were advised to have subsequent cesarean deliveries. In 1980, the National Institute of Child and Human Development and the National Center for Health Care Technology examined the evidence for this practice and outlined recommendations for offering women a TOL. From 1980 to 1996 VBAC rates increased, but from 1996 to 2007 rates steadily declined from 28.5% to 8.3% and have subsequently risen to 20% in 2013 (Curtin, Gregory, Korst, & Uddin, 2015). Interestingly, for those women who choose to have a TOL, the rates of successful VBAC have remained steady at about 74% (Eden et al., 2012).

In 2010 the National Institutes of Health (NIH) addressed the issue of declining availability and low VBAC rates at the Consensus Development Conference on Vaginal Birth After Cesarean. Their recommendation was that institutions offer TOL as an option to women with previous low transverse cesarean sections (LTCS) (NIH, 2010). The American Academy of Family Physicians (King et al., 2015), American College of Nurse-Midwives (2011), and American College of Obstetricians and Gynecologists (ACOG, 2010) have made the same recommendation.

When helping women and families make the decision about their preferred mode of delivery, the practitioner must incorporate principles of informed consent and shared decision making including assessing the woman's desires, her candidacy for TOL, her chances of success, her risk of uterine rupture, and risks and benefits for her and her baby (see Internet resources in section VI). Research shows that a woman's prior birth experience, perceived risk, fear and anxiety, opinions of family and friends, desire for planning and control, knowledge of birth options, and perceived provider preference significantly factor into her decision (Bernstein, Matalon-Grazi, & Rosenn, 2012; Shorten, Shorten, & Kennedy, 2014). It is also important to consider a client's health literacy as well as numeracy when reviewing statistics. It may be helpful to use visual aids such as an icon array (see Internet resources in section VI) to enhance understanding and reduce provider bias (Cox, 2014; Garcia-Retamero & Dhami, 2013). After a decision is made, a consent form should be completed and the process should be documented. Choices may be institution specific and a provider should know who in the obstetric community offers TOL as an option.

II. Risks and benefits of TOL versus repeat cesarean delivery

A. Uterine rupture

The risk of a uterine rupture for a woman choosing a TOL is 0.47% (0.2–0.77%) (Dodd, Crowther, Huertas, Guise, & Horey, 2013; Guise et al., 2010). If a woman has had a previous vaginal birth either before or after her cesarean birth this rate drops (Guise et al., 2010). If the prior cesarean was done within 24 months of the birth, the risk of rupture is slightly higher (Landon et al., 2004). Women with a history of two prior LTCS have about a 2% risk of uterine rupture. If labor is being induced the rate of rupture increases to approximately 1.1–1.5% (NIH, 2010; Rossi & Prefumo, 2015). Labor augmentation with oxytocin does not seem to increase risk of uterine rupture (NIH, 2010; Ouzounian et al., 2011). There have been no reported maternal deaths caused by uterine rupture (NIH, 2010), although it is possible that this is due to underreporting or failure to indicate rupture as the cause of death. Approximately 6% of uterine ruptures result in neonatal death (NIH, 2010).

"Although the literature on uterine rupture is imprecise and inconsistent, existing studies indicate that 370 (study numbers range from 213–1,370) elective caesarean deliveries need to be performed to prevent one symptomatic uterine rupture" (Guise et al., 2004, p. 1).

B. *Risk for future pregnancies*

1. Placenta accreta and hysterectomy

   Women with multiple cesareans have an increased rate of placenta accreta and hysterectomy with each subsequent cesarean birth evidenced by many studies (ACOG, 2012; Marshall, Fu, & Guise, 2011). Some of the best evidence comes from Silver et al. (2006) who cited the incidence of placenta accreta from one previous cesarean to five or more: 0.31%, 0.57%, 2.1%, 2.3%, and 6.7%; and the risk of hysterectomy from one previous cesarean to five or more: 0.42%, 0.90%, 2.41%, 3.49%, and 8.99% (Marshall, Fu, & Guise, 2011; Silver et al., 2006).

2. Placenta previa

   The incidence of placenta previa significantly increases in women with each additional cesarean delivery occurring in 0.9% who have one prior cesarean delivery, 1.7% who have two prior cesarean deliveries, and 3% in women who have three or more cesarean deliveries (NIH, 2010). Women with placenta previa having their third or greater cesarean have a much greater risk of hysterectomy (0.7–4% versus 50–67%) as well as composite maternal morbidity (15% versus 83%) (Marshall, Fu, & Guise, 2011).

C. *Maternal mortality*

Overall numeric estimates of maternal death are 4 per 100,000 for women who undergo a TOL versus 13 per 100,000 for a repeat elective cesarean birth (Dodd et al., 2013; Guise et al., 2010).

D. *Maternal morbidity*

Overall, cesarean deliveries are associated with a 10% risk of morbidity including increased risk of infection (endometritis, urinary tract, or wound); thromboembolism; hysterectomy (2%); larger blood loss and severe postpartum hemorrhage (7.3%); blood transfusion; and surgical injury (e.g., injury to the bladder, ureter, or bowel). Women who have a TOL have a 4.6% risk of infection versus 3.2% in the elective repeat cesarean group, although the repeat cesarean group are more at risk for deep vein thrombosis and pulmonary embolism than the TOL group. The risks of hysterectomy, blood transfusion, and infection are similar in both groups, though evidence is confounding (Guise et al., 2010). In women with increasing numbers of cesarean births, the rates of hysterectomy,

blood transfusions, adhesions, and surgical injury all continued to increase (Marshall, Fu, & Guise, 2011). The long-term effects of urinary incontinence in women who have a VBAC versus cesarean birth are confounding, although mild incontinence may be higher in the short term for women who have a VBAC. Evidence shows lower rates of maternal morbidity in TOL clients with predicted VBAC success rates of greater than 60–70%. (ACOG, 2010; Grobman et al., 2009).

E. *Neonatal mortality*

Studies show that the neonatal mortality rate is higher for TOL at 1.3 per 1,000 compared to elective repeat cesarean at 0.5 per 1,000. The neonatal mortality rate for all first-time mothers is 1 per 1,000 (Guise et al., 2010; Smith, Pell, Cameron, & Dobbie, 2002). Neonatal death rates are higher in settings where rapid emergent cesarean sections cannot be performed.

F. *Neonatal morbidity*

Evidence indicates that infants born by cesarean have higher rates of respiratory distress syndrome, persistent pulmonary hypertension, transient tachypnea of the newborn, and need for oxygen and ventilator support than do infants born vaginally (NIH, 2010). Rates of hypoxic–ischemic encephalopathy in one study were 8 per 10,000 in the TOL group and none in the repeat cesarean group (Landon et al., 2004).

G. *Long-term consequences in offspring*

Evidence suggests that exposure to vaginal flora at birth is associated with the development of a healthy immune response. This is thought to be caused by microflora colonization of the neonatal intestinal tract, adaptive stress of labor and birth, and epigenetic regulation of gene expression, each of which is altered in cesarean birth (Cho & Norman, 2013). Children and adults born by cesarean have a 20% increased risk of developing asthma and a 23% increased risk of developing type 1 diabetes (Cho & Norman, 2013). There is also greater prevalence of allergic rhinitis, food allergies, celiac disease, inflammatory bowel disease, and increased hospitalization for gastroenteritis in these children (Bager, Simonsen, Nielsen, & Frisch, 2012; Cho & Norman, 2013; Decker, Hornef, & Stockinger, 2011). An association between cesarean birth and obesity in childhood and young adulthood has also been cited in many studies (Li, Zhou, & Liu, 2013; Mesquita et al., 2013).

H. *Postpartum period*

Women recover more quickly, have less postpartum pain, and have shorter hospital stays after a vaginal birth versus an operative birth. Mothers who have cesareans not only have a longer recovery but also delayed mother–infant interaction, lower rates of breastfeeding, and more difficulty establishing breastfeeding. Women with cesarean births have less perineal or vaginal trauma and decreased urinary incontinence in the postpartum period. The maternal rehospitalization rate within 30 days is 2.3 times higher in women with a cesarean birth (Declercq et al., 2007). According to Silver (2012), almost 20% of women reported chronic pain 3 months after their surgery, 12% a year after, and 33% had daily incisional pain at their surgery site 2 years after surgery. Pain as well as other morbidity increased with additional numbers of cesarean births (Miller, Hahn, & Grobman, 2013; Silver, 2012).

III. Data collection

A. Subjective: First visit

1. Document the reason for previous cesarean and events surrounding the birth. These include:

   a. Reason for prior cesarean (e.g., emergency cesarean birth for nonreassuring fetal heart tracing, placenta previa, arrest of descent, breech presentation)

   b. Emergent versus nonemergent surgery (emergent more likely to have a classical incision) (see **Table 31-1**)

   c. Gestational age and fetal weight (early preterm more likely to have a classical incision)

   d. Stage of labor (cervical dilation and station) and length of labor

   e. Fetal position, if possible (e.g., posterior)

   f. Where surgery was performed (e.g., small community or major urban hospital)

   g. Type of physician performing surgery (obstetrician, gynecologist, or general practitioner)

   h. Future TOL: Did the physician advise the client whether or not she could attempt a TOL in the future?

   i. Maternal experience of previous labor and birth

2. Note desired family size

TABLE 31-1 VBAC Success Rates

Indication for Prior Cesarean	% Success
Failure to progress	60–65%
Nonrecurring conditions (placenta previa, breech)	74–89%
Fetal intolerance of labor	69–73%
Body mass index > 40	52–70%

See Internet VBAC success calculator for individual risk: http://www.bsc.gwu.edu/mfmu/vagbirth.html

B. Objective

1. Assess type of scar: on physical abdominal examination, assess transverse or vertical skin scar, although skin incision does not reflect uterine incision.

IV. Goals for clinical management/assessment

A. Establish if the client is a candidate for TOL

B. Individualize predicted success rate (Tables 31-1 and 31-2)

C. Establish client's choice using principles of shared decision making

V. Plan

A. Attempt to obtain an operative report (Table 31-3).

1. TOL is not contraindicated with an unknown uterine incision unless there is a high clinical suspicion of a classical scar (ACOG, 2010; Smith et al., 2015).

TABLE 31-2 Factors for VBAC Success

Positive factors
- Maternal age < 40
- Prior vaginal delivery (especially VBAC)
- Favorable cervical factors
- Presence of spontaneous labor
- Nonrecurring indication for previous cesarean (e.g., breech, previa)
- Greater maternal height

Negative factors
- Increased number of prior cesarean deliveries
- Gestational age > 40 weeks
- Birth weight > 4,000 g
- Induction or augmentation of labor (63% success)
- Maternal obesity (body mass index > 30)
- Increased interpregnancy weight gain
- Gestational diabetes
- Maternal disease (e.g., hypertension)

ACOG Practice Bulletin no. 115. (2010). Vaginal birth after previous cesarean delivery. National Institutes of Health Consensus Development Conference statement: Vaginal birth after cesarean: New insights. March 8–10, 2010.

TABLE 31-3 Relative Contraindications for Trial of Labor

- Previous cesarean birth with a uterine incision in the upper part of the uterus ("classical" incision), or low transverse uterine incision with an extension into the upper part of the uterus (active segment)
- Previous transfundal uterine surgery
- Previous uterine rupture
- Medical or obstetric complication that precludes vaginal birth
- Inability to perform emergency cesarean birth

B. Educate on risks and benefits of repeat cesarean versus TOL: consider client desires, factors for success, and previous experience.

C. Establish the client's understanding of benefits and risk.

D. Use principles of shared decision making to ascertain client's choice. See section VI-Internet resources-Six steps of shared decision making.

E. Have the client sign consent for her birth choice (**Figure 31-1**).

FIGURE 31-1 Sample Birth Choices after Cesarean Birth—Client Information and Choice Form

COMMUNITY HEALTH NETWORK
OF SAN FRANCISCO
Birth Choices After Cesarean Birth-Patient Information and Choice Form
Page 1 of 2

NAME _____

DOB _____

MRN _____

PCP _____

Patient ID / Addressograph _____

Even though you had a cesarean birth before, you may choose to try a vaginal birth or choose another cesarean birth for this pregnancy. There are both risks and benefits to trying a vaginal birth or choosing another cesarean. We want you to have the information that you need to make your choice. We want you and your baby to be healthy and we want you to feel good about your choice.

Please read the information below and talk about it with your provider.

1. VAGINAL BIRTH ADVANTAGES
Mothers who have vaginal births usually have less pain after the baby is born. Most recover faster and are able to go home sooner. There is less chance of getting an infection or needing a blood transfusion. Also, babies who go through labor have less breathing problems at birth. Finally, having a vaginal birth avoids the risks of having another cesarean (see number 4).

Many women who had a cesarean can try a vaginal birth. Your chances of being able to have a vaginal birth depend on why you needed a cesarean before. Reasons that had to do with the baby, like breech position (bottom first) or having twins, might not happen again. Reasons that have to do with your body, like a small pelvis, could make a vaginal birth less likely. About 75% of women who had a cesarean before are able to have a vaginal birth with their next pregnancy.

When you are in labor, your family or close friends can be with you. We will give you pain medicine if you want. We will watch you and your baby closely during labor. Sometimes the baby cannot be born through the vagina. If this happens, we will recommend another cesarean. Many women, however, try for a vaginal birth and are successful.

(continues)

FIGURE 31-1 Sample Birth Choices after Cesarean Birth—Client Information and Choice Form *(Continued)*

COMMUNITY HEALTH NETWORK
OF SAN FRANCISCO
Birth Choices After Cesarean Birth-Patient Information and Choice Form
Page 2 of 2

NAME _____

DOB _____

MRN _____

PCP _____

Patient ID / Addressograph _____

2. CESAREAN BIRTH ADVANTAGES

The main advantage of choosing another cesarean is that you have less risk of having the scar on your uterus open during labor which requires an emergency cesarean (see number 3). If you decide to have a cesarean, you avoid the chance of having labor and then still needing a cesarean. This could happen if your labor does not progress or if the baby shows signs of stress during labor. Women who try to have a vaginal birth but then need a cesarean during labor may have more surgical problems than women who choose a cesarean before labor begins. Also, if you choose to have another cesarean, you probably will not have labor pains.

3. VAGINAL BIRTH RISKS

There is a small chance that the scar on your uterus from your cesarean could open up during labor. The risk of this happening depends on where your uterus was cut during your cesarean. If the scar from your cesarean is in the lower part of your uterus, the risk of it opening during labor is less than 1% (1 in 200). If you have had more than one cesarean or if your cesarean was recent (less than 2 years ago), the risk will be slightly increased that the scar could open during labor. If the scar is in the upper part of your uterus, there is much more risk that it could open in labor (as high as 10%). If you have a scar in the upper part of the uterus, we don't think you should try a vaginal birth.

If your provider does not know where your uterus was cut, your risk of the scar opening during labor appears to be the same as those with a scar in the lower part of your uterus (<1%) as most women have cesareans with lower uterine scars. However, it could be as high as 10% if the scar is in the upper part of your uterus.

If the scar on your uterus does open, you might need an emergency cesarean. You could bleed a lot and need a blood transfusion (blood from another person). You also could need a hysterectomy (removal of your uterus). There is a small chance that your baby or you could be injured or die.

4. CESAREAN BIRTH RISKS

If you are able to have a vaginal birth you can avoid some of the risks of a cesarean. For every 100 women who choose a cesarean, about 10 will have a problem. Two women get a wound infection, 6 get a fever, 1 needs a blood transfusion, and less than 1 will have an injury to her intestines, bladder or blood vessels. For every 1,000 women who have a cesarean, about 2 will need a hysterectomy (removal of uterus), usually because of bleeding. The more times you have a cesarean, the more likely you are to have one of these problems.

A cesarean can also cause scarring around the uterus. This scarring can make your next surgery more difficult. In another pregnancy, it can cause problems with the placenta and serious bleeding in a future pregnancy. Rarely, cesareans can weaken the uterus and the scar can open during another pregnancy.

(continues)

FIGURE 31-1 Sample Birth Choices after Cesarean Birth—Client Information and Choice Form (Continued)

COMMUNITY HEALTH NETWORK
OF SAN FRANCISCO
Birth Choices After Cesarean Birth-Patient Information and Choice Form
Page 3 of 3

NAME _____

DOB _____

MRN _____

PCP _____

Patient ID / Addressograph _____

5. I KNOW I CAN CHANGE MY CHOICE AT ANY TIME.

Put your initials next to your choice.

choose to try a vaginal birth _____

choose another cesarean _____

I understand the information on this paper. I talked to my pregnancy care provider about this information. I had all of my questions answered.

Patient signature: _____ _____ Date: _____
                        Print name   Signature

Counseling Provider: _____ _____ Date: _____
                          Print name   Signature

Translator (if applicable): _____ _____ Date: _____
                               Print name   Signature

Courtesy of Community Health Network of San Francisco, Department of Public Health

F. *If the client has an unknown scar, a consultation with a physician may be indicated in your site.*

G. *For those choosing TOL*

1. Discuss with the client the care during her birth (continuous fetal monitoring, intravenous or saline lock). Consult per site guidelines. With induction of labor, the risk of uterine rupture increases and VBAC success decreases. If induction is indicated, the client needs to be recounseled.

H. *For clients choosing a cesarean delivery*

1. Consult with the physician obstetric team to schedule a cesarean at 39 weeks except for those with prior classical scars.
   a. Good dating: 39 weeks
   b. Two prior cesareans: 39 weeks
   c. Known classical scar: early term delivery

VI. Internet resources for providers, clients, and families

A. VBAC Success Calculator (http://www.bsc.gwu.edu/mfmu/vagbirth.html)

Enter data, such as maternal age, height, weight, ethnicity, and historical factors, to calculate the predicted chance of VBAC (based on Grobman et al., 2007).

B. Childbirth Connection (http://www.childbirthconnection.org/):

Organization promoting evidence-based maternity care and helping women and providers make informed decisions. Several sections regarding VBAC decision-making.

C. Pictographs/Icon arrays (http://www.iconarray.com)

Center for Bioethics and Social Sciences in Medicine & Risk Science Center, University of Michigan. Create your own pictographs for use in VBAC counseling.

D. NIH Consensus Development Conference on Vaginal Birth After Cesarean

New insights (http://consensus.nih.gov/2010/vbac.htm).

E. Informed Medical Decisions Foundation: Six steps of shared decision making for health care providers (Wexler, 2012)

http://www.slideshare.net/fimdm/six-steps-of-shared-decision-making.

REFERENCES

American College of Nurse-Midwives. (2011). Care for women desiring vaginal birth after cesarean. *Journal of Midwifery & Women's Health, 56*(5), 517–525.

American College of Obstetricians and Gynecologists. (2010). ACOG practice bulletin no. 115: Vaginal birth after previous cesarean delivery. *Obstetrics & Gynecology, 116*(2, Pt. 1), 450–463.

American College of Obstetricians and Gynecologists. (2012). ACOG committee opinion no. 529: Placenta accreta. *Obstetrics & Gynecology, 120*(1), 207–211.

Bager, P., Simonsen, J., Nielsen, N. M., & Frisch, M.. (2012). Cesarean section and offspring's risk of inflammatory bowel disease: A national cohort study. *Inflammatory Bowel Diseases, 18*(5), 857–862.

Bernstein, S. N., Matalon Grazi, S., & Rosenn, B. M. (2012). Trial of labor versus repeat cesarean: Are clients making an informed decision? *American Journal of Obstetrics and Gynecology, 207*(3), 204–206.

Cho, C. E., & Norman, M. (2013). Cesarean section and development of the immune system in the offspring. *American Journal of Obstetrics and Gynecology, 208*(4), 249–254.

Cox, K. J. (2014). Counseling women with a previous cesarean birth: Toward a shared decision-making partnership. *Journal of Midwifery & Women's Health, 59*(3), 237–245.

Curtin, S. C., Gregory, K. D., Korst, L. M., & Uddin, S. F. G. (2015). *Maternal morbidity for vaginal and cesarean deliveries, according to previous cesarean history: New data from the birth certificate, 201.* (National Vital Statistics Reports, Vol. 64, No. 4). Hyattsville, MD: Centers for Disease Control and Prevention, National Center for Health Statistics, U.S. Department of Health and Human Services.

Decker, E., Hornef, M., & Stockinger, S. (2011). Cesarean delivery is associated with celiac disease but not inflammatory bowel disease in children. *Gut Microbes, 2*(2), 91–98.

Declercq, E., Barger, M., Cabral, H. J., Evans, S. R., Kotelchuck, M., Simon, C., et al. (2007). Maternal outcomes associated with planned primary cesarean births compared with planned vaginal births. *Obstetrics & Gynecology, 109*(3), 669–677.

Dodd, J. M., Crowther, C. A., Huertas, E., Guise, J. M., & Horey, D. (2013). Planned elective repeat caesarean section versus planned vaginal birth for women with a previous caesarean birth. *Cochrane Database of Systematic Reviews, 12*, CD004224-CD004224.

Eden, K. B., Denman, M. A., Emeis, C. L., McDonagh, M. S. Fu, R., Janik, R. K., et al. (2012). Trial of labor and vaginal delivery rates in women with a prior cesarean. *Journal of Obstetric, Gynecologic, and Neonatal Nursing. 41*(5),583–596

Garcia-Retamero, R., & Dhami, M. K. (2013). On avoiding framing effects in experienced decision makers. *Quarterly Journal of Experimental Psychology, 66*(4), 829–842.

Grobman, W. A., Lai, Y., Landon, M. B., Spong, C. Y., Leveno, K. J., Rouse, D. J., et al. (2007). Development of a nomogram for prediction of vaginal birth after cesarean delivery. *Obstetrics & Gynecology, 109*(4), 806–812.

Grobman, W. A., Lai, Y., Landon, M. B., Spong, C. Y., Leveno, K. J., Rouse, D. J., et al. (2009). Can a prediction model for vaginal birth after cesarean also predict the probability of morbidity related to a trial of labor? *American Journal of Obstetrics and Gynecology, 200*(1), 56e1–56e6.

Guise, J., Denman, M. A., Emeis, C., Marshall, N., Walker, M., Fu, R., et al. (2010). Vaginal birth after cesarean: New insights on maternal and neonatal outcomes. *Obstetrics and Gynecology, 115*(6), 1267–1278.

Guise, J. M., McDonagh, M. S., Osterweil, P., Nygren, P., Chan, B. K., & Helfand, M. (2004). Systematic review of the incidence and consequences of uterine rupture in women with previous caesarean section. *British Medical Journal, 329*(7456), 19–25.

Hamilton, B. E., Martin, J. A., Osterman, M. J., & Curtin, S. C. (2015). *Births: Preliminary data for 2014* (National Vital Statistics Reports, Vol. 64, No. 6). Hyattsville, MD: Centers for Disease Control and Prevention, National Center for Health Statistics, U.S. Department of Health and Human Services.

Landon, M. B., Hauth, J. C., Leveno, K. J., Spong, C. Y., Leindecker, S., Varner, M. W., et al. (2004). Maternal and perinatal outcomes associated with a trial of labor after prior cesarean delivery. *New England Journal of Medicine, 351*(25), 2581–2589.

Li, H. T., Zhou, Y. B., & Liu, J. M. (2013). The impact of cesarean section on offspring overweight and obesity: A systematic review and meta-analysis. *International Journal of Obesity, 37*(7), 893–899.

King, V. J., Fontaine, P. L., Atwood, L. A., Powers, E., Leeman, L., Ecker, J. L., et al. (2015). Clinical practice guideline executive summary: Labor after cesarean/planned vaginal birth after cesarean. *Annals of Family Medicine, 13*(1), 80–81.

Marshall, N. E., Fu, R., & Guise, J. (2011). Impact of multiple cesarean deliveries on maternal morbidity: A systematic review. *American Journal of Obstetrics and Gynecology, 205*(3), 262–268.

Mesquita, D. N., Barbieri, M. A., Goldani, H. A., Cardoso, V. C., Goldani, M. Z., Kac, G., et al. (2013). Cesarean section is associated with increased peripheral and central adiposity in young adulthood: Cohort study. *PLoS ONE, 8*(6), e66827–e66827.

Miller, E. S., Hahn, K., & Grobman, W. A. (2013). Consequences of a primary elective cesarean delivery across the reproductive life. *Obstetrics and Gynecology, 121*(4), 789–797.

National Institutes of Health. (2010). NIH Consensus Development Conference statement on vaginal birth after cesarean: New insights. March 8–10, 2010. *Obstetrics & Gynecology, 115*(6), 1279–1295.

Ouzounian, J. G., Miller, D. A., Hiebert, C. J., Battista, L. R., & Lee, R. H. (2011). Vaginal birth after cesarean section: Risk of uterine rupture with labor induction. *American Journal of Perinatology, 28*(8), 593–596.

Rossi, A. C., & Prefumo, F. (2015). Pregnancy outcomes of induced labor in women with previous cesarean section: A systematic review and meta-analysis. *Archives of Gynecology and Obstetrics, 291*(2), 273–280.

Shorten, A., Shorten, B., & Kennedy, H. P. (2014). Complexities of choice after prior cesarean: A narrative analysis. *Birth, 41*(2), 178–184.

Silver, R. M. (2012). Implications of the first cesarean: Perinatal and future reproductive health and subsequent cesareans, placentation issues, uterine rupture risk, morbidity, and mortality. *Seminars in Perinatology, 36*(5), 315–323.

Silver, R. M., Landon, M. B., Rouse, D. J., Leveno, K. J., Spong, C. Y., Thom, E. A., et al. (2006). Maternal morbidity associated with multiple repeat cesarean deliveries. *Obstetrics & Gynecology, 107*(6), 1226–1232.

Smith, D., Stringer, E., Vladutiu, C. J., Zink, A. H., & Strauss R. (2015). Risk of uterine rupture among women attempting vaginal birth after cesarean with an unknown uterine scar. *American Journal of Obstetrics and Gynecology, 213*(1), 80.

Smith, G. C., Pell, J. P., Cameron, A. D., & Dobbie, R. (2002). Risk of perinatal death associated with labor after previous cesarean delivery in uncomplicated term pregnancies. *Journal of the American Medical Association, 287*(20), 2684–2690.

Wexler, R. (2012). Six steps of shared decision making for health care providers. Shared slides. Informed Medical Decisions Foundation. Retrieved from http://www.slideshare.net/fimdm/six-steps-of-shared-decision-making.

COMMON DISCOMFORTS OF PREGNANCY

Cynthia Belew and Jamie Meyerhoff

CHAPTER 32

I. Introduction to common discomforts of pregnancy

Most women suffer considerably during a pregnancy. The normal physiologic changes of pregnancy affect all body systems and can cause symptoms that range from mildly uncomfortable to debilitating. These discomforts very rarely pose a risk to the well-being of the fetus. The degree of discomfort experienced by an individual woman is affected by diet, exercise, genetics, personal self-care habits (e.g., obtaining adequate sleep), mood, body image, level of stress, and social support. A pregnant woman feels more satisfied and confident when her care provider listens to her concerns and treats her respectfully (Avery, Saftner, Larson, & Weinfurter, 2014). Pregnant women calling the Motherisk Helpline regarding common discomforts report that providers trivialize discomforts when attempting to normalize (Madjunkova, Maltepe, & Koren, 2013). A woman is likely to feel less stress when she understands the physiologic basis of her symptoms, knows when she may be reassured of the well-being of her baby, and knows when to seek additional medical evaluation. Knowledge regarding self-care measures to prevent and relieve discomforts may increase her sense of autonomy and control. It is therefore a primary responsibility of the healthcare provider to provide anticipatory guidance regarding the physiologic basis and treatment of common discomforts of pregnancy.

Women with multiple or severe symptoms must be screened for depression and anxiety, as these can each increase symptoms, and conversely, multiple symptoms may increase the risk of developing depression (Kamysheva, Wertheim, Skouteris, Paxton, & Milgrom, 2009).

Poor quality of sleep may also contribute to the development of physical complaints and depressive symptoms and may be correlated with preterm birth (Strange, Parker, Moore, Strickland, & Bliwise, 2009). Providers can help women prioritize adequate sleep and provide education regarding sleep hygiene practices. Poor sleep is a common discomfort of pregnancy (Kizilirmak, Timur, & Kartal, 2012).

II. Poor quality of sleep

Musculoskeletal discomfort, fetal movement, increased frequency of urination, increased appetite, nausea, and increased life stresses all contribute to poor quality of sleep during pregnancy. Women report poor quality of sleep in every trimester of pregnancy, including difficulty falling asleep and staying asleep and frequent waking.

A. Subjective

1. Timing and severity of sleep disturbances
2. Symptoms of depression and anxiety
3. Sources of stress
4. Impact on daily functioning
5. Caffeine and other stimulant intake
6. Current daily habits, including daily exercise and evening routine
7. Self-treatment

B. Goals for clinical management

1. Screen for underlying mood disorders in women with multiple or severe common discomforts.
2. Assess quantity and quality of sleep in pregnant women.
3. Educate pregnant women about sleep hygiene, circadian rhythms, and measures to improve sleep.

C. Management

Treatment approaches begin with education and behavioral changes. There is scant research specific to pregnancy and treatments for insomnia. Moderate exercise, such as daily brisk walking, has been demonstrated to be an effective treatment in other demographic populations (King, Oman, Brassington, Bliwise, & Haskell, 1997). There is some debate regarding whether exercise must occur before evening.

Creation of an evening rhythm that is performed every night before going to sleep including decreased stimulation before time of sleep may be helpful. A pregnant woman can note factors that help her feel drowsy, safe, and relaxed and be encouraged to systemically implement those every evening. Common things that relax include massage, warm baths and showers, low light, warm environment, strolling outside, calming music or scents, reading children's bedtime stories, singing lullabies, and humor.

Chamomile is shown to have effectiveness for anxiety (Amsterdam et al., 2009) and may be helpful for promoting sleep. Other safe herbs include linden, valerian, and passionflower. Catnip specifically helps with an overthinking/overactive mind. These herbs can be taken as a tincture, capsule, or tea.

The pregnant woman should also note individual factors that activate her. Common things that activate/overstimulate are media—movies, television, web surfing; disturbing information, news, charged conversations, topics related to changes, money, or planning; worry. Exposure to screen light from computers, tablets, and cellphones has an impact on circadian rhythms. Control of light/dark exposure patterns can powerfully affect sleep and mood. Evening exposure to blue light, including that from computer, tablet, and cellphone screens, suppresses melatonin production, disrupts sleep quality, and leads to decreased alertness the next morning (Sroykham & Wongsawat, 2013; West et al., 2011). Blocking of late evening blue-light exposure through use of amber-lensed glasses and/or low-blue-light bulbs improves sleep quality and mood (Burkhart & Phelps, 2009). Morning exposure to bright light, either through the use of a light box, blue-light enhanced bulbs, or sunlight, enhances cognitive performance, mood, and well-being (Gabel et al., 2013).

Many small studies in a nonpregnant population have shown acupuncture to be a highly effective treatment for insomnia (Lan et al., 2015). In a blinded randomized clinical trial using "double dummy" technique, the acupuncture cohort slept more and more deeply and also reported significantly better daytime functioning and return of their full energetic state; this concords with Chinese medical theory that "energetic daytime function" and "powerful nocturnal sleep" form a circle. Rupture of this cycle leads to "daytime low spirit" and "nighttime hyperarousal state" (Guo, Wang, Liu, Yi, & Cheng, 2013). In this trial, acupuncture was administered for 30 minutes three times a week. An increasing number of communities have the availability of low-cost acupuncture treatment through community acupuncture clinics (https://www.pocacoop.com).

Pharmacologic treatment of insomnia is discouraged for use in pregnancy due to inadequate safety data and side effects. Antihistamines such as diphenhydramine are Pregnancy Category B and sedating. However, pharmacologic treatment has been shown in meta-analysis to be no superior to behavioral therapy in treating insomnia (Mitchell et al., 2012).

III. Musculoskeletal

Hormonal changes of pregnancy cause relaxation of ligaments throughout the body. The resulting increased mobility of pelvic joints and widening of the sacroiliac and symphyseal joints facilitate childbirth but may lead to pelvic instability and pain. Biomechanical factors also contribute to pregnancy discomforts. The growing uterus moves the center of gravity forward, pulls the spine into lordosis, and strains the lower back. In most cases pain resolves within 4 weeks after delivery.

Two types of lumbopelvic pain are common during pregnancy. Low back pain (LBP) is musculoskeletal pain experienced in the area of the lumbar spine. Pelvic girdle pain (PGP) is musculoskeletal pain experienced in the sacroiliac area, the symphysis pubis, or gluteal area, possibly with radiation to the posterior thigh. LBP and PGP may occur concurrently (Vermani, Mittal, & Weeks, 2009). Both LBP and PGP may be provoked by any sustained posture or activity, including prolonged sitting, standing, or walking. PGP generally is more debilitating than LBP (Gutke, Oberg, & Ostgaard, 2006). Women with PGP may report a "catching" sensation in the leg while walking and may report that pain is aggravated by twisting, standing on one leg, climbing stairs, and turning in bed.

Many treatments target both LBP and PGP; differences in approach are specified next and in **Table 32-1.**

A. Prevention

The woman with strong abdominal, back, gluteal, and pelvic muscles may be less likely to develop lumbopelvic pain of pregnancy (Bewyer, Bewyer, & Messenger, 2009). Several studies show that physical fitness exercises before pregnancy may reduce a woman's risk of developing back pain in pregnancy (Vermani et al., 2009). A tailored exercise program during pregnancy was shown to be effective in preventing LBP (Mørkved, Salvesen, Schei, Lydersen, & Bø, 2007). Individualized exercise programs are generally more effective than group training or no treatment.

Workplace restrictions may significantly affect a woman's risk. Because sustained sitting, standing, or walking may provoke pain, a pregnant woman benefits from the freedom to change activities and positions frequently. Research shows that pregnant women who have job autonomy and the ability to take breaks at work experience less back pain, whereas those working in jobs that necessitate staying in a confined area experience more back pain (Cheng et al., 2009).

TABLE 32-1 Differential Diagnosis and Management of Pelvic Pain and Low Back Pain in Pregnancy

	Subjective	Physical Exam	Imaging	Treatment
Low back pain	Lumbar pain, worse with forward flexion	Negative posterior pelvic pain provocation test	Not indicated	Water aerobics Group exercise for abdominal, back, and pelvic strength Acupuncture Osteopathic manipulation Exercise: pelvic tilt Abdominal support garments
Pelvic girdle pain	Sacroiliac pain May radiate to posterior thigh May involve symphysis pubis or gluteal area	Positive posterior pelvic pain provocation test	Not indicated	Nonelastic pelvic belt to increase stability of sacroiliac joint Individualized pelvic stabilizing and core strengthening exercises
Cauda equina syndrome (severe nerve compression)	Rapid onset of bilateral radiating pain Lower extremity numbness and weakness Numbness of perineum, inner thigh, back of legs Bladder or bowel dysfunction	Supine straight leg raise elicits radiating pain to ipsilateral foot on flexion of hip	Immediate MRI	Orthopedic consultation If stable: bed rest and muscle relaxants If deteriorating: surgery

Data from Smith, M. W., Marcus, P. S., & Wurtz, L. D. (2008). Orthopedic issues in pregnancy. *Obstetrical & Gynecological Survey, 63*(2), 103–111; Vermani, E., Mittal, R., & Weeks, A. (2009). Pelvic girdle pain and low back pain in pregnancy: A review. *Pain Practice, 10*(1), 60–71.

B. Database (may include but is not limited to)

The distribution of pain is the most useful history item for diagnosis. The presence of "red flag" signs and symptoms indicates the possibility of disk herniation and requires immediate consultation and possibly magnetic resonance imaging of the spine (**Table 32-2**).

1. Subjective
   a. Signs or symptoms of preterm labor
   b. Signs or symptoms of pyelonephritis
   c. Events preceding onset
      i. Recent or past history of physical trauma
      ii. History of similar pain
      iii. Anxiety or depression
      iv. Patterns of activity throughout the day
   d. Location and characteristics of pain
      i. Radiation: bilateral or unilateral to thigh or foot
      ii. Pattern of pain: intermittent or constant
      iii. Postures or movements that provoke or alleviate pain
      iv. Quality: sharp, aching, dull; intensity
      v. Level of impact on function and patterns of pacing activity during the day
      vi. Self-treatment, coping strategies, pain beliefs, remedies, and over-the-counter medications

TABLE 32-2 Musculoskeletal Red Flag Symptoms Requiring Consultation or Referral

- Sudden onset of incapacitating back or leg pain, especially pain radiating from the spine along a dermatome bilaterally
- Numbness of perineum, inner thighs, or backs of legs
- Bladder or bowel dysfunction, decreased rectal sphincter tone
- Localized neurologic symptoms (symptoms limited to one nerve root dermatome)
- Decreased muscle strength and sensitivity
- Structural deformity
- Altered deep tendon reflexes
- Localized neurology (symptoms limited to one nerve root dermatome)

2. Objective
   a. Digital cervical examination to rule out preterm labor if indicated (see Chapter 35 on preterm birth management)
   b. Test for costovertebral angle tenderness to rule out pyelonephritis
   c. Observe gait and ability to change positions; observe distress level
   d. Palpate over the sacroiliac, lumbar, symphysis, and gluteal regions (may help to identify pain distribution to differentiate between LBP and PGP; may also rule out structural abnormalities)
   e. Do a posterior pelvic pain provocation test to differentiate PGP from LBP
      i. The patient lies supine with hips flexed to 90 degrees.
      ii. The examiner applies pressure on the flexed knee in the longitudinal axis of the femur while stabilizing the pelvis with the other hand resting on the opposite anterior superior iliac spine.
      iii. If this maneuver produces deep pain in the gluteal region, the test is positive and supports a diagnosis of PGP.
   f. Perform the supine active straight leg raise (SLR) test to identify the possibility of disk herniation with nerve compression. If the SLR elicits pain radiating in a dermatomal pattern or if there is numbness or leg weakness, carry out the following tests: reflexes (Achilles or knee), sensation of lateral and medial sides of feet and toes, and strength testing of the big toe during extension.
   g. Imaging studies, such as magnetic resonance imaging, are recommended only when there are multiple red flags (Albert, Ostgaard, Sturesson, Stuge, & Vleeming, 2008).

3. Differential diagnosis
   a. Pregnancy-related LBP or PGP
   b. Preterm labor
   c. Pyelonephritis
   d. Muscle strain caused by trauma
   e. Sciatica

4. Goals for clinical management
   a. Educate women about physical fitness for prevention of musculoskeletal pain
   b. Assess musculoskeletal pain in pregnant women, ruling out serious pathology
   c. Provide treatment plans, education, and referrals for women with low back pain or pelvic girdle pain during pregnancy

5. Management
   a. Maternity support garments
      i. For PGP, a nonelastic pelvic belt stabilizes the sacroiliac joints and may provide pain relief (Damen, Mens, Snijders, & Stam, 2006). It is most effective when at the level of the greater trocanters.
      ii. Physiotherapists recommend that it be worn for short periods of time rather than continuously (Albert et al., 2008; Chow et al., 2009).
      iii. PGP is less likely than LBP to respond to exercise classes. The abdominal lift garment may be the most beneficial type of maternity support garment for LBP (Albert et al., 2008).
   b. Exercise
      i. Group exercise focused on increasing strength and flexibility and water exercise have been shown to decrease LBP in the second part of pregnancy (Pennick & Liddle, 2013).
      ii. Gentle exercise at home may be helpful, including the pelvic tilt, knee pull, curl-up, lateral SLR, and pelvic floor exercises.
      iii. For PGP, pelvic stabilizing exercises given by a physical therapist are effective (Vleeming, Albert, Ostgaard, Sturesson, & Stuge, 2008).
   c. Workplace modification: a provider's letter to the employer recommending regular rest breaks and movement outside of confined working areas may be beneficial for some women.
   d. Medication for pregnancy-related LBP and PGP
      i. Acetaminophen may not be more effective than placebo for LBP and PGP of pregnancy (Vermani et al., 2009).
      ii. Nonsteroidal anti-inflammatory drugs are not recommended in the last trimester of pregnancy because of risk of premature closure of the ductus arteriosus and risk of oligohydramnios.
      iii. Opioids: Occasional use of small doses of opioids (e.g., codeine) is sometimes indicated in severe cases of pain. Opioid use in late pregnancy can cause respiratory depression in the newborn and, with long-term use, withdrawal effects in the newborn (Vermani et al., 2009).

6. Referrals and self-management resources
   a. European guidelines consider evidence sufficient to recommend the following for PGP:

exercise, individualized physical therapy, massage, acupuncture, osteopathic manipulation, and chiropractic care (Albert et al., 2008).

b. Useful online resources include the Association of Chartered Physiotherapists in Women's Health (www.acpwh.org) and the Pelvic Partnership (http://www.pelvicpartnership.org.uk/).

7. Patient education (adapted from www.acpwh.org)

a. Teach pertinent anatomy and physiology and reassure that pelvic and back pain are a normal part of pregnancy for many women, likely to resolve in the weeks after birth.

b. Provide guidance regarding appropriate pacing of activity and rest.

   i. Be as active as possible within the limits of pain. Staying active can reduce pain and improve function (Krismer & van Tulder, 2007).

   ii. Avoid fatigue by taking frequent rest breaks.

   iii. Avoid being in one posture for a prolonged time.

   iv. Avoid activities that worsen pain. Encourage sitting down to put on pants and shoes.

c. Advise supportive shoes and avoidance of heels.

d. Recommend placement of one pillow between the knees and one under the abdomen when sleeping side-lying

IV. Gastrointestinal tract

Elevated levels of progesterone during pregnancy facilitate maintenance of the pregnancy by relaxing the uterine muscle. However, smooth muscle relaxation decreases gastric and intestinal motility, leading to nausea, dyspepsia, and constipation. Mechanical pressure from the enlarging uterus contributes to heartburn. Management of common gastrointestinal tract discomforts of pregnancy, such as nausea, heartburn, and constipation, proceeds in a stepwise algorithm that begins with lifestyle and dietary modifications and gentle natural remedies. Pharmaceutical treatment is reserved for persistent or severe symptoms. This conservative approach is recommended because of the benign nature of common gastrointestinal tract discomforts of pregnancy.

The Canadian organization Motherisk, a clinical research and teaching program at The Hospital for Sick Children, has an excellent online resource (www.motherisk.org). They provide information both to pregnant and lactating women and to healthcare professionals regarding risks to the fetus from maternal exposure to drugs, chemicals, diseases, radiation, and environmental agents. They maintain several helplines, including one dedicated to questions regarding nausea and vomiting of pregnancy (NVP).

A. Nausea and vomiting of pregnancy

1. Definition and clinical implications

Nausea and vomiting of pregnancy are considered to be a result of hormonal changes. About 50 to 85% of all pregnant women experience NVP. Typically, symptom onset is around 5–7 weeks from the last menstrual period, with resolution at 11–14 weeks gestation. In a subset of women, symptoms may persist until 18 weeks, and 5% of pregnant women have nausea throughout pregnancy. If onset of symptoms occurs at a gestational age of 10 weeks or greater, the etiology is not likely to be pregnancy.

NVP is a normal part of most pregnancies. Although NVP may have a significant impact on a woman's daily life, it is benign. The presence of NVP is associated with a lower risk of miscarriage (Weigel et al., 2006). The reduced maternal nutrient intake that commonly occurs during the first trimester in women with NVP seems to cause complex hormonal and metabolic changes that actually enhance placental growth (Huxley, 2000). It is also proposed that NVP serves a protective evolutionary function, causing women to avoid foods that may cause harm to the embryo (Sherman & Flaxman, 2002). Most women make up for first-trimester weight loss by gaining more weight later in pregnancy.

In contrast, hyperemesis gravidarum (HG) can pose serious risks and is a more debilitating condition. On the continuum from severe NVP to HG, HG is defined as symptoms that lead to weight loss of more than 5% of prepregnancy body weight, hypokalemia, and dehydration or ketonuria. HG may require hospitalization. Holmgren and colleagues reviewed the management of HG (Holmgren, Aagaard-Tillery, Silver, Porter, & Varner, 2008). HG requires medical management because it can be associated with serious sequelae, such as micronutrient deficiency or Wernicke's encephalopathy, if not properly managed (Dodds, Fell, Joseph, Allen, & Butler, 2006).

If heartburn exists concurrent with NVP, pharmacologic treatment of the heartburn is shown to decrease symptoms of NVP (Gill, Maltepe, Mastali, & Koren, 2009).

B. Database

1. Subjective data

   a. Timing of onset, pattern, and frequency of nausea and vomiting

   i. The "PUQE" (pregnancy-unique quantification of emesis/nausea) index may be used to evaluate severity. The woman's subjective experience of the impact of symptoms on her life is an important consideration and may override the PUQE score (King & Murphy, 2009) (**Table 32-3**).

   b. Triggers and coexisting gastric reflux

   c. Eating habits and self-treatment

   d. Red flags for gallbladder disease and HELLP syndrome (hemolysis, elevated liver enzymes, and low platelets)

   i. Epigastric pain, right upper quadrant pain, or coffee grounds emesis

   ii. Upper abdominal pain in a pattern of biliary colic (episodes of sharp, intense pain after meals or at night lasting 30 minutes to 3 hours, or radiation to back or right shoulder) may indicate gallbladder disease.

2. Objective data

   a. Weight loss

   b. Urinalysis: ketones and specific gravity

   c. Signs of dehydration: tachycardia, dry mucosa, and sunken eyes

   d. If severe symptoms are present: order an electrolyte panel and an obstetric ultrasound to rule out twin gestation or trophoblastic disease (molar pregnancy)

   e. If onset of symptoms occurs in third trimester: rule out HELLP syndrome with complete blood count (CBC) and platelets even if symptoms are not severe

   f. If symptoms suggest gallbladder disease: CBC, lipase, liver enzymes, and abdominal ultrasound

3. Differential diagnosis

   a. Dehydration

   b. Ketonuria

   c. Electrolyte imbalance

   d. HG

   e. Gallbladder, liver, or pancreatic disease

   f. HELLP syndrome (third trimester)

   g. Fatty liver of pregnancy (rare)

4. Goals for clinical management

   a. Differentiate normal nausea and vomiting of pregnancy (NVP) from hyperemesis and other serious pathology.

   b. Provide comprehensive education for women with NVP about dietary and lifestyle changes to minimize symptoms.

   c. Provide evidence-based information about safe alternative and complementary treatments for NVP.

   d. Provide evidence-based pharmacotherapy for treatment of NVP.

   e. Assess results of treatment and provide intravenous rehydration as needed.

5. Treatment

   Women commonly find that one therapeutic measure works well for a few days but then becomes less

---

TABLE 32-3 Pregnancy-Unique Quantification of Emesis and Nausea Index

1. On an average day, for how long do you feel nauseated or sick to your stomach?

> 6 hr	4–6 hr	2–3 hr	≤ 1 hr	Not at all
(5 points)	(4 points)	(3 points)	(2 points)	(1 point)

2. On an average day, how many times do you vomit or throw up?

≥ 7	5–6	3–4	1–2	None
(5 points)	(4 points)	(3 points)	(2 points)	(1 point)

3. On an average day, how many times do you have retching or dry heaves without bringing anything up?

≥ 7	5–6	3–4	1–2	None
(5 points)	(4 points)	(3 points)	(2 points)	(1 point)

Total score (sum of replies to 1, 2, and 3): mild NVP, ≤ 6; moderate NVP, 7–12; severe NVP, ≥ 13.

Reprinted from Lacasse, A., Rey, E., Ferreira, E., Morin, C., & Bérard, A. (2008). Validity of a modified Pregnancy-Unique Quantification of Emesis and Nausea (PUQE) scoring index to assess severity of nausea and vomiting of pregnancy. *American Journal of Obstetrics and Gynecology, 198*(1), 71.e3; with permission from Elsevier.

effective. Knowledge about multiple treatments is beneficial to switch tactics as needed.

6. Education

Reassure that mild to moderate symptoms do not have a negative effect on fetal growth and development. Discuss dietary and lifestyle changes.

7. Hydration and nutrition

a. Avoid dehydration by sipping small amounts of water frequently (as little as an ounce every 15 minutes). Large volumes of fluid may provoke nausea.

b. Drink cold fluids between meals instead of with meals.

c. Eat small amounts of food that include protein every 1–2 hours. Low blood sugar provokes nausea. Eat a high-protein snack at bedtime.

d. Keep dry crackers at the bedside and eat a few before rising in the morning.

e. Avoid spicy or fatty foods.

8. Trigger avoidance: triggers are highly individual but may include

a. Strong odors, stuffy rooms, or bus travel.

b. The sight or smell of certain foods.

c. Brushing teeth. Avoid brushing teeth within 1–2 hours after eating. Use a child's size toothbrush and small amounts of a low-foaming toothpaste or brush without toothpaste.

d. Multivitamins: continue to take multivitamin if possible, because it may decrease symptoms, but if taking multivitamin aggravates nausea, discontinue and replace with 600 mcg of folic acid. Resume multivitamin at a later gestational age when NVP resolves. A multivitamin without iron may be more easily tolerated.

9. Therapeutic

a. Alternative and complementary

   i. The Canadian Motherisk reports that 61% of women with NVP report use of complementary and alternative remedies but only 8% of women had discussed these remedies with their healthcare provider (Hollyer, Boon, Georgousis, Smith, & Einarson, 2002)

   ii. Ginger, chamomile, fennel seed, raspberry leaf, and mint are all used traditionally in a tea or tincture for gastric upset. These herbs are regarded as safe by the Canadian Motherisk group (Mills, Duguoa, Perri, & Koren, 2006) and the German Commission E (Blumenthal, Goldberg, & Brinckmann, 2000). Both are authoritative expert panels dealing with the topic of herb safety.

b. Evidence exists supporting the effectiveness and safety of the following therapies:

   i. Acupressure wrist bands (Seabands, Travel-Eze) worn continuously over the P6 acupuncture point (Can Gürkan & Arslan, 2008).

   ii. Ginger capsules, 250 mg orally four times a day (Bryer, 2005)

   iii. Vitamin B$_6$, 25 mg orally three times a day. Avoid excessive doses, which may cause peripheral neuropathy (Keller, Frederking, & Layer, 2008).

c. Intravenous fluid therapy: Intravenous fluid therapy with normal saline, alone or in combination with pharmaceuticals, typically causes an improvement of symptoms for several days. Some women choose it as a primary management strategy, receiving hydration every few days as needed (King & Murphy, 2009). Avoid dextrose-containing fluids, because they may precipitate Wernicke's encephalopathy, a rare but serious complication, in a woman with thiamine deficiency. The addition of thiamine is recommended for the prevention of Wernicke's encephalopathy. Potassium chloride may be added as needed. Consultation is necessary for persistent nausea and vomiting with dehydration, and intravenous vitamins and minerals may be required.

10. Pharmacotherapy (see **Table 32-4**)

a. Antihistamines

Diclegis, delayed release (doxylamine 10 mg, combined with pyridoxine 10 mg) is the only drug approved by the Food and Drug Administration (FDA) for nausea and vomiting during pregnancy. A large body of evidence supports both the safety and effectiveness of the combination. Years of widespread use of this medication in Canada and in the United States in the 1980s contribute to its high safety profile (Nuangchamnong & Niebyl, 2014). Diclegis is taken as a daily prescription, rather than as needed.

b. Dopamine antagonists

Metoclopramide has been a drug of choice for many providers in treating severe NVP and HG. Recent research examining more than 3,400 first-trimester exposures found no association with any of several adverse outcomes (Matok et al., 2009). In a comparison of promethazine and metoclopramide, Tan and colleagues found similar efficacy but metoclopramide had fewer side effects (Tan, Khine, Vallikkannu, & Omar, 2010). In a small study on treatment

TABLE 32-4 Pharmacotherapy for NVP

Generic Name (trade name)	Dosage	Major Side Effects
Antihistamines		
Doxylamine succinate-pyroxidine hydrochloride (Diclegis®)	10 mg doxylamine combined with 10 mg of pyridoxine, delayed release 4 tablets daily: 2 at night, 1 in the morning, 1 in the afternoon	Mild drowsiness
Diphenhydramine	50–100 mg q 4–6 hr PO/IM/IV For treatment of dystonic reaction: 50 mg IV	Drowsiness
Trimethobenzamide	200 mg IM/PR q 6–8 hr	Drowsiness
Dopamine antagonists		
Metoclopramide	1–2 mg/kg IV (dilute in 50 mL IVF) or 5–10 mg q 8 hr PO/PR/IM	Agitation, anxiety, acute dystonic reactions*
Prochlorperazine	5–10 mg PO/IV/IM q 6–8 hr or 25 mg rectal suppository BID/prn for breakthrough vomiting with other medications	Sedation, anticholinergic effects, EPS
Promethazine	12.5–25 mg PO/IV/IM/PR q 4–6 hr	Sedation, anticholinergic effects, dystonic reactions*
Serotonin (5-HT3) antagonists		
Ondansetron Publisher note	4–8 mg PO q 6–8 hr 4–8 mg IV q 12 hr, given over 15 min	Headache. Do not use during the first trimester
Other		
Pyridoxine (vitamin B$_6$)	25 mg TID. Consider combining with doxylamine	
Zingiber officinale (ginger)	Capsules: 250–500 mg TID-QID Not to exceed 1.5 g in 24 hr	

* Give 50 mg diphenhydramine before dose to prevent extrapyramidal reactions

Modified from King, T. L., & Murphy, P. A. (2009). Evidence-based approaches to managing nausea and vomiting in early pregnancy. *Journal of Midwifery & Women's Health, 54*(6), 435; with permission from Elsevier.

of hyperemesis gravidarum, metoclopramide had similar efficacy with increased side effects compared to ondansetron (Abas, Tan, Azmi, & Omar, 2014). Metoclopramide was associated with increased dizziness, dry mouth, headache, diarrhea, and palpitations. Despite these side effects, it remains a reasonable treatment choice.

c. Phenothiazines
Promethazine and prochlorpemazine may be as effective as ondansetron and have no evidence of being teratogenic, although there is less human data than for metoclopramide and Diclegis (Briggs, Freeman, & Yaffe, 2015). These drugs cause significant sedation, making them difficult for women to tolerate.

d. 5-Hydroxytryptamine 3-receptor antagonists
Ondansetron has been used increasingly in treatment of NVP. However, two large studies have recently found statistically significant increases in fetal cardiac anomalies associated with use of ondansetron in the first trimester (Danielsson, Wikner, & Källén, 2014). Ondansetron should not be used during the first trimester. The FDA has issued warnings about serious maternal dysrhythmias associated with use of ondansetron (Koren, 2014). Additionally, there have been 33 case reports of rare but life-threatening intestinal obstruction in which ondansetron was the sole associated pharmaceutical, one of which was in a pregnant patient (Cohen et al, 2014).

11. Follow-up
    a. Send to labor and delivery for rehydration and medication as needed.
    b. Consider increasing the frequency of prenatal visits to once or twice weekly until symptoms diminish.
    c. Assessing and Treating Women with Nausea in Pregnancy.

V. Heartburn

A. Definition

Heartburn, also known as gastroesophageal reflux disease, is a normal part of most pregnancies. Symptoms are usually mild to moderate. Lifestyle and dietary modifications accompanied by safe home remedies and simple antacids often are effective in providing relief. Pregnancy seems to be protective against esophagitis and gastric ulcer disease, and these conditions are uncommon during pregnancy (Cappell, 2003). Even severe symptoms of gastroesophageal reflux disease usually resolve soon after birth.

B. Database (may include but is not limited to)

Red flag symptoms and signs (listed next in section 1b) help in the differentiation of benign heartburn from more serious medical conditions. Gallbladder disease, pancreatitis, and, in the third trimester, HELLP syndrome must be ruled out. Red flag symptoms and signs require immediate consultation.

1. Subjective
   a. Typical symptoms of gastric acid reflux during pregnancy include
      i. Burning in the upper abdomen or midchest.
      ii. Discomfort associated with eating or with a recumbent position.
      iii. Typically worsens as the pregnancy progresses.
      iv. Relieved by antacids.
   b. Red flag symptoms of include:
      i. Gallbladder disease: episodes of biliary colic
      ii. HELLP: Right upper quadrant, midepigastrium, or retrosternal pain, nausea, vomiting, and malaise. HELLP may occur without hypertension.
      iii. Pancreatitis: acute onset of persistent, severe epigastric pain.
2. Objective
   a. Physical examination
      i. Assess for red flag signs of HELLP
      ii. Right upper quadrant or midepigastrium tenderness

   b. Laboratory tests
      i. Serum amylase and lipase as indicated to rule out pancreatitis
      ii. Liver enzymes as indicated to rule out liver disease
      iii. Liver enzymes and platelets as indicated to rule out HELLP
3. Assessment
   a. Normal gastric reflux of pregnancy. This diagnosis is based on symptoms alone.
   b. Rule out liver disease, gallbladder disease, and, if in third trimester, HELLP
4. Goals of clinical management
   a. Assess reflux during pregnancy and rule out serious pathology.
   b. Select pharmaceutical treatments for reflux that have the minimum adverse effects.
   c. Educate women about the adverse effects of proton pump inhibitors and H2 agonists.
   d. Educate women about lifestyle and dietary modifications to minimize symptoms of reflux during pregnancy.
5. Management (see **Table 32-5**)
   Stomach acid is necessary for absorption of essential nutrients, destruction of ingested pathogens, and maintenance of a beneficial gastrointestinal microbiome, all key functions for maintenance of optimal health. Suppression of stomach acid, especially the profound and long-lasting suppression of proton pump inhibitors (PPIs), is linked with a number of adverse effects. A stepwise approach to gastroesophageal reflux disease (GERD) is advised, starting with lifestyle and dietary modifications, moving to raft-forming or simple antacids and then to sucralfate, reserving histamine-2 receptor antagonists (H2RA) and PPIs for persistent severe symptoms. Adverse effects of H2RAs and PPIs are addressed later. The detrimental effects of PPIs may not be seen with antacids because antacids affect gastric acidity to a lesser degree and for a shorter duration of time. Rebound acid hypersecretion occurs after use of PPIs but not after use of H2RAs (Waldum, Qvigstad, Fossmark, Kleveland, & Sandvik, 2010).

   Expert opinion and traditional use support the benefit and safety of marshmallow root (Althea) and the inner bark of slippery elm (Ulmas rubra) for heartburn and gastritis (Romm, 2010). They contain mucilage (insoluble polysaccharides), which absorbs acid and sooths irritated or inflamed mucosa (Deters et al., 2010).

   Raft-forming antireflux medications (Gaviscon) combine a low dose of antacid (magnesium and aluminum salts) with alginic acid and may be more

TABLE 32-5 Management for Heartburn During Pregnancy

Lifestyle Modifications

- Eat small frequent meals rather than two large meals (Jarosz & Taraszewska, 2014)
- Avoid frequent consumption of mint tea (Jarosz & Taraszewska, 2014)
- Do not drink large amounts of liquid with meals
- Take a walk after dinner (Karim et al., 2011)
- Do not recline after meals (Karim et al., 2011)
- Do not gain more than the recommended weight during pregnancy
- Eat in a slow and relaxed manner (Yamamichi et al., 2012)
- Identify and avoid triggers, which may include carbohydrates (Austin, Thiny, Westman, Yancy, & Shaheen, 2006), tobacco, alcohol, and chocolate (Kaltenbach, Crockett, & Gerson, 2006)

Remedies (Romm, 2010)

- Raw almonds (8–10 at a time) chewed slowly, as frequently as needed
- Slippery elm lozenges 2–4 PRN, or slippery elm powder (one teaspoon stirred into applesauce, juice, or water)
- Marshmallow root: one ounce of dried herb steeped for at least 30 minutes in one quart of hot water, strain, sip throughout the day as needed, up to three cups daily.
- Strong tea of chamomile, fennel, ginger, linden, alone or in combination.
- Dandelion root tea (one to three cups sipped throughout the day) or tincture (20–40 drops diluted in a small amount of water three times daily); contraindicated if there are painful gallstones (acute biliary colic) or cholecystitis.

Antacids

Avoid sodium bicarbonate, bismuth, AlkaSeltzer (Mahadevan & Kane, 2006)

Medication	Considerations
Gaviscon (Quartarone, 2013)	- Avoid high doses in pregnancy - Generally well tolerated - For maximum effect, take 30 minutes after meals and maintain upright position.
Calcium- or magnesium-containing antacids (Tytgat et al., 2003)	- Excessive use of calcium carbonate (> 2 g/day) can result in milk alkali syndrome (hypercalcemia and alkalosis, which can cause renal damage). - Magnesium-containing antacids may cause diarrhea. - Avoid excessive doses of aluminum salts. - Although some advocate the benefits of calcium carbonate as an antacid because it also provides supplemental calcium, in reality calcium carbonate contains only 40% elemental calcium and has poor bioavailability (Sipponen & Härkönen, 2010).
Sucralfate	Adverse effects unlikely

Histamine-2 receptor antagonists (H2RA)

Cimetidine or ranitidine are preferred (Mahadevan & Kane, 2006).	- A decrease in effectiveness to H2RA treatment may occur within 2–6 weeks of initiation of therapy (Komazawa et al., 2003). - The safety of H2RAs during the first trimester has not been established (Gilboa, Ailes, Rai, Anderson, & Honein, 2014).

Proton Pump Inhibitors

Omeprazole (Prilosec®) is recommended as the PPI of choice (Mahadevan & Kane, 2006).	- The use of PPIs during pregnancy is not associated with an increased risk of birth defects, perinatal mortality, or morbidity (Matok et al., 2012). - Adverse effects include impaired micronutrient absorption, increased risk of enteric infections including gastroenteritis and *Clostridium difficile* infection, increased risk of community-acquired pneumonia, disrupted gastrointestinal microbiome, and an association with increased risk of allergic disease in the offspring (see text).

effective than antacids alone (De Ruigh, Roman, Chen, Pandolfino, & Kahrilas, 2014; Rohof, Bennink, Smout, Thomas, & Boeckxstaens, 2014). Alginate forms a viscous foam that floats on the surface of the gastric pool, providing a mechanical barrier to reflux. If reflux occurs the nonacidic foam rather than the acidic stomach content moves into the esophagus. Research has demonstrated alginate-containing ant-acids to be highly effective and safe during pregnancy (Quartarone, 2013).

a. Adverse effects of acid inhibitors:
  i. Micronutrient absorption

  A dramatic decrease in absorption of vitamin B_{12} is seen after only 2 weeks of treatment with a PPI (Marcuard, Albernaz, & Khazanie, 1994), and use of both H2RA and PPI is significantly associated with the presence of vitamin B_{12} deficiency (Lam, Schneider, Zhao, & Corley, 2014). The FDA has issued warnings regarding the correlation of PPI use with hypomagnesemia (FDA, 2011; Markovits et al., 2014). PPIs are also linked with hypocalcemia and hypokalemia (Luk, Parsons, Lee, & Hughes, 2013). The implications of PPI-induced hypomagnesemia and hypocalcemia and low B_{12} levels during pregnancy have not been explored. Adequate magnesium and calcium levels are important for normal fetal bone development, and the link between low calcium intake and risk of gestational hypertension is well described (Dodd, O'Brien, & Grivel, 2014). The theoretical link between PPI use and increased risk of calcium-deficiency disorders such as preeclampsia has not been investigated.

  ii. Risk of infection

  PPI use is associated with increased susceptibility of food-borne and enteric infection including *Salmonella*, invasive strains of *Escherichia coli*, *Listeria*, and *Clostridium difficile* infection (CDI) (Bavishi & Dupont, 2011). Outpatients prescribed PPIs have as much as a threefold increased risk of CDI compared with matched controls (Freedberg, Lebwohl, & Abrams, 2014). The FDA has issued a drug alert regarding the connection of PPI use with CDI (FDA, 2012) and has recommended that PPIs be prescribed at the lowest dose and shortest duration possible.

  iii. Alternations in the microbiome

  Use of acid-suppressing drugs rapidly alters the microbiome in the stomach, esophagus, and small intestine, shifting the population toward inflammatory flora (Freedburg et al., 2014) and causing small intestinal bacterial overgrowth (Del Piano et al., 2014). Researchers are exploring the role of selected probiotic supplements to negate the harmful effect of PPIs on the microbiome (Del Piano et al., 2014). The disruption in microbiome might explain the association of prenatal use of acid-suppressive drugs with an increased risk of allergic disease in the offspring (Mulder et al., 2014).

6. Follow-up
  a. Increase frequency of visits based on response to treatment
  b. Nutritionist referral
  c. Physician consultation for persistent severe symptoms unresponsive to treatment

REFERENCES

Abas, M. N., Tan, P. C., Azmi, N., et al. (2014). Ondansetron compared with metoclopramide for hyperemesis gravidarum: A randomized controlled trial. *Obstetrics and Gynecology, 123*(6), 1272–1279.

Albert, H. B., Ostgaard, H. C., Sturesson, B., Stuge, B., & Vleeming, A. (2008). European guidelines for the diagnosis and treatment of pelvic girdle pain. *European Spine Journal, 17*(6), 794–819.

Austin, G. L., Thiny, M. T., Westman, .E C., Yancy, W. S. Jr., & Shaheen, N. J. (2006). A very low-carbohydrate diet improves gastroesophageal reflux and its symptoms. *Digestive Diseases and Sciences, 51*(8), 1307–1312.

Avery, M. D., Saftner, M. A., Larson, B., & Weinfurter, E. V. (2014). A systematic review of maternal confidence for physiologic birth: Characteristics of prenatal care and confidence measurement. *Journal of Midwifery & Women's Health, 59*(6), 586–595.

Bavishi, C., & Dupont, H. L. (2011). Systematic review: The use of proton pump inhibitors and increased susceptibility to enteric infection. *Alimentary Pharmacology & Therapeutics, 34*(11–12), 1269–1281.

Bewyer, K. J., Bewyer, D. C., & Messenger, D. (2009). Pilot data: Association between gluteus medius weakness and low back pain during pregnancy. *Iowa Orthopaedic Journal, 29*, 97–99.

Blumenthal, M., Goldberg, A., & Brinckmann, J. (2000). *Herbal medicine: Expanded Commission E monographs.* Newton, MA: Integrative Medicine Communications.

Briggs, G. G., Freeman, R. K., & Yaffe, S. J. (2015). *Drugs in pregnancy and lactation: A reference guide to fetal and neonatal risk* (10th ed.). Philadelphia: Wolters Kluwer/Lippincott Williams & Wilkins Health.

Bryer, E. (2005). A literature review of the effectiveness of ginger in alleviating mild-to-moderate nausea and vomiting of pregnancy. *Journal of Midwifery & Women's Health, 50*(1), e1–e3.

Burkhart, K., & Phelps, J. R. (2009). Amber lenses to block blue light and improve sleep: A randomized trial. *Chronobiology International, 26*(8), 1602–1612.

Can Gürkan, O., & Arslan, H. (2008). Effect of acupressure on nausea and vomiting during pregnancy. *Complementary Therapy Clinical Practice*, *14*(1), 46–52.

Cappell, M. S. (2003). Gastric and duodenal ulcers during pregnancy. *Gastroenterology Clinics of North America*, *32*(1), 263–308.

Cheng, P. L., Pantel, M., Smith, J. T., Dumas, G. A., Leger, A. B., Plamondon, A., et al. (2009). Back pain of working pregnant women: Identification of associated occupational factors. *Applied Ergonomics*, *40*(3), 419–423.

Chow, D. H., Chung, J. W., Ho, S., Lao, T., Li, Y., & Yu, W. (2009). Effectiveness of maternity support belts in reducing low back pain during pregnancy: A review. *Journal of Clinical Nursing*, *18*(11), 1523–1532.

Cohen, R., Shlomo, M., Dil, D. N., Dinavitser, N., Berkovitch, M., & Koren, G. (2014). Intestinal obstruction in pregnancy by ondansetron. *Reproductive Toxicology*, *50*, 152–153.

Damen, L., Mens, J. M., Snijders, C. J., & Stam, H. J. (2006). The mechanical effect of a pelvic belt in patients with pregnancy-related pelvic pain. *Clinical Biomechanics*, *21*(2), 122–127.

Danielsson, B., Wikner, B. N., & Källén, B. (2014). Use of ondansetron during pregnancy and congenital malformations in the infant. *Reproductive Toxicology*, *50*, 134–137.

De Ruigh, A., Roman, S., Chen, J., Pandolfino, E., & Kahrilas, P. J. (2014). Gaviscon Double Action Liquid (antacid & alginate) is more effective than antacid in controlling post-prandial oesophageal acid exposure in GERD patients: A double-blind crossover study. *Alimentary Pharmacology & Therapeutics*, *40*(5), 531–537.

Dehlink, E., Yen, E., Leichtner, A. M., Hait, E. J., & Fiebiger, E. (2009). First evidence of a possible association between gastric acid suppression during pregnancy and childhood asthma: A population-based register study. *Clinical and Experimental Allergy*, *39*(2), 246–253.

Del Piano, M., Pagliarulo, M., Tari, R., Carmagnola, S., Balzarini, M., Lorenzini, P., et al. (2014). Correlation between chronic treatment with proton pump inhibitors and bacterial overgrowth in the stomach: Any possible beneficial role for selected lactobacilli? *Journal of Clinical Gastroenterology*, *48*(Suppl. 1), S40–S46.

Deters, A., Zippel, J., Hellenbrand, N., Pappai, D., Possemeyer, C., & Hensel, A. (2010). Aqueous extracts and polysaccharides from marshmallow roots (*Althea officinalis* L.): Cellular internalisation and stimulation of cell physiology of human epithelial cells in vitro. *Journal of Ethnopharmacology*, *127*(1), 62–69.

Dodd, J. M., O'Brien, C., & Grivell, R. M. (2014). Preventing pre-eclampsia—Are dietary factors the key? *BMC Medicine*, *12*, 176. doi:10.1186/s12916-014-0176-4.

Dodds, L., Fell, D. B., Joseph, K. S., Allen, V. M., & Butler, B. (2006). Outcomes of pregnancies complicated by hyperemesis gravidarum. *Obstetrics & Gynecology*, *107*(2), 285–292.

Food and Drug Administration. (2011). FDA Drug Safety Communication: Low magnesium levels can be associated with long-term use of Proton Pump Inhibitor drugs (PPIs). Retrieved from http://www.fda.gov/Drugs/DrugSafety/ucm245011.htm.

Food and Drug Administration. (2012). FDA Drug Safety Communication: *Clostridium difficile*-associated diarrhea can be associated with stomach acid drugs known as proton pump inhibitors (PPIs). Retrieved from http://www.fda.gov/drugs/drugsafety/ucm290510.htm.

Freedberg, D. E., Lebwohl, B., & Abrams, J. A. (2014). The impact of proton pump inhibitors on the human gastrointestinal microbiome. *Clinics in Laboratory Medicine*, *34*(4), 771–785.

Gabel, V., Maire, M., Reichert, C. F., Chellappa, S. L., Schmidt, C., Hommes, V., et al. (2013). Effects of artificial dawn and morning blue light on daytime cognitive performance, well-being, cortisol and melatonin levels. *Chronobiology International*, *30*(8), 988–997.

Gilboa, S. M., Ailes, E. C., Rai, R. P., Anderson, J. A., & Honein, M. A. (2014). Antihistamines and birth defects: A systematic review of the literature. *Expert Opinion on Drug Safety*, *13*(12), 1667–1698.

Gill, S. K., Maltepe, C., Mastali, K., & Koren, G. (2009). The effect of acid-reducing pharmacotherapy on the severity of nausea and vomiting of pregnancy. *Obstetrics and Gynecology International*, Epub July 1, 2009, 585269, 1–4.

Guo, J., Wang, L. P., Liu, C. Z., Zhang, J., Wang, G. L., Yi, J. H., et al. (2013). Efficacy of acupuncture for primary insomnia: A randomized controlled clinical trial. *Evidence-Based Complementary and Alternative Medicine*, 2013, 163850.

Gutke, A., Oberg, B., & Ostgaard, H. C. (2006). Pelvic girdle pain and lumbar pain in pregnancy: A cohort study of the consequences in terms of health and functioning. *Spine*, *31*(5), e149–e155.

Hollyer, T., Boon, H., Georgousis, A., Smith, M., & Einarson, A. (2002, May 17). The use of CAM by women suffering from nausea and vomiting during pregnancy. *BMC Complementary and Alternative Medicine*, 2, 5.

Holmgren, C., Aagaard-Tillery, K. M., Silver, R. M., Porter, T. F., & Varner, M. (2008). Hyperemesis in pregnancy: An evaluation of treatment strategies with maternal and neonatal outcomes. *American Journal of Obstetrics and Gynecology*, *198*(1), 56.e1–e4.

Huxley, R. (2000). Nausea and vomiting in early pregnancy—Its role in placental development. *Obstetrics & Gynecology*, *95*(5), 779–782.

Jarosz, M., & Taraszewska, A. (2014). Risk factors for gastroesophageal reflux disease: The role of diet. *Przeglad Gastroenterologiczny*, *9*(5), 297–301.

Kaltenbach, T., Crockett, S., & Gerson, L. B. (2006). Are lifestyle measures effective in patients with gastroesophageal reflux disease? An evidence-based approach. *Archives of Internal Medicine*, *166*(9), 965–971.

Kamysheva, E., Wertheim, E. H., Skouteris, H., Paxton, S. J., & Milgrom, J. (2009). Frequency, severity, and effect on life of physical symptoms experienced during pregnancy. *Journal of Midwifery & Women's Health*, *54*(1), 43–49.

Karim, S., Faryal, A., Majid, S., Majid, S., Salih, M., Jafri, F., et al. (2011). Regular post dinner walk; can be a useful lifestyle modification for gastroesophageal reflux. *Journal of the Pakistan Medical Association*, *61*(6), 526–530.

Keller, J., Frederking, D., & Layer, P. (2008). The spectrum and treatment of gastrointestinal disorders during pregnancy. *Nature Clinical Practice Gastroenterology & Hepatology*, *5*(8), 430–443.

King, T. L., & Murphy, P. A. (2009). Evidence-based approaches to managing nausea and vomiting in early pregnancy. *Journal of Midwifery & Women's Health*, *54*(6), 430–444.

King, A. C., Oman, R. F., Brassington, G. S., Bliwise, D. L., & Haskell, W. L. (1997). Moderate-intensity exercise and self-rated quality of sleep in older adults. A randomized controlled trial. *JAMA*, *277*(1), 32–37.

Kizilirmak, A., Timur, S., & Kartal, B. (2012). Insomnia in pregnancy and factors related to insomnia. *ScientificWorldJournal*, 2012, 197093.

Komazawa, Y., Adachi, K., Mihara, T., Ono, M., Kawamura, A., Fujishiro, H., et al. (2003). Tolerance to famotidine and ranitidine treatment after 14 days of administration in healthy subjects without *Helicobacter pylori* infection. *Journal of Gastroenterology and Hepatology*, *18*(6), 678–682.

Koren, G. (2014). Treating morning sickness in the United States—Changes in prescribing are needed. *American Journal of Obstetrics and Gynecology, 211*(6), 602–606.

Koren, G., Clark, S., Hankins, G. D., Caritis, S. N., Umans, J. G., Miodovnik, M., et al. (2015, March 18). Maternal safety of the delayed-release doxylamine and pyridoxine combination for nausea and vomiting of pregnancy; a randomized placebo controlled trial. *BMC Pregnancy and Childbirth, 15*, 59.

Krismer, M., & van Tulder, M. (2007). Strategies for prevention and management of musculoskeletal conditions: Low back pain (non-specific). *Best Practice & Research Clinical Rheumatology, 21*(1), 77–91.

Lacasse, A., Rey, E., Ferreira, E., Morin, C., & Bérard, A., (2008). Validity of a modified Pregnancy-Unique Quantification of Emesis and Nausea (PUQE) scoring index to assess severity of nausea and vomiting of pregnancy. *American Journal of Obstetrics and Gynecology, 198*(1), 71.e1–e7.

Lam, J. R., Schneider, J. L., Zhao, W., & Corley, D. A. (2013). Proton pump inhibitor and histamine 2 receptor antagonist use and vitamin B12 deficiency. *JAMA, 310*(22), 2435–2442.

Lan, Y., Tan, H. J., Xing, J. J., Wu, N., Xing, J. J., Wu, F. S., et al. (2015). Auricular acupuncture with seed or pellet attachments for primary insomnia: A systematic review and meta-analysis. *BMC Complementary and Alternative Medicine, 15*, 103. doi: 10.1186/s12906-015-0606-7

Luk, C. P., Parsons, R., Lee, Y. P., & Hughes, J. D. (2013). Proton pump inhibitor-associated hypomagnesemia: What do FDA data tell us? *Annals of Pharmacotherapy, 47*(6), 773–780.

Madjunkova, S., Maltepe, C., & Koren, G. (2013). The leading concerns of American women with nausea and vomiting of pregnancy calling Motherisk NVP Helpline. *Obstetrics and Gynecology International, 2013*, 752980.

Mahadevan, U., & Kane, S. (2006). American Gastroenterological Association institute technical review on the use of gastrointestinal medications in pregnancy. *Gastroenterology, 131*(1), 283–311.

Marcuard, S. P., Albernaz, L., & Khazanie, P. G. (1994). Omeprazole therapy causes malabsorption of cyanocobalamin (vitamin B12). *Annals of Internal Medicine, 120*(3), 211–215.

Markovits, N., Loebstein, R., Halkin, H., Bialik, M., Landes-Westerman, J., Lomnicky, J., et al. (2014). The association of proton pump inhibitors and hypomagnesemia in the community setting. *Journal of Clinical Pharmacology, 54*(8), 889–895.

Matok, I., Gorodischer, R., Koren, G., Sheiner, E., Wiznitzer, A., & Levy, A. (2009). The safety of metoclopramide use in the first trimester of pregnancy. *New England Journal of Medicine, 360*(24), 2528–2535.

Matok, I., Levy, A., Wiznitzer, A., Uziel, E., Koren, G., & Gorodischer, R. (2012). The safety of fetal exposure to proton-pump inhibitors during pregnancy. *Digestive Diseases and Sciences, 57*(3), 699–705.

Mills, E., Duguoa, J., Perri, D., & Koren, G. (2006). *Herbal medicines in pregnancy and lactation: An evidence-based approach.* New York: Taylor & Francis.

Mitchell, M. D., Gehrman, P., Perlis, M., et al. (2012). *Comparative effectiveness of cognitive behavioral therapy for insomnia: A systematic review.* BMC family practice.

Mørkved, S., Salvesen, K. A., Schei, B., Lydersen, S., & Bø, K. (2007). Does group training during pregnancy prevent lumbopelvic pain? A randomized clinical trial. *Acta Obstetricia et Gynecologica Scandinavica, 86*(3), 276–282.

Mulder, B., Schuiling-Veninga, C. C., Bos, H. J., De Vries, T. W., Jick, S. S., & Hak, E. (2014). Prenatal exposure to acid-suppressive drugs and the risk of allergic diseases in the offspring: A cohort study. *Clinical and Experimental Allergy, 44*(2), 261–269.

Nuangchamnong, N., & Niebyl, J. (2014). Doxylamine succinate-pyridoxine hydrochloride (Diclegis) for the management of nausea and vomiting in pregnancy: An overview. *International Journal of Women's Health, 6*, 401–409.

Pennick, V., & Liddle, S. D. (2013). Interventions for preventing and treating pelvic and back pain in pregnancy. *Cochrane Database of Systematic Reviews, 8*, CD001139.

Quartarone, G. (2013). Gastroesophageal reflux in pregnancy: A systematic review on the benefit of raft forming agents. *Minerva Ginecologica, 65*(5), 541–549.

Rohof, W. O., Bennink, R. J., Smout, A. J., Thomas, E., & Boeckxstaens, G. E. (2013). An alginate-antacid formulation localizes to the acid pocket to reduce acid reflux in patients with gastroesophageal reflux disease. *Clinical Gastroenterology and Hepatology, 11*(12), 1585–1591; quiz e90.

Romm, A. (2010). *Botanical medicine for women's health.* St. Louis, MO: Churchill Livingstone Elsevier.

Sherman, P. W., & Flaxman, S. M. (2002). Nausea and vomiting of pregnancy in an evolutionary perspective. *American Journal of Obstetrics and Gynecology, 186*(Suppl. 5), S190–S197.

Sipponen, P., & Härkönen, M. (2010). Hypochlorhydric stomach: A risk condition for calcium malabsorption and osteoporosis. *Scandinavian Journal of Gastroenterology, 45*(2), 133–138.

Smith, M. W., Marcus, P. S., & Wurtz, L. D. (2008). Orthopedic issues in pregnancy. *Obstetrical & Gynecological Survey, 63*(2), 103–111.

Smith, M. T., Perlis, M. L., Park, A., Smith, M. S., Pennington, J., Giles, D. E., et al. (2002). Comparative meta-analysis of pharmacotherapy and behavior therapy for persistent insomnia. *American Journal of Psychiatry, 159*(1), 5–11.

Sroykham, W., & Wongsawat, Y. (2013). Effects of LED-backlit computer screen and emotional selfregulation on human melatonin production. *IEEE Engineering in Medicine and Biology Society Conference Proceedings, 2013*, 1704–1707.

Strange, L. B., Parker, K. P., Moore, M. L., Strickland, O. L., & Bliwise, D. L. (2009). Disturbed sleep and preterm birth: A potential relationship? *Clinical and Experimental Obstetrics & Gynecology, 36*(3), 166–168.

Tan, P. C., Khine, P. P., Vallikkannu, N., & Omar, S. Z. (2010). Promethazine compared with metoclopramide for hyperemesis gravidarum: A randomized controlled trial. *Obstetrics and Gynecology, 115*(5), 975–981.

Tytgat, G. N., Heading, R. C., Müller-Lissner, S., Kamm, M. A., Schölmerich, J., Berstad, A., et al. (2003). Contemporary understanding and management of reflux and constipation in the general population and pregnancy: A consensus meeting. *Alimentary Pharmacology & Therapeutics, 18*(3), 291–301.

Untersmayr, E., & Jensen-Jarolim, E. (2008). The role of protein digestibility and antacids on food allergy outcomes. *Journal of Allergy and Clinical Immunology, 121*(6), 1301–1308; quiz 1309.

Vermani, E., Mittal, R., & Weeks, A. (2009). Pelvic girdle pain and low back pain in pregnancy: A review. *Pain Practice, 10*(1), 60–71.

Vleeming, A., Albert, H. B., Ostgaard, H. C., Sturesson, B., & Stuge, B. (2008). European guidelines for the diagnosis and treatment of pelvic girdle pain. *European Spine Journal, 17*(6), 794–819.

Waldum, H. L., Qvigstad, G., Fossmark, R., Kleveland, P. M., & Sandvik, A. K. (2010). Rebound acid hypersecretion from a physiological, pathophysiological and clinical viewpoint. *Scandinavian Journal of Gastroenterology, 45*(4), 389–394.

Weigel, M. M., Reyes, M., Caiza, M. E., Tello, N., Castro, N. P., Cespedes, S., et al. (2006). Is the nausea and vomiting of early pregnancy really feto-protective? *Journal of Perinatal Medicine, 34*(2), 115–122.

West, K. E., Jablonski, M. R., Warfield, B., Cecil, K. S., James, M., Ayers, M. A., et al. (2011). Blue light from light-emitting diodes elicits a dose-dependent suppression of melatonin in humans. *Journal of Applied Physiology, 110*(3), 619–626.

Yamamichi, N., Mochizuki, S., Asada-Hirayama, I., Mikami-Matsuda, R., Shimamoto, T., Konno-Shimizu1, M., et al. (2012). Lifestyle factors affecting gastroesophageal reflux disease symptoms: A cross-sectional study of healthy 19864 adults using FSSG scores. *BMC Medicine, 10*, 45. doi:10.1186/1741-7015-10-45.

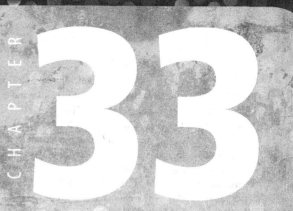

GESTATIONAL DIABETES MELLITUS: EARLY DETECTION AND MANAGEMENT IN PREGNANCY

Maribeth Inturrisi

I. Introduction and general background

Normal pregnancy can be viewed as a progressive condition of insulin resistance, hyperinsulinemia, and mild postprandial hyperglycemia. The mild postprandial hyperglycemia serves to increase the amount of time that maternal glucose levels are elevated above the basal glucose levels after a meal, thereby increasing the flux of ingested nutrients from mother to the fetus and enhancing fetal growth.

During the fasting state (5 hours after food intake), the metabolic processes are relatively the same as the nonpregnant state except that they proceed at an accelerated rate. By 10 weeks gestation, placental hormones begin to alter maternal carbohydrate metabolism (**Table 33-1**).

Early in pregnancy estrogen and human placental lactogen (hPL) tend to dominate such that during weeks 8–15 insulin resistance is low, resulting in lower glucose levels, especially in women with type 1 diabetes mellitus (DM). The fasting blood sugar in the normal pregnant woman is lower than in a nonpregnant woman, averaging about 65 mg/dL (Parretti et al., 2001). However, in the fed state, these same hormones cause a resistance to the cellular uptake of glucose by insulin-sensitive tissue, muscle, and fat. This pattern of insulin resistance tends to parallel the growth of the fetal–placental unit and the levels of hormones secreted by the placenta. In normal pregnant women, pancreatic β cells respond to insulin resistance by increasing their insulin secretion, resulting in normal circulating glucose levels (Barbour et al., 2007).

The fetus does most of its growing in the third trimester of pregnancy. During this time, the fetus is constantly "feeding"

TABLE 33-1 Major Placental Hormones and Their Impact on Maternal Carbohydrate Metabolism in All Pregnancies—Normal and with Diabetes

Placental Hormone	Effect on Carbohydrate Metabolism
Estrogen	Increases insulin binding to cells (insulin sensitivity) in early pregnancy, but this effect is cancelled out by increases in progesterone and cortisol in the second half of pregnancy.
Progesterone	Decreases insulin binding to cells, thus increasing insulin resistance.
Human Placental Lactogen (hPL)	Induces insulin release from the pancreas but may also contribute to peripheral insulin resistance (in muscle and fat cells).
Human Placental Growth Hormone (hPGH)	Causes severe peripheral insulin resistance.
Tumor Necrosis Factor (TNFα)	Has the greatest effect of increasing insulin resistance. Changes in insulin sensitivity correlate specifically with increasing TNFα secretion from 22–35 weeks gestation.
	TNFα is a cytokine, a proinflammatory agent, which impairs insulin's action of moving glucose from the bloodstream into cells (fat and muscle). In women with gestational diabetes mellitus, this downregulation of insulin action is increased
Cortisol	Causes gluconeogenesis from the liver increasing glucose in the bloodstream. In addition, it diminishes insulin secretion from the pancreas.

Data from Barbour et al. (2007). Cellular mechanisms for insulin resistance in normal pregnancy and gestational diabetes. *Diabetes Care*, 30 Suppl 2.

but the mother is alternately fasting and feeding. Glucose is transported across the placenta from the mother by facilitated diffusion. The concentration of glucose within the fetus is only slightly lower than maternal glucose.

Insulin does not cross the placenta. The fetus synthesizes its own insulin starting at about 9 weeks of gestation. The fetal β cells respond to both an increase in glucose and amino acids. Spikes in maternal glucose cause spikes in fetal insulin production.

A. Gestational diabetes mellitus: definition and overview

Gestational diabetes mellitus (GDM) is defined as any degree of glucose intolerance with first recognition during pregnancy with glucose intolerance resolving after delivery of the placenta (World Health Organization [WHO], 2013). This suggests that women who develop gestational diabetes have some defect in carbohydrate metabolism that does not result in hyperglycemia unless exacerbated by a greater demand for insulin production. Women with GDM cannot overcome the insulin resistance mediated by placental hormones. Pregnancy demands a doubling to tripling of insulin output. It is estimated that women with an abnormal oral glucose tolerance test (OGTT) in pregnancy have at baseline (nonpregnant) impaired function in at least 30–50% of their β cells and thus cannot respond to the increased pregnancy need for insulin secretion.

Their fetuses produce insulin in response to the circulating glucose levels. Fetal β cells, in turn, hypertrophy in utero initiating a cascade of abnormal metabolic processes resulting in fetal overgrowth and fetal hyperinsulinemia in the short term and in the long term insulin resistance leading to type 2 diabetes (Hillier et al., 2007).

Treatment of mild hyperglycemia during pregnancy, aka GDM, has been shown to reduce serious perinatal morbidity (Crowther et al., 2005; Landon et al., 2009). In both of these prospective randomized controlled trials, the rate of large for gestational age newborns and the incidence of preeclampsia were cut in half when women were treated for GDM versus not treated. Newborn intensive care admissions were decreased, as were shoulder dystocias. These outcomes were achieved without an increase in labor inductions, cesarean delivery, or small for gestational age newborns. In the Crowther study, women in the treatment group had a 50% decrease in weight gain during the treatment period and had less postpartum depression than women in the untreated group.

GDM is optimally managed by referral to a multidisciplinary health education team trained and skilled in the management of diabetes during pregnancy. Consultation with a registered dietitian is strongly recommended (American College of Obstetricians and Gynecologists [ACOG], 2013; Crowther et al., 2005).

B. Prevalence and incidence

Approximately 9.2% of all pregnancies in the United States are documented to be complicated by diabetes (DeSisto, Kim, & Sharma, 2014). Although 90% of these pregnant women have GDM, a growing number of women (more than 8%) have preexisting type 2 diabetes mellitus (Baptiste-Roberts et al., 2009). The ongoing epidemic of obesity and the increased ethnic diversity in the United States (African-American, Asian/Pacific Islander, East Indian, Hispanic, and Native American populations) has led to more type 2 diabetes in women of childbearing age (ACOG, 2005). The number of women entering pregnancy with undiagnosed type 2 diabetes has increased. In addition, it is estimated that 23% of women of childbearing age in the United States have prediabetes, aka glucose intolerance (DeSisto et al., 2014). Two out of three individuals with prediabetes do not know they have it (DeSisto et al., 2014). This translates to women entering pregnancy with undiagnosed diabetes and prediabetes potentially placing the fetus at risk for adverse outcomes including miscarriage, birth defects, macrosomia, and fetal demise.

II. Database (may include but is not limited to)

In March 2010, the International Association of Diabetes and Pregnancy Study Groups (IADPSG) set forth global recommendations to change the way GDM is diagnosed (Metzger et al., 2010). These recommendations are based on data from the prospective double-blinded (patients and providers), epidemiologic study Hyperglycemia and Adverse Pregnancy Outcomes (HAPO) (Metzger et al., 2008). The research subjects were 25,000 pregnant women from around the world who were given a 75-g OGTT at 24–28 weeks gestation to determine at what glucose level adverse outcomes for the fetus occurred. Removal from the study and treatment occurred only if the glucose level reached those consistent with overt diabetes. The Carpenter and Coustan (1982) 3-hour OGTT was designed to determine which women were at increased risk to develop type 2 diabetes in the future, not outcomes for the fetus/newborn. The HAPO study showed that there was a continuous relationship between increasing maternal blood glucose levels and fetal fat deposition and fetal hyperinsulinemia. The proposed glucose values for a positive test were selected when the odds ratio reached 1.75. These blood glucose values conveyed a 75% increased risk for adverse fetal/neonatal outcomes such as macrosomia, hypoglycemia, and cesarean birth (Metzger et al., 2008, 2010).

The IADPSG Consensus Panel translated the results into a one-step clinical practice guideline for the diagnosis of GDM at 24–28 weeks. Ideally all women, but definitely all women with risk factors, should be screened for type 2 diabetes in the first trimester using one of the standard diagnostic criteria for diagnosing diabetes in the nonpregnant population (Metzger et al., 2010). If a woman is found to have a fasting blood glucose (BG) of > 125 mg/dL or an A1C of > 6.4%, or a random blood glucose of > 199 mg/dL, she should receive a diagnosis of overt, not gestational, diabetes (American Diabetes Association [ADA], 2015). According to the IADPSG recommendations, type 2 diabetes can be diagnosed during pregnancy and management can be instituted early in order to limit the adverse effects of undiagnosed hyperglycemia.

The World Health Organization, the American Diabetes Association, and most countries outside the United States have adopted IADPSG recommendations (ADA, 2015; WHO, 2013). The American College of Obstetricians and Gynecologists (ACOG) did not adopt these guidelines and is awaiting further studies (ACOG, 2013). The National Institutes of Health (NIH) recommended further cost-effective studies and studies in which the improved outcomes could be related to the specific IADPSG testing recommendations (Mission, Ohno, Cheng, & Caughey, 2011). The NIH agreed that we need to adopt a worldwide approach to the diagnosis of GDM to be able to study GDM for best practice management guidelines (Van Dorsten et al., 2013).

Both the 2010 IADPSG method (using one step) and the 1982 Carpenter and Coustan method (using two steps) of diagnosing gestational diabetes are presented here and are used in current practice (ACOG, 2013; ADA, 2015).

A. Subjective

The risk factors (ADA, 2015) for type 2 diabetes, prediabetes, and GDM are the same because they share the same pathophysiology of increased insulin resistance and diminish insulin secretion. All women should be asked about risk factors at the first prenatal visit (see **Table 33-2**).

B. Objective/Assessment

In the presence of any *one* of these high-risk factors, ADA recommends that women be tested for undiagnosed type 2 diabetes or prediabetes at the first prenatal visit (ADA, 2015; Metzger et al., 2010). Some providers use the convenience of an A1C, which does not require fasting and can easily be added to the prenatal panel. However, any method to diagnose diabetes or prediabetes in the nonpregnant woman can be used (ADA, 2015).

ACOG (2013) suggests using a 1-hour 50-g glucose challenge test (GCT) as an early screen in the first or second trimester. If any early screening is negative, the IADPSG, ADA, ACOG, and U.S. Preventive Services Task Force (USPSTF, 2014) recommend universal screening at 24–28 weeks by either a one-step method (ADA, 2015; WHO, 2013) or two-step method (ACOG, 2013; Van Dorsten et al., 2013) (**Tables 33-3** and **33-4**).

III. Goals of clinical management

A. *Identify women at risk and screen for and diagnose both type 2 and gestational diabetes (GDM).*

B. *Reduce adverse fetal and neonatal outcomes through treatment of women with GDM.*
   Incorporate an interdisciplinary approach including nutrition and psychosocial and medical interventions to help women with GDM successfully achieve normal blood glucose levels and decrease perinatal morbidity.

C. *Educate women with GDM regarding testing for overt diabetes every 1–3 years and about early testing in subsequent pregnancies.*

D. *Encourage women with GDM to continue healthy eating and to be active as well as to reduce weight if overweight or obese to prevent future GDM or overt diabetes.*

IV. Plan

Educate all women with GDM concerning healthy lifestyle behaviors that can result in pregnancy outcomes that closely match those of women without hyperglycemia in pregnancy (American Association of Diabetes Educators [AADE], 2010).

A. *AADE's 7 Healthy Lifestyle Behaviors*

TABLE 33-2 Risk Factors for Type 2 Diabetes

History of insulin-resistant conditions: prediabetes, gestational diabetes, obesity (body mass index > 30), and polycystic ovary syndrome
Obstetric and gynecological history: macrosomia, unexplained stillbirth, malformed infant
Medications: any medications that adversely affect glucose levels: e.g., corticosteroids, progesterone, and atypical antipsychotics such as Seroquel
Family history of overt diabetes among first-degree relatives: mother, father, sister, brother, child
Belonging to a high-risk ethnic group: African-American, American Indian, Hispanic/Latina, Asian/Pacific Islander, Southeast Asian, and East Indian, Native American

Data from American College of Obstetricians and Gynecologists (2013); American Diabetes Association (2015); Waters, Schultz, Mercer, & Catalano (2009).

TABLE 33-3 Criteria for the Diagnosis of Diabetes or Prediabetes in the Nonpregnant Population

Test	Overt Diabetes	Prediabetes
A1C The test should be performed in a laboratory using a method that is NGSP-certified and standardized to the Diabetes Control and Complications Trial assay.*	≥ 6.5%	≥ 5.7%–≤ 6.4%
Fasting plasma glucose Fasting is defined as no caloric intake for at least 8 hours.*	≥ 126 mg/dL	≥ 100 mg/dL–≤ 125 mg/dL
2-h plasma glucose during an OGTT The test should be performed as described by the WHO, using a glucose load containing the equivalent of 75 g anhydrous glucose dissolved in water.*	≥ 200 mg/dL	≥ 140 mg/dL–≤ 199 mg/dL
Random plasma glucose In a patient with classic symptoms of hyperglycemia or hyperglycemic crisis	≥ 200 mg/dL	

*In the absence of unequivocal hyperglycemia, result should be confirmed by repeat testing.

Data from American Diabetes Association. (2015). Classification and diagnosis of diabetes. Position statement: Gestational diabetes mellitus. *Diabetes Care, 38* (Suppl. 1), S13–S14.

TABLE 33-4 Methods to Diagnose Gestational Diabetes

One-Step IADPSG Method*

- After an 8–12 hour fast, obtain fasting blood glucose (FBG).
- Administer a 2-hour 75-g OGTT. The patient should remain seated.

If *any one* of the following values are reached or exceeded, the test may be terminated at that time and considered positive.

- FBG: 92 mg/dL; 1-hr: 180 mg/dL; 2-hr: 153 mg/dL

*Note: this method *does not* include a 50-g glucose challenge test (GCT) (ADA, 2015; WHO, 2013)

Two-Step Method

Step 1: Administer a 50-g nonfasting GCT.

- If the result of the GCT is equal to or greater than 180 mg/dL–199 mg/dL, order fasting blood glucose (FBG).
- If the FBG value is less than 95 mg/dL, perform the 3-hour oral glucose tolerance test (OGTT).
- If FBG value is equal to or greater than 95 mg/dL, do not perform the OGTT. Elevated FBG of equal to or greater than 95 mg/dL is diagnostic of GDM.

Step 2: If the result of the GCT is 140–179 mg/dL, proceed to step 2, a fasting 3-hour 100-g OGTT.

- **Two values** equal to or above the following = GDM
  - FBG: 95 mg/d: 1-hr: 180 mg/dL; 2-hr: 155 mg/dL; 3-hr: 140 mg/dL
  - Any one value 200 or above on the OGTT is diagnostic of GDM.

Data from American Diabetes Association (2015); World Health Organization (2013); American College of Obstetricians and Gynecologists (2013).

1. Healthy eating
   a. Healthy eating is the cornerstone of diabetes management (AADE, 2010). Focus on carbohydrate control using the plate method for gestational diabetes (California Diabetes and Pregnancy Program [CDAPP], 2012).
   b. For a healthy eating plan that incorporates pregnancy and diabetes principles, refer to a registered dietitian who can follow up every 2–3 weeks.
   c. Encourage weight gain within the Institute of Medicine (IOM, 2009) recommendations,

which have been associated with optimum outcomes for mother and baby (Cheng et al., 2008).

   d. Prepregnancy body mass index should be determined at first visit. Weight gain recommendations are determined according to prepregnancy BMI (see Figure 28-6). Weight gain should be followed closely and plotted on the appropriate IOM weight graphs (ACOG, 2005; IOM, 2009).

2. Being active

   a. Exercise increases insulin sensitivity (ACOG, 2002; ADA, 2015).

   b. Exercise after meals can help keep blood glucose in target range and reduce the need for medication.

   c. Recommend regular exercise of at least 30 minutes per day, such as brisk walking (ACOG, 2002; ADA, 2015; Metzger et al., 2007).

3. Monitoring blood glucose (BG)

   a. Maintaining near normal BG during pregnancy is associated with reduced macrosomia, preeclampsia, and neonatal hypoglycemia (Crowther et al., 2005; Landon et al., 2009).

   b. Maternal hyperglycemia during pregnancy has been associated with obesity and type 2 diabetes in their adolescent and adult offspring (Baptiste-Robert et al., 2009; Dabelea et al., 2008).

   c. Target blood glucose of fasting < 90 mg/dL; 1 hour after start of meal < 130 mg/dL is associated with a lower risk for adverse perinatal outcomes (Ehrlich, Crites, Hedderson, Darbinian, & Ferrara, 2010; Metzger et al., 2008).

   d. Women who used daily self-monitoring of blood glucose using home glucometer, test strips, and finger-sticking devices had less macrosomia than women who had their BG checked by weekly lab testing only (Hawkins et al., 2009).

   e. Documenting food records and blood glucose results that were reviewed by the providers at each visit was associated with improved blood glucose levels (CDAPP, 2012; Parkin & Davidson, 2009).

4. Healthy coping

   a. Individuals with diabetes are at greater risk for depression as are pregnant women in general (ACOG, 2006; Kozhimannil, Pereira, & Harlow, 2009).

   b. Use a standardized depression screening tool for pregnant women (e.g., Edinburgh Postnatal Depression Scale in the early third trimester) (American Academy of Pediatrics, 2015; ACOG, 2006).

   c. Have women rate their level of stress, discuss coping strategies, refer to mental health providers as needed.

5. Problem solving

   a. Help women to strategize behaviors that are successful in achieving normal blood glucose levels. Help them make associations between food choices and blood glucose levels and understand what they can control (AADE, 2010).

   b. Teach signs and symptoms of hyperglycemia and how to avoid it. When women are taking secretagogues or insulin, teach them to recognize hypoglycemia, how to prevent, and how to treat it (ADA, 2015; CDAPP, 2012).

6. Reducing risks

   a. Review habits, such as smoking, alcohol, and drugs.

   b. Educate concerning tests of fetal well-being such as kick counts, nonstress tests (NST), ultrasounds, and amniotic fluid index (AFI) as needed (CDAPP, 2012).

   c. If clinically indicated (size greater than dates, poor blood glucose control, refusal of medication), obtain ultrasound at 32–35 weeks for fetal growth (CDAPP, 2012).

   d. For women with GDM A1 (achieves BG control with diet and exercise alone), NSTs are not indicated unless there is increased blood pressure, macrosomia, history of intrauterine fetal demise, or decreased fetal movement. Women with GDM A1 may continue pregnancy beyond 40 weeks with biweekly NST/AFI testing (CDAPP, 2012).

   e. For women with GDM A2 (requires the addition of medication to control blood glucose), NST/AFI may be started weekly at 32 weeks and biweekly beginning at 36 weeks (CDAPP, 2012). Women with GDM can be allowed a trial of labor for fetus weighing less than 4,500 g (ACOG, 2013). Induction of labor should optimally occur after 39 weeks but before 40 weeks (ACOG, 2013). After 40 completed weeks, studies show that woman with GDM A2 have increased risk of shoulder dystocia and larger babies (Witkop, Neale, Wilson, Bass, & Nicholson, 2009).

7. Taking medications

   a. Once diet and exercise have been optimized, if blood glucose values exceed targets (fasting elevations three times or greater in a week or post meal six times or more in a week), consider adding medication (CDAPP, 2012). When medication is added to treatment, the type of GDM is GDM A2.

b. Oral agents (metformin or glyburide) are often effective in managing mild hyperglycemia such as GDM (Balani, Hyer, Rodin, & Shehata, 2009; Dhulkotia, Ola, Fraser, & Farrell, 2010; Langer, 2000; Moore, 2007; Rowan, Hague, Gao, Battin, & Moore, 2008).

c. If insulin is needed in multiple daily injections, referral to a high-risk program may be necessary (CDAPP, 2012; Mathiesen et al., 2012).

d. Medical management is beyond the scope of this chapter; therefore, insulin management will not be covered. However, hyperglycemia associated with GDM can often be managed with oral medications as follows:

   i. Metformin

     a. Bioavailability: 40–60%

     b. GI absorption complete in 6 hours, peaks in 40 minutes

     c. No metabolites, few interactions with other drugs (cimetidine, vitamin B_{12}, guar gum)

     d. No liver metabolism, disposed of by the kidney, excreted in 4 hours, half-life 8–12 hours (5% of dose). Administer every 8 or 12 hours.

     e. Synergistic action with glyburide and insulin

     f. May have GI side effects such as stomach upset, diarrhea, and constipation. Generally, if side effects occur they resolve after a few days. Starting with a low dose (500 mg) reduces side effects.

   ii. Metformin and pregnancy

     a. Concentrations of metformin are lower in pregnancy than nonpregnancy due to increased renal clearance during mid and late pregnancy.

     b. Fetal dose is from negligible to as high as maternal dose

     c. Breastfed neonate receives < 0.5% of mother's dose.

     d. Not associated with prenatal hypoglycemia

     e. Use is associated with less neonatal hypoglycemia after birth.

     f. Not associated with lactic acidosis when there is normal renal function.

     g. Extended release not as effective as regular metformin

   iii. Metformin protocol for pregnancy

     a. Begin with 500 mg once or twice daily with AM meal or at bedtime with snack depending on the pattern of hyperglycemia.

     b. Increase dose by 500 mg every 3–7 days as limited by GI side effects, until targets reached.

     c. Obtain serum creatinine if any suspicion of renal disease. Metformin is cleared entirely by the kidney.

   iv. Glyburide

     a. A secretagogue (forces insulin out of the beta cells)

     b. May lead to pancreatic exhaustion.

     c. Two major metabolites may cross the placenta and result in hypoglycemia and macrosomia in the fetus (Castillo et al., 2015).

     d. 5 mg peaks in 2–4 hours; take 60 minutes before meal

     e. Half-life is 2–4 hours.

     f. Can be taken TID rather than BID in pregnancy

     g. Associated with hypoglycemia

   v. Glyburide protocol for pregnancy

     a. Begin with 1.25 mg/day (wt. < 200 lbs.)

     b. Begin with 2.5 mg/day (wt. > 200 lbs.)

     c. To control post meal elevations, take 60 minutes before meal.

     d. To control fasting BG, take at 10 pm–11 pm.

     e. Increase by 1.25 to 2.5 mg every 3–7 days until targets reached or max dose of 20 mg/day

     f. Watch for weight gain

     g. Teach the "rule of 15" to manage hypoglycemia

       i. If symptoms of hypoglycemia, check BG

       ii. If BG < 70 mg/dL, take 15 g fast-acting (liquid) carbohydrate such as 4 oz of juice or 8 oz milk

       iii. Check BG in 15 minutes

       iv. BG should increase by 15 mg/dL

       v. If not, repeat the 15 g fast-acting carbohydrate

     If either of these oral agents cannot control the fasting BG, a single dose of basal insulin, e.g., Levemir (long acting) or NPH (intermediate acting), at bedtime may be indicated.

B. Postpartum management of GDM A1 and GDM A2

1. Encourage women to continue healthy eating and being active.

2. Strongly encourage breastfeeding to help reduce the risk for future obesity and diabetes in both the mother

and the newborn (Feig, Lipscombe, Tomlinson, & Blumer, 2011).

3. Encourage women to get to a normal BMI before conceiving again because obesity confers the same adverse outcomes as diabetes and it increases the risk for GDM and overt diabetes (Roman et al., 2011).

4. Encourage avoidance of pregnancy at least for 2 years to allow the pancreas to "rest" from insulin resistance. Progesterone-only birth control methods, such as medroxyprogesterone (Depo-Provera), etonogestrel, and progesterone-only pills, have been found to increase the conversion rate of GDM to type 2 diabetes in Hispanic women who were breastfeeding (Kjos et al., 1998). Pregnancy will confer greater insulin resistance than progesterone; therefore, the risks must outweigh the benefits when considering birth control methods. The intrauterine device may be an excellent choice for its effectiveness and length of use. Mirena®, despite using progesterone, has only a local effect on the uterus and has not been shown to increase insulin resistance (Damm, Mathiesen, Petersen, & Kjos, 2007).

5. Reclassify glucose tolerance with the nonpregnant 75-g OGTT (fasting plus 2 hr postprandial) at 6–12 weeks (ACOG, 2009, 2013; ADA, 2015).

6. Educate women to get checked for diabetes every 1–3 years using the baby's birthday as a reminder. If prediabetes is identified, or age 40 is reached, then obtain a test for diabetes annually (Bellamy, Casas, Hingorani, & Williams, 2009; Ratner et al., 2008).

7. Obtain an early screen (first visit) for diabetes in future pregnancies (Bentley-Lewis, 2009).

8. About 5% of women with GDM have overt diabetes when tested after pregnancy and another 15% have prediabetes. If either is identified, the woman should be referred to a primary care provider or to a diabetes program with educational classes for prediabetes and diabetes. Metformin was shown to reduce the conversion to type 2 diabetes by 58% in women with previous GDM in the Diabetes Prevention Program Trial (Ratner et al., 2008).

C. Resources for professionals

The prenatal weight gain charts forms are located at the California Department of Public Health (CDPH) website: http://www.cdph.ca.gov/pubsforms/forms/Pages/MaternalandChildHealth.aspx

- CDPH 4472 B1 Prenatal Weight Gain Grid: Prepregnancy Underweight Range
- CDPH 4472 B2 Prenatal Weight Gain Grid: Prepregnancy Normal Weight Range
- CDPH 4472 B3 Prenatal Weight Gain Grid: Prepregnancy Overweight Range
- CDPH 4472 B4 Prenatal Weight Gain Grid: prepregnancy Obese Weight Range

D. Resources for women with GDM

1. American Diabetes Association: 800-342-2383, www.diabetes.org

2. American Association of Diabetes Educators: 800-338-DMED, www.diabeteseducator.org/

3. Centers for Disease Control and Prevention. Division of Diabetes Translation: 877-232-3422, www.cdc.gov/diabetes

4. California Diabetes and Pregnancy Program: Sweet Success: www.cdappsweetsuccess.org/

REFERENCES

American Academy of Pediatrics. (2015). Edinburgh postnatal depression scale. Retrieved from www2.aap.org/sections/scan/practicingsafety/toolkit_resources/module2/epds.pdf.

American Association of Diabetes Educators (2010). *AADE 7 self-care behaviors.* Retrieved from www.diabeteseducator.org/ProfessionalResources/AADE7.

American College of Obstetricians and Gynecologists. (2002). ACOG Committee opinion. Number 267, January 2002: Exercise during pregnancy and the postpartum period. *Obstetrics & Gynecology, 99*(1), 171–173.

American College of Obstetricians and Gynecologists. (2005). ACOG Committee opinion Number 315, September 2005. Obesity in pregnancy. *Obstetrics & Gynecology, 106*(3), 671–675.

American College of Obstetricians and Gynecologists. (2006). ACOG Committee opinion no. 343: Psychosocial risk factors: Perinatal screening and intervention. *Obstetrics & Gynecology, 108*(2), 469–477.

American College of Obstetricians and Gynecologists. (2009). ACOG Committee opinion no. 435: Postpartum screening for abnormal glucose tolerance in women who had gestational diabetes mellitus. *Obstetrics & Gynecology, 113*(6), 1419–1421.

American College of Obstetricians and Gynecologists. (2013). ACOG practice bulletin. Clinical management guidelines for obstetrician-gynecologists. Number. 137 August 2013. Gestational diabetes mellitus. *Obstetrics & Gynecology, 2013, 122*:406–16.

American Diabetes Association. (2015). Classification and diagnosis of diabetes. Position statement: Gestational diabetes mellitus. *Diabetes Care, 38* (Suppl. 1), S13–S14.

Balani, J., Hyer, S. L., Rodin, D. A., & Shehata, H. (2009). Pregnancy outcomes in women with gestational diabetes treated with metformin or insulin: A case-control study. *Diabetic Medicine, 26*(8), 798–802.

Baptiste-Roberts, K., Barone, B. B., Gary, T. L., Golden, S. H., Wilson, L. M., Bass, E. B., et al. (2009). Risk factors for type 2 diabetes among women with gestational diabetes: A systematic review. *American Journal of Medicine, 122*(3), 207–214, e4.

Barbour, L. A., McCurdy, C. E., Hernandez, T. L., Kirwan, J. P., Catalano, P. M., & Friedman, J. E. (2007). Cellular mechanisms for insulin resistance in normal pregnancy and gestational diabetes. *Diabetes Care, 30*(Suppl. 2), S112–S119.

Bellamy, L., Casas, J. P., Hingorani, A. D., & Williams, D. (2009). Type 2 diabetes mellitus after gestational diabetes: A systematic review and meta-analysis. *Lancet, 373*(9677), 1773–1779.

Bentley-Lewis, R. (2009). Gestational diabetes mellitus: An opportunity of a lifetime. *Lancet, 373*(9677), 1738–1740.

California Diabetes and Pregnancy Program (CDAPP). (2012). *Guidelines for care.* Retrieved from www.cdappsweetsuccess.org/Professionals/CDAPPSweetSuccessGuidelinesforCare.aspx.

Carpenter, M. W., & Coustan, D. R. (1982). Criteria for screening tests for gestational diabetes. *American Journal of Obstetrics and Gynecology, 144,* 768–773.

Castillo, W. C., Boggess, K., Stürmer, T., Brookhart A., Benjamin, D. K., & Jonsson Funk, M. (2015). Association of adverse pregnancy outcomes with glyburide vs insulin in women with gestational diabetes. *JAMA Pediatrics, 169*(5), 452–458. doi:10.1001/jamapediatrics.2015.74

Cheng, Y. W., Chung, J. H., Kurbisch-Block, I., Inturrisi, M., Shafer, S., & Caughey, A. B. (2008). Gestational weight gain and gestational diabetes mellitus: Perinatal outcomes. *Obstetrics and Gynecology, 112*(5), 1015–1022.

Crowther, C., Hiller, J., Moss, J., McPhee, A., Jeffries, W., & Robinson, J. (2005). Effect of treatment of gestational diabetes mellitus on pregnancy outcomes from the Australian carbohydrate intolerance study in pregnant women (ACHOIS) trial. *New England Journal of Medicine, 352*(24), 2477–2486.

Dabelea, D., Mayer-Davis, E. J., Lamichhane, A. P., D'Agostino, R. B., Jr., Liese, A. D., Vehik, K. S., et al. (2008). Association of intrauterine exposure to maternal diabetes and obesity with type 2 diabetes in youth: The SEARCH Case-Control Study. *Diabetes Care, 31*(7), 1422–1426.

Damm, P., Mathiesen, E. R., Petersen, K. R., & Kjos, S. (2007). Contraception after gestational diabetes. *Diabetes Care, 30*(Suppl. 2), S236–S241.

DeSisto, C. L., Kim, S. Y., & Sharma, A. J. (2014). Prevalence estimates of gestational diabetes mellitus in the United States. Pregnancy Risk Assessment Monitoring System (PRAMS), 2007–2010. *Preventing Chronic Disease, 11,* 130415. Retrieved from www.cdc.gov/pcd/issues/2014/13_0415.htm.

Dhulkotia, J. S., Ola, B., Fraser, R., & Farrell, T. (2010). Oral hypoglycemic agents vs insulin in management of gestational diabetes: A systematic review and meta analysis. *American Journal of Obstetrics & Gynecology, 203*(5), 457.e1–9.

Ehrlich, S. F., Crites Y. M., Hedderson M. M., Darbinian J. A., & Ferrara, A. (2011). The risk of large for gestational age across increasing categories of pregnancy glycemia. *American Journal of Obstetrics & Gynecology, 204*(3), 240.e1–6.

Feig, D. S., Lipscombe, L. L., Tomlinson, G., & Blumer, I. (2011). Breastfeeding predicts the risk of childhood obesity in a multi-ethnic cohort of women with diabetes. *Journal of Maternal-Fetal & Neonatal Medicine, 24*(3), 511–515.

Hawkins, J. S., Casey, B. M., Lo, J. Y., Moss, K., McIntire, D. D., & Leveno, K. J. (2009). Weekly compared with daily blood glucose monitoring in women with diet-treated gestational diabetes. *Obstetrics & Gynecology, 113*(6), 1307–1312.

Hillier, T. A., Pedula, K. L., Schmidt, M. M., Mullen, J. A., Charles, M. A., & Pettitt, D. J. (2007). Childhood obesity and metabolic imprinting:

The ongoing effects of maternal hyperglycemia. *Diabetes Care, 30*(9), 2287–2292.

Institute of Medicine. (2009). *Weight gain during pregnancy: Re-examining the guidelines.* Washington, DC: National Academies Press.

Kjos, S. L., Peters, R. K., Xiang, A., Thomas, D., Schaefer, U., & Buchanan, T. A. (1998). Contraception and the risk of type 2 diabetes mellitus in Latina women with prior gestational diabetes mellitus. *JAMA, 280*(6), 533–538.

Kozhimannil, K. B., Pereira, M. A., & Harlow, B. L. (2009). Association between diabetes and perinatal depression among low-income mothers. *JAMA, 301*(8), 842–847.

Landon, M. B., Spong, C. Y., Thom, E., Carpenter, M. W., Ramin, S. M., & Casey, B. (2009). A multicenter, randomized trial of treatment for mild gestational diabetes. *New England Journal of Medicine, 361*(14), 1339–1348.

Langer, O., Conway, D. L., Berkus, M. D., Xenakis, E. M., & Gonzales, O. (2000). A comparison of glyburide and insulin in women with gestational diabetes mellitus. *New England Journal of Medicine, 343,* 1134–1138.

Mathiesen, E. R., et al. (2012). Maternal efficacy and safety outcomes in a randomized, controlled trial comparing insulin detemir with NPH insulin in 310 pregnant women with type 1 diabetes. *Diabetes Care, 35*(10), 2012–2017.

Metzger, B. E., Gabbe, S. G., Persson, B., Buchanan, T. A., Catalano, P. A., Damm, P., et al. (2010). International association of diabetes and pregnancy study groups (IADPSG) recommendations on the diagnosis and classification of hyperglycemia in pregnancy. *Diabetes Care, 33*(3), 676–682.

Metzger, B. E., Buchanan, T. A., Coustan, D. R., de Leiva, A., Dunger, D. B., Hadden, D. R., et al. (2007). Summary and recommendations of the Fifth International Workshop-Conference on Gestational Diabetes Mellitus. *Diabetes Care, 30*(Suppl. 2), S251–S260.

Metzger, B. E., Lowe, L. P., Dyer, A. R., Trimble, E. R., Chaovarindr, U., Coustan, D. R., et al. (2008). Hyperglycemia and adverse pregnancy outcomes. *New England Journal of Medicine, 358*(19), 1991–2002.

Mission, J. F., Ohno, M. S., Cheng, Y. W., & Caughey, A. B. (2012). Gestational diabetes screening with the new IADPSG guidelines: A cost-effectiveness analysis. *American Journal of Obstetrics and Gynecology, 207*(4), 326.e1–e9.

Moore, T. R. (2007). Glyburide for the treatment of gestational diabetes. A critical appraisal. *Diabetes Care, 30*(Suppl. 2), S209–S213.

Parkin, C. G., & Davidson, J. A. (2009). Value of self-monitoring blood glucose pattern analysis in improving diabetes outcomes. *Journal of Diabetes Science Technology, 3*(3), 500–508.

Parretti, E., Mecaci, F., Papini, M., Cioni, R., Carignani, L., Mignosa M., et al. (2001). Third-trimester maternal blood glucose levels from diurnal profiles in nondiabetic pregnancies. Correlation with sonographic parameters of fetal growth. *Diabetes Care, 24,* 1319–1323.

Ratner, R. E., Christophi, C. A., Metzger, B. E., Dabelea, D., Bennett, P. H., Pi-Sunyer, X., et al. (2008). Prevention of diabetes in women with a history of gestational diabetes: Effects of metformin and lifestyle interventions. *Journal of Clinical Endocrinology and Metabolism, 93*(12), 4774–4779.

Roman, A. S., et al. (2011). The effect of maternal obesity on pregnancy outcomes in women with gestational diabetes. *Journal of Maternal. Fetal & Neonatal Medicine, 24*(5), 723–727.

Rowan, J. A., Hague, W. M., Gao, W., Battin, M. R., & Moore, M. P. (2008). Metformin versus insulin for the treatment of gestational diabetes. *New England Journal of Medicine, 358*(19), 2003–2015.

U.S. Preventive Services Task Force. (2014). Final recommendation statement: Gestational diabetes: Screening. http://www.uspreventiveservicestaskforce.org/Page/Document/RecommendationStatementFinal/gestational-diabetes-mellitus-screening.

Van Dorsten, J. P., et al. (2013, March 4–6). *Diagnosing gestational diabetes mellitus. National Institutes of Health Consensus Development Conference Statement* (NIH Consensus State Statements Vol. 29, No. 1). Bethesda, MD: National Institutes of Health, U.S. Department of Health and Human Services.

Waters, T. P., Schultz, B. A. H., Mercer, B. M., & Catalano, P. M. (2009). Effect of 17alpha-hydroxyprogesterone caproate on glucose intolerance in pregnancy. *Obstetrics and Gynecology, 114*(1), 45–49.

Witkop, C., Neale, D., Wilson, L. M., Bass, E. B., & Nicholson, W. K. (2009). Active compared with expectant delivery management in women with gestational diabetes: A systematic review. *Obstetrics and Gynecology, 113*(1), 206–217.

World Health Organization. (2013). *Diagnostic criteria and classification of hyperglycaemia first detected in pregnancy.* Geneva: Author.

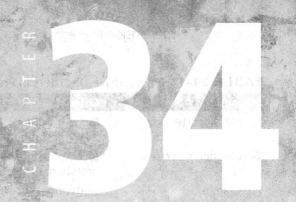

HYPERTENSION IN PREGNANCY: PREECLAMPSIA–ECLAMPSIA

Kim Q. Dau and Jenna Shaw-Battista

CHAPTER 34

I. Introduction and general background

Preeclampsia–eclampsia is typically characterized by hypertension and proteinuria occurring after 20 weeks gestation with an impact on multiple organ systems and likelihood of disease progression over time (American College of Obstetricians and Gynecologists [ACOG], 2013). Preeclampsia occurs in 3–6% of pregnancies in the United States (Ananth, Keyes, & Wapner, 2013) and is a significant risk factor for adverse perinatal outcomes. Approximately 17% of maternal deaths are related to hypertensive disorders in pregnancy (Druzin, Shields, Peterson, & Cape, 2014), including preeclampsia–eclampsia, which has a disparate racial impact for reasons not yet well defined. African-Americans have a rate of preeclampsia that is 1.65 times greater than Caucasians in the United States (Henderson et al., 2014; Tanaka et al., 2007). Hypertensive disorders in pregnancy are outlined in **Table 34-1** and include chronic hypertension with superimposed preeclampsia and HELLP (hemolysis, elevated liver enzymes, and low platelets) syndrome. These diagnoses are beyond the scope of this chapter, which is focused on the diagnosis and evidence-based management of preeclampsia–eclampsia.

Preeclampsia typically includes the finding of both hypertension and proteinuria, but the presence of proteinuria is not required for diagnosis. In the absence of proteinuria, preeclampsia can be diagnosed in the setting of hypertension plus end-organ involvement indicating severe disease and evidenced by abnormal laboratory values (thrombocytopenia, elevated liver enzymes, or elevated serum creatinine), physical examination findings, or client symptomatology. Preeclampsia must be differentiated from gestational hypertension, which occurs after 20 weeks gestation and is defined as a systolic blood pressure greater than or equal to 140 mmHg and/or diastolic blood pressure greater than or equal to 90 mmHg, observed on at least two occasions at a minimum of 4 hours apart in the absence of proteinuria or end-organ involvement.

The etiology of preeclampsia–eclampsia is largely unknown but multifactorial with suspected genetic and immunologic pathways and several identified predisposing risk factors. The pathophysiology of preeclampsia involves abnormal development of placental vascularization and impaired implantation, which often contributes to reduced perfusion and uteroplacental insufficiency. Placental ischemia triggers the release of inflammatory and oxidative stress factors that cause endothelial dysfunction resulting in the classic manifestations of preeclampsia, including hypertension. Preeclampsia typically progresses in severity as pregnancy advances with a variable rate that cannot be reliably predicted. The disease can be resolved only through birth of the infant and placenta but recovery does not occur immediately; symptoms may present or worsen in the first 24–48 hours postpartum, and new diagnoses have been reported up to 6 weeks later (ACOG, 2013; Ananth et al., 2013; Henderson et al., 2014; Sibai, 2012).

There is no reliable predictive model for preeclampsia and few preventative measures with demonstrable efficacy (ACOG, 2013). Daily low-dose aspirin therapy (81 mg) beginning late in the first trimester may reduce the risk of preeclampsia by 10–24% in high-risk populations of clients reviewed in **Table 34-2** (Henderson et al., 2014). Women living in low-income countries are more likely to have low dietary intake of calcium than those living in high-income countries (Hofmeyr et al., 2014). Oral calcium supplementation may reduce preeclampsia incidence among women with low dietary intake (< 600 mg/day) and should be considered for clients with a history of diagnosis in prior pregnancies, keeping in mind that excessive calcium may be harmful (Hofmeyr et al., 2014; Rath & Fischer, 2009; Schoenaker, Soedamah-Muthu, & Mishra, 2014; Sibai, 1998, 2005). Preeclampsia prevention with supplemental vitamins C, E, and D remains controversial and lacks strong evidence to support routine or targeted recommendations (ACOG, 2013; Dodd, O'Brien, & Grivell, 2014; Weinert & Silveiro, 2015). A prepregnancy diet low in these vitamins may increase the risk of preeclampsia, and physical activity may be protective (ACOG, 2013). Thus, health education

313

TABLE 34-1 Hypertensive Disorders in Pregnancy

Diagnosis	Criteria
Chronic hypertension	Blood pressure ≥ 140/90 (two measurements at least 4 hours apart) with onset prior to 20 wk gestation; typically predates the pregnancy.
Gestational hypertension	Blood pressure ≥ 140/90 (two measurements at least 4 hours apart) with onset after 20 wk gestation; no proteinuria; resolves by 6 weeks postpartum.
Preeclampsia	Gestational hypertension in the presence of proteinuria (at least 1+ on urine dipstick OR ≥ 0.3 mg/dL on spot protein/creatinine ratio OR ≥ 300 mg in 24-hour urine collection), OR Gestational hypertension in the absence of proteinuria AND presence of at least one of the following: • Pulmonary edema • Cerebral or visual symptoms • Thrombocytopenia (platelets < 100,000/mL) • ≥ 1.1 mg/dL or a doubling of serum creatinine concentration • Twice the normal concentration of aspartate aminotransferase (AST) or alanine aminotransferase (ALT)
Preeclampsia with severe features	Presence of preeclampsia with any of the following: • Blood pressure ≥ 160/110 (two measurements at least 4 hours apart) • Pulmonary edema • Cerebral or visual symptoms • Thrombocytopenia (platelets < 100,000/mL) • ≥1.1 mg/dL or a doubling of serum creatinine concentration • Twice the normal concentration of AST or ALT
Chronic hypertension with superimposed preeclampsia	Chronic hypertension in the setting of: New onset or increased proteinuria • Sudden increase in blood pressure • Sudden manifestation or worsening of lab abnormalities • Onset of severe headaches, cerebral or visual symptoms, pulmonary edema, right upper quadrant pain
HELLP syndrome	Considered preeclampsia subtype; characterized by hemolysis, elevated liver enzymes, low platelets
Postpartum preeclampsia	Preeclampsia occurring in the postpartum period prior to 6 months postpartum
Eclampsia	New-onset grand mal seizures with preeclampsia in pregnancy or postpartum

Data from American College of Obstetricians and Gynecologists. (2013). *Hypertension in pregnancy*. Washington, DC: American College of Obstetricians and Gynecologists.

focused on nutrition and exercise may be particularly helpful before conception and in early pregnancy.

In the absence of severe features, preeclampsia diagnosed and treated at or near term is unlikely to be associated with significant perinatal complications (Sibai, 2005). However, maternal and neonatal morbidities are likely to result from severe gestational hypertension or preeclampsia, particularly prior to 34 weeks of gestation. Timely recognition and treatment are necessary to prevent progression to eclampsia, which is diagnosed when maternal grand mal seizures occur and is strongly associated with adverse outcomes including maternal and fetal death (Sibai, 2005). Maternal morbidity resulting from preeclampsia with severe features is rare and includes

placental abruption, stroke, pulmonary edema, myocardial infarction, and coagulopathy. Fetal and neonatal sequelae of severe disease may include fetal growth restriction and stillbirth. Preeclampsia also contributes to the iatrogenic preterm birth rate because management includes facilitating delivery with induction of labor or cesarean delivery prior to labor in the case of severe disease with rapid progression.

Early detection and management can reduce adverse perinatal outcomes and may improve long-term maternal cardiovascular health (Druzin et al., 2014; Sibai, 2005). Preeclampsia–eclampsia is associated with a two- to threefold increased risk of cardiovascular disease overall and increased relative risks for chronic hypertension, ischemic heart disease,

TABLE 34-2 Clinical Risk Assessment for Preeclampsia and Use of Low-Dose Aspirin

Risk Level	Risk Factors	Recommendation
High†	• History of preeclampsia, especially when accompanied by an adverse outcome • Multifetal gestation • Chronic hypertension • Type 1 or 2 diabetes • Renal disease • Autoimmune disease (systemic lupus erythematosus, antiphospholipid syndrome)	Recommend low-dose aspirin if the patient has ≥ 1 of these high-risk factors
Moderate‡	• Nulliparity • Obesity (body mass index > 30 kg/m²) • History of preeclampsia in mother or sister • Sociodemographic characteristics (African-American race, low socioeconomic status) • Age ≥ 35 years • Personal history factors (e.g., low birthweight or small for gestational age, previous adverse pregnancy outcome, > 10-year pregnancy interval)	Consider low-dose aspirin if the patient has several of these moderate-risk factors
Low	Previous uncomplicated full-term delivery	Do not recommend low-dose aspirin

†Single risk factors that are consistently associated with the greatest risk for preeclampsia. The preeclampsia incidence rate would be approximately ≥ 8% in a pregnant woman with ≥ 1 of these risk factors.

‡ A combination of multiple moderate-risk factors may be used by clinicians to identify women at high risk for preeclampsia. These risk factors are independently associated with moderate risk for preeclampsia, some more consistently than others.

Reproduced from U.S. Preventative Services Task Force. (2014). *Final Recommendation Statement: Low Dose Aspirin to Prevent Preeclampsia: Preventive Medication.* Retrieved from http://www.uspreventiveservicestaskforce.org/Page/Document/RecommendationStatementFinal /low-dose-aspirin-use-for-the-prevention-of-morbidity-and-mortality-from-preeclampsia-preventive-medication#tab

venous thromboembolism, stroke, and mortality 5–15 years after the affected pregnancy (Bellamy, Casas, Hingorami, & Williams, 2007). Clients with preeclampsia in pregnancy are also at greater risk for postpartum depression and posttraumatic stress disorder following childbirth (Senden et al., 2012).

II. **Database** (may include but is not limited to)

A. *Subjective*

Assess for the presence of risk factors and symptoms. Clients presenting with vague symptoms such as headache, visual disturbances, abdominal pain, shortness of breath, generalized swelling, and complaints of "I just don't feel right" should be evaluated for atypical preeclampsia presentations and severe disease features due to the variable presentation of this serious complication of pregnancy (Sibai & Stella, 2009).

1. Past health history

    a. Medical history:

      Body mass index > 35, diabetes, or chronic hypertension, renal, vascular, or autoimmune disease, such as systemic lupus erythematosus or antiphospholipid syndrome.

    b. Obstetric and gynecological history:

      First pregnancy, maternal age > 40 years, multiple gestation, in vitro fertilization, or history of preeclampsia, placental abruption, or fetal growth restriction.

2. Family history:

    a. Mother or sister with hypertensive disorder in pregnancy

3. Review of systems:

    a. Constitutional signs and symptoms:

      Decreased fetal movement, report of feeling unwell, e.g., fatigued, malaise, dizzy, light headed, anxious, or confused.

    b. Skin:

      Unexplained ecchymosis.

c. Eyes:
Visual disturbances including blurred vision, "spots," "stars," "flashing lights," or blindness (indicative of retinal detachment).

d. Respiratory and cardiovascular:
Shortness of breath or dyspnea (may indicate concomitant pulmonary edema); increased swelling, particularly facial or periorbital.

e. Gastrointestinal:
Epigastric pain or pain in the right upper quadrant of the abdomen, heartburn, nausea, or vomiting.

f. Genitourinary:
Decreased urinary output, vaginal bleeding (may indicate abruptio placentae resulting from severe hypertension).

g. Neurologic:
Paresthesia of hands, feet, or extremities (may accompany significant edema); report of seizure; change in mental status or loss of consciousness. Headaches, particularly with new onset or increased severity or frequency. Headaches associated with preeclampsia are often frontal or occipital and do not respond to conservative treatment, e.g., over-the-counter medication such as acetaminophen.

B. Objective

1. Vital signs

   a. Blood pressure greater than or equal to 140 mmHg systolic and/or 90 mmHg diastolic on at least two occasions more than 4 hours apart. If blood pressure is greater than or equal to 160 mmHg systolic and/or 110 mmHg diastolic, confirm with repeat measurement within minutes to ensure timely management of severe hypertension (see **Table 34-3**).

   b. Rapid and excessive weight gain (> 2 pounds per week)

2. Skin examination: Petechiae, ecchymosis, or jaundice (may be present with hemolysis or thrombocytopenia).

3. Cardiovascular examination: Generalized edema, particularly facial or periorbital, with or without pitting.

4. Abdominal examination:

   a. Liver may be enlarged

   b. Right upper quadrant abdominal pain

   c. Fundal height; if less than expected for gestational age, ultrasound imaging may be indicated to assess for oligohydramnios or fetal growth restriction, which may result from maternal hypertension.

   d. Fetal heart tones

5. Genitourinary: Proteinuria of greater than or equal to 1+ protein on macrourinalysis with a clean, midstream sample. Refer to Table 34-1 for subsequent proteinuria measurement options and diagnostic criteria.

6. Neurologic examination: Hyperreflexia, with or without clonus.

III. Assessment

A. Determine the diagnosis

1. Criteria for preeclampsia diagnosis: Gestational hypertension and either proteinuria or evidence of severe features with end-organ involvement. In the absence of proteinuria, preeclampsia is diagnosed in the setting of gestational hypertension and at least one of the following: pulmonary edema; cerebral or visual symptoms, thrombocytopenia (platelets < 100,000/mL); at least 1.1 mg/dL or a doubling of serum creatinine concentration; or twice the normal concentration of aspartate AST or ALT, as described in Table 34-1.

TABLE 34-3 Steps for Obtaining Accurate Blood Pressure Measurements

To Assure an Accurate Blood Pressure Measurement:
• Obtain correct size cuff that encircles 80% of the arm
• Assess for caffeine or nicotine consumption within 30 minutes
• Be sure patient is sitting or semi-reclining with back supported and feet flat on floor (not dangling)
• Place cuff on bare upper arm without restrictive clothing, with arm supported at heart level
• Auscultation is most accurate. If auscultating: use first audible sound (Korotkoff I) as systolic pressure and use disappearance of sound (Korotkoff V) as diastolic pressure
• For accuracy, a second reading should be taken within 15 minutes in the same position and the highest reading recorded
• If reading is greater than or equal to 140/90 on repeat, further evaluation for preeclampsia is warranted
• Documentation should include the arm in which the blood pressure was taken

2. Differential diagnosis: If criteria are not met, the differential diagnosis should include but is not limited to impending preeclampsia, chronic or gestational hypertension, liver or renal disease, and substance use (Sibai & Stella, 2009). Similarly, HELLP syndrome should be considered, especially when hemolysis (H), elevated liver enzyme levels (EL), or low platelet counts (LP) are observed.

B. Severity

In 2013 the American College of Obstetricians and Gynecologists described the following severe features of preeclampsia:

1. Blood pressure of at least 160 mmHg systolic or 110 mmHg diastolic on two occasions at least 4 hours apart while the client is on bed rest.

2. New-onset cerebral or visual disturbances

3. Pulmonary edema

4. Impaired liver function (twice normal concentration of ALT or AST)

5. Thrombocytopenia (< 100,000/mL)

6. Renal insufficiency: Elevated serum creatinine (> 1.1 mg/dL or a doubling of serum creatinine concentration)

IV. Goals of clinical management

A. Screening

Screen all pregnant women for risk factors at the first prenatal visit and with blood pressure checks at each prenatal visit.

B. Prevention

Treat women at high risk with low-dose aspirin therapy.

C. Identification

Order appropriate diagnostic laboratory tests when blood pressure is elevated and educate all pregnant women of preeclampsia symptoms.

D. Maternal and fetal well-being

Assure maternal and fetal well-being with blood pressure, urine, and symptom monitoring, fetal surveillance methods, and growth ultrasounds. Plan for induction of labor at appropriate gestational age for diagnosis.

V. Plan

A. Diagnostic tests

1. Repeat blood pressure assessment after a 10–30 minute rest period with the client in an upright or sitting position, using an appropriately sized sphygmomanometer cuff. Proper blood pressure assessment is essential and outlined in Table 34-3. Gestational hypertension is diagnosed when two or more elevated readings are observed greater than 4 hours apart. In case of hypertensive emergency in pregnant or postpartum clients, it is not advisable to wait for at least two elevated blood pressure readings in 4 hours before initiating treatment. In case of acute onset or persistent (lasting 15 minutes or more) and severe systolic (≥ 160 mmHg) and/or diastolic (≥ 110 mmHg) hypertension, treat with antihypertensives within 30–60 minutes if blood pressures remain elevated 15 minutes after the initial severe finding (ACOG, 2015).

2. Obtain a clean midstream urine sample to assess for protein on standardized laboratory macrourinalysis if not previously done. Inconsistencies in qualitative assessment of macrourinalysis via dipstick suggest this method of diagnosis should be avoided, but in low-resource settings, a urine dipstick reading of 1+ is sufficient for diagnosis of proteinuria if found on two or more occasions, at least 4 hours apart (Druzin et al., 2014). Consider urine culture and sensitivity to rule out urinary tract infection if proteinuria is present because asymptomatic infection is common in pregnancy and could confound the diagnosis.

3. Initiate 24-hour urine collection or spot urine protein/creatinine ratio to assess for proteinuria if the client has gestational hypertension or 1+ protein on urine dipstick. The 24-hour urine collection for protein measurement remains the gold standard for proteinuria diagnosis but the spot protein/creatinine ratio provides a reliable estimate and is recommended as a less burdensome proxy (Papanna, Mann, Kouids, & Glantz, 2008). A protein/creatinine ratio greater than or equal to 0.3 mg/dL OR a 24-hour urine collection with protein levels equal to or greater than 300 mg is diagnostic of preeclampsia in a hypertensive pregnant client (ACOG, 2013).

4. Order serum testing: complete blood count (CBC) with platelets, and liver function panel including AST, ALT, serum protein, and creatinine. Note that alkaline phosphatase is typically elevated in pregnancy and is not indicative of preeclampsia. Although commonly ordered, uric acid has a 33% positive predictive value and is not a useful diagnostic tool (ACOG, 2013). Lactate dehydrogenase (LDH) and bilirubin levels may be useful in detecting hemolysis associated with HELLP syndrome, in addition to thrombocytopenia assessment (Druzin et al., 2014).

B. Treatment and follow-up of gestational hypertension or preeclampsia without severe features

1. Delivery is recommended after 37 weeks gestation after physician consultation; comanagement may be appropriate.

2. If less than 37 weeks gestation, stable clients may receive outpatient care with maternal and fetal surveillance to identify disease progression and development of severe features (ACOG, 2013; Druzin et al., 2014).

   a. Fetal surveillance and management

      i. Twice-weekly biophysical profile (BPP) or nonstress test (NST) plus amniotic fluid index (AFI) is recommended.

      ii. Ultrasound assessment of fetal growth is recommended upon diagnosis and at 3-week intervals.

   b. Maternal surveillance and management (ACOG, 2013; Druzin et al., 2014)

      i. Blood pressure, proteinuria, and signs/symptom review (severe headache, visual changes, epigastric or right upper quadrant pain, shortness of breath) should be evaluated twice weekly, to monitor for development of severe features.

      ii. Laboratory testing may be repeated weekly or with worsening symptomatology: CBC, ALT/AST, serum creatinine (ACOG, 2013).

      iii. There is no compelling evidence that bed rest reduces disease progression or improves perinatal outcomes. However, the left lateral recumbent position may optimize uterine, placental, and fetal circulation and should be encouraged, particularly if significant edema is present.

      iv. Consider home blood pressure monitoring and recording if clients with nonsevere preeclampsia are being managed on an outpatient basis.

      v. During return visits, complete a review of systems and physical exam as previously described. Discuss parameters for acute reevaluation and ensure client has appointments for subsequent fetal and maternal surveillance.

   c. Ongoing medical consultation about evolving client condition and collaborative management plan.

C. Treatment and follow-up of *severe preeclampsia*

1. Treatment and follow-up of severe preeclampsia requires immediate physician consultation and probable referral to obstetrician or perinatology services.

2. If less than 34 weeks gestation, clients should be admitted to a tertiary facility. Corticosteroids should be considered to enhance fetal lung development during expectant management, which is recommended in the absence of indications for immediate delivery. Severe cases at early gestational ages are more likely to progress rapidly with worse outcomes than later cases, necessitating ongoing surveillance and anticipatory guidance for the family.

3. Delivery is recommended at 34 or more weeks gestation.

4. To minimize risk of maternal stroke, antihypertensives should be administered as soon as possible for those individuals with blood pressure greater than or equal to 160 mmHg systolic or above 105 mmHg diastolic (Druzin et al., 2014).

D. Client education in the setting of suspected or confirmed preeclampsia

1. Advise the client to immediately report signs of severe preeclampsia: Severe headache, visual changes, epigastric or right upper quadrant pain, or shortness of breath.

2. Teach the client how to perform fetal kick counts twice daily after 28 weeks gestation. Instruct the client to notify providers if fewer than 10 fetal movements are felt in a 2-hour period, preferably when client is at rest following a meal.

3. If home blood pressure monitoring is initiated, teach the client how to use the machine and record values. Instruct the client to immediately report critical values ($\geq 160/105$ mmHg).

4. Discuss self-care including nutrition, hydration, exercise, stress management, and relaxation.

5. Provide anticipatory guidance about disease progression and both immediate and long-term sequelae.

6. Clearly document the follow-up plan and include the client in the decision-making process.

7. Provide anticipatory guidance regarding the recommendation of induction of labor in the setting of severe and nonsevere preeclampsia (ACOG, 2013). Encourage individualized care planning with medical providers, taking into consideration the client's own values and judgments (ACOG, 2013).

E. Consultation and referral

Refer to Chapter 30, Guidelines for Medical Consultation, Interprofessional Collaboration, and Transfer of Care During Pregnancy and Childbirth. Physician consultation is indicated for suspected or documented preeclampsia of any severity. Gestational hypertension and nonsevere preeclampsia may be managed by nurse practitioners or nurse-midwives with physician consultation, or collaboratively managed on either an inpatient or outpatient basis. Severe preeclampsia at any gestational age warrants evaluation by an obstetrician as soon as possible, and typically requires referral to obstetrical care or a maternal–fetal medicine service.

F. Postpartum and preconception considerations (ACOG, 2013; Druzin et al., 2014)

1. Postpartum follow-up is recommended to monitor blood pressure at 72 hours and 7–10 days postpartum.

2. Preeclampsia is associated with greater risk of lifelong cardiovascular disease, which may be lessened with healthy lifestyle changes.

3. Any client with a history of preeclampsia should be advised of the risk of recurring preeclampsia in subsequent pregnancy and the availability of low-dose aspirin therapy to reduce the risk of recurrence.

4. In the preconception period, clients with obesity, chronic hypertension, renal disease, diabetes, or autoimmune disease should be advised of the potential risk of preeclampsia and be provided support to improve health and reduce risks of pregnancy complications.

REFERENCES

American College of Obstetricians and Gynecologists. (2013). *Hypertension in pregnancy*. Washington, DC: American College of Obstetricians and Gynecologists.

American College of Obstetricians and Gynecologists. (2015). ACOG Committee Opinion No. 623: Emergent therapy for acute-onset, severe hypertension with preeclampsia or eclampsia. *Obstetrics and Gynecology, 125*(2), 521–525.

Ananth, C. V., Keyes, K. M. & Wapner, R. J. (2013). Pre-eclampsia rates in the United States, 1980-2010: Age-period-cohort analysis. *BMJ, 347*(15), f6564. doi: 10.1136/bmj.f6564.

Bellamy, L., Casas, J. P., Hingorami, A. D., & Williams, D. (2007). Preeclampsia and risk of cardiovascular disease and cancer in later life: Systematic review and meta-analysis. *British Medical Journal (Clinical Research Edition), 335*(7627), 974–982.

Dodd, J. M., O'Brien, C., & Grivell, R. M, (2014). Preventing pre-eclampsia are dietary factors the key? *BMC Medicine, 12*, 176. doi:10.1186/s12916-014-0176-4

Druzin, M. L., Shields, L. E., Peterson, N. L., & Cape, V. (2013). *Preeclampsia toolkit: Improving health care response to preeclampsia (California Maternal Quality Care Collaborative toolkit to transform maternity care)*. Stanford, CA: California Maternal Quality Care Collaborative.

Henderson, J. T., Whitlock, E. P., O'Connor, E., Senger, C. A., Thompson, J. H., & Rowland, M. G. (2014). Low-dose aspirin for prevention of morbidity and mortality from preeclampsia: A systematic evidence review for the U.S. Preventive Services Task Force. *Annals of Internal Medicine, 10*, 695–703.

Hofmeyr, G. J., Belizan, J. M., von Dadelszen, P., & Calcium and Pre-eclampsia Study Group. (2014). Low-dose calcium supplementation for preventing pre-eclampsia: A systematic review and commentary. *British Journal of Obstetrics and Gynaecology, 8*, 951–957.

Ogedegbe, G., & Pickering, T. (2010). Principles and techniques of blood pressure measurement. *Cardiology Clinics, 28*(4), 571–586.

Papanna, R., Mann, L. K., Kouids, R. W., & Glantz, J. C. (2008). Protein/creatinine ratio in preeclampsia. *Obstetrics & Gynecology, 112*(1), 135–144.

Peters, R. M. (2008, October-November). High blood pressure in pregnancy. *Nursing for Women's Health*, pp. 410–422.

Rath, W., & Fischer, T. (2009). The diagnosis and treatment of hypertensive disorders of pregnancy: New findings for antenatal and inpatient care. *Deutsches Ärzteblatt International, 106*(45), 733–738.

Schoenaker, D., Soedamah-Muthu, S. S., & Mishra, G. D. (2014). The association between dietary factors and gestational hypertension and pre-eclampsia: A systematic review and meta-analysis of observational studies. *BMC Medicine, 1*, 157.

Senden, I. P., Duivenvoorden, H. J., Filius, A., DeGroot, C. J., Steegers, E. A., & Passchier, J. (2012). Maternal psychosocial outcome after early onset preeclampsia and preterm birth. *Journal of Maternal Fetal Neonatal Medicine, 25*, 272–276.

Sibai, B. M. (1998). Prevention of preeclampsia: A big disappointment. *American Journal of Obstetrics & Gynecology, 179*, 1275–1278.

Sibai, B. M. (2005). Diagnosis, prevention, and management of eclampsia. *Obstetrics & Gynecology, 105*(2), 402–410.

Sibai, B. M. (2012). Etiology and management of postpartum hypertension-preeclampsia. *American Journal of Obstetrics and Gynecology, 203*(6), 470–475.

Sibai, B. M., & Stella, C. L. (2009). Diagnosis and management of atypical preeclampsia-eclampsia. *American Journal of Obstetrics and Gynecology, 200*(5), e481–e487.

Tanaka, M., Jaamaa, G., Kaiser, M., Hills, E., Soim, A., Zhu, M., et al. (2007). Racial disparity in hypertensive disorders of pregnancy in New York State: A 10-Year longitudinal population-based study. *American Journal of Public Health, 97*(1), 163–170. doi:10.2105/AJPH.2005.068577.

U.S. Preventive Services Task Force. (2014). Final recommendation statement. Low dose aspirin to prevent preeclampsia: Preventive medication. Retrieved from www.uspreventiveservicestaskforce.org/Page/Document/RecommendationStatementFinal/low-dose-aspirin-use-for-the-prevention-of-morbidity-and-mortality-from-preeclampsia-preventive-medication.

Weinert, L. S., & Silveiro, S. P. (2015). Maternal-fetal impact of vitamin D deficiency: A critical review. *Maternal and Child Health Journal, 19*(1), 94–101. doi: 10.1007/s10995-014-1499-7.

PRETERM LABOR MANAGEMENT

Mary Barger

I. Introduction and general background

Twelve percent of births in the United States occur before 37 weeks. Preterm birth is the leading cause of neonatal mortality (American College of Obstetrics and Gynecology [ACOG], 2012). The birth of a premature infant can lead to long-term health consequences such as cerebral palsy and lung, hearing, and vision problems, and new evidence shows an increase in adult diseases such as cardiovascular disease and diabetes. Unfortunately, there are large differences in the burden of prematurity by race/ethnicity with African-Americans having the highest rate. Premature births (PTB) have a large economic impact, averaging more than $54,000 in medical costs per premature infant and 10 times the medical expenses in the first year of life compared to term infants (Behrman & Butler, 2006).

A. Definition

A PTB is any birth that occurs after 20 weeks gestation and prior to 37 completed weeks of gestation (36 6/7 weeks). Preterm births are further classified into:

1. extremely preterm (< 28 weeks)
2. very preterm (28 to < 32 weeks)
3. moderate to late preterm (32 to < 37 weeks).

B. Prevalence/Incidence

The current rate of premature birth is 11.7%, an 11% decrease from 2006 but still higher than the Healthy People 2020 goal of 9.6% and higher than that in European nations (Martin, Hamilton, & Osterman, 2014). Recent progress in preventing iatrogenic late preterm births is one reason for the decrease. The number of multiple births has remained stable, which is good news because the vast majority are born prematurely. Significant sociodemographic differences in prematurity still exist. African-Americans have a 65% higher rate than Asians who have the lowest rate (16.5% and 10%, respectively), and uninsured women have a rate of nearly 20%.

Two-thirds of preterm births are spontaneous and the other one-third are for indicated reasons. It has been noted that, as the rate of indicated late preterm births increased, the rate of stillbirths has decreased.

II. Database (may include but it not limited to)

A. Subjective

1. Reproductive history
   a. Prior spontaneous preterm birth (sPTB) (singleton live birth at 16 0/7–36 6/7 weeks gestation or stillbirth before 24 weeks presenting as labor, ruptured membranes, advanced cervical dilatation)—this is the most important risk factor for sPTB.
   b. Risk of PTB in a subsequent pregnancy after one prior sPTB in a singleton pregnancy is 15%; this risk increases to 33% with two prior sPTBs and is 24% if a woman had a term pregnancy followed by a sPTB (Adams, Elam-Evans, Wilson, & Gilbertz, 2000).
   c. Spontaneous abortions if recurrent and in second trimester
2. Gynecological history
   a. Presence of a uterine malformation (müllerian anomalies)
   b. Previous cervical cone biopsy or excision with loop electrosurgical excision procedure (LEEP)
3. Medical history (puts a woman more at risk for indicated preterm birth)
   a. Type 1 diabetes—not well controlled especially preconception

b. Hypertension

c. Renal disease

d. Autoimmune disease (systemic lupus erythematous)

4. Pregnancy history and personal habits this pregnancy

a. Multiple gestation

b. Placental abnormalities (placenta previa or abruption)

c. Polyhydramnios or oliogohydramnios

d. Abdominal surgery after 18 weeks gestation or cervical surgery

e. Vaginal bleeding in more than one trimester

f. Pregnancy the result of assisted reproductive technology (ART)

g. Presence of a fetus with a congenital anomaly

h. Short interpregnancy interval of less than 6 months

i. Body mass index (BMI) < 19/poor nutritional status

j. Smoking more than 10 cigarettes a day

k. Cocaine use

l. Febrile illness/systemic infection

m. High social stress

n. Occupational/ environmental exposures

o. Cervical length on midtrimester ultrasound less than 25 mm

5. Presence of signs or symptoms of preterm labor

a. Uterine contractions that are frequently painless

b. Back pain—constant or intermittent

c. Menstrual-type cramping

d. Pelvic pressure

e. Change in vaginal discharge

f. Vaginal spotting/bleeding (bloody show)

B. Objective

1. Palpate abdomen/uterus for tenderness and place uterine contraction and fetal heart rate monitor

2. Perform speculum exam to obtain fetal fibronectin (fFN) specimen (this must be done before any digital exam of the cervix and other vaginal/cervical cultures)

3. Check cervix for position, consistency, dilation, effacement (length), and station of presenting part

III. Assessment

A. At risk for preterm labor

B. Threatened preterm labor

IV. Goals of clinical management

A. Identification

Determine through screening and history women at risk for preterm labor.

B. Prevention

Reduce preterm labor and birth rates by using interventions aimed at individual identified risk factors.

C. Treatment

Refer women with previous PTB for progesterone supplementation and serial cervical length assessments. Identify preterm labor early and refer to hospital birth unit to ensure betamethasone treatment to aid in fetal lung maturity.

V. Plan

A. Women at risk for preterm labor

1. Screen all pregnant women for asymptomatic bacteriuria at initial presentation and treat if positive urine culture to prevent pyelonephritis

2. Avoid poor nutrition:

a. If BMI < 19, ensure the woman knows recommended weight gain in pregnancy and refer to nutritionist if needed.

b. Ensure that women eat a Mediterranean-type diet low in fat and processed food, rich in fruits and vegetables, and two servings of fatty fish a week or take omega-3 supplements of 1–1.5 grams a day (Khoury, Henriksen, Christophersen, & Tonstad, 2005).

3. Ensure that women have adequate levels of vitamin D (greater than 20 ng/mL). There is moderate evidence of a relationship between vitamin D levels and risk of spontaneous and indicated preterm birth (Bodnar et al., 2014; Robinson et al., 2013; Wei, Qi, Luo, & Fraser, 2013).

4. Refer women who smoke to a smoking cessation program. Educate women to avoid secondhand smoke.

5. Refer women using cocaine and other substances for drug treatment.

6. Evaluate personal/family resources and potential barriers to accessing care.

7. Consult after the first prenatal visit regarding progesterone supplementation for the prevention of preterm delivery in women with a history of a prior

sPTB in a singleton pregnancy (singleton live birth at 16 0/7–36 6/7 weeks gestation or stillbirth before 24 weeks) (ACOG, 2012; Iams, 2014).

   a. Measure transvaginal cervical length every 14 days from 16–24 weeks for high-risk women. If the cervical length is less than 30 mm increase to weekly. Transvaginal cervical length less than 25 mm before 24 week of gestation: Cerclage should be considered especially if the patient had prior sPTB at less than 28 weeks or if membranes are seen.

8. Consider a cervical length at the time of the second trimester ultrasound (anatomical survey) (18 to 20 weeks) in women without a history of preterm delivery. Consult if cervix less than 25 mm. Consider progesterone supplementation for the prevention of preterm delivery if cervical length less than 20 mm before 24 weeks (ACOG, 2012; Iams, 2014).

B. Women with signs and symptoms of preterm labor (less than 37 weeks gestation)

NOTE: Assessment depends on logistics of your practice site. Sites remote from a hospital or where transportation issues are great may choose to monitor women over a period of time before referral to a hospital; more urban sites may refer directly.

1. Obtain a clean catch urine and dipstick and send for urinalysis to rule out urinary tract infection.

2. Perform an abdominal exam for contractions and tenderness; use toco monitor to detect the presence of contractions.

3. Assess fetal well-being with assessment of fetal heart tones.

4. Depending on setting:

   a. Either refer to a birthing unit for further evaluation OR

   b. If observation in the ambulatory setting:

      i. First, obtain a posterior fornix sample for fetal fibronectin (fFN).

      ii. Obtain a sample for group B *Streptococcus*, if not previously obtained, and other samples, as indicated, for vaginal infections.

      iii. Assess the status of placental membranes and presence of vaginal bleeding. If membranes are ruptured or bleeding is present, the woman should be referred immediately to the hospital.

      iv. Then, perform a digital cervical exam, if membranes intact and no bleeding and no placenta previa on ultrasound.

      v. Observe the woman for 1 to 2 hours and recheck her cervix.

         a. If she meets the criteria for preterm labor, refer her to birthing unit for further evaluation with fFN swab that was obtained.

         b. Diagnostic criteria for preterm labor:

            i. Gestational age 20–36 6/7 weeks AND

            ii. Documented regular contractions AND

            iii. One of the following: documented cervical change OR cervical dilation $\geq$ 2 cm OR cervical effacement $\geq$ 80%.

         c. If no cervical change and no uterine contractions after a 2-hour observation, then educate regarding the signs and symptoms of preterm labor and criteria for calling the healthcare provider.

REFERENCES

Adams, M. M., Elam-Evans, L. D., Wilson, H. G., & Gilbertz, D. A. (2000). Rates of and factors associated with recurrence of preterm delivery. *JAMA, 283*, 1591–1596.

American College of Obstetricians and Gynecologists. (2012). ACOG Practice Bulletin No. 130. Prediction and prevention of preterm birth. *Obstetrics and Gynecology, 120*, 964–973.

Behrman, R., & Butler A. S. (Eds.). (2007). *Preterm birth: Causes, consequences, and prevention*. Institute of Medicine Committee on Understanding Premature Birth and Assuring Healthy Outcomes. Washington, DC: National Academies Press.

Bodnar, L. M., Klebanoff, M. A., Gernand, A. D., Platt, R. W., Parks, W. T, Catov, J. M., et al. (2014). Maternal vitamin D status and spontaneous preterm birth by placental histology in US Collaborative Perinatal Project. *American Journal of Epidemiology, 178*, 168–176.

Iams, J. D. (2014). Prevention of preterm parturition. *New England Journal of Medicine 370*, 254–261.

Khoury, J., Henriksen, T., Christophersen, B., & Tonstad, S. (2005). Effect of a cholesterol-lowering diet on maternal, cord, and neonatal lipids, and pregnancy outcome: A randomized clinical trial. *American Journal of Obstetrics and Gynecology, 193*, 1292–1301.

Martin, J. A., Hamilton, B. E., & Osterman, M. J. K. (2014). *Births in the United States, 2013*. (NCHS Data Briefs No. 175). Hyattsville, MD: National Center for Health Statistics, Centers for Disease Control and Prevention.

Robinson, C. J., Wagner, C. L., Hollis, B. W., et al. (2013). Association of maternal vitamin D and placenta growth factor with the diagnosis of early onset severe preeclampsia. *American Journal of Perinatology, 30*(3), 167–72.

Wei, S. Q., Qi, H. P., Luo, Z. C., & Fraser, W. D. (2013). Maternal vitamin D status and adverse pregnancy outcomes: A systematic review and meta-analysis. *Journal of Maternal, Fetal, and Neonatal Medicine, 26*, 889–899.

URINARY TRACT INFECTION PREVENTION AND MANAGEMENT IN PREGNANCY

CHAPTER **36**

Mary Barger

I. Introduction and general background

A. Physiologic and anatomic changes of the urinary tract in pregnancy predispose lower urinary tract infections (UTIs) to ascend and become upper tract infections, i.e., pyelonephritis, which is a risk factor for preterm labor.

B. Asymptomatic bacteriuria (ASB) is the presence of bacteria in the urine without symptoms and occurs in 2–9% of pregnant women (Nicolle et al., 2005). In pregnancy, 25–40% of women with untreated ASB will develop pyelonephritis; therefore, it is treated with antibiotics, unlike for nonpregnant women in whom it is left untreated.

C. Maternal consequences from pyelonephritis in pregnancy can be life threatening and may include sepsis, acute respiratory distress syndrome, acute renal or heart failure, need for transfusion, and possibly death (Dotters-Katz, Heine, & Grotegut, 2013).

II. Database (may include but is not limited to)

A. Subjective

1. Medical history
   a. Urinary tract infection—number, precipitating factors, e.g., associated with coitus
   b. Pyelonephritis
   c. Urinary tract abnormality, e.g., single kidney, displaced kidneys
   d. Diabetes
   e. Immunosuppression

2. Reproductive history
   a. Gestational age
   b. Parity
   c. Pyelonephritis in a prior pregnancy
   d. Urinary tract infection in prior pregnancy

3. Presence of signs or symptoms of cystitis
   a. Abrupt onset of urinary frequency and hesitancy and dysuria
   b. Suprapubic or low back pain
   c. Flank pain (unusual)
   d. Presence of vaginal discharge or irritation (decreases the likelihood of cystitis)

4. Presence of signs of pyelonephritis
   a. Signs of cystitis PLUS/OR
   b. Fever (> 38° C) and chills
   c. Nausea and vomiting
   d. Costovertebral tenderness
   e. Gross hematuria (not required)
   f. Diarrhea (rare)

5. Presence of signs or symptoms of preterm labor, e.g., contractions, low back pain, increased vaginal discharge, pelvic pressure

B. Objective

1. For diagnosis of ASB—culture urine on all pregnant women at 12–16 weeks or with initial prenatal visit if later (Lin, Fajarado, & U.S. Preventive Services Task Force, 2008).

2. Women presenting with UTI symptoms
   a. Assess temperature, blood pressure, maternal pulse, and respiratory rate. Immediately refer women whose vital signs indicate possible pyelonephritis.
   b. Dipstick urine for nitrites, leukocytes, and blood
   c. Laboratory evidence of anemia (if anemic with pyelonephritis diagnosis, increased risk

of preterm birth—Dotters-Katz, Grotegut, & Heine, 2013)

   d. Send urine for culture and sensitivity (C&S)

   e. Check for costovertebral angle (CVA) tenderness

   f. Palpate abdomen/uterus for tenderness and presence of contractions

   g. Depending on history, perform speculum exam to rule out urethritis from a vaginal infection

   h. Consider vaginal exam if any suspicion of concomitant preterm labor signs

III. Assessment

A. Asymptomatic bacteriuria

B. Possible UTI

C. Possible pyelonephritis

IV. Goals of Clinical Management

A. Identify patients at risk for UTI during pregnancy

B. Diagnose both asymptomatic and symptomatic UTI

C. Individualized treatment: Use medication that is sensitive, well tolerated, and low cost with the lowest number of treatment days and reduced daily dosing

D. Prevent recurrent infections and/or pyelonephritis:

   1. Establish efficacy of treatment by repeat urine culture and sensitivity after treatment and each trimester of pregnancy.

   2. Prescribe suppression for women with more than one UTI or pyelonephritis during pregnancy.

E. Educate women with UTI regarding signs and symptoms of pyelonephritis

V. Plan

A. Women without ASB on initial culture do not need to be rescreened later in pregnancy unless they have a urinary tract anomaly or history of pyelonephritis.

B. Women with ASB or acute cystitis

   1. Treat with appropriate antibiotic for 3–7 days after initial C&S results available (Widmer, Gulmezoglu, Mignini, & Roganti, 2011). (See **Table 36-1**.)

   2. If treating acute cystitis presumptively, follow up on urine culture results to ensure bacteria are sensitive to the prescribed antibiotic. If not, change to antimicrobial-sensitive agent.

   3. Repeat urine C&S 1 week after treatment.

TABLE 36-1 Medications for Urinary Infections in Pregnancy

Principles

- Contraindicated in pregnancy: fluoroquinolones and tetracyclines.
- Avoid in first trimester: nitrofurantoin and sulfonamides (ACOG Committee on Obstetric Practice, 2011; Crider et al., 2009) and trimethoprim (folic acid antagonist) because of increased birth defect risk.
- Avoid using sulfonamides and nitrofurantoin near time of birth because of theoretical increased risk of jaundice.

Recommended treatment regimens, if microorganism susceptible

Medication	Oral Dose	Frequency per Day	Duration in Days	ASB	Cystitis
Amoxicillin	500 mg	Twice	3–7	x	
Amoxicillin-clavulanate	500 mg	Twice	3–7	x	x
Cefpodoxime	100 mg	Twice	3–7		x
Cephalexin	500 mg	Twice	3–5	x	
Fosfomycin	3 g	Twice	Once	x	x
Nitrofurantoin	100 mg	Twice	3–5	x	x

4. If culture is positive, then re-treat for 7–10 days with antimicrobial sensitive agent.

5. Rescreen each trimester or monthly.

6. Initiate suppressive therapy for women with two or more urinary tract infections in pregnancy; typically nitrofurantoin 50–100 mg at bedtime; alternative is cephalexin 250–500 mg at bedtime.

C. Women with suspected pyelonephritis

1. Refer to birthing unit for assessment and parenteral treatment. Most pregnant women with pyelonephritis will receive inpatient IV treatment until they are afebrile for at least 24 hours and then be discharged on a 14-day oral antibiotic course. They will also be monitored for premature labor.

2. Repeat urine C&S follow-up test of cure after 2-week antibiotic course is complete.

3. Ensure woman receives UTI suppressive therapy for remainder of the pregnancy.

D. Women on suppressive therapy do not need monthly cultures but a repeat C&S in early third trimester (~ 32 weeks) to ensure adequacy of suppression.

REFERENCES

ACOG Committee on Obstetric Practice. (2011). Committee opinion no. 494: Sulfonamides, nitrofurantoin, and risk of birth defects. *Obstetrics and Gynecology, 117*, 1484–1485.

Crider, K. S., Cleves, M. A., Reefhuis, J., Berry, R. J., Hobbs, C. A., & Hu, D. J. (2009). Antibacterial medication use during pregnancy and risk of birth defects: National Birth Defect Prevention Study. *Archives of Pediatric and Adolescent Medicine, 163*, 978–985.

Dotters-Katz, S. K., Grotegut, C. A., & Heine, R. P. (2013). The effects of anemia on pregnancy outcome in patients with pyelonephritis. *Infectious Diseases in Obstetrics and Gynecology, 2013*, 780960.

Dotters-Katz, S. K., Heine, R. P., & Grotegut, C. A. (2013). Medical and infectious complications associated with pyelonephritis among pregnant women at delivery. *Infectious Diseases in Obstetrics and Gynecology, 2013*, 124102.

Lin, K., Fajardo, K., & U.S. Preventive Services Task Force. (2008). Screening for asymptomatic bacteriuria in adults: Evidence for the U.S. Preventive Services Task Force reaffirmation recommendation statement. *Annals of Internal Medicine, 149*, W20–W24.

Nicolle, L. E., Bradley, S., Colgan, R., Rice, J. C., Schaeffer, A., & Hooton, T. M. (2005). Infectious Diseases Society of America guidelines for the diagnosis and treatment of asymptomatic bacteriuria in adults. *Clinical Infectious Diseases, 40*, 643–645.

Widmer, M., Gulmezoglu, A. M., Mignini, L., & Roganti, A. (2011). Duration of asymptomatic bacteriuria during pregnancy. *Cochrane Database of Systematic Reviews, 12*, CD000491.

ADULT HEALTH MAINTENANCE AND PROMOTION

Helen R. Horvath and Hattie C. Grundland

CHAPTER 37

I. Introduction and general background

Health maintenance and promotion, also called preventive health care and healthcare maintenance, aim to prevent and minimize disease and promote health. Preventive healthcare interventions include counseling, immunizations, preventive medications (chemoprophylaxis), and screening. This chapter focuses on recommendations for adults for primary and secondary prevention, or measures to prevent disease and to detect asymptomatic conditions. It should be noted that older adolescents often receive care in adult clinic settings. For these patients, preventive service recommendations specific to adolescent populations may be more appropriate. These recommendations can be found in chapter of this book.

The U.S. Preventive Services Task Force (USPSTF), an independent group of national experts in prevention and evidence-based medicine, evaluates existing peer-reviewed evidence regarding preventive services. The task force then grades the quality of the evidence and makes recommendations based on these grades. These recommendations, along with supporting resources for providers and patients, can be found at the website of the USPSTF, www.uspreventiveservicestaskforce.org. The Centers for Disease Control and Prevention (CDC) publishes immunization schedules based on recommendations of the Advisory Committee on Immunization Practices, a group of medical and public health experts. The 2015 Recommended Adult Immunization Schedule is included in **Figure 37-1**. The schedule is available in many formats from the CDC website, www.cdc.gov/vaccines/. See **Figure 37-2** for guidance on scheduling pneumococcal vaccines.

Many professional associations, such as the American Heart Association, the American Cancer Society, and the American Geriatrics Society (AGS), also make recommendations for preventive health care specific to their areas of focus. These guidelines may conflict with each other and with the USPSTF recommendations. The provider must use clinical judgment to assess which preventive interventions are most appropriate for the patient.

Despite strong evidence for effective and cost-effective preventive healthcare interventions, many of these measures remain underused among the U.S. population. A 2007 analysis by the National Commission on Prevention Priorities found that increasing the uptake of just five recommended prevention measures (aspirin to prevent heart disease, tobacco screening and intervention, colorectal cancer screening, influenza vaccination, and breast cancer screening) could save more than 100,000 lives in the United States each year (Partnership for Prevention, 2007).

How, then, do we increase use of these services? The Community Preventive Services Task Force, in collaboration with the CDC and the Agency for Healthcare Research and Quality, conducts systematic reviews and makes evidence-based recommendations for implementing programs and systems to improve the delivery of preventive health care. Examples of interventions that have been evaluated by the task force and recommended include client reminders, one-on-one education, and provider reminders for breast, cervical, and colon cancer screening. Task force findings and recommendations can be found at their website, www.thecommunityguide.org.

II. Individualizing screening decisions in the geriatric population

A key concept in the care of older adults is the notion that decisions about screening for preventable illnesses need to be individualized rather than based solely on age. (see **Figure 37-3**) The large heterogeneity of comorbidities, life expectancy, and goals of treatment in this population means that decisions based simply on age could lead to both over- and undertreatment and potential harm. Screening adults whose life expectancy is shorter than the time it would take them to benefit from a screening intervention subjects them to the potential harms of screening without the potential

Recommended Adult Immunization Schedule—United States — 2016

Note: These recommendations must be read with the footnotes that follow
containing number of doses, intervals between doses, and other important information.

Figure 1. Recommended immunization schedule for adults aged 19 years or older, by vaccine and age group[1]

VACCINE ▼ / AGE GROUP ►	19-21 years	22-26 years	27-49 years	50-59 years	60-64 years	≥ 65 years
Influenza[*,2]	1 dose annually					
Tetanus, diphtheria, pertussis (Td/Tdap)[*,3]	Substitute Tdap for Td once, then Td booster every 10 yrs					
Varicella[*,4]	2 doses					
Human papillomavirus (HPV) Female[*,5]	3 doses					
Human papillomavirus (HPV) Male[*,5]	3 doses					
Zoster[6]					1 dose	
Measles, mumps, rubella (MMR)[*,7]	1 or 2 doses depending on indication					
Pneumococcal 13-valent conjugate (PCV13)[*,8]					1 dose	
Pneumococcal 23-valent polysaccharide (PPSV23)[8]	1 or 2 doses depending on indication					1 dose
Hepatitis A[*,9]	2 or 3 doses depending on vaccine					
Hepatitis B[*,10]	3 doses					
Meningococcal 4-valent conjugate (MenACWY) or polysaccharide (MPSV4)[*,11]	1 or more doses depending on indication					
Meningococcal B (MenB)[11]	2 or 3 doses depending on vaccine					
Haemophilus influenzae type b (Hib)[*,12]	1 or 3 doses depending on indication					

*Covered by the Vaccine Injury Compensation Program

■ Recommended for all persons who meet the age requirement, lack documentation of vaccination, or lack evidence of past infection; zoster vaccine is recommended regardless of past episode of zoster

■ Recommended for persons with a risk factor (medical, occupational, lifestyle, or other indication)

□ No recommendation

Report all clinically significant postvaccination reactions to the Vaccine Adverse Event Reporting System (VAERS). Reporting forms and instructions on filing a VAERS report are available at www.vaers.hhs.gov or by telephone, 800-822-7967.

Information on how to file a Vaccine Injury Compensation Program claim is available at www.hrsa.gov/vaccinecompensation or by telephone, 800-338-2382. To file a claim for vaccine injury, contact the U.S. Court of Federal Claims, 717 Madison Place, N.W., Washington, D.C. 20005; telephone, 202-357-6400.

Additional information about the vaccines in this schedule, extent of available data, and contraindications for vaccination is also available at www.cdc.gov/vaccines or from the CDC-INFO Contact Center at 800-CDC-INFO (800-232-4636) in English and Spanish, 8:00 a.m. - 8:00 p.m. Eastern Time, Monday - Friday, excluding holidays.

Use of trade names and commercial sources is for identification only and does not imply endorsement by the U.S. Department of Health and Human Services.

The recommendations in this schedule were approved by the Centers for Disease Control and Prevention's (CDC) Advisory Committee on Immunization Practices (ACIP), the American Academy of Family Physicians (AAFP), the America College of Physicians (ACP), the American College of Obstetricians and Gynecologists (ACOG) and the American College of Nurse-Midwives (ACNM).

Figure 2. Vaccines that might be indicated for adults aged 19 years or older based on medical and other indications[1]

VACCINE ▼ / INDICATION ►	Pregnancy	Immuno-compromising conditions (excluding HIV infection)[4,6,7,8,13]	HIV infection CD4+ count (cells/µL)[4,6,7,8,13] < 200	HIV infection CD4+ count (cells/µL) ≥ 200	Men who have sex with men (MSM)	Kidney failure, end-stage renal disease, on hemodialysis	Heart disease, chronic lung disease, chronic alcoholism	Asplenia and persistent complement component deficiencies[8,11,12]	Chronic liver disease	Diabetes	Healthcare personnel
Influenza[*,2]	1 dose annually										
Tetanus, diphtheria, pertussis (Td/Tdap)[*,3]	1 dose Tdap each pregnancy	Substitute Tdap for Td once, then Td booster every 10 yrs									
Varicella[*,4]	Contraindicated			2 doses							
Human papillomavirus (HPV) Female[*,5]	3 doses through age 26 yrs			3 doses through age 26 yrs							
Human papillomavirus (HPV) Male[*,5]	3 doses through age 26 yrs			3 doses through age 21 yrs							
Zoster[6]	Contraindicated			1 dose							
Measles, mumps, rubella (MMR)[*,7]	Contraindicated			1 or 2 doses depending on indication							
Pneumococcal 13-valent conjugate (PCV13)[*,8]	1 dose										
Pneumococcal polysaccharide (PPSV23)[8]	1, 2, or 3 doses depending on indication										
Hepatitis A[*,9]	2 or 3 doses depending on vaccine										
Hepatitis B[*,10]	3 doses										
Meningococcal 4-valent conjugate (MenACWY) or polysaccharide (MPSV4)[*,11]	1 or more doses depending on indication										
Meningococcal B (MenB)[11]	2 or 3 doses depending on vaccine										
Haemophilus influenzae type b (Hib)[*,12]	3 doses post-HSCT recipients only	1 dose									

*Covered by the Vaccine Injury Compensation Program

■ Recommended for all persons who meet the age requirement, lack documentation of vaccination, or lack evidence of past infection; zoster vaccine is recommended regardless of past episode of zoster

■ Recommended for persons with a risk factor (medical, occupational, lifestyle, or other indication)

□ No recommendation

■ Contraindicated

These schedules indicate the recommended age groups and medical indications for which administration of currently licensed vaccines is commonly recommended for adults aged ≥19 years, as of February 2016. For all vaccines being recommended on the Adult Immunization Schedule: a vaccine series does not need to be restarted, regardless of the time that has elapsed between doses. Licensed combination vaccines may be used whenever any components of the combination are indicated and when the vaccine's other components are not contraindicated. For detailed recommendations on all vaccines, including those used primarily for travelers or that are issued during the year, consult the manufacturers' package inserts and the complete statements from the Advisory Committee on Immunization Practices (www.cdc.gov/vaccines/hcp/acip-recs/index.html). Use of trade names and commercial sources is for identification only and does not imply endorsement by the U.S. Department of Health and Human Services.

CDC U.S. Department of Health and Human Services
Centers for Disease Control and Prevention

FIGURE 37-1 Recommended Adult Immunization Schedule—United States—2016 *(Continues)*

Reproduced from U.S Department of Health and Human Services, Centers for Disease Control and Prevention. (2016). *Recommended adult immunization schedule—United States—2016.* Retrieved from http://www.cdc.gov/vaccines/schedules/downloads/adult/adult-combined-schedule.pdf

Footnotes—Recommended Immunization Schedule for Adults Aged 19 Years or Older: United States, 2016

1. Additional information
- Additional guidance for the use of the vaccines described in this supplement is available at www.cdc.gov/vaccines/hcp/acip-recs/index.html.
- Information on vaccination recommendations when vaccination status is unknown and other general immunization information can be found in the General Recommendations on Immunization at www.cdc.gov/mmwr/preview/mmwrhtml/rr6002a1.htm.
- Information on travel vaccine requirements and recommendations (e.g., for hepatitis A and B, meningococcal, and other vaccines) is available at wwwnc.cdc.gov/travel/destinations/list.
- Additional information and resources regarding vaccination of pregnant women can be found at www.cdc.gov/vaccines/adults/rec-vac/pregnant.html.

2. Influenza vaccination
- Annual vaccination against influenza is recommended for all persons aged ≥6 months. A list of currently available influenza vaccines can be found at http://www.cdc.gov/flu/protect/vaccine/vaccines.htm.
- Persons aged ≥6 months, including pregnant women, can receive the inactivated influenza vaccine (IIV). An age-appropriate IIV formulation should be used.
- Intradermal IIV is an option for persons aged 18 through 64 years.
- High-dose IIV is an option for persons aged ≥65 years.
- Live attenuated influenza vaccine (LAIV [FluMist]) is an option for healthy, non-pregnant persons aged 2 through 49 years.
- Recombinant influenza vaccine (RIV [Flublok]) is approved for persons aged ≥18 years.
- RIV, which does not contain any egg protein, may be administered to persons aged ≥18 years with egg allergy of any severity; IIV may be used with additional safety measures for persons with hives-only allergy to eggs.
- Health care personnel who care for severely immunocompromised persons who require care in a protected environment should receive IIV or RIV; health care personnel who receive LAIV should avoid providing care for severely immunosuppressed persons for 7 days after vaccination.

3. Tetanus, diphtheria, and acellular pertussis (Td/Tdap) vaccination
- Administer 1 dose of Tdap vaccine to pregnant women during each pregnancy (preferably during 27–36 weeks' gestation) regardless of interval since prior Td or Tdap vaccination.
- Persons aged ≥11 years who have not received Tdap vaccine or for whom vaccine status is unknown should receive a dose of Tdap followed by tetanus and diphtheria toxoids (Td) booster doses every 10 years thereafter. Tdap can be administered regardless of interval since the most recent tetanus or diphtheria-toxoid-containing vaccine.
- Adults with an unknown or incomplete history of completing a 3-dose primary vaccination series with Td-containing vaccines should begin or complete a primary vaccination series including a Tdap dose.
- For unvaccinated adults, administer the first 2 doses at least 4 weeks apart and the third dose 6–12 months after the second.
- For incompletely vaccinated (i.e., less than 3 doses) adults, administer remaining doses.
- Refer to the ACIP statement for recommendations for administering Td/Tdap as prophylaxis in wound management (see footnote 1).

4. Varicella vaccination
- All adults without evidence of immunity to varicella (as defined below) should receive 2 doses of single-antigen varicella vaccine or a second dose if they have received only 1 dose.
- Vaccination should be emphasized for those who have close contact with persons at high risk for severe disease (e.g., health care personnel and family contacts of persons with immunocompromising conditions) or are at high risk for exposure or transmission (e.g., teachers; child care employees; residents and staff members of institutional settings, including correctional institutions; college students; military personnel; adolescents and adults living in households with children; nonpregnant women of childbearing age; and international travelers).
- Pregnant women should be assessed for evidence of varicella immunity. Women who do not have evidence of immunity should receive the first dose of varicella vaccine upon completion or termination of pregnancy and before discharge from the health care facility. The second dose should be administered 4–8 weeks after the first dose.
- Evidence of immunity to varicella in adults includes any of the following:
  — documentation of 2 doses of varicella vaccine at least 4 weeks apart;
  — U.S.-born before 1980, except health care personnel and pregnant women;
  — history of varicella based on diagnosis or verification of varicella disease by a health care provider;
  — history of herpes zoster based on diagnosis or verification of herpes zoster disease by a health care provider; or
  — laboratory evidence of immunity or laboratory confirmation of disease.

5. Human papillomavirus (HPV) vaccination
- Three HPV vaccines are licensed for use in females (bivalent HPV vaccine [2vHPV], quadrivalent HPV vaccine [4vHPV], and 9-valent HPV vaccine [9vHPV]) and two HPV vaccines are licensed for use in males (4vHPV and 9vHPV).
- For females, 2vHPV, 4vHPV, or 9vHPV is recommended in a 3-dose series for routine vaccination at age 11 or 12 years and for those aged 13 through 26 years, if not previously vaccinated.
- For males, 4vHPV or 9vHPV is recommended in a 3-dose series for routine vaccination at age 11 or 12 years and for those aged 13 through 21 years, if not previously vaccinated. Males aged 22 through 26 years may be vaccinated.
- HPV vaccination is recommended for men who have sex with men through age 26 years who did not get any or all doses when they were younger.
- Vaccination is recommended for immunocompromised persons (including those with HIV infection) through age 26 years who did not get any or all doses when they were younger.
- A complete HPV vaccination series consists of 3 doses. The second dose should be administered 4–8 weeks (minimum interval of 4 weeks) after the first dose; the third dose should be administered 24 weeks after the first dose and 16 weeks after the second dose (minimum interval of 12 weeks).

- HPV vaccines are not recommended for use in pregnant women. However, pregnancy testing is not needed before vaccination. If a woman is found to be pregnant after initiating the vaccination series, no intervention is needed; the remainder of the 3-dose series should be delayed until completion or termination of pregnancy.

6. Zoster vaccination
- A single dose of zoster vaccine is recommended for adults aged ≥60 years regardless of whether they report a prior episode of herpes zoster. Although the vaccine is licensed by the U.S. Food and Drug Administration for use among and can be administered to persons aged ≥50 years, ACIP recommends that vaccination begin at age 60 years.
- Persons aged ≥60 years with chronic medical conditions may be vaccinated unless their condition constitutes a contraindication, such as pregnancy or severe immunodeficiency.

7. Measles, mumps, rubella (MMR) vaccination
- Adults born before 1957 are generally considered immune to measles and mumps. All adults born in 1957 or later should have documentation of 1 or more doses of MMR vaccine unless they have a medical contraindication to the vaccine or laboratory evidence of immunity to each of the three diseases. Documentation of provider-diagnosed disease is not considered acceptable evidence of immunity for measles, mumps, or rubella.

Measles component:
- A routine second dose of MMR vaccine, administered a minimum of 28 days after the first dose, is recommended for adults who:
  — are students in postsecondary educational institutions,
  — work in a health care facility, or
  — plan to travel internationally.
- Persons who received inactivated (killed) measles vaccine or measles vaccine of unknown type during 1963–1967 should be revaccinated with 2 doses of MMR vaccine.

Mumps component:
- A routine second dose of MMR vaccine, administered a minimum of 28 days after the first dose, is recommended for adults who:
  — are students in a postsecondary educational institution,
  — work in a health care facility, or
  — plan to travel internationally.
- Persons vaccinated before 1979 with either killed mumps vaccine or mumps vaccine of unknown type who are at high risk for mumps infection (e.g., persons who are working in a health care facility) should be considered for revaccination with 2 doses of MMR vaccine.

Rubella component:
- For women of childbearing age, regardless of birth year, rubella immunity should be determined. If there is no evidence of immunity, women who are not pregnant should be vaccinated. Pregnant women who do not have evidence of immunity should receive MMR vaccine upon completion or termination of pregnancy and before discharge from the health care facility.

Health care personnel born before 1957:
- For unvaccinated health care personnel born before 1957 who lack laboratory evidence of measles, mumps, and/or rubella immunity or laboratory confirmation of disease, health care facilities should consider vaccinating personnel with 2 doses of MMR vaccine at the appropriate interval for measles and mumps or 1 dose of MMR vaccine for rubella.

8. Pneumococcal vaccination
- General information
  — Adults are recommended to receive 1 dose of 13-valent pneumococcal conjugate vaccine (PCV13) and 1, 2, or 3 doses (depending on indication) of 23-valent pneumococcal polysaccharide vaccine (PPSV23).
  — PCV13 should be administered at least 1 year after PPSV23.
  — PPSV23 should be administered at least 1 year after PCV13, except among adults with immunocompromising conditions, anatomical or functional asplenia, cerebrospinal fluid leak, or cochlear implant, for whom the interval should be at least 8 weeks; the interval between PPSV23 doses should be at least 5 years.
  — No additional dose of PPSV23 is indicated for adults vaccinated with PPSV23 at age ≥65 years.
  — When both PCV13 and PPSV23 are indicated, PCV13 should be administered first; PCV13 and PPSV23 should not be administered during the same visit.
  — When indicated, PCV13 and PPSV23 should be administered to adults whose pneumococcal vaccination history is incomplete or unknown.
- Adults aged ≥65 years (immunocompetent) who:
  — have not received PCV13 or PPSV23: administer PCV13 followed by PPSV23 at least 1 year after PCV13.
  — have not received PCV13 but have received a dose of PPSV23 at age ≥65 years: administer PCV13 at least 1 year after PPSV23.
  — have not received PCV13 but have received 1 or more doses of PPSV23 at age <65 years: administer PCV13 at least 1 year after the most recent dose of PPSV23. Administer a dose of PPSV23 at least 1 year after PCV13 and at least 5 years after the most recent dose of PPSV23.
  — have received PCV13 but not PPSV23 at age <65 years: administer PPSV23 at least 1 year after PCV13.
  — have received PCV13 and 1 or more doses of PPSV23 at age <65 years: administer PPSV23 at least 1 year after PCV13 and at least 5 years after the most recent dose of PPSV23.
- Adults aged ≥19 years with immunocompromising conditions or anatomical or functional asplenia (defined below) who:
  — have not received PCV13 or PPSV23: administer PCV13 followed by PPSV23 at least 8 weeks after PCV13. Administer a second dose of PPSV23 at least 5 years after the first dose of PPSV23.
  — have not received PCV13 but have received 1 dose of PPSV23: administer PCV13 at least 1 year after the PPSV23. Administer a second dose of PPSV23 at least 8 weeks after PCV13 and at least 5 years after the first dose of PPSV23.

FIGURE 37-1 Recommended Adult Immunization Schedule—United States—2016 *(Continued)*

Reproduced from U.S Department of Health and Human Services, Centers for Disease Control and Prevention. (2016). *Recommended adult immunization schedule—United States—2016.* Retrieved from http://www.cdc.gov/vaccines/schedules/downloads/adult/adult-combined-schedule.pdf

Footnotes—Recommended Immunization Schedule for Adults Aged 19 Years or Older: United States, 2016

— have not received PCV13 but have received 2 doses of PPSV23: administer PCV13 at least 1 year after the most recent dose of PPSV23.

— have received PCV13 but not PPSV23: administer PPSV23 at least 8 weeks after PCV13. Administer a second dose of PPSV23 at least 5 years after the first dose of PPSV23.

— have received PCV13 and 1 dose of PPSV23: administer a second dose of PPSV23 at least 8 weeks after PCV13 and at least 5 years after the first dose of PPSV23.

— If the most recent dose of PPSV23 was administered at age <65 years, at age ≥65 years, administer a dose of PPSV23 at least 8 weeks after PCV13 and at least 5 years after the last dose of PPSV23.

— Immunocompromising conditions that are indications for pneumococcal vaccination are: congenital or acquired immunodeficiency (including B- or T-lymphocyte deficiency, complement deficiencies, and phagocytic disorders excluding chronic granulomatous disease), HIV infection, chronic renal failure, nephrotic syndrome, leukemia, lymphoma, Hodgkin disease, generalized malignancy, multiple myeloma, solid organ transplant, and iatrogenic immunosuppression (including long-term systemic corticosteroids and radiation therapy).

— Anatomical or functional asplenia that are indications for pneumococcal vaccination are: sickle cell disease and other hemoglobinopathies, congenital or acquired asplenia, splenic dysfunction, and splenectomy. Administer pneumococcal vaccines at least 2 weeks before immunosuppressive therapy or an elective splenectomy, and as soon as possible to adults who are newly diagnosed with asymptomatic or symptomatic HIV infection.

• Adults aged ≥19 years with cerebrospinal fluid leaks or cochlear implants: administer PCV13 followed by PPSV23 at least 8 weeks after PCV13; no additional dose of PPSV23 is indicated if aged <65 years. If PPSV23 was administered at age <65 years, at age ≥65 years, administer another dose of PPSV23 at least 5 years after the last dose of PPSV23.

• Adults aged 19 through 64 years with chronic heart disease (including congestive heart failure and cardiomyopathies, excluding hypertension), chronic lung disease (including chronic obstructive lung disease, emphysema, and asthma), chronic liver disease (including cirrhosis), alcoholism, or diabetes mellitus, or who smoke cigarettes: administer PPSV23. At age ≥65 years, administer PCV13 at least 1 year after PPSV23, followed by another dose of PPSV23 at least 1 year after PCV13 and at least 5 years after the last dose of PPSV23.

• Routine pneumococcal vaccination is not recommended for American Indian/Alaska Native or other adults unless they have an indication as above; however, public health authorities may consider recommending the use of pneumococcal vaccines for American Indians/Alaska Natives or other adults who live in areas with increased risk for invasive pneumococcal disease.

9. Hepatitis A vaccination

• Vaccinate any person seeking protection from hepatitis A virus (HAV) infection and persons with any of the following indications:

— men who have sex with men;

— persons who use injection or noninjection illicit drugs;

— persons working with HAV-infected primates or with HAV in a research laboratory setting;

— persons with chronic liver disease and persons who receive clotting factor concentrates;

— persons traveling to or working in countries that have high or intermediate endemicity of hepatitis A (see footnote 1); and

— unvaccinated persons who anticipate close personal contact (e.g., household or regular babysitting) with an international adoptee during the first 60 days after arrival in the United States from a country with high or intermediate endemicity of hepatitis A (see footnote 1). The first dose of the 2-dose hepatitis A vaccine series should be administered as soon as adoption is planned, ideally 2 or more weeks before the arrival of the adoptee.

• Single-antigen vaccine formulations should be administered in a 2-dose schedule at either 0 and 6–12 months (Havrix), or 0 and 6–18 months (Vaqta). If the combined hepatitis A and hepatitis B vaccine (Twinrix) is used, administer 3 doses at 0, 1, and 6 months; alternatively, a 4-dose schedule may be used, administered on days 0, 7, and 21–30 followed by a booster dose at 12 months.

10. Hepatitis B vaccination

• Vaccinate any person seeking protection from hepatitis B virus (HBV) infection and persons with any of the following indications:

— sexually active persons who are not in a long-term, mutually monogamous relationship (e.g., persons with more than 1 sex partner during the previous 6 months); persons seeking evaluation or treatment for a sexually transmitted disease (STD); current or recent injection drug users; and men who have sex with men;

— health care personnel and public safety workers who are potentially exposed to blood or other infectious body fluids;

— persons who are aged <60 years with diabetes as soon as feasible after diagnosis; persons with diabetes who are aged ≥60 years at the discretion of the treating clinician based on the likelihood of acquiring HBV infection, including the risk posed by an increased need for assisted blood glucose monitoring in long-term care facilities, the likelihood of experiencing chronic sequelae if infected with HBV, and the likelihood of immune response to vaccination;

— persons with end-stage renal disease (including patients receiving hemodialysis), persons with HIV infection, and persons with chronic liver disease;

— household contacts and sex partners of hepatitis B surface antigen–positive persons, clients and staff members of institutions for persons with developmental disabilities, and international travelers to regions with high or intermediate levels of endemic HBV infection (see footnote 1); and

— all adults in the following settings: STD treatment facilities, HIV testing and treatment facilities, facilities providing drug abuse treatment and prevention services, health care settings targeting services to injection drug users or men who have sex with men, correctional facilities, end-stage renal disease programs and facilities for chronic hemodialysis patients, and institutions and nonresidential day care facilities for persons with developmental disabilities.

• Administer missing doses to complete a 3-dose series of hepatitis B vaccine to those persons not vaccinated or not completely vaccinated. The second dose should be administered at least 1 month after the first dose; the third dose should be administered at least 2 months after the second dose (and at least 4 months after the first dose). If the combined hepatitis A and hepatitis B vaccine (Twinrix) is used, give 3 doses at 0, 1, and 6 months; alternatively, a 4-dose Twinrix schedule may be used, administered on days 0, 7, and 21–30, followed by a booster dose at 12 months.

• Adult patients receiving hemodialysis or with other immunocompromising conditions should receive 1 dose of 40 mcg/mL (Recombivax HB) administered on a 3-dose schedule at 0, 1, and 6 months or 2 doses of 20 mcg/mL (Engerix-B) administered simultaneously on a 4-dose schedule at 0, 1, 2, and 6 months.

11. Meningococcal vaccination

• General information

— Serogroup A, C, W, and Y meningococcal vaccine is available as a conjugate (MenACWY [Menactra, Menveo]) or a polysaccharide (MPSV4 [Menomune]) vaccine.

— Serogroup B meningococcal (MenB) vaccine is available as a 2-dose series of MenB-4C vaccine (Bexsero) administered at least 1 month apart or a 3-dose series of MenB-FHbp (Trumenba) vaccine administered at 0, 2, and 6 months; the two MenB vaccines are not interchangeable, i.e., the same MenB vaccine product must be used for all doses.

— MenACWY vaccine is preferred for adults with serogroup A, C, W, and Y meningococcal vaccine indications who are aged ≤55 years, and for adults aged ≥56 years: 1) who were vaccinated previously with MenACWY vaccine and are recommended for revaccination or 2) for whom multiple doses of vaccine are anticipated; MPSV4 vaccine is preferred for adults aged ≥56 years who have not received MenACWY vaccine previously and who require a single dose only (e.g., persons at risk because of an outbreak).

— Revaccination with MenACWY vaccine every 5 years is recommended for adults previously vaccinated with MenACWY or MPSV4 vaccine who remain at increased risk for infection (e.g., adults with anatomical or functional asplenia or persistent complement component deficiencies, or microbiologists who are routinely exposed to isolates of *Neisseria meningitidis*).

— MenB vaccine is approved for use in persons aged 10 through 25 years; however, because there is no theoretical difference in safety for persons aged >25 years compared to those aged 10 through 25 years, MenB vaccine is recommended for routine use in persons aged ≥10 years who are at increased risk for serogroup B meningococcal disease.

— There is no recommendation for MenB revaccination at this time.

— MenB vaccine may be administered concomitantly with MenACWY vaccine but at a different anatomic site, if feasible.

— HIV infection is not an indication for routine vaccination with MenACWY or MenB vaccine; if an HIV-infected person of any age is to be vaccinated, administer 2 doses of MenACWY vaccine at least 2 months apart.

• Adults with anatomical or functional asplenia or persistent complement component deficiencies: administer 2 doses of MenACWY vaccine at least 2 months apart and revaccinate every 5 years. Also administer a series of MenB vaccine.

• Microbiologists who are routinely exposed to isolates of *Neisseria meningitidis*: administer a single dose of MenACWY vaccine; revaccinate with MenACWY vaccine every 5 years if remain at increased risk for infection. Also administer a series of MenB vaccine.

• Persons at risk because of a meningococcal disease outbreak: if the outbreak is attributable to serogroup A, C, W, or Y, administer a single dose of MenACWY vaccine; if the outbreak is attributable to serogroup B, administer a series of MenB vaccine.

• Persons who travel to or live in countries in which meningococcal disease is hyperendemic or epidemic: administer a single dose of MenACWY vaccine and revaccinate with MenACWY vaccine every 5 years if the increased risk for infection remains (see footnote 1); MenB vaccine is not recommended because meningococcal disease in these countries is generally not caused by serogroup B.

• Military recruits: administer a single dose of MenACWY vaccine.

• First-year college students aged ≤21 years who live in residence halls: administer a single dose of MenACWY vaccine if they have not received a dose on or after their 16th birthday.

• Young adults aged 16 through 23 years (preferred age range is 16 through 18 years): may be vaccinated with a series of MenB vaccine to provide short-term protection against most strains of serogroup B meningococcal disease.

12. *Haemophilus influenzae* type b (Hib) vaccination

• One dose of Hib vaccine should be administered to persons who have anatomical or functional asplenia or sickle cell disease or are undergoing elective splenectomy if they have not previously received Hib vaccine. Hib vaccination 14 or more days before splenectomy is suggested.

• Recipients of a hematopoietic stem cell transplant (HSCT) should be vaccinated with a 3-dose regimen 6–12 months after a successful transplant, regardless of vaccination history; at least 4 weeks should separate doses.

• Hib vaccine is not recommended for adults with HIV infection since their risk for Hib infection is low.

13. Immunocompromising conditions

• Inactivated vaccines (e.g., pneumococcal, meningococcal, and inactivated influenza vaccines) generally are acceptable and live vaccines generally should be avoided in persons with immune deficiencies or immunocompromising conditions. Information on specific conditions is available at www.cdc.gov/vaccines/hcp/acip-recs/index.html.

FIGURE 37-1 Recommended Adult Immunization Schedule—United States—2016 *(Continued)*

Reproduced from U.S Department of Health and Human Services, Centers for Disease Control and Prevention. (2016). *Recommended adult immunization schedule—United States—2016.* Retrieved from http://www.cdc.gov/vaccines/schedules/downloads/adult/adult-combined-schedule.pdf

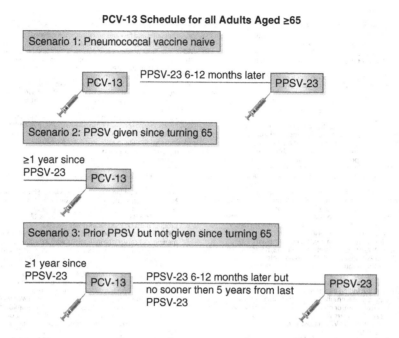

PCV-13 Schedule for all Adults Aged ≥65

Scenario 1: Pneumococcal vaccine naive

PCV-13 — PPSV-23 6-12 months later → PPSV-23

Scenario 2: PPSV given since turning 65

≥1 year since PPSV-23 — PCV-13

Scenario 3: Prior PPSV but not given since turning 65

≥1 year since PPSV-23 — PCV-13 — PPSV-23 6-12 months later but no sooner then 5 years from last PPSV-23 → PPSV-23

FIGURE 37-2 Pneumococcal Vaccine Scheduling

Reproduced from Black, C.L., Yue, X., Ball, S.W. et al (2014). Influenza vaccination coverage among healthcare personnel – United States, 2013–14 influenza season. *Morbidity and Mortality Weekly Report, 63*(37), 805–828. Retrieved from http://www.cdc.gov/mmwr/preview/mmwrhtml/mm6337a4.htm.

benefits. Conversely, not screening an individual based on their age who would be expected to live long enough to benefit from the intervention would deny them the potential benefit of screening (Lee, Leipzig, & Walter, 2013). The difficulty for the clinician arises when the time-to-benefit and the estimated life expectancy are similar and it is not clear whether potential harms or potential benefits are greater. In these cases, what can guide the clinician is the individual's values and preferences regarding healthcare interventions (Walter & Covinsky, 2001; Yourman, Lee, Schonberg, Widera, & Smith, 2012). The following section provides the clinician with a framework for making clinical decisions about offering screening to older adults.

Decision making about individualized screening requires three elements: (1) estimating the patient's life expectancy, (2) estimating the time-to-benefit of the proposed intervention or screening procedure, and (3) evaluating the patient's preferences around the potential harms and benefits of the intervention (Lee, Leipzig, & Walter, 2013).

A core principle in geriatrics is that incorporating a person's comorbidities and functional status with their age can provide a more accurate picture of life expectancy than age alone (Walter & Covinsky, 2001; Yourman et al., 2012). Those with fewer comorbidities and higher functional ability can be expected to live longer than the average, whereas those with more comorbidities and lower functional ability will have a shorter-than-average life expectancy.

Prognosis indices have been developed based on single dominant terminal conditions, such as dementia, cancer, heart failure, or coronary artery disease (Levy et al., 2006; Mitchell et al., 2010; Xie, Brayne, & Matthews, 2008). Other indices have been developed to address prognosis among older adults who do not have a dominant terminal illness. A systematic review of the literature for this population has led to the development of a web and mobile device calculator called ePrognosis (ePrognosis.ucsf.edu), which can help to estimate life expectancy (Yourman et al., 2012). Along with age, this calculator incorporates such factors as location of the patient (community, skilled nursing facility, hospital), functional ability, and comorbidities to pair the clinical question with the appropriate index. As with other clinical decisions, one must assess whether the population studied is like the patient one is addressing.

When considering screening, the provider should evaluate how long it would take the patient to benefit from the screening. Time-to-benefit, or "lag time to benefit," estimation seeks to answer the question, "When will it help?" Unfortunately, these data are rarely reported directly in clinical trials. Some current research is attempting to fill this gap. A 2013 meta-analysis found that the lag time to benefit for breast and colorectal cancer screening is 10 years (Lee, Boscardin, et al., 2013). Treatment for osteoporosis can be clinically significant at 1 year (Black et al., 2000; Pham, Datta, Weber, Walter, & Colón-Emeric, 2011) and statin use for primary prevention of myocardial infarction (MI) is significant at

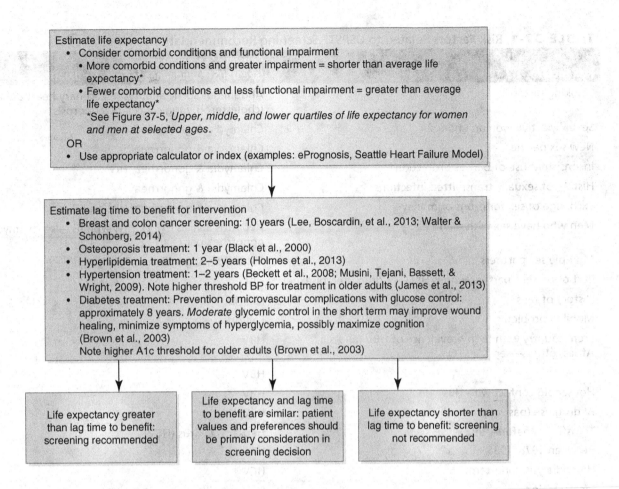

FIGURE 37-3 Individualizing Screening Decision Making for Older Adults

Data from Lee, S. J., Leipzig, R. M., & Walter, L. C. (2013). Incorporating lag time to benefit into prevention decisions for older adults. *JAMA, 310*(24), 2609–2610. doi:10.1001/jama.2013.282612

2–5 years (Holmes et al., 2013). In older adults with diabetes, microvascular complications of diabetes are reduced only after 8 years of glycemic control, whereas treatment of hypertension and dyslipidemia shows benefits in 2–3 years (Brown, Mangione, Saliba, & Sarkisian, 2003). These timelines should be considered when deciding whether or not to screen a patient for one of these conditions.

In addition to the potential benefits of screening interventions, it is necessary to evaluate how a particular intervention fits with an individual's values, preferences, and goals of treatment. Harms to be considered include overdiagnosis (the identification and subsequent treatment of disease that would not have become clinically significant during the patient's lifetime), false positives leading to additional diagnostic procedures with potential complications, and physical and psychologic discomfort from screening. Discussions of screening should include information on treatments that would be expected to follow a positive screening result. General treatment goals for a particular patient may include longevity, preserving function, comfort, or some combination of the three. Clarifying how a particular screening intervention fits within the patient's goals can help facilitate decision making.

III. Database

A. Subjective

1. Symptoms that would trigger diagnosis/management rather than screening

2. Risk factors for diseases (see **Table 37-1**) that can be appropriately screened for:
    a. Behavioral characteristics
    b. Past medical history
    c. Family history

TABLE 37-1 Risk Factors Related to USPSTF Screening Recommendations

Risk Factor	Consider Screening for: (see USPSTF guidelines for greater detail)
Smoking history	Abdominal aortic aneurysm, coronary heart disease (cholesterol), lung cancer, osteoporosis
Sexually active woman under 24	Chlamydia & gonorrhea
New sex partner	Chlamydia & gonorrhea
Inconsistent use of barrier protection	Chlamydia & gonorrhea, HIV
History of sexually transmitted infections	Chlamydia & gonorrhea
Exchange of sex for drugs or money	Chlamydia & gonorrhea, HIV, syphilis
Men who have sex with men	Hepatitis B virus (HBV), HIV, syphilis (also chlamydia & gonorrhea per CDC)
Multiple sex partners	Chlamydia & gonorrhea, HIV
Past or present partner who is HIV+, IV drug user, bisexual	HIV
History of falls	Fall risk
Mobility problems	Fall risk
From country with high prevalence of HBV (all Asia, Africa, others—see USPSTF)	HBV
HIV+	HBV
Household contact with HBV	HBV
IV drug use (past or present)	HBV, HIV
Transfusion before 1992	Hepatitis C virus (HCV)
between 1978–1985	HIV
Hemodialysis, long-term	HCV
Incarceration	HCV, syphilis
Intranasal drug use	HCV
Unregulated tattoos	HCV
Born to HCV+ mother	HCV
Born between 1945 and 1965	HCV
Diabetes	Coronary heart disease (CHD) (cholesterol)
History of CHD or noncoronary atherosclerosis	CHD (cholesterol)
Family history of CHD in men ≤ 50 and women ≤ 60	CHD (cholesterol)
Hypertension	CHD (cholesterol)
Body mass index ≥ 30	CHD (cholesterol)
History of fracture	Osteoporosis
Parent with history of hip fracture	Osteoporosis
History of glucocorticoid use for > 3 months	Osteoporosis
History of rheumatoid arthritis	Osteoporosis
Alcohol ≥ 3 units per day	Osteoporosis
Family history of breast, ovarian, tubal, peritoneal cancer	Breast cancer (BRCA)
Over 65 years and limited prior cervical cancer screening	Cervical cancer

Data from U.S. Department of Health and Human Services. (2014). *The guide to clinical preventive services.* Retrieved from http://www.ahrq.gov /clinic/pocketgd1011/gcp10s1.htm; U.S. Preventive Services Task Force (2014). *About the USPSTF.* Retrieved from www.uspreventiveservicestaskforce .org/Page/Name/about-the-uspstf.

3. Functional status (as a contributor to life expectancy and ability to undergo screening/treatment)

4. Behavioral factors affecting ability to make healthy lifestyle changes

5. Patient values/preferences related to illness prevention and health care

B. Objective

1. Demographics (age, gender)

2. Initial screening physical exam assessments to consider:

   a. Blood pressure (USPSTF, 2014)

   b. Body mass index (USPSTF, 2014)

   c. Clinical breast exam for women over 40 (Barton, Harris, & Fletcher, 1999)

   d. Timed-Up-and-Go or other balance/mobility exam for older adults (see **Figure 37-4**) (USPSTF, 2014)

IV. Assessment

A. Establish what currently undiagnosed conditions patient is at risk for based on subjective and objective characteristics.

B. Consider patient's values, preferences, and stage of development related to recommended measures, particularly if life expectancy and lag time to benefit are similar.

C. Evaluate patient's ability and desire to engage in recommended measures to prevent illness (see **Box 37-1**).

V. Goals of clinical management

A. Primary prevention—prevent injury and disease by minimizing risk factors.

1. Counseling (e.g., behavioral counseling for those at risk for sexually transmitted infections)

2. Immunizations (e.g., influenza, pneumococcal, human papilloma virus)

3. Chemoprophylaxis (e.g., aspirin for prevention of myocardial infarction and stroke)

4. Screening for modifiable risk factors for disease (e.g., screening for hypertension, obesity, and hyperlipidemia as risk factors for cardiovascular disease)

B. Secondary prevention—identify asymptomatic disease when treatment can stop it from progressing. Be sure to weigh risks and benefits of secondary prevention screening and anticipate management of positive screens before initiating screening.

1. Screening for cancer (e.g., mammogram for breast cancer, Pap smear for cervical cancer)

2. Screening for other conditions (e.g., depression, abdominal aortic aneurism, sexually transmitted infections)

C. Tertiary prevention—interventions to minimize complications of disease once it is diagnosed. (Not addressed in this chapter—see chapters dedicated to particular conditions for prevention of disease-specific complications).

VI. Plan

A. Select and order appropriate screening, immunizations, chemoprophylaxis, and counseling based on risk.

1. Use evidence-based recommendations from USPSTF, CDC, or other appropriate source (see Figure 37-1, **Table 37-2** and **37-3**).

2. Consider life expectancy and lag time to benefit of intervention (see **Figures** 37-3 and **37-5**).

B. Consider and order health maintenance interventions related to previously diagnosed conditions (see Table 37-1) following evidence-based guidelines (USPSTF, 2014).

C. Provide education and counseling as appropriate (see Box 37-1).

VII. Self-management tools and resources for health professionals

See USPSTF "Clinical Considerations" section for each recommendation for suggested tools and resources. See also **Table 37-4**.

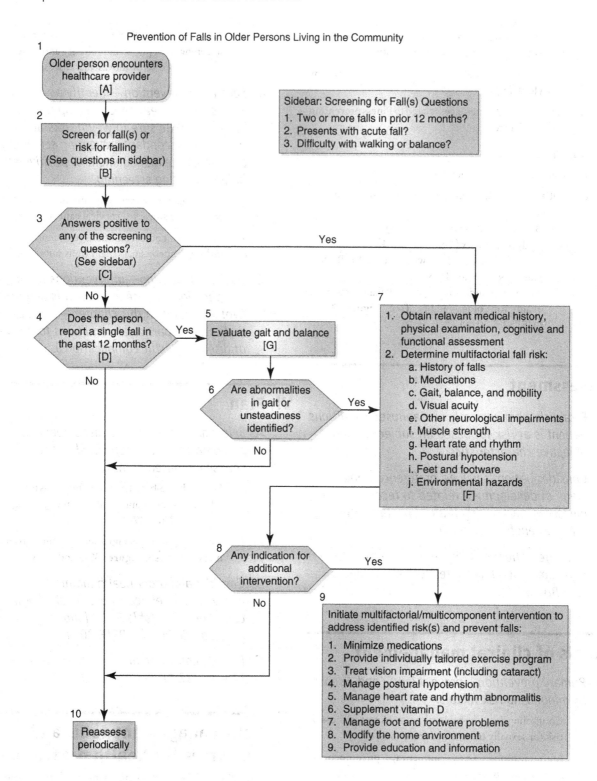

FIGURE 37-4 Fall Prevention

FIGURE 37-4 Fall Prevention. *(Continued)*

Annotation A: *Older Adult Encounters with Healthcare Provider.* This guideline algorithm is to be used in the clinical setting for assessment and intervention to reduce falls in community-residing older persons (≥65). The guideline algorithm is not intended to address fall injuries per se or falls that occur in the hospital.

Annotation B: *Screen for Falls or Risk for Falling.* The screening for falls and risk for falling is aimed at preventing or reducing fall risk. Any positive answer to the screening questions puts the person screened in a high-risk group that warrants further evaluation. All older adults who are under the care of a health professional (or their caregivers) should be asked at least once a year about falls, frequency of falling, and difficulties in gait or balance.

Annotation C: *Screen Positive for Falls or Risk for Falling.* Persons at higher risk of falling, identified by screening, should be assessed for known risk factors. A multifactorial fall risk assessment should be performed for community-dwelling older persons who report recurrent (≥2) falls, report difficulties with gait or balance, or seek medical attention or present to the emergency department because of a fall.

Annotation D: *Report of a Single Fall in the Past 12 Months.* A (first) single fall may indicate difficulties or unsteadiness in walking or standing. In older individuals, a fall may be a sign of problems in gait or balance that was not present in the past.

Annotation E: *Evaluation of Gait and Balance.* Gait and balance deficits should be evaluated in older individuals reporting a single fall as a screen for identifying individuals who may benefit from a multifactorial fall risk assessment. For persons who screen positive for falls or fall risk, evaluation of balance and gait should be part of the multifactorial fall risk assessment. Frequently used tests of gait or balance include the Get Up and Go Test;[9] Timed Up and Go Test,[10] the Berg Balance Scale,[11] and the Performance-Oriented Mobility Assessment.[5,12]

Annotation F: *Determination of Multifactorial Fall Risk.* A multifactorial fall risk assessment can reveal the factors that put an older adult at risk of falling and can help identify the most appropriate interventions. A multifactorial fall risk assessment followed by intervention to modify any identified risks is a highly effective strategy to reduce falls and the risk of falling in older persons.

Reproduced from Panel on Prevention of Falls in Older Persons, American Geriatrics Society and British Geriatrics Society. (2011). Summary of the updated American Geriatrics Society/British Geriatrics Society clinical practice guideline for prevention of falls in older persons. *Journal of the American Geriatrics Society, 59*(1), 148–157. doi:10.1111/j.1532-5415.2010.03234.x

---

BOX 37-1 Assessing a Patient's Readiness for Behavior Change

Counseling interventions regarding patient lifestyle and healthy behaviors begin with an assessment of the patient's recognition of unhealthy behavior and an assessment of the patient's readiness to make health-directed changes. Readiness to change is one of many frameworks designed to help the primary care provider choose an interviewing approach that will be most meaningful to the patient. The Transtheoretical Model defines behavior change as a process that occurs in stages. These stages, often referred to as "stages of change," help the clinician understand why certain patients are more or less successful at changing behavior and which motivational interviewing strategies may help the patient move closer to changing unhealthy behaviors (Walley & Roll, 2007).

Stage of Change	Definition	Patient Approach
Precontemplation	The patient has not recognized the behavior as unhealthy or the patient is not ready to change the behavior	• Inform and educate the patient about the unhealthy behavior and health consequences

BOX 37-1 *Assessing a Patient's Readiness for Behavior Change* (Continued)

Stage of Change	Definition	Patient Approach
Contemplation	The patient understands his or her behavior is unhealthy but is ambivalent about making a change	• Elicit reasons for ambivalence • Weigh the pros and cons and address the patient's concerns • Individualized feedback on negative effects of the unhealthy behavior
Preparation	The patient makes a decision to change	• Commend the decision to change the behavior
Action	The patient is active in some change of the behavior	• Support the changes made and provide encouragement to sustain the changes
Maintenance	The patient has made behavior change and is stable	• Recognize the patient's commitment and continued struggle to maintain the healthy behavior • Anticipate difficulties that may challenge maintenance • Address relapse

Data from Prochaska, J. O., Norcross, J. C., & Diclemente, C. C. (1994). *Changing for good.* New York, NY: Avon Books; Walley, A. Y., & Roll, F. J. (2007). Principles of caring for alcohol and drug users. In T. E. King & M. B. Wheeler (Eds.). *Medical management of vulnerable and underserved patients: Principles, practice and populations* (pp. 341–350). New York, NY: McGraw-Hill.

TABLE 37-2 Chemoprophylaxis Recommended by USPSTF for Prevention

Chemoprophylaxis	Population	Comments
Aspirin	Men 45–79 whose risk of MI is greater than risk of gastrointestinal (GI) bleed with aspirin. Women 55–79 whose risk of ischemic stroke is greater than risk of GI bleed with aspirin.	This 2009 recommendation is in the process of being updated as of June 30, 2015. See USPSTF for details on comparing risks. USPSTF-recommended stroke risk calculator is not functional. Consider Framingham calculator. https://www.framinghamheartstudy.org/risk-functions/stroke/stroke.php
Folic acid	All women planning or capable of pregnancy should take a daily supplement containing 0.4 to 0.8 mg to prevent neural tube defects.	This 2009 recommendation is in the process of being updated as of June 30, 2015.
Breast cancer risk-reducing medications (tamoxifen, raloxifene)	Women at increased risk of breast cancer	Shared, informed decision making with consideration of risk for adverse effects of medication.
Vitamin D	Community-dwelling adults 65 years and older who are at increased risk for falls.	The American Geriatrics Society (2011) recommends 800 IU daily.

Data from U.S. Department of Health and Human Services. (2014). *The guide to clinical preventive services.* Retrieved from http://www.ahrq.gov/clinic/pocketgd1011/gcp10s1.htm; and U.S. Preventive Services Task Force (2014). *About the USPSTF.* Retrieved from www.uspreventiveservicestaskforce.org/Page/Name/about-the-uspstf; AGS. (2011). Summary of the Updated American Geriatrics Society/British Geriatrics Society clinical practice guideline for prevention of falls in older persons. *Journal of the American Geriatrics Society, 59*(1), 148–57. doi:10.1111/j.1532-5415.2010.03234.x.

TABLE 37-3 USPSTF Screening and Counseling Recommendations

Screening Recommendation	Whom to Screen	Screening Test and Frequency	Additional Considerations and Counseling Recommendations
Abdominal aortic aneurysm	Men aged 65–75 who have ever smoked	Ultrasonography One-time screening	Smoking history of at least 100 cigarettes in lifetime
Alcohol misuse	All adults	Many screening tools available (i.e., AUDIT, CAGE). Resources can be found at the USPSTF website and the National Institutes of Health Institute for Alcohol Abuse and Alcoholism website: www.niaaa.nih.gov/. The best interval for screening is unknown.	Provide counseling for those with risky or hazardous drinking. See USPSTF website for resources. Risky/hazardous drinking: > 7 drinks/wk or > 3 drinks per occasion for women and > 14 drinks/wk or > 4 drinks per occasion for men
BRCA risk assessment and genetic counseling/ testing	Women ≥ 18 years of age with ≥ 1 family member with breast, ovarian, or other types of BRCA-related cancer	A number of risk assessment tools are available to help establish which women should be referred for genetic counseling (e.g., B-RST available at www.breastcancergenescreen.org). Consider periodic (every 5–10 years) review of family history to identify increased risk.	Genetic counseling or BRCA mutation testing when access to health professionals trained to provide genetic counseling is available.
Breast cancer	Women aged 50–74	Mammography Every 2 years	There is insufficient evidence to recommend for or against yearly clinical breast examination. Teaching breast self-examination is not recommended. Individualize screening decision for women > 74 and for those ≤ 74 with significant functional impairments and/ or comorbidities (Lee, Leipzig, & Walter, 2013; Siu, 2016; Walter & Covinsky, 2001; Walter & Schonberg, 2014).
Breast cancer risk	Women ≥ 35 years without a prior diagnosis of breast cancer, ductal carcinoma in situ (DCIS), or lobular carcinoma in situ (LCIS)	If a family history of breast cancer or a personal history of breast biopsy, atypical hyperplasia or other nonmalignant high-risk breast lesions, or extremely dense breast tissue, consider further assessment with a breast cancer risk assessment tool such as the National Cancer Institute Breast Cancer Risk Assessment Tool (www.cancer.gov /bcrisktool/)	If increased risk, provider should engage in shared, informed decision making regarding risk-reducing medication such as tamoxifen or raloxifene. See USPSTF website for resources.
Cervical cancer	Women aged 21–65	In women aged 21–65, screen with Pap smear every 3 years. For women 30–65 who desire longer intervals between screening, screen with a combination of Pap and human papillomavirus (HPV) test every 5 years.	May discuss discontinuing screening in females > 65 if adequate recent screening was normal (i.e., 3 consecutive negative cytology results or 2 consecutive negative HPV results within 10 years before cessation of screening, with the most recent test occurring within 5 years) (Saslow et al., 2012).

(continues)

TABLE 37-3 USPSTF Screening and Counseling Recommendations *(Continued)*

Screening Recommendation	Whom to Screen	Screening Test and Frequency	Additional Considerations and Counseling Recommendations
Chlamydia and gonorrhea infection	Women ≤ 24 years of age who are sexually active and older women at increased risk CDC recommends screening for men who have sex with men (MSM) (Workowski & Berman, 2010)	Nucleic acid amplification test (NAAT) (urine or vaginal or cervical swab for both) (CDC, 2014). For details on testing sites for MSM, see CDC info: www.cdc.gov/std/treatment/2010/specialpops.htm, heading "MSM" (Workowski & Berman, 2010). Base screening frequency on individual risk.	Risk factors include new or multiple sex partners, inconsistent condom use, history of sexually transmitted infections, exchange of sex for drugs or money. There is insufficient evidence to recommend routine screening for men. For MSM, see CDC info: www.cdc.gov/std/treatment/2010/specialpops.htm, heading "MSM" (Workowski & Berman, 2010).
Colorectal cancer*	Men and women 50–75 years of age	Annual high-sensitivity fecal occult blood testing (FOBT) [guaiac-based FOBT or fecal immunochemistry test (FIT)] or sigmoidoscopy every 5 years combined with high-sensitivity FOBT every 3 years or colonoscopy every 10 years.	Individualize screening decision for those > 75 years of age and for those < 75 years of age with significant functional impairments and/or comorbidities (Lee, Leipzig, & Walter, 2013; Walter & Covinsky, 2001).
Depression*	All adults if appropriate diagnosis, treatment, and follow-up can be offered	Many screening tools available [e.g., Patient Health Questionnaire (PHQ)]. See USPSTF website for resources. The best interval for screening is unknown.	Screening by asking two questions may be as effective as formal screening tools: "Over the past 2 weeks, have you felt down, depressed, or hopeless?" "Over the past 2 weeks, have you felt little interest or pleasure in doing things?"
Diabetes, type 2*	All adults with sustained blood pressure > 135/80 (whether treated or untreated)	Fasting plasma glucose, hemoglobin A1c, or 2-hour postload plasma glucose. The best interval for screening is unknown.	Fasting plasma glucose has more reproducible results and is easier and faster to perform than other tests. The threshold for treating older adults for diabetes should be individualized. Reasonable A1c targets: 7.0–7.5% in healthy older adults with long life expectancy, 7.5–8.0% in those with moderate comorbidity and a life expectancy < 10 years, and 8.0–9.0% in those with multiple morbidities and shorter life expectancy (Kirkman et al., 2012).
Fall risk	Community-dwelling adults ≥ 65 years of age	A prior fall and/or mobility problems in addition to a Timed Up-and-Go test. The best interval for screening is unknown. Consider annual screening in individuals at increased risk of falls.	Risk factors include: age ≥ 65, history of falls, mobility problems, poor performance on the Timed Up-and-Go test. If at increased risk, refer to exercise and/or PT and supplement with vitamin D 800IU daily (American Geriatrics Society, 2011). See Figure 37-4.
Hepatitis B virus (HBV)	All adults at risk for HBV	Hepatitis B surface antigen (HBsAg) Positive result indicates acute or chronic infection. Test for antibodies to HBsAg (anti-HBs) and hepatitis B core antigen (anti-HBc) during screening to establish acute versus chronic infection. Use clinical judgement to establish screening interval.	Increased risk includes those from countries with high prevalence of HBV infection (all Asia and Africa, others; see USPSTF website), HIV+ persons, injection drug users, men who have sex with men, and household contacts of individuals with HBV infection.

TABLE 37-3 USPSTF Screening and Counseling Recommendations *(Continued)*

Screening Recommendation	Whom to Screen	Screening Test and Frequency	Additional Considerations and Counseling Recommendations
Hepatitis C	All adults born between 1945–1965 and those at increased risk	Hepatitis C antibody (HCab) One-time screen for those born between 1945–1965. Consider repeat screening for those with additional risk factors.	Increased risk includes past or present IV drug use, transfusion before 1992, incarceration, intranasal drug use, unregulated tattoo(s), those born to an HCV+ mother.
High blood pressure*	All adults ≥ 18 years of age	Sphygmomanometer measurement every 2 years if blood pressure ≤ 120/80 and annually if systolic 120–139 or diastolic 80–90	Hypertension defined as blood pressure ≥ 140/90 found on 2 or more visits over a period of 1 to several weeks. In adults ≥ 60 years of age consider a target BP ≤ 150/90 (James et al., 2013).
High cholesterol*	All men ≥ 35 and 20–35 years of age if at increased risk for coronary heart disease (CHD). Women ≥ 20 years of age if at increased risk for CHD.	Total cholesterol and high-density lipoprotein fasting or nonfasting. Screen every 5 years or with increased frequency if lipid levels close to levels requiring treatment; may decrease frequency of screening if repeated screening levels are normal.	Increased risk for CHD: diabetes, prior history of CHD or noncoronary atherosclerosis, family history of CHD in men ≤ 50 and women ≤ 60 years of age, tobacco use, hypertension, and body mass index ≥ 30
HIV infection	All adolescents and adults aged 15–65, > 65 if at increased risk	Enzyme immune assay followed by confirmatory Western blot or immunofluorescent assay or rapid HIV antibody. The best interval for screening is unknown.	Increased risk: those who have or request testing for other STIs; men who have sex with men; active IV drug users; multiple sex partners with inconsistent use of barrier methods; exchange of sex for drugs or money; past or present sex partner who is HIV+, bisexual, IV drug user; blood transfusion between 1978 and 1985.
Intimate partner violence (IPV)	Women of childbearing age	There are several screening tools available such as the four-item HITS tool (Hurt, Insult, Threaten, Scream). See USPSTF website for resources. The best interval for screening is unknown.	IPV describes physical, sexual, or psychologic harm by a current or former partner or spouse
Lung cancer	Adults aged 55–80 with a smoking history	Low-dose computed tomography (LDCT) of the lung annually in current smokers aged 55–80 with a 30 pack-year-history or who have quit in the last 15 years.	Discontinue screening in those who have not smoked for >15 years or in those with comorbidities that limit life expectancy or who would not want/tolerate treatment for lung cancer.
Obesity and overweight	All adults	Body mass index (BMI) The best interval for screening is unknown.	Obesity defined as BMI ≥ 30, overweight as BMI 25.0–29.9. Offer or refer overweight or obese adults who have additional risk factors for cardiovascular disease (hypertension, hyperlipidemia, diabetes, tobacco use) to intensive behavioral counseling about healthful diet and physical activity. Offer or refer obese patients to intensive, multicomponent behavioral interventions.

(continues)

TABLE 37-3 USPSTF Screening and Counseling Recommendations *(Continued)*

Screening Recommendation	Whom to Screen	Screening Test and Frequency	Additional Considerations and Counseling Recommendations
Osteoporosis	All women ≥ 65 years of age and younger women whose 10-year osteoporotic fracture risk ≥ 9.3%.	Dual-energy x-ray absorptiometry (DEXA) measured at the hip and lumbar spine. The best interval for screening is unknown.	The Fracture Risk Assessment (FRAX) tool can be used to calculate an individual's 10-year risk for osteoporotic fracture (www.shef.ac.uk/FRAX/index.aspx). Note: In determining risk for women < 65, the bone mineral density field in the FRAX tool may be left empty. See instructions at tool web page.
Sexually transmitted infection (STI) risk	All adults	Risk factors for STI: Multiple sexual partners History of STI within last year	Adults at risk for STI should receive intensive behavioral counseling to prevent STI. See USPSTF website for resources.
Skin cancer risk	Adults ≤ 24 years of age	Fair skin type as evaluated by eye and hair color, freckling, history of frequent sunburn.	Those at increased risk should be counseled about minimizing exposure to ultraviolet radiation to prevent skin cancer. See USPSTF website for resources.
Syphilis*	Adults at increased risk	Venereal Disease Research Laboratory (VDRL) or Rapid Plasma Reagin (RPR) The best interval for screening is unknown.	Increased risk: men who have sex with men, those who engage in high-risk sex behavior, those who exchange sex for drugs or money, and adults in correctional facilities.
Tobacco use*	All adults	Ask about tobacco use.	Tobacco cessation interventions should be provided to those who use tobacco. Consider assessing readiness for behavior change (Figure 37-1). See USPSTF website for resources.

* Update in progress as of July 2, 2015.

Sources (unless otherwise noted):

AGS. (2011). Summary of the Updated American Geriatrics Society/British Geriatrics Society clinical practice guideline for prevention of falls in older persons. *Journal of the American Geriatrics Society*, *59*(1), 148–157. doi:10.1111/j.1532-5415.2010.03234.x; James, P. A, Oparil, S., Carter, B. L., Cushman, W. C., Dennison-Himmelfarb, C., Handler, J., et al. (2013). 2014 evidence-based guideline for the management of high blood pressure in adults: Report from the panel members appointed to the Eighth Joint National Committee (JNC 8). *JAMA*, *1097*, 1–14. doi:10.1001/jama.2013.284427; Kirkman, M. S., Briscoe, V. J., Clark, N., Florez, H., Haas, L. B., Halter, J. B., et al. (2012). Diabetes in older adults: A consensus report. *Journal of the American Geriatrics Society*, *60*(12), 2342–2356. doi:10.1111/jgs.12035; Lee, S. J., Leipzig, R. M., & Walter, L. C. (2013). Incorporating lag time to benefit into prevention decisions for older adults. *JAMA*, *310*(24), 2609–2610. doi:10.1001/jama.2013.282612; Saslow, D., Solomon, D., Lawson, H. W., Killackey, M., Kulasingam, S. L., Cain, J. M., et al. (2012). American Cancer Society, American Society for Colposcopy and Cervical Pathology, and American Society for Clinical Pathology screening guidelines for the prevention and early detection of cervical cancer. *Journal of Lower Genital Tract Disease*, *16*(3), 175–204. doi:10.1097/LGT.0b013e31824ca9d5; U.S. Department of Health and Human Services. (2014). *The guide to clinical preventive services*. Retrieved from www.ahrq.gov/clinic/pocketgd1011/gcp10s1.htm; U.S. Preventive Services Task Force. *Published recommendations*. Retrieved from www.uspreventiveservicestaskforce.org/BrowseRec/Index; Walter, L. C., & Covinsky, K. E. (2001). Cancer screening in elderly patients: A framework for individualized decision making. *JAMA*, *285*(21), 2750–2756. Retrieved from www.ncbi.nlm.nih.gov/pubmed/11386931; Walter, L. C., & Schonberg, M. A. (2014). Screening mammography in older women: A review. *JAMA*, *311*(13), 1336–1347. doi:10.1001/jama.2014.2834; Workowski, K. A., & Berman, S. (2010). Sexually transmitted diseases treatment guidelines, 2010. *MMWR. Recommendations and Reports*, *59*(RR-12), 1–110.

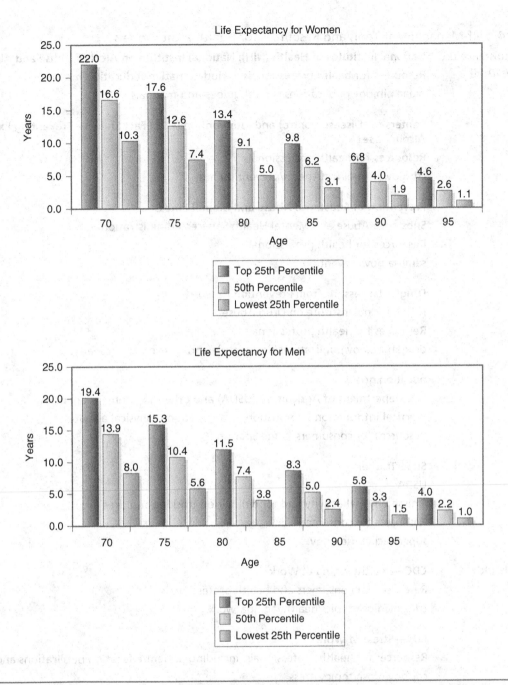

FIGURE 37-5 Upper, Middle, and Lower Quartiles of Life Expectancy for Women and Men at Selected Ages

Data from Walter, L. C., & Schonberg, M. A. (2014). Screening mammography in older women. *JAMA: The Journal of the American Medical Association, 311*(13), 1336–47. doi:10.1001/jama.2014.2834

TABLE 37-4 Self-Management Tools and Resources for Health Professionals

Alcohol and substance use disorders prevention	**National Institutes of Health (NIH): National Institute on Alcohol Abuse and Alcoholism** Resources for health professionals, including patient education materials niaaa.nih.gov/publications/clinical-guides-and-manuals **Centers for Disease Control and Intervention (CDC) Fact Sheets—Preventing Excessive Alcohol Use** Resources for health professionals cdc.gov/alcohol/fact-sheets/prevention.htm **Prevention of Substance Abuse and Mental Illness** Substance Abuse and Mental Health Services Administration Resources for health professionals samhsa.gov/prevention **DrugFacts: Lessons from Prevention Research** NIH: National Institute on Drug Abuse Resources for health professionals drugabuse.gov/publications/drugfacts/lessons-prevention-research
Nutrition	**nutrition.gov** U.S. Department of Agriculture (USDA) and other government agencies Practical information on nutrition, healthy eating, physical activity Resources for consumers, some Spanish **SuperTracker** USDA Online physical activity and food/nutrition tracking site, free Resources for consumers supertracker.usda.gov
Occupational health	**CDC—Healthy Aging at Work** Resources for consumers and health professionals cdc.gov/niosh/topics/healthyagingatwork **CDC—Stress at Work** Resources for health professionals, including patient education publications and videos cdc.gov/niosh/topics/stress **CDC—Occupational Violence** Resources for health professionals cdc.gov/niosh/topics/violence
Physical activity	**Physical Activity Basics** CDC Resources for consumers cdc.gov/physicalactivity/everyone/guidelines/adults.html

TABLE 37-4 Self-Management Tools and Resources for Health Professionals *(Continued)*

Sexually transmitted infection prevention	**Sexually Transmitted Diseases (STDs): Prevention** CDC Resources for consumers Includes fact sheets on individual STIs in multiple languages cdc.gov/std/prevention
Skin cancer prevention	**National Council on Skin Cancer Prevention** Resources for consumers and health professionals skincancerprevention.org **CDC—Skin Cancer** Resources for consumers and health professionals, including printable patient education materials in English and Spanish. cdc.gov/cancer/skin
Suicide prevention	**Suicide Prevention** National Institute of Mental Health Resources for consumers and health professionals nimh.nih.gov/health/topics/suicide-prevention
Tobacco use and cessation	**smokefree.gov** **espanol.smokefree.gov** (Spanish) U.S. Department of Health and Human Services, NIH, National Cancer Institute, and USA.gov Resources for consumers and health professionals **Five Major Steps to Intervention (The "5 As")** Agency for Health Research and Quality Resource for health professionals ahrq.gov/professionals/clinicians-providers/guidelines-recommendations/tobacco/5steps.html
Violence Prevention	**CDC Injury Prevention & Control: Division of Violence Prevention** Resources for consumers and health professionals, including consumer fact sheets on topics including Understanding Intimate Partner Violence, Understanding Elder Abuse, Understanding Sexual Violence, Understanding Suicide cdc.gov/violenceprevention

REFERENCES

American Geriatrics Society. (2011). Summary of the Updated American Geriatrics Society/British Geriatrics Society clinical practice guideline for prevention of falls in older persons. *Journal of the American Geriatrics Society, 59*(1), 148–157. doi:10.1111/j.1532-5415.2010.03234.x

Barton, M. B., Harris, R., & Fletcher, S. W. (1999). Does this patient have breast cancer? *JAMA, 282*(13), 1270. doi:10.1001/jama.282.13.1270

Beckett, N. S., Peters, R., Fletcher, A. E., Staessen, J. A., Liu, L., Dumitrascu, D., et al. (2008). Treatment of hypertension in patients 80 years of age or older. *New England Journal of Medicine, 358*(18), 1887–1898. doi:10.1056/NEJMoa0801369

Black, D. M., Thompson, D. E., Bauer, D. C., Ensrud, K., Musliner, T., Hochberg, M. C., et al. (2000). Fracture risk reduction with alendronate in women with osteoporosis: The Fracture Intervention Trial. FIT Research Group. *Journal of Clinical Endocrinology and Metabolism, 85*(11), 4118–4124. doi:10.1210/jcem.85.11.6953

Brown, A. F., Mangione, C. M., Saliba, D., & Sarkisian, C. A. (2003). Guidelines for improving the care of the older person with diabetes mellitus. *Journal of the American Geriatrics Society, 51* (5 Suppl. Guidelines), S265–S280. doi:10.1046/j.1532-5415.51.5s.1.x

Centers for Disease Control and Prevention. (2014). Recommendations for the laboratory-based detection of chlamydia trachomatis and neisseria gonorrhoeae — 2014. *Morbidity and Mortality Weekly Report,*

63(2), 1-22. Retrieved at http://www.cdc.gov/mmwr/pdf/rr/rr6302.pdf.

Holmes, H. M., Min, L. C., Yee, M., Varadhan, R., Basran, J., Dale, W., et al. (2013). Rationalizing prescribing for older patients with multimorbidity: Considering time to benefit. *Drugs & Aging, 30*(9), 655–666. doi:10.1007/s40266-013-0095-7

James, P. A, Oparil, S., Carter, B. L., Cushman, W. C., Dennison-Himmelfarb, C., Handler, J., et al. (2013). 2014 evidence-based guideline for the management of high blood pressure in adults: Report from the panel members appointed to the Eighth Joint National Committee (JNC 8). *JAMA, 1097,* 1–14. doi:10.1001/jama.2013.284427

Kirkman, M. S., Briscoe, V. J., Clark, N., Florez, H., Haas, L. B., Halter, J. B., et al. (2012). Diabetes in older adults: A consensus report. *Journal of the American Geriatrics Society, 60*(12), 2342–2356. doi:10.1111/jgs.12035

Lee, S. J., Boscardin, W. J., Stijacic-Cenzer, I., Conell-Price, J., O'Brien, S., & Walter, L. C. (2013). Time lag to benefit after screening for breast and colorectal cancer: Meta-analysis of survival data from the United States, Sweden, United Kingdom, and Denmark. *BMJ, 346,* e8441.

Lee, S. J., Leipzig, R. M., & Walter, L. C. (2013). Incorporating lag time to benefit into prevention decisions for older adults. *JAMA, 310*(24), 2609–2610. doi:10.1001/jama.2013.282612

Levy, W. C., Mozaffarian, D., Linker, D. T., Sutradhar, S. C., Anker, S. D., Cropp, A. B., et al. (2006). The Seattle Heart Failure Model: Prediction of survival in heart failure. *Circulation, 113*(11), 1424–1433. doi:10.1161/CIRCULATIONAHA.105.584102

Mitchell, S. L., Miller, S. C., Teno, J. M., Kiely, D. K., Davis, R. B., & Shaffer, M. L. (2010). Prediction of 6-month survival of nursing home residents with advanced dementia using ADEPT vs hospice eligibility guidelines. *JAMA, 304*(17), 1929–1935. doi:10.1001/jama.2010.1572

Musini, V. M., Tejani, A. M., Bassett, K., & Wright, J. M. (2009). Pharmacotherapy for hypertension in the elderly. *Cochrane Database of Systematic Reviews, 4,* CD000028. doi:10.1002/14651858.CD000028.pub2.

Partnership for Prevention. (2007). *Preventive care: A national profile on use, disparities, and health benefits.* Retrieved from www.rwjf.org/content/dam/farm/reports/reports/2007/rwjf13325.

Pham, A. N., Datta, S. K., Weber, T. J., Walter, L. C., & Colón-Emeric, C. S. (2011). Cost-effectiveness of oral bisphosphonates for osteoporosis at different ages and levels of life expectancy. *Journal of the American Geriatrics Society, 59*(9), 1642–1649. doi:10.1111/j.1532-5415.2011.03571.x

Pilkinton, M. A., & Talbot, H. K. (2015). Update on vaccination guidelines for older adults. *Journal of the American Geriatrics Society, 63*(3), 584–588.

Prochaska, J. O., Norcross, J. C., & Diclemente, C. C. (1994). *Changing for good.* New York, NY: Avon Books.

Rapsomaniki, E., Shah, A., Perel, P., Denaxas, S., George, J., Nicholas, O., et al. (2014). Prognostic models for stable coronary artery disease based on electronic health record cohort of 102 023 patients. *European Heart Journal, 35*(13), 844–852. doi:10.1093/eurheartj/eht533

Saslow, D., Solomon, D., Lawson, H. W., Killackey, M., Kulasingam, S. L., Cain, J. M., et al. (2012). American Cancer Society, American Society for Colposcopy and Cervical Pathology, and American Society for Clinical Pathology screening guidelines for the prevention and early detection of cervical cancer. *Journal of Lower Genital Tract Disease, 16*(3), 175–204. doi:10.1097/LGT.0b013e31824ca9d5.

Siu AL, on behalf of the U.S. Preventive Services Task Force (2016). Screening for breast cancer: U.S. Preventive Services Task Force recommendation statement. Ann Intern Med. doi:10.7326/M15-2886.

U.S. Department of Health and Human Services. (2014). *The guide to clinical preventive services.* Retrieved from www.ahrq.gov/clinic/pocketgd1011/gcp10s1.htm.

U.S. Preventive Services Task Force (2014). *About the USPSTF.* Retrieved from www.uspreventiveservicestaskforce.org/Page/Name/about-the-uspstf.

Walley, A. Y., & Roll, F. J. (2007). Principles of caring for alcohol and drug users. In T. E. King & M. B. Wheeler (Eds.). *Medical management of vulnerable and underserved patients: Principles, practice and populations* (pp. 341–350). New York: McGraw-Hill.

Walter, L. C., & Covinsky, K. E. (2001). Cancer screening in elderly patients: A framework for individualized decision making. *JAMAn, 285*(21), 2750–2756.

Walter, L. C., & Schonberg, M. A. (2014). Screening mammography in older women. *JAMA, 311*(13), 1336–1347. doi:10.1001/jama.2014.2834

Workowski, K. A., & Berman, S. (2010). Sexually transmitted diseases treatment guidelines, 2010. *MMWR. Recommendations and Reports, 59*(RR-12), 1–110.

Xie, J., Brayne, C., & Matthews, F. E. (2008). Survival times in people with dementia: Analysis from population based cohort study with 14 year follow-up. *BMJ, 336*(7638), 258–262. doi:10.1136/bmj.39433.616678.25

Yourman, L. C., Lee, S. J., Schonberg, M. A., Widera, E. W., & Smith, A. K. (2012). Prognostic indices for older adults: A systematic review. *JAMA, 307*(2), 182–192. doi:10.1001/jama.2011.1966

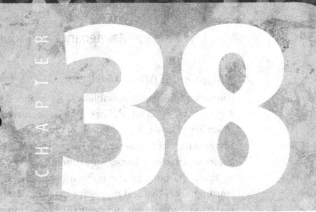

CHAPTER 38

HEALTHCARE MAINTENANCE FOR ADULTS WITH DEVELOPMENTAL DISABILITIES

Geraldine Collins-Bride and Clarissa Kripke

I. Introduction and general background

Individuals with developmental disabilities (DDs) experience health disparities across a number of domains. In the context of disability, a healthcare disparity is a population with a difference in health status not directly attributable to the condition leading to or associated with the disability. Disparities are caused in part by inadequate access to appropriate medical care, accommodations, services, and supports. They are compounded by intersectional issues with social determinants of health such as poverty, social exclusion, and implicit racial bias (Andresen et al., 2013; Horner-Johnson, Dobbertin, & Lee, 2013).

The current healthcare system presents an array of structural deficits that severely limit its ability to provide appropriate care for this vulnerable population. These deficits include:

- Lack of clinicians who are knowledgeable and skilled in the treatment of adults with DDs
- Lack of regular health assessment and care
- Lack of coordination among provider teams
- Limited availability of services in places where patients with DDs live and reside
- Lack of access to health-related, long-term care services and supports
- Exclusion from research and proven care guidelines (Autistic Self Advocacy Network, 2014; Feldman, Bossett, Collet, & Burnham-Riosa, 2014)

Life expectancy and quality of life have improved significantly over the past several decades as people with DDs moved from institutional settings to community-based care. The life expectancy of younger adults with DDs approaches that of the general population (Coppus, 2013). With the rise in life expectancy comes the increased risk for chronic diseases. Many of the chronic illnesses acquired by elders with DDs are similar to those seen in the general population, such as cardiovascular disease, cancers, pulmonary disease, diabetes, and renal diseases. Although individuals with DDs do have an increased incidence of respiratory, gastrointestinal, and musculoskeletal problems, it is imperative that the healthcare practitioner not focus solely on these conditions and perform routine screening for other chronic diseases as well as for secondary conditions that some patients with disabilities may be at increased risk of developing such as hearing loss, dental caries, and contractures.

People with developmental disabilities have a higher prevalence of chronic medical conditions such as epilepsy and neurologic disorders, dermatologic problems, fractures and orthopedic problems, gastrointestinal disorders, cardiovascular disorders, and mental health concerns. They are at risk for secondary conditions such as pressure sores, constipation, and injuries. To access healthcare services and manage their health, they may need support or accommodations for communication, decision making, mobility, sensory processing, personal care, or behavior (Anderson et al., 2013).

Currently, most adults with DDs live in the community in their own homes, with their families, or in group homes. Some lead very independent lives and others require a variety of services. Supports can include, but are not limited to, healthcare advocates, independent living coaches, vocational coaches, and case managers. They can also include personal assistants including direct support professionals, paid or unpaid family members, home health workers, and board and care home staff.

Transition of care from the child-oriented to an adult healthcare system is a particularly challenging and vulnerable time for patients, families, and clinicians. Clinicians who serve children have accumulated a wealth of information about the individual and often have a well-established, trusting relationship with the patient and the family or caregivers. Clinicians who serve adults are rarely trained in this field and often do not have the resources to provide the range of services required for comprehensive care. It is not uncommon for pediatric healthcare providers to continue to provide care for individuals with DDs well beyond the age of 21 (American Academy of Pediatrics, American Academy of Family Physicians, & American College of Physicians, 2011; Kripke, 2014).

A. Definition of DD

The Developmental Disabilities Assistance and Civil Rights Act of 2000 defines DD as a severe, chronic disability caused by physical or mental impairments manifesting before the age of 22 that is expected to continue indefinitely. These impairments cause limitations in three or more of the following categories: self-care, learning, receptive and expressive language, mobility, self-direction, capacity for independent living, and economic self-sufficiency (Developmental Disabilities Assistance and Bill of Rights Act, 2000). Many states define DD according to specific diagnoses or function and have different age cutoffs. To receive Medicaid funding, states must have a mechanism of delivering supports and services to individuals meeting the state eligibility requirements for DD, although the structure of each system varies by state. Both federal and state statutes have been established to determine when an individual is eligible for services and supports. When a clinician is faced with a patient who has high support need, it is important to note that one cannot accurately separate individuals with intellectual disability (ID; defined as IQ less than 70 on a standardized IQ test) from those with borderline intelligence (IQ 70–85) or individuals with severe learning disabilities. Clinicians should be very careful about labelling a person as having ID without clear documentation and appropriate testing.

Clinicians can refer individuals to the local or regional developmental resource center for an eligibility consultation or determination of changes to their individual program plan as their needs evolve.

There is a strong self-advocacy movement and the disability rights community has fought hard to dispel the old notion that individuals with disabilities are limited in their capacity to contribute meaningfully and be fully included in society. People with disabilities have the same rights to lead productive, independent lives as other citizens, and communities benefit from diversity including having people with developmental disabilities integrated into school, work, religious, and social organizations. The Americans with Disabilities Act guarantees people with disabilities the right to access healthcare services although many physical, financial, and programmatic barriers still exist.

B. Overview of common syndromes seen in primary care

1. Intellectual disability (ID) (formerly mental retardation)

   ID is a "disability characterized by significant limitations both in intellectual functioning (reasoning, learning, problem solving) and in adaptive behavior, which covers a range of everyday social and practical skills. This disability originates before the age of 18" (American Association on Intellectual and Developmental Disabilities, 2010, para. 1). Etiologies of ID include genetic conditions; intrauterine factors (asphyxia, maternal infections, and substance use); perinatal factors (hypoxic ischemic encephalopathy, sepsis, and prematurity); and postnatal causes, such as childhood infections, environmental toxins, trauma, and severe malnutrition. Alcohol exposure during pregnancy is the toxin most clearly linked to ID. Intellectual disabilities are complex neurodevelopmental conditions that typically affect many areas of life function. The prevalence of ID is approximately 2% and covers a wide range of cognitive traits and characteristics. The majority of adults (80%) have mild ID. Regardless of functional ability, people with intellectual disabilities benefit from exposure to rich life experiences. Clinicians should presume competence, which means to assume that all people communicate and all people have the capacity to learn and grow and improve skills. It is important not to make assumptions about people's intellect when it cannot be accurately assessed because of limitations in expressive communication. People with profound expressive communication problems can have normal receptive language. Individuals with more severe functional limitations and communication challenges are at particular risk for not receiving regular preventive health screening and lifestyle counseling. Counseling, health education, and information should be delivered directly to patients and their supporters using plain language, pictures, or other visual supports and demonstrations regardless of whether the patient's understanding of the messages can be confirmed. Patients with intellectual disabilities often understand far more than is apparent from their facial expressions, body movements, or other responses.

2. Cerebral palsy

   Cerebral palsy (CP) is a term used to describe a group of chronic conditions affecting body movement and muscle coordination. It is caused by differences in one or more specific areas of the brain, usually occurring during fetal development; before, during, or shortly after birth; or during infancy. Thus, these conditions are not caused by problems in the muscles or nerves. Instead, damage to motor areas in the brain affect the brain's ability to control movement and posture. The diagnosis of CP is not appropriate for individuals with motor impairments caused by spinal cord injuries, peripheral nerve injuries, myopathies, or any other etiology that is not brain based. Historically, individuals with a physical exam consistent with CP were given the diagnosis only if the brain abnormalities or injuries occurred within the first 1–2 years of life—the period associated with the greatest amount of brain development. The time frame for applying the CP diagnosis has loosened over the last several years because of the recognition that the brain continues to develop throughout childhood. Children with brain damage secondary to central nervous system infections or nonaccidental or accidental trauma that causes motor impairments meet criteria for a CP diagnosis, even if the injury occurs after 2 years of age. There is no longer an exact age cutoff for applying the diagnosis; clinical judgment is used to identify children with clear brain-related motor limitations

"Cerebral" refers to the brain and "palsy" to muscle weakness and difficulty with control. Because people may not be able to voluntarily control muscles, this can have an impact on the ability to speak, gesture, or type. Cerebral palsy itself is not progressive (i.e., brain changes do not evolve); however, secondary conditions such as muscle spasticity can develop, which may get better over time, get worse, or remain the same. Cerebral palsy is not communicable. It is not a disease and should not be referred to as such. Although cerebral palsy is not "curable" in the accepted sense, training, therapy, adaptive equipment, and an accommodating physical and social environment and access to education, employment, and services can greatly improve function and quality of life (United Cerebral Palsy, 2011).

The prevalence of CP is 2.1–3.3 per 1,000 live births with higher rates seen in males and African Americans (Yeargin-Allsopp, 2010). The greatest risk factor for CP is prematurity. An estimated one in three very-low-birth-weight children (< 1,500 g) are eventually diagnosed with CP. CP occurs as a consequence of the perinatal course. Spastic diplegia (greater involvement in the legs than the arms) is the type of CP most commonly associated with prematurity with hallmark findings of periventricular leukomalacia commonly seen on CT. Hemiplegic (one side of the body) CP is almost always caused by an in-utero or perinatal stroke, which should raise concerns about possible familial hypercoagulable disorders. Other etiologies for CP include chromosomal and brain anomalies, genetic and metabolic conditions, infection, and trauma.

Individuals with CP frequently have problems with spasticity, seizures, mobility, dystonia, dysarthria, swallowing, constipation, and gastroesophageal reflux (Peterson, 2013). People with cerebral palsy have a wide range of intellect so it is important not to make assumptions about people's intellect based on their method of expressive communication. Many people with CP have normal intelligence, even if they have difficulty producing clear speech

and controlling their bodies (Yin Foo, Guppy, & Johnston, 2013). Performing clinical interviews with nonverbal patients requires special techniques or adaptive equipment. For video models of appropriate interview techniques, visit https://www.mededportal.org/icollaborative/resource/904. The impairments that result from CP may "become more disabling as the person ages or they may accelerate the aging process" (Svien, Berg, & Stephenson, 2008). Symptoms of fatigue, depression, impaired mobility, and musculoskeletal problems frequently worsen with aging. Individuals with CP have high rates of cardiovascular and respiratory disease with aspiration pneumonia as the leading cause of death across all age groups (Frisch & Msall, 2013; Svien et al., 2008).

3. Autism spectrum disorders

Autism spectrum disorders (ASDs) are heterogeneous neurodevelopmental conditions of unclear etiology that are classified according to the *Diagnostic and Statistical Manual 5* (DSM-5) criteria to include atypical development in two major areas: (1) communication used for social purposes, and (2) restricted, repetitive patterns of interests, behaviors, or activities. The hallmark of ASDs is atypical social interaction, resulting from sensory-motor or movement differences or problems with language or social understanding. In addition, current DSM-5 criteria require deficits in the use of nonverbal communication (e.g., quality of eye contact, use of gestures, odd facial expressions, misreading other people's facial expressions, tone of voice) and difficulties with establishing meaningful relationships with peers. Other criteria include a series of highly focused interests over their lifetime that are either unusual or highly focused, need for routines and rituals and distress with change, and repetitive motor mannerisms (hand-flapping, finger flicking, or shuddering, occurring most often when the individual is happy or distressed). Although it has long been recognized that people with ASD react in atypical ways to various sensory input, ranging from extreme negative reactions to sounds, smells, or touch to fascination or soothing related to sounds, visual stimuli, or movement, it was not until the publication of the DSM-5 that sensory issues were included in the diagnostic criteria for ASDs. It is extremely important for the clinician to understand the particular sensory issues that the individual with autism experiences in order to deliver good care.

People on the autism spectrum have a wide range of strengths and challenges, which is one of the reasons that the condition is considered to be a spectrum. Language skills range from nonverbal to normal or advanced language skills. However, even individuals with average to advanced expressive and receptive language skills may demonstrate deficits in how to use language for social purposes (referred to as "pragmatic" language). Problems with motor planning and coordination, sometimes affecting speech, are increasingly being recognized in persons with ASDs.

Some people on the autism spectrum are highly verbal or skilled in writing and mechanical skills. Some have challenges with communication and motor skills including difficulty with articulation and controlling and coordinating movements. Sensory processing differences combined with communication and motor planning problems and lack of accommodation and understanding can lead to difficulties with social interaction, misinterpreted behavior, and developing friendships and peer relationships. They can also lead to the behaviors seen in ASD as described previously or regulating "stims" (self-stimulating behaviors), narrow focus on specific interests or activities, and difficulties with changes to routine, environments, or transitions

The prevalence of people diagnosed with ASD continues to rise but how much of the increase can be attributed to changes in diagnostic criteria, access to services, and reclassification of individuals with other DDs continues to be a subject of debate. Most studies show that somewhere between 30% and70% of the increase is due to the aforementioned issues. However, that leaves at least 30% of the increased incidence of ASDs that may be attributed to a true increase in the condition.

ASDs are diagnosed in boys four times more frequently than girls. The incidence of intellectual impairment is much lower than previously estimated once appropriate testing is done. Many individuals with ASD experience sensory integration problems and may be extremely sensitive to sounds or stimuli in the environment. Sensory processing differences should be explored to learn how to increase the comfort of people with autism in medical environments and during the physical examination. Many people with autism also have seizure disorders and associated mental health conditions. Anxiety almost always accompanies ASDs with depression being quite common as the individual approaches the teenage and adult years. Although individuals with ASD may experience the same range of health problems as the general population, the communication and behavioral features of this condition often require accommodations to deliver high-quality care in primary care settings. These accommodations might include preparation about the visit or examination ahead of time and the use of a timer to indicate the start and stop of the examination (Nicolaidis, Kripke, & Raymaker, 2014).

4. Genetic disorders

A comprehensive genetics work-up, including a microarray test that looks at the entire genome for duplications and deletions, can reveal the causes of DD in many individuals (estimates range from roughly 30% to 60%). One of the most common and well characterized of these genetic conditions is Down syndrome, a chromosomal disorder with an estimated incidence of 1 in 691. The risk for Down syndrome rises with increasing maternal age (Parker et al., 2010). The distinguishing characteristics of Down syndrome include facial dysmorphology (dysmorphic indicates an abnormal appearance), muscle hypotonia, and ID of varying degrees. Numerous medical problems are seen with Down syndrome including visual and hearing impairments, obesity, sleep apnea, hypothyroidism, cardiac and respiratory diseases, and early-onset Alzheimer disease. There are healthcare guidelines for following individuals with Down syndrome (Ross & Olsen, 2014; Sullivan et al., 2011).

When genetic syndromes are suspected or the etiology of a developmental disability is unclear, referral to genetics can be helpful. Given the advances in today's genetic testing, it may be helpful to refer adults with unidentified ID for a genetics evaluation for further diagnostic testing. References for learning about other common (fragile X and Klinefelter syndromes) and less common genetic syndromes can be found at the end of this chapter.

5. Epilepsy

Epilepsy refers to a group of conditions that are characterized by the recurrent disturbance of cerebral function (seizures) caused by excessive neuronal discharges in the brain occurring in a paroxysmal manner. An epileptic seizure occurs when the cerebral cortex is rendered hyperexcitable (because of an increase in excitatory neurotransmission, a decrease in inhibitory neurotransmission, or a disturbance in brain circuitry) by any of a number of causes including metabolic disturbances, injuries, strokes, tumors, and developmental abnormalities. For further discussion of epilepsy, see Chapter 55.

II. Database (may include but is not limited to)

A. Subjective

It can be challenging to obtain an accurate and comprehensive history on individuals with DDs, especially when the individual has communication or cognitive impairments. In order to gather a comprehensive and accurate understanding of the patient, start by collecting information directly from the patient. Historical data can be obtained from a variety of sources including caregivers, case managers, ID and DD nurses, and medical record review.

In some systems, a structured health interview and examination tool is being used to collect and document important past and current health issues. An example of such a tool can be found at www.cddh.monash.org /disability-health-assessment.html. This yearly health assessment form is a component of many healthcare delivery models for adults with DDs throughout the world, although not consistently in use in the United States. These health assessment forms have been well studied and capture key information on functional, behavioral, developmental, and psychosocial issues pertinent to adults with DDs (Robertson, Hatton, Emerson, & Baines, 2014). Regardless of the type of data collection tool used for the history and physical examination, when possible, the healthcare provider should allow extra time for appointments when seeing individuals with DDs. It can also be helpful to schedule visits at regular or more frequent intervals to address the complexities of the patient's healthcare issues. Flexibility and creativity are often required to ensure a successful office visit. Home visits or visits in community settings can be very effective ways to provide care. Such strategies as desensitization, telephone conferences with caregivers, and obtaining assistance from health advocates or case managers can allow the visit to proceed more smoothly. Always attempt to prepare the individual for the appointment and enlist support from a trusted caregiver. For severely agitated patients, sedation with a low dose of benzodiazepines, such as lorazepam, 0.5–1 mg, may be indicated. A test dose of the medication can be tried at home first to determine the timing of peak effect and dose and because some patients have been known to experience a paradoxical reaction where agitation actually increases rather than decreases. Multidisciplinary telemedicine consultation has been shown to be an effective option for addressing difficult behavioral, medical and psychiatric issues in some patients with complex DD disorders www.uctv/show /telemdicine-assessment-and-Consultation-Team- TACT-Caring-for-Individuals-with-Complex-Developmental Disabilities-in-Rural-Northern-California-28909.

1. Pertinent past medical history, as outlined in Chapter 37 (Adult Health Maintenance and Promotion), with a focus on the following additional data
   a. Etiology of DD with review of pediatric records and medical summary when possible. Note previous developmental and genetic evaluations (Sullivan et al., 2011). Note any history of institutionalizations.
   b. Previous medical illnesses, noting history of
      i. Epilepsy: frequency of seizures, medications, use of seizure tracking logs, and emergency management plan.
      ii. Gastroesophageal reflux disease: previous work-up, treatment, and *Helicobacter pylori* testing.
      iii. Constipation: unrecognized or untreated constipation can be a significant cause of morbidity and mortality. Note previous work-up and treatment.
      iv. Visual impairment: use of eyeglasses or contact lenses and date of last ophthalmology examination.
      v. Hearing impairment: use of hearing devices and date of last audiology examination.
      vi. Sensory perceptual differences: note processing of sounds, touch, taste, and sensation, which may affect the physical examination or interpretation of pain behavior. Document recommendations from patients, caregivers, family, and others about accommodations, strategies and the best methods of approaching individuals with sensory integration differences.
   c. Communication: document the patient's usual method of communication (verbal, written, sign language, behaviors, or gestures) and use of augmentative devices.
   d. Mobility and neuromotor function: note if the patient is ambulatory or nonambulatory, use of adaptive equipment, and how much time per day is spent using the equipment. Note how the person transfers if non–weight bearing and what assistance is needed for transfers (equipment, such as a Hoyer lift; staff or family and how many are needed). Note fine and gross motor skills, spasticity, and changes in motor tone, either increased or decreased.
   e. Swallowing and feeding: episodes of choking or coughing with eating, history of aspiration, pneumonia, last swallowing study, and speech therapy treatments.
   f. Bowel and bladder function: constipation, urinary incontinence or retention, and use of diapers or other incontinence supplies.
   g. Dental health issues: caries, periodontal disease, and gingival hyperplasia. Identification of risk factors for dental disease is important to avoid effects of premature demineralization. Often, patients have undiagnosed conditions of gastric reflux resulting in dental erosion or medication induced xerostomia, which leaves the oral cavity hyperacidic and prone to premature

demineralization. Checking for adequate and healthy saliva can help minimize effects of dental disease. Prevention strategies of neutralizing the acids in the mouth through sodium bicarbonate rinses, increasing hydration, and possible fluoride varnishes or sealants (Marinho et al., 2013) can prevent dental caries. Inquire about ongoing dental care, cleanings, and need for sedation before dental visits.

h. Mental health issues: depression, posttraumatic stress disorder, and anxiety are the most common disorders with rates similar to the general population. There is a much lower incidence of psychotic disorders, although antipsychotic medication is often overprescribed to control behavior. Ask specifically how symptoms manifest themselves. Some patients may be capable of verbally expressing mood symptoms and others may express symptoms as a change in behavior. Behavior needs to be interpreted developmentally. For example, a person with an intellectual disability may have imaginary friends and tantrums when frustrated. This behavior is appropriate to the person's intellectual development and is not an indication of a mental illness.

i. Medications: polypharmacy is a significant issue, with multiple medications often used to treat the same health problem. This is an especially common, ineffective and harmful practice used in the treatment of aggressive or other problem behaviors. It is important to note the indications and duration of use for all medications with attention to any side effects, drug interactions, and medication efficacy.

j. Immunization status: in addition to the primary vaccination series and scheduled boosters, note if the patient has received vaccines for hepatitis A and B, pneumococcal, and seasonal flu.

k. History of injuries or falls

l. History of abuse or victimization. This is especially prevalent in those individuals with IDs but it is also seen with high frequency in all individuals with disabilities (Sobsey & Doe, 1991).

m. History of resistive or challenging behavior. *Behavior is often a form of communication* but can easily be misinterpreted, especially in disabilities that affect sensory processing and movement. Difficult behaviors are not part of the disability but rather a means of communication for a patient with neurocognitive disorders. Difficult behaviors that are new or a change from the individual's usual level of functioning may signify an undiagnosed medical or psychiatric problem or may be a sign of a mismatch between a person's needs and the services and supports they are receiving or the environments in which they live and work. *New behaviors always warrant a medical evaluation.* Additionally, new behaviors or significant change in behaviors can indicate the individual has experienced abuse or neglect; therefore, assessment specific to this is also important. Note previous medical and psychiatric evaluations of behavior change. Document behavioral, environmental, and pharmacologic therapies used for treatment.

2. Family history, with emphasis on developmental and genetic disorders

3. Occupational history: people with DDs work in a variety of settings. Inquire about a job coach or other personnel support present at work. Obtain specific details about job tasks to screen for repetitive motion injuries. Ask about job satisfaction and relationships with coworkers.

4. Personal and social history
   a. Housing status and supports: note if the patient lives independently and what support is required for independent living, such as in-home support services, independent living coaches, or case management support. Include type of housing (apartment, family, or residential group home), noting how many individuals live in the home and ratio of staff/caregivers needed to provide a safe environment.
   b. Relationships and social support network: note significant relationships with family, friends, sexual and life partners. Inquire about the quantity and quality of social contact and relationships.
   c. Future goals: note desired future personal, educational, and occupational goals.

5. Habits
   a. Nutrition
   b. Exercise and activity
   c. Tobacco, alcohol, and substance use
   d. Sleep
   e. Sexual activity

6. Interdisciplinary healthcare team members: note each team member's name and contact information, which may include a case manager, nurse, dentist, behavior specialist, pharmacist, physical therapist, occupational therapist, speech and language therapist, psychotherapist, and medical specialists (**Figure 38-1**).

B. Objective

1. Perform an annual physical examination with blood pressure, height, weight, and body mass index (Sullivan et al., 2011). The physical examination is

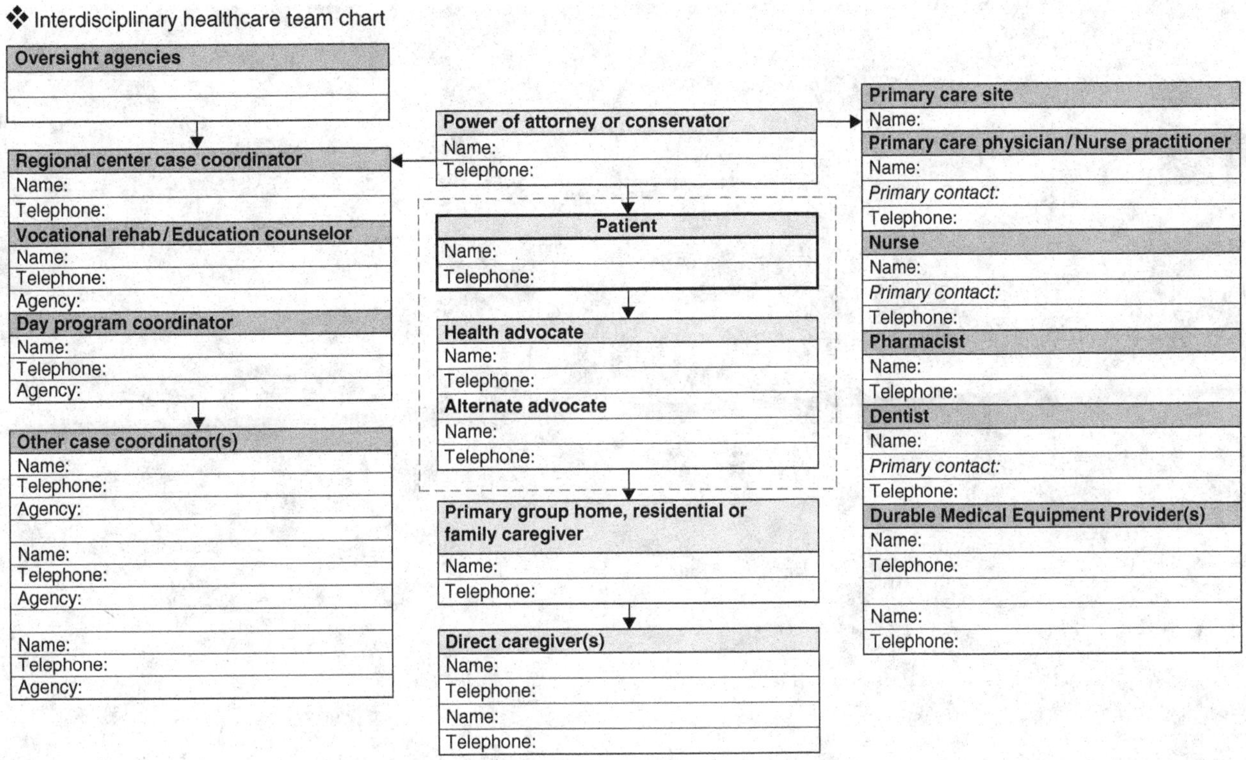

❖ Interdisciplinary healthcare team chart

FIGURE 38-1 Interdisciplinary Healthcare Team Chart
Reproduced from Office of Developmental Primary Care, University of California, San Francisco. http://odpc.ucsf.edu.

particularly important for patients with cognitive and communication impairments, where subjective symptoms may be difficult to elicit (**Figure 38-2**).

2. Pay particular attention to a careful oral examination given the frequency of dental disease (National Institute of Dental and Craniofacial Research, 2009; Sullivan et al., 2011).

3. Perform annual office-based vision and hearing screening examinations (Sullivan et al., 2011).

4. Document the patient's baseline, typical behavior, and method of communication.

5. Schedule a separate appointment dedicated solely to the gynecologic examination. Extra time is needed for the pelvic examination because these examinations can be challenging for providers and for women with disabilities (**Figure 38-3**).

III. Assessment

A. Identify the patient's general and specific health risk profile. If the cause of the DD is unknown or unclear, consider a referral to genetics for an evaluation (Sullivan et al., 2011).

B. Recognize health habits that benefit from lifestyle modification.

C. Ascertain additional members of the interdisciplinary health team that would be beneficial to improve the healthcare plan (Figure 38-1).

D. Determine the support needed for medical decision making and informed consent for

FIGURE 38-2 Exam Room Etiquette

You may need to provide support to communicate with a patient with a developmental disability. Communication may take more thought and planning. Assess whether your patient uses spoken language; if not, he or she may use other forms of language, such as sign language, written language, or augmentative and alternative communication. Even people who do not use language can communicate through behavior, facial expressions, and sounds. Listening to your patient may require using more of your senses. The following are some ideas, but ask your patient and caregivers what works best for them.

- Order an interpreter if spoken English is not the patient's primary language.
- Use person-first or identity-first language for the autistic, deaf, and blind communities (unless your patient prefers something else).
- Talk directly to your patient in an adult voice and listen attentively for your patient to respond and to finish. If your patient appears to be thinking, wait quietly.
- A patient may have better receptive than expressive language. Use plain language without jargon.
- If your patient is not using words to communicate, then try nonverbal communication strategies, such as demonstrations, pictures, touch, gestures, and facial expressions.
- Get your patient's attention before speaking to him or her.
- Check for understanding by repeating and asking your patient to repeat.
- If necessary, use short, concrete questions that require yes or no answers.
- If necessary, ask questions that can be answered nonverbally. For example, "Show me how you say yes."
- Sit at eye level and treat wheelchairs as personal space. Don't touch a wheelchair without permission.
- Before helping, offer assistance, and wait for a response and instructions.
- Offer to shake hands even if your patient has limited use of hands or an artificial limb.
- Identify yourself and others to people with visual disabilities and indicate to whom you are speaking.
- It is okay to use common idioms that refer to vision or hearing such as, "Have you heard about ..." or "See the light ..."

Used with permission from the Office of Developmental Primary Care, Department of Family & Community Medicine, University of California, San Francisco.

diagnostic testing and procedures. Document whether the individual has a power of attorney or a legal decision maker for healthcare decisions. Although many individuals with IDs and DDs require the support of families and caregivers for decision making, it is important to remember that people with IDs and DDs have the right to make decisions about their lives and their health care. For individuals who lack capacity for decision making even with support and have no identified power of attorney for health care, the state developmental disability service can be contacted for procedures to support medical decision making for diagnostic, treatment, or emergency decisions.

E. Assess the patient and caregiver's assets, barriers, and resources needed for implementing recommendations.

IV. Plan

A. Diagnostics (screening and secondary prevention tests)

1. Screen for diseases and conditions based on the patient's risk profile.

2. Screen for diseases and conditions specific to the patient's underlying DD or known specific developmental syndrome. For specific screening and diagnostic test recommendations see **Table 38-1**.

FIGURE 38-3 Tips for a Successful Pelvic Exam

For some women with disabilities, pelvic exams can be frightening and potentially uncomfortable. If the situation permits, focus the first visit on history and relationship building alone. The following may be helpful to reduce both the patient's and the provider's anxiety about the pelvic examination:

- Get to know your patient before attempting a pelvic exam.
- Educate the patient and caregivers about the exam.
- Don't assume that a pelvic exam will be any more difficult or uncomfortable for a person with a disability than for anyone else. You don't know until you try.
- Women with disabilities, including those with intellectual disabilities, can and do have sex.
- Use anatomy models with visual demonstration before the visit.
- Allow extra time (this is a must!).
- Encourage your patient to bring a supportive person to the appointment.
- If needed, locate the cervix manually.
- The anatomy of women with disabilities is often normal. However, it may be helpful to have several different pediatric and adult-sized speculums available.
- Pelvic exams can be done in a variety of positions. You may need assistants to hold a flashlight or help the patient maintain a comfortable position.
- Use a soothing voice, deep breathing, visualization, and praise.
- Consider pelvic ultrasound if bimanual exam is not possible.
- Consider using a short-acting benzodiazepine for sedation before a pelvic exam for women who have anxiety, spasticity, or agitation. Obtain consent from the patient or decision maker. Consider a test dose at home prior to the visit. Ask the caregiver to carefully document the patient's reaction, as well as the peak action of the medication.
- Consider doing the exam under conscious sedation or general anesthesia especially if the patient has a scheduled surgical or dental procedure under anesthesia. Other exams, such as echocardiograms, labs, EKG, hearing tests, etc., can be coordinated at the same time.

Used with permission from the Office of Developmental Primary Care, Department of Family & Community Medicine, University of California, San Francisco.

B. Treatment

1. For general health guidelines, see Chapter 37, Adult Health Maintenance and Promotion.

2. For recommendations targeted toward individuals with DDs, see Table 38-1.

3. For immunizations: see the Centers for Disease Control and Prevention Recommended Adult Immunization Schedule at www.cdc.gov/vaccines/schedules/index.html.

4. For bone health: advise adequate calcium (1,500 mg per day) and vitamin D (400–800 IU per day) supplementation for those patients with a high-risk profile for osteoporosis (mobility impairments, long-term use of antiepileptic or antipsychotic medications, Down syndrome, CP, Prader-Willi syndrome, history of fractures, history of amenorrhea, and cigarette smoking).

5. For mental health: review common stress management strategies with patients and caregivers (Hwang & Kearney, 2013). Prompt referral for psychologic counseling or psychiatry for signs and symptoms of mental illness.

6. For oral health: to reduce dental caries and gingival disease an expert dental panel recommends:

   a. Brushing teeth twice daily for 2 minutes with a fluoridated toothpaste containing triclosan.

   b. Using xylitol for 5 minutes, three times per day. If the patient tolerates chewing, use chewing gum. If chewing is not possible, use a dissolved lozenge, spray, mint, or lollipop.

TABLE 38-1 Healthcare Maintenance Guidelines for Adults with Developmental Disabilities

Health Problem	Who to Screen	Test & Frequency	Special Considerations
Abuse & Neglect	All adults	• Screen yearly with history & physical exam looking for unexplained physical and/or behavioral signs and symptoms such as unexplained bruising, falls, injuries, oral trauma, weight loss, depression, and behavior changes[16]	• Risk factors include caregiver stress
Alcohol & Substance Abuse	• All adults	• Screen yearly with history (although best screening interval is unknown).	• Traditional screening tools such as the CAGE & AUDIT have not been well tested in this population[13]
Breast Cancer	• Women aged 50–74	• Mammography every 2 years[17] • Clinical breast exam (CBE) yearly[19]	• Although the U.S. Preventive Services Task Force (USPSTF) notes that there is insufficient evidence to recommend for or against the CBE, women with ID/DD may not understand the significance of breast changes or have the skills to communicate changes they notice. • Also, women with sensory or neuromuscular problems may have difficulty performing any physical exam & some are not able to tolerate a mammogram[19]
	• Women > 74	• Individualize screening decision depending on life expectancy and comorbidities[18]	
	• Women > 18 with a family history of breast, ovarian, or other types of BRCA1 or BRCA2 gene mutations	• A number of risk assessment tools are available to help establish which women should be referred for genetic counseling (e.g., B-RST available at: www.breastcancergenescreen.org). • Periodic (every 5–10 years) review of family history to identify increased risk.	• Consider referral for genetic counseling and evaluation.

Comments

Family history is often difficult to obtain in this population. Individual decision making is critical. Inform women and caregivers of potential benefits and consequences of breast cancer screening.

TABLE 38-1 Healthcare Maintenance Guidelines for Adults with Developmental Disabilities *(Continued)*

Health Problem	Who to Screen	Test & Frequency	Special Considerations
Cervical Spine Atlanto-Axial Instability	Adults with Down syndrome	• Perform an annual neurologic examination for signs and symptoms of spinal cord injury for patients with Down syndrome & previous negative C spine films.[1] • Order cervical spine x-ray with lateral flexion and extension if symptoms develop, such as changes in behavior or activity, changes in hand preference or urinary incontinence. If this is the first C-spine film, also order an anteroposterior view.[1]	Consider screening cervical spine films prior to participation in athletics & before elective intubation for surgery.[2]
Cervical Cancer (Women)			
	• Women ages 21–65 with average risk	• Perform pap smear every 3 years • May use a combination of cytology and HPV testing every 5 years in women under 30 years old who prefer less frequent testing[15]	
	• Women over 65	• Stop pap screening if three consecutive negative cytology tests or two consecutive negative cytology plus HPV negative tests within 10 years[15]	
	Comments	Individualized decision making depending on patient risk and sexual history. See "Tips for a Successful Pelvic Exam": http://odpc.ucsf.edu/sites/odpc.ucsf.edu/files/pdf_docs/Tips%20for%20a%20Successful%20Pelvic%20Exam.pdf	
Chlamydia	• Sexually active women through age 24 & older women at increased risk	• Nucleic acid amplification test (NAAT) (urine or vaginal or cervical swab for both)[5]	• High risk includes multiple sex partners, h/o sexually transmitted infections, and inconsistent condom use. • USPSTF notes insufficient evidence to screen men although the CDC recommends screening men who have sex with men
	Comments	*Patients may not reliably report sexual activity or symptoms.*	

(continues)

TABLE 38-1 Healthcare Maintenance Guidelines for Adults with Developmental Disabilities *(Continued)*

Health Problem	Who to Screen	Test & Frequency	Special Considerations
Cholesterol & Lipid Disorders	• Men ≥ 35 • Women ≥ 45 with increased coronary heart disease (CHD) risk	• Order a fasting or nonfasting total cholesterol and HDL every 5 years.[17]	• Risk factors for CHD include previous h/o CHD or noncoronary atherosclerosis, diabetes, FHx of CVD ≤ age 55 in first-degree male relative or age 65 in first-degree female relative, tobacco use, hypertension, & obesity • More frequently if patient is taking atypical antipsychotic medications or has diabetes.[17]
Colorectal Cancer	• All adults ages 50–75	• At age 50, screen with one of the following strategies: 1. Annual fecal occult blood test (FOBT) or fecal immunochemical test or 2. Flexible sigmoidoscopy every 5 years along with FOBT 3. Colonoscopy every 10 years.[17]	

Comments

Depending on the patient's comorbidities, anesthesia risk may outweigh the benefits of colonoscopy.

Patients with mobility disorders, spasticity, and/or cognitive impairment may require hospital admission the day prior to testing with colonoscopy and sigmoidoscopy for professional assistance with the bowel preparation.

| Dental Disease | • All adults | • Perform an annual oral exam.
• Refer to dentist for regular dental care including cleaning every 6 months or as recommended by the dentist
• **Check for adequate saliva flow and amount (should be watery and abundant, not bubbly, stringy, or thick)** | • Pay special attention to dental and gum health in persons with certain syndromes, such as Cornelia de Lange, cerebral palsy, Down, Prader-Willi, Turner, Rett, Williams, and tuberous sclerosis.[16]
• USPSTF recommends application of fluoride varnish on individuals with high caries risk[9,17]. |

Comments

Patients with developmental disabilities are at high risk for periodontal disease and dental caries for numerous reasons, including: difficulty maintaining hygiene, lack of access to regular dental care, syndrome-specific susceptibilities, and medication side effects (xerostomia).

In some patients unable to tolerate office exams and treatment, hospital dentistry under anesthesia may be indicated. Other necessary diagnostic testing should be considered while patient is sedated.

TABLE 38-1 Healthcare Maintenance Guidelines for Adults with Developmental Disabilities *(Continued)*

Health Problem	Who to Screen	Test & Frequency	Special Considerations
Depression	• All adults[16]	• Screen annually or sooner for behaviors or emotions that may indicate depression.[11,14,16]	*Patients with developmental disabilities may have difficulty recognizing and communicating symptoms such as depressed mood, anxiety, and sadness. Mental health symptoms are often expressed in physical or behavioral changes. It is critical that healthcare providers obtain information about the patient's usual level of functioning, skills, and behavior in order to assess the potential for mental health disorders.* • *See Diagnostic Manual-Intellectual Disabilities for more in-depth discussion on assessment.[7]*
Fall Risk	• All adults	• Evaluate as part of the annual physical examination including an evaluation of the medication profile for drugs that may affect balance and/or gait. Screen more frequently if there is a change in gait/balance or for individuals at high risk, such as those who have a history of two or more falls in the previous year.[16] • For patients with no previous mobility impairments who report one or more falls, consider performing the Get-Up and Go Test: www.ncbi.nlm.nih.gov/pubmed/3487300. Patients having difficulty with this test should be referred to a physical/occupational therapist for a full fall evaluation.	• If the patient has had an increase in falls or a decline in function, a medical evaluation of the cause is warranted.
HIV	• All individuals 15–65 years old	• Enzyme immune assay followed by confirmatory Western blot or immunofluorescent assay or rapid HIV antibody test • Screen at least once & more frequently depending on risk. • Exact screening interval is unknown.[17]	Sexual history is often overlooked in people with ID/DD. Remember to do a periodic sexual history.[11,16,20]

(continues)

TABLE 38-1 Healthcare Maintenance Guidelines for Adults with Developmental Disabilities *(Continued)*

Health Problem	Who to Screen	Test & Frequency	Special Considerations
Hearing	• All adults	• Screen annually subjectively or objectively with office-based testing (Whisper Test).[16] • Refer to audiology at regular intervals. • Refer to audiology for hearing assessment every 5 years after age 45 (every 3 years throughout life for patients with Down syndrome).[2,6,16]	• Reevaluate hearing if problems are reported or changes in behavior are noted.[16]

Comments

Other syndromes associated with hearing impairments include Cornelia de Lange, Noonan, Usher, and Smith-Magenis.[16]

Methods for testing may include the following:

Method (years)	Applicable for Developmental Age
OtoAcoustic Emissions (OAE)	> 0
Auditory Brainstem Responses (ABR)	> 0
Behavioral observation audiometry	> 0
Pure tone audiometry with visual reinforcement	> 1
Whispered speech	> 3
Pure tone (play) audiometry	> 3–4

Health Problem	Who to Screen	Test & Frequency	Special Considerations
Hypertension	• All adults	Sphygmomanometer measurement every 2 years if blood pressure ≤ 120/80 and annually if systolic 120–139 or diastolic 80–90.[8]	• *For patients with spasticity/contractures, may need to do a wrist or thigh blood pressure measurement. Document type of measurement used.*
Immunizations	• See Centers for Disease Control and Prevention Recommended Adult Immunization Schedule: www.cdc.gov/vaccines/schedules/index.html		
Obesity	• All adults	• Measure height and weight annually.[14,16]	• *Consider weight on home scale in more familiar setting.* • *Accommodations for patients unable to stand include using a Lift Team, a wheelchair scale, Hoyer Lift, and/or hospital bed that includes a scale.*
Osteoporosis	• Women ≥ age 65 & younger women whose 10-year fracture risk is ≥ 9.3%[17] • All adults with ID/DD at high risk.[12]	• Bone mineral density (BMD) screening with dual-energy x-ray absorptiometry (DEXA) testing at the spine and hip earlier and at regular intervals for high-risk patients • Recommended screening interval is unknown.[12,20]	• *The typical sites for DEXA scans (lumbar spine & hip) may be very difficult for some individuals with mobility impairments &/or spasticity. Alternate testing methods are needed.*[12]
	–	• Although the age to begin screening is unclear, some authors suggest age 40 for patients residing in institutions and age 45 for patients residing in the community.[20] • Check serum vitamin D 25 OH levels at regular intervals	

TABLE 38-1 Healthcare Maintenance Guidelines for Adults with Developmental Disabilities *(Continued)*

Health Problem	Who to Screen	Test & Frequency	Special Considerations

Comments

High-risk factors in patients with developmental disabilities include mobility impairments, long-term use of antiepileptic drugs or antipsychotics, nutritional issues, and oral-motor problems. Patients with Down syndrome, cerebral palsy, and Prader-Willi syndrome are also at greater risk.

High-risk factors in the general population include osteopenia on plain films, history of vertebral fractures, early menopause, chronic steroid use, low body weight, cigarette use, and positive family history of osteoporosis.

See FRAX: WHO Fracture Risk Assessment Tool: www.shef.ac.uk/FRAX/. Note that mobility is not calculated in this assessment tool.

Prostate Cancer	–	• Insufficient evidence to recommend routine screening in men under age 75.[17]	• Screening not recommended for men over age 75[17]

Comments

Family history is often difficult to obtain with this population.

Patients at high risk include those with positive family history at an early age and African American men.

Use shared decision-making with the patient and medical decision makers.[17]

Testicular Cancer	• All adolescent & adult males	• Routine screening not recommended. • Prompt assessment and evaluation of testicular problems when young men present with signs and symptoms of testicular disease.[17]	Risk factors for testicular cancer: previous testicular cancer, positive FHx of testicular cancer, cryptorchidism, Klinefelter syndrome

Comments

Clinical exam is especially important in this population who may not be able to report symptoms and may have difficulty with the self-exam technique.

Thyroid Disease	• All adults with DD • Adults with Down syndrome	• Monitor thyroid-stimulating hormone (TSH) regularly. Exact testing interval is unknown.[16] • Check TSH more frequently in patients with Down syndrome.[2,16]	

Comments

Symptoms of thyroid disease are often not elicited due to cognitive impairment and/or communication difficulties in patients with developmental disabilities.

Consider TSH testing if unexplained change in behavior or level of functioning.

Increased risk for thyroid disease seen in patients with Down syndrome and the elderly.

Tuberculosis	All adults with DD	Screen routinely with tuberculin skin test (TST) or gamma release assay (IGRA) based on likelihood of exposure[17])	IGRA if the individual is unlikely to return to have TST read or those who have had previous Bacillus Calmette–Guérin vaccination.

Comments

Consider tuberculin skin testing every 1 to 2 years for patients who live or work in aggregate settings (board and care homes, intermediate care facilities, day programs).

(continues)

TABLE 38-1 Healthcare Maintenance Guidelines for Adults with Developmental Disabilities *(Continued)*

Health Problem	Who to Screen	Test & Frequency	Special Considerations
Vision	• All adults with DD	• Screen annually subjectively or objectively with office-based tests (Snellen test).[14,16,]	
		• Refer to ophthalmology for exam and glaucoma screening at least once before age 40	
		• Refer for ophthalmologic exam and glaucoma screening every 5 years after age 45 or as recommended by ophthalmologist[16]	
	• Adults with Down syndrome	• Refer to ophthalmology for exam and glaucoma screening by age 30 for patients with Down syndrome.[16]	

Comments

Screen more frequently for persons with diabetes, those on long-term psychiatric medication, and those with syndromes associated with vision deficits/ocular abnormalities, such as Cornelia de Lange, Fragile X, Down, Smith-Magenis, tuberous sclerosis, and Velocardiofacial.[16]

Counseling

Lifestyle Modification/ Healthy Quality of Life	**Discuss:**	
	• Adequate calcium and vitamin D supplementation	
	• Dental hygiene	
	• Fall risk assessment and prevention	
	• Nutrition—Excellent resource is the Montana Disability & Health Program: Nutrition for Individuals with Intellectual or Developmental Disabilities, http://mtdh.ruralinstitute.umt.edu/?page_id=813	
	• Physical activity (regular schedule with structured staff training to support & reinforce)[10]	
	• Tobacco and substance abuse cessation	
	• Sexual health, including: contraception, sexually transmitted infection prevention, and healthy relationships	

Comments

Critical to include caregivers, health advocates, and parents/family members to help reinforce teaching concepts.

Advanced directives & end-of-life planning	• Schedule dedicated time for discussion with the individual and support team	
	• Excellent resource: Thinking Ahead Matters (End-of-Life Planning for People with DD, http://coalitionccc.org/tools-resources/people-with-developmental-disabilities/	
Medication Review	• Review medications at regular intervals with patients and caregivers to ensure adherence with regimen and evaluate for side effects and drug interactions.	

Comments

High rates of polypharmacy exist. See medication watch list: http://odpc.ucsf.edu/sites/odpc.ucsf.edu/files/pdf_docs/MedFest-Medical-Watch-List.pdf

TABLE 38-1 Healthcare Maintenance Guidelines for Adults with Developmental Disabilities *(Continued)*

Health Problem	Who to Screen	Test & Frequency	Special Considerations
Safety		• Review safety practices per individual circumstance, such as stranger and street safety for patients who live independently; prevention of head trauma in patients with frequent seizures; and street safety for patients with unpredictable behavior.	

©2015 Geraldine Collins-Bride, MS, ANP, FAAN. Non-commercial use with attribution is permitted.

References

1. American Academy of Pediatrics Committee on Sports Medicine and Fitness. (1995). Atlantoaxial instability in Down syndrome: Subject review. *Pediatrics. 96*, 151–154.

2. Bull, M. J., & the Committee on Genetics. (2011). Clinical report—Health supervision for children with Down syndrome. *Pediatrics, 128*(2), 393–406.

3. Carmeli, E., & Imam, B. (2014). Health promotion and disease prevention strategies in older adults with intellectual and developmental disabilities. *Frontiers in Public Health, 2*, 31. doi: 10.3389/fpubh.2014.00031.

4. Centers for Disease Control and Prevention. (2015). Immunization recommendations. Retrieved from www.cdc.gov/vaccines/schedules /index.html.

5. Centers for Disease Control and Prevention. (2014).Recommendations for the Laboratory-Based Detection of *Chlamydia trachomatis* and *Neisseria gonorrhea*, MMWR March 14, 2014. Retrieved from www.cdc.gov/mmwr/preview/mmwrhtml/rr6302a1.htm.

6. Cohen, W. I. (Ed.). (1999). *Health care guidelines for individuals with Down syndrome: 1999 revision*. Down Syndrome Research Foundation.

7. Fletcher, R., Loschen, E., Stavrakaki, C., & First, M. (Eds.). (2007). *Diagnostic manual—Intellectual disability: A textbook of diagnosis of mental disorders in persons with intellectual disability*. Kingston, NY: NADD Press. *This was published by the National Association for Dual Diagnosis and the American Psychiatric Association.*

8. James, P. A., Oparil, S., Carter, B. L., Cushman, W. C., Dennison-Himmelfarb, C., Handler, J., et al. (2013). 2014 evidence-based guideline for the management of high blood pressure in adults: Report from the panel members appointed to the Eighth Joint National Committee (JNC 8). *JAMA, 1097*, 1–14.

9. Marinho, V. C., Worthington, H. V., Walsh, T., & Clarkson, J. E. (2013). Fluoride varnishes for preventing dental caries in children and adolescents. *Cochrane Database of Systematic Reviews, 7*, CD002279.

10. Marks, B., Sisirak, J., & Chang, Y. C. (2013). Efficacy of the HealthMatters program train-the-trainer model. *Journal of Applied Research in Intellectual Disabilities, 26*(4), 319–334.

11. Massachusetts Department of Developmental Services. (2012). Preventive health recommendations for adults with intellectual disability. Retrieved from www.mass.gov/eohhs/docs/dmr /reports/health-screening-brochure.pdf.

12. Petrone, L. R. (2012). Osteoporosis in adults with intellectual disabilities. *Southern Medical Journal, 105*(2), 87–92.

13. Pezzoni, V., & Kouimtsidis, C. (2015). Screening for alcohol misuse within people attending intellectual disability community service. *Journal of Intellectual Disability Research, 59*(4), 353–359.

14. Prasher, V., & Janicki, M. (Eds.). (2002). *Physical health of adults with intellectual disabilities (International Association for the Scientific Study of Intellectual Disabilities)*. Oxford, UK: Blackwell Publishing.

15. Sawaya, G., Kulasingam, S., Denberg, T., & Quaseem, A. (2015). Cervical cancer screening in average-risk women: Best practice advice from the Clinical Guidelines Committee of the American College of Physicians. *Annals of Internal Medicine, 162*(12), 851–860.

16. Sullivan, W. F., Berg, J. M., Bradley, E., Cheetham, T., Denton, R., Heng, J., et al. (2011). Primary care of adults with developmental disabilities: Canadian consensus guidelines for primary health care of adults with developmental disabilities. *Canadian Family Physician, 57*, 541–553.

17. U.S. Preventive Services Task Force. (2014). Guide to clinical preventative services. U.S. Department of Health and Human Services. Retrieved from www.ahrq.gov/professionals/clinicians -providers/guidelines-recommendations/guide/index.html.

18. Walter, L. C., & Schonberg, M. A. (2014). Screening mammography in older women: A review. *JAMA, 311*(13), 1336–1347. doi:10.1001/ jama.2014.2834

19. Wilkinson, J. E., & Cerreto, M. C. (2008). Primary care for women with intellectual disabilities. *Journal of the American Board of Family Medicine, 21*(3), 215–s22.

20. Wilkinson, J. E., Culpepper, L., & Cerreto, M. (2007). Screening tests for adults with intellectual disabilities. *Journal of the American Board of Family Medicine, 4*, 399–407.

c. Consulting with a dentist regarding fluoride varnishes, rinses, and chlorhexidine rinses (National Institute of Dental and Craniofacial Research, 2009)

C. Patient education

1. Primary focus should be on developing a trusting relationship with the patient and caregivers (**Figure 38-4**).

2. Provide lifestyle modification counseling to promote a healthy and happy quality of life (Table 38-1, counseling section).

3. Provide information on community resources to support patients, caregivers, and families.

4. Review safety practices for prevention of accidents and victimization.

V. Self-management resources and tools

A. Healthcare provider resources

1. Office of Developmental Primary Care, University of California, Department of Family & Community Medicine, http://odpc.ucsf.edu

2. Health care for Adults with Intellectual and Developmental Disabilities: Toolkit for Primary Care Providers, http://vkc.mc.vanderbilt.edu/etoolkit/

3. Society for the Study of Behavioural Phenotypes (information on specific genetic syndromes and specific health risks), www.ssbp.org.uk/syndromes .html

---

FIGURE 38-4 Communicating with Patients with Developmental Disabilities

Person-first language was developed by disability advocates to educate the community at large. It emphasizes the individual before the disability. For example, "Tom has Down syndrome." Some people, especially those in the autistic, blind, and deaf communities, view their disability as an integral part of who they are. They may use identity-first language such as "autistic man" or "blind person." Language evolves and the disability community is diverse. It is always appropriate to inquire about and use the language your patient prefers.

Avoid describing people with disabilities as overly courageous, brave, or special merely for having a disability. It is not unusual for people with disabilities to accomplish significant things and participate in and manage activities of daily living despite functional limitations. It is always appropriate to celebrate the achievement of personal goals and milestones.

Also, avoid describing people with disabilities as overly pitiful and unfortunate. Most people with disabilities do not consider their lives tragic. They rate their quality of life far higher than many nondisabled people estimate.

Likewise, don't assume that people are unhappy or heroic simply because they are caring for a relative or friend who has a disability. It is helpful to inquire what challenges they face and assistance they need. Most caregivers appreciate empathy and assistance if they struggle with discrimination or lack of respite and accommodation.

Instead of...	Use ...
Afflicted with ... suffers from ...	She has Down syndrome
Confined to a wheelchair/wheelchair-bound	Uses a wheelchair
Caretaker	Caregiver, or person who cares for, advocates for, or serves people ...
Handicapped parking	Accessible parking
Mentally retarded	Person with an intellectual disability
"Normal" or "healthy"	Nondisabled/typical/neurotypical

Used with permission from the Office of Developmental Primary Care, Department of Family & Community Medicine, University of California, San Francisco.

4. Health assessment forms, yearly health checks, and other information, www.cddh.monash.org/disability -health-assessment.html

5. AASPIRE Healthcare Toolkit: Primary Care Resources for Adults on the Autism Spectrum and Their Primary Care Providers, http://autismandhealth.org/

6. American Academy of Developmental Medicine and Dentistry: resources for clinicians and students on neurodevelopmental disorders and health care for adults with DDs, www.aadmd.org

7. Developmental Disability Nurses Association (resources for healthcare providers and families), www.ddna.org

8. Coalition for Compassionate Care of California: Addressing the needs of the intellectual and developmentally disabled community when preparing for the end of life, http://coalitionccc.org/tools -resources/people-with-developmental-disabilities/

B. Patient and caregiver resources

1. State of California Regional Center System, www.dds .ca.gov/RC/Home.cfm

2. Support for Families, www.supportforfamilies.org

3. Family Voices, www.familyvoices.org
   Always presume competence. This means assume that all people deserve dignity, privacy, autonomy, access, and respect. Assume all people have the potential to learn. Do not assume that someone who doesn't speak cannot understand. Assume all people communicate, all lives are meaningful and valuable and all people can learn, grow, and benefit from inclusion and opportunity. Speak directly to patients in a normal, adult tone of voice. Offer accommodations to help, but ask before assisting.

   Not all disabilities are visible and many people develop skills or find ways to accommodate their disabilities that make them less apparent to others. However, this does not mean that those individuals do not have significant challenges.

REFERENCES

Academic Autistic Spectrum Partnership in Research and Education. (2015). *AASPIRE healthcare toolkit: Primary care resources for adults on the autism spectrum and their primary care providers.* Retrieved from www.autismandhealth.org/.

American Academy of Pediatrics, American Academy of Family Physicians, & American College of Physicians. (2011). Supporting the health care transition from adolescence to adulthood in the medical home. *Pediatrics, 128*(1), 182–200. Retrieved from http://pediatrics .aappublications.org .

American Association on Intellectual and Developmental Disabilities. (2010). *Definition of intellectual disability.* Retrieved from www.aamr .org/content_100.cfm?navID=21.

Anderson, L. L., Humphries, K., McDermot, S., Marks, B., Sisirak, J., & Larson, S. (2013). The state of the science of health and wellness for adults with intellectual and developmental disabilities. *Intellectual and Developmental Disabilities, 51*(5), 385–398.

Andresen, E. M., Peterson-Besse, J. J., Krahn, G. L., Walsh, E. S., Horner-Johnson, W., & Iezzoni, L. I. (2013). Pap, mammography, and clinical breast examination screening among women with disabilities: A systematic review. *Women's Health Issues, 23*(4), e205–e214.

Autistic Self Advocacy Network, Office of Developmental Primary Care. (2014). *Our lives, our health care: Self-advocates speaking out about our experiences with the medical system.* Retrieved from http://odpc .ucsf.edu/sites/odpc.ucsf.edu/files/pdf_docs/Our%20Lives%20 Our%20Health%20Care%20Final_0.pdf.

Coppus, A. M. (2013). People with intellectual disability: What do we know about adulthood and life expectancy? *Developmental Disabilities Research Reviews, 18*(1), 6–16.

Developmental Disabilities Assistance and Bill of Rights Act of 2000. Public Law 106-402. Retrieved from www.acl.gov/Programs/AIDD /DDA_BOR_ACT_2000/Index.aspx.

Feldman, M. A., Bossett, J., Collet, C., & Burnham-Riosa P. (2014). Where are persons with intellectual disabilities in medical research? A survey of published clinical trials. *Journal of Intellectual Disability Research, 58*(9), 800–809.

Frisch, D., & Msall, M. E. (2013). Health, functioning, and participation of adolescents and adults with cerebral palsy: A review of outcomes research. *Developmental Disabilities Research Reviews, 18*(1), 84–94.

Horner-Johnson, W., Dobbertin, K., & Lee, J. (2013). Disparities in chronic conditions and health status by type of disability. *Disability and Health Journal, 6*(4), 280–286.

Hwang, Y. S., & Kearney, P. (2013). A systematic review of mindfulness intervention for individuals with developmental disabilities: Long-term practice and long lasting effects. *Research in Developmental Disabilities, 34*(1), 314–326.

Kerr, S., Lawrence, M., Darbyshire, C., Middleton, A. R., & Fitzsimmons L. (2013). Tobacco and alcohol-related interventions for people with mild/moderate intellectual disabilities: A systematic review of the literature. *Journal of Intellectual Disability Research, 57*(5), 393–408.

Kripke C. C. (2014). Primary care for adolescents with developmental disabilities. *Primary Care, 41*(3), 507–518.

Marinho, V. C., Worthington, H. V., Walsh, T., & Clarkson, J. E. (2013). Fluoride varnishes for preventing dental caries in children and adolescents. *Cochrane Database of Systematic Reviews, 7*, CD002279.

National Institute of Dental and Craniofacial Research. (2009). *Practical oral care for people with intellectual disability.* Bethesda, MD: National Institutes of Research. Retrieved from www .nidcr.nih.gov/oralhealth/Topics/DevelopmentalDisabilities /PracticalOralCarePeopleIntellectualDisability.htm.

Nicolaidis, C., Kripke, C., & Raymaker, D. (2014). Primary care for adults on the autism spectrum. *Medical Clinics of North America, 98*(5), 1169–1191.

Office of Developmental Primary Care. (n.d.). *Interdisciplinary healthcare team chart.* Retrieved from http://odpc.ucsf.edu/odpc/html/for _clinicians/charts_forms_c.htm.

Parker, S. E., Mai, C. T., Canfield, M. A., Rickard, R., Wang, Y., Meyer, R. E., et al. (2010). Updated national birth prevalence estimates for selected birth defects in the United States, 2004–2006. *Birth Defects Research. Part A, Clinical and Molecular Teratology, 88*(12), 1008–1016.

Peterson, M. D., Gordon, P. M., & Hurvitz, E. A. (2013). Chronic disease risk among adults with cerebral palsy: The role of premature sarcopoenia, obesity and sedentary behavior. *Obesity Reviews, 14*(2), 171–182.

Robertson, J., Hatton, C., Emerson, E., & Baines, S. (2014). The impact of health checks for people with intellectual disabilities: An updated systematic review of evidence. *Research in Developmental Disabilities, 35*(10), 2450–2462.

Ross, W. T., & Olsen, M. (2014). Care of the adult patient with Down syndrome. *Southern Medical Journal, 107*(11), 715–721.

Sobey, D., & Doe, T. (1991). Patterns of sexual abuse and assalt. *Sexuality and Disability, 9*(3), 243–259.

Sullivan, W. F., Berg, J. M., Bradley, E., Cheetham, T., Denton, R., Heng, J., et al. (2011). Primary care of adults with developmental disabilities: Canadian consensus guidelines. *Canadian Family Physician, 57,* 541–553.

Svien, L. R., Berg, P., & Stephenson, C. (2008). Issues in aging with cerebral palsy. *Topics in Geriatric Rehabilitation, 24*(1), 26–40.

United Cerebral Palsy. (2011). United Cerebral Palsy organization. Retrieved from www.ucp.org.

Vanderbilt Kennedy Center for Excellence in Developmental Disabilities. (n.d.). *Healthcare for adults with intellectual and developmental disabilities: Toolkit for primary care providers.* Nashville, TN: Vanderbilt University. Retrieved from http://vkc.mc.vanderbilt.edu/etoolkit/.

Yeargin-Allsopp, M. (2010, March 12). *Trends in the epidemiology of cerebral palsy.* Keynote lecture at the Annual Update on Developmental Disabilities Conference at University of California, San Francisco, San Francisco, California.

Yin Foo, R., Guppy, M., & Johnston, L. M. (2013). Intelligence assessments for children with cerebral palsy: A systematic review. *Developmental Medicine and Child Neurology, 55*(10), 911–918.

HEALTHCARE MAINTENANCE FOR TRANSGENDER INDIVIDUALS

Melissa Wong and Kathryn Wyckoff

I. Introduction and general background

Transgender people living in the United States are a marginalized and medically underserved community. Compared to 62% of the general population, only 40% of transgender individuals who are employed have access to employer-based insurance. Unemployment rates among transgender people are twice the national average, and 27% report annual incomes of less than $20,000 (National Gay and Lesbian Taskforce, 2009). Social stigmatization affects access to work, poverty contributes to housing instability, and institutional barriers make accessing health care difficult, if not impossible, for many transgender patients. In fact, 30–40% of transgender persons in the United States rely on urgent care and emergency departments for their immediate healthcare needs (Feldman & Bockting, 2003). Those who do access care report difficulties finding compassionate providers with transgender health experience (Sanchez, Sanchez, & Danoff, 2009). Nearly a third of transgender patients surveyed in multiple studies report discrimination, hostility, and outright refusal of medical care, resulting in a reluctance to seek routine and even urgent care (Herbst et al., 2008; Minter & Daley, 2003). As a result, the rates of preventable illnesses, such as HIV, are higher in the transgender community than in any other population (Centers for Disease Control and Prevention, 2015). However, it has been demonstrated that routine medical care focusing on healthcare maintenance for transgender individuals can be delivered in the primary care setting safely and compassionately, without the need for specialty or psychiatric referrals (Davidson et al., 2013).

A. Transgender identity

1. Definition and overview

    Data collection and epidemiologic estimates concerning the transgender community in the United States have been challenging because of lack of inclusive survey or data collection forms, lack of reliability due to fear of stigma or discrimination from self-identification and overgeneralization of the term "transgender." Four of the nation's largest, most comprehensive population-based surveys collected data on sexual orientation but failed to explicitly measure gender identity outside of male or female (Gates, 2014). Worldwide data suggest 1 in 30,000 people identify as transwoman (MTF) and 1 in 100,000 people as transman (FTM) (Center of Excellence for Transgender Health, 2014). These numbers, however, are likely underestimated. As data collection methods become more inclusive, these ratios will decrease.

    The terms "transgender" or "trans" are broadly used terms to describe people whose gender identities, expression, and behaviors differ from their birth sex, irrespective of their physical appearance or sexual orientation (Feldman & Bockting, 2003; Kenagy, 2005). Included in the *Diagnostic and Statistical Manual of Mental Disorders* (DSM) as of 1980, the term gender identity disorder has been reclassified as gender dysphoria in the current DSM-V guidelines. Labeling transgender patients with a mental disorder can be controversial and might be offensive to some individuals. For transgender patients who have concerns with the gender dysphoria diagnosis, an alternative diagnosis of endocrine disorder NOS is appropriate. However, a clinical diagnosis is often necessary to receive insurance coverage for hormone therapy and/or surgical procedures. It is important to recognize that gender is seen by many as more than a binary concept. **Figure 39-1** is a graphic representation of the spectrum of gender identity and expression.

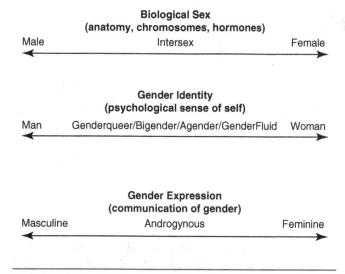

FIGURE 39-1 The Spectrum of Gender Identity and Expression

Modified from Center for Gender Sanity. (2009).

2. Definitions

Male-to-female (MTF): transwoman, persons who were assigned male at birth who identify as female

Female-to-male (FTM): transman, persons who were assigned female at birth who identify as male

Gender-variant, bigendered, or gender-queer, gender nonconforming, agender, gender-fluid: individuals who may be biologic males, females, or intersex individuals who choose to identify as both or neither male or female or somewhere in between the conventional male and female categories.

Cisgender men/woman: individuals whose gender expression is congruent with sex assigned at birth.

II. Database (may include but is not limited to)

A. Subjective

**Always use a transgender patient's chosen name and preferred pronoun (Appendix 39-A).*

1. Pertinent past medical history, as outlined in the chapter Healthcare Maintenance of the Adult and Older Adult with focus on the following additional data:

    a. Previous medical illnesses, with emphasis on a history of coronary disease and/or thromboembolic events

    b. Sexually transmitted infection (STI) history and HIV status, including date of last screening tests

    c. Surgeries, with emphasis on any feminization or masculinization procedures, such as breast augmentation (for MTFs) or mastectomy (for FTMs). Other surgeries include facial feminization and tracheal shaving (MTF) and sexual reassignment surgeries, such as metoidioplasty and phalloplasty (FTM) and vaginoplasty (MTF).

    d. Cosmetic procedures, including those done by nonlicensed laypersons, such as silicone injections

    e. Previous psychiatric hospitalizations and/or any suicide attempts

    f. Medications, with emphasis on hormonal therapy, including names of medications, dosage, route, and source (i.e., Internet, Mexico, buying from friends, and so forth)

    g. Immunization status, with emphasis on hepatitis A, B, and human papillomavirus (HPV) vaccines

    h. Hepatitis C risk factors and antibody status

    i. History of injuries, with emphasis on screening for abuse and intimate partner violence

2. Family history, with emphasis on cardiovascular disease and cardiac risk factors

3. Occupational history: screen for paid sex work and source of income to appropriately identify risk factors and need for support

4. Personal and social history including:

    a. Legal status of name and gender identity (important for billing and documentation)

    b. Citizenship/immigration status

    c. History of alcohol, tobacco, and drug use

    d. History of depression, anxiety, bipolar disorder, trauma, or suicidal ideation or attempts

    e. Relationships and social support network, intimate partner violence screening, social issues (being out at work/school/or to family).

    f. Housing status

    g. Future goals for feminization or masculinization, such as gender reassignment (or gender affirmation) surgery, hormone therapy, or neither. Some transgender patients may choose not to have surgery or take hormones, so it is important to establish each patient's goal.

    h. Successes and failures with gender reassignment, including issues currently concerning the patient about appearance and any issues being out to family, classmates, coworkers, etc.

B. Objective

Physical examination may be deferred until strong clinician–patient relationship is established, unless review of symptoms warrants immediate examination. The patient should be prepared for the need for a physical examination in advance and given an opportunity to discuss feelings about being examined. Guidelines suggest implementing physical exams, screening and healthcare maintenance needs based on the anatomy that is present, regardless of patient's self-identification (Center of Excellence for Transgender Health, 2014).

1. Genital, rectal, and breast/chest examinations may cause particular distress for patients. Discuss with the patient in advance the rationale for the examination and ascertain how the patient would like one to refer to their anatomy (i.e., genitals, instead of penis or vagina, chest instead of breasts).

2. For patients who have had gender reassignment surgery, the clinician must become familiar with the particular surgical technique used and screen for applicable complications.

3. For patients who have had silicone injections, the clinician should carefully examine the patient for signs of cellulitis or tissue deformity.

4. Thyroid physical examination and lab values, as cross-sex hormone use may cause endocrine imbalances.

III. Assessment

A. The current risk factors and health status of the patient should be identified, the patient's motivation to change unhealthy habits should be assessed, and the patient's ability to successfully accomplish adult developmental milestones should be determined as outlined in the chapter Healthcare Maintenance of the Adult.

B. Identify the patient's gender reassignment goals and barriers to the goals.

Assess for benefits of hormonal gender reassignment therapy and undesirable side effects, such as weight gain and increased cardiovascular risk.

C. Identify psychosocial needs of the patient.

IV. Plan

A. Diagnostics (screening and secondary prevention tests)

1. Screen for diseases and conditions based on the patient's risk profile. Note that normal laboratory values are often gender specific. There are no established guidelines for determining normal laboratory values for transgender patients, but the general rule is to use the biologic gender-normal values until 2 years of hormone therapy have been completed, then use the normal values of the assigned gender (Feldman & Goldberg, 2007).

2. Similar healthcare maintenance and screening needs as general populations. **Table 39-1** outlines healthcare maintenance guidelines and special considerations for MTF and FTM trans patients (Center of Excellence for Transgender Health, 2014).

B. Treatment

1. Immunization recommendations are not sex specific. Follow general guidelines but transgender patients who have sex with cisgender men may benefit from hepatitis A and meningococcal vaccines (Center of Excellence for Transgender Health, 2014).

2. For prescribing/furnishing/drug ordering guidelines for hormonal therapy, see **Tables 39-2** and **39-3**. Use the appropriate drug interaction database when prescribing hormone therapy to avoid adverse drug interactions, especially for patients taking HIV antiretroviral, antidepressant, and anticonvulsant medications.

3. Discuss fertility issues and childbearing plans with any patient considering hormonal therapy as cross-sex hormones may interfere with fertility (Center of Excellence for Transgender Health, 2014).

   Figure 39-2 can be used as a starting point to identify appropriate feminizing therapies based on patient goals. **Figure 39-3** outlines goals of masculinizing therapies. Note that the use of hormones for gender reassignment is off label and the provider should obtain informed consent before initiating therapy.

4. **MTF patients:** Most MTF patients can be successfully transitioned with the use of estrogen and spironolactone alone. Progesterone can also be used;

TABLE 39-1 Healthcare Maintenance Guidelines for the Transgender Patient

MTF	FTM
Prostate cancer (CA) screening per general population (prostate-specific antigen can be low, use digital rectal exam if necessary to evaluate based on review of systems)	Cervical CA screening per general population with the following considerations:
Breast CA screening by mammography in presence of other risk factors (estrogen/progestin use > 5 yrs, family history, body mass index ≥ 35)	*if patient has had total hysterectomy and has prior hx of high-grade cervical dysplasia → do pap of vaginal cuff until 3 normal, then q 2–3 yrs*
Pap smears not required if patient has neovagina but do visual inspection to look for genital warts or other lesions.	*if patient has had ovaries removed but uterus/cervix is intact, follow guidelines for biologic females*
Blood pressure (BP) screening prior to hormone initiation with pretestosterone goal of < 130/90 mm Hg then q 1–3 month monitoring	*note that vaginal atrophy from testosterone use can mimic dysplasia*
Annual fasting lipid panel with low-density lipoprotein goal of < 135 mg/dL or < 96 mg/dL in high-risk patients	Uterine Cancer:
Consider liver function tests (LFTs) if on hormones AND higher risk (increased alcohol use, weight gain, or at risk for hep C)	*evaluate all spontaneous vaginal bleeding that cannot be explained by missed or changes in hormone dosing*
Sexual health screening at every visit. Based on sexual practices and may include HIV and sexually transmitted infection testing, hepatitis B & C screening and prevention.	Annual chest wall/axillary exam
Screen for depression/suicidality at every visit	Complete blood count, LFTs every 6 months when on hormone therapy
	Screen for depression/suicidality at every visit

however, it may not be as effective as spironolactone in suppressing testosterone (Gooren & Tangpricha, 2015). **Table 39-4** outlines clinical considerations to estrogen use. Always limit estrogen to one type and use the lowest effective dose. Baseline labs for the MTF patient considering feminizing hormone therapy should include fasting lipids and glucose levels and creatinine and potassium levels in patients considering spironolactone. Recheck laboratory tests after 3 months of therapy or after dose increases and then after 1 year on a stable dose. Some providers may elect to check labs at baseline, 3 months, 6 months, and then 1 year. Monitoring prolactin levels is important, as levels can increase with the use of estradiol. Check LFTs after 1 year of therapy if patient has liver disease risks. Consider adding additional antiandrogen drugs if beard growth is not adequately suppressed or if patient becomes hypotensive on spironolactone. Finasteride may also be used to help prevent male pattern baldness. Checking testosterone levels can help with titration of antiandrogen medications. Orally dosed estrogen should be avoided in patients over 40 years old or with cardiovascular/thromboembolic risks. Patients who have had an orchiectomy or gender

reassignment surgery require only estrogen to maintain a feminine appearance.

5. **FTM patients:** Most FTM patients can be successfully transitioned with the use of testosterone alone. Baseline labs for the FTM patient considering masculinizing hormone therapy should include a complete blood count, complete metabolic profile, and fasting lipids. Check a trough level of testosterone the day before the next injection is due to determine the testosterone level at its lowest. Recheck laboratory tests after 3 months of therapy or after dose increases and then 1 year after starting. *Patients should be educated that it takes approximately 2 years to transition regardless of the dosage of hormone.* Increasing the dose of hormone therapy will not hasten the transitioning process. Discuss contraceptive use in FTM patients having receptive vaginal sex with male partners as testosterone does not reduce fertility and advise patients that it may take up to 6 months for menses to cease once on testosterone therapy. Testosterone dose should not necessarily be reduced after hysterectomy or sex reassignment surgery. Testosterone therapy should be continued even after maximum masculinization for osteoporosis protection.

TABLE 39-2 Feminizing Hormone Options

Estrogen Preparations	Dosage	Precautions	Contraindications	Interactions
Estradiol	Starting: 2–3 mg daily Typical: 4 mg daily Max: 8 mg daily	Deep venous thrombosis, pulmonary embolism, other thromboembolism, thrombophlebitis, hypertension, impotence, prolactinoma, diabetes, nausea or vomiting, migraine or headache, gallbladder disease, abnormal liver function tests, mood disorder or depression, melasma (skin darkening), acne, lipid abnormalities, hypertriglyceridemia, increased risk of heart attack, increased risk of breast cancer, hepatitis, stroke, or other cancers	**Individualize treatment decision based on risk and benefit** Presence of estrogen-dependent cancer **Caution with:** history of thromboembolism or severe thrombophlebitis, tobacco smoking, seizure disorder, CAD, DM, CHF	CYP 3A4, 1A2 inhibitors/inducers
Conjugated	Starting: 1.25–2.5 mg daily			
Equine Estrogens (Premarin®)	Typical: 5 mg daily Max: 10 mg daily			
Estradiol Valerate (Delestrogen)	Starting: 20–40 mg IM/Q2 wk Typical: 40 mg IM/Q2 wk Max: 40–80 mg IM/Q2 wk			
Estradiol Patch (Climara®, Estraderm®, Alora®, Vivelle®)	Starting 0.1 mg/24 hr Typical: 5 mg daily Max: 10 mg daily			

Antiandrogens	Dosage	Precautions	Contraindications/ Considerations	Interactions
Spironolactone	Starting: 25–50 mg BID Typical: 50 mg BID Max: 200 mg BID	Hyperkalemia and other electrolyte imbalances, impotence, mild diuresis	Renal insufficiency Potassium > 5.5	Digoxin, angiotensin-converting enzyme inhibitor, angiotensin receptor blocker, K-sparing diuretics
Finasteride	Starting: 1 mg daily Max: 5–10 mg daily	Metabolized in the liver—use with caution in patients with liver abnormalities	Good alternative for patients who cannot tolerate spironolactone	
GnRH Agonists (Nafarelin, Goserelin Leuprorelin)	Refer to Hembree et al. (2009) for dosing recommendations		Recommended treatment for the adolescent trans patient as pubertal development will be thwarted, but results are fully reversible (Hembree et al., 2009). Another advantage is the lack of thromboembolic risks	
Progesterone	Typical: 5–10 mg daily		Suppresses gonadotropin and testosterone secretion. Less effective than spironolactone.	

Modified from *Tom Waddell Health Center protocols for hormonal reassignment of gender*. (2013).

TABLE 39-3 Masculinizing Hormone Options

Testosterone Preparations	Dosage	Precautions	Contraindications	Interactions
Testosterone Cypionate	Starting: 50–100 mg IM Q2 wk or 25–50 mg/wk Typical: 200 mg Q2 wk Max: 400 mg Q2 wk	Increased BP, erythrocytosis, abnormal hepatic enzymes, dyslipidemia, increased aggressiveness, skin irritation with patch or gels *Allergy warning— injectable testosterone may be in base of cottonseed, sesame, or peanut oils	**Absolute:** Pregnancy, h/o testosterone responsive cancers **Caution with:** erythrocytosis, cardiac, hepatic, renal, or vascular disease with edema, sleep apnea d/t obesity, dyslipidemia, chronic lung disease.	Warfarin Cyclosporine Insulin
Testosterone Patch (Androderm®) Testosterone Gel 1% (Androgel®)	Starting: 2–2.5 mg/24 hr Typical: 5 mg/24 hr Max: 7.5 mg /24 hr Starting: 2.5 mg Q am Typical: 5 mg Q am Max: 10 mg Q am			

Modified from *Tom Waddell Health Center protocols for hormonal reassignment of gender.* (2013).

FIGURE 39-2 Feminizing Therapy

Anti-Androgens	Estrogen
decreased facial/body hair, male pattern baldness	breast development
decreased libido	redistribution of body fat
decreased erections	softening of skin
mild breast growth	suppression of testosterone production
decreased BPH	shrinkage of testes
	decreased libido
Therapies: Spirololactone, finasteride, GnRH agonists	*Therapies: transdermal estrogen, estradiol valerate injection, conjugated equine estrogens*

FIGURE 39-3 Masculinizing Therapy

Androgens
changes/deepening of voice pitch
increased libido
increased muscle mass & strength
more hair growth on face, chest, extremities
cessation of menses
redistribution of body fat
clitoral enlargement
Therapies: Testosterone – intramuscular, transdermal

TABLE 39-4 Contraindications (Individualize Risk vs Benefit) of Estrogen Use

History of, or current thrombophlebitis, or venous thromboembolic disorders—pulmonary embolism, deep vein thrombosis
History of, or active arterial thromboembolic disease—myocardial infarction, cerebrovascular accident
Estrogen-dependent tumor
Hepatic dysfunction
Protein C or protein S antithrombin deficiency
Thrombophilic disorders

Data from Lexicomp. (2015); Center for Excellence for Transgender Health. (2016). *Feminizing medications for transgender clients.* Retrieved from http://transhealth.ucsf.edu/pdf/protocols/Sample_3_Feminizing%20 Medications.pdf; Vancouver Coastal Health Transgender Health Information Program. (2016). *Feminizing hormones.* Retrieved from http:// transhealth.vch.ca/medical-options/hormones/feminizing-hormones.

6. Particular emphasis should be placed on smoking cessation strategies for patients receiving estrogen therapy because of the increased risk of thromboembolus. Aspirin 81 mg may be added for cardiovascular protection.

7. Consider referring HIV-positive patients for care at a specialty clinic, unless the provider is trained in HIV/AIDS.

8. Consider a psychiatric or mental health referral for patients who have mental illnesses, such as depression. Routine referral for psychiatric care is not otherwise warranted and may alienate patients, but note that one or more psychosocial assessments is often a prerequisite for patients considering gender transition surgery.

C. Surgical Options

1. If patient is interested in surgical intervention, assess risks and benefits. Provide patient with surgical options and education. (See **Table 39-5** for common surgical options.)

TABLE 39-5 Surgical Options for the Transgender Patient

Male to Female (MTF)	Female to Male (FTM)
Breast Augmentation/Implants: saline or silicone implants to create larger, female-appearing breasts.	**Mastectomy:** Also called "top surgery," this is the removal of female breast tissue with alteration and reconstruction of surrounding area to create a male-appearing contoured chest
Facial Feminization: a range of aesthetic plastic surgery procedures that can augment proportions of a male face for more feminine facial features. May include brow lift, rhinoplasty, cheek implants, and lip augmentation.	**Hysterectomy:** removal of uterus and/or total removal of uterus and cervix
Thyroid chondroplasty (chondrolaryngoplasty): sometimes referred to as "tracheal shaving," this is the surgical reduction of the thyroid cartilage to reduce appearance of an "Adam's apple," associated with male characteristics.	**Salpingo-Oophorectomy:** removal of fallopian tubes and ovaries. This procedure results in irreversible infertility unless embryo banking has been done prior to surgery.
Orchiectomy: Surgical removal of testicles which results in reduced levels of testosterone in body. Results in irreversible infertility unless sperm banking done prior to surgery.	**Vaginectomy:** Removal of the vagina
Penectomy: Surgical removal of penis with relocation of urethral opening to allow for urination in sitting position.	**Colpocleisis:** Surgical closure of the vagina, often performed when patients choose metoidioplasty or phalloplasty procedures.
Vaginoplasty: Surgical creation of vaginal canal. Goal of surgery is to create a neovagina that has sensation and is wide enough and long enough for sexual penetration.	**Metoidioplasty:** Surgical creation of a phallus using existing genital tissue. Expected phallus size is smaller than average male penis but testosterone use for 2+ years prior to surgery may help add length to new phallus. Successful metoidioplasty results in some level of retained sensation and erectile capability.
Labiaplasty: Surgical creation of labia minora and majora using skin from existing penis and scrotum.	**Scrotoplasty:** Surgical creation of scrotum using existing tissue from genital area and testicular implants.
Clitoroplasty: Surgical creation of clitoris	**Phalloplasty:** Highly complex surgical construction of a penis using skin from abdomen, forearm, or inner thigh. Differs from metoidioplasty in that new phallus length is closer to average male penis and erections are possible only through permanently implanted rod or use of implanted pump.

*Note that patients may choose different levels of surgery and that many of the surgery options may be completed at the same time for optimal results. Refer to the San Francisco Department of Public Health Trans Health Services reference for more detail.

Modified from San Francisco Department of Public Health Transgender Health Services Resources.

2. The primary care provider can adequately manage hormone therapy and medications during the postoperative periods for patients who have undergone transition surgery (either in United States or abroad). Follow-up surgical care is managed by the surgeon.

3. Collaborate with mental health providers and other specialists to support patient during surgical process.

4. Advocate for patients seeking insurance approval for surgery.

D. Patient education

1. Primary focus should be on developing a trusting relationship with the patient and assisting the patient to overcome previous negative experiences with healthcare providers.

2. Provide health counseling with particular attention to HIV prevention.

3. Harm reduction as needed based on findings of subjective and objective assessments

4. Provide information on community resources, such as legal advice, housing assistance, and mental health counseling.

5. Periodic health counseling as outlined in the chapter Healthcare Maintenance of the Adult and Older Adult.

E. Self-management resources and tools

1. University of California, San Francisco's Center of Excellence for Transgender Health provides education, advocacy, and current research around transgender health needs for both trans individuals and providers (http://transhealth.ucsf.edu/).

2. Vancouver Coastal Health Clinic has excellent resources for both providers and patients on a variety of topics related to transgender health promotion, mental health, and other topics (www.transhealth.vch.ca)

3. World Professional Association for Transgender Health conducts academic research and development of evidence-based medicine for transsexual, transgender, and gender nonconforming individuals (www.wpath.org/).

4. Transgender Law Center advocates for individuals who have faced discrimination based on their gender identity of expression (http://transgenderlawcenter.org/).

5. National Center for Transgender Equality is an advocacy organization working to advance equality of transgender individuals (http://transequality.org/).

6. Project Health focuses on advocacy, education, and leadership for transgender health. They host a national online trans medical consultation service for healthcare providers (http://project-health.org).

7. *Trans Bodies, Trans Selves* (Erickson-Schroth, 2014) is a comprehensive book written by and for the transgender community. Trans patients and healthcare providers can benefit from the personal essays and practical overview of trans people's medical and psychosocial needs.

REFERENCES

Centers for Disease Control and Prevention. (2015). HIV among transgender people. Retrieved from www.cdc.gov/hiv/risk/transgender/index.html.

Center for Gender Sanity. (2009). Diagram of sex and gender. Retrieved from www.gendersanity.com/diagram.html.

Center of Excellence for Transgender Health. (2014). General prevention and screening. Retrieved from http://transhealth.ucsf.edu/trans?page=protocol-screening.

Davidson, A., Francivich, J., Freeman, M., Lin, R., Martinez, L., Monihan, M., et al. (2013). *Tom Waddell Health Center protocols for hormonal reassignment of gender.* Retrieved from https://www.sfdph.org/dph/comupg/oservices/medSvs/hlthCtrs/TransGendprotocols122006.pdf.

Erickson-Schroth, L. (Ed.). (2014). *Trans bodies, trans selves: A resource for the transgender community.* New York: Oxford University Press.

Feldman, J., & Bockting, W. (2003). Transgender health. *Minnesota Medicine, 86*(7), 25–32.

Feldman, J., & Goldberg, J. (2006). *Transgender primary medical care: Suggested guidelines for physicians in British Columbia.* Retrieved from http://lgbtqpn.ca/wp-content/uploads/woocommerce_uploads/2014/08/Guidelines-primarycare.pdf.

Feldman, J. L., & Goldberg, J. M. (2007). Transgender primary medical care. *International Journal of Transgenderism, 9*(3/4), 3–34.

Gates, G. J. (2014). *LGB/T demographics: Comparisons among population-based surveys.* Los Angeles, CA: Williams Institute, UCLA School of Law.

Gender Neutral Pronouns. (n.d.). Retrieved from http://forge-forward.org.

Gooren, L. J., & Tangpricha, V. (2015). Treatment of transsexualism. Up To Date. Retrieved from www.uptodate.com/contents/treatment-of-transsexualism.

Hembree, W., Cohen-Kettenis, P., Delemarre-van de Waal, H., Gooren, L., Meyer, W., Spack, N., et al. (2009, January 1). *Endocrine treatment of transsexual persons: An Endocrine Society clinical practice guideline.* Retrieved from https://www.endocrine.org/~/media/endosociety/Files/Publications/Clinical Practice Guidelines/Endocrine-Treatment-of-Transsexual-Persons.pdf.

Herbst, J. H., Jacobs, E. D., Finlayson, T. J., McKleroy, V. S., Neumann, M. S., & Crepaz, N. (2008). Estimating HIV prevalence and risk behaviors of transgender persons in the United States: A systematic review. *AIDS and Behavior, 12*(1), 1–17.

Kenagy, G. P. (2005). Transgender health: Findings from two needs assessment studies in Philadelphia. *Health & Social Work, 30*(1), 19–26.

Lombardi, E. (2001). Enhancing transgender health care. *American Journal of Public Health, 91*(6), 869–872.

Minter, S., & Daley, C. (2003). *Trans realities: A legal needs assessment of San Francisco's transgender communities*. San Francisco, CA: Transgender Law Center and National Center for Lesbian Rights.

National Gay and Lesbian Taskforce. (2009). National transgender discrimination survey: Preliminary findings. Retrieved from www.thetaskforce.org/downloads/reports/fact_sheets/transsurvey_prelim_findings.pdf.

San Francisco Department of Public Health. (n.d.). Transgender health services. Retrieved from https://www.sfdph.org/dph/comupg/oprograms/THS/procedures.asp.

Sanchez, N. F., Sanchez, J. P., & Danoff, A. (2009). Health care utilization, barriers to care, and hormone usage among male-to-female transgender persons in New York City. *American Journal of Public Health, 99*(4), 713–719.

Sobralske, M. (2005). Primary care needs of patients who have undergone gender reassignment. *Journal of the American Academy of Nurse Practitioners, 17*(4), 133–138.

APPENDIX A:
A GUIDE TO COMMON GENDER-NEUTRAL PRONOUN CHOICES AMONG THE TRANS COMMUNITY

Subjective	Objective	Possessive Adjective	Possessive Pronoun	Reflexive
She	Her	Her	Hers	Herself
He	Him	His	His	Himself
Ze	Zim	Zir	Zirs	Zirself
Sie/Zie	Hir	Hir	Hirs	Hirself
Zie	Zir	Zir	Zirs	Zirself
Ey	Em	Eir	Eirs	Eirself
Per	Per	Pers	Pers	Persself
They	Them	Their	Theirs	Themself

Modified from Gender Neutral Pronouns (n.d.). Retrieved from http://forge-forward.org.

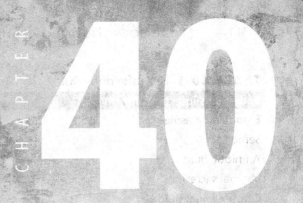

POSTEXPOSURE PROPHYLAXIS FOR HIV INFECTION

Barbara Newlin and Brooke Finkmoore

CHAPTER 40

I. Introduction and general background

Postexposure prophylaxis (PEP) for human immunodeficiency virus (HIV) infection is the use of antiretroviral (ARV) medications after an exposure to HIV has occurred in order to prevent infection with HIV. PEP is the term used when the exposure is occupational (occurs while a person is working at a job). When the exposure occurs at any other time (away from work), the prophylaxis is called nonoccupational postexposure prophylaxis (nPEP).

The advent of HIV infection in the 1980s brought with it widespread anxiety about the risks of infection in health care and other settings. As soon as antiretroviral medications were approved for use in HIV-infected individuals in the 1990s, the concept of using them in people with known exposures arose (PEP). There are an estimated 400,000 occupational exposures to HIV per year in the United States. By 2001, there were 57 confirmed and 138 possible HIV seroconversions caused by occupational exposures (Henderson, 2001).

Antiretrovirals have been used for occupational (PEP) and increasingly for nonoccupational exposures (nPEP). Empiric evidence about the effectiveness of PEP, however, is in short supply. The first attempted randomized trial of zidovudine monotherapy for PEP was closed early because of enrollment difficulties. The best evidence for efficacy is a Centers for Disease Control and Prevention case-control study that suggests 81% reduction in risk of HIV infection with use of zidovudine only (Cardo et al., 1997). Randomized controlled trials of PEP are not feasible, but experts agree that the concept of giving antiretroviral medication to arrest infection before it is able to take hold makes sense and that PEP should be offered to individuals with high-risk exposures to HIV. As such, organizations have developed comprehensive guidelines for the use of PEP (New York State Department of Health AIDS Institute, 2014; World Health Organization, 2005).

A. When should PEP be considered?

Best evidence suggests that the riskiest exposures to HIV occur when large amounts of infectious fluids (**Table 40-1**) are injected directly into the body or contacted by nonintact skin or mucous membranes. **Table 40-2** shows the risks of contracting HIV infection through various routes of exposure. The most recent guidelines from the United States Public Health Service (USPHS) eliminate the necessity to establish the level of risk in order to determine the number of drugs to use for PEP (Kuhar et al., 2013). The guidelines agree that any exposure of open skin or mucous membranes to probable HIV-infected blood, bloody body fluid, or other potentially infected materials warrants the initiation of three drug PEP. The testing of the source patient, recommended PEP regimen, and testing schedule for the infected health worker differ slightly between guidelines. **Table 40-3** is a summary of the differences between the USPHS and the New York State Department of Health (NYSDOH) AIDS Institute guidelines. The drugs recommended for PEP and nPEP have been chosen due to their proven effectiveness in HIV infection, ease of administration (most are once daily dosing), and lower incidence of and milder side effects. All HIV medications, however, have side effect risks and warrant strict adherence because of the danger of developing resistance if doses are skipped.

Special attention must be paid to the source patient's viral load and history of antiretroviral use. If the source has a high viral load and/or has taken or is on antiretrovirals, it is prudent to use HIV medications that the source has never taken for PEP. However, not all HIV medications are appropriate for PEP (**Table 40-4**). As such, all cases where PEP is recommended require expert consultation (see end of chapter for resources).

The guidelines agree that the timing of PEP is crucial. It must be started as soon as possible after exposure and within 72 hours in order to give the best chance for

375

TABLE 40-1 HIV Infectious Fluids

Body fluids infectious for HIV
Blood and plasma
Semen
Amniotic fluid
Vaginal secretions
Cerebrospinal fluid
Synovial fluid
Pleural fluid
Peritoneal fluid
Pericardial fluid
Body fluids noninfectious for HIV
Saliva
Tears
Sweat
Nonbloody urine or feces

Data from Medical Care Criteria Committee, New York State Department of Health AIDS Institute. (2008). HIV prophylaxis following occupational exposure. Retrieved from www.hivguidelnes.org.

TABLE 40-2 Risk of HIV Transmission by Exposure Route

Exposure Route	Risk Per 10,000 Exposures to an Infected Source
Blood transfusion	9,250
Needle-sharing injection-drug use	63
Receptive anal intercourse	138
Percutaneous needle stick	23
Receptive penile-vaginal intercourse	8
Insertive anal intercourse	11
Insertive penile-vaginal intercourse	4
Receptive oral intercourse	low
Insertive oral intercourse	low

Modified from Centers for Disease Control and Prevention. (2015). HIV risk behaviors. Retrieved from http://www.cdc.gov/hiv/risk/estimates/riskbehaviors.html

TABLE 40-3 Occupational Exposure to HIV: Comparison of NYSDOH and USPHS

NYSDOH AI Recommendations (2014)*	USPHS Recommendations (2013)†
Indication for PEP	**Indication for PEP**
Percutaneous or mucocutaneous exposure with blood or visibly bloody fluid or other potentially infectious material.	Percutaneous injury or contact of mucous membrane or nonintact skin with blood, tissue, or potentially infectious body fluids, such as semen, vaginal secretions, and visibly bloody fluids *and* reasonable suspicion that the source patient is HIV infected.
HIV Testing of the Source Patient	**HIV Testing of the Source Patient**
If HIV serostatus of the source is unknown, voluntary HIV testing of the source should be sought. Rapid testing is strongly recommended for the source patient, and for those organizations subject to Occupational Safety and Health Administration regulations, rapid testing of the source patient is mandated for occupational exposures. When the source patient's rapid test result is negative, and the clinician has ascertained that the source patient could have possibly been exposed to HIV in the previous 6 weeks, a plasma HIV RNA assay should be used in conjunction with the rapid HIV antibody test. In these situations, PEP should be initiated and continued until results of the plasma HIV RNA assay are available. In New York State, when the source patient has the capacity to consent to HIV testing, specific informed consent is required.	Although concerns have been expressed regarding HIV-negative sources being in the window period for seroconversion, no case of transmission involving an exposure source during the window period has been reported in the United States. Rapid HIV testing of source patients can facilitate making timely decisions regarding use of HIV PEP after occupational exposures to sources of unknown HIV status.

TABLE 40-3 Occupational Exposure to HIV: Comparison of NYSDOH and USPHS *(Continued)*

NYSDOH AI Recommendations (2014)*	USPHS Recommendations (2013)†
Recommendations for Number of Drugs in PEP Regimen	**Recommendations for Number of Drugs in PEP Regimen**
A three-drug PEP regimen is the preferred option for all significant-risk occupational exposures.	A regimen containing three (or more) antiretroviral drugs is recommended for all occupational exposures. Clinicians facing challenges associated with a three-drug regimen might consider a two-drug regimen in consultation with an expert.
Recommended PEP Regimen	**Recommended PEP Regimen**
Tenofovir 300 mg PO daily + Emtricitabine 200 mg PO daily *or* Lamivudine 300 mg PO daily plus Either Raltegravir 400 mg PO twice daily *or* Dolutegravir 50 mg PO daily	Tenofovir 300 mg PO daily + Emtricitabine 200 mg PO daily plus Raltegravir 400 mg PO twice daily
Duration of PEP: 4 weeks	**Duration of PEP:** 4 weeks
HIV Antibody Testing of Healthcare Worker • Baseline • 1 month postexposure • 3 months postexposure	**HIV Antibody Testing of Healthcare Worker** • Baseline • 6 weeks postexposure • 12 weeks postexposure • 6 months postexposure Alternatively, if the clinician is certain that a fourth-generation antibody/antigen combination assay is being used, then HIV testing could be performed at baseline, 6 weeks, and concluded at 4 months post exposure.
Timing of Initiation of PEP	**Timing of Initiation of PEP**
When a potential occupational exposure to HIV occurs, every effort should be made to initiate PEP as soon as possible, ideally within 2 hours. A first dose of PEP should be offered to the exposed worker while the evaluation is under way. In addition, PEP should not be delayed while awaiting information about the source or results of the exposed individual's baseline HIV test. Decisions regarding initiation of PEP beyond 36 hours post exposure should be made on a case-by-case basis with the understanding of diminished efficacy when timing of initiation is prolonged.	PEP should be initiated as soon as possible, preferably within hours of exposure. Initiation of PEP should not be delayed while awaiting the results of a source patient's HIV test, nor should it be delayed during consultation with experts to determine ideal PEP regimens.

*Reproduced from New York State Department of Health AIDS Institute. (2014). UPDATE: HIV Prophylaxis Following Occupational Exposure. Retrieved from www.hivguidelines.org.

†Kuhar, D. T., Henderson, D. K., Struble, K. A., Heneine, W., Thomas, V., Cheever, L. W., et al. (2013). Updated U.S. Public Health Service guidelines for the management of occupational exposures to HIV and recommendations for postexposure prophylaxis. *Infection Control and Hospital Epidemiology*, 34, 875–892. Retrieved from http://stacks.cdc.gov/view/cdc/20711.

infection to be halted before becoming established (Kuhar et al., 2013). The New York state guidelines encourage providers to seek expert advice before starting PEP if more than 36 hours have passed since the exposure (New York State Department of Health AIDS Institute, 2012). There is agreement that PEP should be continued for 28 days to maximize effectiveness (Kuhar et al., 2013; New York State Department of Health AIDS Institute, 2014; World Health Organization, 2005). The steps for evaluating and managing an occupational exposure to HIV are summarized by the New York Department of Health in **Figure 40-1**.

Nonoccupational postexposure prophylaxis (nPEP) for HIV has been used increasingly. **Figure 40-2** summarizes the evaluation and management of nPEP.

TABLE 40-4 Antiretroviral Drugs to Avoid as PEP Components

Drug(s) to Avoid	Rationale
Efavirenz (EFV)	• Poor adherence anticipated due to central nervous system (CNS) side effects, which are common • CNS side effects may impair work after the initial and subsequent doses • EFV should be avoided in first 6 weeks of pregnancy and in women of childbearing potential who are not using effective contraception • Substantial EFV resistance in community HIV isolates
Nevirapine	Contraindicated for use in PEP due to potential for severe hepatotoxicity
Abacavir	Potential for hypersensitivity reactions
Stavudine, didanosine	Possibility of toxicities
Nelfinavir, indinavir	Poorly tolerated
CCR5 coreceptor antagonists	Lack of activity against potential CXCR4 tropic virus

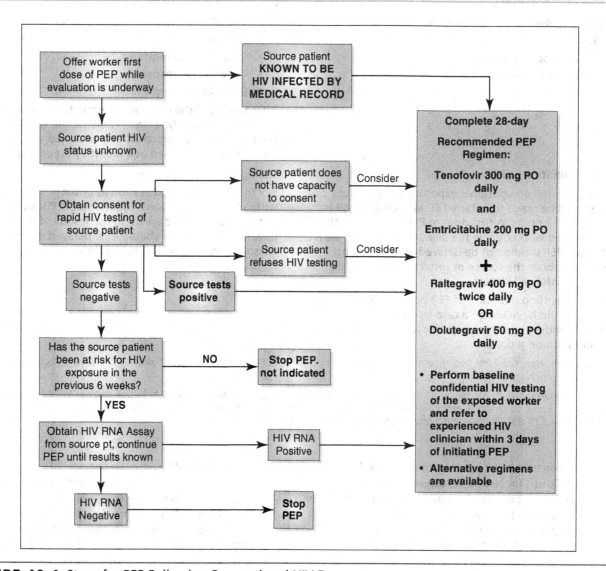

FIGURE 40-1 Steps for PEP Following Occupational HIV Exposure

Modified from New York State Department of Health AIDS Institute. (2015). UPDATE: HIV Prophylaxis Following Occupational Exposure. Retrieved from www.hivguidelines.org.

STEP 1: Evaluation of exposure: Is nPEP indicated?

LOWER-RISK EXPOSURES:
- Oral-vaginal contact (receptive and insertive)
- Oral-anal contact (receptive and insertive)
- Receptive penile-oral contact with or without ejaculation
- Insertive penile-oral contact with or without ejaculation

See Table 1 for factors that may increase risk. If PEP is indicated, go to Step 2.

HIGHER-RISK EXPOSURES:
- Receptive and insertive vaginal or anal intercourse with HIV+ or unknown source
- Needle sharing with HIV+ or unknown source
- Injuries with exposure to blood or other potentially infected fluids from HIV+ or unknown source (including needlesticks with a hollow-bore needle, human bites, accidents)

EXPOSURES THAT DO NOT WARRANT nPEP:
- Oral-to-oral contact without mucosal damage (kissing or mouth-to-mouth resuscitation)
- Human bites not involving blood
- Exposure to solid-bore needles or sharps not in recent contact with blood
- Mutual masturbation without skin breakdown or blood exposure

Provide risk-reduction counseling and offer HIV test.

STEP 2: Is patient presenting within 36 hours?

YES[a]

STEP 3: Initiate first dose of nPEP regimen

28-DAY REGIMEN — Recommended PEP Regimen:[b, c]

Tenofovir 300 mg PO qd + Emtricitabine[d] 200 mg PO qd
plus
Raltegravir[e] 400 mg PO bid or Dolutegravir[e] 50 mg PO qd

See Tables 4 and 5 for alternative regimens

STEP 4: Baseline testing

BASELINE TESTING OF EXPOSED PERSON:
- HIV test*
- Pregnancy test for women
- GC/CT NAAT (based on site of exposure)
- RPR for syphilis

*nPEP should not be continued in those who decline baseline HIV testing

See Section IX for hepatitis B and C post-exposure management.

+

SOURCE TESTING, *if source is available:*
- Obtain consent for HIV testing
- Obtain HIV test with turnaround time < 1 hour
- If the test results are not immediately available, continue exposed person's nPEP while awaiting results
- If the source person's HIV screening test result is negative but there may have been exposure to HIV in the previous 6 weeks, obtain plasma HIV RNA assay
- Continue exposed person's nPEP until results of the plasma HIV RNA assay are available

STEP 5: Provide risk-reduction counseling

- Provide risk-reduction and primary prevention counseling
- Refer for mental health and/or substance use programs when indicated; consider need for intensive risk-reduction counseling services
- Discuss future use of PrEP with persons with ongoing risk behavior (see Appendix C for AI-funded referral sources)

[a]Decisions to initiate nPEP beyond 36 hours post-exposure should be individualized, with the realization of diminished efficacy when timing of initiation is prolonged; assess for hepatitis B and C; recommend serial HIV testing at 0, 4, and 12 weeks; provide risk-reduction counseling.
[b]If the source is known to be HIV-infected, information about his/her viral load, ART medication history, and history of antiretroviral drug resistance should be obtained when possible to assist in selection of a PEP regimen.[67] **Initiation of the first dose of PEP should not be delayed while awaiting this information and/or results of resistance testing.** When this information becomes available, the PEP regimen may be changed if needed in consultation with an experienced provider.
[c]See Appendix A for dosing recommendations in patients with renal impairment.
[d]Lamivudine 300 mg PO qd may be substituted for emtricitabine. A fixed-dose combination is available when tenofovir is used with emtricitabine (Truvada 1 PO qd).
[e]See Appendix A for drug-drug interactions, dosing adjustments, and contraindications associated with raltegravir and dolutegravir.

FIGURE 40-2 Steps for Evaluating and Managing Nonoccupational Exposures to HIV

Reproduced from New York State Department of Health AIDS Institute. (2015). UPDATE: HIV prophylaxis following non-occupational exposure. Retrieved from www.hivguidelines.org.

B. Weighing the risks and benefits of PEP and nPEP

The clinician must decide what to recommend to potentially exposed clients. Because of the lack of empiric data, a cost/benefit analysis of PEP is impossible. Factors to weigh include route of exposure; amount of infectious fluid involved; HIV serostatus and stage of disease of the source (including viral load); overall health and pregnancy status of the recipient; mental state of the recipient; and possibility of adverse reactions to the antiretrovirals. After carefully reviewing all the information, the clinician and the client can together make a decision about whether or not PEP will be initiated.

Pregnancy and breastfeeding status of the patient are especially important considerations. Given the fact that acute HIV infection during pregnancy or breastfeeding greatly increases the risk of infection in the baby (due to very high viral loads during this time) and that the majority of recommended PEP drugs are considered safe in pregnancy and breastfeeding (see exceptions in **Table 40-5**), PEP is highly recommended for pregnant and breastfeeding women with risky exposures. Both HIV and PEP drugs will be present in breast milk. It may be recommended that breastfeeding women stop breastfeeding while on PEP and/or when risk for primary infection is present (Antiretroviral Pregnancy Registry, 2015; Kuhar et al., 2013 New York State Department of Health AIDS Institute, 2014).

1. Depending on the test used, the window period may be shorter than 6 weeks. Clinicians should contact appropriate laboratory authorities to determine the window period for the test that is being used.

2. If the source is known to be HIV infected, information about his/her viral load, ART medication history, and history of antiretroviral drug resistance should be obtained when possible to assist in selection of a PEP regimen. *Initiation of the first dose of PEP should not be delayed while awaiting this information and/or results of resistance testing.* When this information becomes available, the PEP regimen may be changed if needed in consultation with an experienced provider.

Be sure to adjust dosages for renally impaired patients.

a. Decisions to initiate nPEP beyond 36 hours post-exposure should be individualized, with the realization of diminished efficacy when timing of initiation is prolonged; assess for hepatitis B and C; recommend serial HIV testing at 0, 4, and 12 weeks; provide risk-reduction counseling.

b. If the source is known to be HIV-infected, information about his/her viral load, ART medication history, and history of antiretroviral drug resistance should be obtained when possible to assist in selection of a PEP regimen. *Initiation of the first dose of PEP should not be delayed while awaiting this information and/or results of resistance testing.* When this information becomes available, the PEP regimen may be changed if needed in consultation with an experienced provider.

c. See www.hivguidelines.org for dosing recommendations in patients with renal impairment.

d. Lamivudine 300 mg PO qd may be substituted for emtricitabine. A fixed-dose combination is available when tenofovir is used with emtricitabine (Truvada 1 PO qd).

e. See www.hivguidelines.org for drug toxicities. Interactions and alternative regimens.

II. Database (may include but is not limited to)

A. Subjective

1. History of exposure
   a. When did the exposure occur (exact time and date)
   b. What type of exposure (skin, mucous membrane, percutaneous, or sexual; route of exposure if sexual [vaginal, anal, or oral])
   c. Other details about exposure: trauma involved, deep or shallow, and amount and type of fluid involved
   d. Information about the exposure source
      i. Known HIV positive? Able to document? Stage of illness? Type of antiretrovirals

TABLE 40-5 PEP Drugs to Avoid During Pregnancy

Drug(s) to Avoid	Toxicity
Efavirenz	Teratogenicity
Combination of stavudine and didanosine	Mitochondrial toxicity
Nevirapine	Hepatotoxicity
Unboosted indinavir in the second or third trimester	Substantially lower antepartum indinavir plasma concentrations; risk for nephrolithiasis

taken now and in the past? Viral load (HIV RNA) at present time?

ii. If HIV status is unknown or documented negative, are there risk factors for HIV infection present? Does the source have signs or symptoms of primary HIV infection (fever, rash, or flulike symptoms) (**Table 40-6**)? Can the source be located and can a rapid HIV test be obtained?

TABLE 40-6 Signs and Symptoms of HIV Primary Infection (Acute Retroviral Syndrome)

Symptom/Sign	Percentage of Patients with Symptom/Sign
Fever	96%
Lymphadenopathy	74%
Pharyngitis	70%
Rash Erythematous maculopapular with lesions on face, trunk, and sometimes extremities, including palms and soles; mucocutaneous ulceration involving mouth, esophagus, or genitals	70%
Myalgia or arthralgia	54%
Diarrhea	32%
Headache	32%
Nausea and vomiting	27%
Hepatosplenomegaly	14%
Weight loss	13%
Thrush	12%
Neurologic symptoms Meningoencephalitis or aseptic meningitis, peripheral neuropathy or radiculopathy, facial palsy, Guillain-Barré syndrome, brachial neuritis, or cognitive impairment or psychosis	12%

Data from Centers for Disease Control and Prevention. Antiretroviral postexposure prophylaxis after sexual, injection-drug use, or other nonoccupational exposure to HIV in the United States: recommendations from the U.S. Department of Health and Human Services. *Morbidity and Mortality Weekly Report* 2005; 54 (No. RR-2); Smith et al., 2005.

2. Patient history, including but not limited to:

a. Any history of HIV infection or use of antiretrovirals, previous exposures to HIV, previous PEP, previous HIV testing, other HIV risk factors; liver or kidney disease (especially hepatitis A, B, or C); allergies or adverse reactions to medications; previous sexually transmitted infections; surgeries

b. General health history: any chronic disease

c. Social history: sexual history, pregnancy, relationships, social support, living circumstances, and health habits

3. Review of systems

Complete review of systems is appropriate with emphasis on mouth, skin, liver, gastrointestinal, kidney, genitalia, neurologic (especially headache and peripheral neuropathy history), and psychiatric symptoms.

B. Objective

1. Physical examination

a. Examine area of exposure and assess for trauma, lesions, bruising excoriations, or other breaks in the integrity of skin or mucous membranes, and cleanliness.

b. Skin: baseline to identify existing lesions or rashes

c. Head: baseline for headaches or sinus tenderness

d. Mouth: baseline for lesions or periodontal disease

e. Abdomen: baseline liver and spleen size and tenderness, general state of abdomen

f. Neurologic: baseline general neurology (especially deep tendon reflexes and sensory examination)

g. Genital and anal examination for sexual exposures

2. Diagnostic testing

Figures 40-1 and 40-2 delineate the basic initial testing needed before initiation of PEP or nPEP. The clinician may want to add more testing for individual patients, depending on the health state and problems.

See **Tables 40-7** and **40-8** for recommendations for initial and follow-up testing of patients on PEP and nPEP. An additional crucial consideration is the testing of the source patient (see Figures 40-1 and 40-2). Remember that hepatitis B and C testing and sexually transmitted infection (STI) testing may also be important in patients with exposures risky for HIV infection.

TABLE 40-7 Monitoring Recommendations After Initiation of PEP Regimens Following Occupational Exposure[a]

	Baseline	Week 1	Week 2	Week 3	Week 4	Week 12
Clinic Visit	√	√ Or by telephone	√ Or by telephone	√ Or by telephone	√	
Pregnancy Test	√					
Serum liver enzymes, BUN, creatinine, CBC[b]	√		√		√	
HIV test[c]	√				√	√

[a] For postexposure management for hepatitis B and C, see Section XI: *Occupational Exposures to Hepatitis B and C.*

[b] Complete blood count (CBC) should be obtained for all exposed workers at baseline. Follow-up CBC is indicated only for those receiving regimen containing zidovudine.

[c] Recommended even if PEP is declined.

Reproduced from New York State Department of Health AIDS Institute. (2014). *UPDATE: HIV prophylaxis following occupational exposure.* Retrieved from www.hivguidelines.org.

TABLE 40-8 Monitoring Recommendations After Initiation of PEP Regimens Following Nonoccupational Exposures

	Baseline	Week 1	Week 2	Week 3	Week 4	Week 12
Clinic Visit	√	√ Or by telephone	√ Or by telephone	√ Or by telephone	√	
Pregnancy Test	√					
Serum liver enzymes, blood urea nitrogen (BUN), creatinine, CBC[a]	√		√		√	
HIV test[b]	√				√	√
STI Screening (*for exposures unrelated to sexual assault*)[b]: • Nucleic Acid Amplification Testing for Gonorrhea and Chlamydia (GC/CT NAAT) (based on site of exposure) • Rapid Plasma Reagin (RPR) See *HIV Prophylaxis for Victims of Sexual Assault* for recommendations in cases of sexual assault.	√		√ (consider)			
Hepatitis B and C[a]	For postexposure management for hepatitis B and C, see Section IX: *Nonoccupational Exposures to Hepatitis B and C*					

[a] CBC should be obtained for all exposed persons at baseline. Follow-up CBC is indicated only for those receiving a zidovudine-containing regimen.

[b] Recommended even if PEP is declined.

Reproduced from New York State Department of Health AIDS Institute. (2014). *UPDATE: HIV prophylaxis following non-occupational exposure.* Retrieved from www.hivguidelines.org.

III. Assessment

A. Determine the diagnosis and its significance

1. Determine the level of risk for HIV exposure and weigh the benefits of treatment.

2. Determine the significance of possible exposure to the patient and significant others, noting the amount of psychologic distress present.

3. Assess the motivation and ability of the patient to follow through with the treatment plan.

4. Note the amount of social support to help with coping during this stressful time.

IV. Plan

A. Diagnostic tests (See Figures 40-1 and 40-2, and Tables 40-7 and 40-8)

B. Management

1. The area of exposure should be washed gently with soap and water (for skin) or rinsed liberally with clean water or saline solution (for mucous membranes). Genitals and anal area may be gently bathed with mild soapy water, but douching is not recommended. Any trauma should be appropriately treated. Avoid squeezing, scrubbing, or otherwise traumatizing the area of exposure.

2. PEP recommended
   a. If PEP or nPEP is recommended, follow the algorithms and testing schedules (see Figures 40-1 and 40-2, and Tables 40-7 and 40-8).
   b. Follow-up should ideally be referred to an HIV specialist, and when no specialist is available, expert consultation should be sought. Every case should be discussed with an expert (see resources listed at end of chapter—immediate phone consultation is always available). The client should be seen in follow-up at least after the first 3 weeks, or earlier if they are experiencing any problems (drug side effects), especially symptoms of HIV primary infection (see Tables 40-6, 40-7, and 40-8).
   c. Supportive counseling to ensure adherence to the medication regimen and alleviate anxiety is highly recommended (**Table 40-9**).

TABLE 40-9 Counseling for Any Person Having Experienced Exposure to HIV is recommended (whether taking PEP or nPEP or not)

Exposed person should be advised to use precautions (e.g., avoid blood or tissue donations, breastfeeding, or pregnancy) to prevent secondary transmission, especially during the first 6–12 weeks postexposure.

For exposures for which PEP or nPEP is prescribed, patient should be informed regarding

- possible drug toxicities and the need for monitoring,
- possible drug interactions, and
- the need for adherence to PEP regimens.

Consider reevaluation of exposed person 72 hours postexposure, especially after additional information about the exposure or source person becomes available.

Data from Centers for Disease Control and Prevention. Updated U.S. Public Health Service guidelines for the management of occupational exposures to HIV and recommendations for Postexposure Prophylaxis. *Morbidity and Mortality Weekly Report* 2005; 54 (No. RR-9); Panlilio et al., 2005.

3. PEP or nPEP not recommended
   a. If significant exposure has not occurred, counsel patient on why PEP is not recommended and how to avoid further exposures.
   b. Advise patient to follow up if experiencing any problems, especially symptoms of HIV primary infection (Table 40-6).

C. Patient education

Mechanism of HIV infection, possible medication toxicities, strict adherence to medications regimen, mechanism of resistance development, strategies for not infecting others, and signs and symptoms of primary infection (Table 40-6).

D. Reporting requirements

Remember to follow the requirements of your institution and your state on reporting and data keeping for occupational exposures and injuries, including requirements for worker's compensation reporting.

V. Clinician and patient resources

A. HIV Warmline: 800-933-3413

B. PEP Line: 888-HIV-4911

C. National HIV/AIDS Clinicians' Consulting Center: www.nccc.ucsf.edu.

A comprehensive website including links to many HIV-related guidelines, including PEP. It is advisable to check frequently for updates to these guidelines.

REFERENCES

Antiretroviral Pregnancy Registry Steering Committee. (2015). Antiretroviral pregnancy registry international interim report for 1 January 1989 through 31 July 2015. Wilmington, NC: Registry Coordinating Center. Retrieved at www.APRegistry.comhttp://www.apregistry.com/forms/interim_report.pdf

Cardo, D. M., Culver, D. H., Ciesielski, C. A., Srivastava, P. U., Marcus, R., Abiteboul, D., et al. (1997). A case-control study of HIV seroconversion in healthcare workers after percutaneous exposure. Centers for Disease Control and Prevention Needlestick Surveillance Group. *New England Journal of Medicine, 337*(21), 1485–1490.

Centers for Disease Control and Prevention (2014). HIV risk behaviors. Retrieved at http://www.cdc.gov/hiv/risk/estimates/riskbehaviors.html

Henderson, D. K. (2001). HIV postexposure prophylaxis in the 21st century. *Emerging Infectious Diseases, 7*(2), 254–258

Kuhar, D. T., Henderson, D. K., Struble, K. A., Heneine, W., Thomas, V., Cheever, L. W., et al. (2013). Updated U.S. Public Health Service guidelines for the management of occupational exposures to HIV and recommendations for postexposure prophylaxis. *Infection Control and Hospital Epidemiology, 34*, 875–892.

Medical Care Criteria Committee. (2008). *HIV prophylaxis following occupational exposure.* New York: New York State Department of Health AIDS Institute. Retrieved from www.hivguidelines.org.

New York State Department of Health AIDS Institute. (2014). *Update: HIV prophylaxis following occupational exposure.* Retrieved from www.hivguidelines.org/clinical-guidelines/post-exposure-prophylaxis/hiv-prophylaxis-following-occupational-exposure/.

Smith, D. K., Grohskopf, L. A., Black, R. J., Auerbach, J. D., Veronese, F., Struble, K. A., et al. (2005). Antiretroviral postexposure prophylaxis after sexual, injection-drug use, or other nonoccupational exposure to HIV in the United States: Recommendations from the U.S. Department of Health and Human Services. *Morbidity and Mortality Weekly Report, 54*(RR-2), 1–20.

World Health Organization. (2005). *Post-exposure prophylaxis to prevent HIV infection: Joint WHO/ILO guidelines on post-exposure prophylaxis (PEP) to prevent HIV infection.* Retrieved from http://www.who.int/hiv/pub/guidelines/PEP/en/

PREEXPOSURE PROPHYLAXIS FOR HIV

Barbara Newlin and Brooke Finkmoore

CHAPTER 41

I. Introduction and general background

Preexposure prophylaxis (PrEP) is the daily use of antiretroviral (ARV) drugs by HIV-uninfected persons to prevent the acquisition of HIV from nonoccupational exposures. In July 2012, the Food and Drug Administration approved the use of Truvada as PrEP (Food and Drug Administration, 2012). Truvada is a fixed-dose combination pill of two ARV drugs, tenofovir disoproxil fumarate (TDF) and emtricitabine (FTC), that has been used as a part of combination antiretroviral therapy (ART) for HIV-infected individuals since 2004 (Gilead Sciences, 2013). PrEP is indicated for adult men and women who have a substantial risk of acquiring HIV either through sex or and intravenous drug use (IDU) (U.S. Public Health Service, 2014a). The presence of PrEP in the bloodstream and other tissues can stop HIV from establishing infection because it blocks important pathways for viral replication (U.S. Public Health Service, 2014a). If PrEP is taken every day, it reaches its maximum protection in blood at 20 days, in rectal tissue at about 7 days, and in vaginal tissues at about 20 days (U.S. Public Health Service, 2014a). Clinicians are encouraged to offer PrEP to at-risk patients as part of a comprehensive prevention strategy that also includes sexual-risk reduction counseling, condom provision, treatment of sexually transmitted infections (STIs), ART for HIV-infected partners, and referrals to drug treatment and mental health services when indicated.

In 2014, the United States Public Health Service (USPHS) published a clinical practice guideline and a clinical provider supplement on PrEP (U.S. Public Health Service, 2014a, 2014b). Increasing the use of and adherence to HIV prevention strategies is a public health priority because there are approximately 50,000 new cases of HIV infection diagnosed annually in the United States (Centers for Disease Control and Prevention, 2012). These documents orient clinicians to an evidence-based HIV risk assessment, clinical eligibility for PrEP, and safe management practices for patients who are on

PrEP. The information included in this chapter reflects the USPHS recommendations.

A. Evidence for PrEP

1. Efficacy and effectiveness

Randomized controlled trials investigating the efficacy of PrEP have been conducted among various high-risk populations and in a number of settings. Among four PrEP trials published as of August 2013, a 74% and 92% reduction in HIV risk was found among HIV-uninfected men and women who consistently used PrEP; the reduction in HIV risk was lower and more variable, between 40% and 80%, for those who did not consistently use PrEP (Baeten et al., 2012; Choopanya et al., 2013; Grant et al., 2010; Thigpen et al., 2012). Analyses of PrEP trial data found that participants who took PrEP 7 days a week were 99% protected against infection, whereas those who took the pill 4 days a week were 96% protected and those who took the pill 2 days a week were 76% protected (U.S. Public Health Service, 2014a). Overall, these data demonstrate that PrEP provides protection against HIV acquisition and that daily adherence is needed to achieve maximal prophylactic benefit.

Studies on the effectiveness of PrEP in real-life clinical practice have favorable results. For example, a study that randomized 545 high-risk men who have sex with men (MSM) to either immediate initiation of PrEP or delayed initiation, found a 86% relative reduction in HIV acquisition among those who immediately initiated PrEP compared with those delayed PrEP for 1 year and there was not an increase in STIs among immediate PrEP users (McCormack & Dunn, 2015).

The optimal number of drugs for PrEP is unknown. TDF alone was found to reduce the risk of HIV acquisition among IDUs, and the protective effects of TDF/FTC and TDF alone were similar among serodiscordant heterosexual couples (Baeten et al., 2012;

Choopanya et al., 2013). Currently, the USPHS recommends daily oral PrEP with TDF/FTC or TDF alone for IDUs at substantial risk and TDF/FTC for all other populations (U.S. Public Health Service, 2014a).

2. Safety

TDF/FTC has an excellent safety profile and is well tolerated by HIV-infected individuals (Gallant, DeJesus, Arribas, et al., 2006; Gallant, Staszewski, Pozniak, et al., 2004). The PrEP trials found TDF alone or in combination with FTC to be safe and well tolerated when used by HIV-uninfected individuals (Grant et al., 2010; Grohskopf et al., 2013). The initiation of TDF/FTC is associated with self-limited start-up symptoms including nausea, vomiting, and dizziness (U.S. Public Health Service, 2014a).

In one PrEP trial, study subjects randomly assigned to the TDF/FTC group had greater declines in bone mass density compared with those in the placebo group but not a difference in the rate of fractures (Thigpen et al., 2012). In the iPrex study, TDF/FTC use was associated with mild but significant decrease in kidney function but not proximal tubular dysfunction (Solomon et al., 2014). The majority of elevations in serum creatinine occurred by the fourth week of TDF/FTC use and elevations were self-limited; all elevations resolved with discontinuation of TDF/FTC (Solomon et al., 2014). Routine monitoring of serum creatinine is recommended to manage the development of renal insufficiency in individuals on TDF or TDF/FTC for PrEP (U.S. Public Health Service, 2014a).

Although there have been concerns about the selection of viral mutations that confer resistance to TDF or FTC if PrEP fails, instances of seroconversion with resistant virus were extremely rare in the PrEP trials. TDF or FTC resistant virus was not detected among study participants who seroconverted after study enrollment except in one study that was stopped early due to low adherence (Van Damme et al., 2012). Otherwise, viral resistance to TDF or FTC was found only in patients with existing and unrecognized HIV at the time of PrEP initiation (U.S. Public Health Service, 2014a).

None of the PrEP trials studied the effects of PrEP on a developing fetus. TDF/FTC, pregnancy category B, is recommended for serodiscordant couples trying to conceive in combination with ART in the infected partner (Panel on Treatment of HIV-Infected Pregnant Women and Prevention of Perinatal Transmission, 2014).

B. Indications for PrEP

PrEP is indicated for individuals at a substantial risk of acquiring HIV who meet the clinical eligibility criteria.

1. Individuals at substantial risk of acquiring HIV
   a. Men who have sex with men who have any of the following: an HIV-infected sexual partner, a recent bacterial STI, a high number of sex partners, a history of inconsistent or no condom use, current participation in commercial sex work.
   b. Heterosexual men and women who have any of the following: an HIV-infected sexual partner, a recent bacterial STI, a high number of sex partners, a history of inconsistent or no condom use, current participation in commercial sex work in high-prevalence area or network.
   c. Injection drug users who have any of the following: an HIV-infected injecting partner, a practice of sharing injection equipment, recent drug treatment (but currently injecting).

2. Clinical eligibility for PrEP
   a. Individuals at substantial risk of acquiring HIV are clinically eligible for PrEP if they have a negative HIV test at the time they start PrEP, do not have signs or symptoms suggesting acute (primary) HIV infection (see **Figure 41-1: Documenting HIV Status**) and they have normal renal function (estimated creatinine clearance [eCrCl] $\geq$ 60 mL/min).
   b. Patients are not clinically eligible for PrEP if they have signs or symptoms suggestive of acute HIV even if their HIV antibody test is negative because the administration of Truvada alone in the setting of unrecognized HIV infection can select for drug-resistant virus.
   c. Any person with an eCrCl < 60 mL/min should not be prescribed PrEP with TDF/FTC. TDF is associated with acute and chronic kidney disease and there are no safety data on TDF in individuals with an eCrCl < 60 mL/min. There are no approved PrEP regimens for individuals with baseline renal insufficiency.
   d. Age is also a consideration: PrEP is currently approved only for adults because there are insufficient data on the safety and efficacy of PrEP for those under 18 years of age.

II. Database (may include but is not limited to)

A. Subjective

1. Patient history

   Obtaining a thorough history of sexual and drug use behaviors is necessary to determine whether a patient is at substantial risk of acquiring HIV infection.

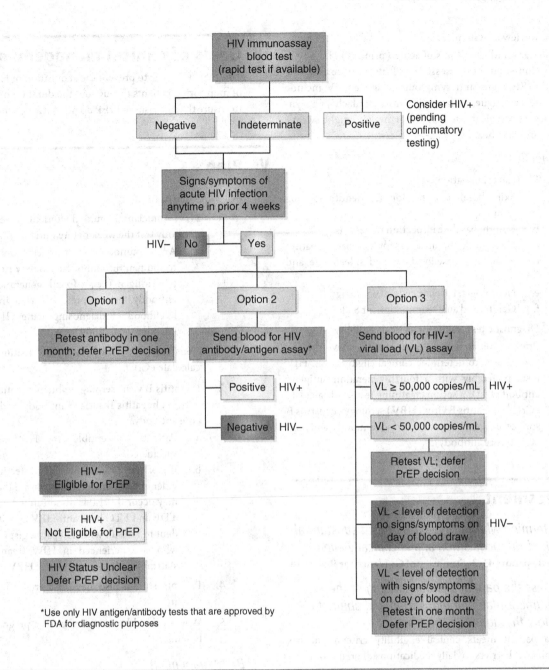

FIGURE 41-1 Documenting HIV Status

Reproduced from U.S. Public Health Service. (2014). *Preexposure prophylaxis for the prevention of HIV infection in the United States—2014 Clinical Practice Guideline.*

The USPHS guidelines contain a set of behavioral risk assessment questions for MSM, heterosexual men and women, and IDU (see **Appendix 41-1: Behavioral Risk Assessment Questions**). The questions assess key sexual and drug use practices identified in epidemiologic studies and PrEP trials that are associated with a high risk of HIV acquisition. A clinical screening tool for MSM has also been developed (see **Appendix 41-2: Screening Tool for MSM**). Clinicians may consider STIs or pregnancy in the past 6 months as evidence of unprotected sex and potential exposure to HIV. If a patient reports a sexual or parenteral exposure to HIV in the previous 72 hours, evaluation for postexposure prophylaxis (PEP) should be started without delay (see Chapter 40, Postexposure Prophylaxis for HIV Infection).

2. Review of systems

Signs and symptoms of acute (primary) HIV infection should be assessed in all patients considering PrEP. Signs and symptoms of acute HIV include fever, fatigue, malaise, skin rash, headache, pharyngitis, cervical adenopathy, arthralgia, night sweats, and diarrhea.

B. Objective

1. Physical examination

   a. Skin: baseline inspection to identify existing lesions or rashes

   b. Mouth: baseline inspection for lesions

   c. Head, neck, throat: assess for lymphadenopathy

   d. Abdomen: baseline liver and spleen size and tenderness

   e. Neurologic: baseline general neurology

   f. Genital and anal examination for STIs

2. Diagnostic test results for clinical eligibility

   Prior to initiating PrEP patients must have the following tests to determine clinical eligibility: an HIV test (preferably with a fourth-generation antigen/antibody test); a serum creatinine test (and calculate eCrCl); hepatitis B virus (HBV) serology (hepatitis B surface antigen, hepatitis B surface antibody, and hepatitis B core antibody).

III. Assessment

A. Determine whether the patient is at substantial risk of HIV acquisition and is clinically eligible
See **Appendix 41-3: Summary of Guidance for PrEP Use.**

B. Assess the patient's understanding of the treatment plan and motivation and ability to follow through with the plan

If a patient meets clinical eligibility criteria but has significant barriers to daily medication adherence or if the provider is unable to develop an appropriate follow-up plan with the patient, the provider should consider delaying PrEP initiation.

C. Weigh the risks and benefits of PrEP with the patient

This should take into account the patient's level of HIV risk, kidney function, and HBV status. If the patient is pregnant or planning to conceive, refer the patient to an obstetrician and/or HIV specialist to discuss risks and benefits of PrEP in pregnancy.

IV. Goals of clinical management

The goal of PrEP is to prevent the acquisition of HIV. The goal of monitoring patients throughout the duration of PrEP use is to ensure that the risks of PrEP do not outweigh the benefits.

V. Plan

A. Diagnostic tests

1. HIV: clinicians should document a negative HIV antibody test the week before initiating PrEP.

   a. An immunoassay that detects both antibody to human immunodeficiency virus and HIV p24 antigen (i.e., a fourth-generation antigen/antibody test) is preferred as it increases the likelihood of diagnosing acute HIV infection (Pandori et al., 2009).

2. Renal function: obtain a serum creatinine test and calculate eCrCl.

3. Hepatitis B virus serology: obtain hepatitis B surface antigen, hepatitis B surface antibody, and hepatitis B core antibody.

   a. Patients susceptible to HBV should be vaccinated.

   b. If a patient has chronic HBV infection, the provider and patient should be aware that a flare-up may occur if PrEP is discontinued because both TDF and FTC have anti-HBV activity. It is prudent to consult with a hepatologist or a clinician who is experienced in HBV treatment when starting a patient with chronic HBV on PrEP.

4. Patients should also have bacterial STI testing at baseline.

5. Women should submit urine for a pregnancy test at baseline.

B. Management

1. Prescribing PrEP

   a. Patients who are initiating PrEP should be given a prescription for a 300 mg TDF coformulated with 200 mg of FTC (Truvada), or 300 mg of TDF alone for IDUs opting for one-drug PrEP.

   b. Prescriptions should be written as oral, daily, and continuous.

   c. A 90-day supply or less is recommended to encourage patients to return for the recommended monitoring.

2. Monitoring patients on PrEP

   a. Patients on PrEP should be seen by their provider at least every 3 months for repeat HIV testing, medication adherence counseling, behavioral risk reduction support, and assessment of side effects of PrEP.

   b. The pregnancy intent and status of women on PrEP should be assessed every 3 months.

   c. A renal panel should be checked 3 months after PrEP initiation and then again every 6 months (providers can consider monitoring renal function more closely in patients with other risk factors for renal disease including hypertension or diabetes).

   d. Testing for bacterial STIs should be conducted every 6 months or more frequently as needed.

3. Discontinuing PrEP

   a. PrEP should be discontinued if a patient's CrCl drops below 60 mL/min. However, PrEP should not be discontinued if the serum creatinine rises above that patient's baseline and the CrCl remains ≥ 60 mL/min. Yet, a referral to a nephrologist should be made for any patient with a CrCl that is steadily declining even if it remains ≥ 60 mL/min.

   b. PrEP should be discontinued if a patient tests positive for HIV during follow-up.

   c. Patients may choose to discontinue PrEP for other reasons including personal choice, cessation of HIV risk behaviors, and intolerable side effects.

   d. Upon discontinuation for any reason, the provider should document the following: HIV status, reason for PrEP discontinuation, recent medication adherence, and reported sexual risk behavior.

C. Patient Education

TDF/FTC is associated with self-limited start-up symptoms including nausea, vomiting, and dizziness. Providing anticipatory guidance that these symptoms are common and typically resolve in 1 month may prevent patients from discontinuing PrEP. Encourage patients to take PrEP with food and use over-the-counter headache medicines or a prescription antiemetic to reduce symptoms.

The PrEP Clinical Provider's Supplement contains a template of a patient and provider checklist for initiating PrEP (see **Appendix 41-4: Provider Checklist**). Following this checklist and reviewing it closely with patients will ensure that they have been educated about the following key points: daily adherence is needed to achieve maximal efficacy of PrEP; frequent monitoring is needed to maximize safety of PrEP; and PrEP does not completely eliminate the possibility of acquiring HIV and thus condom use is still highly recommended.

VI. Resources for clinicians

A. PrEPline

Clinicians may call the PrEPline at 1-855-PrEP for expert advice on PrEP initiation or management from the Clinicians' Consultation Center (www.nccc.ucsf.edu).

B. Updates to the USPHS guidelines

As new data become available, recommendations may change. Revised recommendations may be posted on the CDC website (www.cdc.gov/hiv/pdf/guidelines/PrEPguidelines2014.pdf). Revised recommendations may also be found at the AIDS Info website (www.aidsinfo.nih.gov).

REFERENCES

Baeten, J. M., Donnell, D., Ndase, P., Mugo, N. R., Campbell, J. D., Wangisi, J., et al. (2012). Antiretroviral prophylaxis for HIV prevention in heterosexual men and women. *New England Journal of Medicine, 367*(5), 399–410. doi: 10.1056/NEJMoa1108524

Centers for Disease Control and Prevention. (2012). *Estimated HIV incidence in the United States, 2007–2010* (HIV Surveillance Supplemental Report 2012, Vol. 17, No. 4). Atlanta, GA: Author. Retrieved from www.cdc.gov/hiv/pdf/statistics_hssr_vol_17_no_4.pdf.

Choopanya, K., Martin, M., Suntharasamai, P., Sangkum, U., Mock, P. A., Leethochawalit, M., et al. (2013). Antiretroviral prophylaxis for HIV infection among people who inject drugs in Bangkok, Thailand (the Bangkok Tenofovir Study): A randomised, double-blind, placebo-controlled phase 3 trial. *Lancet, 381*(9883), 2083–2090. doi: 10.1016/S0140-6736(13)61127-7.

Food and Drug Administration (2012). FDA approves first medication to reduce HIV risk. Retrieved from www.fda.gov/ForConsumers/ConsumerUpdates/ucm311821.htm.

Gallant, J. E., DeJesus, E., Arribas, J. R., Pozniak, A. L., Gazzard, B., Campo, R. E., et al. (2006). Tenofovir DF, emtricitabine, and efavirenz vs. zidovudine, lamivudine, and efavirenz for HIV. *New England Journal of Medicine, 354*(3), 251–260.

Gallant, J. E., Staszewski, S., Pozniak, A. L., DeJesus, E., Suleiman, J. M., et al. (2004). Efficacy and safety of tenofovir DF vs. stavudine in combination therapy in antiretroviral-naïve patients: A 3-year randomized trial. *JAMA, 292*(2), 191–201.

Gilead Sciences. (2013). Truvada [package insert]. Retrieved from www.gilead.com/pdf/truvada_pi.pdf.

Grant, R. M., Lama, J. R., Anderson, P. L., McMahan, V., Liu, A. Y., Vargas, L., et al. (2010). Preexposure chemoprophylaxis for HIV prevention in men who have sex with men. *New England Journal Medicine, 363*(27), 2587–2599. doi:10.1056/NEJMoa1011205

Grohskopf, L.A., Chillag, K. L., Gvetadze, R., Liu, A. Y., Thompson, M., Mayer, K. H., et al. (2013). Randomized trial of clinical safety of daily oral tenofovir disoproxil fumarate among HIV-uninfected men who have sex with men in the United States. *Journal of Acquired Immune Deficiency Syndromes, 64*(1), 79–86. doi: 10.1097/QAI.0b013e31828ece33.

Jenness, S. M., Neaigus, A., Murrill, C. S., Wendel, T., Forgione, L., & Hagan, H. (2007). Estimated HIV incidence among high-risk heterosexuals in New York City. *Journal of Acquired Immune Deficiency Syndromes, 56*(2), 193–197. doi: 10.1097/QAI.0b013e318202a9c4.

LaLota, M., Beck, D., Metsch, L., Brewer, T. H., Forrest, D. W., Cardenas, G. A., et al. (2011). HIV seropositivity and correlates of infection among heterosexually active adults in high-risk areas in South Florida. *AIDS Behavior, 15*(6), 1259–1263. doi: 10.1007/s10461-010-9856-z

McCormack, S., & Dunn, D. (2015). Pragmatic pen-label Randomised Trial of Preexposure Prophylaxis: The PROUD Study. Retrieved from www .croiconference.org/sessions/pragmatic-open-label-randomised-trial -preexposure-prophylaxis-proud-study.

Neaigus, A., Miller, M., Gyarmathy, V. A., & Friedman, S. R. (2011). HIV heterosexual sexual risk from injecting drug users among HIV-seronegative noninjecting heroin users. *Substance Use and Misuse, 46* (2–3), 208–217. doi: 10.3109/10826084.2011.521473

Pandori, M. W., Hackett, J., Jr., Louie, B., Vallari, A., Dowling, T., Liska, S., et al. (2009). Assessment of the ability of a fourth-generation immunoassay for human immunodeficiency virus (HIV) antibody and p24 antigen to detect both acute and recent HIV infections in a high-risk setting. *Journal of Clinical Microbiology, 47*(8), 2639–2642.

Panel on Treatment of HIV-Infected Pregnant Women and Prevention of Perinatal Transmission. (2014). Recommendations for use of antiretroviral drugs in pregnant HIV-1-infected women for maternal health and interventions to reduce perinatal HIV transmission in the United States. Retrieved from http://aidsinfo.nih.gov/contentfiles/lvguidelines /PerinatalGL.pdf.

Peterson, L., Taylor, D., Roddy, R., Belai, G., Phillips, P., Nanda, K., et al. (2007). Tenofovir disoproxil fumarate for prevention of HIV infection in women: A phase 2, double-blind, randomized, placebo-controlled trial. *PLoS Clinical Trials, 2*(5), e27. doi: 10.1371/journal.pctr.0020027

Smith, D. K., Pals, S. L., Herbst, J. H., Shinde, S., & Carey, J. W. (2012). Development of a clinical screening index predictive of incident HIV infection among men who have sex with men in the United States. *Journal of Acquired Immune Deficiency Syndromes, 60*(4), 421–427. doi: 10.1097/QAI.0b013e318256b2f6.

Solomon, M. M., Lama, J. R., Glidden, D. V., Mulligan, K., McMahan, V., Liu, A.Y., et al. (2014). Changes in renal function associated with oral emtricitabine/tenofovir disoproxil fumarate use for HIV pre-exposure prophylaxis. *AIDS, 28*(6), 851–859. doi: 10.1097/QAD.0000000000000156

Thigpen, M. C., Kebaabetswe, P. M., Paxton, L. A., Smith, D. K., Rose, C. E., Segolodi, T. M., et al. (2012). Antiretroviral preexposure prophylaxis for heterosexual HIV transmission in Botswana. *New England Journal of Medicine, 367*(5), 423–434. doi: 10.1056/NEJMoa1110711

U.S. Public Health Service (2014a). *Preexposure prophylaxis for the prevention of HIV infection in the United States—2014 clinical practice guideline.* Retrieved from www.cdc.gov/hiv/pdf/prepguidelines2014.pdf.

U.S. Public Health Service (2014b). *Preexposure prophylaxis for the prevention of HIV infection in the United States—2014 provider supplement.* Retrieved from www.cdc.gov/hiv/pdf/prepprovidersupplement 2014.pdf.

Van Damme, L., Corneli, A., Ahmed, K., Agot, K., Lombaard, J., Kapiga, S., et al. (2012). Preexposure prophylaxis for HIV infection among African women. *New England Journal of Medicine, 367*(5), 411–422. doi: 10.1056/NEJMoa1202614

APPENDIX 41-1:
BEHAVIORAL RISK ASSESSMENT QUESTIONS

RISK BEHAVIOR ASSESSMENT FOR MSM

In the past 6 months:

- Have you had sex with men, women, or both?

- (*if men or both sexes*) How many men have you had sex with?

- How many times did you have receptive anal sex (you were the bottom) with a man who was not wearing a condom?

- How many of your male sex partners were HIV-infected?

- (*if any positive*) With these HIV-infected male partners, how many times did you have insertive anal sex (you were the top) without you wearing a condom?

- Have you used methamphetamines (such as crystal or speed)?

RISK BEHAVIOR ASSESSMENT FOR HETEROSEXUAL MEN AND WOMEN

In the past 6 months:

- Have you had sex with men, women, or both?

- (*if opposite sex or both sexes*) How many men/women have you had sex with?

- How many times did you have vaginal or anal sex when neither you nor your partner wore a condom?

- How many of your sex partners were HIV-infected?

- (if any positive) With these HIV-infected partners, how many times did you have vaginal or anal sex without a condom?

Reproduced from U.S. Public Health Service. (2014). *Preexposure prophylaxis for the prevention of HIV infection in the United States—2014 clinical practice guideline.*

APPENDIX 41-2:
SCREENING TOOL FOR MSM

	MSM Risk Index[25]		
1	How old are you today?	If <18 years, score 0 If 18-28 years, score 8 If 29-40 years, score 5 If 41-48 years, score 2 If 49 years or more, score 0	_____
2	In the last 6 months, how many men have you had sex with?	If >10 male partners, score 7 If 6-10 male partners. score 4 If 0-5 male partners, score 0	_____
3	In the last 6 months, how many times did you have receptive anal sex (you were the bottom) with a man without a condom?	If 1 or more times, score 10 If 0 times, score 0	_____
4	In the last 6 months, how many of your male sex partners were HIV-positive?	If >1 positive partner, score 8 If 1 positive partner, score 4 If <1 positive partner, score 0	_____
5	In the last 6 months, how many times did you have insertive anal sex (you were the top) without a condom with a man who was HIV-positive?	If 5 or more times, score 6 If 0 times, score 0	_____
6	In the last 6 months, have you used methamphetamines such as crystal or speed?	If yes, score 6 If no, score 0	_____
		Add down entries in right column to calculate total score	_____
			TOTAL SCORE*

* If score is 10 or greater, evaluate for intensive HIV prevention services including PrEP.
If score is below I0, provide indicated standard HIV prevention services.

Reproduced from Smith, D. K., Pals, S. L., Herbst, J. H., Shinde, S., & Carey, J. W. (2012). Development of a clinical screening index predictive of incident HIV infection among men who have sex with men in the United States. *Journal of Acquired Immune Deficiency Syndromes, 60*(4), 421–427. doi: 10.1097/QAI.0b013e318256b2f6.

APPENDIX 41-3:
SUMMARY OF GUIDANCE FOR PrEP USE

TABLE 41-1 Summary of Guidance for PrEP Use

	Men Who Have Sex with Men	Heterosexual Women and Men	Injection Drug Users
Detecting substantial risk of acquiring HIV infection	HIV-positive sexual partner Recent bacterial STI High number of sex partners History of inconsistent or no condom use Commercial sex work	HIV-positive sexual partner Recent bacterial STI High number of sex partners History of inconsistent or no condom use Commercial sex work In high-prevalence area or network	HIV-positive injection partner Sharing injection equipment. Recent drug treatment (but currently injecting)
Clinically eligible	Document negative HIV test result before prescribing PrEP No signs/symptoms of acute HIV infection Normal renal function; no contraindicated medications Documented hepatitis B virus infection and vaccination status		
Prescription	Daily, continuing oral doses of TDF/FTC (Truvada), ≤90-day supply		
Other services	Follow-up visits at least every 3 months to provide the following: HIV test, medication adherence counseling, behavioral risk reduction support, side effect assessment, STI symptom assessment At 3 months and every 6 months thereafter, assess renal function Every 6 months, test for bacterial STIs		
	Do oral/rectal STI testing	Assess pregnancy intent Pregnancy test every 3 months	Access to clean needles/syringes and drug treatment services

STI, sexually transmitted infection.

Reproduced from U.S. Public Health Service. (2014). *Preexposure prophylaxis for the prevention of HIV infection in the United States—2014 clinical practice guideline.*

APPENDIX 41-4: PROVIDER CHECKLIST

Organization/Clinic Name

CHECKLIST FOR INITIATING PREEXPOSURE PROPHYLAXIS (PrEP)

_____   _____
Print name of provider   Print name of patient

_____
Today's date (month/day/year)

Provider Section

I have provided this patient with the following: (check all as completed):

- ☐ Assessment for possible acute HIV infection
- ☐ Indicated laboratory screening to determine indications for these medications
- ☐ An HIV risk assessment to determine whether PrEP is indicated for this patient
- ☐ A medication fact sheet listing dosing instructions and side effects
- ☐ Counseling or a referral for counseling on condom use and any other HIV risk-reduction methods this patient may need
- ☐ Advice on methods to help the patient to take medication daily as prescribed
- ☐ Information about PrEP use during conception and pregnancy (when indicated)
- ☐ A prescription for Truvada (300 mg tenofovir disoproxil fumarate, 200 mg emtricitabine)
- ☐ A follow-up appointment date

As the provider, I will:

- Limit refill periods to recommended intervals for repeat HIV testing (at least every 3 months)
- Conduct follow-up visits at least every 3 months that include the following:
  - Assessment of HIV status (including signs or symptoms of acute HIV infection)
  - Assessment of side effects and advice on how to manage them
  - Assessment of medication adherence and counseling to support adherence
  - Assessment of STI symptoms, HIV risk behavior and counseling support for risk-reduction practices
- Inform the patient of any new information about PrEP and respond to questions

Patient Section

It has been explained to me that:

- Taking a dose of PrEP medication every day may lower my risk of getting HIV infection
- This medicine does not completely eliminate my risk of getting HIV infection, so I need to use condoms during sex
- This medicine may cause side effects so I should contact my provider for advice by calling _____ if I have any health problems
- It is important for my health to find out quickly if I get HIV infection while I'm taking this medication, so
  - I will contact my provider right away if I have symptoms of possible HIV infection (fever with sore throat, rash, headache, or swollen glands)
- My provider will test for HIV infection at least once every 3 months

Therefore, I will:

- Try my best to take the medication my provider has prescribed every day
- Talk to my provider about any problems I have in taking the medication every day
- Not share the medication with any other person
- Attend all my scheduled appointments
- Call_____to reschedule any appointments I cannot attend

Give one copy to patient

ABSCESS MANAGEMENT

Rosalie D. Bravo

CHAPTER 42

I. Introduction and general background

Cutaneous abscesses are a subcategory of skin and soft tissue infections (SSTIs) that involve the dermis and subcutaneous skin tissue (Stevens et al., 2014). They are inflamed, localized soft tissue masses that are encapsulated collections of pus (Baddour, 2014; Rogers & Perkins, 2006; Stevens et al., 2005). Furuncles and carbuncles are also purulent SSTIs that involve the hair follicles and form small abscesses in the surrounding tissues. Carbuncles are a collection of furuncles that become an inflamed, confluent purulent mass (Baddour, 2014). The etiology of purulent SSTIs is usually bacterial infection, of which methicillin-resistant *Staphylococcus aureus* (MRSA) and methicillin-susceptible S. *aureus* are the most common causative organisms (Frazee et al., 2005; Moran et al., 2006). Bacteria enter the dermis and deeper subcutaneous tissues as a result of a break in the integrity of the skin surface. These minor skin traumas may occur from shaving, abrasions, insect bites, splinters, or other foreign bodies. Abscesses may also occur spontaneously in healthy individuals without predisposing conditions. They begin as localized erythema and tenderness on the skin, and as they develop they enlarge and may become firm and indurated. The center of the abscess softens and is filled with purulent exudate or pus consisting of leukocytes, protein, and bacteria. A pustular point or head may develop. This softened area is known as the area of fluctuance. Characteristically, abscesses are painful, warm, well circumscribed, indurated, and erythematous. They are often located on the buttocks, axillae, or the extremities but they may occur anywhere on the skin. Treatment of an abscess is directed at evacuating the collection of pus by incision and drainage. An abscess may have surrounding cellulitis where the adjacent subcutaneous tissue is inflamed, warm, and tender. The presence of cellulitis in the setting of an abscess presents added complexity and may require antibiotic therapy in addition to incision and drainage (Fitch, Manthey, McGinnis, Nicks, & Pariyadath, 2007; Rogers & Perkins, 2006). The subset of patients with weakened immune systems is at risk of developing abscesses of increased frequency and/or severity due to a decreased ability to fight infection.

II. Database (may include but is not limited to)

A. Subjective

1. Risk factors for MRSA
   a. Injection drug use
   b. Immunosuppression
   c. Incarceration in prison
   d. Sharing sports equipment
   e. Recent hospitalization or antibiotic therapy
   f. Men having sex with men (Gorwitz, Jernigan, Powers, & Jernigan, 2006)

2. Precipitating factors
   a. Recent minor skin trauma
   b. Insect stings
   c. Mechanical manipulation of ingrown hairs or comedones (blackheads or whiteheads)
   d. Other foreign bodies, such as splinters or sutures

3. Past health history
   a. Screen for history of abscesses or soft tissue infections
   b. Medical illnesses: immunosuppression, valvular heart disease, diabetes mellitus, or cancer
   c. Medication history: steroid use or recent antibiotic therapy
   d. Vaccination history: Date of last tetanus vaccination

4. Family or relative history of abscesses or soft tissue infections

5. Personal and social history: health-related behaviors, recent travel, and injection drug use

6. Review of systems
   a. Constitutional systemic symptoms: fevers, chills, regional adenopathy, malaise
   b. Skin: Localized skin symptoms of pain, erythema, warmth, induration, purulent drainage, history of trauma or foreign body
   c. Gastrointestinal: Nausea, vomiting, anorexia

B. Objective

1. General appearance: Body habitus (e.g., obese, cachetic, or temporal wasting) and/or general level of distress

2. Vital signs: temperature, pulse, respiratory rate, and blood pressure

3. Careful skin examination
   a. Note location and dimensions of erythema; dimensions of induration; visible abrasions or puncture wounds; presence of central fluctuance; and purulent, serous, or sanguineous drainage.
   b. Observe for erythematous streaking from the primary abscess site

4. Examine proximal lymph nodes for adenopathy

5. Cardiac: auscultation for murmurs because patients with valvular heart disease or prosthetic valves are at risk for bacteremia (Rogers & Perkins, 2006)

III. Assessment

A. Determine the diagnosis

Diagnosis in the ambulatory care setting is a clinical decision based on the history and the physical examination findings. Differentiate between abscesses requiring incision and drainage alone versus incision and drainage with antibiotics (e.g., abscess with evidence of cellulitis and/or sepsis). Determine if there is evidence of systemic involvement by considering abnormal vital signs that meet systemic inflammatory response syndrome criteria (see **Table 42-1**). It is important to consider host factors, such as diabetes, immunosuppression, valvular heart disease, or cancer, because comorbid conditions may also change the treatment plan to include antibiotic therapy and hospital admission. Determine the need for specialty consultation by considering the location of the purulent SSTI and the underlying structures such as veins, arteries, and nerves.

B. Differential diagnosis

1. Simple cutaneous abscess without surrounding cellulitis
2. Cutaneous abscess with surrounding cellulitis
3. Cutaneous abscess in the setting of patients at risk for bacteremia
4. Furuncle, an abscess involving a hair follicle and the adjacent soft tissue
5. Carbuncle, a larger abscess involving a group of hair follicles
6. Arteriovenous malformation
7. Hidradenitis suppurativa, abscesses that involve the apocrine sweat glands located in the axillary or groin area
8. Epidermoid cyst

C. Complications

1. Bacteremia
2. Endocarditis
3. Osteomyelitis
4. Tenosynovitis
5. Septic thrombophlebitis

IV. Goals of clinical management

A. Implement an appropriate, safe, and cost-effective treatment plan that enables patients' compliance.

B. Relieve symptoms.

C. Prevent systemic infection.

D. Prevent recurrence and disfigurement.

TABLE 42-1 The Systemic Inflammatory Response Syndrome (SIRS)

Two or more of the following:

- Temperature > 38 degrees Celsius or < 36 degrees Celsius
- Heart rate > 90 beats/minute
- Respiratory rate > 20 breaths/minute or $PaCO_2$ < 32 torr
- White blood cell count > 12,000 cell/mm^3, < 4,000 cells/mm^3, or > 10% immature (band) forms

Reproduced from American College of Chest Physicians/Society of Critical Care Medicine Consensus Conference: Definitions for sepsis and organ failure and guidelines for the use of innovative therapies in sepsis. (1992). *Critical Care Medicine, 20*(6), 864–874.

V. Plan

A. Diagnostics

1. Ultrasound if readily available may determine the presence of a fluid collection and the size and depth of the abscess.

2. For mild or moderate purulent SSTIs aerobic and anaerobic wound cultures can be obtained from spontaneous wound drainage or obtained during the incision and drainage procedure (Stevens et al., 2014).

3. Additional testing based on the severity of systemic signs and symptoms, such as fevers, rigors, and malaise, may include complete blood count with differential, metabolic panel, and blood cultures. Blood tests are not necessary for a healthy patient with a simple abscess.

B. Management (includes treatment, consultation, referral, and follow-up care)

Treatment is based on the Practice Guidelines for the Diagnosis and Management of Skin and Soft Tissue Infections: 2014 Update by the Infection Disease Society of America (see **Figure 42-1**).

1. Warm moist compresses if the furuncle or abscess is small and firm without fluctuance (Stevens et al., 2005).

2. Tetanus prophylaxis if the patient has not had a tetanus vaccination within 10 years.

3. Incision and drainage for fluctuant abscesses and all carbuncles.

4. Antimicrobial therapy in addition to incision and drainage if there is a surrounding cellulitis. Antibiotics are unnecessary for immunocompetent patients who have a simple cutaneous abscess without surrounding cellulitis (Hankin & Everett, 2007; Rajendran et al., 2007; Stevens et al., 2014). Prescribe antibiotics for patients who have abscesses with surrounding cellulitis and for patients who are diabetic, immunocompromised, have valvular heart disease, or who have other comorbid conditions that increase the risk of bacteremia. Select antibiotics that are effective in treating MRSA and group A streptococcus. Be familiar with regional guidelines for MRSA treatment. Duration of antibiotic therapy should be based on the resolution of symptoms (Baddour, 2014; Hepburn et al., 2004).
   a. Trimethoprim–sulfamethoxazole, 160 mg/800 mg DS (double strength) (one to two tablets based on weight) every 12 hours
   b. Doxycycline, 100 mg twice daily
   c. Clindamycin 300–450 mg orally every 6 hours
   d. Give prophylactic antibiotics 60 minutes before incision and drainage *only* for high-risk patients with prosthetic heart valves, unrepaired congenital heart defects, implantable cardiac devices, or prior history of infective endocarditis (Rogers & Perkins, 2006). Antibiotic prophylaxis can be delivered with a single dose of a cephalosporin. For severe penicillin allergies, give a single dose of intravenous vancomycin 1 g.

5. Analgesic therapy—local anesthetic and drainage of pus will reduce pain. Over-the-counter pain medications may be recommended for the first 48 hours and prior to repacking the wound.

C. Incision and drainage procedure

1. Description: incision and drainage is a surgical procedure in which an incision is made into the fluctuant area of an abscess to drain the purulent contents of an abscess. The incision is then left open to promote further drainage.

2. Indication: the presence of a cutaneous abscess where there is evidence of a collection of purulent exudate or pus.

3. Contraindications to incision and drainage in the outpatient setting
   a. Cellulitis without an underlying abscess.
   b. The location of the abscess is such that the incision may cause a disfiguring defect.
   c. Abscesses in locations that pose a risk for complications or those requiring specialty consultation such as those located on the hands or plantar surfaces; those located over arteries or large blood vessels such as those on the neck or over the antecubital fossa; and those on or around the nasolabial folds or orbital region of the face.
   d. For large or deep abscesses that require more pain management than a local anesthetic and/or if the patient requires conscious sedation or general anesthesia to tolerate the procedure.

4. Preprocedure
   a. Counsel the patient about risks of the potential for discomfort, bleeding, scarring, damage to surrounding structures, systemic spread of infection, and incomplete or unsuccessful drainage.
   b. Discuss the benefits and risks of undergoing incision and drainage versus the benefits and risks of watchful waiting and conservative management.
   c. Obtain informed consent from the patient or proxy if the patient is unable to give consent.

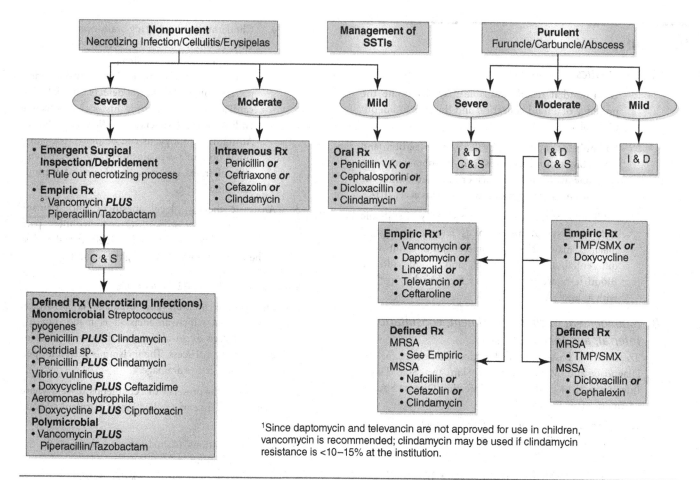

FIGURE 42-1 Management of SSTIs

Reproduced from Stevens, D. L., Bisno, A. L., Chambers, H. F., Dellinger, E. P., Goldstein, E. J., Gorbach, S. L., et al. (2014). Practice guidelines for the diagnosis and management of skin and soft tissue infections: 2014 update by the Infectious Diseases Society of America. *Clinical Infectious Diseases: An Official Publication of the Infectious Diseases Society of America, 59*(2), e10–52.

5. Procedure
   a. Materials
      i. Gown, gloves, face shield, and one pair of sterile gloves
      ii. One bottle of povidine iodine or chlorhexidine solution
      iii. Eight to 10 packs of sterile 4 × 4s and alcohol wipes
      iv. One #11 or #15 blade scalpel
      v. One small curved hemostat for blunt dissection
      vi. One 10-cc syringe
      vii. One 22-gauge needle for drawing up the local anesthetic
      viii. One 25-gauge needle for infiltrating lidocaine
      ix. Lidocaine 1% or bupivacaine 0.5%
      x. One irrigation kit or a 30- to 60-mL syringe and splash guard
      xi. One 1-L bottle of sterile water or normal saline solution
      xii. Swabs for bacterial culture and sterile basin
      xiii. 0.25- or 0.50-in plain or iodoform coated wound packing material, top dressings, and tape
      xiv. Cotton-tip swabs or blunt-edged forceps
   b. Incision and drainage procedure
      i. Wash your hands and observe universal precautions.
      ii. Identify the patient by asking his or her name and assess the patient's allergy history.
      iii. Consider premedication with an anxiolytic or analgesic medication.
      iv. Position the patient so that the abscess is easily accessible.
      v. Put on gloves and a face shield.
      vi. Cleanse the skin with povidine iodine or chlorhexidine in a circular motion starting

from the center of the abscess and working outward. Allow the cleaning solution to dry.

vii. Cover the surrounding area with sterile drapes so that the abscess is exposed.

viii. Infiltrate the intradermal tissue under the surface of the wound with a local anesthetic agent, such as lidocaine or bupivacaine, using a 22- or 25-gauge needle. The maximum dose of lidocaine 1% solution without epinephrine is 4 mg/kg (Hsu, 2014). Bupivacaine without epinephrine should not exceed a dose of 1–2 mg/kg (Hsu). Neither bupivacaine or lidocaine with epinephrine is indicated for the incision and drainage procedure because local vasoconstriction is not necessary. Plain bupivacaine and lidocaine both provide a minimum duration of anesthesia for 30 minutes, which is sufficient to complete the procedure. If the patient is allergic to lidocaine, then conscious sedation should be considered. Inject parallel to the skin surface. Do not inject perpendicular to the skin surface (i.e., into the deeper tissues) because this may spread the infection. An alternative method is to inject in a field block pattern where the anesthetic agent is injected around the entire peripheral field surrounding the abscess but not directly over the site to be incised.

ix. Put on sterile gloves.

x. Palpate for the most fluctuant part of the abscess and make a small incision with a #11 blade scalpel over the center, then extend the incision to form a line. The depth and length of the incision are variable and should be based on the size and location of the abscess. If possible make the incision along the Langer's lines or skin-tension lines to promote optimal cosmetic results. The incision should not puncture the back wall of the abscess capsule. The goal of the incision is to provide an opening large enough to allow for drainage of the abscess and insertion of packing material. In addition, the incision should be large enough to insert the curved hemostat into the incision to break up loculations. This is called blunt dissection, which allows for further drainage of pus. Gently compress the outer sides of the abscess to express more drainage. Insert the curved hemostats and explore the abscess cavity, and open the hemostats to break up loculations.

xi. Collect a culture of the wound using aerobic and anaerobic culture medium. Cultures are beneficial if it is a first abscess, if the abscess worsens after incision and drainage, or if there has been a history of antibiotic treatment failure.

xii. Irrigate the incised abscess with normal saline solution using the large syringe and splash guard. An 18-gauge angiocatheter may be attached without the needle to the syringe. Irrigate until the drainage is clear or slightly serous.

xiii. Insert the 0.25- or 0.50-in packing gauze into the abscess taking care to loosely pack into the entire wound cavity. The goal is to keep the wound open to promote drainage and prevent closure of the wound. Closure of the wound without adequate drainage may lead to reformation of the abscess.

xiv. Cover the wound with a sterile top dressing and paper tape. For additional information and a streaming video of the incision and drainage procedure, visit www.nejm.org (Fitch et al., 2007).

6. Follow-up

a. The patient should return within 48–72 hours for a wound check.

b. Remove the packing and assess the amount of drainage. If the drainage is minimal, then warm soaks should be initiated and continued until the wound is healed. If the wound continues to have purulent drainage, then the wound should be irrigated with normal saline, explored again to assess for any unbroken loculations, and then repacked with new gauze. The patient should return again in 48 hours (Fitch et al., 2007; Kronfol, 2009).

7. Criteria for hospital admission or referral for specialty consultation either at the time of initial evaluation or at follow up

a. Patients with signs of systemic toxicity, such as fevers, rigors, or unstable vital signs, should be admitted for parenteral antibiotics.

b. Patients who have failed appropriate initial treatment.

c. The location of the abscess is such that the incision may cause a disfiguring defect. Refer immediately to a dermatologist or plastic surgeon.

d. Abscesses located on the hands or plantar surfaces should be immediately referred to an orthopedic or plastic surgeon.

e. Abscesses located over arteries or large blood vessels on the neck or over the antecubital fossa or inguinal areas should be immediately referred to an otolaryngologist or vascular surgeon.

f. Abscesses on or around the nasolabial folds may pose the risk of septic cavernous venous thrombosis and the patient should be immediately referred to an otolaryngologist.

D. Patient education

1. Instruct the patient in the signs and symptoms of worsening infection (fevers or chills, increasing pain, redness or swelling, and increasing purulent drainage or recurrent abscess).

2. Instruct the patient to be rechecked right away if these symptoms develop. Inform the patient of expected outcomes. The wound will likely heal in 7–10 days but may take longer. There will likely be a scar from the incision. This may be minimized by limiting direct sun exposure and wearing sun block if the scar is in an exposed area.

REFERENCES

American College of Chest Physicians/Society of Critical Care Medicine Consensus Conference: Definitions for sepsis and organ failure and guidelines for the use of innovative therapies in sepsis. (1992). *Critical Care Medicine, 20*(6), 864–874.

Baddour, L. M. (2014). Skin abscesses, furuncles, and carbuncles. Retrieved from www.uptodate.com/contents/skin-abscesses-furuncles-and-carbuncles.

Fitch, M. T., Manthey, D. E., McGinnis, H. D., Nicks, B. A., & Pariyadath, M. (2007). Videos in clinical medicine: Abscess incision and drainage. Retrieved from www.nejm.org/doi/full/10.1056/NEJMvcm071319.

Frazee, B. W., Lynn, J., Charlebois, E. D., Lambert, L., Lowery, D., & Perdreau-Remington, F. (2005). High prevalence of methicillin-resistant staphylococcus aureus in emergency department skin and soft tissue infections. *Annals of Emergency Medicine, 45*(3), 311–320.

Gorwitz, R. J., Jernigan, D. B., Powers, J. H., Jernigan, J. A., & Participants in the CDC-Convened Experts' Meeting on Management of MRSA in the Community. (2006). *Strategies for clinical management of MRSA in the community: Summary of an experts' meeting convened by the centers for disease control and prevention.* Retrieved from www.cdc.gov/mrsa/pdf/MRSA-Strategies-ExpMtgSummary-2006.pdf.

Hankin, A., & Everett, W. W. (2007). Are antibiotics necessary after incision and drainage of a cutaneous abscess? *Annals of Emergency Medicine, 50,* 48.

Hepburn, M. J., Dooley, D. P., Skidmore, P. J., Ellis, M. W., Starnes, W. F., & Hasewinkle, W. C. (2004). Comparison of short-course (5 days) and standard (10 days) treatment for uncomplicated cellulitis. *Archives of Internal Medicine, 164*(15), 1669–1674.

Hsu, D. (2014). Infiltrative anesthetics. Retrieved from www.uptodate.com/contents/infiltration-of-local-anesthetics.

Kronfol, R. (2014). Retrieved from www-uptodate-com.ucsf.idm.oclc.org/contents/technique-of-incision-and-drainage-for-skin-abscess?source=search_result&search=technique+of+incision+and+drainage&selectedTitle=1%7E150

Moran, G. J., Krishnadasan, A., Gorwitz, R. J., Fosheim, G. E., McDougal, L. K., Carey, R. B., et al. (2006). Methicillin-resistant *S. aureus* infections among patients in the emergency department. *New England Journal of Medicine, 355*(7), 666–674.

Rajendran, P. M., Young, D., Maurer, T., Chambers, H., Perdreau-Remington, F., Ro, P., et al. (2007). Randomized, double-blind, placebo-controlled trial of cephalexin for treatment of uncomplicated skin abscesses in a population at risk for community-acquired methicillin-resistant *Staphylococcus aureus* infection. *Antimicrobial Agents Chemotherapy, 51*(11), 4044.

Rogers, R. L., & Perkins, J. (2006). Skin and soft tissue infections. *Primary Care: Clinics in Office Practice, 33,* 697.

Stevens, D. L., Bisno, A. L., Chambers, H. F., Dellinger, E. P., Goldstein, E. J., Gorbach, S. L., et al. (2014). Practice guidelines for the diagnosis and management of skin and soft tissue infections: 2014 update by the infectious diseases society of America. *Clinical Infectious Diseases, 59*(2), e10–e52.

Stevens, D. L., Bisno, A. L., Chambers, H. F., Everett, E. D., Dellinger, P., Goldstein, E. J., et al. (2005). Practice guidelines for the diagnosis and management of skin and soft-tissue infections. *Clinical Infectious Diseases, 41*(10), 1373–1406.

ANEMIA

Michelle M. Marin and Laurie Jurkiewicz

CHAPTER 43

I. Introduction and general background

Anemia is defined as a decrease in the red blood cell (RBC) number, hemoglobin (Hgb) concentration, or the volume of packed red blood cells (hematocrit) in the blood. The World Health Organization defines anemia by laboratory definition as hemoglobin of less than 13 g/dL for adults, less than 12 g/dL for menstruating females, and less than 11 g/dL for pregnant females (Beutler & Waalen, 2006). However, data from the Scripps-Kaiser and National Health and Nutrition Examination Survey study recommend that lower limits of hemoglobin be stratified based on gender and race (black men ages 20–59: 12.9 g/dL; black men > 60 years: 12.7 g/dL; black women ages 20–49: 11.5 g/dL; black women > 50 years: 11.5 g/dL; white men ages 20–59: 13.7 g/dL; white men > 60 years: 13.2 g/dL; white women ages 20–49: 12.2 g/dL; white women > 60 years: 12.2 g/dL) (Beutler & Waalen, 2006).

Erythropoiesis is the regulated process of RBC production through a series of steps (National Anemia Action Council, 2002). In adults, this process occurs in the bone marrow of the sternum, ribs, vertebrae, and pelvis. The process begins when pluripotent stem cells are dedicated and the hematopoietic precursor cells mature with growth factors and hormones. The key to erythropoietin production is the availability of oxygen, which is carried to the tissues bound to the hemoglobin. When oxygen is low, then erythropoietin (90% from the kidney) triggers the red cell production to meet tissue demand. This production feedback system can occur only when all the needed substrates are in place: normal renal production of erythropoietin, a functioning bone marrow, and an adequate support of substrates of hemoglobin synthesis (National Anemia Action Council, 2002).

Normally, **anemia is seen during pregnancy**, because the blood volume increases by about 50% to meet the demands of increased circulation of the placenta and maternal fetal tissue.

This increase in intravascular volume starts at 6 weeks, peaks at about 28–34 weeks, and levels off during the last 6 weeks of pregnancy. Because plasma volume expansion is faster and greater than red blood cell production, there is a lowering of the Hgb and hematocrit referred to as "physiologic anemia." If there is no significant blood loss during the intrapartal period, the Hgb and hematocrit typically return to normal at about 6 weeks postpartum. Severe anemia in pregnancy is associated with an increased risk of spontaneous abortion, low birth weight, preterm birth, and fetal death (Brabin, Hakimi, & Pelletier, 2001). Persistent severe anemia increases the risk of maternal mortality (Sifakis & Pharmakides, 2000).

Otherwise, anemia is a sign and consequence of disease or treatments. It can be caused by a variety of systemic disorders and diseases and by a primary hematologic disorder. As a result, most individuals' physical symptoms and signs reflect the underlying illness rather than the anemia itself. Correct identification of the underlying disease is essential for appropriately directed treatment.

Anemia classification is based on (1) excessive RBC loss, (2) inadequate or ineffective RBC production, (3) abnormal RBC destruction, or (4) morphologic characteristics. These characteristics of cell size are microcytic, normocytic, and macrocytic (**Table 43-1**). Common microcytic anemias are iron deficiency, thalassemia, lead poisoning, and sideroblastic anemia. The most common causes of normocytic anemias include anemia of chronic disease, hemolytic anemia (may see elevated mean cell volume [MCV] due to reticulocytosis), bone marrow failure or infiltration, endocrine disorders, and renal disease. Common macrocytic anemias are vitamin B_{12} and folate deficiencies. Multiple etiologies of anemia can coexist together requiring a stepwise diagnostic approach critical to not missing a treatable cause. Outside of the usual categories of anemia lies a unique group of poorly diagnosed anemias that occurs in the geriatric population, accounting for 43% of hypoproliferative anemia (Makipour, Kanapuru, & Ershler, 2008) (**Table 43-2**).

TABLE 43-1 Separating Anemia by MCV

Hypochromic Microcytic MCV < 80 fL	Iron deficiency	Thalassemia	Sideroblastic	Hemoglobinopathies	Lead poisoning
Normochromic/ Normocytic MCV 80–100 fL	Acute hemorrhage	Acute hemolysis	Early iron deficiency, folate, and vitamin B$_{12}$ deficiency	Anemia of chronic disease Chronic inflammation Acute and chronic infections Cancer Kidney disease	Myelodysplastic syndromes: bone marrow failure, pregnancy
Macrocytic MCV > 100 fL	Megaloblastic: vitamin B$_{12}$ and folate deficiencies and drug induced	Reticulocytosis: intense red blood cell stimulation caused by acute hemolysis or hemorrhage (reticulocytes are large and young red blood cells)	Chronic liver disease	Myelodysplastic syndromes: bone marrow failure or infiltration	Endocrinopathies Postsplenectomy

Reproduced from Collins-Bride, G., & Saxe, J. (Eds.). (1998). *Nurse practitioner/physician collaborative practice: Clinical guidelines for ambulatory care.* San Francisco, CA: UCSF Nursing Press. Used with permission from the UCSF Nursing Press.

A. Microcytic anemias

1. Iron deficiency anemia

   a. Definition and overview: Iron deficiency is a microcytic and hypochromic (decrease in hemoglobin concentration) anemia. It occurs when the bone marrow iron stores are less than what is needed to produce RBCs. Common causes of iron deficiency are:

      i. Pregnancy accounts for about 75% of non-physiologic anemia in the childbearing woman (American College of Obstetricians and Gynecologists [ACOG], 2008). The physiology is described by an increased demand on iron stores during pregnancy not only for Hgb synthesis but also for fetal liver storage to meet the needs of the infant in the first 6 months of life. The demand for iron increases in the second half of the pregnancy because of the increased red cell mass and the demands of the growing fetus

      ii. Low-iron diets caused by inadequate intake or rapid growth during prolonged growth.

      iii. Poor absorption seen with gastric atrophy, achlorhydria

      iv. Blood loss caused by menstrual bleeding, large intra-abdominal or joint bleeding, or occult gastrointestinal and genitourinary bleeding. Of note, it takes 20 mL/day of blood for the usual stool hemoccult test to become positive (Umbreit, 2005). One milliliter of blood loss is equivalent to the loss of 0.5 mg of iron (Tables 43-1 and 43-2).

   b. Prevalence and incidence: Iron deficiency anemia is the most common nutritional deficiency (Umbreit, 2005). It affects more than 3 million people according to the National Heart, Lung,

TABLE 43-2 Differentiating Anemias

	MCV	RDW	Retics	Iron	TIBC	% Sat	Ferritin
Iron deficiency	D	I	D	D	I	D	D
Iron depletion	N	N	N	N	I	D	D
β-Thalassemia	DQ	D	I	N	N	N	N
Sideroblastic	D	H	I	NII	NID	NII	N
Chronic disease	D or N	N	NID	D	N/D	N/I/D	N
Lead poisoning	D	N	I	N	N	N	N

I, increased; D, decreased; DQ, decreased greater than expected in iron deficiency; N, normal; II, increased significantly.

and Blood Institute. Iron deficiency results in increased pediatric and maternal mortality; decreased work production; delayed childhood development; and with mild to moderate deficiency, an increased risk for developing infectious diseases. There are estimates that 4% of U.S. women between the ages of 20 and 49 years have iron deficiency anemia with the higher rates in Mexican-American women (Killip, Bennett, & Chambers, 2007). African-American women, adolescents, and women of low socioeconomic status are at increased risk for iron and folic acid deficiencies (Laubach & Bendell, 2008). The incidence of anemia increases with age with 10% seen in the 65 years and older age group (Schrier, 2010). This increase is associated with a significant increase in morbidity and mortality, impaired cognition, decrease in exercise tolerance, and decrease in quality of life measures.

2. Thalassemia
   a. Definition and overview: Thalassemia syndromes are a group of inherited autosomal-recessive anemias classified by defects in the synthesis of one or more of the hemoglobin globin chain subunits. These defects can occur either in the α or β globin chains of hemoglobin. The combined imbalances of globin and inadequate hemoglobin production result in a variety of clinical manifestations. The former causes hypochromia and microcytosis; the latter leads to ineffective erythropoiesis. Both types cause hemolysis (Giardina & Forget, 2008). The diagnosis of thalassemia is made by a hemoglobin electrophoresis test (**Table 43-3**).
      i. α-Thalassemia trait: loss of one α gene, not anemic but mean cell volume may be low.
      ii. α-Thalassemia minor: loss of two genes of α globin, hematocrit is low and MCV is 60–75 fL.
      iii. Hemoglobin H: loss of three α genes, moderate microcytic anemia.
      iv. β-Thalassemia minor: mild microcytic anemia, asymptomatic.
      v. β-Thalassemia intermedia: severe anemia often requiring RBC transfusion.
      vi. β-Thalassemia major: condition is life threatening requiring chronic transfusions and possibly hematopoietic cell transplantation.
      vii. Hg E/β-Thalassemia: combined (Yaish, 2013).
   b. Prevalence and incidence: Thalassemias are the most common single genetic disorders known. They are encountered in every ethnic group and geographic location, although they are most common in the Mediterranean basin and tropic and subtropic areas of Asia and Africa. Thalassemia in these regions ranges from 2.5 to 15%. In the United States, 15% of African-Americans are silent carriers of α-thalassemia, with 3% carrying the trait; 1–15% of those of Mediterraneans origin carry the trait. For β-thalassemia, 10–15% of Mediterraneans and 0.8% of African-Americans in the United States are affected (Hoffman et al., 2008). In a world of immigration and intermarriage, new patterns of thalassemia have emerged. In southeastern Asians, Hb E and β-thalassemia combined, making this combination most common in many parts of the world (Yaish, 2013).

3. Sideroblastic anemia
   a. Definition and overview: Sideroblastic anemias are a group of disorders with ringed iron-laden

TABLE 43-3 Thalassemia Percent of Abnormal Hgb and Degrees of Anemia

	HgbA	HgbA2	HgbF	Comments
Normal	97–99%	1–3%	<1%	
β-Thalassemia (minor)	80–95%	4–8%	1–5%	MCV 55–75 fL, Hematocrit (Hct) 28–40%, peripheral smear mildly abnormal, heterozygous trait
β-Thalassemia (intermediate)	0–30%	0–10%	6–100%	Moderate anemia
β-Thalassemia (major)	0%	4–10%	90–96%	Homozygous trait, marked microcytosis with severe anemia
α-Thalassemia trait	Normal	Normal	Normal	Heterozygous trait, 2/4 genes normal, MCV 60–70 fL, Hct 28–40%, diagnosis of exclusion

Reproduced from Collins-Bride, G., & Saxe, J. (Eds.). (1998). *Nurse practitioner/physician collaborative practice: Clinical guidelines for ambulatory care*. San Francisco, CA: UCSF Nursing Press. Used with permission from the UCSF Nursing Press.

sideroblasts in the bone marrow accompanied by moderate to severe microcytic anemia. The classification of sideroblastic anemias is distinguished between diseases of the heme synthesis pathway and those diseases of mitochondrial DNA or those with defects in the nuclear DNA. There are two primary X-linked inherited forms that are recognized early in life. Acquired types are caused by exposures from toxins or drugs (alcohol, lead, or zinc). Once the offending toxin is removed, recovery occurs within 1–2 weeks (Gehrs & Friedberg, 2002). Others are associated with ringed sideroblasts, the myelodysplastic syndrome of refractory anemia.

b. Prevalence and incidence: The incidence of sideroblastic anemia is low. Acquired types are more prevalent than hereditary types. Many individuals are stable for years but in a subset of patients who belong to the myelodysplastic syndrome category, 5% go on to develop leukemia. Acquired sideroblastic anemias are not fully established because of the multiple triggers and clinical presentations (Schwartz, 2007).

B. Normocytic anemias

1. Definition and overview: The MCV is within normal limits but hemoglobin and hematocrit are decreased mildly to moderately. Individuals are generally asymptomatic. Nearly all anemias are normocytic in their initial stages (Brill & Baumgardner, 2000).

2. Anemia of chronic disease and anemia of chronic inflammation (ACD).

   a. Definitions and overview: This is an anemia of underproduction of RBCs often associated with chronic inflammatory disease. A decreased life span of the RBC and inhibition of hematopoiesis, deregulation of iron absorption and transport, and decreased erythropoietin production defines this anemia (Gardner & Benz, 2008). Hepcidin, an iron regulatory peptide produced by the liver, is thought to be the central regulator in iron metabolism and is controlled by the erythropoietic activity in the bone (Kemna, 2008). ACD is usually seen as normocytic, normochromic, or mildly microcytic with a low reticulocyte count. Iron stores may be normal or increased. The most common causes are usually multifactorial.

      i. Chronic systemic diseases, such as diabetes, congestive heart failure, and chronic obstructive pulmonary disease

      ii. Chronic inflammation, such as rheumatoid arthritis and inflammatory bowel disease

      iii. Neoplasm

      iv. Chronic liver and kidney disease

      v. Chronic infection, such as HIV/AIDS

      vi. Endocrine deficiencies, such as hypothyroidism, diabetes, adrenal or pituitary insufficiencies, and hypogonadism

      vii. Uncompensated blood loss

      viii. Hypersplenism

   b. Prevalence and incidence: This is the second most common form of anemia worldwide, second to iron deficiency. In a review of hospitalized patients, estimated prevalence is 20–40% for ACD (Tefferi, 2007).

3. Hemolytic anemia

   a. Definition and overview: Hemolytic anemia is a normocytic, normochromic anemia where there is a premature destruction of RBCs for which the bone marrow cannot compensate. This occurs when RBC survival is less than normal (120 days) or when the bone marrow is impaired (Linker, 2007). This can be seen congenitally with recognition early in life as in sickle cell disease or later in life when exposed to a stressor, such as G6PD (glucose-6-phosphate dehydrogenase) deficiency. The acquired type usually occurs in adulthood, in those persons older than 40 years of age and in those with mechanical hemolysis, paroxysmal nocturnal hemolysis, or warm and cold reactive antibodies.

   b. Prevalence and incidence: Hemolytic anemia represents 5% of all anemias (Schick, 2010). Autoimmune hemolytic anemia occurs in 10% of systemic lupus erythematosus, most occurring in women older than 65 years of age (Schwartz, 2007). The underlying disorder and etiology of hemolysis dictates survival.

C. Macrocytic anemias

Macrocytosis can be seen without megaloblastic changes in liver disease, hypothyroidism, aplastic anemia, autoimmune hemolytic anemia, and some forms of myelodysplasia. Megaloblastic anemias are a group of diverse anemias that share the failure in the synthesis and assembly of DNA resulting in ineffective erythropoiesis. Findings of MCV greater than 100 suggest megaloblastic anemia, but with MCV greater than 110 it is much more likely to be present. The most common causes of megaloblastosis are vitamin B_{12} and folate deficiencies. Deficiencies of one of these vitamins can cause malabsorption of the other vitamin. Megaloblastic disease, especially when combined with microcytic anemia, can be present as normocytic.

1. Vitamin B_{12} deficiency

   a. Definitions and overview: Vitamin B_{12} (cobalamin) deficiency is a problem of either inadequate intake over several years or of inadequate absorption.

Lifelong subclinical vitamin B_{12} deficiency, 50% with normal vitamin B_{12} levels, when challenged with abnormal absorption or altered metabolism can tip individuals into symptomatic deficiency (Langan & Zawistoski, 2011). Low levels of vitamin B_{12} elevate homocysteine, which is associated with cardiovascular disease (CVD); however, replacement with vitamin B_{12} does not change CVD risk (Elmadfa & Singer, 2009; Langan & Zawistiski, 2011). Consider screening high-risk individuals for megaloblastic anemia.

Common causes are:

i. Pernicious anemia associated with autoimmune disorders, atrophic gastritis.

ii. Gastrectomy, bariatric surgery, and intestinal surgeries.

iii. Small-bowel disorders, such as inflammatory bowel disease, bacterial overgrowth, tapeworms, enteritis, sprue, and celiac disease all affecting the terminal ileum.

iv. Long-term vegan diets without dairy products or eggs.

v. Medications inhibiting absorption, such as metformin, proton pump inhibitors, and histamine 2 blockers.

vi. Food: cobalamin malabsorption syndrome when nutritional intake is adequate and there is no evidence of other causes of malabsorption or pernicious anemia.

b. Prevalence and incidence: Determining the frequency of vitamin B_{12} deficiency anemia is difficult because the etiologies are diverse. It is estimated that vitamin B_{12} deficiency occurs in 5.3% of those older than 60 years. In the elderly, rates increase from 5 to 20%. Those 31–51 years old have 3.5% incidence and have a subclinical presentation (Centers for Disease Control and Prevention [CDC], 2009). Although usually seen in adults older than 40 of Scandinavian or Northern European ancestry, it can also be seen in any population. Nutritional deficiency is seen worldwide; however, in affluent countries, inadequate absorption is most common.

2. Folic acid deficiency

a. Definitions and overview: Folic acid is present in most fruits and vegetables. A typical diet of 50 mg/d should be adequate. Folic acid stores of 5–20 mg last about 4 months. Common causes of folic acid deficiency include:

i. Inadequate diet of fruits and vegetables.

ii. Inflammatory bowel disease, such as sprue.

iii. Cultural or ethnic cooking destroying folate, as in prolonged stewing.

iv. Medications interfering with absorption, such as methotrexate, phenytoin, acyclovir, oral contraceptives, colchicine, and trimethoprim.

v. Increased demand in pregnancy and lactation; hyperemesis gravidarum; and intrinsic hematologic disease, such as malignancy infiltration in the bone marrow.

b. Prevalence and incidence: The United States Food and Drug Administration mandated that folic acid be added to enriched grain products in 1998, which resulted in a significant decrease in folate deficiency. In temperate zones, folate deficiency is most common in alcoholics. Tropical sprue, which is endemic near the equator, results in malabsorption of this critical vitamin.

II. Database (may include but is not limited to)

A. Subjective: microcytic

1. Iron deficiency anemia, thalassemia, and sideroblastic anemia

a. Past health history

i. Medical illnesses: recurrent iron deficiency anemia, anorexia, gastrointestinal or genitourinary malignancy, celiac disease, atrophic gastritis, *Helicobacter pylori*, helminthic infections, and chronic inflammatory conditions

ii. Surgical history: partial or total gastroenterostomy, gastric resection, or splenectomy

iii. Obstetric and gynecological history: heavy menses, multiparty, recent pregnancy, and parturition

iv. Medication history: nonsteroidal anti-inflammatory drugs, steroids, chemotherapy, iron or multivitamins, salicylates, antacids that block iron absorption, and health food products

v. Exposure history: toxic exposures, such as lead poisoning (exposure to lead-based paint, lead-contaminated dust, and lead-contaminated residential soil) and potent marrow toxic agents

b. Family history

i. Anemia

ii. Chronic inflammatory diseases

iii. Malignancy

iv. Lead poisoning

c. Personal and social history
   i. Diet inadequate in iron, dairy, or animal products
   ii. Heavy alcohol use
   iii. Intravenous drug use and sharing needles
   iv. Travel to sub-Sahara Africa exposing the person to *Schistosoma*, such as *Trichuris* infections, and malarial zones
   v. Regular blood donations

2. Thalassemia
   a. Past health history
      i. Medical illnesses: chronic microcytic anemia and iron overload.
      ii. Surgical history: splenectomy or hematopoietic stem cell transplant.
      iii. Obstetric history: pregnancy or stillborn fetus caused by hydrops fetalis.
      iv. Medication history: chelation therapy and RBC transfusions.
   b. Family history
      i. Thalassemia and hemoglobinopathies
      ii. Ethnicity: Mediterranean, Southeast Asian, Chinese, and African-American descent

3. Sideroblastic anemia
   a. Past health history
      i. Medical illness: copper deficiency, vitamin B_6 deficiency, and myelodysplastic syndrome
      ii. Medication history: excessive use of zinc supplements, antibiotics, copper chelating agents, antituberculosis agents, and chemotherapy
      iii. Exposure history: lead poisoning and prolonged exposure to cold
   b. Family history
      i. Sideroblastic anemia
      ii. Mitochondrial disease
   c. Personal and social history
      i. Chronic excessive alcohol intake
      ii. Coin ingestion

4. Review of systems for microcytic anemias
   a. Constitutional: degree of symptoms depends on the degree and rate of anemia development. Marked fatigue and decreased exercise tolerance may be the earliest symptoms along with weakness, postural faintness, headache, and weight loss. Pica, especially eating ice, is common.
   b. Skin and nails: pallor; bruising; koilonychia (spoon nails); and brittle nails.
   c. Ears, nose, and throat: bleeding, fissures at corners of mouth, and painful mouth.
   d. Neck: swollen neck glands.
   e. Pulmonary: cough, shortness of breath, and hemoptysis.
   f. Cardiac: chest pain, palpitations, and tachycardia
   g. Abdomen: tenderness, masses, changes in bowel habits, bleeding hemorrhoids, hematemesis, melena or bright red blood per rectum, distention, and difficulty swallowing.
   h. Genitourinary: bloody urine
   i. Gynecological: heavy and or irregular menses, pregnancy, and multiple pregnancies
   j. Skeletal: bone tenderness

B. Subjective: normocytic anemias

1. Anemia of chronic disease
   a. Past health history
      i. Medical illness: anemia; chronic diseases, such as renal disease; inflammatory bowel disease; autoimmune disorders; malignancies; sickle cell disease; and liver disease
      ii. Surgical history: cholecystectomy, prosthetic cardiac valves, and stem cell transplant
      iii. Medication history: penicillin, quinine, and quinidine
      iv. Exposure history: parvovirus B19
   b. Family history
      i. G6PD deficiency
      ii. Sickle cell disease
      iii. Hereditary anemia disorders
      iv. Autoimmune disorders
      v. Renal or liver disease
   c. Personal and social history
      i. Diet including fava beans

2. Hemolytic anemia
   a. Past medical history
      i. Medical illnesses: previous hemolysis, chronic hemolytic anemia, systemic lupus erythematosus, rheumatoid arthritis, chronic lymphocytic leukemia, non-Hodgkin's lymphoma, various carcinomas, idiopathic thrombocytopenic purpura and thrombotic thrombocytopenic purpura, G6PD deficiency, malaria, and cold agglutinin disease
      ii. Surgical: prosthetic heart valves, patches, and vascular grafts
      iii. Medications: antimalarials, sulfonamides, nitrofurantoin, sulfonylureas, quinine, quinidine, interferon, phenacetin, high-dose penicillin, and blood transfusions
      iv. Exposures: infectious agents, such as parasites; viruses, such as Epstein-Barr or cytomegalovirus; measles; syphilis; enteric bacteria; spider bites and snake venom; copper; and organic compounds

b. Family history
  i. G6PD deficiency
  ii. Autoimmune hemolytic anemia
  iii. Red cell membrane disorders
c. Personal and social history
  i. Aggressive exercise causing microvascular trauma

3. Review of symptoms for normocytic anemia and anemia of chronic disease and hemolysis
a. Constitutional: fatigue, weakness, postural faintness, poor exercise tolerance, and abrupt or gradual onset.
b. Skin: rash, yellowing color, bruising, petechiae, pale skin, and nails
c. Neck: swollen lymph nodes.
d. Pulmonary: shortness of breath
e. Cardiac: palpitations, tachycardia, and chest pain
f. Abdominal: right upper quadrant pain, abdominal fullness, and decreased appetite
g. Extremities: leg ulcers and edema
h. Joints: swollen painful joints
i. Bladder: dark or bloody urine

C. Subjective: macrocytic and megaloblastic

1. Vitamin B_{12} deficiency
a. Past health history
  i. Medical history: autoimmune thyroid disease, type I diabetes mellitus, Addison's disease, idiopathic hypoparathyroidism, autoimmune hemolytic diseases, tropical sprue, atrophic gastritis, regional enteritis, or gastric cancer
  ii. Surgical: gastrectomy, bariatric surgery, or intestinal surgery
  iii. Medications: metformin, thyroid replacement, colchicine, cholestyramine, histamine 2 blockers, proton pump inhibitors, and azidothymidine
  iv. Exposures: intestinal tape worm infestation and repeated and prolonged (> 6 hr) nitrous oxide inhalation especially in the elderly (Longo, 2009)
b. Family history
  i. Pernicious anemia
  ii. Autoimmune disorders, such as diabetes mellitus type 1 and thyroid disorders, vitiligo, hypoparathyroidism, and Addison's disease.
c. Personal and social history
  i. Vegan diet, high folate intake
  ii. Alcohol use

2. Folate deficiency
a. Past health history
  i. Medical history: vitamin B_{12} deficiency, chronic hemolytic anemia, sprue, atrophic gastritis, small bowel disease, psoriasis, epilepsy, and chronic hemodialysis
  ii. Obstetric and gynecological history: pregnancy
  iii. Medications: methotrexate, pentamidine, trimethoprim, cancer chemotherapy, triampterene, phenytoin, primadone, phenobarbital, cholestyramine, and sulfasalazine
b. Family history
  i. Hereditary disorders
  ii. Gluten sensitivities
c. Personal and social history
  i. Alcohol abuse
  ii. Narcotic addiction
  iii. Inadequate diet

3. Review of systems: macrocytic or megaloblastic anemia, vitamin B_{12} or folic acid deficiency.
a. Constitutional: fatigue, decreased exercise tolerance, weakness, and weight loss
b. Skin: yellow skin, pallor, vitiligo, and rashes.
c. Mouth: cheilosis, stomatitis, sore smooth tongue, and atrophic glossitis
d. Neck: sense of fullness in the thyroid region
e. Pulmonary: shortness of breath
f. Cardiac: tachycardia, chest pain, palpitations.
g. Abdominal: diarrhea, pain, anorexia, nausea, constipation, bowel incontinence, and sense of fullness
h. Bladder: incontinence
i. Neurologic: paresthesias, balance problems, and difficulty walking
j. Extremities: edema
k. Neuropsychiatric: depression, irritability, dementia, and insomnia

D. Physical examination

1. Evaluate weight and height.
2. Complete vital signs: postural blood pressure and pulse, respiratory rate, and temperature.
3. See **Table 43-4** for physical examination findings seen in anemia.

III. Assessment

A. Determine the diagnosis

After the health history and physical examination. Guide the workup based on the clues found. Review previous complete blood cell count (CBC) to evaluate what might be the individual's trend of blood counts.

TABLE 43-4 Physical Examination Findings Seen with Anemia

Location	Finding	Implication
Skin and nails	Pallor	Decreased number of red blood cells
	Petechiae	Thrombocytopenia, leukemia, disseminated intravascular coagulation
	Telangiectasia and spider angiomas	Liver disease
	Jaundice, icterus	Hemolytic and megaloblastic anemia, liver disease
	Decreased elasticity of skin, brittle nails	Long-standing anemia
	Koilonychia (spoon nails)	Long-standing anemia, especially iron deficiency
	Hair loss	
	Rash	Systemic lupus erythematosis
Neck	Thyromegaly or masses	Endocrinopathies
Mucous membranes	Pallor, cheilosis, and stomatitis	Leukemia, pernicious anemia, or severe iron deficiency
	Smooth red tongue and atrophic glossitis	Vitamin B_{12} deficiency
Lymph nodes	Lymphadenopathy	Leukemia, lymphoma, HIV
Heart	Tachycardia, loud murmurs, decreased PMI, congestive heart failure, functional murmurs, hypertension	Severe anemia, pregnancy, renal disease
Pulmonary	Tachypnea	Severe anemia
Abdomen	Splenomegaly, hepatomegaly, or hepatic tenderness	Leukemia, lymphoma, hemolytic anemia, liver disease, autoimmune disease
Central nervous system	Decreased vibratory and position sense/ataxia, and decreased vibration of 256-degree tuning fork	Pernicious anemia Lead poisoning causing ringed sideroblasts
Skeletal	Bone tenderness, swollen joints	Hematologic disease, rheumatoid arthritis, autoimmune disorders
Rectal	Guiaic-positive stool, or bright red blood per rectum	Gastrointestinal bleeding
Extremities	Edema	Heart failure, renal failure, cirrhosis, hepatitis
	Leg ulcers	Chronic hemolytic anemia, iron deficiency

B. **Differentiate the anemia and assess the severity of the disease.**

1. Microcytic anemias
   a. Iron deficiency anemia
      i. CBC: white cell and platelet abnormalities give clues about bone marrow malfunction, such as myelodysplastic or myeloproliferative disorder.
      ii. Assess anemia based on the MCV (Table 43-1).
      iii. Order iron studies: ferritin, iron, total iron binding capacity, and reticulocyte count with a peripheral blood smear (**Table 43-5**).
      iv. Determine the type of microcytic anemia. If iron deficiency, order stool guaiac and urinalysis to rule out blood loss from the gastrointestinal and genitourinary tracts, respectively. It is critical not to miss an occult gastrointestinal lesion, frequently a malignancy. Refer patients older than age 50, or younger than age 50 with a positive family history of colon cancer, to gastroenterology for endoscopy and colonoscopy. Young patients with iron deficiency anemia, weight loss, and persistent abdominal discomfort should also be referred to gastroenterology.

TABLE 43-5 Red Blood Cell Morphology

Description of Red Blood Cell		Associated with Disease
Anisocytosis	Excessive number of red blood cells of various sizes	Larger size = vitamin B_{12} or folate deficiency, drug effect
		Smaller size = iron deficiency
Hypochromia (decreased hemoglobin content in the red blood cell)	Central pallor	Iron deficiency
Macro-ovalocytes	Oval red blood cell	Vitamin B_{12} or folate deficiency, liver disease, myelodysplastic syndrome
Polychromasis	Wright's stain: large grayish blue with pink	Reticulocytes
		Increased levels in a peripheral smear are a result from a variety of anemias or from damage to the bone marrow
Poiklocytosis	Abnormal red blood cell shapes, such as:	(the following is not inclusive list)
	Acanthocytes (spur cells)	Severe liver disease
	Echinocytes (burr cells)	Uremia, red blood cell volume loss
	Schistocytes (schizocytes)	Microangiopathic or macroangiopathic hemolytic anemia
	Spherocytes	Autoimmune hemolytic anemia, G6PD deficiency, hereditary spherocytosis
	Target cells	Thalassemia, liver disease, hemoglobin C, sickle cell disease
	Teardrop cells	Myelofibrosis, infiltrative processes of marrow
	Rouleaux formation	Paraproteinemia, such as multiple myeloma
Red blood cell inclusions		(the following is not inclusive list)
	Basophilic stippling	Lead poisoning, thalassemia, myelofibrosis
	Pappenheimer (iron) bodies	Sideroblastic anemia, lead poisoning
	Parasites	Malaria, babesiosis
Hypersegmentation	Neutrophil nuclei with more than seven lobes	Vitamin B_{12} or folate deficiency, drug effects

v. Pregnant women and young menstruating women who are asymptomatic and otherwise healthy likely have iron deficiency anemia caused by menses or increased iron demands from a growing fetus in the context of inadequate dietary iron intake (ACOG, 2008).

vi. A therapeutic trial of iron reevaluating the results can be helpful because only an iron-deficient state will (see the treatment section) will improve with iron supplementation.

b. Thalassemia anemia

i. If iron studies are normal and abnormal peripheral smear is reported, consider thalassemia based on the individual's history. Milder forms of thalassemia need to be distinguished from iron deficiency and more severe forms need to be distinguished from other hemoglobinopathies.

ii. Thalassemias are congenital. Compare current CBC to previous CBCs. Microcytosis is usually significant, whereas the RBC count is normal or elevated.

iii. If no diagnosis, order hemoglobin A_2, globin chain synthesis ratio, and hemoglobin electrophoresis including Hgb H (Table 43-3).

iv. If a pregnant woman is thought to be a carrier, the father of the baby should be tested. A CBC and hemoglobin electrophoresis should be done.

c. Sideroblastic anemia

    i. Review the CBC and iron studies; iron overload is suggestive of congenital or acquired clonal sideroblastic anemia.

    ii. A bone marrow biopsy with appropriate staining ultimately is the gold standard for this diagnosis.

d. Lead poisoning

    i. Review the CBC and iron studies.

    ii. Consider getting a zinc protoporhyrin or free erythrocyte protoporphyrin (an elevated level suggests lead poisoning or iron deficiency anemia) as either test can be used as an indication of lead exposure over the past 3 months.

    iii. Obtain a serum lead level.

2. Normocytic anemia

  a. Anemia of chronic disease. This is a diagnosis of exclusion when CBC and iron stores are normal. Identify potential causes of this anemia.

    i. Consider ordering an erythrocyte sedimentation rate and a C-reactive protein to look for chronic inflammatory states, both elevated in infection and inflammation.

    ii. Rule out liver disease with liver functions tests, thyroid disease with a thyroid-stimulating hormone level and thyroid function tests, and renal disease with a serum creatinine and urinalysis.

  b. Hemolytic anemia

    i. With a careful health and medication history and physical examination, look at the normocytic anemia MCV for reticulocytosis.

    ii. Order an indirect bilirubin and lactate dehydrogenase blood test.

    iii. Consider ordering a direct antiglobin test or Coombs to confirm immune-mediated hemolysis. Order a G6PD blood test 1–2 months after acute hemolysis.

    iv. Consider ordering a cold agglutinin titer.

3. Macrocytic and megaloblastic anemias

  a. Vitamin B_{12} deficiency

    i. CBC with elevated MCV and a peripheral smear with macro-ovalocytes and hypersegmented polymorphonuclear cells are seen with vitamin B_{12} and folate deficiency.

    ii. Order a vitamin B_{12} and a folate level to differentiate the common causes of megaloblastic anemia. Consider screening high-risk individuals especially those with health conditions resulting in a high cell turnover as after a prolonged or critical illness and

normal MCV (Bryan, 2010; Langan & Zawistoski, 2011).

    iii. Consider serum methylmalonic level, which has increased sensitivity and specificity for confirming vitamin B_{12} deficiency. Additional serologic testing for gastrin and intrinsic factor (IF) are used to diagnose pernicious anemia (Oberly & Yang, 2013).

    iv. Low cobalamin distinguishes vitamin B_{12} from myelodysplastic syndrome.

  b. Folate deficiency: with normal vitamin B_{12} level, low serum folate level, normal methylmalonic level, and elevated homocysteine, folate deficiency is the probable diagnosis.

IV. Goals of clinical management

A. *Choose a cost-effective approach for diagnosing anemia.*

B. *Choose a treatment plan that normalizes serum RBC level and minimizes the risk of anemia relapse (**Table 43-6**).*

C. *Select an approach that maximizes the patient's short- and long-term adherence to treatment.*

V. Plan

A. *Microcytic anemias*

  1. Iron deficiency anemia

    a. Encourage intake of iron-rich foods: lean red meat, poultry, egg yolks, beans, dried fruit, dark leafy greens, broccoli, asparagus, or infusion of dried nettle.

    b. Review foods that interfere with iron absorption: coffee, tea, soda, dairy, and antacids.

    c. Ferrous sulfate therapy, 325 mg (65 mg elemental iron) daily to twice daily, depending on severity of anemia treatment. In pregnancy, this should be given in addition to prenatal vitamins (CDC, 1998; Graves & Barger, 2001). A 4-week trial of iron supplementation for mild anemia before a definitive diagnosis of iron deficiency anemia with iron studies is an acceptable initial intervention. If the follow-up complete blood count (CBC) is normal, it is reasonable to assume the anemia was caused by a deficiency in iron. Plan to give iron 1–2 months for anemia correction then an additional 4–5 months to replenish iron stores (ferritin level to 50 mcg/mL).

TABLE 43-6 Laboratory Tests with Normal Values
*Note each lab has their own result standards.

Test	Normal	Comment
Complete blood count Hgb Hct	Hemoglobin: F: 12–15.5 g/dL M: 13.6–17.5 g/dL Hematocrit: F: 35–49% M: 39–49	Physiologic variation because of age, smoking, and altitude. Hemogloblin reflects amount of oxygen carrying protein. Hematocrit measures percentage of Hgb in blood
Red blood cell indices		
Red blood count	F: 3.5–5.2 10 × 6th/mcL M: 4.3–6 10 × 6th/mcL	Elevated in dehydration, lung disease, smoking, polycythemia vera
Mean cell volume	80–100 fL	Reflects size of red cell
Mean cell hemoglobin concentration	31–36 g/dL	Increased with spherocytosis, hemolysis; decreased in other anemias
Mean cell Hgb	26–34 pg	Is calculation of average amount of Hgb in RBC
Red cell distribution width	11.5–14.5%	Is calculation of variation of red blood cell size; decreased in iron deficiency
White blood cell count	4.5–11 10 × 3rd/mcL	
Platelets	15,000–450,000 µL	
Reticulocyte count	33–137 10 × 3rd/mcL > 400 reflects RBC loss or destruction < 200 reflects low production, macrocytosis, ACD, or myelodysplastic disease	Expect increase of two to three times in 10 days after anemia starts if normal erythropoietin and bone marrow
Iron supply studies	50–175 mcg/dL	
Serum iron, total iron binding capacity	250–460 mcg/dL	Is decreased in iron deficiency anemia
% transferring saturation	25–50%	low in iron deficiency < 16%
Ferritin	M: 10–300 µg/mL F: 10–200 µg/mL	Most useful in separating iron deficiency from ACD, thalassemia; lowest levels correlate with depleted bone marrow
Haptoglobin	4–316	High levels helpful in ruling out significant intravascular hemolysis
Folate	165–760 ng/mL	
Vitamin B$_{12}$	140–820 pg/mL	

Data from Gomella, L., & Haist, S. (2007). *The famous scut monkey handbook: Clinician's pocket reference* (11th ed.). New York, NY McGraw-Hill; Nicoll, D., McPhee, S., Pignone, M., & Lu, C. (2007). *Pocket guide to diagnostic tests* (5th ed.). New York, NY. McGraw-Hill Medical.

d. Discuss ways to increase iron intake and absorption: take with juice with vitamin C and in-between meals.

e. Review side effects of supplementation: constipation, nausea, bloating, almost dark, charcoal-colored stool, and abdominal cramps.

f. If iron is poorly tolerated because of side effects, consider switching to ferrous fumarate, 325 mg, or ferrous gluconate, 325 mg.

g. *Keep iron tablets out of reach of children, because they can be fatal if ingested in quantities of only 10–20 pills.*

h. If the patient has mild anemia, consider intermittent dosing (120 mg elemental iron one to two times weekly).

i. Consider informing the patient of the availability in health food stores of Floridex Liquid Iron Supplement. Floridex has very little elemental iron and thus is better tolerated. However, it may not be as effective in treating anemia.

j. Elemental iron interferes with zinc absorption, so consider zinc supplementation (25 mg, which is the amount found in prenatal vitamins) is recommended in pregnant patients (Graves & Barger, 2001).

k. Repeat CBC and reticulocyte count in 2–4 weeks after initiation of treatment. An increased reticulocyte count confirms that the patient is taking iron supplementation.

l. Although medication nonadherence is the most common cause of response failure, having the incorrect diagnosis has to be considered.

m. Plan for patient follow-up with laboratory values at 1, 2, 4, and 6 months to ensure full recovery.

n. In pregnancy, obtain medical consultation if severe anemia (Hgb is less than 9 g/dL) despite initiation of therapy or if anemia is chronic.

2. Thalassemia

a. Individuals with mild disease should be identified to prevent repeated unnecessary diagnostic anemia evaluations and to prevent patients from taking iron unnecessarily.

b. For those with hemoglobin H disease, 1 mg of folate daily should be prescribed.

c. Individuals who have severe anemia and need to be treated with red cell transfusions and chelation therapy should be referred to a hematologist.

d. Pregnant women who are found to be carriers and whose partner is also a carrier of either a thalassemia or sickle cell trait should have genetic counseling because of the risk of fetal hemoglobinopathy. Women who either have a thalassemia or sickle cell disease may have profound anemia with considerable neonatal morbidity and therefore should be cared for by a specialist in obstetrics and hematology (ACOG, 2008).

3. Sideroblastic anemia

a. If medically stable, no treatment is needed. Patients often do not respond to erythropoietin therapy.

b. Occasionally, these patients need RBC transfusions. A hematologist should be managing their anemia.

4. Lead poisoning

a. Further investigate the patient's possible lead exposures: exposure to lead-based paint, lead-contaminated dust, lead-contaminated residential soil (U.S. Environmental Protection Agency, 2010).

b. Refer patient to the public health department to help with investigation of lead exposure.

c. Consult with a hematologist to evaluate for a plan of treatment (e.g., need for therapeutic administration of a chelating agent).

B. *Normocytic anemias*

1. Anemia of chronic disease

a. Treat underlying conditions.

b. In most cases, correction of anemia is not indicated. However, erythropoietin can be effective for those individuals with renal failure, cancer, and inflammatory disorders.

2. Hemolytic anemias

a. Treat illness and discontinue drugs that may have triggered this anemia.

b. Prednisone is the standard initial treatment in autoimmune hemolytic anemia. Symptomatic individuals should receive transfusions. In those who fail remission or cannot sustain remission, a splenectomy is recommended. Immunosuppressive agents are used in those persons who fail to respond with splenectomy.

c. Instruct patients to take 1 mg of folate daily. In those individuals with G6PD deficiency, avoid giving oxidant medications (e.g., sulfamethoxazole). In those susceptible to hemolysis, avoid giving medications known to trigger hemolytic anemia.

d. Hematology evaluation and management are indicated.

e. For pregnant patients with sickle cell trait, the father of the baby should be tested (CBC and Hgb electrophoresis). If the father is found to be a sickle cell trait carrier, refer to genetics for counseling regarding the risk of sickle cell disease in the neonate. Urine culture and sensitivity screening every trimester should be done, because pregnant women who are a carrier for sickle cell trait have an increased risk of urinary tract infection (Pastore, Savitz, & Thorp, 1999).

f. For pregnant patient with a child with sickle disease, refer to genetics for counseling.

C. *Macrocytic and megaloblastic anemias*

1. Vitamin B_{12} deficiency anemia

a. Administer cobalamin, 1,000 mg, parenterally daily for 1 week, then weekly for 1 month, then monthly lifelong. In severe anemia, serum potassium and hematocrit may drop with initial treatment with cobalamin.

b. Oral cobalamin, 1,000–2,000 mcg daily, can be substituted with equal effect as parental administration (Vidal-Alaball, Butler, Cannings-John, & Goringe, 2009). Follow-up serum vitamin B_{12} levels need to be monitored to ensure there is adequate absorption. Lifelong compliance is critical, especially for the elderly who are more prone to have atrophic gastritis. Treat subclinical deficiency with 500 mcg to 1g dose, just enough to correct the deficiency.

c. It is important to appropriately investigate macrocytosis. All patients with suspected myelodysplastic disease need a hematologic evaluation.

d. Those individuals who do not respond to vitamin B_{12} treatment, who are medically unstable, or whose vitamin B_{12} and folic acid levels are normal should be referred to a hematologist.

2. Folate deficiency anemia

a. Avoid treating patients with potential cobalamin deficiency with folate alone unless vitamin B_{12} deficiency anemia has been ruled out and treated because this may lead to progressively severe neuropsychiatric disease caused by untreated vitamin B_{12} deficiency.

b. Administer folate, 1 mg daily. In 1 week, the patient should begin to have a sense of improvement with increase in reticulocytes. CBC corrects in 2 months, and then the patient may be tapered to folate, 0.5 mg/d long term.

D. Client education

1. Provide verbal and written information regarding

a. The disease process, including signs and symptoms and underlying etiologies.

b. Diagnostic tests that include a discussion about preparation, actual procedures, and follow-up care.

c. Management plan: rationale, action, use, side effects, and cost of therapeutic interventions, and the need for adhering to the long-term treatment plans.

VI. Self-management resources and tools

A. *The American Society of Hematology's website is www.bloodthevitalconnection.org. This website provides both an overview of anemia and other links for additional information for patients.*

B. *The National Institutes of Health has a collection of patient information sites that discuss anemia with handouts under links on dietary supplementation: www.nhi.gov.*

REFERENCES

American College of Obstetricians and Gynecologists. (2008). ACOG practice bulletin No. 95: Anemia in pregnancy. *Obstetrics & Gynecology, 112*(1), 201–207.

Beutler, E., & Waalen, J. (2006). The definition of anemia: What *is* the lower limit of normal of the blood hemoglobin concentration? *Blood, 107*(5), 1747–1750.

Brabin, B. J., Hakimi, M., & Pelletier, D. (2001). An analysis of anemia and pregnancy-related maternal mortality. *Journal of Nutrition, 131*, 604S.

Brill, J., & Baumgardner, D. (2000). Normocytic anemia. *American Family Physician, 62*(10), 2255.

Bryan, R. (2010). Are we missing vitamin B12 deficiency in the primary care setting? *Journal of Nurse Practitioners, 6*(7), 519–523.

Centers for Disease Control and Prevention. (2009). Vitamin B 12 deficiency. National Center on Birth Defects and Developmental Disabilities Centers for Disease Control and Prevention. (1998). Recommendations to prevent and control iron deficiency in the United States. *Morbidity and Mortality Weekly Report, 47*, 1–29.

Collins-Bride, G., & Saxe, J. (Eds.). (1998). *Nurse practitioner/physician collaborative practice: Clinical guidelines for ambulatory care.* San Francisco, CA: UCSF Nursing Press.

Elmadfa, I., & Singer, I. (2009). Vitamin B12 and homocysteine status among vegetarians: A global perspective. *American Journal of Clinical Nutrition, 89*(5), 1693S–1698S.

Gardner, L., & Benz, Jr., E. (2008). Anemia of chronic disease. In R. Hoffman, H. Heslop, B. Furie, E. Benz, Jr., P. McGlave, L. Silberstein, & et al. (Eds.), *Hematology: Basic principles and practice* (5th ed., pp. 469–474). Philadelphia, PA: Elsevier Churchill Livingstone.

Gehrs, B., & Friedberg, R. (2002). Autoimmune hemolytic anemia. *American Journal of Hematology, 69*(4), 258–271.

Giardina, P., & Forget, B. (2008). Thalassemia syndromes. In R. Hoffman, H. Heslop, B. Furie, E. Benz, Jr., P. McGlave, L. Silberstein, & et al. (Eds.), *Hematology: Basic principles and practice* (5th ed., pp. 535–563). Philadelphia, PA: Elsevier Churchill Livingstone.

Gomella, L., & Haist, S. (2007). *The famous scut monkey handbook: Clinician's pocket reference* (11th ed.). New York: McGraw-Hill.

Graves, B. W., & Barger, M. K. (2001). A "conservative" approach to iron supplementation during pregnancy. *Journal of Midwifery & Women's Health, 46*(3), 159–160.

Hoffman, R., Benz, E. J., Shatti, S. S., McGlave, P., Silberstein, L. E., & Shattil, S. J. (Eds.). (2008). *Hematology: Basic principles and practice* (5th ed.). Philadelphia, PA: Elsevier Churchill Livingstone.

Kemna, E. H. (2008). Hepcidin: From discovery to differential diagnosis. *Haematologia, 9*(3), 90–97.

Killip, S., Bennett, J., & Chambers, M. (2007). Iron deficiency anemia. *American Family Physician, 75*(5), 671–678.

Langan, R., & Zawistoski, K. (2011). Update of vitamin B12 deficiency. *American Family Physician, 83*(12), 1425–1430.

Laubach, J., & Bendell, J. (2008). Hematologic changes of pregnancy. In R. Hoffman, H. Heslop, B. Furie, E. Benz, Jr., P. McGlave, L. Silberstein, & et al. *Hematology: Basic principles and practice* (5th ed., pp. 2385–2396). Philadelphia, PA: Elsevier Churchill Livingstone.

Linker, C. (2007). Blood. In S. McPhee & M. Papadakis (Eds.), *Current medical diagnosis & treatment* (pp. 493–507). New York, NY: McGraw-Hill.

Longo, D. (2009). Examination of blood smears and bone marrow and red blood cell disorders. In A. Fauci, E. Braunwald, D. Kasper, S. Hauser, D. Longo, J. Jameson, et al. (Eds.), *Harrison's manual of medicine* (17th ed., pp. 321–328). New York, NY: McGraw-Hill.

Makipour, S., Kanapuru, B., & Ershler, W. B. (2008). Unexplained anemia in the elderly. *Seminars in Hematology, 45*(4), 250–254.

Nicoll, D., McPhee, S., Pignone, M., & Lu, C. (2007). *Pocket guide to diagnostic tests* (5th ed.). New York: McGraw-Hill Medical.

Oberly, M. J., & Yang, D. T. (2013). Laboratory testing for cobalamin deficiency in megaloblastic anemia. *American Journal of Hematology, 88*, 522.

Pastore, L. M., Savitz, D. A., & Thorp, J. M., Jr. (1999). Predictors of urinary tract infection at the first prenatal visit. *Epidemiology, 10*, 282.

Schick, P. (2010). Hemolytic anemia, Version 2010. Retrieved from http://emedicine.medscape.com/article/201066-overview.

Schrier, S. (2010). To be old is to be inflamed? *Blood, 115*(18), 3651–3652.

Schwartz, R. (2007). Autoimmune and intravascular hemolytic anemias. In L. Goldman, D. Ausiello, W. Arend, J. Armitage, D. Clemmons, J. Drazen, et al. (Eds.), *Goldman Cecil medicine: Expert consult* (23rd ed., pp. 1194–1202). Philadelphia, PA: W. B. Saunders.

Sifakis, S., & Pharmakides, G. (2000). Anemia in pregnancy. *Annals of the New York Academy of Sciences, 900*, 125.

Tefferi, A. (2007). Nonhemolytic normochromic, normocytic anemias. In L. Goldman, D. Ausiello, W. Arend, J. Armitage, D. Clemmons, J. Drazen, et al. (Eds.), *Goldman Cecil medicine: Expert consult* (23rd ed., pp. 1228–1230). Philadelphia, PA: W. B. Saunders.

Umbreit, J. (2005). Iron deficiency: A concise review. *American Journal of Hematology, 78*, 225–231.

U.S. Environmental Protection Agency. (2010, May 19). *Lead in paint, dust and soil.* Retrieved from www.epa.gov/lead/.

Vidal-Alaball, J., Butler, C., Cannings-John, R., & Goringe, A. (2009). Oral vitamin B_{12} versus intramuscular vitamin B_{12} for vitamin B_{12} deficiency (review). *The Cochrane Collaboration.* Retrieved from www.thecochranelibrary.com.

Yaish, H. (2013). Pediatric thalassemia. *Medscape reference: Drugs, diseases & procedures.* Retrieved from http://emedicine.medscape.com/article/958850-overview.

CHAPTER 44

ANTICOAGULATION THERAPY (ORAL)

Fran Dreier and Linda Ray

I. Introduction and general background

Authors' note: Since the previous publication of this chapter in 2011, treatment options for oral anticoagulation have been broadened by the introduction and the increasingly widespread use of the target-specific oral anticoagulants (TSOACs); these have been approved by the Food and Drug Administration (FDA) for most but not all indications. The new agents have both advantages and disadvantages over warfarin; as clinical experience and research accumulates with the new agents, recommendations for their use will undoubtedly be further refined. Because warfarin continues to be the most widely used and best understood oral anticoagulant, this chapter continues to focus on its use but also includes basic information about the TSOACs. Updated expert clinical practice guidelines are expected to be published by the American College of Chest Physicians (ACCP) within the near future. The 9th (2012) edition of these guidelines was consulted for the preparation of this chapter.

Long-term oral anticoagulation (OAC) with warfarin (Coumadin®) is indicated for numerous conditions (**Table 44-1**). Used for primary and secondary prevention of thromboembolism (TE), OAC requires careful and meticulous management by the clinician to achieve effective and safe outcomes. Although the best practice model for anticoagulation management is a dedicated anticoagulation service, the primary clinician often oversees warfarin therapy. Warfarin management can be complex because the drug possesses what one anticoagulation expert (Ansell, 2009) describes as a "high risk/benefit profile." Warfarin has a narrow therapeutic index and thus requires careful follow-up at regular intervals because what may be a therapeutic dose at one time may be subtherapeutic or supratherapeutic at other times. The discussion that follows is intended to increase clinician comfort with managing warfarin for the patient on OAC.

Warfarin belongs to the class of OAC called vitamin K antagonists (VKA) and of these, it is the most commonly used

(and the only one available in the United States). Whether or not generic warfarin is dispensed, it is often referred to by both clinicians and patients by its trade name Coumadin®. The term "blood thinner" is a useful though misleading way to describe the action of warfarin to patients. In reality it does not make blood more watery. The action of a VKA is to interfere with hepatic synthesis of vitamin K dependent proteins. The net effect is to slow down or delay fibrin clot formation in the systemic circulation. In this way, the ability to easily make harmful thrombi is limited. In most cases, this effect translates to roughly 10–15 seconds delay in clot formation.

A. Monitoring warfarin therapy

The prothrombin time (PT) measures the speed of clot formation but the reagents used to perform the test vary in their sensitivities among manufacturers. The INR is a ratio that corrects for this variation and therefore its interpretation is consistent among laboratories and institutions (Nicoll, McPhee, Pignone, & Lu, 2007). The INR is intended to be used only for warfarin monitoring. Unlike the PT, it is not a measure of liver function. Individuals not on a VKA usually have a baseline INR value between 0.8 and 1.2; under the influence of a VKA, the PT and the INR both rise indicating delay in the onset of clot formation, and the blood is described as being "thinner" than it was at baseline.

B. Target population

Indications associated with increased clot risk are shown in Table 44-1, along with the recommended target INR for that indication; the target INR may be amended to suit the health and safety profile of the individual. For instance, consider the rare patient who develops a clot despite being at their therapeutic target of 2.0–3.0. In such a case the therapeutic target may be raised to 3.0–3.5. A polar opposite example is the patient whose bleeding risk is very high because of high fall risk. In this situation, the INR target may be lowered to as little as 1.5–2.0. Older patients also deserve special consideration. Common barriers to an older patient taking warfarin safely include cognitive

TABLE 44-1 Indications with Therapeutic International Normalized Ratio (INR) Range of 2–3

Indications with Therapeutic INR Range of 2–3	Duration of OAC
Treatment of deep vein thrombosis/pulmonary embolism (DVT/PE), collectively known as venous thromboembolism (VTE)	
Provoked by transient risk factor	3 months
Unprovoked	Reevaluate at 3 months
Recurrent	Long term
Stroke/TIA/systemic arterial embolism, secondary prevention	Long term
Prevention of systemic embolism (acute coronary syndrome, atrial fibrillation, valvular heart disease, severe left ventricular dysfunction [ejection fraction < 30%], postsurgical VTE prophylaxis)	Varies with indication
Pulmonary hypertension	Long term
Mechanical prosthetic valves in the aortic position*	Long term
Indications with Therapeutic INR Range of 2.5–3.5	**Duration of OAC**
Recurrent thromboembolism while on therapeutic warfarin	Long term
Mechanical prosthetic valves in the mitral position or ball and cage valves in any position	Long-term

* Goal INR 2.5–3.5 if patients have additional risk factors (e.g., AF)

Data from Guyatt, G., Akl, E., Crowther, M., Gutterman, D., & Schünemann, H. J. (2012). Executive summary: Antithrombotic therapy and prevention of thrombosis (9th ed.). *Chest, 141*(2, Suppl.), 7S–47S.

impairment, increased fall risk, visual or hearing impairment, or dependency on others for warfarin administration (Evans-Molina, Henault, Regan, & Hylek, 2003).

In patients diagnosed with atrial fibrillation (AF), warfarin is highly effective in preventing complications of TE, particularly stroke, in patients of any age (Wolf, Abbott, & Kannel, 1991). The $CHADS_2$ score (**Table 44-2A**) is a widely used scheme for evaluating stroke risk in patients with lone or nonvalvular AF (Gage et al., 2001). Patients with a score of greater than or equal to 1 are likely to benefit from warfarin, unless risk for bleeding outweighs the potential for clotting. Patients with AF and a score of 0 have traditionally been treated with aspirin (Fang et al., 2008). The $CHA2DS_2$-VASc score (**Table 44-2B**) is a more recently developed risk scheme that has been adopted by the American Heart Association and some other groups. This scheme includes additional risks factors: age 65–74, female gender, and vascular disease. Age 75 years and older gains extra weight, with 2 points. The result is to further subdivide the low-risk group of patients with AF so that anticoagulation is recommended for a greater proportion of the group. However, as pointed out by Fang in 2015, to date it has not been shown that treating these additional AF patients results in improved stroke outcome without unjustified increase in bleeding.

The clinician should keep in mind that an individual's risk of complications of thrombosis versus bleeding risk may change over time and, as such, the assessment of need for OAC treatment should be reexamined from time to time.

C. Associated risk of vitamin K antagonists (VKAs)

The potential for bleeding is the primary side effect of OAC with warfarin. As reported by the Centers for Medicare and Medicaid Services (2009), those at increased risk of bleeding are patients with the following: INR greater than 4.0, labile INR pattern, history of gastrointestinal bleeding, existing cerebrovascular disease, serious heart disease, anemia, malignancy, trauma, renal insufficiency, concomitant drugs, advanced age, and prior stroke. It is axiomatic that the higher the INR, the greater the risk for bleeding complications. However, it is important to point out that an elevated INR is a measure of *risk* of harmful bleeding, which is not the same as *having* harmful bleeding.

D. Treatment duration

The ACCP guidelines include recommendations for treatment duration. Patients who are at high risk of TE need lifelong OAC (Table 44-1). Short-term therapy, which usually lasts 3 months, is appropriate for indications where clot risk is transitory or triggered by a provoking event, such as the case of a single-event deep venous thrombosis after hip replacement.

E. Variables that affect response to warfarin

1. Diet

The most frequent cause for a change in INR in a patient who has been otherwise stable is a change in oral vitamin K intake or absorption. For

TABLE 44-2A CHADS₂ Score for Assessment of Stroke Risk in Patients with Atrial Fibrillation

Congestive Heart Failure*	1 pt
Hypertension	1 pt
Age ≥ 75 years	1 pt
Diabetes	1 pt
Stroke (previous transient ischemic attack [TIA] or cerebrovascular accident [CVA])	2 pts

*Ejection fraction < 25% or have had a heart failure exacerbation in the last 90 days

Risk of events per year without OAC:

   0 points = 1.9%
   1 point = 2.8%
   2 points = 4%
   3 points = 5.9%
   4 points = 8.5%
   5 points = 12.5%
   6 points = 18.2%

Data from Gage, B. F., Waterman, A. D., Shannon, W., Boechler, M., Rich, M. W., & Radford, M. J. (2001). Validation of clinical classification schemes for predicting stroke: Results from the National Registry of Atrial Fibrillation. *JAMA, 285,* 2864–2870.

TABLE 44-2B CHADS₂-VASc Score for Assessment of Stroke Risk in Patients with Atrial Fibrillation

Congestive Heart Failure*	1 pt
Hypertension	1 pt
Age ≥ 75 years	2 pt
Diabetes	1 pt
Stroke (previous TIA or CVA)	2 pts
Vascular Disease (myocardial infarct, aortic plaque, peripheral artery disease)	1 pt
Age 65–74 years	1 pt
Sc Sex category (i.e., female sex)	1 pt

*Ejection fraction < 25% or have had a heart failure exacerbation in the last 90 days

Risk of events per year without OAC:

   0 points = 0.0 low risk
   1 point = 1.3% moderate risk
   2 points = 2.2% high risk
   3 points = 3.2% high risk
   4 points = 4.0% high risk
   5 points = 6.7% high risk
   6 points = 9.8% high risk
   7 points = 9.6% high risk
   8 points = 6.7% high risk
   9 points = 15.2% high risk

Data from Odum, L., Cochran, K., Aistrope, D., & Snella, K. (2012). The CHADS₂ vs the New CHA2DS₂-VASc scoring systems for guiding antithrombotic treatment of patients with atrial fibrillation: review of the literature and recommendations for use. *Pharmacotherapy, 32*(3), 285–296.

example, warfarin effect is enhanced in the presence of decreased appetite or acute diarrhea. For optimal stability, patients should be encouraged to maintain a consistent amount of vitamin K in their diet from week to week. Vitamin K is a nutrient that is present in varying quantities in most foods, and deficiency is rare for the individual who is not starving. The daily value (DV) recommended by the U.S. Department of Agriculture (2001) is 120 mcg for men and 90 mcg for women. Certain foods are very rich in vitamin K, and far exceed the DV in a single serving. *The foods highest in vitamin K are the dark green leafy vegetables, such as kale and spinach.* Several other vegetables are moderately high in vitamin K. A patient's vitamin K intake should be assessed at every visit, and patients should be reminded periodically that it is their responsibility to maintain consistent vitamin K intake. Some common vitamin K–rich foods are listed in **Table 44-3**. A comprehensive list can be found at: U.S. Department of Agriculture, Agricultural Research Service, Nutrient Data Laboratory. (2015). USDA National Nutrient Database for Standard Reference, Release 28. Retrieved from www.ars.usda.gov/nea/bhnrc/ndl.

Supplements, both tablet and liquid forms, and multivitamins may contain significant amounts of

TABLE 44-3 Foods Rich in Vitamin K

Beet greens*	Kale*
Broccoli	Lentils
Brussels sprouts	Lettuce†
Cabbage	Mustard greens*
Cauliflower	Seaweed (nori)
Chard*	Soybean oil‡
Collard greens*	Spinach*
Garbanzo beans	Turnip greens*

* Extremely high in vitamin K.

† Except iceberg.

‡ In large quantities.

Data from U.S. Department of Agriculture, Agricultural Research Service. National Nutrient Database for Standard Reference, Release 27.

vitamin K; clinicians should ask about supplement use at each visit. A change in multivitamin brand or in frequency of use can significantly affect the INR.

2. Alcohol intake

Alcohol can affect the INR unpredictably. Paradoxically, chronic alcohol use tends to lower the INR, whereas acute binge drinking tends to increase the INR. Light to moderate drinking (i.e., up to two servings of alcohol [12 oz of wine, 24 oz of beer, 2 oz of hard liquor] at one time) may be less problematic. Alcohol also increases the likelihood of injury if ingested in excess, may cause bleeding by irritating the upper gastrointestinal tract, and may impair platelet function. Abstention from alcohol does simplify warfarin management (Wittkowsky, 2009b).

3. Comorbidities

An acute illness or a worsening of a chronic illness may affect warfarin stability. Changes in liver, cardiac, or thyroid function are likely to alter usual dose requirements. In general, severe illness tends to increase one's sensitivity to warfarin and necessitates dose reduction to achieve target INR. For reasons not fully understood, fever itself may independently cause an increased response to warfarin (Self, 2000).

4. Interactions

a. Drug interactions and other medications

Many drug interactions with warfarin have been documented. For most agents, there is significant individual variability among patients as to timing and extent of the interaction. Drug interactions may vary both among individuals and within a drug class itself (see **Table 44-4** for a partial list of interactions). It is important that the clinician very clearly educate patients to report any acute illness, new medicines, or change in medicines. It is critical that clinicians maintain meticulous communication to ensure that all members of the healthcare team are aware of new drugs that have been prescribed. If a new medication is recommended for which there is no reasonable alternative and if it is likely to interact, the clinician may choose to preemptively alter warfarin dose or increase the frequency of INR checks. This is often done in consultation with an anticoagulation specialist. A comprehensive list of interactions can be found in the article by Holbrook and colleagues (2005). Fortunately, first-generation penicillins do not interact with warfarin.

Pain medications represent a special category of consideration because the need for acute or chronic analgesia arises so frequently in

TABLE 44-4 Warfarin–Drug Interactions

Increase in INR	Decrease in INR
Alcohol	Alcohol
Amiodarone*	Antiretrovirals (some)[†]
Antiretrovirals (some)[†]	Carbamazepine
Azoles[‡]*	Phenobarbital*
Cimetidine*	Rifampin/rifabutin*
Erythromycin*	Vitamin K (phytonadione)*
Fibrates*	
Fluoroquinolones (some)*	
Phenytoin	
Statins	
Prednisone*	
Allopurinol	
Tramadol	

This is not a comprehensive list. INR should be monitored after initiating or modifying any drug therapy.

* Significant interaction.

[†] The reader is advised to go to literature for specifics of individual drugs of this class.

[‡] Azoles include antifungals, metronidazole, and sulfamethoxazole, a component of Bactrim®/Septra®.

Modified from UCSF Medical Center. (Updated February 2009). Comprehensive Hemostasis and Antithrombotic Service (CHAS).

the primary care setting. Nonsteroidal anti-inflammatory drugs (NSAIDs), both nonselective and selective (cyclooxygenase-2 inhibitors), should be avoided in patients taking warfarin because they increase the risk of gastrointestinal bleeding (Battistella, Mamdani, Juurlink, Rabeneck, & Laupacis, 2005; Cheetham, Levy, Niu, & Bixler, 2009). If a patient must take an NSAID, it is best to take the shortest acting agent, at the smallest dose, for the briefest time. If a patient must be on chronic NSAID therapy, the clinician should consider monitoring stool with fecal occult blood testing (FOBT) Although adding a drug from the class of proton pump inhibitors theoretically confers some protection to the upper gastrointestinal tract, this does not protect the lower gastrointestinal tract.

The safest alternative for a patient requiring short-term pain relief is acetaminophen. Although it does not relieve inflammation, when the dosage does not exceed 2 g/day, there is very small likelihood that an interaction will occur. However, the INR may increase with the use of 4 g/day (Carrier, Grégoire, & Wells, 2009). Tramadol may increase the INR; narcotics do not by themselves alter the INR or platelet function. However in the setting of acute pain, oral intake including vitamin K is likely to decrease and result in a rise in INR.

   b. Interactions and supplements

It has been estimated that 50% of patients are taking some form of nutritional supplement and that up to 60% do not report use of alternative therapies to their healthcare providers (Wittkowsky, 2009a). Although there are relatively few case reports of supplement–warfarin interactions to date and these are poorly documented, potential interactions do exist, either by diminishing platelet activity or by directly affecting the INR (**Table 44-5**). The clinician is advised to check Web-based information systems for further information regarding these products (www.naturaldatabase.com)

F. Issues of dosing and follow-up in OAC

1. OAC is best managed using a systematic approach of patient assessment, addressing dose adjustment, and scheduling the next follow-up interval. The use of a flow sheet or electronic record is strongly advised to help the clinician interpret the visit data in the context of overall INR trends and usual dose patterns (Garcia et al., 2008).

2. At each visit the clinician should assess the patient's overall health status. The clinician should confirm actual dosing at each visit with direct and specific questions:

   a. Based on the 7-day week, tell me what dose you take on what days.

   b. Do you recall having missed any doses recently, particularly in the last 7 days?

Additional areas to cover at each visit are shown in **Table 44-6.**

3. Past guidelines indicated that the stable patient with therapeutic INR readings should undergo follow-up testing every 4 weeks (Ansell, 2009), although there is evidence suggesting that the stable patient without significant comorbidities might be followed less frequently (Witt et al., 2009). ACCP guidelines (2012) suggest (grade 2B) that for stable patients, follow-up may safely be extended up to 12-week intervals. Testing every 1 to 2 weeks is recommended if the INR is not within therapeutic range or if warfarin dose is changed. In certain situations, such as a very high (supratherapeutic) INR, it may be advisable to retest in 1 or 2 days.

G. Managing variations in INR

1. One of the challenges of managing OAC is deciding how to respond to INR variations. Small INR variations occur from visit to visit for even the more stable patient, and not all INR variations require new dose adjustment. The trend of a patient's INR readings is more important than any single INR. Abrupt change in dosing should be avoided, because it is responsible for some of the difficulty that can occur in attempting to maintain INRs within target range.

2. When presented with an INR that is out of target range, the clinician should look for variables that

TABLE 44-5 Warfarin and Commonly Used Dietary Supplements/Herbal Medicines

Herbs and Dietary Supplements	Impact or Effect
American ginseng	May either potentiate warfarin or inhibit warfarin effect
Chinese herbs and medicines	Impact determined by active ingredients
Coenzyme Q-10	Mixed reports on its effects; avoid or monitor closely for 3 months at time of supplement initiation
Echinacea	No case reports of interaction with warfarin
Fish oil and omega-3 fatty acids	Antiplatelet activity; may increase bleeding risk
Garlic	Antiplatelet activity when taken in large quantities
Ginkgo biloba	Antiplatelet activity; may increase bleeding risk (hemorrhagic stroke case reports)
Glucosamine	May increase INR (based on a few isolated case reports)
Multivitamins containing vitamin K	Inhibits warfarin; choose product with ≤ 30 mcg vitamin K

Data from Dennehy, C. (2010, April 9–11). *An evidence based look at popular dietary supplements.* Presented at Clinical Pharmacotherapy 2010, University of California, Davis.

TABLE 44-6 Warfarin Management: Questions to Ask at Follow-up Visits

Current dose and tablet strength?
Any changes in health status?
Any unusual bruising or bleeding?
Any change in diet?
Any new medicines or supplements?
Any change in medicines or supplements?
Any falls?
Any questions?

affect warfarin stability, determine if these variables are transient or continuing, and review or reinforce topics in patient education that may explain the variation in the INR reading. If a subtherapeutic or supratherapeutic value can be explained by a transient change in a variable, the provider should adjust the dose for 1 or 2 days and then resume the prior dose, usually with follow-up in 1 or 2 weeks.

3. Variables affecting warfarin stability (Carrier et al., 2009) include the following
   a. Changes in other medications, including additions or deletions of routine, over-the-counter, and herbal medications and dose changes of current medications
   b. Intercurrent illness, especially febrile or diarrheal illness
   c. Dietary habits (wide swings in amount of intake or type of foods)
   d. Alcohol intake
   e. Travel, which can alter lifestyle habits and dosing schedules
   f. Issues of patient adherence

4. A patient's response to chronic warfarin treatment may vary over time, and occasionally a previously stable patient requires a new weekly warfarin dose in the absence of any clear influencing variables.

5. The degree of response to an INR out of range should also be based on the patient's risk category. For example, a single low value is more concerning for patients with a mechanical mitral valve than it is for one with lone AF. A supratherapeutic value is more concerning when there is a high risk for falls or a past history of gastrointestinal bleeding. Patients at higher risk for complications require closer follow-up than patients at lower risk.

6. Although computer-based programs and warfarin dosing tables are available to aid clinicians in predicting

maintenance dose (e.g., www.warfarindosing.org) these are not likely to take the place of a clinician's familiarity with a patient's case history. Some guidelines for dose adjustments include the following:
   a. Change the total weekly dose by approximately 10–15%, depending on the magnitude of the INR variation and the stability and risk profile of the patient.
   b. Use a single-strength tablet to propose a weekly dose schedule (e.g., two and three tablets alternating) or fractions (e.g., dose reduction from one tablet daily to half a tablet Monday, Wednesday, and Friday, and one tablet the other 4 days). Although dosing with one tablet strength is easier for some patients to manage than using tablets of different strengths, using a combination of 1- and 5-mg tablets offers good dosing flexibility for most patients.
   c. Before changing to a new dose, evaluate the patient's risk for confusion, dose error, practicality and cost of dose adjustment, and patient preference (Wong, Wilson, & Wittkowsky, 1999).

7. Patients with persistently unstable INRs may benefit from switching to brand Coumadin® or dispensing a generic from the same manufacturer each time (Wittkowsky, 2009b).

8. Subtherapeutic INRs
   If an INR is below goal, inquire about recent change in vitamin K intake, along with the possibility of missed doses or an error in dosing. See **Table 44-7** for additional guidelines for evaluating a subtherapeutic INR.

9. Supratherapeutic INRs
   If an INR is above goal, inquire whether the patient has increased bruising or frank bleeding. An INR greater than 4 carries an increased risk of serious bleeding (Beyth, 2005). Inquire about intercurrent illness, acute dose error, recent addition of antibiotics, or reduction in dietary vitamin K intake or in total dietary intake (**Table 44-8**). See **Table 44-9** for specific guidelines for managing supratherapeutic INRs.

TABLE 44-7 Evaluation of Subtherapeutic INR

Dose error? (particularly missed dose)
Increase in vitamin K intake?
New medication or supplement?
Change in medication or supplement?
Improvement in heart or liver function?
Change in usual manufacturer of tablet?

TABLE 44-8 Possible Causes of Supratherapeutic INR

Dose error
Diet change
Change in medicine or supplement
Acute illness
Decrease in liver function
Decrease in cardiac function
Change in usual manufacturer of tablet
Laboratory error

II. Patient education and safety

A. *Patient education is the cornerstone of safe and effective warfarin management.*

This requires that the patient have a basic understanding of the purpose and mechanism of anticoagulation. At the beginning of treatment it should be made clear to patients that although warfarin does slow clotting, it does not initiate bleeding. Warfarin comes in nine strengths; each strength is uniquely color coded, although shape and manufacturer do vary. The coding of color to strength helps to prevent dosing errors and to discover them quickly when they occur.

B. *To promote adherence and minimize error, warfarin dosing should be tailored to the individual patient.*

Some patients achieve their best INR control with one single-strength daily dose, although those less susceptible to confusion or error can manage a variable dose. Equal daily dosing causes less confusion and is associated with lower rates of dose error. However, using the same dose every day may require the patient to have tablets in more than one strength or to split tablets. Although warfarin comes in multiple strengths, many patients need a dose that falls somewhere in between these strengths. In many cases it is not possible to achieve a target INR with 7 days of equal dosing.

C. *The fundamentals of safe warfarin therapy should be reinforced frequently:*

1. Clarify warfarin tablet strength and dosing schedule at each visit. It should be clear to the patient whether the dosing instructions are given in terms of milligrams or tablets. It is most precise to talk with patients about their weekly dosing schedule in terms of specific milligrams per day rather than number of tablets per day. However, many patients know their warfarin only by its color and prefer instructions given in tablets per day. It is critical to patient safety that the patient, caregiver, and clinician have a clear mutual understanding of what dose is being recommended.

TABLE 44-9 Recommendations for the Management of Excessive Oral Anticoagulation or Bleeding

INR supratherapeutic, but < 5 with no significant bleeding	Lower or omit dose, monitor more frequently, resume at lower dose when INR is therapeutic. If only minimally elevated or associated with a transient variable, dose adjustment may not be necessary.
INR > 5 but < 9, no significant bleeding	Omit the next one or two doses, monitor more frequently, resume therapy at adjusted dose when INR is therapeutic. Alternatively, omit dose and give 1–2.5 mg vitamin K orally, particularly for those at increased risk of bleeding. If more rapid reversal is required because the patient needs urgent surgery, give vitamin K ≥ 5 mg orally, expecting INR reduction within 24 hours. If INR remains high, give additional vitamin K of 1–2 mg.
INR > 9, no significant bleeding	Hold warfarin therapy and give a higher dose of vitamin K (2.5–5 mg) orally, expecting INR to reduce significantly within 24–48 hours. Monitor the INR more frequently, give additional vitamin K if needed, and resume therapy at an adjusted dose when the INR is in therapeutic range.
INR therapeutic or elevated with serious or life-threatening bleeding	Hold warfarin therapy and give vitamin K by slow intravenous infusion along with fresh frozen plasma, prothrombin complex concentrate, or recombinant factor VIIa. For life-threatening bleeding, recombinant factor VIIa is supplemented with vitamin K, 10 mg by slow infusion, repeated as necessary.

Data from Guyatt, G., Aki, E., Crowther, M., Gutterman, D., Schünemann, H. (2012). Executive Summary: Antithrombotic therapy and prevention of thrombosis, 9th ed: American College of Chest Physicians Evidence-Based Clinical Practice Guidelines. *Chest*, 141(Suppl. 2), 7S–47S.

2. Reinforce dietary guidelines and the need to report any significant changes.

3. Report any signs of possible warfarin complications, which include unusual bruising, epistaxis, bleeding gums, hematuria, hematochezia, or melena.

4. Report if any medicines or supplements have been started, changed, or discontinued. Avoid aspirin, NSAIDs, and all nonprescription medications unless approved by the clinician.

5. Report any acute illness, especially vomiting or diarrhea, or significant change in health status.

6. Avoid activities that increase risk of injury, particularly contact sports.

7. Call the clinic or go to an acute care setting in case of a fall or serious injury, particularly head trauma. Because the most devastating potential complication of warfarin therapy is intracranial bleeding, even minor head trauma should prompt a call to the clinic or an urgent care visit.

D. Special considerations

1. Multiple providers: it is best to identify a single provider for warfarin management and prescription refills. This simple strategy can help to avoid potentially serious errors in dosing.

2. Women and gynecological issues: women who are of childbearing age must be informed about the teratogenic risks of warfarin. They should be advised to use contraception at all times and to tell their clinician about future plans to become pregnant. They should also be counseled that warfarin may increase menstrual flow and/or duration. Because warfarin can unmask an existing gynecological issue in a woman of any age, patients should report unusual, heavy, or intermenstrual bleeding.

3. Combined warfarin and antiplatelet therapy (often referred to as "dual" or "triple" therapy): some patients, such as those with coronary artery disease, may be prescribed warfarin as well as one or two antiplatelet agents (i.e., aspirin and clopidogrel [Plavix®]). Because the bleeding risk has been shown to be significantly higher in these patients, the need for antiplatelet therapy should be carefully evaluated (Douketis et al., 2008). If the patient does require dual or triple therapy, one option is to lower the INR target within the limits of safety given the patient's indication for warfarin: For example, for a patient with AF and coronary artery disease (CAD) who is on an antiplatelet agent, the usual goal of 2–3 might be lowered to 2–2.5 (Rossini et al., 2008).

4. Planned interruptions of OAC: the relative risk of bleeding during a procedure versus developing a thrombus off anticoagulation determines whether and when an individual may need to interrupt warfarin. In a case of low risk for thrombosis, the dose may be safely stopped 5 days before the procedure and resumed when the clinician performing the procedure deems it safe, usually the day of or day after the procedure. More complicated situations require a decision tree as to whether to bridge the patient with low-molecular-weight heparin (LMWH) or lengthen the time off warfarin. A minority of patients considered high risk may require hospitalization for heparinization preceding and following their procedure. The CHADS$_2$ score can help with risk stratification for patients with AF who need to interrupt OAC treatment. A patient with a CHADS$_2$ score of 5–6 is considered to be high risk for TE when OAC is suspended (**Table 44-10**). Consensus regarding bridging for warfarin interruptions has been favoring not to bridge the AF patient except in certain high-risk situations. In a recent well-designed large study, not bridging was found to be noninferior to bridging and, as expected, bleeding risk was lowered (Douketis et al., 2015).

5. Oral procedures: some oral procedures can be safely performed at an INR of 2. The decision to alter warfarin dosing is based on how much bleeding the procedure may induce. See **Table 44-11** for guidelines for oral procedures.

6. Travel: Diets often change significantly when patients travel. Counsel patients to maintain their intake of vitamin K–rich food at its usual level and to maintain the usual 24-hour dosing interval across changing time zones.

TABLE 44-10 Risk of Thromboembolism for Patients with AF Interrupting Warfarin

Low risk	CHADS$_2$ score of 0–2
	No history of CVA or TIA
Moderate risk	CHADS$_2$ score of 3 or 4
High risk	CHADS$_2$ score of 5–6
	Recent (i.e., within 3 months) stroke or TIA
	Rheumatic valvular heart disease

Data from Douketis, J. D., Spyropoulos, A. C., Spencer, F. A., Mayr, M., Jaffer, A. K., Eckman, M. H., et al. (2012). Perioperative management of antithrombotic therapy: Antithrombotic therapy and prevention of thrombosis, 9th ed: American College of Chest Physicians evidence-based clinical practice guidelines. *Chest, 141*(Suppl. 2), e326S–e350S. doi:10.1378/chest.11-2298.

TABLE 44-11 Guidelines for the Management of Anticoagulation During Oral Surgery

Patients who require interventional or surgical procedures while they are taking anticoagulants can pose a therapeutic dilemma for clinicians. The need for alteration of anticoagulant therapy in patients undergoing general dentistry, periodontal, and oral surgical procedures is dependent on several factors including the intensity of anticoagulation, the type of procedure, and the likelihood of thrombosis versus bleeding. Because of the risk for thromboembolism, patients undergoing invasive procedures who require interruption of their anticoagulant therapy should have it interrupted for the shortest possible time period. The trend to lower intensity of anticoagulation allows many procedures to be performed without interruption of therapy while maintaining the INR at approximately 2.0.

All patients undergoing any procedure associated with a risk for bleeding should have the **INR evaluated within 24 hours before the procedure**. If interruption of therapy is necessary, it must be individualized. When therapy is interrupted, it should usually be resumed the evening of the procedure if hemostasis has been achieved.

Low-Risk or Routine Procedures can usually be performed with an INR of 2–3 and include

    a. Routine hygiene and light scaling.

    b. Routine restorative procedures including fillings performed under local infiltrative anesthesia.

    c. Simple, single extractions. Multiple and surgical extractions may require modification of anticoagulant therapy.

    d. Sockets should be sutured and packed with a local hemostatic agent, such as Gelfoam or Surgicel®.

Moderate-Risk Procedures can be performed with an INR of approximately 1.5.

    a. Procedures requiring mandibular blocks to accomplish adequate local anesthesia.

    b. Deep scaling.

    c. Multiple extractions or other extensive periodontal surgery.

    d. Sockets should be sutured and packed with a local hemostatic agent, such as Gelfoam or Surgicel®.

High-Risk Procedures should be performed only when the INR is normalized. Periprocedural heparinization in the hospital setting may be necessary for some patients, for example those with mechanical heart valves who are at a high risk of both bleeding and development of thrombosis.

    a. Multiple extractions or extraction of impacted teeth.

    b. Major reconstructive procedures.

General Guidelines

    a. Aspirin and other nonsteroidal anti-inflammatory drugs should not routinely be used in most patients for postoperative analgesia because of their antiplatelet effect. An exception is once-daily aspirin, 81–325 mg, when prescribed for patients with a cardiovascular or cerebrovascular indication. This therapy should not be interrupted at any time and should be continued before and after the dental procedure. In addition, therapy with clopidogrel (Plavix®) should not be interrupted when it is used in patients with drug-eluting stents.

    b. A thorough medication history should be obtained before the planned procedure. Keep in mind that herbal medications may also influence hemostasis.

    c. Prophylactic antibiotics are required for patients at risk of bacterial endocarditis. See the American Heart Association guidelines for recommendations.

    d. Patients should be instructed to avoid chewing hard foods, to avoid hot liquids, and to perform vigorous mouth washing for 24–48 hours after procedures. They should use external ice packs and biting pressure on gauze pads to control localized bleeding.

    e. Tranexamic acid mouthwashes have been suggested as an intervention to minimize bleeding after oral surgical procedures. In a well-designed 2003 study, a 5% solution of tranexamic acid used immediately after surgery and four times a day for 2 days was as effective as a 5-day course to reduce bleeding (Carter & Goss, 2003).

    f. Patients undergoing major procedures who have had anticoagulant therapy interrupted should be scheduled for a follow-up anticoagulation clinic appointment within 7–14 days. Patients who have required bridging with low-molecular-weight heparin need earlier follow-up.

References

Carter, G., & Goss, A. (2003). Tranexamic acid mouthwash: A prospective randomized study of a 2-day regimen vs. 5-day regimen to prevent post-operative bleeding in anticoagulated patients requiring dental extractions. *International Journal of Oral and Maxillofacial Surgery, 32*, 504–507.

Carter, G., Goss, A., Lloyd, J., & Tocchetti, R. (2003). Tranexamic acid mouthwash versus autologous fibrin glue in patients taking warfarin undergoing dental extractions: A randomized prospective clinical study. *Journal of Oral and Maxillofacial Surgery, 61*, 1432–1435.

(continues)

TABLE 44-11 Guidelines for the Management of Anticoagulation During Oral Surgery *(Continued)*

References (Continued)

Dalen, J. E., & Hirsh, J. (Eds.). (2008). Eighth ACCP Consensus Conference on Antithrombotic Therapy. *Chest, 133,* 67S–887S.

Douketis, J. D. (2003). Perioperative anticoagulation management in patients who are receiving oral anticoagulant therapy: A practical guide for clinicians. *Thrombosis Research, 108,* 3–13.

Douketis, J. D., Berger, P. B., Dunn, A. S., Jaffer, A. K., Spyropoulos, A. C., Becker, R. C., et al. (2008). The perioperative management of antithrombotic therapy: American College of Chest Physicians evidence-based clinical practice guidelines (8th edition). *Chest Supplement, 133*(6, Suppl.), 299S–339S.

Dunn, A. S., & Turpie, A. G. G. (2003). Perioperative management of patients receiving oral anticoagulants. *Archives of Internal Medicine, 163,* 901–908.

Ferrieri, G. B., Castiglioni, S., Carmagnola, D., Cargnel, M., Strohmenger, L., & Abati, S. (2007). Oral surgery in patients on anticoagulant treatment without therapy interruption. *Journal of Oral and Maxillofacial Surgery, 65,* 1149–1154.

Nishimura, R. A., Carabello, B. A., Faxon, D. P., Freed, M. D., Lytle, B. W., O'Gara, P. T., et al. (2008). ACC/AHA 2008 guideline update on valvular heart disease: Focused update on infective endocarditis. A report of the American College of Cardiology/American Heart Association Task Force on Practice Guidelines. *Circulation, 118,* 887–896.

Wilson, W., Taubert, K. A., Gewitz, M., Lockhart, P. B., Baddour, L. M., Levison, M., et al. (2007). Prevention of endocarditis. Guidelines from the American Heart Association. *Circulation, 116,* 1736–1754.

Addendum: preparation of 5% tranexamic acid mouthwash

Tranexamic acid is freely soluble in water. A 500-mg tablet of tranexamic acid can be crushed and dispersed in 10 mL of water immediately before administration. Alternatively, a liquid can be prepared by mixing crushed tablets with water and then filtering out the insoluble excipients to give a clear solution. A maximum expiry date of 5 days is suggested for this preparation, which has not been formally tested.

Adapted from Kayser, S. R., Kearns, G., & Smith, R. (2009). The Anticoagulation Clinic, Division of Oral Surgery, University of California San Francisco.

7. Discontinuing warfarin: if a patient is at high risk of falls or of dose error (as may occur in dementia), or if the patient is unable or unwilling to adhere to monitoring schedules, the clinician should reevaluate if the risk of bleeding outweighs the possible benefits of treatment. Chronic warfarin treatment should prompt periodic review of the risk/benefit ratio for each individual patient.

8. Self-testing: patients on lifelong anticoagulation sometimes ask about the possibility of self-testing at home with their own point-of-care-testing (POCT) device. This is a viable option for some, and many insurance companies now reimburse for the use of the machine and the testing supplies. Because POCT is not reliable for every patient, it is wise to run at least two simultaneous venipunctures to evaluate for concordance. Some patients show a persistent discordance and, in that case, are not candidates for self-testing. POCT/venipuncture discordance can also be a problem when the clinician is relying on home health POCT reports to evaluate warfarin levels.

9. Specialty referral: patients at higher risk for bleeding (e.g., INR goal of >/= 3.0) or thrombosis (an example of the latter is a patient who has had an arterial clot) may do best with services offering specialty management, such as a hematology or dedicated anticoagulation clinic.

III. Target-specific anticoagulants

No text discussing OAC would be complete without some focus on the recently introduced target-specific oral anticoagulants (TSOACs), also called novel oral anticoagulants (NOACs) and direct oral anticoagulants (DOACs). There are currently two groups of TSOACs approved for use in the United States: direct thrombin inhibitors, dabigatran (Pradaxa®) and factor Xa inhibitors [rivaroxaban (Xarelto®), apixaban (Eliquis®), and edoxaban (Savaysa®)] Both these groups act further down the clotting cascade than warfarin and thus have more predictable pharmacodynamics. Although the prothrombin time (PT) and partial thromboplastin time (PTT) are prolonged with all the TSOACs, this occurs in an unpredictable manner, and so these measures are not useful or reliable for drug activity monitoring.

A. Advantages of the TSOACs:

1. Fixed oral dosing

2. Rapid onset of action

3. Few drug-drug interactions. However, patients *do need* to be screened for these since there are drugs that do interact. See the individual prescribing information (see Hellwig and Gulseth, 2013).

4. Not affected by diet

5. No need for routine coagulation monitoring (This can also be seen as a disadvantage, because there is no validated lab assay for measuring drug effect in patients on active medication.)

B. Disadvantages of TSOACs are:

1. Adherence must be strict due to the short half-lives of these agents

2. Anticoagulant effect cannot be immediately reversed (The development of reversal agents is an area of continuing research.)

3. More difficult to determine whether there is residual anticoagulant effect

4. More costly than warfarin, not always covered by insurance

C. Indications and dosing

Table 44-12 compares indications and dosing of the TSOACs currently approved for use in the United States. It should be noted that these agents are currently contraindicated for patients with prosthetic valves or significant valvular heart disease. Research to date shows noninferiority of the TSOACs to warfarin for approved indications. Bleeding rates are similar, but the TSOACs seem to confer a consistently lower risk for intracranial hemorrhage. The direct thrombin inhibitor dabigatran confers a higher risk of gastrointestinal bleeding compared to warfarin. Again, a major disadvantage to all the TSOACs is the lack of a reversal agent or antidote, although reversal agents are currently in trials.

If a patient has been doing well on warfarin (i.e., has stable therapeutic INRs), it is not recommended that therapy be changed. As always, decisions regarding OAC should be individualized.

D. Appropriate candidates for TSOAC:

1. History of medication adherence

2. History of unstable INRs unrelated to adherence problems

3. Difficulty or hardship with INR monitoring

E. Do not meet the following exclusions:

1. History of medication nonadherence

2. History of underlying bleeding disorder or increased risk for bleeding

3. Creatinine clearance < 15 mL/min. Modified doses have not been well studied to date

4. Low body weight (Use in patients with low body weight has not been well studied.)

5. Severe hepatic dysfunction or any hepatic disease-associated coagulopathy

6. Pregnant or breastfeeding women (insufficient data)

7. Prosthetic heart valve or severe valvular disease

8. Medication interactions (for instance, chronic use of an azole)

9. No prescription insurance or unable to afford the copay

10. Pediatric patients (not FDA approved for pediatric use)

F. Baseline studies recommended for good candidates for TSOAC use:

1. Complete blood count with differential

2. Liver function tests (aspartate aminotransferase, alanine aminotransferase, total bilirubin)

3. Renal function studies (serum creatinine and creatinine clearance)

4. Coagulation studies (PT, PTT)

G. Counseling patients about TSOACs

When discussing and initiating a TSOAC, it is important to remind patients of the need for strict adherence to their dosing schedule. Although warfarin is fairly forgiving of minor dosing errors, this is not the case with the TSOACs. As is the case with warfarin, patients taking TSOACs should carry with them something that identifies them as taking an anticoagulant. There are a few medications that need to be avoided with TSOACS, and the patient should be given a list of these: (a) P-glycoprotein inhibitors/inducers: verapamil, amiodarone, dronedarone, macrolide antibiotics; and (b) CYP3A4 inhibitors/inducers: rifampin, phenytoin, carbamazepine, phenobarbital, St. John's wort, antifungals (econazole, ketoconazole), protease inhibitors.

If a long-term interacting medication is needed, the TSOAC would be contraindicated because currently there is no way to dose adjust for interactions.

As is the case with warfarin, patients on TSOACs should avoid NSAIDs and should not take aspirin (ASA) unless specifically recommended (ASA is often indicated for cardiac protection in CAD).

Any surgery needs to be carefully planned, taking TSOAC use into account. We recommend consulting with an anticoagulation specialist when preparing these patients for treatment interruption. In conclusion, the TSOACs are probably as effective as warfarin for many indications and may result in fewer serious bleeds. However the decision whether to use a TSOAC must take into account in each case the individual patient risk-benefit profile.

TABLE 44-12 Indications and Dosing of TSOACs Approved for Use in the United States

Dabigatran (Pradaxa®) Dosing

Indication	Renal Function (CrCl mL/min)	Recommended Dose
Atrial fibrillation	> 30	150 mg po twice daily
	15–30	75 mg po twice daily
	CrCl < 15 or dialysis	Avoid use
Treatment of DVT/PE	CrCl > 30	150 mg po twice daily after 5–10 days of parenteral therapy
	CrCl < 30 or on dialysis	Avoid

Rivaroxaban (Xarelto®) Dosing

Indication	Renal Function (CrCl mL/min)	Recommended Dose
Atrial fibrillation (stroke prevention)	> 50	20 mg po daily with evening meal
	15–50	15 mg po once daily with evening meal
	< 15	Avoid use
Treatment of DVT/PE	≥ 30	15 mg twice daily with food for 21 days, then 20 mg once daily with food
	< 30	Avoid use
Knee replacement	≥ 30	10 mg once daily for 12–14 days
	< 30	Avoid use
Hip replacement	≥ 30	10 mg once daily for 35 days
	< 30	Avoid use

Apixaban (Eliquis®) Dosing

Indication	Recommended Dose	Dose Adjustments
Atrial fibrillation (stroke prevention)	5 mg twice daily	2.5 mg twice daily if any 2 of the following: • Age ≥ 80 years • Body weight ≤ 60 kg • Serum creatinine ≥ 1.5 mg/dL
Treatment DVT/PE	10 mg twice daily x 7 d Followed by 5 mg twice daily	After 6 months 2.5 mg twice daily
Prophylaxis after total knee arthroplasty/total hip arthroplasty (TKA/THA)	2.5 mg twice daily	TKA 12 days, THA 35 days

Edoxaban (Savaysa) Dosing

Indication	Renal Function (CrCl mL/min)	Recommended Dose
Atrial fibrillation (stroke prevention)	> 50 ≤ 95 Do not use if > 95	60 mg po once daily
	< 50 > 15	30 mg po once daily
Treatment DVT/PE	> 50	60 mg po once daily following 5–10 days parenteral anticoagulation
	15–50 or body weight ≤ 60 kg	30 mg po once daily

Used with permission from Dr. Steve Kayser, anticoagulation pharmacist, University of California, San Francisco.

REFERENCES

Ansell, J. E. (2009). The value of an anticoagulation management service. In J. Ansell, L. Oertel, & A. Wittkowsky (Eds.), *Managing oral anticoagulation therapy* (3rd ed., pp. 1–8). St. Louis, MO: Wolters Kluwer Health.

Battistella, M., Mamdani, M. M., Juurlink, D. N., Rabeneck, L., & Laupacis, A. (2005). Risk of upper gastrointestinal hemorrhage in warfarin users treated with nonselective NSAIDs or COX-2 inhibitors. *Archives of Internal Medicine, 165*, 189–192.

Beyth, R. (2005). Assessing risk factors for bleeding. In J. Ansell, L. Oertel, & A. Wittkowsky (Eds.), *Managing oral anticoagulation therapy* (2nd ed., pp. 1–6). St. Louis, MO: Wolters Kluwer Health.

Carrier, M., Grégoire, L. G., & Wells, P. S. (2009). Factors that influence warfarin effect. In J. Ansell, L. Oertel, & A. Wittowsky (Eds.), *Managing oral anticoagulation therapy* (3rd ed., pp. 183–191). St. Louis, MO: Wolters Kluwer Health.

Centers for Medicare and Medicaid Services. (2009). *Decision memo for prothrombin time (INR) monitor for home anticoagulation management.* Retrieved from www.cms.gov.

Cheetham, C. T., Levy, G., Niu, F., & Bixler, F. (2009). Gastrointestinal safety of nonsteroidal anti-inflammatory drugs and selective cyclooxygenase-2 inhibitors in patients on warfarin. *Annals of Pharmacotherapy, 43*, 1765–1773.

Dennehy, C. (2010, April 9–11). *An evidence based look at popular dietary supplements.* Presented at Clinical Pharmacotherapy 2010, University of California, Davis.

Douketis, J. D., Berger, P. B., Dunn, A. S., Jaffer, A. K., Spyropoulos, A. C., Becker, R. C., et al. (2008). The perioperative management of antithrombotic therapy: American College of Chest Physicians evidence-based clinical practice guidelines (8th ed). *Chest Supplement, 133*, 299S–339S.

Douketis, J., Spyropoulos, A., Kaatz, S., Becker, R. C., Caprini, J. A., Dunn, A. S., et al. (2015). Perioperative bridging anticoagulation in patients with atrial fibrillation. *New England Journal of Medicine, 373*, 823–833. doi: 10.1056/NEJMoa1501035

Douketis, J. D., Spyropoulos, A. C., Spencer, F. A., Mayr, M., Jaffer, A. K., Eckman, M. H., et al. (2012). Perioperative management of antithrombotic therapy: Antithrombotic therapy and prevention of thrombosis, 9th ed.: American College of Chest Physicians evidence-based clinical practice guidelines. *Chest, 141*(2, Suppl.), e326S–e350S.

Evans-Molina, C., Henault, L. E., Regan, S., & Hylek, E. M. (2003). Nurse assessment of warfarin candidacy among geriatric patients with atrial fibrillation referred to an anticoagulation clinic. *Journal of Thrombosis and Thrombolysis, 16*(1–2), E310S.

Fang, M. C. (2015). Implications of the new atrial fibrillation guideline. *JAMA Internal Medicine, 175*(5), 850–851.

Fang, M., Fang, M. C., Go, A. S., Chang, Y., Borowsky, L., Pomernacki, N. K., et al. (2008). Comparison of risk stratification schemes to predict thromboembolism in people with nonvalvular atrial fibrillation. *Journal of the American College of Cardiology, 51*, 810–815.

Gage, B. F., Waterman, A. D., Shannon, W., Boechler, M., Rich, M. W., & Radford, M. J. (2001). Validation of clinical classification schemes for predicting stroke: Results from the National Registry of Atrial Fibrillation. *JAMA, 285*, 2864–2870.

Garcia, D. A., Witt, D. M., Hylek, E., Wittkowsky, A. K., Nutescu, E. A., Jacobson, A., et al. (2008). Delivery of optimized anticoagulant therapy: Consensus statement from the Anticoagulation Forum. *Annals of Pharmacotherapy, 42*, 979–988.

Guyatt, G., Akl, E., Crowther, M., Gutterman, D., & Schünemann, H. J. (2012). Executive summary: Antithrombotic therapy and prevention of thrombosis (9th ed.). *Chest, 141*(2, Suppl.), 7S–47S.

Hellwig, T. & Gulseth, M. (2013). Pharmacokinetic and pharmcodynamic drug interactions with new oral anticoagulants: What do they mean for patients with atrial fibrillation? *Annals of Pharmacotherapy, 47*(1), 478–487.

Holbrook, A. M., Pereira, J. A., Labiris, R., McDonald, H., Douketis, J. D., Crowther, M., et al. (2005). Systemic overview of warfarin and its drug and food interactions. *Archives of Internal Medicine, 165*, 1095–1106.

Nicoll, D., McPhee, S., Pignone, M., & Lu, C. M. (2007). *Pocket guide to diagnostic tests* (5th ed.). Retrieved from http://www.worldcat.org/title/diagnostic-tests/oclc/225863401

Odum, L., Cochran, K., Aistrope, D., & Snella, K. (2012). The CHADS$_2$ vs the New CHA2DS$_2$-VASc scoring systems for guiding antithrombotic treatment of patients with atrial fibrillation: review of the literature and recommendations for use. *Pharmacotherapy, 32*(3), 285–296.

Rossini, R., Musumeci, G., Lettieri, C., Molfiese, M., Mihalcsik, L., Mantovani, P., et al. (2008). Long-term outcomes in patients undergoing coronary stenting on dual oral antiplatelet treatment requiring oral anticoagulant therapy. *American Journal of Cardiology, 102*(12), 1618–1623.

Self, T. H. (2000). *Warfarin and other oral anticoagulants.* Retrieved from www.medscape.com/viewarticle/410539.

U.S. Department of Agriculture, Agricultural Research Service, Nutrient Data Laboratory. (2015). USDA National Nutrient Database for Standard Reference, Release 28. Retrieved from www.ars.usda.gov/nea/bhnrc/ndl.

Witt, D. M., Delate, T., Clark, N. P., Martell, C., Tran, T., & Crowther, M. A.; Warfarin Associated Research Projects and other EnDeavors (WARPED) Consortium. (2009). Outcome and predictors of very stable INR control during chronic anticoagulation therapy. *Blood, 114*, 952–956.

Wittkowsky, A. K. (2009a). Initiation and maintenance dosing of warfarin and monitoring the INR. In J. Ansell, L. Oertel, & A. Wittkowsky (Eds.), *Managing oral anticoagulation therapy* (3rd ed., pp. 173–182). St. Louis, MO: Wolters Kluwer Health.

Wittkowsky, A. K. (2009b). Pharmacology of warfarin and related anticoagulants. In J. Ansell, L. Oertel, & A. Wittkowsky (Eds.), *Managing oral anticoagulation therapy* (3rd ed., pp. 149–160). St. Louis, MO: Wolters Kluwer Health.

Wolf, P. A., Abbott, R. D., & Kannel, W. B. (1991). Atrial fibrillation as an independent risk factor for stroke: The Framingham Study. *Stroke, 22*, 983–988.

Wong, W., Wilson, N. J., & Wittkowsky, A. K. (1999). Influence of warfarin regimen type on clinical and monitoring outcomes in stable patients on an anticoagulation management service. *Pharmacotherapy, 19*, 1385–1391.

ANXIETY

Esker-D Ligon

CHAPTER 45

I. Introduction and general background

Anxiety disorders are commonly encountered, although often not adequately addressed, in the primary care setting. It is estimated that 8% of patients presenting for primary care services have a form of anxiety disorder, and the presence of such disorders may increase the disability of existing chronic medical conditions (Kroenke, Spitzer, Williams, Monahan, & Lowe, 2007). Despite increased awareness of the prevalence of these disorders, less than 40% of patients with anxiety are diagnosed and treated in the primary care setting (Kroenke et al., 2007). Although some providers hold the sentiment that treatment of mental health disorders in the primary care setting is too time consuming, lack of treatment prevents one from being able to adequately address physical health issues. In a study conducted by Weisberg, Beard, Moitra, Dyck, and Keller (2014), 51% of patients with anxiety disorders received pharmacotherapy from a primary care provider. Anxiety disorders can be adequately treated in primary care (Bandelow et al., 2012).

Anxiety disorders contribute to functional impairments, disability, decreased health outcomes, comorbidity, and high use of health services. Given the impact of these disorders and the emerging trend toward the provision of integrated services, primary care providers should be equipped to properly screen and treat patients presenting with anxiety symptoms.

The etiology of anxiety disorders involves environmental, biochemical, psychosocial, and genetic factors. Many types of anxiety disorders exist; however, this guideline focuses on the identification and treatment of the most common anxiety disorders: generalized anxiety disorder, social anxiety disorder, and panic disorder as well as posttraumatic stress disorder (PTSD) (American Psychiatric Association [APA], 2013). The most commonly found anxiety disorder is generalized anxiety, followed by panic disorder and social phobia (Kroenke et al., 2007). With improved screening by primary care providers, PTSD may be found to have higher rates than previously known, especially for persons who are homeless or of low socioeconomic status who may be chronically exposed to violence and other forms of trauma (Bobo, Warner, & Warner, 2007; Meredith et al., 2009).

Diagnosis of anxiety disorders in the primary care setting is often influenced by a number of factors. Many patients present with somatic complaints or problems with sleep. Some patients use substances to self-medicate symptoms. Substance use, although a separate problem, is often a symptom of an underlying disorder. It is imperative that providers adequately assess for such disorders. Cultural factors may also confound the diagnosis of anxiety disorders (Brenes et al., 2008). Each culture or demographic group has a set of norms for addressing mental health disorders, which may be influenced by stigma. Cultural identity involves not only ethnicity, acculturation and biculturalism, and language but also age, gender, socioeconomic status, sexual orientation, religious and spiritual beliefs, disabilities, political orientation, and health literacy, among other factors (APA, 2000).

Anxiety disorders across a spectrum of intensity and clinical relevance may present at any time during the course of a primary care visit. It is normal for patients to feel nervous on first meeting with a stranger, including a new primary care provider. This must not be overinterpreted as a sign of a significant or enduring psychiatric condition for which treatment is indicated. Visiting an unfamiliar treatment center may cause a patient to present as anxious or distressed. Actual or perceived sociocultural differences between the provider and the patient may contribute to a greater chance of initial anxiety. Traditional office settings can be noisy, congested, and stressful environments, often requiring the patient to wait well beyond their appointment time. A sincere apology for causing a patient any inconvenience often goes far to help their situational anxiety subside.

Providers must evaluate anxiety symptoms for the presence of an anxiety disorder. A provider should be aware of his or her personal biases, prejudices, or lack of knowledge pertaining to particular personal issues or cultural standards of a given patient. Privacy must be ensured, and the provider must assume a nonjudgmental tone about anything that the patient may be encouraged to reveal. Even when the provider inquires in a warm, nonjudgmental manner, some topics are inherently difficult for patients to discuss. They may feel embarrassed and guarded, and the interviewer may need to phrase questions in different ways and repeatedly. Throughout any clinical encounter the provider needs to be alert for signs of increased agitation, such as increasing restlessness or pacing, clenched fists, verbal threats or pressured or loud speech. When one detects such agitation, it is advisable to refrain from further discussion of distressing topics that are not germane to the patient's current presentation (Lange, Lange, & Cabaltica, 2000).

II. **Database** (may include but is not limited to)

A. Subjective

1. Symptomatology and relevant supporting data
   Patients may present with a variety of complaints related to anxiety disorders. Providers should inquire about the duration of symptoms, effect of symptoms on patient's functioning, and relationships between symptoms and contributory factors. Providers should assess for the following:
   a. Feelings of nervousness, anxiety, panic, excessive worry, or feeling generally stressed and overwhelmed
   b. Negative thoughts, ruminative or obsessive thinking; unrelenting pessimism, feelings of foreboding, and excessive guilt
   c. Adrenergic effects: irregular heartbeat, tachycardia, and palpitations; shortness of breath, diaphoresis, lightheadedness, paresthesias, and tremor
   d. Sleep disturbances including insomnia, hypersomnia, nightmares, and restless sleep
   e. Marked avoidance of specific situations and social withdrawal
   f. Restlessness, irritability, agitation, and excessive anger
   g. Appetite disturbance
   h. Difficulty with memory or concentration
   i. Persistent sense of fear, foreboding, apprehension, and hypervigilance
   j. Suicidality: ideation, thoughts of being better off dead or that life is not worth living, and planned or attempted suicidal acts
   k. Somatic complaints: headaches, gastrointestinal complaints, back and neck pain, chest pain, and excessive concern with physical health
   l. Precipitating stressors, events, and losses (including community violence and vicarious trauma)
   m. Substance use: changes in types, frequency, and quantity of alcohol or drugs, including street drugs or prescribed medications
   n. Past health history: history of other mental health disorders and medical illnesses causing or exacerbating signs and symptoms of anxiety (e.g., hyperthyroidism, attention deficit hyperactivity disorder [ADHD], major depression, bipolar disorder, and schizophrenia)

B. Objective

1. Appearance and kinetic behavior: restlessness, wringing hands, biting nails, shaking legs or feet, rocking, sitting unusually still, appearing tense, and altered grooming and hygiene.

2. Mental status examination which includes: appearance, mood, affect, speech, thought content, thought process, memory and concentration, and assessment of insight and judgment.

3. Evidence-based screening tools: it is advisable that primary care practice settings adopt a screening tool for early identification of comorbid anxiety disorders:
   a. The Generalized Anxiety Disorder 7-item (GAD-7) scale (see **Figure 45-1**) is a useful anxiety screening tool (Spitzer, Kroenke, Williams, & Lowe, 2006). The tool should be used to screen for the emergence of anxiety disorder symptoms. Screening should be repeated periodically to objectively measure changes after behavioral or psychotherapeutic intervention.
   b. DREAMS mnemonic is a useful interview tool to screen for PTSD (Lange et al., 2000).
      i. **D**etachment (alexithymia) or feeling emotionally numb
      ii. **R**eexperiencing the event via nightmares, flashbacks
      iii. **E**vent with emotional effects, such as distress, feeling unsafe, fear
      iv. **A**voidance of reminder places, activities, or people
      v. **M**onth duration of symptoms or longer
      vi. **S**ympathetic hyperactivity (e.g., tachycardia, tachypnea, and insomnia)

4. Diagnostic studies: include laboratory testing for thyroid disorders, hormonal imbalances, substance intoxication or occult use, electrolyte imbalances, vitamin B_{12} deficiency, hypo- or hyperglycemia.

5. Collateral data: include information from members of a multidisciplinary treatment team when possible. With the permission of the patient, a brief discussion

GAD-7

Over the last 2 weeks, how often have you been bothered by the following problems? *(Use "✓" to indicate your answer)*	Not at all	Several days	More than half the days	Nearly every day
1. Feeling nervous, anxious or on edge	0	1	2	3
2. Not being able to stop or control worrying	0	1	2	3
3. Worrying too much about different things	0	1	2	3
4. Trouble relaxing	0	1	2	3
5. Being so restless that it is hard to sit still	0	1	2	3
6. Becoming easily annoyed or irritable	0	1	2	3
7. Feeling afraid as if something awful might happen	0	1	2	3

Total Score ____ = ____ + ____ + ____

Scoring and Interpretation:

GAD-2 Score	GAD-7 Score
Provisional Diagnosis	**Provisional Diagnosis**
0-2 None	**0-7 None**
3-6 Probable anxiety disorder	**8+ Probable anxiety disorder**
*GAD-2 is the first 2 questions of the GAD-7	

FIGURE 45-1 Generalized Anxiety Disorder 7-Item (GAD-7) Scale

Reproduced from Pfizer. (n.d.). *GAD-7*. Retrieved from www.phqscreeners.com. Developed by Drs. Robert L. Spitzer, Janet B.W. Williams, Kurt Kroenke, and colleagues, with an educational grant from Pfizer Inc. No permission required to reproduce, translate, display, or distribute. Scoring and interpretation table modified from www.lifesolutionsforyou.com.

with family members or friends may yield corroborating or missing information about manifestations of the patient's anxiety or provide perspective on the cause, duration, intensity, and possible remedies of the patient's condition. Collateral contacts may also yield helpful information regarding suicidal statements, failure to eat or function normally, or use of substances.

III. Assessment

A. Determining a diagnosis

Refer to the diagnostic criteria and/or decision trees for anxiety in the *Diagnostic and Statistical Manual of Mental Disorders, 5th Edition,* published by the American Psychiatric Association (2013), or the *DSM-5 Handbook of Differential Diagnosis* (First, 2013). The DSM-5 classification and the specific diagnostic criteria are meant to serve as guidelines to be informed by clinical judgment in the categorization of the patient's conditions and are not meant to be applied in a rote fashion. The following are summarized criteria for anxiety and trauma and stressor-related disorders common to primary care settings. In general, symptoms should not be attributable to the effects of a substance or another medical or psychiatric condition.

1. Panic attack: a feature of many anxiety disorders characterized by the following:
   a. Palpitations or rapid heart rate
   b. Sweating
   c. Trembling or shaking
   d. Shortness of breath
   e. Feeling of choking
   f. Chest pain, pressure, or discomfort
   g. Nausea or stomach upset
   h. Dizziness or lightheadedness
   i. Feelings of unreality or self-detachment
   j. Fear of dying
   k. Numbness or tingling of extremities
   l. Chills or hot flushes

2. Panic disorder: recurrent unexpected panic attacks and at least one of the attacks has been followed by at least a month of one of the following symptoms: persistent worry about having another attack, worry about the consequences of the attack, or significant change in behavior related to attacks.

3. Generalized anxiety disorder: excessive anxiety and worry about a variety of situations. Patients report difficulty controlling the anxiety, and it interferes with their ability to function. Anxiety is associated with at least three of six symptoms as noted previously.

4. Social anxiety disorder: fear of being embarrassed or humiliated in social or performance situations when exposed to unfamiliar people or possible scrutiny by others. Exposure to feared situation provokes anxiety, and in some cases a panic attack. In most cases, the patient recognizes fear is excessive or unreasonable. The feared situation is avoided or experienced with intense anxiety; avoidance may interfere with normal functioning or cause marked distress.

5. Agoraphobia
   a. Fear about being in situations that would be difficult to escape or in which help would not be available if a panic attack was experienced
   b. Significant avoidance of such situations, enduring situations in distress, or requiring a companion to function

6. PTSD
   a. Condition may be acute (lasting > 1 month but < 3 months) or chronic (lasting > 3 months).
   b. Person has been exposed to an event in which they witnessed or experienced something that threatened life, serious injury, or damage to personal integrity; their response included intense fear, helplessness, or horror and lasts for longer than 1 month. The traumatic event is reexperienced in one of four ways:
      i. Intrusive distressing recollections of the event.
      ii. Distressing dreams or nightmares of the event.
      iii. Having a sense of reliving the event, including flashbacks and hallucinations.
      iv. Intense psychologic or physiologic response to triggers and cues reminiscent of the event
   c. Persistent avoidance of stimuli associated with the trauma including avoidance of triggers associated with trauma, inability to remember important details of trauma, anhedonia, isolation, restricted emotions, and sense of shortened lifespan.
   d. Increased state of arousal evidenced by sleep disturbance, irritability, poor concentration, hypervigilance, or becoming easily startled.

B. Functional assessment and severity of illness

1. Consider the patient's current clinical status, psychosocial factors affecting the clinical situation, the patient's highest level of past functioning, and the patient's quality of life.

2. A functional assessment may be useful for assessing strengths and disease severity and should focus on the patient's ability to perform essential activities of daily living. Information gathered may also facilitate the monitoring of treatment by assessing important beneficial and adverse effects of treatment.

IV. Plan

Anxiety disorders are a common and often disabling mental disorder. Treatment is indicated when symptoms of the disorder interfere with functioning or cause significant distress. Effective treatment for anxiety disorders should lead not only to reduction in frequency and intensity of symptoms but should optimally yield full remission of symptoms and return to a premorbid level of functioning. A range of evidence-based psychosocial and pharmacologic interventions exist for treatment of anxiety disorders and should be instituted for all patients requiring treatment.

The treatment plan is ideally collaboration between the patient, the provider, and other members of the treatment team. It should include a combination of biologic and sociocultural interventions to create an integrated treatment plan. Optimally, interventions should encourage recovery from illness through community integration and empower patients to make choices that improve their quality of life. Considerations that guide the choice of an initial treatment modality include patient preference, the risks and benefits of treatment, past treatment history, presence of co-occurring conditions, cost, and treatment availability.

A. Medication selection

When making the decision to use pharmacologic treatments, providers must consider a patient's ability to remain compliant with treatment. Selective serotonin reuptake inhibitors (SSRIs) and serotonin-norepinephrine reuptake inhibitors (SNRIs) are regarded as first-line agents for treatment of anxiety disorders. Before selecting a specific medication one must balance the risks associated with the medication against the benefits of treatment and consider the following: potential side effects, potential drug interactions or contraindications, pharmacologic properties, co-occurring medical and psychiatric conditions, and the strength of the evidence for the particular medication in treatment of anxiety disorders. With regard to co-occurring psychiatric conditions, it is imperative that the potential for bipolar disorder be assessed. Treatment with certain agents can precipitate mania.

Please refer to the chapter on depression for a list of medications commonly used to treat anxiety and depression. The use of benzodiazepines is often a controversial issue. Additionally, the treatment of PTSD is often complex and may require a specialty referral.

Benzodiazepines are appropriate as monotherapy only in the absence of a co-occurring mood disorder and may be preferred (as monotherapy or in combination with antidepressants) for patients with very distressing or impairing symptoms in whom rapid symptom control is critical. The benefit of rapid response must be balanced against the potential for depressive and sedative side effects and physiologic dependence that may lead to difficulty discontinuing the medication. Addition of benzodiazepines to an SSRI or SNRI is a common augmentation strategy to target residual symptoms. They are also commonly used to treat severe presentations initially with another agent, followed by a gradual taper of the benzodiazepine. When the goal is to prevent panic attacks rather than reduction of symptoms after an attack has occurred, a regular dosing schedule rather than an "as needed" schedule is preferred. In such instances, agents with a longer half-life, such as clonazepam, may provide better coverage than short half-life agents, such as lorazepam.

PTSD may manifest with a variety of physical and psychiatric symptoms, which must be addressed to successfully treat this disorder. Treatment often requires a multidisciplinary approach, including polypharmacy in some cases (Bobo et al., 2007). Severe cases should be referred to a psychiatric or mental health clinician. Refer to **Table 45-1** for possible pharmacotherapeutic options to treat PTSD.

B. Medication management

1. Educate patients about the likely course of treatment associated with a particular medication. Pharmacotherapy should generally be continued for 1 year or more after acute response to promote further symptom reduction and decrease risk of recurrence.

2. Patients with anxiety disorders can be sensitive to medication side effects; thus, low starting doses of medications are recommended with a gradual increase to a full therapeutic dose over several days and as tolerated by the patient. Underdosing of antidepressants is common in treatment of anxiety disorders and is a frequent source of partial response or nonresponse.

3. Medication monitoring involves assessment of the change in symptoms, such as frequency and intensity of panic attacks, level of anticipatory anxiety, degree of agoraphobic avoidance, quality of sleep, persistence of somatic symptoms, and severity of interference and distress related to anxiety disorders.

   a. Patients typically require monitoring every 1–2 weeks when first starting a new medication, then every 2–4 weeks until the dose is stabilized.

   b. Less frequent monitoring is required after stabilization and reduction of symptoms.

4. Discontinuation of medication should be performed in a gradual and collaborative manner. This allows for continual assessment of the effects of the taper, the patient's response to any changes that emerge, and, if required, treatment may be reinitiated at a previously effective dose. However, medications can be discontinued much more quickly in urgent conditions, such as pregnancy. Before advising a

TABLE 45-1 Pharmacotherapeutic Options for Treating PTSD

Medication	Starting Dose (mg)	Effective Dose (mg)	Maximum Dose/Day
First line			
Fluoxetine (Prozac®)	20 mg/day	20–40 mg/day	200 mg/day
Paroxetine (Paxil®)	20 mg/day	20–50 mg/day	50 mg/day
Sertraline (Zoloft®)	50 mg/day	50–200 mg/day	80 mg/day
Citalopram (Celexa®)	20 mg/day	20–40 mg/day	60 mg/day
Escitalopram (Lexapro®)	10 mg/day	10–20 mg/day	20 mg/day
Fluvoxamine (Luvox®)	50 mg/day	50–300 mg/day	300 mg/day
Non-SSRI antidepressants			
Venlafaxine, Venlafaxine ER (Effexor®)	37.5–75 mg BID	75–225 mg Most people use venlafaxine ER	Varies from 225–375 mg/day depending on the targeted condition and the medication preparation
Mirtazapine (Remeron®)	15 mg q.h.s.	15–45 mg q.h.s.	45 mg/day
Trazodone (Desyrel®)	25–50 mg q.h.s.	25–150 mg q.h.s.	200 mg/day
Amitriptyline (Elavil®, Amitid®, Amitril®)—TCA	25–100 mg q.h.s.	50–150 mg/day	300 mg/day
Doxepin (Adapin®, Sinequen®)—TCA	25 mg q.h.s.	150–300 mg q.h.s.	300 mg/day
Imipramine (Tofranil®, Presamine®, Janimine®)—TCA *off-label use	25 mg q.h.s.	150–300 mg q.h.s.	300 mg/day
Nortriptyline (Pamelor®, Aventyl®)—TCA *off-label use	25 mg q.h.s.	50–150 mg q.h.s.	150 mg/day
Augmenting agents			
Antiadrenergic agents			
Prazosin	1 mg BID	5–20 mg/day	40 mg/day
Clonidine	0.1 mg BID	0.2–1.2 mg/day	2.4 mg/day
Guanfacine	1 mg q.h.s.	1–2 mg/day	3 mg/day
Propranolol (Inderal®)	20–40 mg BID	160–480 mg/day	640 mg/day
Mood stabilizers/anticonvulsants			
*Should refer to a psychiatric specialist if required for treatment			
Lamotrigine (Lamictal®)	25–50 mg/day	50–250 mg BID	500 mg/day
Gabapentin (Neurontin®)	300 mg q.h.s.	300–600 mg TID	3,600 mg/day
Atypical antipsychotics			
*Should refer to a psychiatric specialist if required for treatment			
Risperidone (Risperdal®)	1 mg/day	1–3 mg BID	6 mg/day
Olanzapine (Zyprexa®)	25–5 mg/day	5–20 mg/day	20 mg/day
Quetiapine (Seroquel®)	25 mg/day	150–750 mg/day divided BID–TID	800 mg/day
Miscellaneous agents			
Zolpidem (Ambien®)	5 mg q.h.s.	5–10 mg q.h.s.	10 mg/day
Zaleplon (Sonata®)	5 mg q.h.s.	5–10 mg q.h.s.	20 mg/day
Diphenhydramine (Benadryl®)	25 mg q.h.s.	25–50 mg q.h.s.	50 mg/day
Buspirone (BuSpar)	7.5 mg BID	30 mg/day	60 mg/day

*Hydroxyzine is an additional antihistamine medication that is useful for the treatment of anxiety at doses of 10–100 mg daily, in split doses.

Modified from Bobo, W., Warner, C., & Warner, C. (2007). The management of post traumatic stress disorder (PTSD) in the primary care setting. *Southern Medical Journal, 100*(8), 797–801.

taper of effective pharmacotherapy, one should consider the patient's history of previous mood or anxiety disorder episodes, the duration of symptom remission, the presence of current or impending psychosocial stressors in the patient's life, and the extent to which the patient is motivated to discontinue the medication. This discussion should also include the possible outcomes of taper, including discontinuation symptoms and recurrence of panic symptoms.

C. Psychosocial interventions

Psychosocial treatment is recommended for pregnant women and other patients who prefer nonpharmacologic treatment and can invest the time and effort required to attend weekly sessions. Psychosocial treatments for anxiety disorders should be conducted by professionals with an appropriate level of training and experience in the relevant approach.

1. Cognitive-behavioral therapy (CBT): CBT is a time-limited treatment, generally 10–15 weekly sessions, that yields durable effects. It can be successfully administered individually or in a group format. CBT and other psychosocial treatments are not readily available in some geographic areas. Self-directed forms of CBT may be useful for patients who do not have ready access to a trained CBT therapist. CBT for anxiety disorders generally includes psychoeducation, self-monitoring, countering anxious beliefs, exposure to fear cues, modification of anxiety-maintaining behaviors, and relapse prevention.

2. Combined treatment should be considered for patients who have failed to respond to monotherapy, and may also be used under certain clinical circumstances (e.g., using pharmacotherapy for temporary control of severe symptoms that are impeding the patient's ability to engage in psychosocial treatment). Such treatment may also enhance long-term outcomes by reducing the likelihood of relapse when pharmacologic treatment is stopped.

3. Other group therapies: patient support groups are not recommended as monotherapy, although they may be useful adjuncts to other effective treatments for some patients.

4. Couples or family therapy may be helpful in addressing co-occurring relationship dysfunction. When initiating treatments for anxiety disorders, educate significant others about the nature of the disorder, enlisting their assistance to improve treatment adherence.

5. Complementary and alternative medicine methods, such as tai chi and meditation, and regular exercise regimens have been proven helpful at addressing anxiety in some cases (van der Watt, Laugharne, & Janca, 2008).

D. Referral to specialty care

As a primary care provider, it is important to have the ability to differentiate cases that can be managed in one's own setting from more severe cases that require consultation or referral to dedicated psychiatric care. If response to an adequate trial of a first-line treatment (e.g., CBT, SSRI, or serotonin-norepinephrine reuptake inhibitor) is unsatisfactory, it is appropriate for the provider and the patient to consider a change to another treatment. Decisions about whether and how to make changes depends on the level of response or lack thereof to the initial treatment, the feasibility of other treatment options, and the severity of remaining symptoms and impairment. After first- and second-line treatments and augmentation strategies have been exhausted, either because of lack of efficacy or patient intolerance, providers are encouraged to consult with experienced colleagues or refer the patient to dedicated psychiatric services.

V. Special populations

A. Dually diagnosed patients

There is a high prevalence of self-medication with alcohol and other substances by persons with anxiety disorders (Arch, Craske, Stein, Sherbourne, & Roy-Byrne, 2006). It is often advantageous for patients to receive integrated treatment of both conditions (Mueser, Noordsy, Drake, & Fox, 2003). Patients often decrease their use of substances once the underlying anxiety is effectively addressed (Denning & Little, 2000). Providers should exercise caution when prescribing medications because of potential interactions with substances of abuse. Extreme caution should be used when using benzodiazepines to treat patients using alcohol or opiates. Patients should be educated about the additive effects of the previously mentioned substances.

B. Pregnant women

For women with anxiety disorders who are pregnant, nursing, or planning to become pregnant, psychosocial interventions should be implemented. Pharmacotherapy may be indicated but requires discussion of the potential benefits and risks with the patient and, her obstetrician. Such discussions should also consider the potential risks to the patient and the child of untreated psychiatric illness, including anxiety disorders and any co-occurring psychiatric conditions.

C. Older adults

There are important safety considerations for SSRIs, tricyclic antidepressants, and benzodiazepines, which include increased risk of falls and osteoporotic fractures in patients age 50 and older. Caution and careful monitoring are indicated when prescribing medications to elderly patients, because they may produce sedation, fatigue, ataxia, slurred speech, memory impairment, and weakness. Check the American Geriatrics Society Beers Criteria Medication List at www.dcri.org for potentially harmful medications in the elderly.

D. Children and adolescents

Children and adolescents may present with different symptoms than adults. Please refer to the DSM-5 for further information. There is also a higher risk of suicidality as a potential adverse effect of SSRIs and other antidepressants in this population. Psychotherapy is the first-line treatment for children and adolescents with anxiety disorders.

VI. Self-management resources and tools

A. Patient and client educational handouts and resources

1. Educational handouts for patients and families can be found at www.nimh.nih.gov. Many handouts are available in multiple languages and are updated periodically.

2. *The Anxiety and Phobia Workbook* (Bourne, 2005).

3. National Alliance for the Mentally Ill (NAMI), www.nami.org

4. National Center for PTSD website (www.ptsd.va.gov/) has factsheets and resources for patients and providers.

5. Anxiety Disorders Association of America website (www.adaa.org) has resources for patients and providers.

REFERENCES

American Psychiatric Association. (2013). *Diagnostic and statistical manual of mental health disorders* (5th ed.). Washington, DC: Author.

American Psychiatric Association. (2000). *Diagnostic and statistical manual of mental health disorders* (4th ed.), *text revision*. Washington, DC: Author.

Arch, J., Craske, M., Stein, M., Sherbourne, C., & Roy-Byrne, P. (2006). Correlates of alcohol use among anxious and depressed primary care patients. *General Hospital Psychiatry, 28*, 37–42.

Bandelow, B., Sher, L., Bunevicius, R., Hollander, E., Kasper, S., Zohar, J., et al. (2012). Guidelines for the pharmacological treatment of anxiety disorders, obsessive-compulsive disorder, and posttraumatic stress disorder in primary care. *International Journal of Psychiatry in Clinical Practice, 16*(2), 77–84.

Bobo, W., Warner, C., & Warner, C. (2007). The management of post traumatic stress disorder (PTSD) in the primary care setting. *Southern Medical Journal, 100*(8), 797–801.

Bourne, E. (2005). *The anxiety and phobia workbook* (4th ed.). Oakland, CA: New Harbinger.

Brenes, G., Knudson, M., McCall, W., Williamson, J., Miller, M., & Stanley, M. (2008). Age and racial differences in the presentation and treatment of generalized anxiety disorder in primary care. *Journal of Anxiety Disorders, 22*, 1128–1136.

Denning, P., & Little, J. (2000). *Practicing harm reduction psychotherapy: An alternative approach to addictions.* New York, NY: Guilford.

First, M. (2013). *DSM-5 handbook of differential diagnosis.* Arlington, VA: APA.

Kroenke, K., Spitzer, R., Williams, J., Monahan, P., & Lowe, B. (2007). Anxiety disorders in primary care: Prevalence, impairment, comorbidity, and detection. *Annals of Internal Medicine, 146*(5), 317–325.

Lange, J., Lange, C., & Cabaltica, R. (2000). Primary care treatment of posttraumatic stress disorder. *American Family Physician, 62*(5), 1035–1040, 1046.

Meredith, L., Eisenman, D., Green, B., Basurto-Davila, R., Cassells, A., & Tobin, J. (2009). System factors affect the recognition and management of posttraumatic stress disorder by primary care clinicians. *Medical Care, 47*(6), 686–694.

Mueser, T., Noordsy, D., Drake, R., & Fox, L. (2003). *Integrated treatment for dual disorders: A guide to effective practice.* New York, NY: Guilford.

Spitzer, R. L., Kroenke, K., Williams, J. B. W., & Lowe, B. (2006). A brief measure for assessing generalized anxiety disorder: The GAD-7. *Archives of Internal Medicine, 166*, 1092–1097.

van der Watt, G., Laugharne, J., & Janca, A. (2008). Complementary and alternative medicine in the treatment of anxiety and depression. *Current Opinion in Psychiatry, 21*(1), 37–42.

Weisberg, R. B., Beard, C., Moitra, E., Dyck, I., & Keller, M. B. (2014). Adequacy of treatment received by primary care patients with anxiety disorders. *Depression and Anxiety, 31*(5), 443–450.

ASTHMA IN ADOLESCENTS AND ADULTS

Susan L. Janson

CHAPTER 46

I. Introduction and general background

Asthma is an inflammatory disease of the airways characterized by airflow obstruction that is reversible (at least partially) either spontaneously or with treatment. Airway inflammation and bronchospasm cause recurring symptoms of wheezing, coughing, breathlessness, and the sensation of chest tightness that occurs particularly at night or early morning. The obstruction to airflow in the airways is the result of mucosal inflammation caused by inflammatory cell infiltration with neutrophils, eosinophils, and lymphocytes, in addition to mast cell activation and epithelial cell injury. Airway inflammation contributes to hyperresponsiveness of the airway and airway narrowing caused by bronchoconstriction of airway smooth muscle. In some patients, persistent changes in airway structure occur, resulting in airway remodeling and airflow limitation that are not fully reversible.

A. Pathogenesis

The etiology of asthma is unknown but the strongest predictor for developing asthma is atopy, the genetic predisposition for development of an immunoglobulin (Ig) E–mediated response to common aeroallergens. Viral respiratory infections may also contribute and are the most important cause of asthma exacerbations. There is considerable variability in the pattern of airway inflammation indicating phenotypic differences of expression that may influence response to treatment. Onset of asthma for most people begins early in life with recurrent wheezing, atopic disease, and a history of parental asthma.

Understanding of the pathogenesis of asthma is evolving as genetic and phenotypic variations are identified. Research has focused on an imbalance of Th1 and Th2 cytokines in allergic diseases including asthma that result in either overexpression of Th2 or underexpression of Th1 cells. Th2 cells mediate inflammation, whereas Th1 cells respond to infection. The "hygiene hypothesis" illustrates how this imbalance may occur, as in westernized civilizations, where exposure to infections is limited resulting in persistence of Th2 dominance in genetically susceptible children (Brooks, Pearce, & Douwes, 2013; Busse & Lemanske, 2001).

B. Prevalence

Asthma affects 25 million people in the United States (Centers for Disease Control and Prevention, 2011) and more than 300 million worldwide (World Health Organization, 2007). Early in life the prevalence of asthma is higher in boys, but at puberty the gender ratio shifts toward girls and asthma is seen predominantly in women after puberty. Asthma exacerbations are responsible for more than $37 billion in direct costs annually in the United States (Kamble & Bharmal, 2009). Severe asthma affects approximately 10% of the population with asthma and accounts for 50% of asthma-related health costs (Sullivan et al., 2007).

C. Factors that precipitate or aggravate asthma

1. Allergens: Exposure to aerosolized allergens (aeroallergens) for people who are sensitized to them is an important precipitant of asthma. Outdoor allergens are primarily pollens from trees and plants that occur in seasonal waves. Patients with these sensitivities have more frequent exacerbations during the time of heavy pollination if they are sensitized. Even more important are the perennial indoor allergens (molds, house dust mites, cockroaches, and animal dander) because of the length of time people stay indoors.

2. Irritants: The most important airway irritant exposure is environmental tobacco smoke. Other irritants include bleach, sprays like perfume, strong odors (paint fumes, cooking gas, and wood smoke) and air pollution, with increased exposure in closed, poorly ventilated areas.

3. Medication and drugs: Some medications are known to trigger airway constriction through neural or metabolic pathways. These include β-blockers, aspirin, and nonsteroidal anti-inflammatory drugs.

4. Other factors that can worsen asthma: Sulfites found in beer, wine, and food; strong emotions; cold air; weather changes; exercise; and viral infections are common triggers for asthma symptoms.

5. Comorbid conditions that exacerbate asthma: Among the chronic conditions that make asthma harder to control are gastroesophageal reflux disease (GERD), rhinitis and sinusitis, obesity, and chronic stress and depression. Evidence is stronger for the first two, but efforts should be made to treat and control all of these conditions when present.

II. **Database** (may include but is not limited to)

A. Subjective

1. Symptom description: The most common signs and symptoms of asthma are intermittent dyspnea, cough, and wheezing. These symptoms occur together creating a well-recognized syndrome.
   a. Presenting symptoms: recurrent wheezing, shortness of breath, chest tightness, cough that is worse at night, and sputum production
   b. Pattern of symptoms
      i. Perennial, seasonal, or both
      ii. Continual, episodic, or both
      iii. Onset, duration, and frequency (number of days or nights per week or month)
      iv. Diurnal variations, especially nocturnal and on awakening in early morning
   c. Precipitating or aggravating factors
      i. Viral respiratory infections
      ii. Environmental allergens, indoor (e.g., mold, house dust mite, cockroach, and animal dander or secretions) and outdoor (e.g., pollen)
      iii. Home characteristics (age, location, heating and cooling system, wood-burning stove, humidifier, carpeting over concrete, molds or mildew, floor coverings, and stuffed or upholstered furniture)
      iv. Smoking (patient or others in home or work)
      v. Exercise
      vi. Occupational chemicals or allergens
      vii. Environmental change (relocation or remodeling)
      viii. Irritants (secondhand tobacco smoke, strong odors, air pollutants, dusts, particulates, vapors, gases, and aerosols)
      ix. Emotions (e.g., fear, anger, frustration, hard crying or laughing) or stress
      x. Medications (e.g., aspirin, other nonsteroidal anti-inflammatory drugs, β-blockers)
      xi. Food, food additives, and preservatives (e.g., sulfites)
      xii. Changes in weather and exposure to cold air
      xiii. Endocrine factors (e.g., menses, pregnancy, and thyroid disease)
      xiv. Comorbid conditions (e.g., sinusitis, allergic rhinitis, GERD, and allergic responses to specific foods or alcohol)

2. Past health history
   a. Age of onset of disease
   b. History of emergency department visits, hospitalizations, need for intubation, and mechanical ventilation
   c. Need for systemic or oral corticosteroids and frequency of use
   d. History of exacerbations
      i. Prodromal signs and symptoms
      ii. Rapidity of onset and duration and frequency
      iii. Severity (need for urgent care, hospitalization, or intensive care unit care)
      iv. Impact (number of days missed from work or school, limitation of activities, nocturnal awakening, and economic impact)

3. Family history: Allergies, atopy, or asthma

4. Occupational and environmental history: Work-related exposures, such as vapors, gas, dusts, fumes, isocyanates, or cedar

5. Personal and social history: Tobacco smoking and secondhand tobacco exposure

6. Review of systems
   a. Constitutional signs and symptoms: fatigue caused by sleep disruption.
   b. Ear, nose, and throat: congestion, sneezing, runny nose, sinus headache, and postnasal drip.
   c. Respiratory: recurrent wheezing, cough, breathlessness, chest tightness, and increased mucus production.
   d. Cardiac: palpitations during times of severe breathlessness.
   e. Gastrointestinal: heartburn or dyspepsia.
   f. Psychiatric: anxiety or depression.

B. Objective

1. Physical findings
   a. General appearance: anxious, labored breathing, hyperexpansion of the chest (especially in children), use of accessory muscles, hunched shoulders, and deformed chest
   b. Ear, nose, and throat: pale and boggy nasal mucosa, thin and watery nasal secretions, red

or streaked posterior pharynx, and thrush (associated with inhaled corticosteroid use [ICS])

  c. Lungs: diffuse or scattered expiratory wheezes, prolonged expiration, wheezing with forced exhalation, and decrease in air entry and movement

  d. Cardiac: tachycardia (if hypoxic or if recently used beta-agonists)

  e. Skin: atopic dermatitis or eczema; pallor or cyanosis (if hypoxic)

2. Supporting data from relevant diagnostic tests, such as bronchoprovocation and especially spirometry.

III. Assessment

A. Differential diagnosis

1. Asthma

2. Chronic obstructive pulmonary disease (COPD) (e.g., emphysema and/or chronic bronchitis)

3. Upper airway disease: allergic rhinitis and sinusitis

4. Vocal cord dysfunction

5. Obstructions of large airways (foreign body, tumor, and lymph nodes)

6. Obstructions of small airways (cystic fibrosis, bronchiolitis, and bronchopulmonary dysplasia)

7. Recurrent cough secondary to medications

8. Aspiration

9. Congestive heart failure

B. Asthma severity, control, and response to treatment

1. Classify asthma severity (**Table 46-1**) as intermittent, mild persistent, moderate persistent, or severe persistent. Severity of asthma is the intrinsic intensity of the disease and is most easily determined when the patient is not on long-term treatment. Severity is measured in two domains: impairment and risk. Impairment is assessed by history of symptoms, nocturnal awakenings, short-acting beta$_2$-agonists use for relief of symptoms, activity limitation and by spirometry to assess airway caliber. It is important to assess the quantity and quality of sleep, limits to desired activity, and need for medication to gain a full picture of impairment. If these components are missed in history-taking asthma severity may be misclassified. Risk is assessed by the likelihood of frequent exacerbations, also assessed by history and by forced expiratory volume in 1 second (FEV$_1$). Predictors of asthma exacerbation include severe airflow obstruction, two or more emergency department visits or hospitalizations in the last year, intubation or intensive care unit admission for asthma in the last 5 years, patient report of feeling in danger from asthma, depression, and certain demographic characteristics (female, nonwhite, not using corticosteroid medication, and current smoking).

2. Classify asthma control (**Table 46-2**): Asthma can be classified as well controlled, not well controlled, or very poorly controlled. Asthma control is classified when the patient is currently on a controller medication, considering domains of impairment and risk. Control is the degree to which the symptoms, impairments, and risk are minimized and the goals of therapy are met. Control is assessed by symptoms, night-time awakenings, need for a short-acting β-agonist for relief of symptoms, ability to engage in usual activities and the frequency of exacerbations requiring treatment with oral corticosteroids. Several standardized questionnaires have been developed for the assessment of asthma control as reported by patients.

3. Assess responsiveness to therapy: Responsiveness is the ease with which asthma control is achieved by therapy.

C. Significance and motivation

Assess the significance of asthma to the patient and family, including how much asthma interferes with quality of life, work, and play. Determine willingness and ability to follow the treatment plan and properly inhale medications.

IV. Goals of clinical management to control asthma

A. Reduce impairment

1. Prevent chronic symptoms and night-time awakenings

2. Require only infrequent use of short-acting β-agonist (infrequent use is ≤ 2 d/wk) for quick relief of symptoms

3. Maintain normal (or near normal) lung function

4. Maintain normal activity levels: exercise and attendance at work and school

B. Reduce risk

1. Prevent recurrent exacerbations and minimize need for urgent care

2. Prevent progressive loss of lung function; for youth, prevent reduced lung growth

3. Provide optimal pharmacotherapy with minimal or no adverse effects

TABLE 46-1 Classifying Asthma Severity and Initiating Treatment in Adolescents ≥ 12 Years of Age and Adults

Components of Severity		Intermittent	Classifying of Asthma Severity		
			Persistent		
			Mild	**Moderate**	**Severe**
Impairment Normal FEV₁/FVC: 8–19 yr 85% 20–39 yr 80% 40–59 yr 75% 60–80 yr 70%	Symptoms	≤ 2 d/wk	≥ 2 d/wk but not daily	Daily	Throughout the day
	Nighttime awakenings	≤ 2 times per month	3–4 times per month	> 1 per week but not nightly	Often 7 times per week
	Short-acting β₂-agonist use for symptom control (not prevention of EIB)	≤ 2 d/wk	> 2 d/wk but not daily, and not more than one time on any day	Daily	Several times per day
	Interference with normal activity	None	Minor limitation	Some limitation	Extremely limited
	Lung function	Normal FEV₁ between exacerbations FEV₁ > 80% predicted FEV₁/FVC normal	FEV₁ > 80% predicted FEV₁/FVC normal	FEV₁ > 60% but < 80% predicted FEV₁/FVC reduced 5%	FEV₁ < 60% predicted FEV₁/FVC reduced > 5%
Risk	Exacerbations requiring oral systemic corticosteroids	0–1/yr (see note)	≥ 2/yr (see note) →		
		← Consider severity and interval since last exacerbation. → Frequency and severity may fluctuate over time for patients in any severity category. Relative annual risk of exacerbation may be related to FEV₁.			
Recommended step for initiating treatment		Step 1	Step 2	Step 3	Step 4 or 5
				and consider short course of oral systemic corticosteroids	
		In 2–6 weeks, evaluate level of asthma control that is achieved and adjust therapy accordingly.			

Abbreviations: EIB, exercise-induced bronchospasm; FEV₁, forced expiratory volume in 1 second; FVC, forced vital capacity. ICU, intensive care unit.

The stepwise approach is meant to assist, not replace, the clinical decision making required to meet individual patient needs.

Level of severity is determined by assessment of both impairment and risk. Assess impairment domain by patient's and caregiver's recall of previous 2–4 weeks and spirometry. Assign severity to the most severe category in which any feature occurs.

At present, there are inadequate data to correlate frequencies of exacerbations with different levels of asthma severity. In general, more frequent and intense exacerbations (e.g., requiring urgent, unscheduled care, hospitalization, or ICU admission) indicate greater underlying disease severity. For treatment purposes, patients who had ≥ 2 exacerbations requiring oral systemic corticosteroids in the past year may be considered the same as patients who have persistent asthma, even in the absence of impairment levels consistent with persistent asthma.

Reproduced from National Heart, Lung and Blood Institute, National Asthma Education and Prevention Program, & National Institutes of Health. (2007). *Expert panel report 3: Guidelines for the diagnosis and management of asthma* (Publication No. 08-5846). Bethesda, MD: Author.

V. Plan

A. Diagnostic tests

1. Pulmonary function testing (spirometry) (**Figure 46-1**): Spirometry, which measures airflow obstruction, is needed to diagnose asthma because medical history

and physical examination are not reliable ways to exclude other causes of respiratory impairment. The key measures are FEV₁, forced vital capacity (FVC), and FEV₁/FVC ratio. For those who cannot sustain expiration for the length of time necessary to measure FVC, FEV in 6 seconds is used as a substitute for FVC. Significant reversibility is demonstrated by an

TABLE 46-2 Assessing Asthma Control and Adjusting Therapy in Adolescents ≥ 12 Years of Age and Adults

		Classifying of Asthma Control		
		Well Controlled	Not Well Controlled	Very Poorly Controlled
Impairment	Symptoms	≤ 2 d/wk	> 2 d/wk	Throughout the day
	Nighttime awakenings	≤ 2 times per month	1–3 times per week	≥ 4 times per week
	Interference with normal activity	None	Some limitation	Extremely limited
	Short-acting β$_2$-agonist use for symptom control (not prevention of EIB)	≤ 2 d/wk	> 2 d/wk	Several times per day
	FEV$_1$ or peak flow	> 80% predicted/personal best	60–80% predicted/personal best	< 60% predicted/personal best
	Validated questionnaire	0	1–2	3–4
	ATAQ	≤ 0.75*	≥ 1.5	N/A
	ACQ	≥ 20	16–19	≤ 15
	ACT			
Risk	Exacerbations requiring oral systemic corticosteroids	0–1/yr	≥ 2/yr (see note) →	
		Consider severity and interval since last exacerbation		
	Progressive loss of lung function	Evaluation requires long-term follow-up care		
	Treatment-related adverse effects:	Medication side effects can vary in intensity from none to very troublesome and worrisome. The level of intensity does not correlate to specific levels of control but should be considered in the overall assessment of risk.		
Recommended action for treatment		Maintain current step. Regular follow-ups every 1–6 months to maintain control. Consider step down if well controlled for at least 3 months.	Step up 1 step and Reevaluate in 2–6 weeks. For side effects, consider alternative treatment options.	Consider short course of oral systemic corticosteroids. Step up 1–2 steps, and Reevaluate in 2 weeks. For side effects, consider alternative treatment options.

Abbreviations: EIB, exercise-induced bronchospasm; ICU, intensive care unit.

*ACQ values of 0.76–1.4 are indeterminate regarding well-controlled asthma.

The stepwise approach is meant to assist, not replace, the clinical decision making required to meet individual patient needs.

The level of control is based on the most severe impairment or risk category. Assess impairment domain by patient's recall of previous 2–4 weeks and by spirometry or peak flow measures. Symptom assessment for longer periods should reflect a global assessment, such as inquiring whether the patient's asthma is better or worse since the last visit.

At present, there are inadequate data to correspond frequencies of exacerbations with different levels of asthma control. In general, more frequent and intense exacerbations (e.g., requiring urgent unscheduled care, hospitalization, or ICU admission) indicate poorer disease control. For treatment purposes, patients who had ≥ 2 exacerbations requiring oral systemic corticosteroids in the past year may be considered the same as patients who have not-well-controlled asthma, even in the absence of impairment levels consistent with not-well-controlled asthma.

Validated questionnaires for the impairment domain (the questionnaires do not assess lung function or the risk domain).

ATAQ = Asthma Therapy Assessment Questionnaire® (see sample in "Component 1: Measures of Asthma Assessment and Monitoring").

ACQ = Asthma Control Questionnaire® (user package may be obtained at www.qoltech.co.uk or juniper@qoltech.co.uk).

ACT = Asthma Control Test™ (see sample in "Component 1: Measure of Asthma Assessment and Monitoring").

Minimal important difference: 1.0 for the ATAQ; 0.5 for the ACQ; not determined for the ACT.

Before step up in therapy:

Review adherence to medication, inhaler technique, environmental control, and comorbid conditions.

If an alternative treatment option was used in a step, discontinue and use preferred treatment for that step.

Reproduced from National Heart, Lung and Blood Institute, National Asthma Education and Prevention Program, & National Institutes of Health. (2007). *Expert panel report 3: Guidelines for the diagnosis and management of asthma* (Publication No. 08-5846). Bethesda, MD: Author.

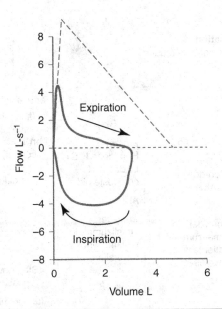

FIGURE 46-1 Flow-Volume Loop Generated by Spirometry

Reproduced from Pellegrino, R., Viegi, G., Brusasco, V., Crapo, R. O., Burgos, F., Casaburi, R., et al. (2005). Interpretive strategies for lung function tests. *European Respiratory Journal, 26*, 948–968. Reprinted with permission from the European Respiratory Society.

increase in FEV_1 or FVC of 200 mL and greater than or equal to 12% change from baseline after inhaling two puffs of albuterol at 90 mcg/puff (Pellegrino et al., 2005). Some patients with the symptoms of asthma do not demonstrate reversibility until they have a 2-week trial of oral corticosteroids.

2. Chest radiograph to exclude other causes of airway obstruction

3. Allergy testing by skin tests or in vitro tests

4. Exhaled nitrous oxide testing to detect inflammation

5. Additional pulmonary function tests that are not routinely necessary but can be useful when considering alternative diagnoses:

   a. Flow–volume loops to assess the presence of inspiratory airflow obstruction

   b. Bronchoprovocation challenge testing with methacholine or cold air may be helpful when asthma is suspected but spirometry is normal or near normal.

   c. Diffusing capacity to assess for emphysema

   d. Total lung volumes to assess for restrictive ventilatory defects.

B. Management

1. Medications: A stepwise approach to pharmacologic therapy is recommended (**Table 46-3**)

   a. Quick relief "rescue" medications are short-acting β_2-agonists. These include albuterol-HFA and levalbuterol-HFA, which are prescribed for any severity of asthma. Patients should be instructed to inhale two puffs every 4–6 hours as needed for symptoms of asthma. They also may be used 20–30 minutes before exercise to prevent exercise-induced bronchospasm.

   b. Long-acting "controller" medications

      i. ICS are the most effective to reduce airway inflammation and control persistent asthma. (See **Table 46-4** showing the estimated comparative daily doses for inhaled corticosteroids.) For patients who have had well-controlled asthma for at least 3 months, it is essential to step down therapy to identify the minimum medication necessary to maintain control.

      ii. Long-acting β_2-agonists (LABA) added if asthma is not controlled with ICS alone. Do not use LABA as monotherapy. Consider discontinuing LABA when control is achieved.

      iii. Consider combined ICS and LABA in one inhaler if asthma is not controlled by ICS alone.

      iv. When initiating therapy monitor at 2- to 4-week intervals to ensure that asthma control is achieved.

      v. Consider adding a leukotriene receptor antagonist (e.g., montelukast [sold as Singulair®] if allergies are a strong component of the asthma.

   c. Anti-IgE therapy: Omalizumab (Xolair®)

      i. Consider for adolescents older than 12 years and adults with severe uncontrolled asthma, skin or in vitro test positive to perennial allergens, and elevated IgE. Omalizumab is given subcutaneously under direct observation.

      ii. Be alert to the possibility of anaphylaxis which has been reported to occur up to 24 hours after giving this medication.

2. Environmental control

   a. Reduce exposure to allergens to which the patient is sensitized and exposed (dust mites, animal dander, mold, cockroach, and pollens).

Intermittent Asthma	Persistent Asthma: Daily Medication Consult with asthma specialist if step 4 care or higher is required. Consider consultation at step 3.

						Step 6 *Preferred:* High-dose ICS+ LABA+oral corticosteroid AND Consider Omalizumab for patients who have allergies	**Step up if needed** (first, check adherence, environmental control, and comorbid conditions)

Step 5
Preferred:
High-dose ICS
+LABA

AND

Consider
Omalizumab for
patients who
have allergies

Step 4
Preferred:
Medium-dose
ICS+LABA

Alternative:
Medium-dose
ICS+either
LTRA,
Theophylline,
or Zileuton

Step 3
Preferred:
Low-dose ICS+
LABA
OR
Medium-dose
ICS

Alternative:
Low-dose ICS+
either LTRA,
Theophylline,
or Zileuton

Step 2
Preferred:
Low-dose ICS

Alternative:
Cromolyn,
LTRA,
Nedocromil, or
Theophylline

Step 1
Preferred:
SABA PRN

Assess control

Step down if
possible

(and asthma is
well controlled at
least 3 months)

Each step: Patient education, environmental control, and management of comorbidities.

Steps 2-4: Consider subcutaneous allergen immunotherapy for patients who have allergic asthma (see notes).

Quick-relief medication for all patients

- SABA as needed for symptoms. Intensity of treatment depends on severity of symptoms: up to 3 treatments at 20-minute intervals as needed. Short course of oral systemic corticosteroids may be needed.

- Use of SABA >2 days a week for symptom relief (not prevention of EIB) generally indicates inadequate control and the need to step up treatment.

TABLE 46-3 Stepwise Approach for Managing Asthma in Adolescents ≥ 12 Years of Age and Adults

Key: **Alphabetical order is used when more than one treatment option is listed within either preferred or alternative therapy.** EIB, exercise-induced bronchospasm; ICS, inhaled corticosteroid; LABA, long-acting inhaled beta$_2$-agonist, LTRA, leukotriene receptor antagonist; SABA, inhaled short-acting beta$_2$-agonist.

Notes:

The stepwise approach is meant to assist, not replace, the clinical decision making required to meet individual patient needs.

If alternative treatment is used and response is inadequate, discontinue it and use the preferred treatment before stepping up.

Zileuton is a less desirable alternative due to limited studies as adjunctive therapy and the need to monitor liver function. Theophylline requires monitoring of serum concentration levels.

In step 6, before oral corticosteroids are introduced, a trial of high-dose ICS + LABA + either LTRA, theophylline, or zileuton may be considered, although this approach has not been studied in clinical trials.

Step 1, 2, and 3 preferred therapies are based on Evidence A; step 3 alternative therapy is based on Evidence A for LTRA, Evidence B for theophylline, and Evidence D for zileuton. Step 4 preferred therapy is based on Evidence B, and alternative therapy is based on Evidence B for LTRA and theophylline and Evidence D zileuton. Step 5 preferred therapy is based on Evidence B. Step 6 preferred therapy is based on Expert Panel Report 3 (EPR3; National Heart, Blood, and Lung Institute, 2007) and Evidence B for omalizumab.

Immunotherapy for steps 2–4 is based on Evidence B for house dust mites, animal dander, and pollens; evidence is weak or lacking for molds and cockroaches. Evidence is strongest for immunotherapy with single allergens. The role of allergy in asthma is greater in children than in adults.

Clinicians who administer immunotherapy or omalizumab should be prepared and equipped to identify and treat anaphylaxis that may occur.

Reproduced from National Heart, Lung and Blood Institute, National Asthma Education and Prevention Program, & National Institutes of Health. (2007). *Expert panel report 3: Guidelines for the diagnosis and management of asthma* (Publication No. 07-4051). Bethesda, MD: Author.

TABLE 46-4 Estimated Comparative Daily Doses: Ages 12 Years and Older

Medication Daily Dose	Low	Medium	High
Beclomethasone MDI	80 to 240 micrograms	more than 240 to 480 micrograms	more than 480 micrograms
40 micrograms per puff	1 to 3 puffs twice a day	4 to 6 puffs twice a day	
80 micrograms per puff	1 puff a.m., 2 puffs p.m.	2 to 3 puffs twice a day	4 or more puffs twice a day
Budesonide DPI	180 to 540 micrograms	more than 540 to 1,080 micrograms	more than 1,080 micrograms
90 micrograms per inhalation	1 to 3 inhalations twice a day		
180 micrograms per inhalation	1 inhalation a.m., 2 inhalations p.m.	2 to 3 inhalations twice a day	4 or more inhalations twice a day
Budesonide Nebules	not applicable	not applicable	not applicable
0.25 mg	not applicable	not applicable	not applicable
0.5 mg	not applicable	not applicable	not applicable
1.0 mg	not applicable	not applicable	not applicable
Ciclesonide MDI	160 to 320 micrograms	more than 320 to 640 micrograms	more than 640 micrograms
80 micrograms per puff	1 to 2 puffs twice a day	3 to 4 puffs twice a day	
160 micrograms per puff		2 puffs twice a day	3 or more puffs twice a day
Flunisolide MDI	320 micrograms	more than 320 to 640 micrograms	more than 640 micrograms
80 micrograms per puff	2 puffs twice a day	3 to 4 puffs twice a day	5 puffs or more twice a day
Fluticasone MDI	88 to 264 micrograms	more than 264 to 440 micrograms	more than 440 micrograms
44 micrograms per puff	1 to 3 puffs twice a day		
110 micrograms per puff		2 puffs twice a day	3 puffs twice a day
220 micrograms per puff		1 puff twice a day	2 or more puffs twice a day
Fluticasone DPI	100 to 300 micrograms	more than 300 to 500 micrograms	more than 500 micrograms
50 micrograms per inhalation	1 to 3 inhalations twice a day		
100 micrograms per inhalation		2 inhalations twice a day	3 or more inhalations twice a day
250 micrograms per inhalation		1 inhalations twice a day	2 or more inhalations twice a day
Mometasone DPI	110 to 220 micrograms	more than 220 to 440 micrograms	more than 440 micrograms
110 micrograms per inhalation	1 to 2 inhalations p.m.	3 to 4 inhalations p.m. or 2 inhalations twice a day	3 or more inhalations twice a day
220 micrograms per inhalation	1 inhalation p.m.	1 inhalation twice a day or 2 inhalations p.m.	3 or more inhalations divided in two doses

Reproduced from National Heart, Lung, and Blood Institute, & National Institutes of Health. (2012). *Asthma care quick reference: Diagnosing and managing asthma.* Retrieved from http://www.nhlbi.nih.gov/health-pro/guidelines/current/asthma-guidelines/quick-reference-html#estimated -comparative-daily-doses.

b. Effective allergen avoidance requires a multi-faceted, comprehensive approach (e.g., carpets harbor dust mites so remove or vacuum often; use allergen-proof mattress and pillow covers to protect against dust mites; wash all bed linens in hot water at least every 2 weeks; eliminate any cockroach infestation and do not leave food or garbage out or exposed; remove mold and mildew; and repair leaks).

c. Avoid exposure to environmental tobacco smoke and other respiratory irritants (wood smoke, perfume, strong odors and fumes, bleach, and cleaning products).

d. Avoid exertion outside when air pollution levels are high.

e. Avoid use of nonselective β-blockers.

f. Avoid sulfite-containing food and foods to which the patient is sensitive.

3. Treat and control comorbid diseases that aggravate asthma

a. Allergic rhinitis or sinusitis (consider leukotriene receptor antagonist, antihistamine, nasal corticosteroid spray, and nasal saline washes).

b. GERD: consider use of a proton pump inhibitor; elevate head of bed at night; no food at bedtime; and decrease use of alcohol and caffeine. See chapter on GERD for further suggestions.

c. Other conditions that make asthma harder to control include obesity, depression, family barriers to self-management, and vocal cord dysfunction.

4. Consider specialty consultation for uncontrolled asthma that has not responded to maximal therapy, when allergy immunotherapy or omalizumab is being considered, or when exacerbations require hospitalizations.

5. Follow-up should be at frequent intervals until control is achieved and then at 3- to 6-month intervals to maintain control. More frequent follow-up is determined by individual characteristics, past history, and psychosocial factors that increase risk.

C. *Patient education and training in self-management of asthma*

1. Elicit the patient's concerns and questions regarding asthma.

BOX 46-1 Instructions for Using a Metered-Dose Inhaler With or Without a Spacer

1. To begin, shake the inhaler five or six times.
2. Remove the mouthpiece cover. If using a spacer, place the spacer over the mouthpiece at the end of the inhaler.
3a. Use of a metered-dose inhaler without a spacer: Put your lips and teeth over the inhaler mouthpiece and breathe in slowly. As you do so, squeeze the top of the canister once. Keep inhaling even after you finish the squeeze. Continue inhaling slowly and deeply.
3b. Use of the metered-dose inhaler with a spacer: Put your lips and teeth over the mouthpiece. Squeeze the top of the canister once and then breathe in slowly. Keep inhaling even after you finish the squeeze. Continue inhaling slowly and deeply.
4. After inhaling, remove the inhaler or spacer from your mouth and hold your breath for up to 10 seconds.
5. Rinse your mouth after using the inhaler.

If you need another dose of medication, repeat the previous steps.

BOX 46-2 Patient Instructions for Using a Dry Powder Disk Inhaler

1. Hold the disk level in one hand. With the other hand, put your thumb in the appropriate notch and push it away from you as far as it goes. The mouthpiece will appear and snap into place.
2. Keep the disk horizontal. Again with your thumb, slide the lever away from you until it clicks. The disk is now ready to deliver medication. Breathe out all the way away from the mouthpiece prior to inhalation from the dry powder inhaler.
3. Put your lips around the mouthpiece. Breathe in quickly and deeply through your mouth—not your nose.
4. After inhaling, remove the disk from your mouth and hold your breath for up to 10 seconds.
5. To close the disk, put your thumb in the notch and slide it back toward you as far as it goes. The disk will click shut, and the lever will automatically return to its original position. The disk is now ready for your next dose.
6. Rinse your mouth after using the inhaler.

Ask your pharmacist for a demonstration when you pick up the medication from the pharmacy.

BOX 46-3 Instructions for Using a Dry Powder Tube Inhaler

Flexhaler®

1. To begin, hold the inhaler in the upright position and twist the cover off and set it down.
2. Next, load the dose of medication. Twist the base grip to the right as far as it will go. Twist it back to the left. You will hear a click, which means it is ready to go.
3. You do not need to shake the inhaler. Breathe out all the away from the mouthpiece prior to inhalation from the dry powder inhaler.
4. Bring the inhaler to your lips in a horizontal position. Put your lips over the tube and take a fast and powerful deep breath. Continue inhaling quickly and deeply.
5. Hold your breath for up to 10 seconds.
6. If you need another dose of medication, repeat the previous steps. The tube inhaler is designed to deliver one dose at a time.
7. Do not blow into your inhaler after loading a dose because the medication will become saturated with condensation and difficult to dispense.
8. When you are finished, place the cover back on the inhaler and twist shut. Keep your inhaler dry and store it at room temperature.
9. Rinse your mouth after using the inhaler.

Asthmanex Twisthaler®

1. To begin, hold the inhaler in the upright position and grip the white cap.
2. Turn the cap counter-clockwise while keeping the inhaler in an upright position, then lift off the cap. As the cap is lifted off, the dose counter counts down.
3. Breathe out all the way away from the inhaler.
4. Bring the inhaler to your lips in a horizontal position. Put your lips over the mouthpiece and take a fast and powerful deep breath. Continue inhaling quickly and deeply. Do not cover the ventilation hole while inhaling.
5. Remove the inhaler from your mouth and hold your breath for about 10 seconds.
6. Wipe the mouthpiece dry and put the cap back on. Turn the cap in a clockwise direction as you gently press down. You will hear a click to let you know the cap is fully closed.
7. Rinse your mouth after using the inhaler.

BOX 46-4 Patient Education Supplement: Peak Expiratory Flow Rate Monitoring

What is a peak expiratory flow rate?

Peak expiratory flow rate is a measurement of the highest speed at which you can blow out air when you exhale as hard and as fast as you can. This measurement tells us how much impediment, or obstruction, there is in your airways. Flow rates decrease when asthma obstructs, or narrows, your airways. Flow rates are normal when there is no, or minimal obstruction of your airways.

What are the steps to measuring a peak expiratory flow rate?

1. Place the indicator at the base of the numbered scale.
2. Stand up or sit up straight with head erect.
3. Take a deep breath.
4. Place the meter in your mouth and close your lips around the mouthpiece.
5. Blow out as hard and as fast as possible.
6. Write down the achieved measurement. This is where the indicator stops.
7. Repeat this process two more times.
8. Record the highest of the three measurements.

When and how often should you measure and record peak flow rates?

You and your provider will plan this during your visits.

Modified from National Heart, Lung, and Blood Institute, National Asthma Education and Prevention Program. (1997). Expert panel report 2: Guidelines for the diagnosis and management of asthma (NIH Publication No. 97-4051). Bethesda, MD: Author.

2. Describe airway inflammation and bronchospasm.
3. Teach the patient how to recognize and avoid individual triggers: explain the cumulative effect of precipitating factors.
4. Instruct the patient not to smoke and to avoid secondhand smoke.
5. Review all of the patient's medications, including the purpose, actions, dosage, side effects, and interactions. Explain how each medication works to relieve, control, or prevent asthma signs and symptoms.

6. Demonstrate the proper use of the metered-dose inhaler or dry powder inhaler and also spacer device for metered-dose, inhaler containing corticosteroid medication (**Boxes 46-1** through **46-3**). Have the patient demonstrate proper use periodically or at each follow-up visit.

7. For patients who meet the criteria for moderate-persistent or severe-persistent asthma, demonstrate the use and rationale of peak flow meters (for use at home or in the office) before the initiation of therapy. See the Patient Education Supplement: Peak Expiratory Flow Rate Monitoring (**Box 46-4**). Recommend daily morning measurements on awakening before inhaling medications. Teach the patient how to measure and interpret the peak flow rate readings (**Box 46-5**). Provide written guidelines for what the patient should do when the readings fall below a specified level.

8. Have a written action plan directing the patient what to do during an exacerbation. Include when the patient should call his or her provider, increase or add medications, or go to the emergency department (**Figure 46-2**).

9. Encourage adequate hydration, proper nutrition, and adequate rest.

10. Encourage the patient to keep regular appointments for follow-up and evaluation, even if the symptoms of asthma are not present.

Step 1, 2, and 3 preferred therapies are based on Evidence A; step 3 alternative therapy is based on Evidence A for LTRA, Evidence B for theophylline, and Evidence D for zileuton. Step 4 preferred therapy is based on Evidence B, and alternative therapy is based on Evidence B for LTRA and theophylline and Evidence D zileuton. Step 5 preferred therapy is based on Evidence B. Step 6 preferred therapy is based on EPR 2 (National Heart, Blood, and Lung Institute, 1997) and Evidence B for omalizumab.

Immunotherapy for steps 2–4 is based on Evidence B for house dust mites, animal danders, and pollens; evidence is weak or lacking for molds and cockroaches. Evidence is strongest for immunotherapy with single allergens. The role of allergy in asthma is greater in children than in adults.

Clinicians who administer immunotherapy or omalizumab should be prepared and equipped to identify and treat anaphylaxis that may occur.

Source: National Heart, Lung, and Blood Institute. (2007). *Expert panel report3: Guidelines for the diagnosis and management of asthma* (NIH Publication No. 07-4051). Bethesda, MD: Author.

D. Asthma education resources

1. American Academy of Allergy, Asthma, and Immunology: www.aaaai.org

2. American Lung Association: www.lung.org

3. Association of Asthma Educators: www.asthmaeducators.org

4. National Heart, Lung, and Blood Institute Information Center: www.nhlbi.nih.gov

5. U.S. Environmental Protection Agency: www.airnow.gov

VI. Future update topics in asthma

A. The National Heart, Lung, and Blood Advisory Council Asthma Expert Working Group

1. The National Heart, Lung, and Blood (NHLB) Advisory Council Asthma Expert Working Group recently released an assessment of potential areas for

---

> ### BOX 46-5 Instructions for Using a Peak Flow Meter
>
> The peak flow meter helps you to monitor your asthma by measuring the maximum airflow you can blow out of your lungs.
>
> Ask your clinician about where to set the color-coded indicators. They can help determine the status of your airflow.
>
> 1. To begin, hold the meter by the handgrip. Slide the measurement arrow to the bottom of the scale, next to the mouthpiece. (One device requires you to shake the arrow to the bottom of the device).
>
> 2. Raise the meter horizontally, inhale deeply from room air, then place your mouth over the mouthpiece and blow forcefully. Make sure your lips act as a seal over the mouthpiece so that no air escapes. Make sure your tongue is not in the mouthpiece.
>
> 3. The measurement arrow will slide up the scale. The number that it stops on is your peak flow reading.
>
> 4. Repeat the test two more times. Each time, remember to slide the measurement arrow back to its start position near the mouthpiece. Remember the highest reading of your three blows.
>
> 5. Record the highest reading, with the date and time. Your clinician will help determine a personalized scale to use with your meter, dependent on your age, height, and gender.

Asthma Action Plan

PROVIDER INSTRUCTIONS

At initial presentation, determine the level of asthma severity

- Level of severity is determined by both impairment and risk and is assigned to the most severe category in which any feature occurs.

At subsequent visits, assess control to adjust therapy

- Level of control is determined by both impairment and risk and is assigned to the most severe category in which any feature occurs.
- Address adherence to medication, inhaler technique, and environmental control measures.
- Sample patient self-assessment tools for asthma control can be found at
  http://www.asthmacontrol.com/index.html
  http://www.asthmacontrolcheck.com

Stepwise approach for managing asthma:

- Therapy is increased (stepped up) if necessary and decreased (stepped down) when possible as determined by the level of asthma severity or asthma control.

Asthma severity and asthma control include the domains of current impairment and future risk.

Impairment: frequency and intensity of symptoms and functional limitations the patient is currently experiencing or has recently experienced.

Risk: the likelihood of either asthma exacerbations, progressive decline in lung function (or, for children, reduced lung growth), or risk of adverse effects from medication.

ASTHMA MANAGEMENT RECOMMENDATIONS:

— Ensure that patient/family receive education about asthma and how to use spacers and other medication delivery devices.

— Assess asthma control at every visit by self-administered standardized test or verbal history.

— Perform spirometry at baseline and at least every 1 to 2 years for patients ≥ 5 years of age.

— Update or review the Asthma Action Plan every 6 to 12 months.

— Perform skin or blood allergy tests for all patients with persistent asthma.

— Encourage patient/family to continue follow-up with their clinician every 1 to 6 months even if asthma is well controlled.

— Refer patient to a specialist if:

- there are difficulties achieving or maintaining control OR
- step 4 care or higher is required (step 3 care or higher for children 0-4 years of age) OR
- immunotherapy or omalizumab is considered OR
- additional testing is indicated OR
- if the patient required 2 bursts of oral systemic corticosteroids in the past year or a hospitalization.

HOW TO USE THE ASTHMA ACTION PLAN:

Top copy (for patient):

- Enter specific medication information and review the instructions with the patient and/or family.
- Educate patient and/or family about factors that make asthma worse and the remediation steps on the back of this form.
- **Complete and sign the bottom of the form and give this copy of the form to the patient.**

Middle copy (for school, childcare, work, etc):

- Educate the parent/guardian on the need for their signature on the back of the form in order to authorize student self-carry and self-administration of asthma medications at school and also to authorize sharing student health information with school staff.
- **Provide this copy of the form to the school/childcare center/work/caretaker or other involved third party. (This copy may also be faxed to the school, etc.)**

Bottom copy (for chart):

- **File this copy in the patient's medical chart.**

FOR MORE INFORMATION:

To access the August 2007 full version of the NHLBI Guidelines for the Diagnosis and Treatment of Asthma (EPR-3) or the October 2007 Summary Report, visit **http://www.nhlbi.nih.gov/guidelines/asthma/index.htm**

©2008, Public Health Institute (RAMP)

FIGURE 46-2 Asthma Action Plan

FIGURE 46-2 Asthma Action Plan *(Continued)*

Key: Alphabetical order is used when more than one treatment option is listed within either preferred or alternative therapy. EIB, exercise-induced bronchospasm; ICS, inhaled corticosteroid; LABA, long-acting inhaled beta$_2$-agonist, LTRA, leukotriene receptor antagonist; SABA, inhaled short-acting beta$_2$-agonist.

Notes:

The stepwise approach is meant to assist, not replace, the clinical decision making required to meet individual patient needs.

If alternative treatment is used and response is inadequate, discontinue it and use the preferred treatment before stepping up.

Zileuton is a less desirable alternative due to limited studies as adjunctive therapy and the need to monitor liver function. Theophylline requires monitoring of serum concentration levels.

In step 6, before oral corticosteroids are introduced, a trial of high-dose ICS + LABA + either LTRA, theophylline, or zileuton may be considered, although this approach has not been studied in clinical trials.

Reproduced from National Heart, Lung and Blood Institute, National Asthma Education and Prevention Program, & National Institutes of Health. (2007). Expert panel report 3: Guidelines for the diagnosis and management of asthma (NIH Publication No. 08-5846). Bethesda, MD: Author.

potential update in the Guidelines of the Diagnosis and Management of Asthma (NHLB Advisory Council Asthma Expert Working Group, 2015). These five topics have the highest priority for new systematic literature review and potential update of the guidelines in the future:

a. Role of adjustable medication dosing in recurrent wheezing and asthma

b. Role of long-acting antimuscarinic agents (LAMAs) in asthma management as add-on to inhaled corticosteroids

c. Role of bronchial thermoplasty in adult severe asthma

d. Role of fractional exhaled nitric oxide (FeNO) in diagnosis, medication selection, and monitoring treatment response in asthma

e. Role of remediation of indoor allergens (house dust mites/pets) in asthma management

REFERENCES

Brooks, C., Pearce, N., & Douwes, J. (2013). The hygiene hypothesis in allergy and asthma: An update. *Current Opinion Allergy Clinical Immunology, 13*(1), 70–77.

Busse, W. W., & Lemanske, R. F., Jr. (2001). Asthma. *New England Journal of Medicine, 344*(5), 350–362.

Centers for Disease Control and Prevention. (2011). Asthma in the U.S. *Vital Signs.* Retrieved from www.cdc.gov/VitalSigns/Asthma/index .html.

Kamble, S., &. Bharmal, M. (2009). Incremental direct expenditure of treating asthma in the United States. *Journal of Asthma, 46*(1), 73–80.

National Heart, Lung, and Blood Advisory Council Asthma Expert Working Group. (2015). *Needs assessment for potential update of the Expert Panel Report-3 (2007): Guidelines for the diagnosis and management of asthma.* Retrieved from www.nhlbi.nih.gov/sites/www.nhlbi.nih.gov/files /Asthma-Needs-Assessment-Report.pdf.

National Heart, Lung, and Blood Institute. (2012). Estimated comparative daily doses: Inhaled corticosteroids for long–term asthma control. In *Asthma care quick reference: Diagnosing and managing asthma guidelines from the National Asthma Education and Prevention Program: Expert Panel Report 3.* Retrieved from www .nhlbi.nih.gov/health-pro/guidelines/current/asthma-guidelines /quick-reference-html#estimated-comparative-daily-doses.

National Heart, Lung, and Blood Institute. (1997). *Expert panel report 2: Guidelines for the diagnosis and management of asthma* (Publication No. 97-4051). Bethesda, MD: Author.

National Heart, Blood, and Lung Institute. (2007). *Expert panel report 3: Guidelines for the diagnosis and management of asthma* (Publication No. 07-4051). Bethesda, MD: Author.

Pellegrino, R., Viegi, G., Brusasco, V., Crapo, R. O., Burgos, F., Casaburi, R., et al. (2005). Interpretative strategies for lung function tests. *European Respiratory Journal, 26*, 948–968.

Sullivan, S. D., Rasouliyan, L., Russo, P. A., Kamath, T., Chipps, B. E., & TENOR Study Group (2007). Extent, patterns, and burden of uncontrolled disease in severe or difficult-to-treat asthma. *Allergy, 62,* 126–133.

World Health Organization. (2007). Global surveillance, prevention and control of chronic respiratory diseases: A comprehensive approach. Retrieved from www.who.int/gard/publications/GARD%20Book%20 2007.pdf.

BENIGN PROSTATIC HYPERPLASIA

Jean N. Taylor-Woodbury

CHAPTER 47

I. Introduction and general background

The prostate is a muscular gland roughly triangular in shape and located in the lower abdomen between a man's bladder and rectum. According to some anatomic descriptions it has a median lobe and two lateral lobes and physically surrounds the neck of the bladder and the urethra (Venes, 2013). Other sources, such as the classification system of Lowsley, attribute five lobes to the prostate: (1) anterior, (2) posterior, (3) media, (4) right lateral, and (5) left lateral (Tanagho & Lue, 2013). Partly muscular and partly glandular, the prostate has ducts opening into the prostatic portion of the urethra. Normally the prostate is roughly 2 × 4 × 3 cm and weighs approximately 20 g; it is enclosed in a fibrous capsule containing smooth muscle fibers in its inner layer. Muscle fibers also separate the glandular tissue and encircle the urethra. The gland secretes a thin, opalescent, slightly alkaline fluid that forms part of the seminal fluid (Venes, 2013). The gland is responsible for secreting liquid that then mixes with additional fluids secreted by the seminal vesicles and with the sperm produced by the testicles.

A. Benign prostatic hyperplasia

1. Definition and overview

   Benign prostatic hyperplasia (BPH) is generally considered to be a progressive disease and is considered to be the most common benign tumor in men (Meng, Walsh, & Chi, 2014). The etiology of BPH is not known, but it is believed to be multifactorial with testicular androgens being the most probable controlling factor for the prostatic enlargement (Barry, 2009; Meng et al., 2014).

   Hyperplasia of the prostate occurs in a nodular pattern, increasing the cell numbers and occurring in varying amounts in the stroma or epithelium and glandular tissue of the prostate (Barry, 2009; Meng et al., 2014). The hyperplasia begins in the area around the urethra and gradually increases in nodules

over a period of years. As BPH progresses, the affected individual may or may not develop lower urinary tract symptoms (LUTS), which may include urinary frequency, hesitancy, urgency, nocturia, decreased force of stream, intermittent stream, incomplete bladder emptying, and incontinence or dribbling.

Prostatic enlargement may cause obstruction of the bladder outlet and compression of the urethra. If this occurs, compromised urinary flow and deterioration of the upper urinary tract and renal failure can result (Emberton et al., 2008).

Does BPH increase the risk for development of prostatic carcinoma? Most current clinical research suggests that although BPH may not result in prostatic carcinoma, pathologic changes that are associated with BPH may be associated with prostatic carcinoma (Bushman, 2009). An extensive study by Negri et al. (2005) concluded that the development of BPH seemed to be increased in those with a family history of bladder cancer but not with those having a family history of prostatic carcinoma. Some studies have indicated an association between chronic inflammation and both BPH and prostatic carcinoma (Abdel-Meguid, Mosli, & Al-Maghrabi, 2009) and have found that prostatic cancer develops in 83% of prostate glands where BPH is also found (Bostwick et al., 1992). A study conducted by Hammarsten and Högstedt (2002) suggests that fast-growing BPH is a factor that increases the risk of developing clinical prostate cancer. The authors note that these findings support the hypothesis of an association between the development of BPH and clinical prostate cancer. The association between BPH and prostate cancer is complicated and controversial. To date, no clear-cut answers exist as to the actual association and risk.

2. Prevalence and incidence

   BPH is very common, beginning around age 45 with development of accompanying symptoms by the age of 65 in whites and 60 in blacks (Longo et al., 2014).

It affects up to 80% of men 80 years or older (Barnard & Aronson, 2009). Not all men, however, who have histologic BPH are symptomatic with lower urinary tract symptoms (LUTS). Twenty-five percent of men age 55 and 50% age 75 report signs and symptoms (Meng et al., 2014). Up to 80% of men 80 years of age and older report being affected by BPH (Barnard & Aronson, 2009).

It is difficult to predict who will develop BPH because the risk factors are poorly understood, although some studies have indicated racial differences and some have indicated a genetic link. Age is considered a correlate to likelihood of BPH and its progression. For those who progress early, findings have suggested that approximately half of all men younger than age 60 who require surgical intervention for BPH may have an inherited form of BPH that is an autosomal-dominant trait. According to Meng, Walsh, and Chi (2014), the first-degree male relatives of those with the heritable form of BPH have a fourfold increased relative risk of developing BPH.

More recent studies have also indicated that diabetes and obesity increase the risk of BPH and BPH symptom progression, whereas exercise and moderate alcohol consumption seem to decrease the risk of BPH and BPH progression (Parsons, 2007; Platz et al., 1998; Sea, Poon, & McVary, 2009).

II. Database (may include but is not limited to)

A. Subjective

1. BPH
   a. Current symptoms and severity: The American Urological Association (McVary et al., 2010) offers effective tools for screening symptoms and severity (**Appendices 47-1** and **47-2**).
   b. Past health history
      i. Medical illnesses: any prostatic disease, renal disease, renal infection, or renal calculi; and any bladder disease, dysfunction, or recurrent infections.
      ii. Sexual history to include practices and any history of infection.
      iii. History of diabetes mellitus and obesity.
      iv. History of physical trauma to the bladder or the urethra.
      v. History of neurologic disease or injury.
      vi. Any history of cancer.
      vii. Surgical history: bladder surgery, urethral surgery, or penile surgery.
      viii. Trauma history: brain trauma including infarct or hemorrhagic stroke; trauma to bladder, urethra, or penis
      ix. Exposure history: any prior chemical or radioactive exposures to the lower genito-urinary tract or perineal area.
      x. Medication history: medications and supplements that may affect urinary flow or retention (e.g., antihistamine and decongestant use). Note any history of use of medications or supplements for treatment of existing or prior genitourinary disorders or disease or prostatic disease.
      xi. A history of eye disease or cataracts should also be evaluated. Boehringer Ingelheim and the Food and Drug Administration notified healthcare professionals of revisions to the precautions and adverse reactions sections of the prescribing information for tamsulosin (Flomax®), indicated for the treatment of the signs and symptoms of BPH. A surgical condition termed "intraoperative floppy iris syndrome" (IFIS) has been observed during phacoemulsification cataract surgery in some patients treated with α_1 blockers including Flomax®. Most of these reports were in patients taking the α_1 blocker when IFIS occurred, but in some cases the α_1 blocker had been stopped before surgery. It is recommended that male patients being considered for cataract surgery, as part of their medical history, be specifically questioned to ascertain whether they have taken Flomax® or other α_1 blockers. If so, the patient's ophthalmologist should be prepared for possible modifications to their surgical technique that may be warranted should IFIS be observed during the procedure (U.S. Food and Drug Administration, 2005).
   c. Family history
      i. Prostatic disease, particularly in first-degree relatives, includes age of onset of disease
      ii. Diabetes
      iii. Neurologic disorders
      iv. Cancer
   d. Occupational and environmental history
      i. Work-related exposures, such as chemical or radiation exposures
      ii. Degree of access to appropriate facilities for voiding
   e. Personal and social history
      i. Recreational drug use, including methamphetamines, and tobacco
      ii. Dietary intake and caffeine

f. Review of systems

   i. Abdomen: suprapubic pain (suggestive of acute urinary retention) and flank pain.

   ii. Genitourinary: urethral discharge; dysuria; irritative symptoms (urgency, frequency, or nocturia); or obstructive symptoms (hesitancy, decreased or intermittent stream flow, sensation of incomplete void, and dribbling incontinence).

   iii. Neurologic: focal neurologic findings suggestive of neurologic etiology of the presenting urinary symptoms, such as lower extremity weakness or radiculopathic or neuropathic symptoms (e.g., saddle anesthesia).

B. Objective

1. Physical examination findings

   a. An abdominal examination may demonstrate a palpable, distended bladder, which may be asymptomatic if LUTS are otherwise mild or absent.

   b. Absence of costovertebral angle pain

   c. Absence of urethral discharge or other genital findings suggestive of infection or sexually transmitted infection as a source of the LUTS

   d. A digital rectal examination should be done and may reveal an enlarged prostate, which may be focal or diffuse. However, the size of the prostate correlates poorly with either the symptoms or the signs of BPH.

   e. A focused neurologic examination should be accomplished to rule out a neurogenic bladder.

2. Supporting data from relevant diagnostic tests

   a. Urinalysis by either dipstick or microscopic examination to evaluate for hematuria or urinary tract infection.

   b. Measurement of the serum prostate-specific antigen (PSA) should be considered for those patients with at least a 10-year life expectancy and for whom the knowledge of prostate cancer would change symptom or disease management and for those whose PSA level might change the management of their LUTS (McVary et al., 2010).

III. Assessment

A. Determine the diagnosis

1. BPH

2. Prostatitis

3. Prostatic neoplasms (benign or malignant)

4. Other conditions that may explain the patient's presentation

   a. Diabetes mellitus

   b. Urethral stricture

   c. Bladder neck contracture

   d. Bladder stone

   e. Neurogenic bladder

B. Assess the severity of the disease

1. The American Urological Association's Symptom Index for Benign Prostatic Hyperplasia and the Disease Specific Quality of Life Question (Appendices 47-1 and 47-2) are helpful tools for assessing the severity of the condition.

C. Assess the significance of the problem to the patient and significant others

IV. Goals of clinical management

A. Choose a cost-effective approach for screening or diagnosing BPH

B. Select a treatment plan that returns the client to a symptom-free state in a safe and effective manner

C. Select an approach that maximizes client adherence

V. Plan

A. Screening

1. There are no screening tests for BPH. Examination is usually done in response to complaints of symptoms, although prostatic hyperplasia may be detected during a routine digital rectal examination.

B. Diagnostic tests (see **Box 47-1** for a description of relevant diagnostic studies and **Figure 47-1** for the suggested approach for BPH diagnosis and treatment)

C. Management (includes treatment, consultation, referral, and follow-up care)

1. If symptoms are mild (American Urological Association Symptom Scale of less than or equal to 7 or no bothersome symptoms), then watchful waiting is indicated.

2. If symptoms are moderate to severe, then discuss treatment options with the patient.

BOX 47-1 Description of Relevant Diagnostic Studies

Common prostate studies may include, but are not limited to the following:

1. Urinalysis (may be done by dipstick testing or microanalysis). According to the American Urological Association, routinely measuring the serum creatinine levels in the initial assessment of men with lower urinary tract symptoms is not indicated (McVary et al., revised 2010).

2. The U.S. Preventive Services Task Force (USPSTF) recommends against routine prostate cancer and prostate-specific antigen screening, citing that risk of harm outweighs the benefits of screening. However, the American Urological Association continues to recommend digital rectal exam and PSA screening in asymptomatic males aged 40 years and older with a life expectancy of more than 10 years. Other agencies, such as the American Cancer Society and the American College of Preventive Medicine recommend education-based informed decision making regarding the risks and benefits of screening men 50 years or older (USPSTF, 2012).

3. Urine cytology may be considered if there is a predominance of irritative (versus obstructive) symptoms and if the patient has a history of smoking or other significant risk factors for bladder carcinoma.

4. Optional tests for men with moderate to severe urinary symptoms include test of postvoid residual and urinary flow. If there is significant postvoid residual volume, transabdominal kidney ultrasound or intravenous urography by radiograph may be helpful in evaluating for hydronephrosis (American College of Radiology, 1995, revised 2014).

Data from American College of Radiology. (1995, last reviewed 2014). *ACR appropriateness criteria®: Lower urinary tract symptoms: Suspicion of benign prostatic hyperplasia.* Retrieved from https://acsearch.acr.org/docs/69368/Narrative/.; McVary, K. T., Roehrborn, C. G., Avins, A. L., Barry, M. J., Bruskewitz, R., Donnell, R. F., et al. (2010). *Management of benign prostatic hyperplasia (BPH)* (rev. ed.). Baltimore, MD: American Urological Association Education and Research, Inc.

---

guideline for the management of BPH [McVary, et al., 2010], there is insufficient evidence to support the use of either phenoxybenzamine or prazosin for the treatment of LUTS with BPH)

   c. Alfuzosin, 10 mg orally daily

   d. Doxazosin, 1–8 mg orally daily

   e. Tamsulosin, 0.4 or 0.8 mg orally daily

   f. Terazosin, 1–10 mg orally daily

   g. Silodosin, 8 mg orally daily

   h. In using α-blockers, a gradual upward titration is recommended to minimize the risk of orthostatic hypotension that may occur with the use of this class of medications

   i. 5α-Reductase inhibitors (used for individuals with prostates > 40 mL by ultrasonographic examination) (Meng et al., 2014)

      i. Dutasteride, 0.5 mg orally daily

      ii. Finasteride, 5 mg orally daily

      iii. Combination therapy: α-blocker and 5α-reductase inhibitor

   j. Dietary supplements

      i. Based on expert panel recommendations, and noted in the American Urological Association guideline for the management of benign prostatic hyperplasia (McVary et al., 2010), phytotherapeutics and other dietary supplements—e.g., saw palmetto (*Serenoa repens*), African prune tree (*Pygeum africanum*), and rye pollen (*Secale cereale*)—are not currently recommended for the treatment of LUTS with BPH (Barry et al., 2011; Dedhia & McVary, 2008; Dreikorn, 2002).

   k. If the patient desires invasive therapy, refer to the urology service.

      i. The specialist may consider additional optional diagnostic tests, such as pressure flow, urethrocystoscopy, or prostate ultrasound.

      ii. Minimally invasive surgical options include transurethral laser-induced prostatectomy, transurethral needle ablation of the prostate, transurethral electrovaporization of the prostate, and hyperthermia.

      iii. Conventional surgical therapy includes transurethral resection of the prostate, transurethral incision of the prostate, and open simple prostatectomy.

3. If patient chooses noninvasive therapy, may choose watchful waiting or the following medical therapy.

   a. Phenoxybenzamine, 5–10 mg orally twice daily

   b. Prazosin, 1–5 mg orally twice daily (according to the current American Urological Association

4. Adverse effects of treatment

Regardless of treatment approach, patient education around both desired and the potential for undesired or adverse effects of the treatment should be thorough. The adverse effects depend on the treatment

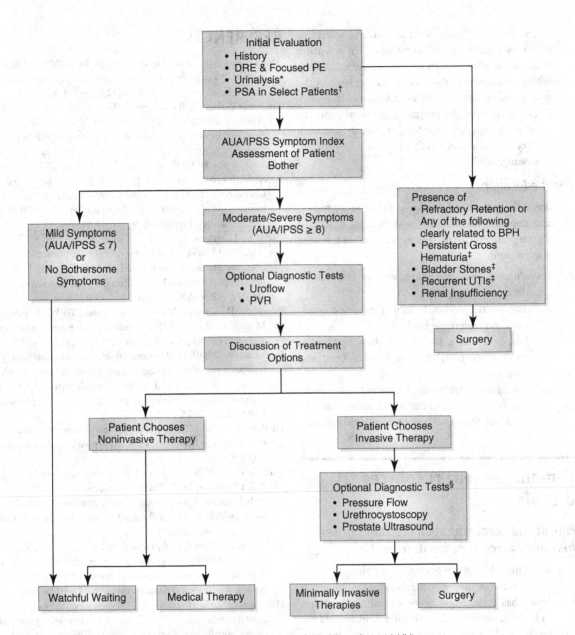

*In patients with clinically significant prostatic bleeding, a course of a 5 alpha-reductase inhibitor
 may be used. If bleeding persists, tissue ablative surgery is indicated.
†Patients with at least a 10-year life expectancy for whom knowledge of the presence of prostate
 cancer would change management or patients for whom the PSA measurement may change the
 management of voiding symptoms.
‡After exhausting other therapeutic options as discussed in detail in the text.
§Some diagnostic tests are used in predicting response to therapy. Pressure-flow studies are
 most useful in men prior to surgery.
AUA, American Urological Association; DRE, digital rectal exam; IPSS, International Prostate
Symptom Score; PE, physical exam; PSA, prostate-specific antigen; PVR, postvoid residual urine;
UTI, urinary tract infection.

FIGURE 47-1 Benign Prostatic Hyperplasia (BPH) Diagnosis and Treatment

Reproduced from McVary, K. T., Roehrborn, C. G., Avins, A. L., Barry, M. J., Bruskewitz, R.C., Donnell, R. F., et al.
(2010). *American Urological Association: Management of benign prostatic hyperplasia (BPH)* (rev. ed.). Baltimore,
MD: American Urological Association Education and Research, Inc.

course and may range from no adverse effects to either asymptomatic or symptomatic hypotension with the use of α-blockers to more severe side effects with surgical intervention. For example, beyond the risk of immediate surgical complications, transurethral resection of the prostate has the potential to result in retrograde ejaculation, erectile dysfunction, urinary incontinence, inability to void, and infection (DuBeau, 2009).

D. Client education

1. Assist the patient and significant others in expressing and coping with concerns and feelings related to the respective prostate disease process and disease management.

2. Provide oral and, preferably, written information regarding:

   a. The disease process, including signs and symptoms and underlying etiologies.

   b. Diagnostic tests, including a discussion about preparation, cost, the actual procedures, and aftercare.

   c. Management (rationale, action, use, side effects, and cost of therapeutic interventions; and the need for adhering to long-term treatment plans).

VI. Self-management resources and tools

A. Patient and client education brochures or frequently asked question documents:

1. The National Institutes of Health's website (www.nlm.nih.gov/medlineplus/prostatediseases .html) has patient and client education brochures and frequently asked question documents in English and Spanish. The documents include visual resources and include a link to a number of other resources, including to the American Urological Association Foundation Urology Care Foundation website (www.urologyhealth.org).

2. The Merck Medicus Resource Library (Merck Sharp & Dohme Corp., now called univadis, 2001–2014) provides a range of patient information and patient teaching resources for BPH, which include a high-quality interactive 3-D human atlas. For more information go to www.merckmedicus.com/.

3. Johns Hopkins Medical School offers a Health Alerts electronic subscription service for BPH, which provides regular updates on BPH and treatments.

REFERENCES

Abdel-Meguid, T., Mosli, H., & Al-Maghrabi, J. (2009). Prostate inflammation. Association with benign prostatic hyperplasia and prostate cancer. *Saudi Medical Journal, 30*(12), 1563–1567.

American College of Radiology. (1995, last reviewed 2014). *ACR appropriateness criteria®: Lower urinary tract symptoms: Suspicion of BPH.* Retrieved from https://acsearch.acr.org/docs/69368/Narrative/.

Barnard, R. J., & Aronson, W. J. (2009). Benign prostatic hyperplasia: Does lifestyle play a role? *Physician and Sportsmedicine, 37*(4), 141–146.

Barry, M. J. (2009). Approach to benign prostatic hyperplasia. In A. H. Goroll & A. G. Mulley, *Primary care medicine: Office evaluation and management of the adult patient* (6th ed.) (pp. 974–979). Philadelphia: Wolters Kluwer/Lippincott, Williams & Wilkins.

Barry, M. J., Meleth, S., Lee, J. Y., Kreder, K. J., Avins, A. L., Nickel, J. C., et al. (2011). Effect of increasing doses of saw palmetto on lower urinary tract symptoms: A randomized trial. *JAMA, 306*(12), 1344–1351. doi:10.1001/jama.2011.1364 Retrieved from www.ncbi.nlm.nih.gov /pmc/articles/PMC3326341/.

Bostwick, D., Cooner, W., Denis, L., Jones, G. W., Scardino, P. T., & Murphy, G. P. (1992). The association of benign prostatic hyperplasia and cancer of the prostate. *Cancer, 70*(Suppl. 1), 291–301.

Bushman, W. (2009). Etiology, epidemiology, and natural history of benign prostatic hyperplasia. *Urologic Clinics of North America, 36*(4), 403–415.

Dedhia, R. C., & McVary, K. T. (2008). Phytotherapy for lower urinary tract symptoms secondary to benign prostatic hyperplasia. *Journal of Urology, 179*(6), 2119–2125.

Dreikorn, K. (2002). The role of phytotherapy in treating lower urinary tract symptoms and benign prostatic hyperplasia. *World Journal of Urology, 19*(6), 426–435.

DuBeau, C. E. (2009). Chapter 50. Benign prostate disorders. In J. B. Halter, J. G. Ouslander, M. E. Tinetti, S. Studenski, K. P. High, & S. Asthana (Eds.), *Hazzard's geriatric medicine and gerontology* (6th ed.). New York: McGraw-Hill. Retrieved from http://accessmedicine.mhmedical.com /book.aspx?bookID=371.

Emberton, M., Cornel, E. B., Bassi, P. F., Fourcade, R. O., Gómez, J. M., & Castro, R. (2008). Benign prostatic hyperplasia as a progressive disease: A guide to the risk factors and options for medical management. *International Journal of Clinical Practice, 62*(7), 1076–1086.

Hammarsten, J., & Högstedt, B. (2002). Calculated fast-growing benign prostatic hyperplasia—a risk factor for developing clinical prostate cancer. *Scandinavian Journal of Urology and Nephrology, 36*(5), 330–338.

Longo, D. L., Fauci, A. S., Kasper, D. L., Hauser, S. L., Jameson, J., & Loscalzo, J. (2014). Urinary tract obstruction. In D. L. Longo, A. S. Fauci, D. L. Kasper, S. L. Hauser, J. Jameson, & J. Loscalzo (Eds.), *Harrison's Manual of Medicine* (18th ed.). New York: McGraw-Hill. Retrieved from http://accessmedicine.mhmedical.com/book .aspx?bookID=1140.

McVary, K. T., Roehrborn, C. G., Avins, A. L., Barry, M. J., Bruskewitz, R. C., Donnell, R. F., et al. (2010). *Management of benign prostatic hyperplasia (BPH)* (rev. ed.). Baltimore, MD: American Urological Association Education and Research, Inc. Retrieved from https://www.auanet.org /education/guidelines/benign-prostatic-hyperplasia.cfm.

Meng, M. V., Walsh, T. J., & Chi, T. D. (2014). Urologic disorders. In M. A. Papadakis, S. J. McPhee, & M. W. Rabow (Eds.), *Current medical diagnosis & treatment 2015.* Retrieved from http://accessmedicine .mhmedical.com/book.aspx?bookID=1019.

Negri, E., Pelucchi, C., Talamini, R., Montella, M., Gallus, S., Bosetti, C., et al. (2005). Family history of cancer and the risk of prostate cancer and benign prostatic hyperplasia. *International Journal of Cancer, 114*(4), 648–652.

Parsons, J. (2007). Modifiable risk factors for benign prostatic hyperplasia and lower urinary tract symptoms: New approaches to old problems. *Journal of Urology, 178,* 395–401.

Platz, E., Kawachi, I., Rimm, E., Colditz, G., Stampfer, M., Willett, W., et al. (1998). Physical activity and benign prostatic hyperplasia. *Archives of Internal Medicine, 158*(21), 2349–2356.

Sea, J., Poon, K., & McVary, K. (2009). Review of exercise and the risk of benign prostatic hyperplasia. *Physician and Sportsmedicine, 37*(4), 75–83.

Tanagho, E. A., & Lue, T. F. (2013). Chapter 1. Anatomy of the genitourinary tract. In J. W. McAninch & T. F. Lue (Eds.), *Smith and Tanagho's general urology* (18th ed.). New York: McGraw-Hill. Retrieved from http://accessmedicine.mhmedical.com/book.aspx?bookID=508.

U.S. Food and Drug Administration. (2005). *Tamsulosin: Safety warning /recommendation statement.* Retrieved from www.fda.gov/Safety /MedWatch/SafetyInformation/SafetyAlertsforHumanMedicalProducts /ucm151211.htm.

U.S. Preventive Services Task Force. (2012). *Final recommendation statement: Prostate cancer: Screening, May 2012.* Retrieved from http://www .uspreventiveservicestaskforce.org/Page/Document/Recommendation StatementFinal/prostate-cancer-screening#recommendations-of-others.

Venes, D. (Ed.). (2013). *Taber's cyclopedic medical dictionary* (22nd ed.). Philadelphia, PA: F.A. Davis Company.

APPENDIX 47-1:
THE AMERICAN UROLOGICAL ASSOCIATION (AUA) SYMPTOM INDEX FOR BENIGN PROSTATIC HYPERPLASIA (BPH) AND THE DISEASE SPECIFIC QUALITY OF LIFE QUESTION

Patient Name: _____   Date of birth: _____   Date completed _____

	Not at All	Less than 1 in 5 Times	Less than Half the Time	About Half the Time	More than Half the Time	Almost Always	Your Score
1. Over the past month, how often have you had a sensation of not emptying your bladder completely after you finished urinating?	0	1	2	3	4	5	
2. Over the past month, how often have you had to urinate again less than 2 hours after you finished urinating?	0	1	2	3	4	5	
3. Over the past month, how often have you stopped and started again several times when you urinated?	0	1	2	3	4	5	
4. Over the past month, how often have you found it difficult to postpone urination?	0	1	2	3	4	5	
5. Over the past month, how often have you had a weak urinary stream?	0	1	2	3	4	5	
6. Over the past month, how often have you had to push or strain to begin urination?	0	1	2	3	4	5	
	None	1 Time	2 Times	3 Times	4 Times	5 or More	
7. Over the past month, how many times did you most typically get up to urinate from the time you went to bed at night until the time you got up in the morning?	0	1	2	3	4	5+	

Total Symptom Score

Score: 1–7: *Mild* 8–19: *Moderate* 20–35: *Severe*

The possible total runs from 0 to 35 points with higher scores indicating more severe symptoms. Scores less than seven are considered mild and generally do not warrant treatment.

The International Prostate Symptom Score uses the same seven questions as the AUA Symptom Index (presented here) with the addition of the following Disease Specific Quality of Life Question (bother score) scored on a scale from 0 to 6 points (delighted to terrible): "If you were to spend the rest of your life with your urinary condition just the way it is now, how would you feel about that?"

Reproduced from McVary, K. T., Roehrborn, C. G., Avins, A. L., Barry, M. J., Bruskewitz, R. C., Donnell, R. F., et al. (2010). *Management of benign prostatic hyperplasia (BPH)* (rev. ed.). Baltimore, MD: American Urological Association Education and Research, Inc.

APPENDIX 47-2:
BENIGN PROSTATIC HYPERPLASIA (BPH) IMPACT INDEX ("BOTHER" SCORE)

Patient Name: _____	DOB: _____ ID: _____ Date of assessment _____
Initial Assessment ❑ Monitor during: _____	Therapy ❑ after: _____ Therapy/surgery ❑ _____

	BPH Impact Index
1. Over the past month how much physical discomfort did any urinary problems cause you?	None ❑ Only a little ❑ Some ❑ A lot ❑
2. Over the past month, how much did you worry about your health because of any urinary problems?	None ❑ Only a little ❑ Some ❑ A lot ❑
3. Overall, how bothersome has any trouble with urination been during the past month?	Not at all bothersome ❑ Bothers me some ❑ Bothers me a little ❑ Bothers me a lot ❑
4. Over the past month, how much of the time has any urinary problem kept you from doing the kind of things you would usually do?	None of the time ❑ Most of the time ❑ A little of the time ❑ All of the time ❑ Some of the time ❑
	Total Score: (Scoring based on 0-4 point scale)

Reproduced from McVary, K. T., Roehrborn, C. G., Avins, A. L., Barr, M. J., Bruskewitz, R. C., Donnell, R. F., et al. (2010). *Management of benign prostatic hyperplasia (BPH)* (rev. ed.). American Urological Association Education and Research, Inc.

CANCER SURVIVORSHIP IN ADULT PRIMARY CARE

Tara D. Lacey and Sheila N. Lindsay

I. Introduction and background

A. Definition and overview

There are an estimated 14.5 million cancer survivors currently living in the United States, and that number is expected to increase by 31% to approximately 19 million by 2024 (American Cancer Society [ACS], 2014). This represents an increase of more than 4 million cancer survivors over 10 years (DeSantis et al., 2014).

The concept of "cancer survivorship" is relatively young, dating back to a 1985 *New England Journal of Medicine* article by Fitzhugh Mullan, a physician and cancer survivor, in which he wrote, "The challenge in overcoming cancer is not only to find therapies that will prevent or arrest the disease quickly, but also to map the middle ground of survivorship and minimize its medical and social hazards" (Mullan, 1985, p. 273). In 1986 the National Coalition for Cancer Survivorship (NCCS) formalized the first definition of the term and laid the foundation for the current definition developed by the National Cancer Institute (NCI). The definition states that the term survivor applies to "an individual from the time of diagnosis, through the balance of his or her life. Family members, friends, and caregivers are also impacted by the survivorship experience and are therefore included in this definition" (Hewitt, Greenfield, & Stoval, 2006, p. 29). In 2006, the seminal report from the Institute of Medicine (IOM) titled *From Cancer Patient to Cancer Survivor: Lost in Transition* (Hewitt et al., 2005) highlighted the importance of cancer survivorship and the multifaceted aspects of caring for those affected by cancer. The IOM report outlined essential components of survivorship care including (1) prevention and detection of new and recurrent cancers; (2) surveillance for cancer spread, recurrence, or second cancers; (3) intervention for consequences of cancer and its treatment; and (4) coordination between specialists and primary care providers to ensure that all of a person's health needs are met (Hewitt et al., 2005). The American Society for Clinical Oncology (ASCO) further defined high-quality cancer survivorship care by recommending that providers address psychosocial effects of cancer diagnosis, provide health education, promote a healthy lifestyle including diet and exercise guidance, provide resources for financial hardships, and empower cancer survivors to be their own healthcare advocate (McCabe et al., 2013).

Oncology providers have historically been responsible for coordinating cancer survivorship care. The projected increase in the number of survivors requiring follow-up care will place a serious burden on oncology providers. There is evidence to suggest that the increased time pressure on healthcare providers and the shrinking oncology workforce will make it difficult for practicing oncologists to adequately manage this increasing number of cancer survivors and meet the goal of delivering high-quality cancer survivorship care. These pressures in combination with increased access to care through the Affordable Care Act will compound the burden of oncology providers (Chandak et al., 2014; Edwards et al., 2014). This growing burden signals the need for a multidisciplinary approach that includes primary care providers is warranted to ensure continuity and complete cancer survivorship care.

Many models of care for survivorship have been identified including shared care nurse-led, primary care, and oncology provider led (Hewitt, Bamundo, Day, & Harvey, 2007; Keesing, McNamara, & Rosenwax, 2014; Rowland, Hewitt, & Ganz, 2006). There is no consensus across institutions on the optimal model of healthcare delivery to cancer survivors at this time, but because of the growing demands on oncology specialists, it is evident that primary care providers will be key members of the cancer survivors, care team.

Figure 48-1 shows the Cancer Care Trajectory taken from the IOM report *From Cancer Patient to Cancer Survivor: Lost in Transition* (Hewitt et al., 2005).

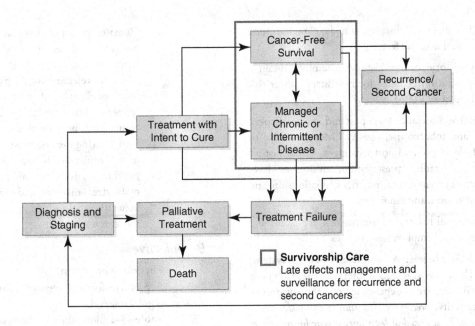

FIGURE 48-1 Cancer Care Trajectory

Reproduced from Institute of Medicine and National Research Council of the National Academies. *From Cancer Patient to Cancer Survivor: Lost in Transition*. M. Hewitt, S. Greenfield, and E. Stovall (Eds.). Washington, DC: The National Academies Press.

B. Epidemiology

In 2014, the Surveillance, Epidemiology, and End Results (SEER) database showed that 46% of survivors were 70 years or older. Only 5% of survivors were under the age of 40. The three most common cancers in males were prostate (43%), colorectal (9%), and melanoma (8%). In women, the three most common cancers were breast (41%), uterine corpus (8%), and colorectal (8%). Survival rates and survivor ages vary between cancer types. In all cancer sites, the relative 5-year cancer survival rate is estimated at 66% (DeSantis et al., 2014; Howlader et al., 2014). The largest group of survivors, about 36%, are less than 5 years from diagnosis, 10% are 15 to 20 years from diagnosis, and only 5% are more than 30-year cancer survivors (De Santis et al., 2014). The number of cancer survivors who are living 5 or more years beyond their diagnosis is projected to increase by 37%, reaching nearly 12 million over the next decade (de Moor et al., 2013).

II. Database

The clinical assessment of the cancer patients in the survivorship phase of care should include the following:

A. Subjective

1. Cancer history: specific site and type, stage at diagnosis, and histology; age at diagnosis

2. Cancer treatment history:
   a. Chemotherapy: therapeutic agents used including dose, date initiated and completed
   b. Radiotherapy: region treated, radiation dose, date initiated and completed
   c. Surgery: Surgical procedure, date of surgical procedure, pathology, and surgical complications
   d. Hereditary risk and genetic testing: Assess if genetic counseling was completed including results. Follow screening guidelines for moderate-to high-risk cancer survivors (Wood et al., 2012).
   e. Complications from treatment course: hospitalizations, toxicities during treatment, ongoing toxicity at completion of treatment, and functional and performance status

3. Medications: current medications for ongoing cancer therapy, current medications for cancer treatment sequelae, complementary and alternative medicine practices.

4. Past medical history: Comorbid conditions both pre and post cancer diagnosis, gynecologic and obstetric history including menstrual history, contraception,

sexually transmitted diseases, gravida/para, hormone replacement use, and fertility.

5. Family history: cancer history in family. Obtain a three-generation pedigree for hereditary cancer risk (Rowland et al., 2006).

6. Personal and social history: past and current alcohol intake and tobacco use, obesity history, exercise or activity level pre and post treatment, sexual history including fertility preservation, desire to have children, current sexual practices, relationship and living situation, and ethnicity

7. Occupational history: environmental exposures and cancer-related employment changes

8. Review of systems: A complete review of systems should be assessed at regular intervals. These intervals are individualized depending on the diagnosis. Generally it is *recommended that a complete review of systems be assessed at least once a year for all cancer survivors.*

   a. Constitutional: weight gain or loss, fatigue, fevers, sweats, pain, changes or limitations in exercise ability

   b. Skin and integument: treatment-related skin changes from radiotherapy, surgery, or chemotherapy; skin changes including fibrosis, telangiectasia, or thinning of skin; hair loss.

   c. Head, eyes, ear, nose, throat, and mouth: vision or hearing changes, dental problems, jaw pain or nonhealing sores, and xerostomia.

   d. Pulmonary: cough, hemoptysis, shortness of breath or dyspnea on exertion

   e. Cardiovascular: signs or symptoms of congestive heart failure, palpitations, coronary ischemia, pleural or pericardial chest pain, claudication or vascular ischemic symptoms, Reynaud's phenomenon, hypertension.

   f. Breast: new lumps or bumps, nipple or skin changes, nipple discharge.

   g. Gastrointestinal: diarrhea, constipation, nausea, emesis, abdominal pain, ostomy site problems, hepatitis, and cirrhosis.

   h. Genitourinary: incontinence, dysuria, hematuria, urinary frequency or hesitancy, erectile dysfunction.

   i. Gynecologic: premature menopause, vasomotor symptoms.

   j. Endocrine, reproductive, and sexual functioning: symptoms of hypothyroidism, metabolic syndrome, vaginal dryness, dyspareunia, decreased libido, body image issues, decreased sexual functioning, and vasomotor changes.

   k. Hematologic and lymphatic: bleeding, easy bruising, and recurrent or chronic infections, lymphedema.

   l. Musculoskeletal: chronic pain, height changes, joint swelling, and joint stiffness, decreased range of motion, new lumps or bumps.

   m. Neurologic: peripheral neuropathy, neuropathic pain, hearing loss, decreased cognitive function, mental acuity, and headaches.

   n. Psychiatric/psychosocial: depression, posttraumatic stress disorder, and cancer related changes in health, relationships, and finance, fear of recurrence or new cancers.

B. Objective

1. Physical examination
   A problem-focused physical exam should occur at regular intervals.
   Table 48-1 shows the late effects of both radiotherapy and chemotherapy on organ systems including specific chemotherapy drugs as a reference for physical exam findings.

2. Diagnostics

   a. Diagnostic testing should be based on the following: Review of systems and physical exam findings, surveillance tests based on specific cancer history and hereditary risk factors, and standard of care cancer screening and prevention (Smith et al., 2014).

   b. Immunizations: influenza vaccine (only inactive or recombinant) for all cancer survivors, pneumococcal vaccine, Tdap, human papillomavirus in survivors aged 26 or younger. Zoster vaccine (a live attenuated vaccine) in survivors aged 60 or older without active or ongoing immunodeficiency, no history of cellular immunodeficiency or hematopoietic stem cell transplant, or who have not received chemotherapy or radiotherapy in the past 3 months (National Comprehensive Cancer Network [NCCN], 2014).

III. Assessment

The NCI guidelines and NCCN clinical practice guidelines in oncology for survivorship recommend that a provider see an adult cancer survivor at regular intervals. These intervals are driven by individual cancer history and follow-up recommendations (NCCN, 2014). At each visit, the differential diagnosis is based on the survivor's symptoms. The guidelines recommend addressing the following subjects at regular

TABLE 48-1 Late Effects for Cancer Treatment

Organ/System	Late Effects of Radiotherapy	Late Effects of Chemotherapy	Some of the Drugs Responsible
Cardiovascular	Pericardial effusion, pericarditis, coronary artery disease	Cardiomyopathy, congestive heart failure, hypertension	Anthracyclines (doxorubicin, daunorubicin, epirubicin, mitoxantrone), cyclophosphamide, monoclonal antibodies (trastuzumab & pertuzumab)
Central Nervous System	Cognitive deficits, structural changes, hemorrhage, increased risk of stroke, hearing loss, psychiatric and psychosocial distress	Cognitive deficits, seizure, hemiplegia, hearing loss, psychiatric and psychosocial distress	Methotrexate Cisplatin
Gastrointestinal	Malabsorption, stricture, liver abnormalities	Abnormal liver function tests, hepatic fibrosis/failure, cirrhosis	Methotrexate, carmustine (BCNU®)
Genitourinary	Bladder fibrosis, contractures	Bladder fibrosis, hemorrhagic cystitis, urination dysfunction and malignancy	Cyclophosphamide, ifosfamide
Hematology/Lymph	Cytopenias, myelodysplasia	Myelodysplastic syndrome, acute myeloid leukemia	Alkylating agents, platinum agents (cisplatin, carboplatin, & oxaliplatin)
Musculoskeletal/ Soft Tissue	Fibrosis, atrophy, osteonecrosis, secondary malignancies, cosmetic changes, lymphedema	Avascular necrosis, osteoporosis, pain	Steroids, methotrexate, aromatase inhibitors (letrozole, anastrozole, exemestane)
Ophthalmologic	Cataracts, retinopathy, double vision	Cataracts	Steroids, tamoxifen, busulfan
Oral Health	Poor enamel and root formation, xerostomia	Xerostomia, increased incidence of caries	All chemotherapies
Peripheral Nervous System	Peripheral neuropathy	Peripheral neuropathy, hearing loss	Cisplatin, taxanes (paclitaxel, docetaxel, & albumin bound paclitaxel), vinca alkaloids (vincristine, vinorelbine), proteasome inhibitors (thalidomide)
Pulmonary	Pulmonary fibrosis, decreased lung volumes	Pulmonary fibrosis, interstitial pneumonitis	Bleomycin, BCNU, methotrexate, anthracyclines (doxorubicin, daunorubicin, epirubicin, mitoxantrone), MTOR/PI3K inhibitors (temsirolimus & everolimus)
Renal	Decreased creatinine clearance, hypertension	Decreased creatinine clearance, increased serum creatinine	Methotrexate, nitrosoureas, ifosfamides, Platinum agents (cisplatin, carboplatin, & oxaliplatin)
Reproductive	Men: risk of sterility, Leydig cell dysfunction Women: ovarian failure, premature menopause	Men: sterility, deficient or insufficient testosterone Women: sterility, premature menopause	Alkylating agents (cyclophosphamide and ifosfamide), procarbazine, antiestrogen therapies (tamoxifen, anastrozole, letrozole, and exemestane), platinum agents
Endocrine	Hypothyroidism, nodules, growth hormone deficiencies, pituitary deficiencies		

Data from Ganz, P. A. (2001). Late effects of cancer and its treatment. *Seminars in Oncology Nursing*, *17*(4), 241–248. doi: http://dx.doi.org/10.1053/sonu.2001.27914; Oeffinger, K. C., Hudson, M. M., & Landier, W. (2009). Survivorship: Childhood cancer survivors. *Primary Care, 36*(4), 743–780. doi: 10.1016/j.pop.2009.07.007.

SURVIVORSHIP BASELINE ASSESSMENT
(Patient version)

Please answer the following questions regarding possible symptoms that you may have experienced over the past 4 weeks:

Survivorship Concerns	Survivorship Care Survey
Anxiety and Depression	1. Do you often feel nervous or do you worry? Yes/No 2. Do you often feel sad or depressed? Yes/No 3. Have you lost interest in things you used to enjoy? Yes/No
Cognitive Function	4. Do you have difficulties with multitasking or attention? Yes/No 5. Do you have difficulties with remembering things? Yes/No 6. Does your thinking seem slow? Yes/No
Fatigue	7. Do you feel persistent fatigue despite a good night's sleep? Yes/No 8. Does fatigue interfere with your usual activities? Yes/No 9. How would you rate your fatigue on a scale of 0 (none) to 10 (extreme) over the past month? 0-10
Pain	10. Are you having any pain? Yes/No 11. How would you rate your pain on a scale of 0 (none) to 10 (extreme) over the past month? 0-10
Sexual Function	12. Are you dissatisfied with your sexual function? Yes/No 13. Do you have any concerns regarding sexual function or sexual activity? Yes/No
Sleep Disorder	14. Are you having problems falling asleep or staying asleep? Yes/No 15. Are you experiencing excessive sleepiness (ie, sleepiness or falling asleep in inappropriate situations or sleeping more during a 24-hour period than in the past)? Yes/No
Physical Activity	16. Are you exercising or doing some physical activity for less than 150 minutes a week? Yes/No 17. Do you have any limitations to participating in the physical activities that you enjoy? Yes/No
Immunizations and Infections	18. Have you received your flu vaccine this year? Yes/No 19. Have you received any vaccinations recently? Yes/No

Note: All recommendations are category 2A unless otherwise indicated.
Clinical Trials: NCCN believes that the best management of any cancer patient is in a clinical trial. Participation in clinical trials is especially encouraged.

FIGURE 48-2 NCCN Survivorship Baseline Assessment Guideline

Reproduced from National Comprehensive Cancer Network. (2014). *NCCN clinical practice guidelines in oncology™: Survivorship* (v.2.2014). Retrieved from www.nccn.org/professionals/physician_gls/f_guidelines .asp#survivorship.

intervals to see if there are contributing and/or reversible factors affecting health, current disease status, performance status, medications, comorbid conditions, and cancer history (NCCN, 2014). **Figure 48-2** is the NCCN survivorship baseline assessment guideline (NCCN, 2014).

IV. Goals of clinical management

The 2005 IOM report created the foundation of survivorship care and its essential components (Hewitt et al., 2005). These principles of cancer survivorship care have been used as the backbone for subsequent discussions and represent the overarching goals of management of the cancer survivor: (1) prevention and detection of new cancers and recurrent cancer, (2) surveillance for cancer spread and secondary cancers, (3) intervention for the consequences of cancer and its treatment, and (4) coordination between specialists and primary care providers to ensure health needs are met.

Many factors including lifestyle, environment, hereditary risks and the late effects of cancer treatment contribute to the development of secondary malignancies or disease recurrence in cancer survivors (Wood et al., 2012). It is important to identify those at higher risk and employ lifestyle interventions that mitigate risks including counseling on smoking cessation and alcohol usage, increasing physical activity, improving nutrition, and limiting sun exposure (NCCN, 2014).

The timing and patterns of local regional recurrence and metastatic disease are disease-site specific, and surveillance must be highly individualized. The NCCN has created disease specific guidelines that can help the primary care provider navigate the care of the cancer survivor (Morgan & Denlinger, 2014). In addition, interventions to prevent new cancers including standard age-appropriate cancer screening should be considered (Smith et al., 2014).

Cancer is more than just a disease of the body. The consequences of cancer and the downstream effects of a cancer diagnosis and its often multimodal treatments affect each individual patient and family differently. Cancer can leave its mark on all aspects of patients' lives including their physical condition, psychosocial and financial well-being, employment status, and interpersonal relationships. The late effects of treatment can be long lived and contribute to chronic physical and psychosocial changes such as fatigue, pain, anxiety, depression, and fear of recurrence. Regular assessments of these areas are essential and profoundly affect the quality of life of the cancer survivor. Cancer survivorship requires a multidisciplinary team of specialists who along with the primary care provider can help navigate the transition from patient to survivor. A physical exam should be completed at every visit, and sites of previous cancers should be assessed (Wood et al., 2012). In addition, appropriate screening guidelines should be implemented at each visit.

ASCO and the American College of Surgeons Commission on Cancer Program Standard for 2012 recommend treatment summaries and survivorship care plans for all cancer survivors to enhance both communication between the oncology team and the primary care provider and patient–provider communication (McCabe et al., 2013). The survivorship care plan should consist of two components: the treatment summary and follow-up plan. Together, these two components help to facilitate continuity of care and promote high-quality survivorship care.

The treatment summary should include the malignant diagnosis, stage at diagnosis (including histology), specific treatment modalities, ongoing toxicities of all treatments, and genetic or hereditary risk factors. The specific treatment modalities include surgical procedures, individually listed chemotherapy names and end date of chemotherapy, and radiotherapy treatment including anatomic location, duration, total dose, and end date (Mayer et al., 2014).

The follow-up plan should include oncology team members' names and contact information, ongoing need for adjuvant therapy with planned duration, schedule for follow-up visits, recommended surveillance tests for recurrence, cancer screening for new cancers, and other periodic testing needed as applicable. The patient should be given a list of symptoms concerning recurrence and a list of clinically significant late or long-term effects of treatment. The plan should end with a general statement educating the patient about healthy lifestyle including diet and exercise plans and a list of resources to address ongoing psychosocial, financial, employment, or parenting issues (Mayer et al., 2014). **Figure 48-3** is the ASCO survivorship care plan template.

V. Plan

A. Diagnostic tests

Diagnostic testing is based on the specific cancer history, symptoms at presentation, and subjective and objective findings. These diagnostic tests can include laboratory tests including tumor markers and/or imaging studies, which may include CT scan, bone scan, or PET scan. The NCCN and ASCO guidelines outline specific follow-up recommendations based on cancer diagnosis, stage at presentation, and risk. These guidelines are widely available and useful to all providers managing cancer survivors (ASCO, n.d.; NCCN, 2014). Included in these guidelines are recommendations for ongoing cancer screening and preventative imaging studies for cancer survivors, including screening tests for breast, prostate, cervical, colorectal, and lung cancer (Smith et al., 2014).

B. Patient education

It is important for survivors to be reminded that recovery takes time. They need to understand that their journey is not completed at the end of acute treatment but continues throughout their lives. Cancer survivors should be provided information about their individual care plan, symptoms to watch for, and lifestyle modifications that can aid in managing long-term effects and reduce risks for a second malignancy.

1. Lifestyle interventions

   Cancer survivors often request information and advice from providers about what they can do to improve their quality of life following cancer treatment and increase survival. Healthcare providers have a significant opportunity to counsel cancer survivors

ASCO Treatment Summary and Survivorship Care Plan

General Information	
Patient Name:	Patient DOB:
Patient phone:	Email:

Healthcare Providers (Including Names, Institution)

Primary Care Provider:
Surgeon:
Radiation Oncologist:
Medical Oncologist:
Other Providers:

Treatment Summary

Diagnosis

Cancer Type/Location/Histology Subtype:	Diagnosis Date (year):
Stage: ☐ I ☐ II ☐ III ☐ Not applicable	

Treatment

Surgery ☐ Yes ☐ No	Surgery Date(s) (year):
Surgical procedure/location/findings:	

Radiation ☐ Yes ☐ No	Body area treated:	End Date (year):

Systemic Therapy (chemotherapy, hormonal therapy, other) ☐ Yes ☐ No

Names of Agents Used	End Dates (year)

Persistent symptoms or side effects at completion of treatment: ☐ No ☐ Yes (enter type(s)) :

Familial Cancer Risk Assessment

Genetic/hereditary risk factor(s) or predisposing conditions:

Genetic counseling: ☐ Yes ☐ No	Genetic testing results:

Need for ongoing (adjuvant) treatment for cancer ☐ Yes ☐ No

Additional treatment name	Planned duration	Possible Side effects

Schedule of clinical visits

Coordinating Provider	When/How often

FIGURE 48-3 ASCO Survivorship Care Plan Template

Reproduced from American Society of Clinical Oncology. (2016). *ASCO Cancer Treatment and Survivorship Care Plans.* Retrieved from www.cancer.net.

ASCO Survivorship Care Plan

Updated based on consensus conference held on 9.27.13 and the ASCO Survivorship Committee

Cancer surveillance or other recommended related tests	
Coordinating Provider	What/When/How Often

Please continue to see your primary care provider for all general health care recommended for a (man) (woman) your age, including cancer screening tests. Any symptoms should be brought to the attention of your provider:

1. Anything that represents a brand new symptom;
2. Anything that represents a persistent symptom;
3. Anything you are worried about that might be related to the cancer coming back.

Possible late- and long-term effects that someone with this type of cancer and treatment may experience:

Cancer survivors may experience issues with the areas listed below. If you have any concerns in these or other areas, please speak with your doctors or nurses to find out how you can get help with them.

- ☐ Emotional and mental health ☐ Fatigue ☐ Weight changes ☐ Stopping smoking
- ☐ Physical Functioning ☐ Insurance ☐ School/Work ☐ Financial advice or assistance
- ☐ Memory or concentration loss ☐ Parenting ☐ Fertility ☐ Sexual functioning
- ☐ Other

A number of lifestyle/behaviors can affect your ongoing health, including the risk for the cancer coming back or developing another cancer. Discuss these recommendations with your doctor or nurse:

- ☐ Tobacco use/cessation ☐ Diet
- ☐ Alcohol use ☐ Sun screen use
- ☐ Weight management (loss/gain) ☐ Physical activity

Resources you may be interested in:

Other comments:

Prepared by: Delivered on:

- This Survivorship Care Plan is a cancer treatment summary and follow-up plan is provided to you to keep with your healthcare records and to share with your primary care provider.
- This summary is a brief record of major aspects of your cancer treatment. You can share your copy with any of your doctors or nurses. However, this is not a detailed or comprehensive record of your care.

FIGURE 48-3 ASCO Survivorship Care Plan Template (*Continued*)

Reproduced from American Society of Clinical Oncology. (2016). *ASCO Cancer Treatment and Survivorship Care Plans.* Retrieved from www.cancer.net.

on lifestyle modifications that may decrease their risk of recurrence, manage cancer treatment effects, and improve overall quality of life. The lifestyle modifications that have shown to make the greatest benefit are increased physical activity, weight management, and nutrition (Pekmezi & Demark-Wahnefried, 2011).

a. The current physical activity recommendations from both ACS and NCCN are that cancer survivors engage in regular physical exercise with the goal of 150 minutes of moderate to vigorous aerobic exercise per week. In addition, they recommend 2 days a week of resistance or strength training and that exercise programs are tailored to individual needs (NCCN, 2014; Rock et al., 2012).

b. Nutrition and dietary choices have also been shown to play a role in cancer recurrence risk, improved quality of life after cancer treatment, and overall survival (Pekmezi & Demark-Wahnefried, 2011). Though more data are needed to further investigate the role nutrition and weight management play in cancer survivorship, current recommendations follow those of the general population. It is recommended that cancer survivors maintain a healthy weight with body mass index < 25 and consume a plant-based diet high in vegetables, fruits, and whole grains (Kushi et al., 2012; Rock et al., 2012). Many studies have attempted to include supplements from isolated nutrients as chemoprevention from cancer or recurrence. Unfortunately, to date, there are no trials that have confirmed additional supplementation to be beneficial in cancer prevention. Some of these trials have revealed high-dose isolated nutrients can actually be detrimental. Evidence for supplementation in cancer is not supported, with best advice currently being portion-controlled consumption of whole foods to obtain nutrients (Kushi et al., 2012). The recommendations for alcohol consumption are no different from the general population guidelines.

C. Consultations and Referrals

The care of the adult cancer survivor is complex. Each survivor has his or her own specific cancer story and follow-up recommendations. It is imperative to consult the oncology team with any questions or concerns regarding surveillance and possible recurrence. The open line of communication will ensure high-quality care.

In addition, the mental, psychosocial, and financial health of the cancer survivor should not be overlooked. Referrals to psycho-oncology, psychology, psychiatry, and social work should be used to address those needs.

VI. Self-management resources

Cancer survivors are a unique population. They have medical needs that reach beyond physical well-being, and navigating those needs can be challenging. The survivorship care plan is an individualized road map for providers to help facilitate and direct follow-up care. It is also a tool for cancer survivors and families to help them understand their individualized history and risks, and it empowers them to be active members in their follow-up care. As the cancer survivor population increases it will be essential that both oncology and primary care providers work together as the cancer survivorship care team to ensure continued, coordinated, and high-quality care for this unique population.

A. Educational resources

www.cancer.org/treatment/survivorshipduringandafter treatment/index
www.canceradvocacy.org
http://cancercontrol.cancer.gov/ocs/index.html
http://journeyforward.org
www.cancer.net/survivorship
www.cdc.gov/cancer/survivorship
www.livestrong.org/we-can-help/healthy-living-after-treatment/
www.mskcc.org/cancer-care/integrative-medicine/about-herbs-botanicals-other-products

B. Community support groups

1. ACS provides a resource link where survivors can look up local support groups based on location: www.cancer.org/treatment/supportprogramsservices/app/resource-search.

2. Cancer Care is a national organization that provides free, professional support services and information to help survivors manage the emotional, practical, and financial challenges of cancer. They provide online, telephone, and face-to-face support groups: www.cancercare.org/support_groups.

REFERENCES

American Cancer Society. (2014). *Cancer facts & figures 2014*. Atlanta: American Cancer Society.

American Society of Clinical Oncology. (n.d.). Practice guidelines. Retrieved from www.instituteforquality.org/practice-guidelines.

Chandak, A. N., Loberiza, F. R., Deras, M., Armitage, J. O., Vose, J. M., & Stimpson, J. P. (2014). Estimating the state-level supply of cancer care providers: Preparing to meet workforce needs in the wake of healthcare reform. *Journal of Oncology Practice*. [Epub 2014, Nov. 12] doi: 10.1200/JOP.2014.001565.

de Moor, J. S., Mariotto, A. B,, Parry, C., Alfano, C. M., Padgett, L., Kent, E. E., et al. (2013). Cancer survivors in the United States: Prevalence across the survivorship trajectory and implications for care. *Cancer Epidemiology, Biomarkers and Pprevention, 22*(4), 561–570. doi: 10.1158/1055-9965.EPI-12-1356. [Epub 2013 Mar 27].

DeSantis, C. E., Lin, C. C., Mariotto, A. B., Siegel, R. L., Stein, K. D., Kramer, J. L., et al. (2014). Cancer treatment and survivorship statistics, 2014. *CA: A Cancer Journal for Clinicians, 64*(4), 252–271. doi: 10.3322/caac.21235

Edwards, B. K., Noone, A. M., Mariotto, A. B., Simard, E. P., Boscoe, F. P., Henley, S. J., et al. (2014). Annual report to the nation on the status of cancer, 1975–2010, featuring prevalence of comorbidity and impact on survival among persons with lung, colorectal, breast, or prostate cancer. *Cancer, 120*(9), 1290–1314. doi: 10.1002/cncr.28509

Ganz, P. A. (2001). Late effects of cancer and its treatment. *Seminars in Oncology Nursing, 17*(4), 241–248. doi: http://dx.doi.org/10.1053/sonu.2001.27914

Ganz, P. A. (2006). Monitoring the physical health of cancer survivors: A survivorship-focused medical history. *Journal of Clinical Oncology, 24*(32), 5105–5111. doi: 10.1200/jco.2006.06.0541

Hewitt, M., Greenfield, S., & Stoval, E. (2005). *From cancer patient to cancer survivor—Lost in transition.* Washington, DC: National Academies Press.

Hewitt, M. E., Bamundo, A., Day, R., & Harvey, C. (2007). Perspectives on post-treatment cancer care: Qualitative research with survivors, nurses, and physicians. *Journal of Clinical Oncology, 25*(16), 2270–2273. doi: 10.1200/jco.2006.10.0826

Howlader, N., Noone, A. M., Krapcho, M., Garshell, J., Miller, D., Altekruse, S. F., et al. (Eds.). (2014). *SEER cancer statistics review 1975–2011.* Bethesda, MD: National Cancer Institute. Retrieved from http://seer.cancer.gov/archive/csr/1975_2011/.

Keesing, S., McNamara, B., & Rosenwax, L. (2014). Cancer survivors' experiences of using survivorship care plans: A systematic review of qualitative studies. *Journal of Cancer Survivorship, 9*(2), 1–9. doi: 10.1007/s11764-014-0407-x

Kushi, L. H., Doyle, C., McCullough, M., Rock, C. L., Demark-Wahnefried, W., Bandera, E. V., et al. (2012). American Cancer Society guidelines on nutrition and physical activity for cancer prevention: Reducing the risk of cancer with healthy food choices and physical activity. *CA: A Cancer Journal for Clinicians, 62*(1), 30–67. doi: 10.3322/caac.20140

Mayer, D. K., Nekhlyudov, L., Snyder, C. F., Merrill, J. K., Wollins, D. S., & Shulman, L. N. (2014). American Society of Clinical Oncology clinical expert statement on cancer survivorship care planning. *Journal of Oncology Practice, 10*(6), 345–351. doi: 10.1200/jop.2014.001321

McCabe, M. S., Bhatia, S., Oeffinger, K. C., Reaman, G. H., Tyne, C., Wollins, D. S., et al. (2013). American Society of Clinical Oncology statement: Achieving high-quality cancer survivorship care. *Journal of Clinical Oncology, 31*(5), 631–640. doi: 10.1200/jco.2012.46.6854

Morgan, M. A., & Denlinger, C. S. (2014). Survivorship: Tools for transitioning patients with cancer. *Journal of the National Comprehensive Cancer Network, 12*(12), 1681–1687.

Mullan, F. (1985). Seasons of survival–Reflections of a physician with cancer. *New England Journal of Medicine, 313*(4), 270–273. doi: 10.1056/nejm198507253130421

National Comprehensive Cancer Network. (2014). *NCCN clinical practice guidelines in oncology: Survivorship* (v.2.2014). Retrieved from www.nccn.org/professionals/physician_gls/f_guidelines.asp#survivorship.

Oeffinger, K. C., Hudson, M. M., & Landier, W. (2009). Survivorship: Childhood cancer survivors. *Primary Care, 36*(4), 743–780. doi: 10.1016/j.pop.2009.07.007

Pekmezi, D. W., & Demark-Wahnefried, W. (2011). Updated evidence in support of diet and exercise interventions in cancer survivors. *Acta Oncologica, 50*(2), 167–178. doi: 10.3109/0284186X.2010.529822. [Epub 2010 Nov 24.]

Rock, C. L., Doyle, C., Demark-Wahnefried, W., Meyerhardt, J., Courneya, K. S., Schwartz, A. L., et al. (2012). Nutrition and physical activity guidelines for cancer survivors. *CA: A Cancer Journal for Clinicians, 62*(4), 243–274. doi: 10.3322/caac.21142

Rowland, J. H., Hewitt, M., & Ganz, P. A. (2006). Cancer survivorship: A new challenge in delivering quality cancer care. *Journal of Clinical Oncology, 24*(32), 5101–5104. doi: 10.1200/jco.2006.09.2700

Smith, R. A., Manassaram-Baptiste, D., Brooks, D., Cokkinides, V., Doroshenk, M., Saslow, D., et al. (2014). Cancer screening in the United States, 2014: A review of current American Cancer Society guidelines and current issues in cancer screening. *CA: A Cancer Journal for Clinicians, 64*(1), 31–51. doi: 10.3322/caac.21212

Wood, M. E., Vogel, V., Ng, A., Foxhall, L., Goodwin, P., & Travis, L. B. (2012). Second malignant neoplasms: Assessment and strategies for risk reduction. *Journal of Clinical Oncology, 30*(30), 3734–3745. doi: 10.1200/jco.2012.41.8681

CHRONIC OBSTRUCTIVE PULMONARY DISEASE

Lynda A. Mackin

I. Introduction and general background

Chronic obstructive pulmonary disease (COPD) is an umbrella name for two major pulmonary obstructive disorders: chronic bronchitis and emphysema. Although each disorder has its own distinctive pathophysiology, many COPD patients have a combination of chronic bronchitis and emphysema.

A. COPD

1. Definition and overview

   COPD is defined as "a common preventable and treatable disease, characterized by persistent airflow limitation that is usually progressive and associated with an enhanced chronic inflammatory response in the airways and the lung to noxious particles and gases. Exacerbations and comorbidities contribute to the overall severity in individual patients" (Global Initiative for Chronic Obstructive Lung Disease [GOLD], 2015, p. 2).

   The main pathophysiologic problem in COPD is expiratory airflow limitation. In the case of chronic bronchitis, loss of structural integrity and bronchospasm in the larger airways, plus excess mucous production, are the cause of expiratory airflow limitation. The classic definition of chronic bronchitis is a productive cough for 3 months for 2 successive years (American Thoracic Society, 1962). In emphysema, smaller, more distal airways and alveoli are damaged, resulting in loss of structural integrity plus destruction of the alveolar–capillary membrane. The small airway changes result in early collapse during expiration, causing airflow limitation. Additionally, the loss of surface area at the alveoli–capillary level impairs gas exchange. Smoking is recognized to be the most common cause of COPD. Environmental toxin exposures, including outdoor and indoor air pollution, are also known

   causes. Exposure to fumes from cooking and burning of biomass is recognized as a significant risk in developing countries. Occupational exposures can also cause COPD (GOLD, 2014). Examples include but are not limited to silica, coal dust, cotton dust, grain dust, toxic chemicals, secondhand smoke, biomass smoke, diesel exhaust, welding flames, and wood finishing fumes (Balmes & Speizer, 2015).

   Several comorbidities are associated with COPD: cardiovascular disease, osteoporosis, metabolic syndrome, diabetes mellitus, bronchiectasis, lung cancer, anxiety, and depression (GOLD, 2014). Additionally, COPD is recognized as a systemic disease evidenced by nutritional depletion and skeletal muscle dysfunction (Decramer, De Benedetto, Del Ponte, & Marinari, 2005; Maltais et al., 2014). An asthma-COPD overlap syndrome (ACOS) has also been described (Global Initiative for Asthma [GINA], 2014).

2. Prevalence and incidence

   According to U.S. National Center for Health Statistics data collected between 2007 and 2012, 14.7% of adults aged 40–79 reported some degree of lung obstruction (including COPD and asthma), with adults aged 60–79 having a higher prevalence (17%) compared to younger adults aged 40–59 (13.6%) (Tilert, Paulose-Ram, & Brody, 2015). Currently, COPD is the third leading cause of death in the United States (Centers for Disease Control and Prevention [CDC], 2015a). According to the CDC (2015a), COPD deaths among men have declined: 57.0 per 100,000 in 1999 falling to 47.6 per 100,000 in 2010 There has not been a similar decline in death rates in women (35.3 per 100,000 in 1999 and 36.4 per 100,000 in 2010) (CDC, 2015a). U.S. state-level data reported in 2012 revealed that people living in the Ohio and Mississippi River valleys had the highest incidence of COPD (CDC, 2012).

II. Database

A. Subjective

1. COPD

   COPD is symptomatically characterized by chronic, progressive cough, dyspnea, and sputum production that can vary from day to day (GOLD, 2014). The clinician should elicit information about these key symptoms, as well as query progression of symptoms over time. The comprehensive history should also include the following:

   a. Past health history
      i. Medical illnesses: asthma, allergies, nasal polyps, sinusitis, gastroesophageal reflux disease, childhood respiratory infections, adult respiratory illnesses, hospitalizations and other respiratory diseases. Elicit if there has been any pattern to symptom development over time.
      ii. Surgical history: chest or lung
      iii. Exposure history: environmental tobacco smoke exposure, occupational dusts and fume exposures toxins; indoor and outdoor air pollution, cooking fumes, and biomass fuel combustion fumes (GOLD, 2014)
      iv. Medication history: medications taken to relieve symptoms currently and in the past (oral or inhaled bronchodilators and oral or inhaled steroids)

   b. Family history: obstructive pulmonary disease (COPD, asthma, bronchiectasis)

   c. Occupational and environmental history
      i. Work-related exposures: toxins and fumes
      ii. Exposure to home cooking or biomass fuel fumes

   d. Personal and social history
      i. History of or current smoking; impact of symptoms on physical function and occupational activities.
      ii. Diet: caloric intake
      iii. Exercise capacity
      iv. Social support resources.

   e. Review of systems
      i. Constitutional signs and symptoms: fatigue, activity intolerance, weight change, and fevers; impact of symptoms on activities of daily living and occupational and recreational pursuits
      ii. Ear, nose, and throat: allergic rhinitis, sinus symptoms, and postnasal drip
      iii. Respiratory: chronic cough (with or without sputum production; may be intermittent); chronic sputum production; and progressive, persistent dyspnea (worsens with activity or on exertion), wheezing, hemoptysis
      iv. Cardiac: chest pain, fluid retention and peripheral edema, and dysrhythmias
      v. Gastrointestinal: heartburn, reflux, cough with meals

B. Objective

The GOLD Guidelines (GOLD, 2014) recommend that assessment focus on an objective determination of disease severity and impact on functional and personal activities and determine risk of future events such as hospitalizations, exacerbations, and death.

1. Physical examination findings (**Table 49-1**).

2. Spirometry: Spirometry is an important tool in classifying the severity of chronic airflow limitation and is particularly useful as a confirmatory test. Key spirometric values are the forced vital capacity (FVC) and the forced expiratory volume in 1 second (FEV_1), percentage predicted and is performed before and after inhaled bronchodilator administration. A postbronchodilator FEV_1/FVC ratio of less than 0.7 confirms airflow limitation. Classification of airflow limitation severity is further defined by FEV_1 value. See **Table 49-2** (GOLD, 2014) for GOLD classification of severity of airflow obstruction in COPD.

3. Combined assessment of COPD: The GOLD Guidelines recommend the combination of spirometric data, objective symptom measurement, and frequency of exacerbation be considered together to determine risk. Based on these data,

TABLE 49-1 Classic Physical Examination Findings in Chronic Bronchitis and Emphysema

Chronic Bronchitis	Emphysema
Overweight	Thin
Cyanotic but breathing comfortably at rest	Not cyanotic, breathing looks comfortable
Noisy breath sounds, rhonchi, wheezing	Quiet, distant breath sounds
Peripheral edema	No peripheral edema

Note: Most chronic obstructive pulmonary disease patients have clinical characteristics of both chronic bronchitis and emphysema to varying degrees.

TABLE 49-2 Classification of Severity of Airflow Limitation in COPD (Based on Postbronchodilator FEV$_1$)

In patients with FEV$_1$/FVC < 0.70:		
GOLD 1:	Mild	FEV$_1$ ≥ 80% predicted
GOLD 2:	Moderate	50% ≤ FEV$_1$ < 80% predicted
GOLD 3:	Severe	30% ≤ FEV$_1$ < 50% predicted
GOLD 4:	Very Severe	FEV$_1$ < 30% predicted

Reproduced from Global Initiative for Chronic Obstructive Lung Disease (GOLD). (2015). *Pocket guide to COPD diagnosis, management, and prevention*. Available from http://www.goldcopd.org/. Used with permission.

TABLE 49-3 Modified Medical Research Council Questionnaire (mMRC) for Assessing the Severity of Breathlessness

Please check the box that applies to you (one box only)	
mMRC Grade 0. I get breathless only with strenuous exercise.	☐
mMRC Grade 1. I get short of breath when hurrying on the level or walking up a slight hill.	☐
mMRC Grade 2. I walk slower than people of the same age on the level because of breathlessness, or I have to stop for breath when walking on my own pace on the level.	☐
mMRC Grade 3. I stop for breath after walking about 100 meters or after a few minutes on the level.	☐
mMRC Grade 4. I am too breathless to leave the house or I am breathless when dressing or undressing.	☐

Reproduced from Global Initiative for Chronic Obstructive Lung Disease (GOLD). (2015). *Pocket guide to COPD diagnosis, management, and prevention*. Available from http://www.goldcopd.org/. Used with permission.

patients are grouped into one of four groups (A, B, C, D) with groups C and D being at the highest risk. Either the modified British Medical Research Council Questionnaire for Assessing the Severity of Breathlessness (mMRC) (Bestall et al., 1999) or the COPD Assessment Test (CAT) (Jones et al., 2009) can be used to assess symptoms. See **Table 49-3** for the mMRC Scale. The CAT can be accessed at http://www.catestonline.org/. Exacerbation frequency, and specifically if hospitalized, is considered. See **Table 49-4** for the combined assessment of risk matrix.

TABLE 49-4 Combined Assessment of COPD

When assessing risk, choose the **highest risk** according to GOLD grade or exacerbation history.
(One or more hospitalizations for COPD exacerbations should be considered high risk.)

Patient	Characteristic	Spirometric Classification	Exacerbations per year	CAT	mMRC
A	Low Risk Less Symptoms	GOLD 1-2	≤ 1	< 10	0-1
B	Low Risk More Symptoms	GOLD 1-2	≤ 1	≥ 10	≥ 2
C	High Risk Less Symptoms	GOLD 3-4	≥ 2	< 10	0-1
D	High Risk More Symptoms	GOLD 3-4	≥ 2	≥ 10	≥ 2

Reproduced from Global Initiative for Chronic Obstructive Lung Disease (GOLD). (2015). *Pocket guide to COPD diagnosis, management, and prevention*. Available from http://www.goldcopd.org/. Used with permission.

4. Chest radiograph: Does not confirm diagnosis of COPD but may demonstrate hyperinflation and flattened diaphragms and may reveal other conditions. In the absence of obstruction on pulmonary function tests, chest CT scan can provide evidence of nonobstructive emphysema.

5. Check complete blood count (may see polycythemia in chronic hypoxemia) and complete metabolic panel. When vitamin D25 hydroxy serum levels are low, patients may be more likely to have respiratory symptoms. Hyperthyroid symptoms can sometimes mimic COPD.

6. Pulse oximetry: Saturation is reduced in cases of hypoxemia. Six-minute walk is used to evaluate oxygen need with exercise. Nocturnal oximetry can be ordered through a durable medical equipment (DME) company to evaluate oxygen need with sleep.

7. Consider arterial blood gases: reflects hypoxemia and possible hypercapnia.

8. Consider α_1-antitrypsin deficiency screen (in cases of younger onset of symptoms and more extensive disease).

9. Additional pulmonary function testing (lung volumes, diffusing capacity) and exercise testing may be useful in further differentiating diagnosis. Emphysema is often associated with air trapping (increased TLC and RV) and decreased diffusing capacity.

10. To assess systemic effect of disease, composite assessments such as the BODE Index (Celli et al., 2004) may be useful: the BODE Index is a multidimensional mortality prediction that incorporates body mass index, severity of airflow obstruction, dyspnea, and exercise capacity as measured by 6-minute walk performance.

III. Goals of clinical management of stable COPD (GOLD, 2014)

A. Reduce symptoms

B. Improve activity tolerance
Management of stable COPD focuses on improving activity tolerance and overall health status in addition to reducing symptoms. This goal is achieved through use of pharmacologic and nonpharmacologic therapeutics.

C. Reduce risk
Management of stable COPD also focuses on reducing future risk of the disease. The focus is on strategies to prevent disease progression, prevent and treat exacerbations, and reduce overall mortality. As with symptom reduction, both pharmacologic and nonpharmacologic therapeutics are used.

IV. Plan (components of COPD management)

A. Pharmacologic therapy

1. Pharmacologic therapeutics include short-acting (SA) and long-acting (LA) beta$_2$-agonist or anticholinergic bronchodilators, oral and/or inhaled corticosteroids, phosphodiesterase-4 (PDE-4) inhibitor (for prevention of exacerbation), and in highly selected cases, theophylline or carbocysteine (GOLD, 2014). When clinically indicated, supplemental oxygen should also be used; oxygen flow rate can be determined though an oxygen prescription test with exercise (arranged through a pulmonary function laboratory) and at night (arranged through a DME company).

2. The GOLD Patient Group Classification provides a basis for initial pharmacologic therapy in stable COPD. See **Table 49-5** for an overview of recommended pharmacologic therapy by COPD patient group. See **Table 49-6** for formulations and typical doses of COPD medications

3. General pharmacotherapy recommendations for stable COPD per the GOLD Guidelines (GOLD, 2014) are as follows:

   a. Bronchodilators: Long-acting bronchodilators are preferred, but short-acting bronchodilators may be helpful if symptoms are not sufficiently relieved with long-acting bronchodilators alone. Inhaled bronchodilators are preferred over oral bronchodilators. Theophylline is not recommended unless other agents are not available or unaffordable.

   b. Corticosteroids: A trial of oral corticosteroid to determine steroid responsiveness is not recommended. Long-term treatment with oral or inhaled corticosteroids alone is not recommended. It is not recommended to use inhaled corticosteroids at doses outside typical dose range.

   c. PDE-4 inhibitor: May reduce the frequency of exacerbation in patients with chronic bronchitis, severe or very severe airflow limitation (category 3 or 4), or frequent exacerbations not controlled by a long-acting bronchodilator.

B. Nonpharmacologic therapy

1. Management of stable COPD should incorporate regular exercise, including participation in a formal pulmonary rehabilitation program if available and qualified.

C. Risk reduction strategies

1. Smoking cessation or prevention

2. Eliminate or reduce occupational exposures and indoor and outdoor pollution.

TABLE 49-5 Initial Pharmacologic Management of COPD*

Patient Group	Recommended First Choice	Alternative Choice	Other Possible Treatments**
A	Short-acting anticholinergic prn *Or* Short-acting beta$_2$-agonist prn	Long-acting anticholinergic *Or* Long-acting beta$_2$-agonist *Or* Short-acting beta$_2$-agonist and short-acting anticholinergic	Theophylline
B	Long-acting anticholinergic prn *Or* Long-acting beta$_2$-agonist prn	Long-acting anticholinergic and long-acting beta$_2$-agonist	Short-acting beta$_2$-agonist and/or Short-acting anticholinergic Theophylline
C	Inhaled corticosteroid + long-acting beta$_2$-agonist *Or* Long-acting anticholinergic	Long-acting anticholinergic and long-acting beta$_2$-agonist or Long-acting anticholinergic and phosphodiesterase-4 inhibitor or Long-acting beta$_2$-agonist and phosphodiesterase-4 inhibitor	Short-acting beta$_2$-agonist and/or Short-acting anticholinergic Theophylline
D	Inhaled corticosteroid + long-acting beta$_2$-agonist and/or Long-acting anticholinergic	Inhaled corticosteroid + long-acting beta$_2$-agonist and long-acting anticholinergic or Inhaled corticosteroid + long-acting beta$_2$-agonist and phosphodiesterase-4 inhibitor or Long-acting anticholinergic and long-acting beta$_2$-agonist or Long-acting anticholinergic and phosphodiesterase-4 inhibitor	Carbocysteine *N*-acetylcysteine Short-acting beta$_2$-agonist and/or Short-acting anticholinergic Theophylline

*Medications in each box are mentioned in alphabetical order and therefore not necessarily in order of preference.

**Medications in this column can be used alone or in combination with other options in the Recommended First Choice and Alternative Choice columns.

Reproduced from Global Initiative for Chronic Obstructive Lung Disease (GOLD). (2015). *Pocket guide to COPD diagnosis, management, and prevention.* Available from http://www.goldcopd.org/. Used with permission.

3. Prevent exacerbations from infectious processes through common health promotion measures such as hand washing and crowd avoidance.

4. Vaccination: Both the pneumococcal polysaccharide vaccine (PPSV23) and the pneumococcal conjugate vaccine (PCV-13) are recommended (CDC, 2015b). Annual vaccination against the seasonal flu vaccine is also recommended.

D. Monitoring and follow-up care

1. Continue to monitor exacerbations frequency/severity, symptoms including responsiveness to pharmacotherapy; promote smoking cessation or maintenance of nonsmoking status; promote avoidance of smoke/fumes/toxins/pollution exposure; manage comorbidities; and evaluate disease progression, when indicated, through spirometry.

E. Management of exacerbations

1. Background information
   a. Definition: "An exacerbation of COPD is defined as an acute event characterized by worsening of the patient's respiratory symptoms that is beyond normal day-to-day variations and leads

TABLE 49-6 Formulations and Typical Doses of COPD Medications*

Drug	Inhaler (mcg)	Solution for Nebulizer (mg/mL)	Oral	Vials for Injection (mg)	Duration of Action (hours)
Beta$_2$-agonists					
Short-acting					
Fenoterol	100–200 (MDI)	1	0.05% (Syrup)		4–6
Levalbuterol	45–90 (MDI)	0.21, 0.42			6–8
Salbutamol (albuterol)	100, 200 (MDI & DPI)	5	5 mg (Pill), 0.024%(Syrup)	0.1, 0.5	4–6
Terbutaline	400, 500 (DPI)		2.5, 5 mg (Pill)		4–6
Long-acting					
Formoterol	4.5–12 (MDI & DPI)	0.01			12
Arformoterol		0.0075			12
Indacaterol	75–300 (DPI)				24
Salmeterol	25–50 (MDI & DPI)				12
Tulobuterol			2 mg (transdermal)		24
Anticholinergics					
Short-acting					
Ipratropium bromide	20, 40 (MDI)	0.25–0.5			6–8
Oxitropium bromide	100 (MDI)	1.5			7–9
Long-acting					
Aclidinium bromide	322 (DPI)				12
Glycopyrronium bromide	44 (DPI)				
Tiotropium	18 (DPI), 5 (SMI)				24
Umeclidinium	62.5 (DPI)				24
Combination short-acting beta$_2$-agonist plus anticholinergic in one inhaler					
Fenoterol/ ipratropium	200/80 (MDI)	1.25/0.5			6–8
Salbutamol/ ipratropium	100/20 (SMI)				6–8
Combination long-acting beta$_2$-agonist plus anticholinergic in one inhaler					
Formoterol/ aclidinium	12/340 (DPI)				12
Indacaterol/ glycopyrronium	85/43 (DPI)				24
Vilanterol/ umeclidinium	25/62.5 (DPI)				24
Methylxanthines					
Aminophylline			200–600 mg (Pill)	240	Variable, up to 24
Theophylline (SR)			100–600 mg (Pill)		Variable, up to 24

(continues)

TABLE 49-6 Formulations and Typical Doses of COPD Medications* *(Continued)*

Drug	Inhaler (mcg)	Solution for Nebulizer (mg/mL)	Oral	Vials for Injection (mg)	Duration of Action (hours)
Inhaled corticosteroids					
Beclomethasone	50–400 (MDI & DPI)	0.2–0.4			
Budesonide	100, 200, 400 (DPI)	0.20, 0.25, 0.5			
Fluticasone	50–500 (MDI & DPI)				
Combination long-acting beta₂-agonists plus corticosteroids in one inhaler					
Formoterol/ beclometasone	6/100 (MDI)				
Formoterol/ budesonide	4.5/160 (MDI) 9/320 (DPI)				
Formoterol/ mometasone	10/200, 10/400 (MDI)				
Salmeterol/ fluticasone	50/100, 250, 500 (DPI)				
Vilanterol/ fluticasone furoate	25/100 (DPI)				
Systemic corticosteroids					
Prednisone			5–60 mg (Pill)		
Methyl-prednisolone			4, 8, 16 mg (Pill)		
Phosphodiesterase-4 inhibitors					
Roflumilast			500 mcg (Pill)		24

MDI = metered dose inhaler; DPI = dry powder inhaler; SMI = soft mist inhaler

*Not all formulations are available in all countries; in some countries, other formulations may be available.

† Formoterol nebulized solution is based on the unit dose vial containing 20 mcg in a volume of 2.0 mL.

Reproduced from Global Initiative for Chronic Obstructive Lung Disease (GOLD). (2015). *Pocket guide to COPD diagnosis, management, and prevention.* Available from http://www.goldcopd.org/. Used with permission.

to a change in medication" (GOLD, 2014, p. 40). Additionally, exacerbations are recognized to reduce physical function and objective pulmonary function, accelerate disease progression, have a negative impact on quality of life, and cause considerable morbidity and increased risk of mortality (GOLD, 2014).

b. Most exacerbations are caused by lower respiratory tract infection or air pollution. Symptoms may overlap with other illnesses such as pneumonia, pulmonary embolism, pleural effusion, pneumothorax dysrhythmia, and heart failure.

c. Etiology can be viral or bacterial. Most common bacterial etiologies are *Haemophilus Influenzae, Streptococcus pneumoniae,* and *Moraxella catarrhalis.*

d. Key history: acute change in symptoms of COPD—dyspnea, fatigue, cough, and sputum production/sputum character including duration of symptoms. Determine frequency/pattern of exacerbations. Individuals who have two or more exacerbations per year are considered "frequent exacerbators" (Hurst et al., 2010). Elicit if required hospitalizations in past and if required intubation. Consider comorbidities, especially in older adults. Review current medications (including adherence to regimen) as breaks in maintenance therapy has been associated with exacerbations. Severity of airflow limitation at baseline must be kept in consideration when in exacerbation (GOLD, 2014).

e. Physical examination: body temperature; tachypnea; tachycardia; blood pressure and pulse (hemodynamic instability is a serious sign); pulse oximetry; altered mental status (serious sign); increased work of breathing; use of accessory muscles, poor air entry; wheezing; rhonchi; new or worsening peripheral edema; progressive new or worsening cyanosis (serious sign). If possible, sputum should be observed by the clinician.

f. Diagnostic studies

   i. Arterial blood gas: PaO_2 less than 60 or Spo_2 less than 90%; moderate to severe acidosis (pH < 7.36) plus hypercapnia ($PaCO_2$ 45–60) in the patient with respiratory failure indicates the need for mechanical ventilation.

   ii. Chest radiograph: identify alternative diagnosis (pneumonia, heart failure).

   iii. Electrocardiogram: look for right ventricular hypertrophy, arrhythmias, and ischemia. Others: sputum culture, metabolic panel, and complete blood count (may not be necessary for outpatient treatment but should be considered). Spirometry is not considered helpful in the midst of exacerbation.

2. Exacerbation treatment

   The discussion that follows here applies only to mild exacerbations that can be safely treated as an outpatient. The reader is directed to the GOLD Guidelines (GOLD, 2014) for detailed guidance and recommendations for management of exacerbations in moderate and severe cases and recommendations for emergency department and hospital treatment.

   a. Determine appropriate treatment site: Strongly consider hospitalization for the following: sudden/significant increase in symptoms, severe airflow limitation at baseline, changes in mental status, new physical examination findings (edema, cyanosis), self-care/functional impairment, inadequate home support, uncertain diagnosis, inadequate outpatient response to treatment, inability to eat or sleep due to symptoms, worsening hypoxemia and hypercapnia, high-risk comorbidity (pneumonia, dysrhythmias, heart failure, diabetes mellitus, or renal or liver failure) (GOLD, 2014)

   b. Outpatient treatment of exacerbation: summary of GOLD Guidelines, Chapter 5: Management of Exacerbations (GOLD 2014). *Limited to outpatient management. See GOLD Guidelines for management of urgently/severely/critically ill.*

      i. Increase short-acting bronchodilator: Beta$_2$-agonist and/or anticholinergic short-acting bronchodilators through a metered dose inhaler or via nebulizer are recommended; a spacer device is optional.

      ii. Oral corticosteroids: prednisone 40 mg PO for 5 days is recommended. Oral prednisolone is preferable; nebulized budesonide can also be used in place of oral prednisone.

      iii. Antibiotic treatment: Controversial; in outpatient setting sputum culture not helpful. Antibiotics recommended when all three cardinal symptoms of infection are present: increased dyspnea, increased sputum volume, and more purulent sputum. The following antibiotic are recommended, but antibiotic selection should take into consideration local bacterial resistance patterns: aminopenicillin (with or without clavulanic acid), tetracycline, or macrolide.

      iv. Patient/family education and follow-up: smoking cessation (if actively smoking); medication side effects, dosing and dosing schedule; when to expect symptoms to improve; signs and symptoms of worsening; when to call provider or seek emergency evaluation. Provide written instructions. The patient should be reappointed to see the provider again in 2–3 days or sooner as needed.

V. Care from a population health perspective

A. Smoking cessation

Smoking cessation is by far the most important preventative strategy; smokers should be counseled and supported in achieving and maintaining cessation at all clinical encounters. All adjuncts to cessation should be employed and care should support cessation indefinitely.

B. Promotion and advocacy for disease awareness, screening, and access to spirometry for identification and clinical monitoring

C. Risk reduction by working for clean air and environmental issues at a public health level

D. Active management of comorbidities in addition to COPD symptoms, especially in older adults.

REFERENCES

American Thoracic Society. (1962). Chronic bronchitis, asthma and pulmonary emphysema: A statement by the Committee on Diagnostic Standards for Nontuberculous Respiratory Diseases. *American Review of Respiratory Disease, 85,* 762–768.

American Thoracic Society-European Respiratory Society. (2004). Standards for the diagnosis and management of patients with COPD. Retrieved from www.thoracic.org/clinical/copd-guidelines/index.php.

Balmes, J. R., & Speizer, F. E. (2015). Chapter 311: Occupational and environmental lung disease. In D. L. Kasper, A. S. Fauci, S. L. Hauser, D. L. Longo, J. L. Jameson, & J, Loscalzo (Eds.), *Harrison's principles of internal medicine* [Electronic version]. Retrieved from http://accessmedicine.mhmedical.com.ucsf.idm.oclc.org/ViewLarge.aspx?figid=79744941.

Bestall, J. C, Paul, E. A., Garrod, R., Garnham, R., Jones, P. W., & Wedzicha, J. A. (1999). Usefulness of the Medical Research Council (MRC) dyspnea scale as a measure of disability in patients with chronic obstructive pulmonary disease. *Thorax, 54,* 581–586.

Celli, B. R., Cote, C. G., Marin, J. M., Casanova, C., Montes de Oca, M., Mendez, R. A., et al. (2004). The body-mass index, airflow obstruction, dyspnea and exercise capacity index in chronic obstructive pulmonary disease. *New England Journal of Medicine, 350,* 1005–1012.

Centers for Disease Control and Prevention. (2012). Chronic obstructive pulmonary disease among adults—United States, 2011. *Morbidity and Mortality Weekly Report, 61*(46), 938–943.

Centers for Disease Control and Prevention. (2015a). COPD statistics. Retrieved from www.cdc.gov/copd/data.htm.

Centers for Disease Control and Prevention. (2015b). Pneumococcal vaccination. Retrieved from www.cdc.gov/vaccines/vpd-vac/pneumo/default.htm.

Decramer, M., De Benedetto, F., Del Ponte, A., & Marinari, S. (2005). Systemic effects of COPD. *Respiratory Medicine, 99,* S3–S10.

Global Initiative for Asthma. (2014). Diagnosis of diseases of chronic airflow limitation: Asthma, COPD and Asthma-COPD Overlap Syndrome (ACOS). Retrieved from www.goldcopd.org/asthma-copd-overlap.html.

Global Initiative for Chronic Obstructive Lung Disease. (2015). *Global strategy for the diagnosis, management, and prevention of chronic obstructive pulmonary disease. Update 2015.* Retrieved from www.goldcopd.org/guidelines-global-strategy-for-diagnosis-management.html.

Hurst, J. R, Vestbo, J., Anzueto, A., Locantore, N., Mullerova, H., Tal-Singer, R., et al. (2010). Susceptibility to exacerbation in chronic obstructive pulmonary disease. *New England Journal of Medicine, 363,* 1128–1138.

Jones, P. W., Hardy, G., Berry, P., Wiklund, I., Chen, W. H., & Lines Leidy, N. (2009). Development of the first validation of the COPD Assessment Test. *European Respiratory Journal, 34,* 648–654.

Maltais, F., Decramer, M., Casaburi, R., Barrioer, E., Burelle, Y., Debigare, R., et al. (2014). An official American Thoracic Society/European Respiratory Society statement: Update on limb muscle dysfunction in chronic obstructive pulmonary disease. *American Journal of Respiratory and Critical Care Medicine, 189*(9), e15–e62.

Tilert, T., Paulose-Ram, R., & Brody, D. J. (2015). Lung obstruction among adults aged 40–79: United States, 2007–2012 (NCHS Data Brief No. 180). Hyattsville, MD: National Center for Health Statistics. Retrieved from www.cdc.gov/nchs/data/databriefs/db180.pdf.

CHRONIC NONMALIGNANT PAIN MANAGEMENT

JoAnne M. Saxe, Nicole Una, and Kellie McNerney

I. Introduction and general background

In this chapter, the authors examine nonpharmacologic treatments, nonopioid medications, and the use of chronic opioid medication for the management of chronic nonmalignant pain (CNP). If nonpharmacologic agents and nonopiates fail to relieve pain, the subsequent use of opioids may be indicated. According to the 2009 American Pain Society Guidelines, "evidence is limited, but chronic pain can be effectively treated with chronic opioid therapy" (Chou et al., 2009, p. 1).

We also discuss patient selection concerns related to chronic opioid therapy; risk evaluation, a strategy to initiate and monitor chronic opioid therapy; and related informed consent and safety issues. One difficulty of managing opioid therapy for CNP patients is that clients may present with a history of risk behaviors or a potential for or history of substance abuse (Passik & Weinreb, 2000). Definitions of substance use, including dependence, addiction, pseudoaddiction, substance abuse, physical dependence, and tolerance are important for review and are included in **Figure 50-1** (Federation of State Medical Boards of the United States, 2004). Patients with substance abuse history do have chronic pain, perhaps at a higher prevalence than the general population, but there are few studies that document this (Rosenblum et al., 2003). This chapter provides guidelines based on the American Pain Society (Chou et al., 2009) and the Medical Board of California (2014) recommendations for chronic opioid therapy, so that patients in higher risk populations, including those with histories of substance abuse, can be safely treated.

The goal of therapy for the clinician is to provide adequate management of CNP in a timely, safe, and effective manner for the patient. The goals of therapy for many individuals with CNP often includes maximizing self-care strategies for pain management and control, optimizing function, and preventing untoward outcomes related to chronic pain (Caudill, 2009; Saxe et al., 2009, Saxe, Smith, & McNerney, 2013).

A. Definition and overview

The International Association for the Study of Pain defines pain as "an unpleasant sensory and emotional experience associated with actual or potential tissue damage, or described in terms of such damage. Pain is always subjective. Each individual learns the application of the word through experiences related to injury in early life" (IASP, 2012, para. 2). IASP further describes the subjective nature of pain as "Many people report[ing] pain in the absence of tissue damage or any likely pathophysiological cause; usually this happens for psychological reasons" (IASP, 2012, para 1). "If they regard their experience as pain and if they report it in the same ways as pain caused by tissue damage, it should be accepted as pain. This definition avoids tying pain to the stimulus" (IASP, 2012, para 2).

Chronic pain is generally defined as "pain which persists beyond the normal tissue healing time" With nonmalignant pain, three months is the most convenient point of division between acute and chronic pain" (IASP, 2014, p. 4). Some authors, however, use 6 months as the duration needed to meet the definition of chronic pain (Barclay & Nghiem, 2008; Bedard, 1997; Chou et al., 2009). Chronic pain may occur in the context of numerous diseases and syndromes. For the purpose of this guideline, all chronic pain disorders outside of cancer pain are referred to as CNP.

Chronic pain syndrome is a condition in which a client's pain "consumes and incapacitates his/her life to the point that the pain and suffering becomes his/her main focus" (Saxe et al., 2009, p. 1). Anxiety and depression are common comorbidities, and the client often has difficulty with work and personal life (Saxe, Smith, & McNerney, 2013; Yalcin & Barrot, 2014). Examples of CNP include but are not limited to osteoarthritis, rheumatoid arthritis, trigeminal and postherpetic neuralgia, fibromyalgia, myofascial pain, low back pain, peripheral neuropathy, phantom limb pain, reflex sympathetic dystrophy, sickle cell disease, temporomandibular joint dysfunction,

FIGURE 50-1 Definition of Terms

Addiction is "a primary, chronic disease of brain reward, motivation, memory and related circuitry. Dysfunction in these circuits leads to characteristic biological, psychological, social and spiritual manifestations. This is reflected in an individual pathologically pursuing reward and/or relief by substance use and other behaviors. Addiction is characterized by inability to consistently abstain, impairment in behavioral control, craving, diminished recognition of significant problems with one's behaviors and interpersonal relationships, and a dysfunctional emotional response. Like other chronic diseases, addiction often involves cycles of relapse and remission. Without treatment or engagement in recovery activities, addiction is progressive and can result in disability or premature death" (American Society of Addiction Medicine, 2011).

Pseudoaddiction is the "iatrogenic syndrome resulting from the misinterpretation of relief seeking behaviors as though they are drug-seeking behaviors that are commonly seen with substance use disorders. The relief seeking behaviors resolve upon institution of effective analgesic therapy" (Federation of State Medical Boards of the United States, 2004).

Physical dependence "is a state of biologic adaptation that is evidenced by a class-specific withdrawal syndrome when the drug is abruptly discontinued or the dose rapidly reduced, and/or by the administration of an antagonist."

Signs of substance abuse and dependence may include some or all of following:

- Manipulative or abusive behavior directed at caregivers, including intimidation or coercion and aimed at acquisition and continuance of the substance abuse
- Evidence of compulsive drug use, such as unsanctioned dose increases or unapproved uses despite side effects
- Chaotic psychosocial history
- Involvement with the law
- Diversion for sale or misuse of controlled substances
- Urine drug screening with aberrancies from prescribed medications (Medical Board of California, 2014)
- Signs of poor personal habits, activities of independent living, or social dysfunction
- Physical or emotional deterioration and deconditioning
- *Tolerance* "is a state of physiologic adaptation in which exposure to a drug induces changes that result in diminution of one or more of the drug's effects over time. Tolerance is common in opioid treatment, has been demonstrated following a single dose of opioids, and is not the same as addiction."

Data from Federation of State Medical Boards of the United States. (2004).

---

chronic abdominal pain from such conditions as Crohn's disease or chronic pancreatitis, and headaches, including cluster, tension, and migraine.

B. Prevalence and costs

The prevalence of chronic pain in the general population of the United States has been estimated at between 10% and 35% or 70–105 million people (Rosenblum et al., 2003; Turk, 2006). Chronic pain affects about 100 million American adults, more than the total affected by heart disease, cancer and diabetes combined (Institute of Medicine [IOM], 2011). An international survey of chronic pain revealed an overall prevalence of chronic pain as 22% of the population (Rosenblum et al., 2003). Significant financial burden is attributed to this syndrome because of loss of productivity and disability and the direct cost of physician visits and medication treatment

(Turk, 2006). Costs associated with chronic pain have been estimated to be $635 billion each year in medical treatment and lost productivity (IOM, 2011).

II. Database (may include but is not limited to)

A. Subjective

1. History of the presenting complaint

   The history of the presenting symptom should include the identification of pain: its source onset, location, radiation, duration, characteristics, alleviating factors, aggravating factors, treatments tried, and the response to treatments. The significance of

FIGURE 50-2 CNP Client Pain Questionnaire

1. Please tell us about your pain:

   - Where is your pain? _____
   - When did it start? _____
   - How often do you have this pain? _____
   - What do you think caused your pain? _____
   - How would you rate your pain on a scale of 1 to 10 (1 being mild pain and 10 being the worst pain ever)?

     _____

   - Describe your pain (check all that apply):

     ❑ Stabbing   ❑ Throbbing   ❑ Aching   ❑ Burning

     ❑ Pins and needles   ❑ Other _____

2. What helps your pain? _____

3. Does your pain interfere with any of the following activities (check all that apply)?

   ❑ Work   ❑ Household chores   ❑ Exercising   ❑ Shopping

   ❑ Self-care activities (bathing, dressing, preparing food)   ❑ Sex

   ❑ Relationships with family and friends   ❑ Recreational activities

   ❑ Other _____

4. Please check all of the activities below that are limited because of your pain:

   ❑ Standing   ❑ Walking   ❑ Sitting   ❑ Turning/twisting

   ❑ Raising your arms/legs   ❑ Repeated arm/hand use (using a computer, etc.)

   ❑ Other _____

5. Does your pain interfere with your energy level?   ❑ Yes   ❑ No

6. How many hours do you sleep at night? _____ During the day? _____

7. What treatments have you received for your pain?

8. What medications have you taken for your pain, including ones you are taking now?

9. What tests have you had to find out the cause of your pain?

Reproduced from Hockenberry, M. J., & Wilson, D. (2009). *Wong's essentials of pediatric nursing* (9th ed.). St. Louis, MO: Mosby. Used with permission. Copyright Mosby.

pain (i.e., impact on work, relationships, and activities of daily living) should also be assessed. Pain and functional scales can be helpful in measuring the subjective report of pain (**Figure 50-2**). Note: Because pain and related functional assessments are challenging to assess in nonverbal individuals, such as persons affected by advanced dementia, behavioral pain assessment tools or surrogate pain reports will need to be used (Herr et al., 2006). See the Objective section for additional details.

2. Past health history
    a. Medical and psychiatric illnesses, surgical history, hospitalizations, and physical and psychological trauma in relation to the pain syndrome
    b. Medications: current and history of medications
    c. Medication allergies and drug interactions
3. Family history of chronic pain and mental health disorders.
4. Occupational history: if pain occurred as a result of a job injury, note any related litigation issues, present ability to work, and goals for work in the future.
5. Psychosocial history: to include substance abuse screening. A tool, such as the CAGE-AID (Brown & Rounds, 1995) or equivalent tool, may be used. The CAGE-AID can be downloaded from www.cqaimh.org/pdf/tool_cageaid.pdf.
6. Review of systems
    a. Constitutional signs and symptoms: fatigue or weight gain
    b. Skin: scar tissue including trauma or surgical scars
    c. Cardiac: chest pain or arrhythmias (assessing risk for side effects or contraindication to medications including opiates)
    d. Respiratory: shortness of breath and sleep apnea (assessing risk for side effects or contraindications to opiates)
    e. Gastrointestinal: constipation
    f. Musculoskeletal: joint erythema, swelling and/or warmth, pain, decreased range of motion, arthralgias, myalgias, stiffness, and muscle wasting
    g. Neurologic: paresthesias, dysthesias, abnormal gait, muscle strength, symmetry, mood disorders, depression, and anxiety

B. Objective

1. The physical examination: focus on the areas affected, which typically includes the completion of musculoskeletal and neurologic examinations. The initial examination should also include a baseline cardiopulmonary examination, especially if opioids will be considered in the future.
2. Diagnostics
    a. Pain assessment includes behavioral, functional, mood, and substance use and abuse and opioid risk assessment tools. For example:
        i. Pain and function assessment: CNP Client Pain Questionnaire (see Figure 50-2) is especially useful during an initial evaluation. The PEG (pain intensity [P], interference with enjoyment of life [E], and interference with general activity [G]) Scale (Krebs et al., 2009) is valuable for repeated and brief pain assessments. All items are weighted on a scale of 0 (no pain or major interference, respectively) to 10 (severe to major interference, respectively). The PEG Scale can be accessed at https://openi.nlm.nih.gov/detailedresult.php?img=2686775_11606_2009_981_Fig1_HTML&req=4.

For elderly individuals who are nonverbal, assessment tools have been developed to evaluate their pain (Herr et al., 2006). One such tool is the Pain Assessment Scale for Seniors with Severe Dementia that includes an assessment of facial expressions, social/personality/mood indicators, activity/body movement, and physiological indicators/eating/sleeping changes/vocal behaviors (Fuchs-Lacelle & Hadjistavropoulos, 2004). For depression screening, use the Patient Health Questionnaire–9 (Spitzer, Kroenke, & Williams, 1999) or equivalent resource. (The Patient Health Questionnaire–9 can be accessed at http://www.integration.samhsa.gov/images/res/PHQ%20-%20Questions.pdf.)
        ii. Substance use and abuse risk: CAGE-AID (Can be accessed at www.cqaimh.org/pdf/tool_cageaid.pdf.)
        iii. Opioid risk assessment: Opioid Risk Tool (Webster & Webster, 2005) (see **Figure 50-3**)
    b. Obtain a baseline electrocardiogram for QTc interval measurement before methadone administration (Cohen & Mao, 2009; Krantz, Martin, Stimmel, Metha, & Haigney, 2009).
    c. Review pertinent laboratory studies and imaging or other radiologic examinations.
    d. Review any other relevant past medical documents or diagnostic tests.

III. Assessment

A. Determine the diagnosis with appropriate International Classification of Diseases –10 codes (www.icd10data.com/) (e.g., chronic primary osteoarthritis of the right hip: M16.11)

Date_____

Patient Name_____

OPIOID RISK TOOL

		Mark each box that applies	Item Score If Female	Item Score If Male
1. Family History of Substance Abuse	Alcohol	☐	1	3
	Illegal Drugs	☐	2	3
	Prescription Drugs	☐	4	4
2. Personal History of Substance Abuse	Alcohol	☐	3	3
	Illegal Drugs	☐	4	4
	Prescription Drugs	☐	5	5
3. Age (Mark box if age 16–45)		☐	1	1
4. History of Preadolescent Sexual Abuse		☐	3	0
5. Psychological Disease	Attention Deficit Disorder, Obsessive Compulsive Disorder, Bipolar, Schizophrenia	☐	2	2
	Depression	☐	1	1
	TOTAL		_____	_____

Total Score Risk Category
Low Risk 0–3
Moderate Risk 4–7
High Risk ≥ 8

FIGURE 50-3 Opioid Risk Tool

Reproduced from Webster, L.R., & Webster, R. (2005). Predicting aberrant behaviors in opioid-treated patients: preliminary validation of the Opioid Risk Tool. *Pain Med* 6(6):432.

B. *Severity*

Assess severity of symptoms (e.g., "moderate pain with frequent episodes of severe pain related to activity interfering with sleep and ability to work").

C. *Significance and motivation*

Assess significance of diagnosis in relation to functional capacity, mood, and support systems. Determine the client's strengths, ability to follow the treatment plan, and risk for nonadherence and/or substance misuse

IV. Goals of clinical management

Focus on the patient's desired goals and expected outcomes, which may include but are not limited to:

A. *Improve and maximize functioning in relationships, at work, or at home*

B. *Decrease related depression and anxiety*

C. *Minimize pain and pain-related distress and disability*

D. Minimize adverse effects and/or associated risks from pain management strategies

V. Plan (interventions and ongoing approach to care)

A. Nonmedication strategies include but are not limited to:

1. Cognitive behavioral therapy
   a. Stress reduction
   b. Relaxation techniques
   c. Attention diversion
   d. Goal setting
   e. Pain and symptom diary

2. Physical activity and physical therapy

3. Transcutaneous electrical nerve stimulation unit for neuropathic pain

4. Heat and cold therapies

5. Pain support group

6. Acupuncture

7. Massage

8. Guided imagery techniques

9. Laugh therapy and laugh yoga (Barclay & Nghiem, 2008; Buckhardt et al., 2005; Caudill, 2009; Keefe, Somers, & Kothadia, 2009)

B. Nonopiate medication strategies (Barclay & Nghiem, 2008; Caudill, 2009)

1. Acetaminophen: for mild to moderate pain 325 mg one to two tablets, four times daily, not to exceed 3 g/day; 2g/day for the elderly. Caution with liver disease, alcohol use, hepatitis, and use of other medications metabolized by the liver.

2. Nonsteroidal anti-inflammatory drugs (NSAIDs): for mild to moderate pain, may use in conjunction with acetaminophen. Examples include ibuprofen, 400–800 mg every 6–8 hours yet not to exceed a total of 2,400 mg per 24 hours; diflunisal, 500–1,000 mg twice daily; or naproxen, 250–500 mg twice daily. If one class fails, consider switching to another class of NSAIDs (e.g., switching from a nonselective cyclooxygenase inhibitor (e.g., ibuprofen) to a salicylic acid derivative (e.g., trilisate propionic acids) or a selective cyclooxygenase inhibitor (e.g., celecoxib). It is important to review the specific medication because dose and timing vary depending on the medication. Note the precautions associated with hypertension, coronary artery disease, diabetes, benign prostatic hypertrophy, and individuals older than 50 years of age. NSAIDs are contraindicated in patients with a history of gastrointestinal ulcer disease and chronic kidney disease.

3. Topical analgesic creams and patches: Appropriate for mild to moderate pain; may be used in conjunction with acetaminophen and NSAIDs. Dose varies and is dependent on analgesia desired and person's response. Examples include lidocaine 5% patches, up to three patches to the affected area at once for 12 hours within a 24-hour period; and lidocaine 4% cream or capsaicin cream 0.025–0.075%, applied to the affected area up to three to four times daily.

4. Antidepressants: chronic pain can cause depression or may worsen depression. Additionally, depression can worsen with chronic pain. As such, antidepressants may be a useful adjunctive therapy.

   Tricyclic antidepressants are helpful for neuropathic pain disorders and associated sleep disturbances. A baseline electrocardiogram is indicated before initiating this classification of medication to assess for any conduction abnormalities because they may cause arrhythmias. Start with a low dose and titrate up over several weeks.

   Serotonin-norepinephrine reuptake inhibitors (SNRIs), e.g., duloxetine and venlafaxine, may also be effective in the management of pain and depression. Because SNRIs may cause an increase in blood pressure, the person's blood pressure should be well controlled before initiating an SNRI. Additionally, duloxetine should not be used in persons with current liver impairment or risk of liver impairment, given reports of fatal hepatotoxicity (eMedExpert, 2007—2014). As with tricyclics, SNRIs should be titrated. They should not be abruptly discontinued given the risk for withdrawal signs and symptoms (may include but not limited to nausea, dizziness, irritability, and insomnia).

   Some antidepressants can change the potency of opiates. Be certain to check for medication interactions.

5. Anticonvulsants: These medications have been used for neuropathic pain, such as diabetic neuropathy and postherpetic neuralgias. Examples include gabapentin, 300–600 mg three times a day. Start at 300 mg at bedtime, titrate up by 300 mg weekly. Use with caution in renal insufficiency. Pregabalin (Lyrica®) can be started at 25–75 mg twice per day dependent on the severity of pain. Pregabalin may be titrated up to 450 mg/day in divided doses. Adjustments for renal impairment are indicated. Refer to reliable drug resources for dosing adjustment guidelines.

6. Other adjunctive medications: muscle relaxants. Examples include baclofen, 10–20 mg three times daily, or cyclobenzeprine, 5–10 mg three times daily. Avoid carisoprodol (Soma®) because of abuse potential and availability of other muscle relaxants.

C. Opiates

1. Standards for prescribing controlled substances
The clinician follows the accepted standards for prescribing controlled substances. For example, in the state of California, nurse practitioners and nurse midwives are expected to follow Standardized Procedures for Controlled Substances (**Figure 50-4**).

2. Starting opiates
The following recommendations for starting opiates, if indicated, are based on the American Pain Society-American Academy of Pain Medicine's clinical guidelines for the use of chronic opioid therapy in chronic noncancer pain (Chou et al., 2009) and the Medical Board of California's (2014) guidelines for prescribing controlled substances for pain.

a. New clients require sufficient visits to complete a full history and physical and to review all prior medical records, pain and functioning questionnaires, depression and substance abuse screenings with appropriate laboratory studies, imaging, and urine drug screen, and if available, a state prescription drug monitoring program (PMP) report. In the state of California, the Department of Justice compiles a record of all Schedule II through IV prescriptions so pharmacists and prescribers can access the database called Controlled Substance Utilization Review and Evaluation System (CURES) (California Department of Justice, 2014). PMPs are increasingly used nationally in pain management and frequently used by providers before initiating a controlled medication prescription. This reporting is designed to prevent individuals from obtaining multiple controlled prescriptions in 1 month, prevent dangerous mixing of medications, and decrease the potential for misuse.

b. A mental health evaluation visit is recommended during the establishment of care. Opiates are not prescribed until these procedures are complete and 30 days have passed. Exceptions can be made if the provider has access to the patient's previous records and, ideally, have been approved by a chronic pain treatment team.

c. Existing patients receiving primary care may be given a trial of opioid therapy before enrolling in the CNP protocol if the primary care provider deems the patient is a candidate for opioid therapy. If the provider believes therapy will be chronic, the provider obtains and completes the same pain questionnaire, depression, substance abuse, and opioid risk screening required for adherence to the protocol (see Figures 50-2 and 50-3).

d. Enrollment in a CNP protocol is indicated if the clinician deems that opioid therapy is appropriate for care. The following matters are discussed with the patient and family in depth, including a signed and agreed-upon CNP treatment agreement plan (see **Figure 50-5**):

i. The prescribed treatment plan, which includes a discussion about associated risks and benefits of opioid treatment, medications to be used, nonopioid therapies to be pursued, and the follow-up interval.

ii. Patient expectations and responsibilities including keeping appointments, adherence to treatment plans, obtaining medications from a single provider, single pharmacy, feedback to provider, and legal issues including diversion.

iii. How to take the medication and importance of dosing and timing of dose and interaction with other medications.

iv. Potential adverse effects of treatment with opioid medication include safety and recommending not driving or operating equipment until the patient is tolerant of the medication regime. Other adverse effects include the potential for altered mentation, respiratory depression, and arrhythmias, and the risk of death if used incorrectly or in conjunction with other substances.

v. Risk of overdose, signs of overdose (see **Figure 50-6**), and a rapid response to an actual and potential overdose.

vi. Prophylactic treatment for constipation caused by opiates, because untreated constipation can worsen back and abdominal pain.

vii. Random urine testing is required for all patients on opioid therapy (at initiation, randomly, or at least annually). Because the interpretation of urine tests is frequently misunderstood, providing interpretation guides and training for all providers is strongly recommended. Gourlay, Heit, and Caplan (2010) have noted important details related to this matter at http://issuu.com/cafamilydocs/docs/udtmonograph.

viii. The procedure for CNP protocol treatment agreement, and minor and major agreement breaks, is reviewed including consequences of breaks (for example, evidence of drug

FIGURE 50-4 *Furnishing and Ordering Controlled Substances from Schedule II–V at the UCSF DCHS Faculty Practices*

I. **POLICY:**

   A. Only approved nurse practitioners with current furnishing licenses and DEA registration for ordering schedule II–V CS may furnish these drugs and devices.

   B. The qualified nurse practitioner may initiate, alter, discontinue, and renew category II–V CS (see addendum) included in the UCSF DCHS Faculty Practices Formulary.

   C. As described in the Policies and in the "Furnishing/Ordering Drugs and Devices by Nurse Practitioners" Standardized Procedure.

II. **PROTOCOL**

   A. Definition: This protocol covers the management of Schedule II–V CS for all adults and children seen in the UCSF DCHS Faculty Practices with the following conditions, illnesses, diseases:

      1. Acute traumatic injuries,

      2. Acute infections (e.g., pyelonephritis),

      3. Acute and chronic musculoskeletal disorders,

      4. Acute and chronic neurological disorders (e.g., migraines),

      5. Chronic psychological disorders (e.g., ADHD),

      6. Acute urological conditions (e.g., renal calculi), and/or

      7. Post-surgical pain.

   B. Subjective Data: Subjective information will include but is not limited to:

      1. Relevant health history to warrant the use of the drug or device.

      2. No allergic history to the drug or device.

      3. No past health, family and/or personal-social history, which are an absolute and/or potential for contra-indication to the use of the drug or device.

   C. Objective: Objective information will include but is not limited to:

      1. A physical examination to indicate/contraindicate the use of the drug and/or device.

      2. Diagnostics: Laboratory tests or procedures to determine the underlying etiology of pain and/or to indicate/contraindicate use of the drug and/or device, if needed.

   D. Assessment: Subjective and objective data supports the use of the drug and/or device. Contraindications, safety issues, and/or cost concerns have been adequately assessed and documented.

   E. Management:

      1. Diagnostics: Ordering relevant laboratory/diagnostic studies.

      2. Treatment:

         a. The following controlled substances may be used:

            i. Opioid agonists (For example but not limited to: Morphine, morphine controlled–release, hydromorphone, levorphanol, meperidine, methadone, oxymorphone, fentanyl, buprenorphine, tramadol, codeine (with or without aspirin or acetaminophen), hydrocodone, oxycodone or oxycodone controlled-release): Use the guidelines noted in the current UCSF DCHS Faculty Practices Formulary Guidelines for drug dosage, frequency, route of administration. Schedule II opioid agonist analgesics should be reserved for severe, incapacitating pain. Schedule III opioid agonists should be used for moderate to severe pain.

            ii. Stimulants (For example but not limited to: Mixed salts of dextroamphetamine and amphetamines, dextroamphetamine sulfate, atomoxetine, methylphenidate, and pemoline): Use the guidelines noted in the current UCSF DCHS Faculty Practices Formulary Guidelines.

      3. Drug/device order: Write a separate drug order for each Schedule II–V CS on anti-fraud prescription form. (Note: Telephone orders are acceptable for Schedule III through V CS.) Each order needs to include:

         a. Name, age, telephone number, and the medical record number of the client,

         b. Name of the medication/device,

         c. Dosage, frequency, route, duration of the use, amount; and number of refills of the drug/device (Note: CS II may not be refilled. Schedule III CS may only be filled 5 times in a 6 month period),

    d.   Brief statement regarding the reason for using the drug/device, and

    e.   Printed name, furnishing number, DEA number and signature of the nurse practitioner

4. Supportive/Adjunctive Therapy:

    a.   Consider using tricyclic antidepressants, sustained-release bupropion, or anticonvulsants for neuropathic pain since these medications may be more effective in managing the pain as compared to opioids.

    b.   Recommend non-pharmacologic therapies (e.g., thermal therapy, massage, physical therapy, chiropractic, acupuncture, and meditation) as indicated since these modalities may be useful in pain management.

5. Client Education:

    a.   Provide the client and/or the client's caregiver with the information and counseling in regards to the action and use of the drug/device. Caution the client and/or the client's caregiver on the pertinent side effects and complications with the chosen drug/device. Advise on how to communicate with the Clinic staff should s/he have any questions/concerns/side effects/complications.

6. Physician Consultation/Referral:

Consult or refer to physician if the client is:

    a.   Unresponsive to the drug/device therapy,

    b.   Demonstrating unusual or unexpected side effects,

    c.   Known to have a history of CS and/or alcohol abuse; and as indicated in the general policy section.

7. Follow-up: In accordance with standard practice or with consulting physician's recommendation.

8. Record keeping: As described in General Policies.

Addendum

Federal Controlled Substance Law

Federal Controlled Substance Law: The Federal Controlled Substances Act of 1970 recognized five schedules of drugs based upon their relative abuse potential (Note: California State regulatory requirements have been added.) The lists of schedules for controlled substances are updated annually and can be accessed at http://www.deadiversion.usdoj.gov/21cfr/cfr/2108cfrt.htm

Class I: Drugs with no current medical application and maximum abuse potential. Examples: Heroin, lysergic acid diethylamide (LSD), marijuana, 3, 4 methylenedioxymethamphetamine (MDMA [Ecstasy]).

Class II: Includes opioid analgesics (e.g., codeine, hydrocodone, morphine, methadone and oxycodone), stimulants (e.g., dextroamphetamine, cocaine, methylphenidate), and depressants (e.g., pentobarbital). Facsimile of Schedule II CS permitted under certain circumstances (e.g., hospice care). Facsimile for emergency dispensing must be followed up with a written and signed transmittal order within 7 days. Refills are prohibited.

Class III: Buprenorphine; codeine (Not more than 1.8 grams of codeine per 100 milliliters or not more than 90 milligrams per dosage unit) and other opioids in lower doses than class II controlled substances along with non-narcotic agents May communicate to pharmacist Schedule III-V CS prescriptions/transmittal orders either orally, in writing, or by facsimile. May refill Schedule III-IV's 5 times in 6 months; and refills of Schedule V's as noted by the practitioner.

Class IV: Benzodiazepines (e.g., Valium®, Ativan®, Xanax®, Klonopin®), stimulants such as phentermine. Written prescription required, up to 5 refills allowed within 6 months of issuance for this class. In August 2014, Tramadol was classified as Schedule IV due to possible abuse potential.

Class V: Low-dose controlled substances containing non-narcotic active medicinal ingredients (e.g., Cough medicines with codeine in low dose (Robitussin-AC®). May refill Schedule III-IV's 5 times in 6 months; and refills of Schedule V's as noted by the practitioner.

IMPORTANT: Refills for schedule II medications or future dated prescriptions are not allowed by the Drug Enforcement Agency.

Data from State of California Board of Registered Nursing, 1998, 2004a, 2004b; University of California San Francisco [UCSF], Department of Community Health Systems [DCHS], 2010, 2015; U.S. Department of Justice, Drug Enforcement Agency, 2014.

FIGURE 50-5 Pain Management Agreement

Glide Health Services
330 Ellis Street
San Francisco, CA 94102

The purpose of this agreement is to prevent misunderstandings about certain medicines you will be taking for pain management or other medical conditions. This agreement will help both you and your provider comply with laws regarding controlled pharmaceuticals.

I. *Client Name* and *Provider Name* have decided together to use a controlled substance for management of pain or other medical condition.

MEDICATION	INSTRUCTIONS	AMOUNT PER WEEK/MONTH

✓ I agree that this medication will only be used by myself and as it is prescribed.

✓ I will not share, sell or trade my medication with anyone.

✓ I will safeguard my medication from loss or theft. Lost or stolen medicine may not be replaced.

✓ If I run out of the medication, Glide Health Services may not refill the prescription early.

✓ I will not seek controlled substances from other medical providers.

✓ I understand that there will be no refills on my medications without a provider visit at Glide.

✓ I agree to share my complete medications history in order to avoid adverse drug interactions.

✓ I will attend all my scheduled appointments, including any referral appointments my clinician has made for me, and follow up as designated in my plan of care.

✓ I agree to bring all unused pain medication to every office visit.

✓ I understand pharmacy records may be reviewed to confirm prescriptions.

✓ I understand I may be required to have random urine or blood testing completed. I agree to this testing, and understand that if I fail to do so, I will be safely tapered off the medication(s).

✓ I understand if I break this agreement, my provider may stop prescribing these pain medicines.

✓ I understand that many pain medicines may cause drowsiness and impair my ability to drive and operate machinery and may impair my thinking and judgment.

✓ I understand that misuse of these drugs or use of these drugs in combination with alcohol, unauthorized prescription medications, or illicit drugs may have serious effects including death.

✓ The prescribing provider has explained that the above medications have possible side effects and may be addictive.

Comments:

_____

_____

_____

_____   _____
Client's Signature   *Date*

_____   _____
Provider Signature   *Date*

FIGURE 50-6 Signs of Opiate Overdose

- Extreme sleepiness with an inability to awaken the person verbally or with vigorous movement (e.g., sternal rubbing)
- Slow respirations (<12 respirations/minute) and/or shallow breathing
- Vomiting
- Cyanosis of the digits and/or lips
- Constricted pupils
- Bradycardia and/or hypotension

treatment completion or 6-month waiting period before being reconsidered to resume opiate management).

3. Subsequent evaluations

Subsequent visits are determined by the clinician but initially may be monthly. More frequent visits may be required at the provider's discretion. Exceptions may be made for low-risk clients with stable housing situations. These low-risk patients should be seen every 2–3 months at a minimum. The provider makes this determination after at least 2 months of contact and assessment.

a. All patients leave a urine sample on monthly or routine follow-up visits, but it is up to the provider to determine if urine toxicology screens are done randomly on that visit (Chou et al., 2009; Saxe et al., 2009).

b. Clinical encounters include an assessment of:
    i. Pain: intensity and response to treatment plan (Figure 50-2)
    ii. Adverse events and side effects of therapy
    iii. Activity and functioning level to evaluate efficacy of treatment plan
    iv. Adherence to essential components of treatment agreement is documented with nonadherence to plan of care and documentation of minor or major agreement break on the problem list. Specific plans for addressing agreement breaks should be discussed and documented. For example, a setting may consider adopting the following approach: any client with more than two major agreement breaks or three minor breaks will be referred for evaluation to a CNP team to determine appropriate action to follow.

c. Refills of medications are documented in the electronic health record or paper chart to include date, name of opiate, dose, instructions for use, quantity prescribed, and number of refills. The patient brings all pain medication bottles to each and every visit at the request of the provider.

d. One primary provider writes prescriptions. In their absence, an alternate or covering provider is determined. This arrangement is reviewed with the patient.

e. Refills on controlled substances should be done during the visit with only enough medication to last until the next visit.

f. Refills are not completed without an appointment or over the telephone.

g. Lost medications or stolen medications should not be replaced and recorded as a major agreement break. With rare exceptions, providers do not routinely refill lost or stolen medications. Exceptions by provider discretion require documentation of the rationale, and the incident must be recorded as a minor agreement break.

h. A treatment plan for addressing adverse effects is discussed and documented.

4. Medication considerations

a. Note contraindications to opioid therapy
    i. Absolute contraindications
        a. Allergy to opiate agents
        b. Coadministration of drug capable of inducing life-threatening drug–drug interaction
        c. Active diversion of controlled substances
        d. Unwillingness or inability to comply with treatment plan
        e. Unwillingness to adjust at-risk activities that may result in serious injury/re-injury
    ii. Relative contraindications (prescribe with caution and more intensive monitoring)
        a. Meets criteria for current substance use disorder (e.g., as noted by the *Diagnostic and Statistical Manual of Mental Disorders*-5 [American Psychological Association, 2013])
        b. Acute psychiatric instability or high suicide risk
        c. History of intolerance, serious adverse effects, or lack of efficacy of opioid therapy
        d. Inability to manage opioid therapy responsibly (i.e., cognitive impairment; without stable and reliable caregiver or social support network)

e. Severe social instability or inability to manage medications safely

f. Client with sleep apnea not on continuous positive airway pressure machine

g. Elderly clients particularly without stable and reliable caregiver or social support network

b. Assess and address common adverse effects of opioid therapy: constipation, nausea and vomiting, itching, sweating, peripheral edema, urinary retention, myoclonus, hyperalgesia, dyspepsia, changes in cognition, perceptual or affective adverse effects, or sexual dysfunction.

c. Short-acting opiates: Short-acting medications should generally not be the mainstay of chronic pain treatment. Short-acting medications are not recommended for chronic pain because of high-risk metabolites (e.g., meperidine/Demerol®); low efficacy (e.g., propoxyphene/Darvocet®); or risk of rebound headaches (e.g., butalbital/Fioricet®). Note: Potency varies considerably; see analgesic comparison tables at www.global-rph.com/narcoticonv.htm for assistance with converting from one opiate to another, and converting short-acting to long-acting opiates (McAuley, 2015). Cost varies considerably; many are now available as a generic. Types of short-acting opiates are noted on **Table 50-1**.

However, short-acting medications for CNP may be appropriate in the following situations:

i. To manage pain until the correct dose of long-acting medications is determined, and then the short-acting medications can be discontinued.

ii. To assist with titrating the patient off of or down from longstanding opiate regimes.

iii. To manage predictable pain flares (long travel or before exercise, dental appointments, and so forth)

iv. To manage chronic pain in patients who do not need high doses of medications (e.g., elderly patients may do well with hydrocodone/acetaminophen, 5/325 mg half a tablet four times daily on a schedule, plus half a tablet as needed for additional pain)

d. Long-acting opiates: Long-acting medications should be the primary therapy for patients using opiates for chronic pain. For all patients (especially the elderly), start with low doses and build up slowly, because sedation and respiratory depression can occur with too-rapid dose escalation. Types of long-acting opiates are provided in **Table 50-2**.

e. Changing from short-acting to long-acting medications: Changing from short-acting to long-acting medications is the standard of care for chronic pain, because short-acting medications have increased dependence, addiction potential, and increased street value with an increased risk of diversion. Short-acting opiates also may not control baseline pain and require a greater total dose of medications to control pain (Chou et al., 2009). Equianalgesic tables provide helpful guidelines with the conversion of dosing

TABLE 50-1 Short-Acting Opiates

Medication	Strengths	Comments
Hydrocodone combined with acetaminophen or ibuprofen	5-, 7.5-, and 10-mg tablets	Caution: keep acetaminophen dose at or under 3,000 mg daily, or 2,000 mg daily in the elderly
Oxycodone combined with acetaminophen or aspirin	2.5-, 5-, 7.5-, and 10-mg	Also available in extended release. Caution: keep acetaminophen dose under 4,000 mg daily, or 2,000 mg in the elderly. Approximately 10% of patients do not metabolize oxycodone well and will not get effective pain relief; consider changing opiates if there is a poor response (Chou et al., 2009).
Codeine combined with acetaminophen	30/300 or 60/300	Caution: keep acetaminophen dose at or under 3,000 mg daily, or 2,000 mg daily in the elderly.
Morphine	15 and 30 mg	Also available in long-acting form.
Hydromorphone	2, 4, and 8 mg	
Fentanyl transmucosal lozenge	100-, 200-, 400-, 600-, and 800-mcg buccal tablets	Typically used for cancer pain because of rapid action, occasionally used for chronic pain. It is expensive.
Oxymorphone	5 and 10 mg	Also available as extended release

TABLE 50-2 Long-Acting Opiates

Medication	Strengths	Comments
Morphine sulfate (sustained/extended release): examples include Kadian® and MS Contin®	Kadian® (sustained-release pellets in capsules): 10-, 20-, 30-, 50-, 60-, 80-, 100, and 200-mg capsules; MS Contin® (sustained-release tablets): 15-, 30-, 60-, 100, and 200-mg tablets	Dose varies by product, generally daily to twice a day. Often preferred by providers because diversion potential is lower.
Methadone	5- and 10-mg tablets	Methadone is an appropriate medication for severe pain for patients with CNP, even in opioid-tolerant patients. Titrate up very slowly because methadone has a very long and "highly variable" half-life (Chou et al., 2009). Get a baseline ECG to measure QTc interval, recommend a repeat in 30 days and an ECG early or more frequently at doses over 100 mg daily, because fatal arrhythmias can occur if patients develop long QTc intervals (Krantz et al., 2009). Safe starting dose for opioid-naive patient is 2.5 mg every 8 hours. Increase medication weekly, not more frequently. Use cautious titration and dosing (e.g., consider starting with half-tablets) in the elderly or patients with renal or hepatic dysfunction (Chou et al., 2009). Although withdrawal symptoms are prevented in daily dosing and the half-life is long, the pain relief is at most 8 hours; dosing must be at least every 8–12 hours when prescribing methadone for pain.
Oxycodone controlled release	10-, 15-, 20-, 30-, 40-, 60-, and 80-mg controlled-release tablets	10% of people do not metabolize this drug well, so they do not feel effective relief (Chou et al., 2009). Consider transition to another opiate for patients who request escalation of dose because of inadequate pain control. Considered to have a high street value.
Fentanyl patch	12, 25, 50, 75, and 100 mcg/h patch	The fentanyl patch is not indicated for opiate-naive patients. Change the patch every 48–72 hours (some patients report difficulty with adherence and pain relief after 48 hours). Start at lower doses and start cautiously because of the long half-life. Initial fentanyl transdermal doses are based on daily total morphine requirements for individuals already on opiates. The total daily dosing is then moderately reduced, usually 25–50% (Chou et al., 2009). Considered to have a high street value.
Hydromorphone	Has numerous strengths with short-acting and extended-release formulations	It is not commonly used in some community clinics.
Buprenorphine/naloxone combo: Suboxone	2- and 8-mg sublingual tablets	This opiate agonist–antagonist is not approved by the Food and Drug Administration for pain, yet some patients with mixed addiction and chronic pain do well on this option. Although prescribed for addiction, it can offer some pain relief for patients with CNP. Requires special Food and Drug Administration license and training.

between different types of opiates, yet they do not play a role in individual patient factors that influence safe dosing (Vissers, Besse, Hans, Devulder, & Morlion, 2010). As such, it has been recommended by notable authorities to reduce dosing on these tables by one-third to two-thirds of the stated dosing (Vissers et al., 2010). A well-referenced web-based opiate conversion chart can be found at http://www.globalrph.com/narcoticonv.htm (McAuley, 2015).

f. Dose Ceiling: Since 2010, several municipalities and clinics have implemented dose ceilings on opiates. These limits were a response to escalating rates of accidental overdose deaths, increased hyperalgesia among individuals receiving chronic opiates, and data revealing limited improvement of functionality with high doses of opiates among treatment recipients during the previous years. There is no national consensus on a precise ceiling dose at which opiates are no longer safe. The Medical Board of California (2014) issued recommendations that above 80 mg of morphine equivalents, a pain management specialist should be consulted before further dose escalation.

g. Indications to stop opiate therapy: Medication nonadherence or noncompliance with the pain agreement

   i. Institutions differ on the definition of agreement breaks and the consequences. At the authors' institution, the number of minor and major agreement breaks that require action is defined (Saxe et al., 2009). Examples of minor agreement breaks include missed appointments, early refill requests, seeking medications from another provider or different pharmacy, and not adhering to treatment agreement plans.

   ii. Major agreement breaks include refusal of urine toxicology screen, lost or stolen medications, drug screening (with high-sensitivity confirmation, such as gas chromatography) indicating that the prescribed medication is absent despite client statements of recent ingestion, client is abusive to staff, pill count discrepancy, or request for pill count is refused.

   iii. The institution has in place consequences of agreement breaks; for example, two major agreement breaks may be grounds for review by a CNP team and consideration for addiction referral and discontinuation of opioid therapy. Unless there

has been fraud or multiple prescribers, consider a standard policy of weaning as opposed to abrupt discontinuation. This increases the chance that the patient will continue to work with the team on other options (complementary treatments, behavioral therapy, and addiction treatment) as opposed to just seeking another provider, and it decreases the likelihood of emergency department visits for withdrawal symptoms. Pharmacies can be instructed to dispense small supplies at a time (a 1-, 3-, or 7-day supply) to assist the weaning plan (Saxe et al., 2009). A recommended weaning strategy is to decrease opiate dose by 10% every 3 days (Medical Board of California, 2014).

   iv. Inappropriate use of alcohol or illicit drugs may be considered a major agreement break or cause for termination. Some institutional flexibility may be spelled out per chronic pain team. For example, rather than termination, the client must agree to a mental health evaluation and commit to a drug treatment cessation program to continue treatment.

   v. Opioid therapy may be discontinued for patients with multiple minor agreement breaks or at the provider's discretion. Otherwise the patient is evaluated by the primary provider frequently until adherence problems have resolved. Final determination to address repetitive agreement breaks is made by a CNP team or medical director (Saxe et al., 2009).

   vi. Opioid therapy is discontinued when the therapy or side effects of the therapy are a greater detriment than benefit as determined by consultation with the client, family, and CNP team.

   vii. Opioid therapy is discontinued if evaluation demonstrates lack of efficacy, the client desires to discontinue therapy, or the cause of pain has resolved.

   viii. Opioid therapy is discontinued when there are serious safety issues as a result of treatment.

   ix. When opioid therapy is discontinued, opioid is tapered and weaned off, unless there is dangerous or illegal behavior. Strategies for tapering and weaning have been suggested by the Medical Board of California (2014). Opioid therapy should be immediately discontinued for unsafe use of medications, diversion of prescription of medication, or alteration or forgery of prescriptions. Provider should treat withdrawal symptoms with noncontrolled medications or refer for addiction counseling (Chou et al., 2009; Saxe et al., 2009).

    x. Clients that have been dismissed from opiate treatment for agreement breaks may not receive prescriptions for controlled substances from other providers at the same institution unless that client is first reviewed by a CNP team and approved for renewal of treatment, with a plan in place to address the previous cause of dismissal, for example, showing successful completion of substance treatment program or after a break of at least 6 months (Saxe et al., 2009).

5. Referral to mental health and substance abuse services for further management is recommended for the following indications:

    a. Patients with a past or current history of behaviors suggestive of substance abuse disorder. It is recommended to include this statement in the patient's treatment agreement.

    b. Patients with psychosocial problems that hinder treatment of pain.

    c. Patients with a diagnosis of depression, anxiety, or other mental health disorders.

    d. Provider's discretion: all patients may benefit from learning cognitive behavioral techniques to improve self-care and function.

6. Consultation with pain specialist or addiction specialist is indicated when:

    a. Patients have significant chronic, substantiated pain that develops addiction behaviors in the context of chronic opioid therapy (IASP, 2009; Saxe et al., 2009).

    b. The patient's pain is not well controlled on current pain treatment plan and/or exceeds the established dose ceiling limits

    c. The provider determines the need for consultation.

    d. All consultation is documented as part of the patient record. Not all patients have access to pain management specialists because of financial, insurance, location, availability, and transportation barriers. In these circumstances, review of the case with a CNP team or review of the case with pain specialists by email or telephone consultation may be appropriate (Saxe et al., 2009).

VI. Patient education

A. *Assist the patient and family in understanding and coping with chronic pain, and steps of care in terms of CNP protocol*

1. Provide verbal and written information regarding chronic pain and nonpharmacologic and pharmacologic treatments.

2. Assist the patient and family in obtaining all prior medical records and diagnostics, and facilitate the request for prior medical records.

B. *Provide self-care strategies as mentioned in nonpharmacologic management of chronic pain*

C. *Discuss management rationale for:*

1. Nonpharmacologic and nonopiate strategies as first-line treatment and progression to opiates as indicated

2. Reasons for a CNP team and protocol

D. *Review the individual treatment agreement if the patient proceeds to the CNP protocol*

1. Discuss medication(s): dose; schedule of dosing; side effects of medications; and safety of activity on medication (e.g., driving or swimming), including risk of death if medications are used incorrectly or combined with substances or dangerous activity.

2. Provide an explanation that one provider prescribes and one pharmacy dispenses, patient responsibility for managing medications safely, keeping appointments, and random urine screening.

3. Provide an overview of and the need for signing the individual treatment plan or pain agreement (Figure 50-5).

4. Discuss overdose prevention that includes ready access to drug and alcohol treatment services and management strategies that include access to emergency medical services and the administration for naloxone. For additional information and educational resources, review the Substance Abuse and Mental Health Services Administration (2014) *Opioid Overdose Toolkit* at http://store.samhsa.gov/shin/content//SMA14 -4742/Overdose_Toolkit.pdf.

5. Discuss the need for documenting the consequences of nonadherence to the treatment plan including discontinuation.

E. *Encourage chronic pain support groups*

F. *Encourage mental health provider evaluation for ongoing support*

VII. Chronic pain support resources and tools

A. *American Pain Society: www.ampainsoc.org*

B. *International Association for Study of Pain: www.iasp.org*

C. *Laughter Yoga International: www.laughteryoga.org*

D. *Self-help book, Managing Pain Before It Manages You (Caudill, 2009)*

E. *Kaiser Permanente Chronic Pain Program and Support Group*

REFERENCES

American Pain Society (2009). *Guideline for the use of chronic opioid therapy in chronic noncancer pain: Evidence review.* Retrieved from http://americanpainsociety.org/uploads/education/guidelines/chronic-opioid-therapy-cncp.pdf.

American Psychological Association. (2013). *Diagnostic and statistical manual of mental disorders-5* (5th ed.). Arlington, VA: American Psychological Association.

American Society of Addiction Medicine (2011). American Society of Addiction Medicine (ASAM). *The definition of addiction.* Chevy Chase, MD: The Society.

Barclay, L., & Nghiem, H. T. (2008). Primary care management of nonmalignant pain reviewed. *Medscape Multispecialty.* Retrieved from www.medscape.org/viewarticle/584508.

Bedard, M. E. (1997). *Fact sheet on chronic non-malignant pain (CNP).* American Society for Action on Pain. Retrieved from www.druglibrary.org/schaffer/asap/factsheet.html.

Brown, R. L., & Rounds, L. A. (1995). Conjoint screening questionnaires for alcohol and other drug abuse: Criterion validity in a primary care practice. *Wisconsin Medical Journal, 94*(3), 135–140.

Buckhardt, C. S., Goldenberg, D., Crofford, L., Gerwin R, Gowens, S., Jackson, K., Kugel, P., McCarberg, W., Rudin, N., Schanberg, L., Taylor, A.G., Taylor, J., & Turk, D. (2005). *Guideline for the management of fibromyalgia syndrome pain in adults and children.* p. 109 (Clinical practice guideline; no. 4). Glenview, IL: American Pain Society.

Caudill, M. A. (2009). *Managing pain before it manages you* (3rd ed.). New York, NY: Guilford Press.

Chou, R., Fanciullo, G., Fine, P., Adler, J. A., Ballantyne, J. C., Davies, P., et al. (2009). Clinical guidelines for the use of chronic opioid therapy in chronic noncancer pain. *Journal of Pain, 10*(2), 113–130.

Cohen, S. P., & Mao, J. (2009). Concerns about consensus guidelines for QTc interval screening in methadone treatment, letters. *Annals of Internal Medicine, 151*(3), 216–217. Retrieved from http://annals.org/article.aspx?articleid=744638.

eMedExpert. (2007–2014). Antidepressants comparison: Effexor versus Cymbalta. Retrieved from www.emedexpert.com/compare/effexor-vs-cymbalta.shtml.

Federation of State Medical Boards of the United States, Inc. (2004). *Model policy for the use of controlled substances for the treatment of pain.* Retrieved from www.painpolicy.wisc.edu/sites/www.painpolicy.wisc.edu/files/model04.pdf.

Federation of State Medical Boards of the United States, Inc. (2013). *Model policy for the use of controlled substances for the treatment of pain controlled substances for the treatment of pain.* Retrieved from http://www.fsmb.org/Media/Default/PDF/FSMB/Advocacy/pain_policy_july2013.pdf

Fuchs-Lacelle, S., & Hadjistavropoulos, T. (2004). Development and preliminary validation of the pain assessment checklist for seniors with limited ability to communicate (PACSLAC). *Pain Management in Nursing, 5*(2), 37–49.

Gourlay, D. L., Heit, H. A., & Caplan, Y. H. (2010). *Urine drug testing in clinical practice* (4th ed.). Baltimore, MD: Johns Hopkins University School of Medicine. Retrieved from http://issuu.com/cafamilydocs/docs/udtmonograph.

Herr, K., Coyne, P. J., Key, T., Manworren, R., McCaffery, M., Merkel, S., et al. (2006). Pain assessment in the nonverbal patient: Position statement with clinical practice recommendations. *Pain Management Nursing, 7*(2), 44–52. Retrieved from http://www.medscape.com/viewarticle/533939_4.

Hockenberry, M. J., & Wilson, D. (2009). *Wong's essentials of pediatric nursing* (8th ed.). St. Louis, MO: Mosby.

International Association for the Study of Pain. (2009). *Recommendations for pain treatment services.* Retrieved from http://www.iasp-pain.org/Education/Content.aspx?ItemNumber=1381.

International Association for the Study of Pain. (2012). *IASP taxonomy.* Retrieved from http://www.iasp-pain.org/Taxonomy#Pain

International Association for the Study of Pain. (2014). *Classification of Chronic Pain, Second Edition (Revised),* Introduction. Retrieved at http://www.iasp-pain.org/PublicationsNews/Content.aspx?ItemNumber=1673

Institute of Medicine. (2011). *Relieving pain in America: A blueprint for transforming prevention, care, education, and research.* Washington, DC: Author. Retrieved from www.iom.edu/~/media/Files/Report%20Files/2011/Relieving-Pain-in-America-A-Blueprint-for-Transforming-Prevention-Care-Education-Research/Pain%20Research%202011%20Report%20Brief.pdf.

Keefe, F. J., Somers, T. J., & Kothadia, S. M. (2009). Coping with pain. *Pain Clinical Update, 17*(5), 1–6.

Krantz, M. J., Martin, J., Stimmel, B., Metha, D., & Haigney, M. C. P. (2009). QTc interval screening in methadone treatment. *Annals of Internal Medicine, 150*(6), 387–399. Retrieved from http://annals.org/article.aspx?articleid=744382.

Krebs, E. E., Lorenz, K. A., Bair, M. J., Damush, T. M., Wu, J., Sutherland, J. M., et al. (2009). Development and initial validation of the PEG, a three-item scale assessing pain intensity and interference. *Journal of General Internal Medicine, 24*(6), 733–738.

McAuley, D. F. (2015). Opioid (narcotic) analgesic converter. Retrieved from http://www.globalrph.com/narcoticonv.htm

Medical Board of California. (2014). *Guidelines for prescribing controlled substances for pain.* Retrieved from www.mbc.ca.gov/Licensees/Prescribing/Pain_Guidelines.pdf.

Passik, S. D., & Weinreb, H. J. (2000). Managing chronic non-malignant pain: Overcoming obstacles to the use of opioids. *Advances in Therapy, 17*(2), 70–80.

Rosenblum, A., Joseph, H., Fong, C., Kipnis, S., Cleland, C., & Portenoy, R. K. (2003). Prevalence and characteristics of chronic pain among chemically dependent patients in methadone maintenance and residential treatment facilities. *JAMA, 289*(18), 2370–2378. Retrieved from http://jama.ama-assn.org/content/289/18/2370.full.

Saxe, J. M., Smith, V. & McNerney, K. (2013). A blueprint to managing multiple chronic conditions and pain. *Journal of Family Practice, 62*(12), S1–S25.

Saxe, J. M., Smith, V., Ligon, E. D., McNerney, K., Hill, K., & Nierman, J. (2009). *Glide Health Services chronic nonmalignant pain management protocol* (unpublished protocol). San Francisco, CA: Glide Health Services.

Spitzer, R. L., Kroenke, K., & Williams, J. B. W. (1999). Validation and utility of a self-report version of PRIME-MD: The PHQ primary care study. *JAMA, 282*(18), 1737–1744.

State of California Board of Registered Nursing. (1998). *An explanation of standardized procedure requirements for nurse practitioner practice.* Retrieved from www.rn.ca.gov/pdfs/regulations/npr-b-20.pdf.

State of California Board of Registered Nursing. (2004a). *Nurse practitioner expanded furnishing authority for schedule II controlled substances, BPC 2836.1.* Retrieved from www.rn.ca.gov/pdfs/regulations/npr-b-51.pdf.

State of California Board of Registered Nursing. (2004b). *Criteria for furnishing number utilization by nurse practitioners.* Retrieved from www.rn.ca.gov/pdfs/regulations/npr-i-16.pdf.

State of California Department of Justice. (2014). *Controlled Substance Utilization Review and Evaluation System (CURES), California Prescription Drug Monitoring Program (PDMP).* Retrieved from http://oag.ca.gov/cures-pdmp.

Substance Abuse and Mental Health Services Administration. (2014). *Opioid overdose prevention toolkit.* Retrieved from http://store.samhsa.gov/product/Opioid-Overdose-Prevention-Toolkit-Updated-2014/SMA14-4742.

Turk, D. (2006). Pain hurts—individuals, significant others and society! *American Pain Society Bulletin, 16*(1).

U.S. Department of Justice. (2014). List of controlled substances. Retrieved from www.deadiversion.usdoj.gov/schedules/index.html.

University of California San Francisco (UCSF), Department of Community Health Systems. (2010; 2015). *Standardized procedures,* unpublished manuscript, San Francisco: UCSF.

Vissers, K. C., Besse, K., Hans, G., Devulder, J., & Morlion, B. (2010). Opioid rotation in the management of chronic pain: Where is the evidence? *Pain Practice, 10*(2), 85–93.

Webster, L. R., & Webster, R. (2005). Predicting aberrant behaviors in opioid-treated patients: Preliminary validation of the Opioid Risk Tool. *Pain Medicine, 6*(6), 432–442.

Yalcin, I., & Barrot, M. (2014). The anxiodepressive comorbidity in chronic pain. *Current Opinion in Anaesthesiology, 27*(5), 520–527.

CHRONIC VIRAL HEPATITIS

Miranda Surjadi

I. Introduction and general background

The liver is the largest solid organ in the body, weighing approximately 1–1.5 kg. The majority of cells in the liver consist of hepatocytes. Hepatocytes are responsible for the synthesis of serum proteins (albumin, coagulation factors, many hormonal and growth factors), the production of bile, the regulation of nutrients, and metabolism and conjugation of lipophilic compounds for excretion in the bile or urine. Although there are many causes of liver diseases, one of the most common is viral hepatitis. Chronic viral hepatitis is defined by the persistence of viral infection for 6 months or more after initial exposure. The primary causes of chronic viral hepatitis are hepatitis B virus (HBV) and hepatitis C virus (HCV). Potential long-term complications of chronic viral hepatitis include cirrhosis, decompensated liver disease, and hepatocellular carcinoma (HCC) and are the leading indication for liver transplantation in the United States (Ghany & Hoofnagle, 2005).

A. Chronic hepatitis B

1. Definition and Overview

   Chronic HBV is defined as persons positive for hepatitis B surface antigen (HBsAg) for more than 6 months. Worldwide, there are 350 million individuals with chronic HBV, and in the United States, there are approximately 1.25 million. HBV is a DNA virus from the hepadnavirus family. It replicates by forming an RNA intermediate, which is copied using reverse transcriptase to generate DNA strands (Lavanchy, 2004; McQuillan et al., 1999).

2. HBV Prevalence/Incidence

   In the United States, the prevalence is approximately 1% of the population. The prevalence is greatest in Alaskan natives, first-generation immigrants from Southeast Asia, injection drug users, and men who have sex with men. After an acute HBV infection, the risk of developing chronic infection varies with age. In an adult, the risk is approximately 10%. In a newborn,

the risk is 90% (without HBV vaccine and HBIG). Risk of acute HBV infection has been dramatically reduced by universal HBV vaccination.

3. HBV Natural History

   Natural history of HBV has stages—initially after infection, patients often have high HBV DNA and HBeAg is present. In late childhood and early adulthood, most patients with chronic infection develop inactive chronic HBV with low-level HBV DNA and normal alanine aminotransferase (ALT) and loss of HBeAg, and later in life it can reactivate with elevated ALT and high-level HBV DNA and can have reactivation of HBeAg. Patients can move between active and inactive HBV, but typically antiviral treatment is used during active phases. High HBV DNA levels increase the risk of cirrhosis and HCC and HCC can develop in the absence of cirrhosis (Lok & McMahon, 2009).

4. HBV Screening

   Screening for HBV with HBsAg is recommended for many demographic groups including Alaskan natives; persons born in endemic areas; first-generation immigrants from Southeast Asia; injection drug users; men who have sex with men; persons with HCV, HIV, and alcohol use; and long-term hemodialysis.

B. Chronic hepatitis C

1. Definition and Overview

   The hepatitis C virus (HCV) is a single-stranded, enveloped RNA virus from the flaviviridae family. Exposure to HCV results in chronic infection in 75–80% of the cases. Persistence of HCV RNA in the serum for 6 months or more after exposure results in chronic HCV infection. HCV replicates with a high mutation rate, thereby resulting in heterogeneity within the HCV genome.

   HCV has six major genotypes (1–6) with subtypes (1a, 1b, 2a, 2b, etc) within the genotypes. Genotype 1 is the most common genotype in the United States, accounting for approximately 70% of the population.

Genotypes 2 and 3 account for 25% of the U.S. population. Genotypes 4, 5, and 6 are rare and account for the remainder. Genotypes do not influence progression of liver disease, but genotype is a major determinant of treatment regimens.

2. HCV Prevalence/Incidence

It is estimated that 180 million people are infected with hepatitis C worldwide. In the United States, it is estimated that there are 3.9 million individuals infected with HCV. The prevalence is highest in people born between 1945 and 1965 and individuals with a history of injection drug use, blood transfusions before 1992, and HIV infection. Incidence has declined since screening for HCV in blood banks and use of needle exchange programs.

3. HCV Natural history

Chronic HCV infection has variable rates of fibrosis progression. It is estimated that cirrhosis develops in 15–30% of cases. On average, cirrhosis will take 20–30 years to develop in immunocompetent adults. Alcohol, HIV, metabolic syndrome, and coinfection with other hepatitis viruses will increase the likelihood of developing cirrhosis and hasten the development of cirrhosis (Ghany et al., 2009). The risk for hepatocellular carcinoma is 1–5% per year in persons with chronic HCV and cirrhosis (Ghany et al., 2009).

4. HCV Screening

It is estimated that 50% of persons with HCV in the United States are unaware of their infection. New recommendations from the Centers for Disease Control and Prevention and the U.S. Preventive Services Task Force are that all persons born between 1945 and 1965 have a one-time HCV antibody test, regardless of risk factor. Additionally, persons with risk factors (e.g., any history of injection drug use even once) should be tested for HCV Ab, and in persons with ongoing risk behaviors, periodic screening should be continuously performed.

II. **Database** (may include but is not limited to)

A. Subjective

1. Chronic Hepatitis B
   a. Past health history
      i. Medical illnesses:
         HIV, coinfection with hepatitis C or D, hepatitis A, nonalcoholic fatty liver disease (NAFLD), diabetes mellitus, hyperlipidemia, obesity, other illnesses which may affect liver enzymes or liver function
      ii. Obstetrical/gynecological history:
         Recent pregnancy may flare HBV; risk of transmission to fetus and efficacy of hepatitis B immunoglobulin (HBIG)/HBV vaccine will depend on level of maternal HBV DNA.
      iii. Exposure history:
         Born in endemic area, parents born in endemic area, healthcare worker, sexual exposure, injection drug use (IDU)
      iv. Medication history:
         a. Medications that can cause flare-up of HBV such as steroids, chemotherapy, biologic agents (TNF-alpha inhibitors)
         b. Hepatotoxic medications, such as tuberculosis (TB) medications, methotrexate, statins, etc.
   b. Family history
      i. Chronic hepatitis B
      ii. Hepatocellular carcinoma
   c. Occupational/environmental history
      i. Work-related exposures: healthcare worker
   d. Personal/social history
      i. Sexual history, illicit drug use, alcohol use
      ii. Household contacts
   e. Review of systems
      i. Constitutional signs and symptoms: Fatigue, weight loss, fevers/chills (acute HBV)
      ii. Skin, hair, and nails: Itching, bruising
      iii. Ear, nose, and throat: Jaundice
      iv. Chest: Gynecomastia
      v. Cardiac: Shortness of breath, chest pain, palpitations
      vi. Abdomen: Abdominal pain, nausea, vomiting, clay-colored stools
      vii. Genitourinary: Dark urine
      viii. Musculoskeletal: Joint pains
      ix. Extremities: Pedal edema
      x. Neurological: Confusion, tremors, sleep/wake cycle disturbances
2. Chronic Hepatitis C
   a. Past health history
      i. Medical illnesses:
         HIV, coinfected with hepatitis B, NAFLD, other illnesses that may affect liver function/enzymes. Cardiopulmonary diseases (if ribavirin is to be used in treatment).
      ii. Obstetrical/gynecological history:
         a. Mother to child transmission is < 5% (except with HIV coinfection, then risk is 20%).
         b. Breastfeeding in HCV-infected mother is safe for the baby.
      iii. Exposure history:
         IDU, blood transfusions, sexual exposure, needlestick exposure

iv. Medication history:
   Hepatotoxic medications such as TB medications, methotrexate, statins etc.
b. Family history
   i. Other viral hepatitis
   ii. Hepatocellular carcinoma
c. Personal/social history
   i. IDU, other illicit drugs, alcohol intake
   ii. Housing, access to phone, refrigerator if needed
   iii. Mental health/psych history: suicidal/homicidal ideation if pegylated interferon will be used as part of HCV treatment
d. Review of systems
   i. Constitutional signs and symptoms: Fatigue, fevers/chills (acute HCV)
   ii. Skin: Jaundiced, itchy, bruising
   iii. Ear, nose, and throat: Jaundiced
   iv. Cardiac: Shortness of breath, chest pain, palpitations
   v. Abdomen: Abdominal pain, nausea, vomiting, clay-colored stools
   vi. Genitourinary: Dark urine
   vii. Musculoskeletal: Joint pains
   viii. Extremities: Pedal edema
   ix. Neurological: Confusion, tremors, sleep/wake cycle disturbances

B. Objective

1. Physical exam findings (see **Table 51-1**)
2. Supporting data from relevant diagnostic tests (see **Tables 51-2, 51-3, and 51-4**)

TABLE 51-1 Physical Examination Findings

Condition	Associated Findings (may or may not include):
Chronic Hepatitis B and C	Assess:
	1. Vital Signs: temperature, heart rate
	2. General Appearance: lethargy (hepatic encephalopathy)
	3. Skin/hair: jaundiced, pruritus, bruising (cirrhosis)
	4. Eyes: icteric sclerae (cirrhosis)
	5. Chest/Lungs: spider nevi, gynecomastia, crackles (from right heart failure due to portal hypertension)
	6. Cardiovascular: increased jugular venous pressure (due to right heart failure from portal hypertension)
	7. Abdomen: ascites, fluid wave, caput medusae, hepatomegaly, splenomegaly (cirrhosis)
	8. Extremities: palmar erythema, pedal edema (cirrhosis)
	9. Neurological: asterixis, tremors, behavioral changes (hepatic encephalopathy)
	10. Genitourinary: testicular atrophy, dark urine (cirrhosis)

TABLE 51-2 HBV Serologic Tests

Test	Clinical Implications	Comments
Hepatitis B surface antigen (HBsAg)	• If positive for 6 months or more, denotes chronic infection	
Hepatitis B core antibody IgG (IgG anti-HBc)	• Past exposure to HBV	
Hepatitis B core antibody IgM (IgM anti-HBc)	• Acute exposure to HBV • Reactivation of chronic infection	
Hepatitis B surface antibody (HBsAb)	• Immunity to HBV	Vaccine induced immunity will not have positive anti-HBc
Hepatitis B DNA (HBV DNA)	• Active viral replication	May be present in inactive disease state, but usually < 2,000 IU/mL
Hepatitis B E antigen (HBeAg)	• Active viral replication	May be negative in those with a precore mutant HBV
Hepatitis B E antibody (HBeAb)	• Low replicative state	
Hepatitis D virus	• RNA virus that needs HBsAg to replicate	Consider ordering if coinfection of HDV is suspected
Hepatitis B genotype and resistance	• Quasispecies of HBV (genotype A responds well to pegylated interferon) • Resistance to antiviral medications based on mutations of HBV	Consider ordering if past resistance to antiviral therapy is suspected or when considering pegylated interferon therapy.

TABLE 51-3 Common Liver Tests

Function	Test	Definition	Clinical Implications	Comments
Marker of hepatocellular injury	Aspartate amino-transferase (AST)	Found mainly in hepatocytes. Released into bloodstream when there is liver injury	• Increased in viral hepatitis • AST:ALT ratio 2:1 in alcoholic hepatitis	Found in liver, heart skeletal muscle, brain
Marker of hepatocellular injury	Alanine amino-transferase (ALT)	Found mainly in hepatocytes. Released into bloodstream when there is liver injury	• Increased in viral hepatitis • ALT > AST in chronic viral hepatitis	Found in liver
Marker of cholestatic injury	Alkaline phosphatase	Canicular enzyme that plays a role in bile production	• Increased in hepatobiliary disease, bone disease, pregnancy, hyperparathyroidism	Found in liver, bone, intestine, and placenta
Marker of cholestatic injury	Bilirubin	Breakdown product of hemolysis. Taken up by liver cells and conjugated to water soluble product. Excreted in bile.	• Elevations may indicate hepatic or extrahepatic disorder	Hepatitis and cirrhosis causes conjugated hyperbilirubinemia
Marker of liver function	Albumin	Major component of plasma proteins. Liver synthesizes albumin	• Decreased in cirrhosis from chronic liver disease. • Also decreased in nephrotic syndrome, malabsorption, protein losing enteropathy	Indication of severity of liver disease
Marker of liver function	Prothrombin time	Liver produces clotting factors I, II, V, VII, and X. Prothrombin time depends on the activity of these clotting factors.	• Increased in cirrhosis from chronic liver disease. • Also increased with coumadin, vitamin K deficiency	Vitamin K is needed to activate some of the clotting factors.

TABLE 51-4 HCV Serologic tests

Test	Definition	Clinical Implications	Comments
Hepatitis C Antibody (HCV Ab)	Detects antibodies to hepatitis C virus	Positive in patients who have been exposed to hepatitis C	Will stay positive even if HCV treatment is successful and sustained virologic response is achieved.
HCV RNA	Determines HCV viral load and determines if HCV RNA is undetectable	Positive in patients with chronic hepatitis C. Useful in monitoring response to HCV therapy.	HCV RNA values will fluctuate. Values do not correlate with liver disease progression.
Hepatitis C genotype	Genotype 1–6 and subtype a or b	Necessary for determining appropriate HCV treatment regimen and duration	

III. Assessment

A. Determine the diagnosis

1. Chronic hepatitis B (see **Tables** 51-2 and **51-5**)

2. Chronic hepatitis C (see Table 51-4)

3. Other conditions that may explain the patient's elevated liver function tests (LFTs)

    a. Autoimmune hepatitis: antinuclear antibody (ANA)/antismooth muscle antibody positive; chronic necroinflammatory liver disease of unknown etiology

    b. Nonalcoholic steatohepatitis (NASH)/ NAFLD: associated with diabetes mellitus, hyperlipidemia, obesity

    c. Primary biliary cirrhosis: antimitochondrial antibody positive in 95%; chronic cholestatic liver disease more common in women age 50 and older

    d. Hemochromatosis: most common genetic disorder in the Caucasian population. The extent of liver injury is associated with the accumulation of hepatic iron.

    e. Wilson's disease: autosomal recessive defect of cellular copper export; decreased ceruloplasmin

    f. Alpha-1 antitrypsin deficiency: genetic disorder that affects lungs and liver

    g. Primary sclerosing cholangitis: chronic biliary duct inflammation; associated with inflammatory bowel disease

B. Severity

Assess the severity of the liver disease and determine if patient has cirrhosis or intact liver function (normal platelets, albumin, total bilirubin, prothrombin time/international normalized ratio). Decompensated liver disease is manifested by history of ascites, pedal edema, encephalopathy, and/or variceal bleeding. These patients should be referred to a liver transplant center for evaluation and treatment. Calculate MELD (Model for End-Stage Liver Disease) score (United Network for Organ Sharing, 2015). Allocation calculators: https://www.unos.org/transplantation/allocation-calculators/). If MELD score is 10 or greater, refer to liver transplant center.

C. Significance

Assess the significance of the problem to the patient and significant others. Discuss transmission and vaccinate appropriately.

D. Motivation and ability

Determine the patient's willingness and ability to follow the treatment plan.

IV. Goals of clinical management

A. Hepatocellular carcinoma (HCC) screening/surveillance

1. Choose a cost-effective approach for screening.

B. Treatment goals

1. Chronic HBV:

    a. Convert HBsAg positive to HBsAg negative (very rare)

    b. Convert HBeAg positive to negative with the development of anti-HBe.

    c. HBV DNA undetectable

    d. Normalization of liver enzymes

2. Chronic HCV:

    a. Goal of hepatitis C therapy is elimination of the virus from the bloodstream, as defined by a sustained virologic response (SVR), considered a virologic cure. SVR is defined by a HCV RNA that becomes undetectable during treatment and remains undetectable 3 months after completion of HCV therapy. Evidence supports that achieving an SVR will significantly reduce the likelihood of progression to cirrhosis, development of hepatocellular carcinoma, and development of end stage liver disease. Patients who achieve SVR will continue to have HCV antibodies but no longer have detectable HCV RNA in their serum, liver tissue, or mononuclear cells. HCV treatment should be considered for all HCV patients, weighing the benefits of potential SVR in light of other medical problems and life expectancy.

TABLE 51-5 Interpretation of Chronic HBV Serologies

CHRONIC HEPATITIS B		
	Replicative Phase	Nonreplicative Phase
HBsAg	+	+
HBsAb	–	–
HBcAb (total)	+	+
HBeAg	+/–	–
HBeAb	–	+/–
ALT	normal or elevated	normal
HBV DNA	≥ 2,000 IU/mL	< 2,000 IU/mL

b. Genotype 1: SVR in 95–100% of patients with 12–24 weeks of HCV therapy.

c. Genotype 2: SVR 94–100% with 12–16 weeks of HCV therapy

d. Genotype 3: SVR 84–97% with 12–24 weeks of HCV therapy

e. Genotype 4: SVR 95–100% with 12–24 weeks of HCV therapy

f. Genotypes 5 and 6: SVR 96–100% with 12 weeks of HCV therapy. Genotypes 4, 5, and 6 are very rare in the United States.

g. Cirrhotic patients and previous nonresponders to HCV therapy tend to have decreased SVR rates.

C. Patient adherence

1. Select an approach that maximizes patient adherence (i.e., all-oral regimen and easy dosing instructions).

V. Plan

A. HCC Screening/ Surveillance

The American Association for the Study of Liver Diseases (AASLD) guidelines recommends screening with abdominal ultrasound every 6 months. Measurement of alpha fetoprotein (AFP) is optional but not necessary for screening, and AFP alone is not recommended as a screening tool, unless in rare cases where imaging is not available. Imaging is the necessary technique for HCC screening. Whom to screen:

1. All patients with cirrhosis

2. All patients with family history of HCC

3. In chronic hepatitis B patients:
   a. All Asian men 40 years and older
   b. All Asian women 50 years and older
   c. All Africans 20 years and older
   d. Patients above 40 years with an elevated ALT and HBV DNA > 2,000 IU/mL should be considered for HCC surveillance.

B. Diagnostic Tests

1. Chronic hepatitis B: The detection of HBsAg at 6 months after time of infection defines chronic HBV. Most patients with HBsAg will also have detectable HBV DNA at some level. Patients with normal ALT and low level HBV DNA (< 2,000 IU/mL) are considered inactive chronic HBV, whereas patients with elevated ALT and higher levels of HBV DNA are considered chronic HBV.
   a. Complete blood count (CBC), complete metabolic panel, coagulation tests (PT/INR)
   b. HBV DNA, HBeAg anti-HBe.

c. HIV

d. Hepatitis serologies: Hepatitis C Ab, HepA total Ab, Hepatitis D Ab (if coinfection is suspected)

e. Other tests to rule out other types of liver diseases if etiology is not certain: ANA, iron studies, antimitochondrial antibody (AMA), antismooth muscle antibody, ceruloplasmin, lipids, glucose (gastroenterology [GI]/hepatology specialist may order these tests)

f. Imaging—see special populations who need HCC surveillance

g. Fibrosis testing—newer and noninvasive tests for fibrosis testing are preferable to liver biopsy if available. Some blood test markers (e.g., Fibrosure) are becoming more widely available. Transient elastography is a technique used to estimate liver stiffness (e.g., Fibroscan) but is not as widely available. Liver biopsy is still considered the gold standard for staging fibrosis but is less often performed than in the past and is rarely required for treatment initiation.

2. Chronic hepatitis C: If HCV antibody is positive, then confirm chronic HCV infection with an HCV RNA test. Formerly, HCV RNA tests were categorized as quantitative or qualitative but as RNA testing has developed greater sensitivity, extremely low levels of RNA are detectable and most assays are able to determine quantitative measurements as well as low-level qualitative virus detection.

   a. If HCV RNA negative, then recheck in 6 months to confirm resolved Hepatitis C. Two negative HCV RNA tests 6 or more months apart will confirm resolved hepatitis C.

   b. If HCV RNA is positive, then you have confirmed chronic HCV. There is no need to use HCV RNA as a monitoring tool for liver disease progression. HCV RNA, both qualitative and quantitative, is used primarily in the setting of HCV therapy.
      i. CBC, complete metabolic panel, coagulation studies
      ii. HCV genotype
      iii. HIV
      iv. AFP
      v. Hepatitis serologies: HepBsAg, HepBsAb, HepBcAb, HepA total Ab (vaccinate for Hep A and Hep B if not immune)
      vi. Other tests to rule out other types of liver diseases if etiology is uncertain: ANA, iron studies, AMA, antismooth muscle antibody, ceruloplasmin, lipids, glucose (GI/hepatology specialist may order these)
      vii. Baseline imaging to look for cirrhosis

TABLE 51-6 Treatment for Chronic HBV Patients

Generic Name	Dose	Resistance Rate
Lamivudine	100 mg daily	14–32% in 1 year
Adefovir	10 mg daily	29% in 5 yrs
*Entecavir	0.5 mg, 1 mg daily	1.2% in 5 yrs
		7.8% in 2 years if lamivudine resistance is present
Telbivudine	600 mg daily	25% in 2 yrs
*Tenofovir	300 mg daily	None
*Pegylated interferon	180 mcg SQ weekly x 48 weeks	None

*Considered first-line treatment.

Entecavir 1 mg used for patients with past treatment experience to lamivudine and decompensated cirrhotic patients.

viii. Liver biopsy for staging or diagnosing of liver disease if indicated to start treatment (usually this is ordered by the GI/hepatology specialist).

C. Management

1. Chronic hepatitis B (see **Table 51-6** for a list of medications for chronic HBV treatment)—Refer chronic HBV patients to specialists when they are in chronic active, replicative phase (see Table 51-5)

   If hepatitis B surface antigen is positive:

   a. Hepatitis B E antigen positive
      i. Alanine aminotransferase (ALT) elevated
      ii. HBV DNA ≥ 20,000 IU/mL
      iii. Refer to specialist for treatment
   b. Hepatitis B E antigen negative
      i. ALT elevated
      ii. HBV DNA ≥ 2,000 IU/mL
      iii. Refer to specialist for treatment
   c. Cirrhotics—Refer all to specialist for treatment despite ALT or HBV DNA level
   d. Coinfection with hepatitis D—Refer to specialist for treatment despite ALT or HBV DNA level
   e. Inactive chronic hepatitis B or isolated positive hepatitis B core antibody who are about to undergo immunosuppressive therapy. Refer to specialist for treatment despite ALT or HBV DNA level
   f. Inactive chronic hepatitis B
      i. ALT normal
      ii. HBV DNA < 2,000 IU/mL
      iii. Followed by primary care provider every 6 months: ALT, HBV DNA
         a. Refer to specialist when ALT becomes abnormal or if HBV DNA

is persistently > 2,000 IU/mL for 6 months or more.
      b. Follow HCC surveillance guidelines for all chronic hepatitis B patients (both active and inactive)
      c. Vaccinate for hepatitis A if not immune

2. Chronic hepatitis C. See **Table 51-7** for a list of medications for the treatment of chronic hepatitis C and **Table 51-8** for an explanation of the classification system and level of evidence noted in Table 51-7.

   a. Who and when to refer to specialist for HCV treatment:
      i. HCV treatment should be considered for all patients. Patients with an urgent need for treatment are those with:
         a. Advanced fibrosis or cirrhosis (liver biopsy stage 3–4 fibrosis by Metavir staging)
         b. Liver transplant recipients
         c. Severe extrahepatic manifestations of HCV
            i. Mixed cryoglobulinemia with end organ manifestations (i.e., vasculitis)
            ii. Proteinuria, nephritic syndrome, or membranoproliferative glomerulonephritis
      ii. The following groups of patients should be considered high priority for HCV treatment:
         a. Stage 2 fibrosis
         b. HIV coinfection
         c. HBV coinfection
         d. Other coexistent liver disease conditions (i.e., NASH/NAFLD)
         e. Debilitating fatigue
      iii. The following group of patients present an elevated risk of increased transmission of HCV and HCV treatment may result in decrease of transmission:
         a. Men who have sex with men with high-risk sexual practices (MSM)
         b. Active IDU
         c. Incarcerated persons
         d. Those on long-term hemodialysis
         e. HCV-infected women of childbearing age
   b. Chronic HCV patients who are being followed by primary care providers (those who are not currently receiving treatment)
      i. Cirrhotic patients:
         a. HCC surveillance
         b. Monitor MELD score every 3–6 months: INR, total bilirubin, albumin, creatinine, AST, ALT, platelets

TABLE 51-7 Initial Treatment of Chronic Hepatitis C: Recommendations from the American Association for the Study of Liver Diseases (AASLD) and the Infectious Diseases Society of America (IDSA) (2015)

Genotype 1a	• Ledipasvir 90 mg/sofosbuvir 400 mg 1 tablet daily for 12 weeks. SVR 97–99% (Class I, Level A). • Paritaprevir 150 mg/ritonavir 100 mg/ombitasvir 25 mg daily plus dasabuvir 250 mg and weight-based ribavirin twice daily for 12 weeks (no cirrhosis, SVR 95%) or 24 weeks (cirrhosis, SVR 95%) (Class I, Level A). • Simeprevir 150 mg daily plus sofosbuvir 400 mg daily with or without weight-based ribavirin for 12 weeks (no cirrhosis, SVR 95%) or 24 weeks (cirrhosis, SVR 100%) (Class IIa, Level B) • Daclatasvir 60 mg plus sofosbuvir 400 mg daily for 12 weeks (no cirrhosis) and 24 weeks (with cirrhosis) with or without weight based ribavirin. SVR 96% Class I, Level B (no cirrhosis); Class IIa, Level B (cirrhosis)
Genotype 1b	• Ledipasvir 90 mg/sofosbuvir 400 mg 1 tablet daily for 12 weeks. SVR 97–99% (Class I, Level A) • Paritaprevir 150 mg/ritonavir 100 mg/ombitasvir 25 mg daily plus dasabuvir 250 mg for 12 weeks (no cirrhosis, SVR 99%). The addition of weight-based ribavirin is recommended for cirrhotic patients, SVR 98.5% (Class I, Level A) • Simeprevir 150 mg daily plus sofosbuvir 400 mg daily with or without weight-based ribavirin for 12 weeks (no cirrhosis, SVR 95%) or 24 weeks (cirrhosis, 100%) (Class IIa, Level B) • Daclatasvir 60 mg plus sofosbuvir 400 mg daily for 12 weeks (no cirrhosis) and 24 weeks (with cirrhosis) with or without weight based ribavirin. SVR 96% Class I, Level B (no cirrhosis); Class IIa, Level B (cirrhosis)
Genotype 2	• Sofosbuvir 400 mg daily plus weight-based ribavirin for 12 weeks. SVR 94% (Class I, Level A). • Sofosbuvir 400 mg daily plus weight-based ribavirin for 16 weeks is recommended in patients with cirrhosis (Class IIb, Level C) • Daclatasvir 60 mg plus sofosbuvir 400 mg daily for 12 weeks is recommended for patients who cannot tolerate ribavirin. SVR 92%. (Class IIa, Level B)
Genotype 3	• Sofosbuvir 400 mg daily plus weight-based ribavirin for 24 weeks. SVR 84% (Class I, Level B). • Sofosbuvir 400 mg daily plus weight-based ribavirin plus weekly pegylated interferon for 12 weeks. SVR 97% (Class IIa, Level A). • Daclatasvir 60 mg plus sofosbuvir 400 mg daily for 12 weeks (no cirrhosis) and 24 weeks (with cirrhosis) with or without weight based ribavirin. SVR 90–97%. Class I, Level A (no cirrhosis); Class IIa, Level C (cirrhosis)
Genotype 4	• Ledipasvir 90 mg/sofosbuvir 400 mg 1 tablet daily for 12 weeks. SVR 95% (Class IIb, Level B). • Paritaprevir 150 mg/Ritonavir 100 mg/ombitasvir 25 mg daily plus weight-based ribavirin for 12 weeks. SVR 100% (Class I, Level B). • Sofosbuvir 400 mg plus weight-based ribavirin for 24 weeks. SVR 100% (Class IIa, Level B).
Genotype 5	• Sofosbuvir 400 mg daily plus weight-based ribavirin plus weekly pegylated interferon for 12 weeks. SVR 100% (Class IIa, Level B).
Genotype 6	• Ledipasvir 90 mg/sofosbuvir 400 mg 1 tablet daily for 12 weeks. SVR 96% (Class IIa, Level B). • Sofosbuvir 400 mg daily plus weight-based ribavirin plus weekly pegylated interferon for 12 weeks. SVR 100% (Class IIa, Level B).

*HIV/HCV coinfected persons should be treated the same as persons without HIV infection after managing potential interactions with antiretroviral medications.

c. Refer to liver transplant/liver specialist when appropriate for evaluation and treatment (if MELD > 12).

d. Vaccinate for hepatitis A and B.

e. Patient education: avoid alcohol, low-salt diet, avoid raw fish/shellfish, avoid nonsteroidal anti-inflammatories, and limit acetaminophen with a maximum of 2,000 mg daily

3. Chronic HCV—no evidence of cirrhosis

a. Monitor ALT/AST every 6–12 months as needed

TABLE 51-8 Classification System and Levels of Evidence

Classification	Description
Class I	Conditions for which there is evidence and/or general agreement that a given diagnostic evaluation, procedure, or treatment is beneficial, useful, and effective
Class II	Conditions for which there is conflicting evidence and/or a divergence of opinion about the usefulness and efficacy of a diagnostic evaluation, procedure, or treatment
Class IIa	Weight of evidence and/or opinion is in favor of usefulness and efficacy
Class IIb	Usefulness and efficacy are less well established by evidence and/or opinion
Class III	Conditions for which there is evidence and/or general agreement that a diagnostic evaluation, procedure, or treatment is not useful and effective or if it in some cases may be harmful

Level of Evidence	Description
Level A	Data derived from multiple randomized clinical trials, meta-analyses, or equivalent
Level B	Data derived from a single randomized trial, nonrandomized studies, or equivalent
Level C	Consensus opinion of experts, case studies, or standard of care

b. HCV RNA monitoring is not necessary unless during treatment and in the 6 months after treatment
c. Vaccinate for hepatitis A and B
d. Patient education: avoid alcohol, support groups
e. Update patients on future HCV therapies and refer when appropriate for treatment of chronic HCV

D. Client education

1. Chronic hepatitis C treatment side effects
   a. All new oral agents for hepatitis C have very few if any side effects. See **Table 51-9** if patients are taking pegylated interferon and/or ribavirin for a list of side effects.
   b. Advice for patients currently undergoing treatment with pegylated interferon and ribavirin:
      i. Drink plenty of clear liquids. Try to drink between 8 and 10 glasses of water or another clear liquid every day. Increase this amount if you are vomiting.
      ii. Avoid drinks that have alcohol, caffeine (coffee, cola, and strong tea) or lots of sugar (most soft drinks).
      iii. Try to get plenty of sleep at night. Take short naps during the day.
      iv. Eat small, nutritious meals. Crackers, clear sodas, and ginger ale can help settle your stomach. Greasy, high-fat foods (including most fast food) can make you feel worse. Try to eat even if you are not very hungry.
      v. Exercise lightly. Walking and lifting light weights are good exercises while you are on treatment.
      vi. Take your medicine before you go to bed, so that you can sleep through the side effects.
      vii. Take any pain relievers recommended by your doctor. Taking a pain reliever about a half hour before your pegylated interferon injection can help make the side effects less severe. Do not take any pain reliever, however, unless your doctor says it is okay.

TABLE 51-9 Side Effects of Pegylated Interferon and Ribavirin

Drug	Side Effects
Pegylated interferon	• Flulike symptoms • Depression/anxiety/irritability • Complete blood count abnormalities: neutropenia, thrombocytopenia • Anorexia, nausea, diarrhea, vomiting (rare) • Alopecia • Skin irritation around shot • Thyroid abnormalities (rare) • Retinal disorders (rare)
Ribavirin	• Anemia • Insomnia • Birth defects (need double contraception) • Rash/pruritus • Numbness/tingling in extremities

viii. Avoid situations or "triggers" that make you feel worse, such as loud noises, bright lights, strong odors, and/or skipped meals.

ix. Do not color or perm your hair until after your treatment is finished.

x. Do not use harsh detergents or soaps that might irritate your skin.

xi. Simple, unscented lotions can help dry, itchy skin. If taking ribavirin gives you a rash, Benadryl lotion might help.

c. For patients who are having mood symptoms on pegylated interferon and ribavirin therapy

i. Talk about your feelings with a family member, friend or someone else that you trust.

ii. Tell people close to you when you are taking your HCV treatment. Tell them that it can affect your moods.

iii. Join a support group.

iv. Avoid things that can make you feel stressed, like too much caffeine, sugar, or nicotine.

v. Learn ways to relax. Meditate or breathe quietly. Go for a walk or do some other light exercise.

vi. Take care of your body. Eat healthy meals, get lots of sleep and drink plenty of water.

vii. If you are taking medicine because you are depressed, be sure not to skip a dose. Keep all of your appointments with your psychiatrist or therapist.

VI. Self-management resources and tools

A. Patient/client education

1. American Association for the Study of Liver Diseases, www.aasld.org

2. National Institute of Diabetes and Digestive and Kidney Diseases, http://www2.niddk.nih.gov/

3. American Liver Foundation, www.liverfoundation.org/

REFERENCES

American Association for the Study of Liver Diseases & Infectious Diseases Society of America. (2015). *HCV guidance: Recommendations for testing, managing, and treating hepatitis C.* Retrieved from www.hcvguidelines .org/full-report/when-and-whom-initiate-hcv-therapy.

Feld, J. J., Kowdley, K. V., Coakley, E., Sigal, S., Nelson, D. R., Crawford, D., et al. (2014). Treatment of HCV with ABT-450/r-ombitasvir and dasabuvir with ribavirin. *New England Journal of Medicine, 370*(17), 1594-1603.

Ghany, M., & Hoofnagle, J. H. (2005). Approach to the patient with liver disease. In D. L. Kasper, A. S. Fauci, D. L. Longo, E. Braunwald, S. L. Hauser, & J. L. Jameson, *Harrison's principles of internal medicine* (pp. 1808–1813). New York: McGraw-Hill.

Ghany, M. G., Strader, D. B., Thomas, D. L., & Seeff, L.B. (2009). Diagnosis, management, and treatment of hepatitis C: An update. *Hepatology, 49*(4), 1335–1374.

Jacobson, I. M., Gordon, S. C, Kowdley, K. V., Yoshida, E. M., Rodriguez-Torres, M. Sulkowski, M. S., et al. (2013). Sofosbuvir for hepatitis C genotype 2 or 3 in patients without treatment options. *New England Journal of Medicine, 368*(20), 1867–1877.

Kowdley, K. V., Gordon, S. C., Reddy, K. R., Rossaro, L., Bernstein, D. E., Lawitz, E., et al. (2014). Ledipasvir and sofosbuvir for 8 or 12 weeks for chronic HCV without cirrhosis. *New England Journal of Medicine, 370*(20), 1879–1888.

Lavanchy, D. (2004). Hepatitis B virus epidemiology, disease burden, treatment, and current and emerging prevention and control measures. *Journal of Viral Hepatitis, 11*(2), 97–107.

Lawitz, E., Mangia, A., Wyles, D., Rodriguez-Torres, M., Hassanein, T., Gordon, S. C., et al. (2013). Sofosbuvir for previously untreated chronic hepatitis C infection. *New England Journal of Medicine, 368*(20), 1878–1887.

Lawitz, E., Poordad, F. F., Pang, P. S., Hyland, R.H., Ding, X., Mo, H., et al. (2014). Sofosbuvir and ledipasvir fixed dose combination with or without ribavirin in treatment naïve and previously treated patients with genotype 1 hepatitis C virus infection (LONESTAR): An open label randomized, phase 2 trial. *Lancet, 383*(9916), 515–523.

Lawitz, E., Sulkowski, M. S., Ghalib, R., Rodriguez-Torres, M., Younossi, Z. M., Corregidor, A., et al. (2014). Simeprevir plus sofosbuvir, with or without ribavirin, to treat chronic infection of hepatitis C virus genotype 1 in non-responders to pegylated interferon and ribavirin and treatment naïve patients: The COSMOS randomized study. *Lancet, 384*(9956), 1756–1765.

Lok, A. S., & McMahon, B. J. (2009). Chronic hepatitis B: Update 2009. *Hepatology, 50*(3), 1–36.

McQuillan, G. M., Coleman, P. J., Kurszon-Moran, D., Moyer, L. A., Lambert, S. B., & Margolis, H. S. (1999). Prevalence of hepatitis B virus infection in the United States: The National Health and Nutrition Examination Surveys. *American Journal of Public Health, 89*(1), 14–18.

Shiffman, R. N., Shekelle, P., Overhage, J. M., Slutsky, J., Grimshaw, J., & Deshpande, A. M. (2003). Standardized reporting of clinical practice guidelines: A proposal from the Conference on Guideline Standardization. *Annals of Internal Medicine, 139*(6), 493–498.

Swain, M. G., Lai, M. Y., Shiffman, M. L., Cooksley, W. G., Zeuzem, S., Dieterich, D. T., et al. (2010). A sustained virologic response is durable in patients with chronic hepatitis C treated with peginterferon alfa-2a and ribavirin. *Gastroenterology, 139*(5), 1593–1601.

United Network for Organ Sharing. (2015). Allocation calculators. Retrieved at https://www.unos.org/transplantation/allocation-calculators/

DEMENTIA

CHAPTER 52

Jennifer Merrilees

I. Introduction and general background

Dementia refers to diseases and conditions characterized by decline in cognitive function that negatively affects a person's abilities to perform daily activities (Alzheimer's Association, 2014). Dementia is typically a slowly progressive disease caused by damage and death of neurons in the brain. The definition of dementia has been recently categorized as a neurocognitive disorder that is either mild (cognitive impairment with no impact on daily function) or major (cognitive impairment that interferes with daily function). Presenting symptoms are varied and can include memory loss, executive dysfunction, speech and language changes, and/or behavioral and emotional symptoms. Common causes of dementia include Alzheimer's disease (AD), vascular dementia, frontotemporal dementia (FTD), and dementia with Lewy bodies (DLB). Other disorders that may be associated with dementia are Huntington's disease, HIV/AIDS, Parkinson's disease, alcoholism, and head trauma. Rapidly progressive dementias are rare and may include Creutzfeldt-Jakob disease. For many individuals (especially those of older age), there are multiple types of pathology present. There is no cure for dementia, although current research aimed at the reversal or prevention of dementia is under way.

There is no single test for dementia and the evaluation is directed at clarifying the nature of the impairment, ruling out reversible conditions, and specifying the likely cause for the dementia (see **Table 52-1**). Approximately 9% of patients have a potentially treatable cause for dementia (e.g., thyroid abnormality, vitamin deficiency, depression, delirium, medication side effects, and excessive use of alcohol). Thus, a comprehensive evaluation is critical to correctly identify and diagnose patients with dementia and to initiate appropriate management.

A. Alzheimer's disease (AD)

1. Definition and overview

   AD is the most common cause of dementia. Although the sites of earliest damage in AD are the hippocampus and entorhinal cortex (areas important to memory function), the disease eventually affects multiple regions of the brain. Neuronal death is caused by the overaccumulation of amyloid plaques and neurofibrillary tangles. The strongest risk factor for AD is advanced age, although prior head injury, family history of AD, and cardiovascular factors, such as hypertension, pose increased risk for development of AD. When AD occurs in a person younger than age 65, it is referred to as presenile, early age onset, younger onset, or early onset AD. Most cases of AD are not familial, although genetic risk increases in presenile AD when a first-degree relative has AD and in the presence of certain genetic mutations.

2. Prevalence

   One in nine people age 65 and older have AD, whereas one in three people age 85 and older have AD. More women than men have AD largely because women typically live longer than men. It is estimated that a growing number of Americans will live into their 80s and 90s, resulting in even greater numbers of people with dementia.

B. Vascular dementia

1. Definition and overview

   Vascular dementia (also called multi-infarct dementia) is caused by cerebrovascular ischemia and lacunar infarcts in the brain (often referred to as white matter disease). Symptoms are similar to AD, although the onset may be more easily identified and the progression of symptoms can be characterized by "stepwise" changes reflecting the occurrence of strokes. Risk factors include strokes, hypertension, hypercholesteremia, and diabetes. Vascular dementia may coexist with AD or DLB.

2. Prevalence

   Vascular dementia is considered the second most common cause for dementia, occurring in approximately 20–30% of people with dementia (Plassman et al., 2007; Rizzi, Rosset, & Roriz-Cruz, 2014).

TABLE 52-1 Possible Causes of Dementia (Partial List)

Neurodegenerative	Alzheimer's disease, Down syndrome, Parkinson's disease, dementia with Lewy bodies, frontotemporal dementia, multisystem atrophy, Huntington disease
Cerebrovascular	Vascular dementia, vasculitis
Prion-associated	Creutzfeldt-Jakob disease, Gerstmann-Straüssler-Scheinker syndrome, fatal familial insomnia
Neurogenetic	Spinocerebellar ataxias, mitochondrial encephalopathies, Wilson's disease
Infectious	Meningitis, encephalitis, leukoencephalopathy, neurosyphilis, Whipple's disease, HIV
Toxic or metabolic	Systemic: thyroid, parathyroid, adrenal, liver, kidney, sarcoidosis, vitamin deficiencies, hypoxia/ischemia, drugs, alcohol, heavy metals
Other	Multiple sclerosis, neoplastic, hydrocephalus

C. Dementia with Lewy bodies (DLB)

1. Definition and overview

   The symptoms of DLB can be similar to AD with several important distinctions. Diagnostic criteria for DLB include the presence of visual hallucinations; Parkinsonian signs (stiffness, slowness of movement, shuffling gait); and fluctuations in alertness and attention (McKeith, 2006). DLB is caused by the accumulation of Lewy bodies containing α-synuclein, which deposit within neurons and affect multiple brain regions.

2. Prevalence

   DLB is considered the third most common cause for dementia. It occurs in 1 out of 25 cases of dementia (Vann Jones & O'Brien, 2014).

D. Frontotemporal dementia (FTD)

1. Definition and overview

   FTD refers to a heterogeneous group of syndromes caused by focal damage to the frontal and anterior temporal lobes of the brain. The focal damage results in behavioral disorders, executive dysfunction, and language deficits. FTD is divided into two major subtypes: behavioral variant frontotemporal dementia (bvFTD) and aphasia syndromes. The aphasia syndromes include a semantic variant and progressive nonfluent aphasia (PNFA). Behavioral variant FTD is the most common clinical subtype typically characterized by social disinhibition, impulsivity, apathy, loss of empathy, and executive dysfunction. Semantic variant is characterized by difficulty naming common objects, people, and words with progressive trouble in identifying the meaning of those items they are trying to name. Complaints about fluency or speech rhythm and pronunciation occur with PNFA. Other FTD-related movement disorders include corticobasal degeneration, progressive supranuclear palsy and motor neuron disease. Tau, TDP-43, and progranulin

are proteins involved in cellular dysfunction and death that occur with FTD. The average age at onset of FTD is between 50 and 60 years of age.

2. Prevalence

   The prevalence of FTD is 81 per 100,000 cases of dementia among people under the age of 65 (Ratnavalli, Brayne, Dawson, & Hodges, 2002).

E. Mixed dementia

1. Definition and overview

   Mixed dementia occurs when more than one type of dementia is present. Common combinations include AD and vascular, AD with DLB, and AD with vascular and DLB.

2. Prevalence

   Advances in research have shown that the presence of mixed pathologies is relatively common. About half of people with dementia have mixed pathology.

II. Database (may include but is not limited to)

A. Subjective (see Table 52-2)

One of the most important steps in the evaluation of a person with suspected dementia is to obtain a description of the symptoms and associated features with the patient and an informant (someone who knows the patient well). It is critical to involve an informant to verify information: patients with dementia may have limited insight and may mask or downplay their deficits. The focus of the interview is aimed at onset and duration of symptoms and whether they represent a change from the patient's baseline abilities. Taking a careful history is critical to determine how the symptoms have progressed and potential temporal relationships of related factors (for example, medical conditions, medications, stroke events). It is

TABLE 52-2 Features of Dementia

Syndrome	Symptoms	Onset	Areas of Brain Affected	Biochemical/ Protein	Possible Associated Symptoms	Progression
Alzheimer's disease	Short-term memory loss, word-finding difficulty, visual–spatial difficulties (getting lost or disoriented)	Gradual; more common after age 65, but can occur earlier	Multiple areas; global atrophy on imaging	Deficits in acetylcholine/ beta amyloid and tau	Apathy, depression, diminished insight over time	Slowly progressive over 7–10 yrs (or longer)
Dementia with Lewy bodies	Recurrent and well-formed visual hallucinations, fluctuating cognition, parkinsonian symptoms, visual–spatial deficits, short-term memory loss	Gradual	Multiple areas; global atrophy on imaging	Deficits in acetylcholine and dopamine/ alpha synuclein	Rapid eye movement sleep behavior disorder, falls, anxiety	Slowly progressive
Vascular dementia	Dependent on the location of ischemia	May be sudden with identifiable onset and proceed in a stepwise manner	Cortical or subcortical changes on imaging		Irritability, apathy	Dependent on management of stroke risk factors
Frontotemporal dementia	Behavior and personality change: apathy, disinhibition, poor judgment, social misconduct, executive dysfunction	Gradual; before age 60	Frontal and anterior temporal lobes (anterior sections of the brain)	Deficits in serotonin/tau, Pick bodies, or TDP-43	Speech and language changes occur in the aphasic variant. Motor deficits occur in progressive supranuclear palsy and corticobasal degeneration, and amyotrophic lateral sclerosis (related disorders), diminished insight early in disease (behavioral variant frontotemporal dementia)	Progressive over 6–8 yrs

important to understand the pattern and character of the deficits. Patients and families can be encouraged to maintain a log or journal to help in the evaluation of the person with suspected cognitive deficits. It can be helpful to start with general questions: "What are you concerned about?" moving to more specific questions, such as "What was the very first thing that was different or caused you concern?" and "How have the symptoms progressed: have they worsened, stayed the same, or improved?"

Most dementia conditions have a slow progression and an onset that can be hard to identify. In contrast, the rapidly progressive dementias (RPDs) can manifest in a much shorter time, sometimes over weeks to months. If RPD is suspected, the evaluation should be completed with referral to a specialist made promptly.

A careful review of medications (prescription and over-the-counter) should be conducted. It is important that the patient bring all medications to the evaluation in order to clarify dosages and expiration dates and the patient's understanding of the purpose, administration, and adherence for the medications.

1. Alzheimer's disease
    a. Patients or families often report deficits in short-term memory although memory loss is not always a primary cognitive deficit. First symptoms can also include nonamnestic symptoms such as problems with word finding, visual–spatial deficits (getting lost), or executive dysfunction (organization and planning). Statements may include: "s/he seems more forgetful," "s/he takes longer to get things done," "s/he is getting lost in familiar places," "s/he repeats the same question multiple times," "s/he cannot multitask as well as before," "s/he cannot come up with the right word to use," or "s/he is having trouble learning new things, such as the computer, cell phone, or television remote control".
    b. Report of personality or behavioral changes: apathy, depression, anger/aggression, or irritability and mood swings. Common complaints may include: "s/he is quieter," "s/he doesn't engage in activities as in the past," or "s/he angers easily now."
    c. Report of functional decline. Examples may include problems with completing tasks at work, paying bills late, forgetting appointments, misplacing personal items, diminished standards in personal hygiene and grooming (e.g., not showering as often, appearance that is unkempt, or wearing the same clothes over again), and problems with driving (e.g., running through stop signs, driving too fast or slow, getting lost, new traffic violations or car accidents, and/or new dents and scrapes on the car).
    d. Report of risk factors for AD. Risk factors include advanced age, family history of AD, history of moderate and severe traumatic brain injury (with loss of consciousness or posttraumatic amnesia), cardiovascular disease risk factors, and mild cognitive impairment.

2. Vascular dementia
    a. Patient or family reports of deficits in short-term memory, finding the right word, navigation, or executive function (organization and planning).
    b. Report of personality or behavioral changes: apathy, depression, irritability, or anxiety.
    c. Report of functional decline. See examples in 1. Alzheimer's disease.
    d. Report of a strokelike event that coincides with the previously mentioned cognitive, behavioral, and functional changes. It may be possible to identify a specific time point that symptoms presented. A medical review may reveal the presence of vascular risk factors (hypertension, hypercholesteremia, or diabetes).

3. Dementia with Lewy bodies (DLB)
    a. Patient or family reports of fluctuating deficits in visual–spatial abilities, navigation, executive function (organization and planning), short-term memory, or finding the right word.
    b. Report of personality or behavioral changes. Visual hallucinations are common (for example, small people or animals, movement in one's peripheral vision) as well as misperceiving objects (for example, mistaking a tree for the figure of a person). Other examples of behavioral changes may include daytime sleepiness, anxiety, apathy, and depression.
    c. Report of functional decline. See examples in 1. Alzheimer's disease.
    d. Report of motor symptoms suggestive of Parkinsonism (shuffling gait or dragging feet more while walking, bradykinesia, stiffness, and falls caused by tripping).
    e. Report of sleep changes suggestive of rapid eye movement behavior disorder. Symptoms may include new onset of thrashing and moving while sleeping, arm and leg movements as if warding off an attack, hitting the bed partner during sleep, or falling out of bed during sleep.

4. Frontotemporal dementia (FTD)
    a. Report of executive dysfunction, poor judgment, speech and language changes that may include loss of object and word meaning, or dysarthria. Common complaints may include: "s/he has been making risky decisions," "s/he cannot seem to organize tasks," "s/he doesn't know what

certain words mean anymore," or "speech is halting and it is hard to get words out."

b. Report of personality and behavioral changes: apathy, disinhibition, impulsivity, social or personal misconduct, unusual eating behaviors, compulsions, and diminished empathy. Common complaints: "s/he has become a different person," "s/he has been yelling at people," "s/he doesn't care about things, doesn't care about me," "s/he says she will do things, but doesn't," "s/he makes suggestive comments to others," "s/he talks to strangers more readily," "s/he has become self-centered," "eating behavior has changed (eats more, carbohydrate cravings, or engaging in food fads)."

c. Report of functional decline. Examples may include trouble with task completion, trouble maintaining a job, diminished abilities in managing financial and legal matters (showing poor judgment, making risky investments, unusual purchases, or giving away money), and diminished standards in hygiene and grooming.

d. Report of motor symptoms suggestive of amyotrophic lateral sclerosis, corticobasal degeneration, or progressive supranuclear palsy (falls, weakness, or diminished ability to control limb movements).

e. Report of a family history suggestive of FTD that may include dementia, behavioral disorders, or psychiatric disorders.

B. Objective

1. Mental status screening and evaluation
   a. Use a reliable and valid instrument. The Montreal Cognitive Assessment (MOCA) provides brief screening of memory, language, executive function, and visual–spatial abilities. It is available in multiple languages and is free of charge.
   b. The MOCA along with administration instructions are available at www.mocatest.org.
   c. Comprehensive neuropsychological testing by a neuropsychologist may be necessary to accurately demonstrate the presence and character of deficits.

2. Functional assessment
   a. A reliable and valid instrument that assists in comparing present with past performance in functional domains can be used in conjunction with the clinical interview.
   b. Functional abilities can be assessed in multiple domains including occupational performance, finances, driving, use of computer, household tasks (e.g., housekeeping and cooking), and personal hygiene.
   c. Examples of functional assessment instruments include the Functional Activities Questionnaire (Pfeffer, Kurosaki, Harrah, Chance, & Filos, 1982) and the Instrumental Activities of Daily Living Scale (Lawton & Brody, 1969). Both tools are easy to administer and have good reliability and validity. A disadvantage of both tools is the reliance on self- or informant report rather than direct observation of functional abilities.
   d. An instrumental activities of daily living scale is available at http://consultgerirn.org.
   e. Direct observation of a person's function can be accomplished with tools such as the Texas Functional Living Scale or the Executive Function Performance Test. In addition, occupational therapists can be helpful in the assessment of mobility, function, self-care, and swallowing.

3. Assessment of mood
   a. Evaluation should include an assessment for depression because mood disorders share similar features with neurodegenerative conditions. Depression can coexist with dementia, although its prevalence decreases with increased dementia severity.
   b. A commonly used screen is the Geriatric Depression Scale. Using a yes/no format, patients answer questions about their mood over the past week. A long version (30 items) and a short version (15 items) are available. Scoring guidelines are provided to rate the severity of depression.
   c. The Geriatric Depression Scale is available at http://consultgerirn.org.
   d. The Patient Health Questionnaires (PHQ) are mental health screening tools designed for use in the office practice setting. They are available at www.phqscreeners.com. For additional details about the PHQ, see Chapter 53, Depression.

4. Physical and neurologic examination
   a. The routine physical examination should be completed to identify the presence of any medical problems (e.g., hypertension or atrial fibrillation).
   b. The neurologic examination should include an assessment of motor abilities, reflexes, coordination, gait and balance, and an assessment for focal neurologic signs.

5. Relevant diagnostic tests
   a. Laboratory screening routinely includes complete blood count (to rule out anemia and infection), serum chemistries, thyroid and liver function, and vitamin B_{12} (to rule out metabolic conditions). Rapid plasma reagin test (RPR)

TABLE 52-3 Common Laboratory Screening in Assessment of Dementia

Laboratory Tests
Complete blood cell count
Serum electrolytes, including magnesium
Serum chemistry panel, including liver function
Thyroid function
Vitamin B$_{12}$
Folate acid level or homocysteine
Methylmalonic acid
Urinalysis
Serologic tests for syphilis*
Toxicology screening*
Human immunodeficiency virus*

* Based on clinical relevance.

and/or folate level or homocysteine and methylmalonic acid may be warranted depending on clinical findings and history. See **Table 52-3** for a summary of routine laboratory screening.

b. Other tests may be indicated based on the history or physical examination (e.g., electrocardiography or electroencephalography).

c. Biomarkers

    i. Brain imaging can help identify the degree and pattern of atrophy and may detect other causes for cognitive deficits (e.g., intracranial bleeding, space-occupying lesions, and hydrocephalus). The most common imaging techniques are magnetic resonance imaging (MRI) and computed tomography (CT). Functional brain imaging such as positron emission tomography (PET) provides information on metabolic activity in the brain, although the data can be difficult to interpret. The Food and Drug Administration has approved newer techniques in PET imaging using florbetapir (binds to beta-amyloid protein). This imaging is not covered by most insurance and current guidelines suggest its use be always in the context of an evaluation by a specialist as the results are difficult to interpret if not in conjunction with an appropriate work-up.

    ii. Proteins in cerebrospinal fluid (CSF): Specialty laboratories can provide analysis of levels of β-amyloid and phosphorylated tau although these results can be inconclusive and difficult to interpret.

d. Genetic testing: may be pursued if there is a family history, a known gene, and a desire for confirmation. The different types of dementia carry varying familial risk. Referral to a genetic counselor is typically indicated in order to clarify the presence of genetic risk and to discuss the implications of genetic testing.

III. Assessment

A. Determine the diagnosis

1. Dementia is diagnosed when there are cognitive or behavioral (neuropsychiatric) symptoms that interfere with usual function, represent a decline from previous levels of performance, and are not explained by delirium or major psychiatric disorder. The cognitive or behavioral impairment involves a minimum of two of the following domains: (a) impairment in ability to remember new information, (b) impaired reasoning and ability to manage complex tasks, (c) impaired visuospatial abilities, (d) impaired language functions, or (e) changes in behavior, personality, or comportment (American Psychiatric Association, 2013).

2. If cognitive impairment is present, and there is no decline in functional abilities, consider a diagnosis of mild neurocognitive disorder or mild cognitive impairment (MCI), terms to describe a condition that may or may not precede the development of dementia. Schedule follow-up testing within 6 months to a year or as needed.

IV. Goals of clinical management

Desired outcomes for the patient with dementia are that (a) s/he remains as independent as possible in an environment that matches his or her functional abilities; and (b) the dementia and comorbid conditions are well managed.

V. Plan

A. Conduct further work-up or referral to specialist as needed.

Referrals are indicated when symptoms are atypical, occurring in a younger patient, are suggestive of a rapidly progressive dementia, or confounded by difficult psychiatric or behavioral disturbances. Referrals may be helpful when a second opinion is desired.

B. Pharmacologic management

1. There are several classes of medications used to treat disease symptoms or improve cognitive function. Currently, there are no agents available to cure dementia.

2. Commonly used medications are outlined in **Table 52-4**. Discuss possible side effects of the acetylcholinesterase inhibitors including gastrointestinal upset and vivid dreams. Slow titration of medication, use of the patch, or administration of medication in the morning and not bedtime are common strategies to prevent these side effects. These medications are not indicated for patients with bradycardia: it may be necessary to obtain an electrocardiogram before initiation of therapy.

3. Review expected and realistic goals of treatment (e.g., treatment is for symptomatic improvement and not a cure or reversal of disease). Expected benefits may be mild improvement in memory function, mood, and alertness. Higher doses are often indicated in DLB. It is recommended that 6–12 months of therapy are needed to adequately assess the benefit of therapy (California Workgroup on Guidelines for Alzheimer's Disease Management, 2008).

4. Dietary supplements and other medications: ginkgo biloba, vitamin E, and estrogen have been considered as treatment for AD, although research has not provided compelling evidence in favor of these medications.

5. If the patient has vascular disease or mixed dementia, they should receive management and education regarding modification of cardiovascular risk factors.

C. Nonpharmacologic management

1. Conduct patient and family education
   a. Discuss implications of diagnosis as it pertains to the patient's occupation and other responsibilities.
   b. Provide education regarding dementia diagnosis, progression, and goals of care in a manner that is consistent with their values, culture, education, and abilities.
   c. Stress the importance of exercise: physical exercise has been linked to improvement of mood, maintenance of mobility, and decrease in the risk for falls, and may improve cognition.
   d. Provide information regarding educational and supportive resources available in the community (see Resources and Tools at end of chapter for suggestions).
   e. Provide information about advance directives and durable power of attorney while the patient is in the early stages of disease and able to articulate his or her wishes. Make referrals for legal and financial advice, especially if there are concerns about the patient's judgment, decision making, or vulnerability. A formal evaluation for capacity may be warranted.
   f. Discuss participation in research. The National Institutes of Health maintains a listing of all clinical trials at www.clinicaltrials.gov.

2. Safety management
   a. Determine whether patient is residing in a setting that best meets his or her functional and cognitive abilities. Types of living situations range from living at home alone, living at home

TABLE 52-4 Medications Used in the Treatment of Dementia

Drug	Indications	Possible Side Effects	Other Considerations
Cholinesterase inhibitors: Donepezil (Aricept®); Galantamine (Razadyne®, Reminyl®); Rivastigmine (Exelon®)	Used primarily in AD and DLB to slow the breakdown of acetylcholine, a neurotransmitter important for memory. May be helpful in managing the hallucinations and fluctuating cognition of DLB.	Gastrointestinal (nausea, vomiting, diarrhea). Contraindicated in patients with bradycardia.	Obtain baseline electrocardiogram before initiation in patients with cardiovascular conditions. Rivastigmine available in patch form.
N-methyl-D-aspartate antagonist: Memantine (Namenda®)	Used to reduce glutamate-mediated excitotoxicity that occurs with cell death. Approved for treatment of advanced AD (Mini-Mental Status Examination scores ≤ 15).	Constipation, dizziness, and headache.	Not effective in FTD.
Selective serotonin reuptake inhibitors	Used to treat mood disorders in dementia as well as the behavioral symptoms in FTD	Gastrointestinal (nausea and diarrhea), agitation.	

with supervision, board and care, assisted living, and memory care units.

b. If wandering or getting lost is a concern, discuss strategies for maintaining safety and refer the patient and family to the MedicAlert +Alzheimer's Association Safe Return program (operated by the Alzheimer's Association). Discuss strategies for ensuring safety concerns (e.g., door alarms and supervision).

c. Patients with dementia and their caregivers are vulnerable to abuse. Refer to Adult Protective Services if there is concern for the well-being of the patient or the caregiver.

d. Driving

   i. Depending on cognitive and motor findings, the patient can be requested to stop driving, complete test of driving abilities through the department of motor vehicles, or be referred to a driver's safety course that will assess driving ability.

   ii. Reporting to the department of motor vehicles of the diagnosis of dementia should be consistent with state laws: some states have mandatory reporting requirements.

3. Management of behavioral symptoms
Behavioral symptoms occur commonly in dementia and contribute to caregiver distress. Behavioral symptoms are caused by structural changes in the brain, a result of neurotransmitter depletion, by changes in how the patient perceives and responds to environmental stimuli, or a combination of all of these factors.

a. The first step in managing these symptoms is to discuss the character, frequency, and severity of the symptoms with the patient and caregiver. Describe the behavior specifically (e.g., not just "sundowning," but "behavior that changes in the evening and includes pacing, repetitive statements that this is not their house, pushes caregiver away, and tries to open front door to leave the house").

b. Identify whether the symptoms are hazardous, annoying, or tolerable. Not all behaviors are problematic. For example, wandering is a beneficial form of exercise as long as the patient can engage in the activity safely. Other behaviors are hazardous, such as agitation and aggression that may be physically dangerous to the patient or the caregiver.

c. Develop an individualized plan of care for managing behavioral symptoms. Strategies for managing behavioral symptoms fall into five categories. In many cases, using a combination of interventions is necessary.

   i. *Environmental* refers to modifying the patient's environment. Examples include providing activities that are enjoyable for the patient and match his/her functional level without overwhelming. For patients vulnerable to sweepstakes offers in the mail, have mail diverted to a post office box where it can be screened before reaching the patient. If the patient is having disturbing visual illusions, remove the stimuli from the environment. Environmental strategies also include the use of communication techniques that match the patient's level of comprehension and that do not provoke an argument.

   ii. *Behavioral* refers to substituting for a behavior that is more tolerable or safer than the current/prior behavior(s). Examples include substitution of sugar-free candy or nonalcoholic beverages for patients with food cravings.

   iii. *Pharmacologic* refers to the use of a medication targeted specifically for the behavior. Examples include a selective serotonin reuptake inhibitor to treat agitation. Antipsychotics can be used for delusions that are frightening and disabling for the patient. Their use is associated with increased risk of death and should be used only in cases of severe agitation, aggression, or psychosis and in conjunction with an assessment for potential medical reasons for the behavior.

   iv. *Physical* refers to the use of a physical restraint or barrier to prevent patient's movement. These strategies should only be considered as a last resort. It may be necessary to move the patient to a more protected and supportive environment such as a memory care unit in which the patient can move about in a secured setting.

   v. *Internal to the caregiver* refers to acknowledgement and acceptance by the caregiver for the behavior. Counseling and education regarding expected disease symptoms, identification of strategies for effective behavior management, and obtaining respite and support from caregiving duties are examples of helpful interventions.

4. Follow-up care

a. Follow-up assessment of the person with dementia is typically every 6 months to a year or sooner if needed and should include:

   i. An assessment of daily function to assess progression of disease and to identify concerns of the patient or family.

  ii. Cognitive status testing to assess progression of disease.

  iii. Review for comorbid physical or neuropsychiatric conditions.

  iv. Review of current medications to assess for therapeutic effectiveness and potential negative side effects.

  v. Physical examination as appropriate.

  vi. Continuation of patient and family education as needed and referrals for education and support as needed.

 5. Preparation for end-of-life care.

  a. Assess the patient's and family's cultural values and preferences (per advance directives if available).

  b. Discuss goals for managing patient care regarding dementia and any comorbid conditions.

  c. Emphasize comfort measures (e.g., simplify medication regimen, maximize comfort for patient, and initiate referral for hospice care as indicated).

VI. Assessment and management of concomitant conditions

There are factors that may negatively affect the status of the patient with dementia and their caregiver. For example, depression has been shown to contribute to excess disability of the patient with dementia. The selective serotonin reuptake inhibitors are the ideal medication for treating depression (Swartz, Barak, Mirecki, Naor, & Weizman, 2000). Sudden changes in the patient's behavior may not be caused by advancing disease but may be delirium, a result of underlying acute medical change, such as pneumonia or urinary tract infection, constipation, or poorly controlled pain. Sudden changes warrant both a medical evaluation and a review of the patient's medications.

VII. Assessment of the status of the family caregiver

Family caregivers provide the bulk of care to people with dementia. Survival of AD is typically 4 to 8 years following diagnosis, although some people live as long as 20 years with the disease. Over the disease trajectory, family caregivers provide an extensive range of assistance. Caregiving responsibilities may include a variety of tasks ranging from management of medications and appointments, decision making, money management, guarding the safety of the patient, locating and arranging for assistance via community resources and programs, hiring and supervising hired help, and assistance with walking, dressing, and other aspects of physical

care. Dementia family caregiving is associated with negative physical and emotional outcomes for the caregiver although many express satisfaction with their roles. Race, ethnicity, financial resources, supportive resources, and preparedness are only a few of the factors that affect the caregiver's experience with this role. Children and teenagers often need support and education. Desired outcomes for family caregivers include the promotion of positive coping and emotional and physical well-being.

A. Assess the caregiver's physical and emotional health concerns

 1. Assess their level of strain: The Modified Caregiver Strain Index (CSI) is a 13-item survey designed to measure strain for certain aspects of caregiving with higher scores indicative of greater strain. The CSI is available at http://consultgerirn.org.

 2. Assess for depression and anxiety. Consider tools such as the Geriatric Depression Scale or the Patient Health Questionnaires (PHQ) as previously noted.

 3. Assess the caregiver's coping strategies for managing the strain of caregiving and promote positive strategies (e.g., exercise, counseling, and so forth).

 4. Assist the caregiver in identifying activities that are pleasurable for them and methods for incorporating these activities into their lifestyle.

 5. Refer to caregiver support groups, counseling, respite care, or other services

B. Provide assistance for children and teenagers dealing with a family member's dementia

 1. There are educational and supportive resources for children and teenagers coping with a family member's dementia:

  a. www.alz.org/living_with_alzheimers_just_for_kids_and_teens.asp

  b. http://www.alzheimers.org.uk/site/scripts/documents

VIII. Resources and tools

A. Resources for all

 1. Alzheimer's Association is a national organization with local offices and can be a resource for all types of dementia (www.alz.org; 1-800-272-3900)

 2. Alzheimer's Disease Education and Referral Center, a service sponsored by the National Institute on Aging (www.alzheimers.org; 1-800-438-4380)

 3. lzheimers.gov: sponsored by the U.S. Department of Health and Human Services

4. Family Caregiver Alliance (https://www.caregiver.org)

5. Get Palliative Care: Palliative care directory (http://getpalliativecare.org)

B. Resources for providers

1. Costa, P., Williams, T., & Somerfield, M. (1996). *Early identification of Alzheimer's disease and related dementias.* Clinical practice guideline, Quick reference guide for clinicians (AHCPR Publication No. 97-0703). Rockville, MD: Author.

2. Guideline for Alzheimer's Disease Management: California Workgroup on Guidelines for Alzheimer's Disease Management. (www.alz.org/socal/images/professional_NATLguideline.pdf).

3. The Hartford Institute for Geriatric Nursing, College of Nursing, New York University. Contains best practice information on the care of older adults and multiple assessment tools with administration and scoring instructions (http://consultgerirn.org or www.hartfordign.org).

REFERENCES

Alzheimer's Association. (2014). 2014 Alzheimer's disease facts and figures. *Alzheimer's & Dementia, 10*(2). Retrieved from www.alz.org/downloads/facts_figures_2014.pdf.

American Psychiatric Association. (2013). *Diagnostic and statistical manual of mental disorders* (5th ed.). Arlington, VA: American Psychiatric Publishing.

Lawton, M., & Brody, E., (1969). Assessment of older people: Self-maintaining and instrumental activities of daily living. *Gerontologist, 9*(3):179–186.

McKeith, I. G. (2006). Consensus guidelines for the clinical and pathologic diagnosis of dementia with Lewy bodies (DLB): Report of the consortium on DLB International Workshop. *Journal of Alzheimer's Disease, 9*(Suppl. 3), 417–423.

Pfeffer, R., Kurosaki, T., Harrah, C., Chance, J., & Filos, S. (1982). Measurement of functional activities in older adults in the community. *Journal of Gerontology, 37*(3), 323–329.

Plassman, B. L., Langa, K. M., Fisher, G. G., Heeringa, S. G., Weir, D. R., Ofstedal, M. B., et al. (2007). Prevalence of dementia in the United States: The aging, demographics, and memory study. *Neuroepidemiology, 29*(1–2), 125–132.

Ratnavalli, E., Brayne, C., Dawson, K., & Hodges, J. R., (2002). The prevalence of frontotemporal dementia. *Neurology, 58*(11), 1615–1621.

Rizzi, L., Rosset, I., & Roriz-Cruz, M., (2014). Global epidemiology of dementia: Alzheimer's and vascular types. *BioMed Research International, 2014,* 908915.

Swartz, M., Barak, Y., Mirecki, I., Naor, S., & Weizman, A. (2000). Treating depression in Alzheimer's disease: Integration of differing guidelines. *International Psychogeriatrics, 12*(3), 353–358.

Vann Jones, S., & O'Brien, J. (2014). The prevalence and incidence of dementia with Lewy bodies: A systematic review of population and clinical studies. *Psychological Medicine, 44*(4), 673–683.

DEPRESSION

CHAPTER 53

Matt Tierney and Beth Phoenix

I. Introduction and general background

A. Definition, overview, and epidemiology

The term "depression" may be used to describe a mood state, a clinical syndrome, or a distinct mental disorder. In a clinical context, "depression" refers to conditions characterized by persistent depressed mood accompanied by additional symptoms (see **Figure 53-1**). Depression can be expressed as discrete major depressive episodes or as persistent depressive disorder (dysthymia), a condition characterized by depressive symptoms of varying severity that continue for at least 2 years. It can also occur as part of a bipolar mood disorder in which depressive episodes alternate with manic or hypomanic episodes or where both manic–hypomanic and depressive symptoms are manifested during the same period of time (mixed episode).

Depression can appear similar to, or accompany, other psychiatric disorders, such as anxiety disorders, thought disorders, and substance abuse disorders. Thus, clinicians should be familiar with the current version of the *Diagnostic and Statistical Manual of Mental Disorders* (DSM) to distinguish depression from other psychiatric illnesses. As with all psychiatric illness, medical causes of depressive symptoms must be ruled out before determining a diagnosis of depression. Therefore, clinical evaluation should involve the assessment of biologic, psychological, and social factors.

The 12-month prevalence of major depressive disorder for U.S. adults has been estimated at 6.9% (see **Figure 53-2**; National Institute of Mental Health [NIMH], n.d.). Lifetime prevalence of major depressive disorder has been estimated at 16.6% (Kessler, Chiu, Demler, Merikangas, & Walters, 2005). The prevalence of depression in primary care settings is estimated to be between 5% and 9% among adults (U.S. Department of Health and Human Services, Depression Guideline Panel, 1993;

Zuithoff et al., 2009), so it is important for the primary care provider to screen for, assess, and treat depression. Although depression is comparable in prevalence to other disorders commonly seen in primary care, it remains underrecognized by primary care providers (Wittkampf et al., 2009). Depression is not only underdiagnosed, it is also undertreated; it is estimated that only about 20% of Americans with depression receive care consistent with treatment guidelines (Gonzalez et al., 2010). Fortunately, initiatives to improve quality of depression care in primary care settings have resulted in the development of a number of diagnostic and treatment planning tools (MacArthur Initiative on Depression & Primary Care, 2009).

Depression is a significant public health problem; the Global Burden of Disease Study 2010 rates depression as the fifth leading cause of U.S. years of health lost to disability (U.S. Burden of Disease Collaborators, 2013). Depression has a significant impact on public health for multiple reasons: it is common and interferes with many aspects of functioning; the typical age of onset is in the teenage or young adult years; and the disorder can easily become chronic, particularly if treatment is not prompt and adequate. If depressive episodes are not adequately treated, the brain becomes sensitized to being in a depressed state, which is then more likely to recur in the future. This phenomenon, called "kindling," may lead to depressive episodes that are more frequent, more severe, and of longer duration, with incomplete recovery between episodes. For this reason, it is important to prevent long-term morbidity through early diagnosis and aggressive treatment with the goal of complete remission.

Inadequately treated depression is problematic not just in and of itself but also because it exacerbates other health problems. Persons with major depressive disorder seen in general medical settings have more pain and physical illness and more impairment in physical, social, and role functioning than other patients (American Psychiatric Association [APA], 2013).

Client Name:
Chart No.
Date:

Over the last 2 weeks, how often have you been bothered by any of the following problems?	Not at all	Several days	More than half the days	Nearly every day
1. Little interest or pleasure in doing things	0	1	2	3
2. Feeling down, depressed, or hopeless	0	1	2	3
3. Trouble falling or staying asleep, or sleeping too much	0	1	2	3
4. Feeling tired or having little energy	0	1	2	3
5. Poor appetite or overeating	0	1	2	3
6. Feeling bad about yourself — or that you are a failure or have let yourself or your family down	0	1	2	3
7. Trouble concentrating on things, such as reading the newspaper or watching television	0	1	2	3
8. Moving or speaking so slowly that other people could have noticed? Or the opposite — being so fidgety or restless that you have been moving around a lot more than usual	0	1	2	3
9. Thoughts that you would be better off dead or of hurting yourself in some way	0	1	2	3

For office coding

0 +_____ + _____ + _____ = Total Score:_____

If you checked off *any* problems, how *difficult* have these problems made it for you to do your work, take care of things at home, or get along with other people?
_ Not difficult at all _ Somewhat difficult _ Very difficult _Extremely difficult

PHQ-9 Scoring
For healthcare professional use

Total Score	Depression Severity
1–4	Minimal Depression
5–9*	Mild Depression
10–14*	Moderate Depression
15–19*	Moderately Severe Depression
20–27*	Severe Depression

* For any score 5 and above offer referral for Behavioral Health Services

FIGURE 53-1 Patient Health Questionnaire-9 (PHQ-9)

Reproduced from Pfizer. (1999). *Patient Health Questionnaire-9 (PHQ-9)*. Retrieved from www.phqscreeners.com. Scoring table reproduced from US Preventative Services Task Force. Retrieved from http://www.uspreventiveservices taskforce.org/Home/GetFileByID/218.

In addition to the significant burden of depression-related disability, depression is also a significant cause of premature mortality from suicide. Many adults who died by suicide visited their primary care provider within 1 month of their deaths; thus, familiarity with suicide risk factors is strongly recommended (Luoma, Pearson, & Martin, 2002). The SAD PERSONS mnemonic (**Table 53-1**) summarizes major risk factors for suicide. The combination of severe depression and excessive alcohol consumption is implicated in a substantial majority of completed suicides in the United States, making substance use assessment a critical part of depression screening.

The U.S. Preventive Services Task Force (USPSTF) recommends depression screening for adults when support services, including the ability to provide follow-up, are in place to accurately diagnose and treat depression.

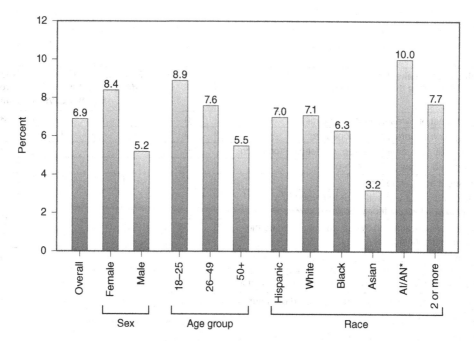

*AI/AN = American Indian/Alaska Native

FIGURE 53-2 12-month Prevalence of Major Depressive Episode Among U.S. Adults

Reproduced from National Institute of Mental Health. (n.d.). *Major depression among adults*. Retrieved from http://www.nimh.nih.gov/health/statistics/prevalence/major-depression-among-adults.shtml

---

USPSTF does not recommend a specific screening instrument. The following two questions, sometimes referred to as the Patient Health Questionnaire (PHQ)-2, are highly effective in identifying most cases of depression (Arroll et al., 2010): "Over the past 2 weeks, have you felt down, depressed, or hopeless?" and "'Over the past 2 weeks, have you felt little interest or pleasure in doing things?"

A positive response to either of these questions warrants a more thorough screening for depression using diagnostic criteria from the DSM (Figure 53-1). The Geriatric Depression Scale may be used to screen for and monitor depressive symptoms in older adults (Greenberg, 2012).

II. Database

A. Subjective (*Table 53-2*)

1. Past health history: depression; anxiety; other psychiatric illness; trauma history including head trauma; chronic medical illnesses (e.g., HIV/AIDS, hepatitis C); physical disability; new serious health diagnosis; obstetric history; medication history, including current medications, medications or supplements taken in the past, and effect on depression

2. Family history: depression, including death by suicide; other psychiatric illness; alcoholism or other substance abuse

TABLE 53-1 SAD PERSONS Mnemonic for Suicide Risk Factors

Sex (male)
Age (elderly or adolescent)
Depression
Previous suicide attempts
Ethanol abuse
Rational thinking loss (psychosis)
Social supports lacking
Organized plan to commit suicide
No spouse (divorced > widowed > single)
Sickness (physical illness)

Modified from Patterson, W. M., Dohn, H. H., Bird, J., & Patterson, G. A. (1983). Evaluation of suicidal patients: The SAD PERSONS scale. *Psychosomatics, 24*(4), 343–349.

TABLE 53-2 Depression Risk Factors

Other serious physical and mental health problems
Concurrent substance abuse or dependence
Family history of depression or suicide
Childhood depression or physical, emotional, or sexual abuse
Long-term use of certain medications
Personality traits, such as having low self-esteem and being overly dependent, self-critical, or pessimistic
Having recently given birth
Unemployment or low socioeconomic group
Female gender
Poor social support
Negative life events, such as bereavement, new onset of illness, institutionalization, financial strain, work-related distress, or experience of discrimination

3. Occupational history: presence or absence of rewarding and meaningful work, work stress

4. Personal and social history: support systems; substance use, including alcohol, nicotine, narcotics, and illicit drugs; relationship status; precipitating factors (stressors and losses)

5. Review of systems: somatic complaints without focal findings, including headaches and other pain; anhedonia, depressed mood, hypersomnia or insomnia, psychomotor agitation or slowing; indecisiveness or decrease in concentration; fatigue or loss of energy; changes in appetite or weight; feeling guilty or poor self-esteem; suicidal thoughts or plans; irritability; pressured speech or thoughts; increase in goal-directed behaviors or risk-taking behaviors or in activities that have a high potential for negative consequences (e.g., buying sprees or sexual indiscretions); expansive or euphoric mood; psychosis including paranoia and auditory or visual hallucinations; and inability to care for activities of daily living.

B. Objective

1. Physical examination findings
   a. Vital signs, including weight
   b. Thyroid examination
   c. Neurologic examination if indicated. Clinical assessment sometimes reveals that depressive symptoms are caused by an organic brain illness. Many discrete neurologic disorders (e.g., Parkinson's disease, Alzheimer's disease, cerebral vascular accidents, multiple sclerosis, traumatic brain and spinal cord injuries, dementias, and epilepsy) are associated with increased risk of depression (Hellman-Regen et al., 2013). Thus, a neurologic examination is often indicated in the physical assessment of depression.
   d. Mental status examination
      i. Appearance and behavior: patient may demonstrate poor hygiene, poor eye contact, and inability to engage with interviewer.
      ii. Motor function: may demonstrate motor slowing or agitation.
      iii. Affect: can vary from anxious or irritable, to depressed with constricted affect.
      iv. Mood: use the patient's own description of mood.
      v. Language: assess flow and volume. Speech may be quiet with few words and slow or may exhibit some nervous pressure.
      vi. Thought process: may be slow, evidenced by increased latency of response.
      vii. Thought content: what are the patient's main concerns? Patient may have suicidal or homicidal thoughts with or without a plan to carry these out (these may indicate an emergency situation and must be carefully evaluated). Depressive symptoms may include obsessions, perseverations, paranoid ideas, feelings of depersonalization or unreality, and morbid thoughts. Psychotic depression may include auditory or visual hallucinations, or delusions.
      viii. Cognition: assess possible changes in all areas, including orientation, concentration, and memory; visuospatial skills; ability to abstract; and executive functioning.
      ix. Insight: rated good, fair, or poor based on the patient's awareness of their depressive symptoms. Patients who are unsure or unaware that symptoms may be caused by depression are rated fair or poor.
      x. Judgment: rated good, fair, or poor based on the patient's ability to gather and organize information to make plans and function well.

2. Data from diagnostic tests. No single test is associated with a definitive diagnosis of depression; however, the following should be considered as part of a basic work-up of depressive symptoms from other causes or of medical problems associated with depression
   a. Complete blood count to rule out anemia
   b. Metabolic panel to rule out possible medical causes of depressive symptoms
   c. Thyroid-stimulating hormone and free T4 to rule out thyroid dysregulation

d. Serum vitamin D, vitamin B$_{12}$, and folic acid levels to rule out vitamin deficiencies

e. Drug of abuse screen to rule out co-occurring substance use disorders

f. Hormone levels (gender specific) to rule out endocrine dysregulation

III. Assessment

A. Determine the diagnosis (DSM-5)

1. Major depressive disorder: presence of five out of nine depressive symptoms, with one of the symptoms being depressed mood or anhedonia, occurring daily for at least 2 weeks.

2. Persistent depressive disorder (dysthymia): presence of three depressive symptoms (including depressed mood) for a duration of at least 2 years, with symptoms present more days than not.

3. Dysthymia with intermittent major depressive episodes ("double depression"): persistent depression with periods of more severe depressive symptoms.

4. Other psychiatric conditions that may explain the patient's presentation

a. Bipolar disorder: if patient currently meets criteria for a depressive episode but also has a history of manic or hypomanic episodes characterized by sustained expansive, euphoric, or irritable mood with pressured speech or thoughts, with increase in goal-directed behaviors or risk-taking activities (e.g., gambling with money that is meant to be used to pay rent) or with reduced need for sleep without feeling fatigue.

b. Thought disorder: presence of psychosis, disorganized thinking, or paranoia.

c. Anxiety disorder: when patient does not meet all criteria for a depressive disorder but may have some of the symptoms accompanied by disabling worry about things that are out of the patient's control.

d. Substance abuse disorder: if depressive symptoms are better accounted for by substance intoxication or withdrawal.

e. Other medical conditions that explain symptoms, including but not limited to thyroid or other endocrine disorders, dementia, anemia, and malnutrition.

f. Medication side effects (**Table 53-3**)

g. Bereavement: persistent feelings of grief associated with loss of a loved one.

TABLE 53-3 Medications That May Cause Depression

Acyclovir	Clonidine	Metoclopramide
Alcohol	Cocaine (withdrawal)	Metrizamide
Amantadine	Contraceptives	Metronidazole
α-Methyldopa	Corticosteroids	NSAIDs
Amphetamines (withdrawal)	Cycloserine	Opiates
Anabolic steroids	Dapsone	Pentazocine
Anticonvulsants	Digitalis	Pergolide
Antihistamines	Disopyramide	Phenylpropanolamine
Antineoplastic agents	Disulfiram	Physostigmine
Antipsychotic medications	Estrogens	Prazosin
Baclofen	Ethambutol	Progestins, implanted
Barbiturates	Fluoroquinolone antibiotics	Reserpine
Benzodiazepines	Guanethidine	Statins
β-Adrenergic blockers	Interferon alfa	Sulfonamides
Bromocriptine	Isotretinoin	Thiazide diuretics
Calcium channel blockers	Levodopa	
Cimetidine	Mefloquine	

Note. NSAIDs = nonsteroidal anti-inflammatory drugs.

Reproduced from Schatzberg, A., & Nemeroff, C. (2009). *The American Psychiatric Publishing textbook of psychopharmacology* (4th ed.). Washington, DC: APA. Reprinted with permission (Copyright 2009). American Psychiatric Publishing, Inc.

5. Specifiers may be used if appropriate
   a. Severity: mild, moderate, or severe, based on the impact depression has on the patient's functional ability, the intensity of distress caused by symptoms of depression, and by the presence of suicidal thoughts
   b. Chronicity: single episode or recurrent
   c. With or without psychotic features, such as nihilistic delusions or ideas of reference
   d. With atypical features: presence of weight gain and hypersomnia. Although "typical depression" is characterized by insomnia and weight loss, "atypical depression" is characterized by hypersomnia and weight gain. This specifier can be misleading, because both types of depression are commonly seen in the primary care setting.
   e. In remission: partial (alleviation of some but not all symptoms) or full (complete alleviation of symptoms); early (< 6 months) or sustained (> 6 months)
   f. Other specifiers, including with anxious distress, with mixed features, with melancholic features, with catatonia, with peripartum onset, and with seasonal pattern. Note: The reader is encouraged to consult the DSM-5 for a description of these specifiers (APA, 2013, pp. 184–188).

B. Significance and motivation

Assess the significance of depression to the patient and significant others, including impact on work, relationships, and activities. Determine the patient's willingness and ability to follow the treatment plan. Assess for presence of social supports and other patient strengths that may influence the ability to recover from depression.

IV. Goals of clinical management

A. Screening and diagnosing depression

Although there is no consensus on screening for depression, the USPSTF notes that "recurrent screening may be most productive in patients with a history of depression, unexplained somatic symptoms, comorbid psychological conditions (e.g., panic disorder or generalized anxiety), substance abuse, or chronic pain. The optimal interval for screening is unknown" (U.S. Department of Health and Human Services, 2009, p. 125).

B. Treatment

Select a treatment plan that leads to sustained full remission of depressive symptoms. Approximately one-third of depressed patients achieve remission with their initial treatment regimen, and approximately another one-third requires several treatment regimens. Another one-third fail to respond to two or more adequate trials of antidepressant monotherapy, which is considered treatment-resistant depression (Gaynes et al., 2009). Treatment resistance is associated with a range of comorbid physical and mental disorders, including substance abuse.

Recovery is likely to begin within 3 months of onset for about 40% of individuals with major depression and about 80% will recover within a year. "Recency of onset is a strong determinant of the likelihood of near-term recovery, and many individuals who have been depressed only for several months can be expected to recovery spontaneously" (APA, 2013, p. 165). Depression can remit without treatment; one model estimates that 23% of cases of untreated depression will remit by 3 months, 32% by 6 months and 53% by 12 months (Whiteford et al., 2013). All patients with depression need to be monitored for changes in condition, and treatment planning should involve not only a consideration of the severity and impact of depression but also the patient's health beliefs as well as adherence to the treatment plan and ability to access components of the care plan.

1. Treatment phases (see **Figure 53-3**)
   a. Acute phase: 0–16 weeks. Plan: initiate treatment and monitor weekly for first month and at least once a month thereafter.
   b. Continuation phase: 16–20 weeks after symptom remission. Plan: continue treatment, monitor every 2–3 months.
   c. Maintenance phase: 6 months symptom free. Plan: continue monitoring and treatment every 2–3 months.
   d. Discontinuation: consider treatment discontinuation only after patient has been symptom free for 6–12 months. Because risk of relapse is highest in the initial 2-month period following discontinuation of treatment, patients should continue to be monitored for several months. Patient education should include a review of the early signs of depression, such as sleep disturbance and loss of interest in normal activities, and emphasize the importance of immediately resuming previously successful treatment in the event of a symptom relapse (APA, 2010).

C. Patient adherence

Select an approach that maximizes patient adherence, including but not limited to cost, frequency of treatment, tolerability of treatment, and patient health beliefs.

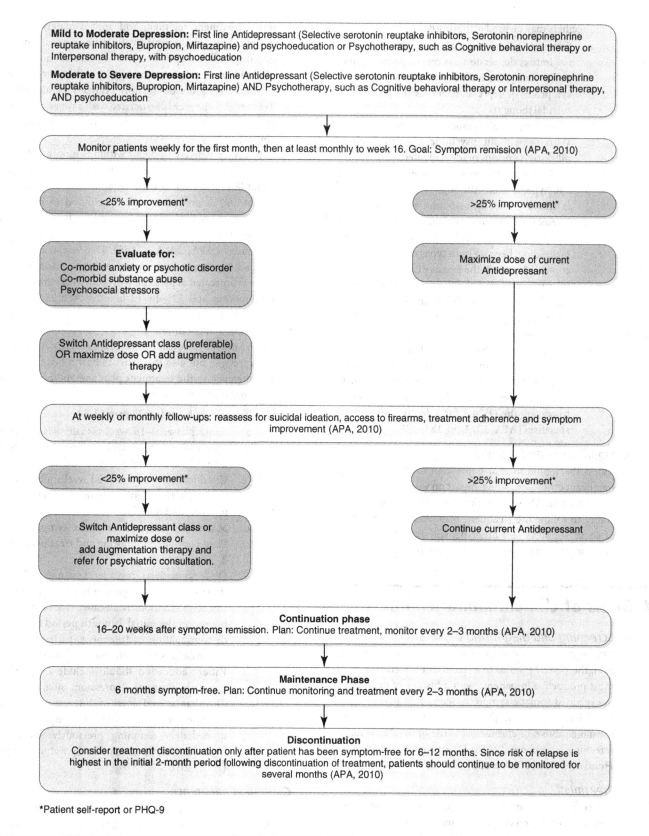

FIGURE 53-3 Primary Care Treatment Algorithm for Depression

Data from Fancher, T., McCarron, R. M., Kukoyi, O., & Bourgeois, J. A. (2009). Chapter 2: Mood disorders—Depression. In R. M. McCarron, G. L. Xiong, & J. A. Bourgeois (Eds.), *Lippincott's Primary Care Psychiatry*, 31. Lippincott Williams & Wilkins.

V. Plan

A. Diagnostic tests to rule out other causes of depressive symptoms

Complete blood count with differential; complete metabolic panel, vitamin B_{12}, folate, thyroid-stimulating hormone, free T4; gamma-glutamyl transferase (GGT) or breathalyzer if alcohol use suspected; consider a drug of abuse screen and a more thorough toxicology screen (e.g., heavy metal screen) if indicated by history. HIV testing if indicated by history.

B. Management (includes treatment, consultation, referral, and follow-up care)

1. Medication management. Medication treatment should always include consideration of the following: patient history of medication treatment for depression, cost and insurance coverage, past or anticipated side effects, and concurrent patient medications (**Tables 53-4**, **53-5**, and **53-6**)

2. Psychotherapy: for mild to moderate depression, psychotherapy has generally been found to be equal in efficacy to pharmacologic treatment (Wolf & Hopko, 2008), and the combination of medication and psychotherapy is more effective than either modality alone. Circumstances under which referral for psychotherapy should be considered as a first-line treatment option include patient preference and pregnancy and lactation. Even brief psychotherapy of 6 to 8 sessions, in particular cognitive behavioral therapy and problem-solving therapy, can be effective in treating depression (Nieuwsma et al., 2012). Behavioral activation, in which patients are encouraged to increase their participation in interesting and enjoyable activities, is easy to administer in primary care settings and has shown efficacy in decreasing depressive symptoms (Gros & Haren, 2011).

3. Combined treatment with antidepressants and psychological treatment is recommended for:
   a. Partial response to either treatment alone
   b. Patients with personality disorders or complex psychosocial problems
   c. Patients with a history of chronic or severe depression

4. Consultation with physician: Confirmed or suspicion of concurrent medical illness and polypharmacy treatment.

5. Referral to mental health or psychiatric specialty for evaluation or management: psychotic symptoms, suspicion of bipolar disorder or thought disorder, current or prior treatment-resistant depression, active suicidal ideation or plan and concurrent psychiatric or neurologic disorder. Additionally, the World Federation of Societies of Biological Psychiatry (WFSBP) recommends that mental health specialists should take responsibility for treating depression that is recurrent, that presents with atypical features or with special risks, or when the patient's dysfunction or risk for mortality is severe (Bauer et al., 2013, p. 342)

C. Client education

1. Information: provide verbal and written information regarding:
   a. The disease process, including but not limited to signs and symptoms and possible causes and risks, including self-harm
   b. The importance of treatment, including non-pharmacologic treatment, with the goal of complete and sustained remission of depression; expected treatment duration; and community resources to manage psychiatric crises
   c. Selection of written educational materials should consider:
      i. Patient educational and reading level
      ii. Availability of materials in patient's preferred language
      iii. Accuracy of information and freedom from commercial bias

2. Counseling
   a. Supportive counseling, focusing on problem solving and use of coping strategies (MacArthur Initiative on Depression & Primary Care, 2009)
   b. Behavioral recommendations: regular exercise, especially aerobic exercise; balanced diet; presence of supportive relationships; increased engagement in pleasurable activities; and sleep hygiene

TABLE 53-4 Overview of Antidepressant Classes

	Selective Serotonin Reuptake Inhibitors (SSRI)	Tricyclic Antidepressants (TCA)	Monoamine Oxidase Inhibitors (MAOI)
Efficacy	First-line treatment in MDD (FDA approved for all except fluvoxamine), dysthymia PD (FDA approved for fluoxetine, paroxetine, and sertraline) OCD (FDA approved for all except citalopram and escitalopram) PTSD (FDA approved for sertraline and paroxetine) Bulimia (FDA approved for fluoxetine) GAD (FDA approved for fluoxetine [Sarafem only], paroxetine [controlled release only], and sertraline)	Second- or third-line agents for MDD (FDA approved for all) Panic disorder OCD (FDA approved for clomipramine) Pain syndromes, migraine prophylaxis Enuresis (FDA approved for imipramine)	Third-line agents for MDD (FDA approved for resistant depression) Social anxiety Panic disorder Second-line agents for Parkinson's disease (selegiline has FDA approval)
Side Effects	GI side effects (nausea, diarrhea, heartburn) Sexual dysfunction (↓ libido, delayed orgasm) Headache Insomnia/somnolence	Dry mouth, constipation, urinary retention, blurred vision, confusion Weight gain Sedation Sexual dysfunction Orthostasis Tachycardia Cardiac conduction abnormalities	Weight gain Orthostasis Sexual dysfunction Dry mouth Insomnia/somnolence Headache
Dosage and Administration	Citalopram, paroxetine, fluoxetine: daily dosing, starting at 10–20 mg, increasing to a maximum of 40 mg (citalopram), 50 mg (paroxetine), and 80 mg (fluoxetine). Escitalopram: daily dosing, starting at 10 mg, increasing to 20 mg after minimum of 1 week. Sertraline: starts at 25–50 mg and is increased, as needed, to 200 mg maximum.	Individualize with low bedtime dosing (25–50 mg) for imipramine and amitriptyline. Increase by 25–50 mg every 3–7 days to target dosage of 150–300 mg/day. (Nortriptyline should be started at 10–25 mg and increased, as needed, to a maximum dosage of 150 mg/day.) Monitor levels and ECGs after dose stabilized.	Phenelzine: start at 15 mg bid or tid and increase by 15 mg per week to target dosage of 60–90 mg/day. Tranylcypromine: start at 10 mg bid or tid and increase by 10 mg per week to target dosage of 40–60 mg/day. Isocarboxazid: start at 10 mg bid and increase dosage, if the drug is tolerated, by 10 mg every 2–4 days to 40 mg/day by end of first week. Maximum recommended dosage is 60 mg/day, administered in divided doses. Selegiline transdermal system (Emsam): start with 6-mg patch daily for 4 weeks and then increase to 9-mg patch for 2 weeks, and then 12-mg patch as needed. No dietary restrictions at 6 mg/day.

TABLE 53-4 Overview of Antidepressant Classes *(Continued)*

	Selective Serotonin Reuptake Inhibitors (SSRI)	Tricyclic Antidepressants (TCA)	Monoamine Oxidase Inhibitors (MAOI)
Discontinuation	Paroxetine, fluvoxamine, sertraline: discontinuation associated with parasthesias, nausea, headaches, flulike symptoms, 1–7 days after sudden discontinuation	Flulike and GI symptoms from cholinergic rebound. Reduce by 25–50 mg every 3 days.	Flulike symptoms, hallucinations, hypomania, and dysphoria reported with sudden discontinuation. Taper dose by 25% per week.
Drug Interactions	MAOI (**contraindicated**): serotonin syndrome ↑ TCA levels (paroxetine, fluoxetine) ↑ Carbamazepine, phenobarbital, phenytoin levels ↑ Haloperidol, clozapine levels (fluvoxamine) ↑ Theophylline levels (fluvoxamine) ↑ Encainide, flecainide levels (**avoid**)	CNS depressants: ↑ sedation, ataxia Anticoagulants: ↑ warfarin levels Antipsychotics: ↑ TCA and antipsychotic levels Cimetidine: ↑ TCA levels Clonidine: hypertensive crisis (**avoid**) L-Dopa: TCAs ↓ absorption MAOIs: serotonin syndrome (avoid clomipramine; imipramine and amitriptyline may be used with close monitoring) Stimulants: ↑ TCA levels Oral contraceptives: ↑ TCA levels Quinidine: ↑ arrhythmias (**avoid**) SSRIs: ↑ TCA levels Sympathomimetics: ↑ arrhythmias, hypertension, tachycardia	Food containing high levels of tyramine, such as aged cheeses or cured or pickled foods (**contraindicated**) hypertensive crisis β-Blockers: ↑ hypotension, bradycardia Oral hypoglycemics: ↑ hypoglycemic effects Bupropion (**contraindicated**): hypertensive crisis, seizure Carbamazepine (**contraindicated**): hypertensive crisis Meperidine (**contraindicated**): serotonin syndrome Nefazodone: possible serotonin syndrome Sympathomimetics: hypertensive crisis SSRIs (**contraindicated**): serotonin syndrome TCAs: clomipramine **contraindicated** Mirtazapine (**contraindicated**): hypertensive crisis SNRIs (**contraindicated**): serotonin syndrome
Safety in Overdose	Generally safe in overdose to 30–90 days' supply; manage with vital sign support, lavage Seizures/status epilepticus (rare)	Lethal in overdose (induces arrhythmias). Lavage and monitor on a cardiac bed for QRS widening.	Can be lethal in overdose. Hypertensive crisis, stroke, and myocardial infarction have been reported. Manage with lavage, emesis induction, and close management of blood pressure and airway.

Notes: CNS = central nervous system; ECG = electrocardiogram; FDA = U.S. Food and Drug Administration; GAD = generalized anxiety disorder; GI = gastrointestinal; MAOI = monoamine oxidase inhibitor; MDD = major depressive disorder; SNRI = serotonin-norepinephrine reuptake inhibitor; OCD = obsessive-compulsive disorder; PD = panic disorder; PMDD = premenstrual dysphoric disorder; PTSD = posttraumatic stress disorder; SSRI = selective serotonin reuptake inhibitor; TCA = tricyclic antidepressant.

Adapted from Schatzberg, A. F., & DeBattista, C. (2015). *Manual of clinical psychopharmacology* (8th ed.). Arlington, VA: American Psychiatric Publishing.

TABLE 53-5 Antidepressant Names, Formulations and Strengths, and Dosages

Generic Name	Brand Name	Formulations & Strengths	Therapeutic Dosage Range (mg/day)[a]
Selective Serotonin Reuptake Inhibitors			
citalopram	Celexa®	Tablets: 10, 20, 40 mg	20–40
		Oral solution: 10 mg/5 mL (240-mL bottle)	
escitalopram	Lexapro®	Tablets: 5, 10, 20 mg	
		Oral solution: 5 mg/5 mL (240-mL bottle)	
fluoxetine	Prozac®	Capsules: 10, 20, 40 mg	20–60
		Capsule (weekly): 90 mg	
		Oral solution: 20 mg/5 mL (120-mL bottle)	
	Luvox®	Tablets: 10, 20 mg	
fluvoxamine	Luvox CR®	Tablets: 25, 50, 100 mg	100–200
		Tablets: 100, 150 mg	
paroxetine	Paxil®	Tablets: 10, 20, 30, 40 mg	20–50
	Paxil-CR® (controlled-release)	Oral suspension: 10 mg/5 mL (250-mL bottle)	
sertraline	Zoloft®	Tablets: 12.5, 25, 37.5 mg	
		Tablets: 25, 50, 100 mg	50–200
		Oral concentrate: 20 mg/mL (60-mL bottle)	
Serotonin Norepinephrine Reuptake Inhibitors			
venlafaxine	Effexor®	Tablets: 25, 37.5, 50, 75, 100 mg	75–375
	Effexor-XR® (sustained-release) and generic	Capsules: 37.5, 75, 150 mg	
desvenlafaxine	Pristiq®	Tablets (extended release): 50, 100 mg	50–100
duloxetine	Cymbalta®	Capsules: 20, 30, 60 mg	60–120
levomilnacipran	Fetzima®	Capsules: 20, 40, 80, 120 mg	40–120
milnacipran[b]	Savella®	Tablets: 12.5, 25, 50, 100 mg	100–200
5-HT$_2$ antagonists			
nefazodone	Generic only	Tablets: 50, 100, 150, 200, 250 mg	300–500
trazodone	Generic only	Tablets: 50, 100, 150,[c] 300[c] mg	150–300
	Oleptro (extended release)	Tablets (scored): 150, 300 mg	150–375
Tricyclics[d]			
amitriptyline	Elavil®	Tablets: 10, 25, 50, 75, 100, 150 mg	150–300
clomipramine	Anafranil®	Capsules: 25, 50, 75 mg	100–250
desipramine	Norpramin®	Tablets: 10, 25, 50, 75, 100, 150 mg	150–300
doxepin	Sinequan®	Capsules: 10, 25, 50, 75, 100, 150 mg	150–300
		Oral solution: 10 mg/mL (120-mL bottle)	
imipramine	Tofranil®	Tablets: 10, 25, 50 mg	150–300
imipramine pamoate	Tofranil-PM[e]	Capsules: 75, 100, 125, 150 mg	150–300
nortriptyline	Aventyl®, Pamelor®	Capsules: 10, 25, 50, 75 mg	50–150
		Oral solution: 10 mg/5 mL (480-mL bottle)	
protriptyline	Vivactil®	Tablets: 5, 10 mg	15–60
trimipramine maleate	Surmontil®	Capsules: 25, 50, 100 mg	150–300

TABLE 53-5 Antidepressant Names, Formulations and Strengths, and Dosages *(Continued)*

Generic Name	Brand Name	Formulations & Strengths	Therapeutic Dosage Range (mg/day)[a]
Tetracyclics[e]			
amoxapine	Asendin®	Tablets: 25, 50, 100, 150 mg	150–400
maprotiline	Ludiomil®	Tablets: 25, 50, 75 mg	150–225
Monoamine Oxidase Inhibitors			
phenelzine	Nardil®	Tablet: 15 mg	45–90
selegiline	Eldepryl®	Capsule: 5 mg	20–50
	Carbex®	Tablet: 5 mg	
	Zelapar®	Orally disintegrating tablet: 1.25 mg	
	Emsam®	Patch: 6 mg/24 hr, 9 mg/24 hr, 12 mg/24 hr	
tranylcypromine	Parnate®	Tablet: 10 mg	30–60
isocarboxazid	Marplan®	Tablet: 10 mg	30–60
Other Antidepressants			
bupropion	Wellbutrin® and generic	Tablets: 75, 100 mg	200–450
	Wellbutrin SR® (sustained-release)	Tablets: 100, 150, 200 mg	
	Wellbutrin XL® (extended-release)	Tablets: 150, 300 mg	
mirtazapine	Remeron®	Tablets: 7.5, 15, 30, 45 mg	15–45
		Soltabs: 15, 30, 45 mg	
vortioxetine	Brintellix®	Tablets: 5, 10, 20 mg	10–20
vilazodone	Viibryd®	Tablets: 10, 20, 40 mg	40

Note. 5-HT$_2$ = serotonin$_2$ receptor.

[a] Dosage ranges are approximate. Many patients respond at relatively low dosages (even dosages below those in the ranges given in table); others may require higher dosages.

[b] Approved for fibromyalgia; doses given are those recommended for that use.

[c] Trazodone also available in 150- and 300-mg divided-dose formulations.

[d] All the tricyclic and tetracyclic antidepressants shown are available generically. Most of the brand name drugs listed have been discontinued.

[e] Sustained release.

Adapted from Schatzberg, A. F., & DeBattista, C. (2015). *Manual of clinical psychopharmacology* (8th ed.). Arlington, VA: American Psychiatric Publishing.

TABLE 53-6 Antidepressant Side Effects

Side effects account for as many as two-thirds of all premature discontinuations of antidepressants. Most side effects are early onset and time limited (e.g., SSRI decreased appetite, nausea, diarrhea, agitation, anxiety, headache). These can be managed by temporary aids to tolerance. Some side effects are early onset and persistent or late onset (e.g., SSRI apathy, fatigue, weight gain, sexual dysfunction) and may require additional medications or a switch in antidepressant.

Strategies for Managing Antidepressant Side Effects:

1. Allow patient to verbalize his/her complaint about side effects.
2. Wait and support. Some side effects (i.e., GI distress) will subside over 1–2 weeks.
3. Lower the dose temporarily.
4. Treat the side effects (discussed next).
5. Change to a different antidepressant.
6. Discontinue medications and start psychological counseling.

(continues)

TABLE 53-6 Antidepressant Side Effects *(Continued)*

Side Effect	SSRIs & Effexor	Tricyclics (nortriptyline, amitriptyline, imipramine)	Bupropion	Mirtazapine	Management Strategy
Sedation	±	++	−	+	Give medication at bedtime. *Increase* Remeron dose. Try caffeine.
Anticholinergic-like symptoms: Dry mouth/eyes, Constipation, Urinary retention, Tachycardia	±	+++	−	±	Increase hydration. Sugarless gum/candy. Dietary fiber. Artificial tears. Consider switching medication.
GI distress Nausea	++	−	+	±	Often improves in 1–2 weeks. Take with meals. Consider antacids or H2 blockers.
Restlessness Jitters/tremors	+	±	++	−	Start with small doses, especially with anxiety disorder. Reduce dose temporarily. Add beta-blocker (propranolol 10–20 mg bid/tid). Consider short trial of benzodiazepine.
Headache	+	−	+	−	Lower dose. Acetaminophen.
Insomnia	+	−	+	−	Trazodone 25–100 mg po qhs (can cause orthostatic hypotension and priapism). Take medication in A.M.
Sexual dysfunction	++	−	−	−	May be part of depression or medical disorders. Decrease dose. Consider a trial of Viagra. Try adding bupropion 100 mg qhs or bid. Try adding buspirone 10–20 mg bid/tid. Try adding cyproheptadine 4 mg 1–2 hrs before sex.
Seizures	−	−	+	±	Discontinue antidepressant.
Weight gain	±	±	±	++	Exercise. Diet. Consider changing medications.
Agranulocytosis	−	−	−	±	Monitor for signs of infection, flulike symptoms. Stop drug, check white blood count.

Key: − Very unlikely; ± Uncommon/mild; + moderate

Courtesy of MacArthur Foundation Initiative on Depression and Primary Care. MacArthur Toolkit—Copyright April 2009 3 CM LLC. Used with permission. Retrieved from http://www.dphhs.mt.gov/Portals/85/amdd/documents/AMDD%20Website%20Migration%20 Documents/13macarthurtoolkit.pdf

VI. Self-management resources and tools

Brief educational or self-management interventions, such as manualized or book-based therapies and the use of interactive web-based or other computer programs based on cognitive-behavioral approaches, have been shown to improve depression outcomes for patients treated in primary care settings (McNaughton, 2009).

A. Educational resources (books and websites)

1. Patient education brochures about depression in English and Spanish can be downloaded or ordered from the National Institutes for Mental Health (http://www.nimh.nih.gov/health/publications /depression/complete-index.shtml). The National Institutes for Mental Health also produced a brief video about depression ("www.nimh.nih.gov/health /publications/depression/complete-index.shtml). The National Institutes for Mental Health also produced a brief video about depression (https:// www.youtube.com/watch?v=mlNCavst2EU).

2. The MacArthur Initiative on Depression and Primary Care (2009) developed patient education materials as part of its Depression Management Tool Kit. The toolkit can be accessed at www.dphhs.mt.gov/Portals/85/amdd /documents/AMDD%20Website%20Migration%20 Documents/13macarthurtoolkit.pdf.

3. Beyond Blue (www.beyondblue.org.au), an organization to address issues related to depression in Australia, has information about depression as well as online communities, a hotline, and online chat. Depression information in multiple languages including Spanish, Chinese, Arabic, and Vietnamese can be found at www .beyondblue.org.au/resources/for-me/multicultural -people.

4. The Antidepressant Skills Workbook, a self-management manual for adults with depression, can be downloaded free from www.comh.ca /antidepressant-skills/adult/.

5. *Feeling Good: The New Mood Therapy* (Burns, 1980) describes a cognitive therapy approach to depression management. It is commonly used as self-guided treatment and in depression treatment programs.

6. A free interactive skills program based on cognitive-behavioral and interpersonal psychotherapy approaches can be found at http://moodgym.anu.edu.au.

B. Community support groups

1. National Alliance on Mental Illness website (www .nami.org). This support, education, and advocacy organization offers a variety of educational materials about depression including fact sheets, podcasts, and video clips.

2. The Depression and Bipolar Support Alliance (www .dbsalliance.org) offers educational brochures about depression and other mood disorders and conducts in-person and online support groups and educational events.

REFERENCES

American Psychiatric Association. (2010, October). *Practice guideline for the treatment of patients with major depressive disorder* (3rd ed.). Retrieved from https://psychiatryonline.org/pb/assets/raw/sitewide/practice _guidelines/guidelines/mdd.pdf.

American Psychiatric Association. (2013). *Diagnostic and statistical manual of mental disorders* (5th ed.). Washington, DC: Author.

Arroll, B., Goodyear-Smith, F., Crengle, S., Gunn, J., Kerse, N., Fishman, T., et al. (2010). Validation of PHQ-2 and PHQ-9 to screen for major depression in the primary care population. *Annals of Family Medicine*, 8(4), 348–353. doi:10.1370/afm.1139.

Bauer, M., Pfennig, A., Severus, E., Whybrow, P. C., Angst, J., & Moller, H-J. (2013). World Federation of Societies of Biological Psychiatry (WFSBP) guidelines for biological treatment of unipolar depressive disorders, Part I: Update 2013 on the acute and continuation treatment of unipolar depressive disorders. *World Journal of Biological Psychiatry*, 14, 334–385. doi: 10.3109/15622975.2013.804195

Burns, D. D. (1980). *Feeling good: The new mood therapy*. New York: William Morrow.

Fancher, T., McCarron, R. M., Kukoyi, O., & Bourgeois, J. A. (2009). Chapter 2: Mood disorders—Depression. In R. M. McCarron, G. L. Xiong, & J. A. Bourgeois (Eds.), *Lippincott's primary care psychiatry* (pp. 17–39). Philadelphia, PA: Wolters Kluwer/Lippincott Williams and Wilkins.

Gaynes, B. N., Warden, D., Trivedi, M. H., Wisniewski, S. R., Fava, M., & Rush, A. J. (2009). What did STAR*D teach us? Results from a large-scale, practical, clinical trial for patients with depression. *Psychiatric Services*, 60(11), 1439–1445.

Gonzalez, H. M., Vega, W. A., Williams, D. R., Taraf, W., West, B. T., & Neighbors, H. W. (2010). Depression care in the United States: Too little for too few. *Archives of General Psychiatry*, 67(1), 37–46.

Greenberg, S. A. (2012). The Geriatric Depression Scale (GDS). In *Try this: Best practices in nursing care to older adults* (No. 4). Retrieved from http://consultgerirn.org/uploads/File/trythis/try_this_4.pdf

Gros, D. F., & Haren, W. B. (2011). Open trial of brief behavioral activation psychotherapy for depression in an integrated Veterans Affairs primary care setting. *Primary Care Companion to CNS Disorders*, 13(4), PCC.11m01136. doi:10.4088/PCC.11m01136

Hellmann-Regen, J., Piber, D., Hinkelmann, K., Gold, S. M., Heesen, C., Spitzer, C., et al. (2013). Depressive syndromes in neurological disorders. *European Archives of Psychiatry and Clinical Neuroscience, 263,* (2, Suppl.), 123–136.

Kessler, R. C., Chiu, W. T., Demier, O., Merikangas, K. R., & Walters, E. E. (2005). Prevalence, severity, and comorbidity of 12-month DSM-IV disorders in the National Comorbidity Survey Replication. *Archives of General Psychiatry, 62*(6), 617–627.

Luoma, J. B., Pearson, J. L., & Martin, C. E. (2002). Contact with mental health and primary care prior to suicide: A review of the evidence. *American Journal of Psychiatry, 159,* 909–916.

MacArthur Initiative on Depression & Primary Care. (2009). *Depression management toolkit.* Retrieved from http://www.dphhs.mt.gov/Portals/85 /amdd/documents/AMDD%20Website%20Migration%20Documents /13macarthurtoolkit.pdf.

McNaughton, J. L. (2009). Brief interventions for depression in primary care: A systematic review. *Canadian Family Physician, 55*(8), 789–796.

National Institute of Mental Health. (n.d.). *Major depression among adults.* Retrieved from http://www.nimh.nih.gov/health/statistics /prevalence/major-depression-among-adults.shtml.

Nieuwsma, J. A., Trivedi, R. B., McDuffie, J., Kronish, I., Benjamin, D., & Williams, J. W. (2012). Brief psychotherapy for depression: A systematic review and meta-analysis. *International Journal of Psychiatry in Medicine, 43*(2), 129–151.

Patterson, W. M., Dohn, H. H., Bird, J., & Patterson, G. A. (1983). Evaluation of suicidal patients: The SAD PERSONS scale. *Psychosomatics, 24*(4), 343–349.

Schatzberg, A. F., & DeBattista, C. (2015). *The manual of clinical psychopharmacology* (8th ed.). Arlington, VA: American Psychiatric Publishing.

Schatzberg, A., & Nemeroff, C. (2009). *The American Psychiatric Publishing textbook of psychopharmacology* (4th ed.). Washington, DC: APA.

U.S. Burden of Disease Collaborators. (2013). The state of U.S. health, 1990–2010: Burden of diseases, injuries, and risk factors. *JAMA, 310*(6), 591–608.

U.S. Department of Health and Human Services, Depression Guideline Panel. (1993). *Clinical practice guideline No. 5, depression in primary care: Vol. 1. Detection and diagnosis.* (AHCPR Publication No. 93-0550). Rockville, MD: Author.

U.S. Department of Health and Human Services. (2009). *Guide to clinical preventive services, 2009 recommendations of the U.S. Preventive Services Task Force* (pocket guide, Abridged version of the recommendations). Retrieved from www.ncbi.nlm.nih.gov/books/NBK37637/.

Whiteford, H. A., Harris, M. G., McKeon, G., Baxter, A., Pennell, C., Barendregt, J. J., et al. (2013). Estimating remission from untreated major depression: a systematic review and meta-analysis. *Psychological Medicine, 43*(8):1569–1585. doi: 10.1017/S0033291712001717.

Wittkampf, K., van Ravesteijn, H., Baas, K., van de Hoogen, H., Schene, A., Bindels, P., et al. (2009). The accuracy of Patient Health Questionnaire-9 in detecting depression and measuring depression severity in high-risk groups in primary care. *General Hospital Psychiatry, 31*(5), 451–459.

Wolf, N. J., & Hopko, D. R. (2008). Psychosocial and pharmacological interventions for depressed adults in primary care: A critical review. *Clinical Psychology Review, 28,* 131–161.

Zuithoff, N. P., Vergouwe, Y., King, M., Nazareth, I., Hak, E., Moons, K. G., et al. (2009). A clinical prediction rule for detecting major depressive disorder in primary care: The PREDICT-NL study. *Family Practice, 26*(4), 241–250.

DIABETES MELLITUS

Carolina Noya and Maureen McGrath

CHAPTER **54**

I. Introduction and general background

Diabetes mellitus (DM) is a metabolic disorder characterized by hyperglycemia that results from decreased insulin secretion, insulin resistance, or both. There are several types of diabetes. The most common types are type 1, type 2, and gestational diabetes.

A. Prevalence and incidence

Approximately 29.1 million children and adults in the United States (9.3% of the population) have diabetes. Of these, 21.0 million are diagnosed and 8.1 million are undiagnosed (Centers for Disease Control and Prevention, 2014). Type 1 diabetes accounts for approximately 5–10% of diagnosed diabetes cases, whereas type 2 makes up the other 90–95% (American Diabetes Association [ADA], 2009b). This number is predicted to increase from 23.6 million in 2009 to 44.1 million in 2034 (Huang, Basu, O'Grady, & Capretta, 2009).

B. Type 1 diabetes

1. Definition and overview

Type 1 diabetes (T1D) is caused by an autoimmune process that destroys the β cells in the pancreas, thereby resulting in little or no insulin production. Individuals with type 1 diabetes cannot live without administration of exogenous insulin. Whereas T1D is usually associated with youth, there is a form of T1D diagnosed in adulthood called latent autoimmune diabetes of the adult or LADA. The presentation of T1D is often acute and approximately 25% of new-onset T1D presents in diabetic ketoacidosis (DKA) (Dabelea et al., 2014).

C. Type 2 diabetes

1. Definition and overview

Type 2 diabetes is usually the result of insulin resistance, although it can also be caused by decreased insulin production. Risk factors for type 2 include age older than 45 years, obesity, sedentary lifestyle, family history of diabetes, history of gestational diabetes, delivery of a baby over 9 lb, and race or ethnicity (African Americans, Latinos, Native Americans, and Asian Americans/Pacific Islanders). Type 2 diabetes is becoming more common in children and adolescents. According to the SEARCH for Diabetes in Youth Study (Dabelea et al., 2014), type 2 diabetes in youth represents 50% of new-onset diabetes in youth. Moreover, ethnic minority youth are at higher risk for type 2 diabetes when compared to their white peers.

D. Gestational diabetes

1. Definition and overview

Gestational diabetes occurs in 3–12% of pregnancies. Pregnancy is an insulin-resistant state. Women with a history of gestational diabetes have a 40–60% chance of developing type 2 diabetes in the next 5–10 years after their pregnancy; therefore, they should have their blood sugar monitored periodically. For more in depth information, see Chapter 33 on gestational diabetes.

II. Database (may include but is not limited to)

A. Subjective

1. History of presenting illness
   a. Age of onset
   b. Presenting signs and symptoms: Assess for classic signs or symptoms—weight gain or loss, polyuria, polydipsia, and/or polyphagia
   c. Growth and developmental history for children and youth
   d. Habits: including nutrition (food diary, meal planning), exercise (type and duration)

e. Review of medication regimens, response to therapy, and adherence issues

f. Assessment of readiness for change, SMART (Specific-Measurable-Attainable-Realistic-Timely) goal attainment, and barriers to self-care

g. Self-glucose monitoring: assess trends of high and low values.

h. Hypoglycemia: assess for awareness, frequency, and cause.

2. Past health history

a. Medical illnesses: hypertension, metabolic syndrome, hyperlipidemia, pancreatitis, pancreatic cancer, cystic fibrosis, hemochromatosis, Cushing's syndrome, acromegaly, glucagonoma, obesity, and pheochromocytoma. Diabetes-related complications: Microvascular disease (retinopathy, nephropathy, neuropathy, including sensory and autonomic). Macrovascular disease: cardiovascular disease (CVD), peripheral artery disease, and cerebrovascular disease.

b. Surgical history: pancreatic surgery and liver surgery

c. Trauma history: pancreatic trauma

d. Obstetric and gynecological history: history of gestational diabetes or delivery of baby weighing more than 9 lb; contraception method

e. Medication history: medications that increase blood glucose levels or interfere with the release of insulin (e.g., glucocorticoids, pentamidine, nicotinic acid, thyroid hormone, phenytoin, atypical antipsychotics, and thiazides). Any over-the-counter or herbal medication (e.g., sweetened cough preparations).

3. Family history

a. DM

b. Metabolic syndrome

c. Obesity

d. Autoimmune disorders

e. Other endocrine disorders

4. Occupational and educational history

a. Education and literacy level

b. Occupation: type, ability to control environment as it relates to food intake, self-monitoring of blood glucose, and rest

c. Days missed from school or work due to illness

5. Personal and social history

a. Tobacco, alcohol, and drug use

b. Diet history and recall

c. Exercise: type and duration

d. Cultural history, living arrangements, housing, presence of food insecurity, and psychosocial supports and problems

e. Sexual history: partners and sexual activity; sexually transmitted infection prevention/condom use

6. Review of symptoms

a. Constitutional signs and symptoms: fatigue, weight loss, and polydipsia

b. Skin, hair, and nails; slowed wound healing

c. Eye, ear, nose, and throat; blurry vision; and gum infections or dental disease

d. Respiratory: shortness of breath

e. Cardiac: chest pain

f. Gastrointestinal: polyphagia and symptoms of gastroparesis

g. Genitourinary: polyuria, recurrent vaginal yeast infections, sexual or erectile dysfunction

h. Neurologic: decreased sensation or tingling and numbness in extremities

i. Psychiatric: anxiety and/or depression

B. Objective

1. Physical examination findings

a. Height, weight, body mass index (BMI > 25 or > 23 in Asians)

b. Vital signs, including orthostatic blood pressure if indicated

c. Skin: acanthosis nigricans; fungal infections of feet or toenails; and cracks in skin or wounds, especially hands and feet; insulin injection sites

d. Head, eyes, ears, nose, and throat: fundoscopic exam to assess for retinopathy, cataracts, vision test for blurry vision, teeth or gum inflammation, and poor dentition

e. Thyroid: thyromegaly

f. Lungs: crackles consistent with cardiovascular sequela

g. Cardiac: irregular heartbeat, cardiomegaly, and murmurs

h. Abdomen: hepatomegaly

i. Vascular: peripheral pulses, bruits, and edema

j. Neurologic: sensory; motor strength; and deep tendon reflexes (patellar and Achilles)

k. Foot examination: inspection (note calluses, lesions, edema, nail integrity, and any structural deformities); pulses in dorsalis pedis and posterior tibial, determination of proprioception, vibration, and monofilament sensation

TABLE 54-1 Diagnostic Criteria for Nongestional Diabetes

1.	HgbA$_{1C}$ ≥ 6.5%
2.	Fasting (minimum of 8 hours without food) plasma glucose ≥ 126 mg/dL
3.	2-hour plasma glucose ≥ 200 mg/dL following a 75-g oral glucose tolerance test
4.	Random plasma glucose 200 mg/dL in patients presenting with signs & symptoms of hyperglycemia

Repeat testing should be done unless test results are clearly unequivocal.

Data from American Diabetes Association. (2015). Standards of medical care in diabetes—2015. *Diabetes Care, 38*(Suppl. 1), S9.

2. Supporting data from relevant diagnostic tests (**Table 54-1**)

III. Assessment

A. Type

1. Type 1 and type 2 diabetes (See Table 54-1 for the criteria of diagnosis and **Table 54-2** for the clinical interpretations of plasma glucose concentrations)

   a. Special tests for T1D may be obtained to assess for beta cell function (e.g., C-peptide) and immune-mediated beta cell destruction (e.g., islet cell autoantibodies and autoantibodies to insulin). Yet, their use in regard to diagnosis is limited because of variable predictive values, availability, and/or cost (ADA, 2015; Patel, & Macerollo, 2010).

2. Gestational diabetes

   a. There are two strategies, but no clinical evidence to support one or the other.

      i. One-step strategy: 2-hour, 75-g oral glucose tolerance test or

      ii. Two-step approach: 1-hour, 50-g (nonfasting) screen followed by a 3-hour, 100-g oral glucose tolerance test for those who screen positive.

   b. Diagnosis of gestational diabetes mellitus (GDM) is made when values exceed:

      i. One step:
         - Fasting ≥ 92 mg/dL
         - 1h: ≥ 180 mg/dL
         - 2h: ≥ 153 mg/dL

      ii. Two step:
         - 1h: ≥ 140 mg/dL, then proceed to step 2
         - 3h: ≥ 140 mg/dL (ADA, 2015, p. S14)

B. Severity

Assess the severity of the disease via the presence or absence of end-organ complications and/or impact on basic and intermediate activities of daily living.

C. Significance

Assess the significance of the problem to the patient and significant others.

D. Motivation and ability

Determine patient's motivation for change, via motivational interviewing techniques, and assess for support and barriers to achieve self-management goals.

TABLE 54-2 Clinical Interpretations of Plasma Glucose Concentrations

Glucose Concentration (mg/dL)	Clinical Interpretation
Fasting	
< 100	Within the reference range
100–125	Impaired fasting glucose/prediabetes
≥ 126	Overt diabetes mellitus
2-hr postchallenge load (75-g oral glucose tolerance test)	
< 140	Within the reference range
140–199	Impaired glucose tolerance/prediabetes
≥ 200	Overt diabetes mellitus

Data from American Diabetes Association. (2015). Standards of medical care in diabetes—2015. *Diabetes Care, 38*(Suppl. 1), S1–S93.

IV. Goals of clinical management

A. Screening or diagnosing diabetes (see Tables 54-1, 54-2, and 54-3)

Choose a cost-effective approach for screening and diagnosing diabetes.

B. Treatment

Select a treatment plan that controls glucose in a safe and effective manner, without causing hypoglycemia. Treatment goals should be adjusted and determined by multiple factors, including risk for hypoglycemia, disease duration, life expectancy, comorbidities, vascular complications, and resources and support systems available to patient (ADA, 2015).

For type 2 diabetes, current guidelines should be used to address dyslipidemia and hypertension therapy goals. Refer to current guidelines (Aronow, 2014; Eckel et al., 2014).

C. Patient adherence

Provide self-management education and support in order to maximize patient adherence. Providers should use motivational interviewing and problem-solving strategies to support patients and create collaborative goals. National standards for diabetes self-management education (DSME) clearly state that goals should be patient centered, personally relevant, and take into account the patient's lived experience (Haas et al., 2012).

D. Prevention of complications

For all types of diabetes, screening of kidney disease, retinopathy, and neuropathies is of primary importance, as glycemic control can reduce microvascular complications. Additionally, for type 2 DM, primary and secondary prevention of cardiovascular risk factors is as important as glycemic control.

V. Plan

A. Primary prevention: criteria screening of high-risk groups (see Table 54-3)

1. Treatment guidelines for prediabetes: Individuals at high risk for developing type 2 diabetes (prediabetes), defined as impaired fasting glucose (IFG) of 100–125 mg/dL, impaired glucose tolerance (IGT) of 140–199 mg/dL 2 hours post glucose load, or an HbA_{1C} of 5.7–6.4%, should be referred to structured programs that emphasize lifestyle changes, including moderate weight loss (7% body weight) and regular physical activity (150 min/wk, strength training 2x/wk) (ADA, 2015). In at-risk individuals with a BMI > 35 kg/m² and younger than 60 years old, metformin therapy should be considered for the

TABLE 54-3 Criteria for Testing for Diabetes or Prediabetes in Asymptomatic Adults

1. Testing should be considered in all adults who are overweight (BMI ≥ 25 kg/m² or ≥ 23 kg/m² in Asian Americans) and have additional risk factors:
   - Physical inactivity
   - First-degree relative with diabetes
   - High-risk race/ethnicity (e.g., African American, Latino, Native American, Asian American, Pacific Islander)
   - Women who delivered a baby weighing > 9 lb or were diagnosed with GDM
   - Hypertension (≥ 140/90 mmHg or on therapy for hypertension)
   - HDL cholesterol level < 35 mg/dL (0.90 mmol/L) and/or a triglyceride level > 250 mg/dL (2.82 mmol/L)
   - Women with polycystic ovary syndrome
   - A1C ≥ 5.7%, IGT, or IFG on previous testing
   - Other clinical conditions associated with insulin resistance (e.g., severe obesity, acanthosis nigricans)
   - History of CVD

2. For all patients, particularly those who are overweight or obese, testing should begin at age 45 years.

3. If results are normal, testing should be repeated at a minimum of 3-year intervals, with consideration of more frequent testing depending on initial results (e.g., those with prediabetes should be tested yearly) and risk status.

Reproduced from American Diabetes Association. (2015). Standards of medical care in diabetes—2015. *Diabetes Care, 38*(Suppl. 1), S10.

prevention of type 2 diabetes. Ongoing monitoring for diabetes should be done at least annually. Modifiable CVD risk factors should be identified and appropriate interventions are recommended (ADA, 2015). Refer to Table 54-3 for criteria of high-risk groups.

B. Diagnostics Care

1. $HgbA_{1C}$ every 3–6 months (depending on control)
2. Annual urine albumin:creatinine ratio
3. Creatinine, eGFR, potassium
4. Annual lipid panel
5. Liver function tests if on thiazolidinedione medications and/or statins

C. Management (includes treatment, consultation, referral, and follow-up care)

Providers must first investigate the cause of the diabetes, especially if it is related to infection or medication use, and treat the patient accordingly. Patients initially presenting with type 1 diabetes may be hospitalized depending on their symptoms and degree of illness (e.g., diabetic keto-acidosis). The goal of treatment is to achieve near-normal blood glucose levels without significant hypoglycemia, attain and maintain reasonable body weight, and normalize lipids and blood pressure as indicated.

1. Medical nutrition therapy (MNT)

    a. Reduction in energy intake is a cornerstone of treatment in type 2 diabetes and may be needed in type 1 diabetes. MNT for both types of diabetes involves distribution of carbohydrates that takes into consideration an individual's pharmacological treatment as well as the person's activity pattern.

    b. Of the macronutrients, carbohydrates (CHO) have the most significant effect on blood glucose levels so patients need to learn to "carb count" or use "experience-based estimation." Recent evidence suggests that there are no ideal percentages for CHO, protein, and fat intake and that the individual MNT plan should be personalized and address current eating patterns as well as personal preference inclusive of cultural traditions. It is advisable that patients obtain most of their carbohydrates from whole foods such as fruit, vegetables, whole grains, legumes, and other low glycemic index foods. Sucrose is allowable but if used on a regular basis will replace more nutrient-dense food. Sugar-containing beverages should be avoided as much as possible because of their immediate effect on blood glucose levels and contribution to nonnutritive calories and may worsen CVD risk profiles.

    c. Fiber, saturated fat, and dietary cholesterol intake are as recommended for the general population. Newer studies show benefit from Mediterranean-style diets that are rich in MUFA—monounsaturated fatty acids (ADA, 2015).

2. Exercise

    a. At least 150 minutes/week of moderate-intensity aerobic physical activity (50–70% of maximum heart rate). For exercise rules and precautions, refer to **Table 54-4**.

    b. Patients with type 2 diabetes without contraindications should perform resistance training at least two times per week (ADA, 2015).

3. Pharmacological therapy

    a. Prophylactic medications

        i. Aspirin, 75–162 mg/day for patients with type 1 or type 2 diabetes at increased cardiovascular risk (most men > 50 years of age and women > 60 years of age who have at least one additional major risk factor [i.e., family medical history of cardiovascular

TABLE 54-4 Exercise Rules and Precautions

Avoid vigorous exercise in the presence of ketosis.
Wear properly fitted footwear.
Before starting, screen for vascular or neurologic complications.
Caution in patients with retinopathy, neuropathy, and peripheral vascular disease.
High-risk patients should start slowly.
Carry identification that includes diagnosis and medication list.
If taking sulfonylureas, meglitinides, or insulin, check glucose before starting and carry carbohydrates.
Check glucose before and after exercise.
Avoid exercise in extreme temperatures and humidity.
Use proper equipment.
Complete proper warm-up and stretching exercises.
Adequate hydration.
Stop for any pain, lightheadedness, or shortness of breath.

Data from American Diabetes Association. (2015). Standards of medical care in diabetes—2015. *Diabetes Care, 38*(Suppl. 1), S9.

disease, hypertension, smoking, dyslipidemia, or albuminuria]) (Handelsman et al., 2015).

        ii. Angiotensin-converting enzyme inhibitors or angiotensin receptor blockers for patients with hypertension or micro-albuminuria (ADA, 2015; Joslin Diabetes Center & Joslin Clinic, 2009b; Handelsman et al., 2015).

    b. Type 1 DM

    For type 1 diabetes management, the mainstay of the treatment plan is insulin, preferably a basal/bolus regimen via injection or insulin pump. Dosing of insulin for type 1 is often 0.4–1.0 units/kg (ADA, 2015). According to the Diabetes Control and Complications Trial (DCCT) and the follow-up Epidemiology of Diabetes Interventions and Complications (EDIC) (National Diabetes Information Clearinghouse, 2009), it is well established that patients with type 1 diabetes check their blood glucose level and base insulin dosing on the amount of carbohydrates eaten and the corresponding blood glucose level. Current therapy for patients with type 1 diabetes usually requires prandial injections of a rapid acting insulin and a once or twice per day long-acting basal insulin. This type of therapy is referred to as basal/bolus therapy and insulin pumps provide an alternate

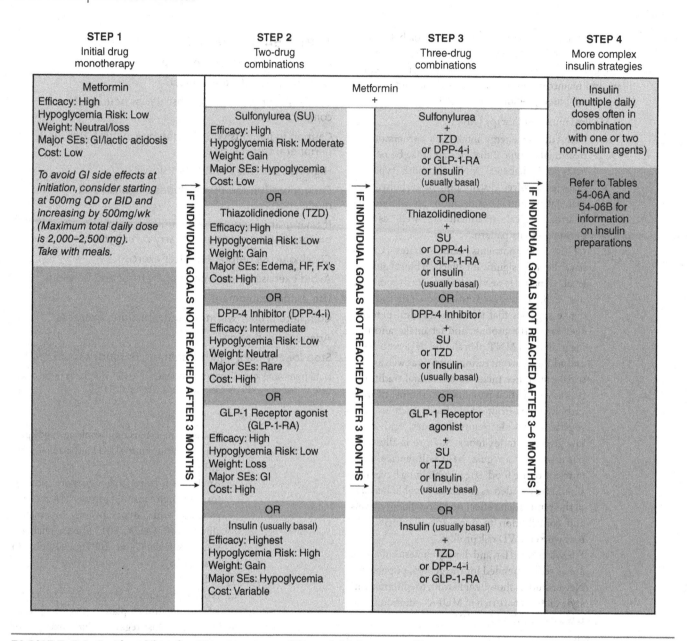

FIGURE 54-1 Algorithm for Management of Type 2 Diabetes Mellitus

Data from Inzucchi , S. E., Bergenstal, R. M., Buse, J. B., Diamant, M., Ferrannini, E., Nauck, M., et al. (2012). Management of hyperglycemia in type 2 diabetes: a patient-centered approach. Position statement of the American Diabetes Association (ADA) and the European Association for the Study of Diabetes (EASD). *Diabetes Care*, 35,1364–1379.

delivery to the minimum of 4–6 injections required for this intensive regimen.

c.   Type 2 DM

Type 2 diabetes management usually begins with lifestyle modification, exercise, and then oral agents. This treatment plan is, however, usually guided by the patient's HgbA$_{1C}$ level, blood glucose levels, and their comorbidities.

If the patient is grossly hyperglycemic at presentation (e.g., HgbA$_{1c}$ > 9%), then insulin is recommended. There are several algorithms for the treatment of type 2 diabetes (American Diabetes Association, 2015; Joslin Diabetes Center & Joslin Clinic, 2009a; Rodbard et al., 2009) (**Figure 54-1**).

d.   Oral agents (**Table 54-5**)

TABLE 54-5 Oral Agents*

Generic	Brand Name	Daily Dose (Min-Max)	Dosing (QD = Daily; BID = twice a day; TID = three times a day)
Sulfonylureas			
Glipizide	Glucotrol®	2.5–40 mg	QD-BID
Glipizide controlled release	Glucotrol XL®	2.5–20 mg	QD
Glimepiride	Amaryl®	1–8 mg	QD
Glyburide	Micronase®, DiaBeta®	1.25–20 mg	QD-BID
Micronized glyburide	Glynase®	0.75–12 mg	QD-BID
Meglitinide analogs			
Repaglinide	Prandin®	0.5–16 mg	BID before meals
D-Phenylalanine derivative			
Nateglinide	Starlix®	120–360 mg	TID before meals
Biguanides			
Metformin	Glucophage®	500–2,000 mg	QD-TID with meals
Metformin extended-release	Glucophage XR® Glumetza®	500–2,000 mg	QD with a meal
Metformin	Riomet® (oral solution)	(5 cc = 500 mg) 500–550 mg	QD-TID with meals
Thiazolidinediones			
Pioglitazone	Actos®	15–45 mg	QD
Rosiglitazone	Avandia®	4–8 mg	QD-BID
Alpha-glucosidase inhibitors			
Acarbose	Precose®	25–300 mg	TID with meals
Miglitol	Glyset®	25–300 mg	TID with meals
DPP-4 inhibitors			
Sitagliptin	Januvia®	100 mg	QD
Saxagliptin	Onglyza®	2.5–5 mg	QD
SLGT-2 inhibitors			
Canagliflozin	Invokana	100–300 mg	QD
Dapagliflozin	Farxiga	5–10 mg	Q am
Empagliflozin	Jardiance	10–25 mg	QD

* Note: There are several combinations of various oral agents that are often available.

e. Injectable (other than insulin)
   i. Exenatide (Byetta): class-incretin mimetic; dose 5–10 mcg taken 60 minutes before a meal (type 2 only)
   ii. Pramlintide (Symlin): class-synthetic hormone; dose for type 1 is 15–60 mcg and for type 2 is 60–120 mcg taken before meals
f. Insulins (**Table 54-6A** and **54-6B**)

4. Self-blood glucose monitoring (SBGM)
According to the Joslin Diabetes Center & Joslin Clinic (2009b), "the frequency of self glucose monitoring is highly individualized and should be based on such factors as glucose goals, exercise, medication changes and patient motivation. Patients with type 1 diabetes should monitor at least three times a day. In patients with type 2 diabetes, the frequency of

TABLE 54-6A Insulins*

Generic Name	Brand Name	Type	Onset	Peak	Duration
Aspart	NovoLog®	Rapid	10–20 min	1–3 hr	3–5 hr
Lispro	Humalog®	Rapid	5–15 min	30–75 min	2–4 hr
Glulisine	Apidra®	Rapid	5–15 min	30–75 min	2–4 hr
Regular insulin	Novolin® R	Short acting	30–60 min	2–4 hr	5–8 hr
	Humulin® R	Same	Same	Same	Same
NPH	Novolin® N	Intermediate	1–3 hr	6–10 hr	16–24 hr
	Humulin® N	Same	Same	Same	Same
Glargine	Lantus®	Long acting	45 min–4 hr	None	24 hr
Detemir	Levemir®	Long acting	45 min–4 hr	None	24 hr

*Inhaled insulins (e.g., glargine u-300 [Toujeo®] and Humulin Regular u-500) are available yet less commonly used than the standard injectable insulins.

TABLE 54-6B Combined Insulins

Premixed	Brand Name
NPH/Regular	Novolin® 70/30
	Humulin® 70/30
	Humulin® 50/50
Lispro protamine/lispro	Humalog® Mix 75/25
Lispro protamine/lispro	Humalog® Mix 50/50
Aspart protamine/aspart	Novolog® Mix 70/30

monitoring is dependent upon such factors as mode of treatment and level of glycemic control" (p. 2).

5. Self-management goals and clinical goals (**Table 54-7**)

6. Healthcare maintenance

    a. Immunizations

        i. Annual influenza vaccine

        ii. Pneumococcal 23-valent polysaccharide vaccine (> 2 years old) and pneumococcal 13-valent conjugate vaccine (> 65 years old)

TABLE 54-7 Clinical Goals

	American Diabetes Association	American Association of Clinical Endocrinologists
Preprandial glucose	80–130	< 110
2-hour postprandial glucose	< 180	< 140
HbA$_{1c}$	< 7% with a less stringent goal of 8% for selected populations	≤ 6.5% for most. Less stringent for people with comorbidities and older adults.
Blood pressure	< 140/90	< 130/80: Individualized based on age, comorbidities, and duration of disease.
Lipids	ADA recommendations are in alignments with the American College of Cardiology (ACC) and American Heart Association (AHA) cholesterol treatment guidelines: The focus on statin therapy should be tailored for cardiovascular risk rather than LDL target therapy (Stone et al., 2014). See Chapter 63, Lipid Disorders, for additional information.	Low-density lipoprotein (LDL) mg/dL: < 100, moderate risk; < 70, high risk
	Triglycerides: < 150 mg/dL	Same
Urine albumin/creatinine ratio	< 30 mg /g alb/creat ratio	Same

Data from American Diabetes Association (2015). Standards of medical care in diabetes—2015. *Diabetes Care, 38*(Suppl. 1), S1–S93; Handelsman, Y., et al. (2015). American Association of Clinical Endocrinologists and American College of Endocrinology—Clinical practice guidelines for developing a diabetes mellitus comprehensive care plan. *Endocrine Practice, 21*(Suppl. 1), 1–87.

iii. Hepatitis B vaccine in adults 19–59 years old if unvaccinated, and consider if > 60 years old (ADA, 2015)

iv. Pap and mammogram for women

v. Smoking cessation counseling at every visit

7. Referrals and monitoring

Patients should be educated about potential complications from diabetes and how to prevent them. With this in mind, all people with diabetes should have the following referrals and monitoring.

a. Patients with diabetes should be referred to an endocrinologist for the following reasons:

i. Starting an insulin pump

ii. Recurrent diabetic ketoacidosis

iii. Recurrent hypoglycemia

iv. Unable to adequately control glucose or erratic blood glucose readings

b. Women of childbearing age should receive preconception counseling and care. Note: combined oral contraceptives should be avoided in patients with DM-related complications and who are over the age of 35 (American College of Obstetricians and Gynecologists, 2000).

c. Mental health referrals should be made as needed: screen for depression, diabetes-related stress, anxiety, eating disorders, and cognitive impairment when self-management is poor.

d. All patients with diabetes mellitus should be referred for diabetes self-management education and support services.

e. Dilated eye examination by an ophthalmologist annually. For people with type 1 DM, first referral should occur after 5 years of disease onset and yearly thereafter. For people with type 2 DM referral should occur at initial visit, if exam is normal it can be followed up every 2 years. Women with GDM should be referred during the first trimester.

f. Foot examination at every primary care provider visit (with 10 g monofilament) and by a podiatrist every 12 months (for patients without complications).

g. Dental examination every 6 months with dentist

8. Patient education

a. Sick-day guidelines

i. Prevent dehydration and ketosis

ii. Adequate fluid and calorie intake

iii. Alert patient to signs and symptoms of hypoglycemia and hyperglycemia

iv. Include patient's family and significant others in the plan

b. Education: diabetes self-management education and support

c. Concerns and feelings

Assist the patient and significant others in expressing and coping with concerns and feelings related to the diagnosis of diabetes, its potential complications, and the management of this disease. Assist the patient to develop strategies to promote behavior change.

d. Information: provide verbal and written information regarding:

i. The diabetes disease process, including signs and symptoms of hyperglycemia and hypoglycemia; pathophysiology of type 1 and type 2 diabetes; and complications of diabetes

ii. Diagnostic tests, including what they mean, frequency, and importance of testing

iii. Medical management

iv. Meal planning and exercise: how to incorporate these into the patient's lifestyle

v. Rationale, action, use, side effects, and cost of therapeutic interventions, including medications

vi. Self-glucose monitoring: what the parameters are and how to interpret the results for self-management decision making (American Diabetes Association, 2014)

vii. Adherence to long-term treatment plans

viii. Prevention of complications, self-management strategies

ix. Travel instructions, medical alert identification, sick-day guidelines, and health maintenance

VI. Self-management resources and tools

There are numerous educational opportunities for individuals with diabetes, either online, by mail, or by telephone.

A. National Diabetes Education Program

The National Diabetes Education Program has publications available by mail or online that are geared toward different age groups (from teenagers to older adults) and ethnic backgrounds and are written in a variety of languages (http://ndep.nih.gov/)

B. American Diabetes Association

The American Diabetes Association's (2009a) website has extensive patient information online, brochures for purchase, and a hotline number for patients who want to speak with someone directly (www.diabetes.org).

C. Joslin Diabetes Center

The Joslin Diabetes Center has patient education online, brochures, and cookbooks for purchase, including some for children and teenagers, and has Spanish and Asian American websites (www.joslin.org).

D. Juvenile Diabetes Research Foundation International

The Juvenile Diabetes Research Foundation International provides online or printed information for adults, teenagers, and children and has links to Facebook, Twitter, and YouTube. In addition, it has links to community events, local chapters, and affiliates around the globe (www.jdrf.org).

E. Community support groups

There are numerous support groups for individuals with diabetes, in addition to those listed previously.

1. Defeat Diabetes Foundation, Inc.
   Find local support groups (www.defeatdiabetes.org/).

2. American Diabetes Association
   Website has a link to community events and programs, including those geared for specific ethnic groups (www.diabetes.org/).

3. Diabetes Health
   Website links to multiple community events (www.diabeteshealth.com/)
   dLife (www.dlife.com)
   GLU (https://myglu.org/)
   TuDiabetes (www.tudiabetes.org/)
   DiabetesMine (www.healthline.com/diabetesmine)
   TCOYD—Taking Control of Your Diabetes (http://tcoyd.org/)
   Behavioral Diabetes Institute (www.behavioraldiabetesinstitute.org/)
   diaTribe (http://diatribe.org/)

REFERENCES

American College of Obstetricians and Gynecologists. (2000). *The use of hormonal contraception in women with coexisting medical conditions* (ACOG Practice Bulletin No. 18). Washington, DC: American College of Obstetricians and Gynecologists. Retrieved from www.guideline.gov/content.aspx?id=10924.

American Diabetes Association. (2009a). *Community events.* Retrieved from www.diabetes.org/in-my-community/.

American Diabetes Association. (2009b). *Diabetes statistics.* Retrieved from www.diabetes.org/diabetes-basics/diabetes-statistics/.

American Diabetes Association. (2014). Standards of medical care in diabetes—2014. *Diabetes Care, 37*(1), S14–S80.

American Diabetes Association. (2015). Standards of medical care in diabetes—2015. *Diabetes Care, 38* (Suppl. 1), S1–S93. Retrieved from care.diabetesjournals.org/content/38/Supplement_1/S4/suppl/DC1

Aronow, W. S. (2014). Eighth Joint National Committee guidelines. *Future Cardiology, 10*(4), 461–463.

Centers for Disease Control and Prevention. (2014). *National diabetes statistics report, 2014.* Retrieved from www.cdc.gov/diabetes/pubs/statsreport14/national-diabetes-report-web.pdf. http://www.cdc.gov/diabetes/pubs/statsreport14/national-diabetes-report-web.pdf

Dabelea, D., Rewers, A., Stafford, J. M., Standiford, D.A., Lawrence, J. M., Saydah, S., et al. (2014). Trends in the prevalence of ketoacidosis at diabetes diagnosis: The SEARCH for Diabetes in Youth Study. *Pediatrics, 133*(4). e938–e945. doi: 10.1542/peds.2013-2795

Eckel, R. H., Jakicic, J. M., Ard, J. D., de Jesus, J. M., Houston Miller, N., Hubbard, V. S., et al. (2014). 2013 AHA/ACC guideline on lifestyle management to reduce cardiovascular risk: A report of the American College of Cardiology/American Heart Association Task Force on Practice Guidelines. *Journal of the American College of Cardiology, 63*(25, Pt. B), 2960–2984.

Haas, L., Maryniuk, M., Beck, J., Cox, C. E., Duker, P., Edwards, L., et al. (2012). National standards for diabetes self-management education and support. *Diabetes Educator, 38*(5), 619–629.

Handelsman, Y., Bloomgarden, Z. T., Grunberger, G., Umpierrez, G., Zimmerman, R. S., Bailey, T. S. et al. (2015). American Association of Clinical Endocrinologists and American College of Endocrinology clinical practice guidelines for developing a diabetes mellitus comprehensive care plan. *Endocrine Practice, 21*(Suppl. 1), 1–87.

Huang, E. S., Basu, A., O'Grady, A., & Capretta, J. C. (2009). Projecting the future diabetes population size and related costs for the U.S. *Diabetes Care, 32*(12), 2225–2229.

Inzucchi, S. E., Bergenstal, R. M., Buse, J. B., Diamant, M., Ferrannini, E., Nauck, M., et al. (2012). Management of hyperglycemia in type 2 diabetes: A patient-centered approach. Position statement of the American Diabetes Association (ADA) and the European Association for the Study of Diabetes (EASD). *Diabetes Care, 35*, 1364–1379.

Joslin Diabetes Center & Joslin Clinic. (2009a). *Clinical guideline for pharmacological management of type 2 diabetes.* Retrieved from www.joslin.org/09_12_2014_Pharma_Guideline_emb_final.pdf

Joslin Diabetes Center & Joslin Clinic. (2009b). *Clinical guidelines for adults with diabetes.* Retrieved from www.joslin.org/joslin_clinical_guidelines.html.

National Diabetes Information Clearinghouse. (2009). *DCCT and EDIC: The diabetes control and complications trial and follow-up study.* Retrieved from http://diabetes.niddk.nih.gov/dm/pubs/control/.

Patel, P., & Macerollo, A. (2010). Diabetes mellitus: Diagnosis and screening. *American Family Physician, 81*(7), 863–870.

Rodbard, H. W., Jellinger, P. S., Davidson, J. A., Einhorn, D., Garber, A. J., Grunberger, G., et al. (2009). Statement by an American Association of Clinical Endocrinologists/American College of Endocrinology consensus panel on type 2 diabetes mellitus: An algorithm for glycemic control. *Endocrine Practice, 15*(6), 540–559.

Stone, N. J., Robinson, J. G., Lichtenstein, A. H., Merz, C. N. B., Blum, C. B., Eckel, R. H., et al. (2014). 2013 ACC/AHA guideline on the treatment of blood cholesterol to reduce atherosclerotic cardiovascular risk in adults: A report of the American College of Cardiology/American Heart Association Task Force on Practice Guidelines. *Circulation, 129*(25, Suppl. 2), S1–S45.

EPILEPSY

Maritza Lopez, Paul Garcia, and M. Robin Taylor

CHAPTER

55

I. Introduction and general background

This chapter provides information to help the primary care provider evaluate a patient with previously diagnosed epilepsy. *Epilepsy* refers to a group of conditions that are characterized by the recurrent risk of disturbances of cerebral function (seizures) because of excessive neuronal discharges in the brain occurring in a paroxysmal manner (Fisher et al., 2014). An epileptic seizure occurs when the cerebral cortex is rendered hyperexcitable (because of an increase in excitatory neurotransmission, a decrease in inhibitory neurotransmission, or a disturbance in brain circuitry) by any of a number of causes, including metabolic disturbances, injuries, strokes, tumors, and developmental abnormalities (Lowenstein, 2008). Depending on the site in the brain that is affected, the disturbance of function may result in a loss or impairment of consciousness, a disturbance of behavior, or an abnormality of motor or sensory function. When the cause of the disturbance is easily reversible (e.g., hyponatremia, hypoglycemia, alcohol withdrawal, medication toxicity, or fever), the seizure is said to be "provoked" and the patient's condition is not considered epilepsy.

When the cause of the seizure is not readily reversible, and seizures have occurred on more than one occasion, the chance for further seizures is high and the patient is said to have epilepsy (Marks & Garcia, 1998). According to the International League Against Epilepsy (ILAE), epilepsy can be diagnosed when two or more unprovoked seizures recur after 24 hours; when a person has one unprovoked seizure but is at high risk of another; or, if the person is diagnosed with an epilepsy syndrome (Fisher et al., 2014).

Epilepsy is a common condition in all medical practices, and almost all practitioners are called on to care for patients with epilepsy. In the United States, an estimated 2.2 million people live with epilepsy and 150,000 new cases are diagnosed each year. About 1 in 26 people will develop epilepsy in his or her lifetime (England, Liverman, Schultz, &

Strawbridge, 2012). People of all ages, genders, and ethnicities are affected by epilepsy. As a group, people with epilepsy face both medical and psychosocial challenges (including employment and educational barriers). The lifetime risk of dying from a seizure-related cause is estimated to be as high as 20% (Hesdorffer & Tomson, 2013). Successful treatment of epilepsy both prolongs life and improves quality of life (Galanopoulou et al., 2012).

II. Database (may include, but is not limited to)

A. Subjective

1. Seizure history
   a. Age of onset
   b. Description of seizures from patient and witnesses
   c. Most recent seizures: characteristics and frequency
   d. Any changes in seizure pattern (including characteristics and frequency)
   e. Triggering events (stress, fatigue, alcohol, sleep deprivation, and menstruation)
   f. Impairment of consciousness
   g. Any recent intervention including paramedics, emergency department visits, or benzodiazepine use
   h. Any previous intervention, including surgery or medications changes
   i. Previous diagnostic work-up, including electroencephalogram (EEG) and magnetic resonance imaging (MRI); last visit with neurologist

2. Antiepileptic drugs (AEDs) and medications
   a. Name, formulation, strength, and dosing schedule. Note recent change from brand to generic or between different generics and adherence to medication.

b. Dose changes: drugs tried in the past, responses (therapeutic and toxic), and tolerability

c. Signs and symptoms of AED toxicity including blurred vision, diplopia, ataxia, somnolence or fatigue, confusion or mental slowing, and gastrointestinal upset

d. Concomitant treatment for other conditions that may interact with AEDs (e.g., nonsteroidal anti-inflammatory drugs, antibiotics, oral contraceptives, and anticoagulants, herbal supplements)

e. Use of rescue medications, such as sublingual lorazepam, buccal midazolam, or rectal diazepam

3. Past medical history

a. Head trauma, developmental and genetic disorders, and neurologic and psychiatric disorders

b. Recent minor illnesses, especially gastrointestinal disorders with vomiting or fever

c. Chronic illnesses (e.g., HIV/AIDS, cerebrovascular disease, and cancer)

4. Family history (query both sides of the family): epilepsy, Alzheimer's disease, neurodegenerative disorders, malignancy, and psychiatric disorders

5. Personal and social history

a. Occupational history

b. Habits: alcohol or illicit drug use

c. Sleep patterns (change in sleep patterns may provoke seizures)

d. Stress and coping: recent stressors (can provoke seizures), coping strategies, and social support

e. Recreational activities and safety: driving, swimming, climbing, other risky activities for patients with ongoing seizures, and use of helmets or other protective devices

6. Review of systems

a. Skin: rash or jaundice

b. Gastrointestinal: signs and symptoms of chemical hepatitis (e.g., nausea, vomiting, anorexia, abdominal pain, or malaise)

c. Neurologic: full review of systems

d. Psychiatric: note affect and symptoms of active psychiatric disease

e. Weight gain or loss

B. Objective

1. Physical examination

a. Temperature and blood pressure

b. Cardiac (rule out cardiac origin)

c. Neurologic examination

i. Cranial nerves (special emphasis on nystagmus)

ii. Cerebellar testing (special emphasis on gait disturbances and Romberg)

iii. Focal motor signs and mental status

d. Skin: rashes, signs of neurocutaneous syndrome (hypo/hyperpigmented macules)

2. Diagnostic testing and work-up

a. Source (should be neurologist or epileptologist)

b. Supporting documentation

i. Abnormal electroencephalogram (EEG) (not always present)

ii. MRI. Though not always revealing, MRI remains the best modality to identify subtle but dangerous structural causes of seizures (e.g., small tumors or vascular malformations). A CT scan can be obtained quickly at most institutions and, thus, is useful for visualizing acute structural causes such as hemorrhages or trauma; however, if CT is unrevealing, MRI is still necessary to exclude subtle structural causes (Ramli, Rahmat, Lim, & Tan, 2015).

III. Assessment

A. Determine the diagnosis: the following diagnoses should be considered for all patients presenting with seizures

1. Epilepsy (**Table 55-1**)

2. Cerebrovascular disease

3. Cardiac arrhythmias with resulting cerebral hypoperfusion

4. Syncope

5. Nonepileptic (i.e., psychogenic) seizure

6. Transient ischemic attack

7. Migraine

8. Alzheimer's and other neurodegenerative disorders (can cause seizures in the geriatric population)

9. Infection, may exacerbate seizures

10. Movement disorder

11. Diabetes

B. Severity

1. Determine if seizures are fully controlled.

2. If seizures are not fully controlled, determine if the patient is at the maximum clinically tolerated dose of medication (regardless of serum levels)

3. Assess for AED toxicity (**Table 55-2**)

TABLE 55-1 Epilepsy Syndromes

	Generalized	Focal
	Seizures begin diffusely throughout the cerebral cortex	Seizures arise from a discrete focus in cerebral cortex or limbic structures (hippocampus or amygdala)
Idiopathic (primary, without clear cause)	**Seizure types:** absence, myoclonic, tonic–clonic **Neurologic examination:** normal **Neuroimaging:** normal **EEG:** normal background with fast (3–6 Hz) generalized spike-and-wave discharges **Common examples:** childhood absence epilepsy, juvenile myoclonic epilepsy, epilepsy with generalized tonic–clonic seizures on awakening **Treatment:** valproate, ethosuximide (effective for absence seizures only), topiramate, lamotrigine, felbamate, levetiracetam, or zonisamide	**Seizure types:** simple partial (focal without impairment of consciousness), complex partial (focal with impairment of consciousness), or secondarily generalized tonic–clonic **Neurologic examination:** normal **Neuroimaging:** normal **EEG:** normal background with focal epileptiform discharges **Common examples:** benign childhood epilepsy with centrotemporal spikes (Rolandic epilepsy); benign epilepsy with occipital paroxysms **Treatment:** often no medical treatment is necessary; all AEDs may be effective except ethosuximide
Symptomatic (secondary; caused by an apparent or assumed brain lesion)	**Seizure types:** atypical absence, myoclonic, tonic, atonic, tonic–clonic **Neurologic examination:** diffuse or multifocal abnormalities **Neuroimaging:** diffuse or multifocal abnormalities common **EEG:** abnormal background with slow (< 3 Hz) generalized or multifocal epileptiform discharges **Common examples:** Lennox-Gastaut syndrome, progressive myoclonus epilepsies **Treatment:** valproate, lamotrigine, levetiracetam, felbamate, rufinamide, topiramate, zonisamide, clobazam, ketogenic diet, or corpus callosotomy, vagus nerve stimulator	**Seizure types:** focal without impairment of consciousness, focal with impairment of consciousness, secondarily generalized tonic–clonic **Neurologic examination:** focal abnormalities or normal **Neuroimaging:** focal abnormalities common **EEG:** normal or abnormal background with focal or multifocal epileptiform discharges **Common examples:** temporal lobe epilepsy, frontal lobe epilepsy **Treatment:** carbamazepine, phenytoin, valproate, gabapentin, pregabalin, lacosamide, lamotrigine, levetiracetam, oxcarbazepine, topiramate, zonisamide, (adjunct therapy— vigabatrin, pregabalin, ezogabine, perampanel, eslicarbazepine) or resective surgery

Modified with permission from "Management of seizures and epilepsy," 1998, *American Family Physician*. Copyright © 1998 American Academy of Family Physicians. All Rights Reserved; Modified from Marks, W. J., Jr., & Garcia, P. A. (1998). Seizures and epilepsy: Current management. *American Family Physician, 57*(7), 1589–1600.

C. *Significance*

Assess the significance of the symptoms and chronic nature of this disorder to the patient and significant others (i.e., burden, quality of life, eagerness for surgical intervention)

D. *Patient adherence*

Assess if the patient is able to adhere to the treatment plan (direct, open-ended inquiry; medication refill history).

IV. Goals of clinical management

A. *Achieve seizure-free status with lowest side effect profile of AED therapy*

B. *Attempt to arrive at AED monotherapy if possible*

TABLE 55-2 Oral Antiepileptic Medications

Generic Name	Brand Name	Strengths Available[1] (mg)	Typical Adult Starting Dose[2]	Typical Increment and Rate of Ascension[3]	Most Common Dose-Related Adverse Effects	Nondose-Related and Idiosyncratic Reactions
Carbamazepine	Tegretol®	100, 200	200 mg BID	200 mg/wk (dose TID-QID)	Dizziness, somnolence, ataxia, nausea, vomiting, diplopia, blurred vision	Hyponatremia, rash, Stevens-Johnson syndrome, leukopenia, aplastic anemia, agranulocytosis, transaminitis, hepatic failure
	Tegretol-XR®	100, 200, 400	200 mg BID	200 mg/wk		
	Carbatrol®	100, 200, 300	200 mg BID	200 mg/wk		
Clobazam	Onfi®	2.5 mg/mL Tablet: 10 mg, 20 mg	10 mg BID	10 mg BID on week 1 then to 20 mg BID	Ataxia, dysarthria, constipation, drooling, lethargy, somnolence, urinary tract infection, cough, fever, aggressive behavior	Stevens-Johnson syndrome
Eslicarbazepine	Aptiom®	200, 400, 600, 800	400 mg daily	Increments of 400 mg/wk to 800–1,200 mg	Nausea, vomiting, ataxia, dizziness, headache, somnolence, fatigue, blurred vision, diplopia	Drug-induced eosinophilia, liver dysfunction, anaphylaxis, angioedema
Ethosuximide	Zarontin®	250	250 mg QD to 250 mg BID	250 mg/wk	Anorexia, nausea, vomiting, drowsiness, headache, dizziness	Rash, Stevens-Johnson syndrome, hemopoietic complications, systemic lupus erythematosus (SLE)
Ezogabine	Potiga®	50, 200, 300, 400	100 mg TID	increase dosage by 50 mg or less 3 times daily (150 mg/day) every week to max 200–400 mg TID	Confusion, dizziness, decrease coordination, memory impairment, somnolence, tremor, vertigo, blurred vision, diplopia, fatigue	Prolonged QT interval, syncope, amnesia, psychotic effects such as hallucinations, renal effects.
Felbamate	Felbatol®	400, 600	1,200 mg/day in 3 to 4 divided doses	600-mg increments every 2 weeks to 2,400 mg/day	Photosensitivity, weight loss, abdominal pain, nausea/vomiting, dizziness, headache, insomnia	Stevens-Johnson syndrome, hematologic abnormalities (i.e., aplastic anemia and leukopenia, hepatic failure
Gabapentin	Neurontin®	100, 300, 400, 600, 800	300 mg TID	300 mg/wk	Somnolence, dizziness, ataxia, fatigue	Rash, weight gain, behavioral changes, extremity edema
Lacosamide	Vimpat®	50, 100, 150, 200	50 mg BID	100 mg/wk to max 400 mg/d	Dizziness, ataxia, vomiting, diplopia, nausea, vertigo	PR interval lengthening

TABLE 55-2 Oral Antiepileptic Medications *(Continued)*

Generic Name	Brand Name	Strengths Available[1] (mg)	Typical Adult Starting Dose[2]	Typical Increment and Rate of Ascension[3]	Most Common Dose-Related Adverse Effects	Nondose-Related and Idiosyncratic Reactions
Lamotrigine	Lamictal® Lamictal-XR®	25, 100, 150, 200 25, 50, 100, 200	25 mg daily only for monotherapy (special considerations for polytherapy not addressed here)	25–50 mg/ 2 wk only for monotherapy (special considerations for polytherapy not addressed here)	Dizziness, ataxia, somnolence, headache, diplopia, blurred vision, nausea, vomiting, rash	Rash, Stevens-Johnson syndrome, transaminitis
Levetiracetam	Keppra® Keppra-XR®	250, 500, 750 500, 750	500 mg BID	1,000 mg/d/ 2 wk to max 3,000 mg	Somnolence, asthenia, infection, dizziness	Depression, irritability
Oxcarbazepine	Trileptal® Oxtellar	150, 300, 600	300 mg BID	600 mg/d/wk to max 2,400 mg	Dizziness, somnolence, diplopia, fatigue, nausea, vomiting, ataxia, abnormal vision, abdominal pain, tremor, dyspepsia, abnormal gait	Stevens-Johnson syndrome, bone marrow suppression, hyponatremia
Perampanel	Fycompa®	2, 4, 6, 8, 10, 12	2 mg orally	Increase by 2 mg daily per week. Max dose 12 mg qhs.	Backache, unsteady gait, ataxia, dizziness, headache, somnolence, psychiatric effects, fatigue	Psychiatric behavior, homicidal, suicidal thoughts
Phenobarbital		15, 30, 60, 100	100 mg QD	15–30 mg/wk	Somnolence, cognitive and behavioral effects	Rash, Stevens-Johnson syndrome, hematopoietic complications, transaminitis, hepatic failure
Phenytoin	Dilantin ®	30, 50, 100	300 mg daily	25–30 mg/wk	Ataxia, diplopia, slurred speech, confusion	Rash, Stevens-Johnson syndrome, hematopoietic complications, gingival hyperplasia, coarsening of facial features, transaminitis, hepatic failure
Pregabalin	Lyrica®	25, 50, 75, 100, 150, 200, 225, 300	75 mg BID or 50 mg TID	300 mg/wk to max 600 mg/day	Dizziness, somnolence, dry mouth, peripheral edema, ataxia, confusion, asthenia, abnormal thinking, blurred vision, incoordination, weight gain	Weight gain Skin rash

(continues)

TABLE 55-2 Oral Antiepileptic Medications *(Continued)*

Generic Name	Brand Name	Strengths Available[1] (mg)	Typical Adult Starting Dose[2]	Typical Increment and Rate of Ascension[3]	Most Common Dose-Related Adverse Effects	Nondose-Related and Idiosyncratic Reactions
Rufinamide	Banzel®	200, 400	400–800 mg/d (BID doses)	400–800 mg/day every 2 days to max 3,200 mg/day	Somnolence, dizziness, ataxia, headache, fatigue, nausea	Multiorgan hypersensitivity, QT interval shortening
Tiagabine	Gabitril®	4, 6, 8, 10, 12, 16	4 mg daily	4 mg/wk (dose BID-QID)	Dizziness, nervousness, asthenia, confusion, tremor	
Topiramate	Topamax 1® Trokendi XR	25, 50, 100, 200 (same as above)	25 mg BID 50 mg daily	50 mg/wk (same as above)	Somnolence, dizziness, ataxia, slurred speech, psychomotor slowing, cognitive problems, word-finding difficulty	Weight loss, transaminitis, nephrolithiasis
Valproate	Depakote® Depakote-ER®	125, 250, 500 250, 500	250 mg TID 500 mg daily	250 mg/wk Same as above	Nausea, vomiting, tremor, thrombocytopenia, weight gain	Transaminitis, hepatic failure, pancreatitis, rash, Stevens-Johnson syndrome, hair damage or loss,
Vigabatrin	Sabril®	500	500 mg orally twice daily	500-mg increments at weekly intervals, depending upon response, up to 1,500 mg twice daily	Weight increase, confusion, decreased coordination, blurred vision, diplopia, infection of ear, aggressive behavior, fatigue	Hepatic failure, visual field defect, psychiatric disorder, suicidal thoughts.
Zonisamide	Zonegran®	25, 50, 100	100 mg/day	200 mg/day for 2 wk to max 400 mg/day	Somnolence, anorexia, dizziness, headache, nausea, agitation/irritability	Stevens-Johnson syndrome, oligohydrosis/hyperthermia, nephrolithiasis

[1]Strengths listed are for tablet or capsule formulations of the brand name agents.

[2]Initiation doses for some agents vary, depending on concomitant medications, body weight, age of patient, and other factors; consult prescribing information for each drug. Doses are for nonurgent initiation of medication; clinical circumstances may necessitate higher initial doses and accelerated titration. See prescribing information for pediatric doses, which are based on body weight and often must be administered more frequently than in adults.

[3]Rate of ascension may need modification, depending on seizure frequency and occurrence of adverse effects. Note that phenytoin may be increased in 25-mg increments by using a halved 50-mg Dilantin® Infatab® tablet or by 30 mg using a 30-mg Dilantin Kapseal® capsule.

[3]For children and adults with swallowing impairments, check with your pharmacy to see whether tablets can be crushed or if oral solutions/suspensions are available.

Data from "Management of seizures and epilepsy," 1998, American Family Physician. Copyright © 1998 *American Academy of Family Physicians.* All Rights Reserved; Marks, W. J., Jr., & Garcia, P. A. (1998). Seizures and epilepsy: Current management. *American Family Physician, 57*(7), 1589–1600. Additional medication information was obtained from: http://www.micromedexsolutions.com/micromedex2/librarian/ © 2015 Truven Health Analytics Inc Reviewed by Brian Alldredge, PharmD UCSF Epilepsy Center. Acknowledgment: Robin Taylor, NP, authored prior edition.

C. Assist the patient to achieve optimal level of functioning with daily activities and quality of life while living with a chronic, often unpredictably relapsing disorder

V. Plan

A. Screening: There are no screening tests or preventive strategies for epilepsy.

B. Diagnostic tests

1. Blood levels of AEDs: to assess for adherence or possible toxicity. Not all AEDs have defined "therapeutic ranges" (e.g., benzodiazepines and all AEDs released subsequent to valproic acid). Note that AED therapeutic ranges are only a rough guide; many patients require levels in the "toxic" range to achieve complete seizure control and tolerate these levels without significant clinical toxicity. Likewise, some patients may have their seizures controlled at blood levels below the usual therapeutic range. Routine blood level monitoring is not useful.

2. Complete blood count: thrombocytopenia, anemia, and leukopenia secondary to AEDs. Obtain a baseline before initiating a new AED and in early phase of treatment or if patient is symptomatic.

3. Liver enzymes and liver function tests: obtain a baseline before initiating a new AED and in early phase of treatment or if patient is symptomatic. Some AEDs can cause elevated liver enzymes, but this is uncommonly clinically significant and usually does not require discontinuation of the AED.

4. Consider other tests if diagnosis is in question (electrolytes, glucose, creatinine, rapid plasma reagin [RPR], EKG, tilt-table [to rule out syncope], video-EEG telemetry)

C. Medication management (**Tables 55-2** and **55-3**)

D. Referral guidelines
Refer to neurologist or epileptologist when:

1. Diagnosis of epilepsy is in question

2. Seizures are uncontrolled on one AED at maximum tolerated dose

3. Complete seizure control, but with bothersome or intolerable AED side effects

4. AED withdrawal: Consider after 2–3 years of seizure control

5. Pregnant woman with a seizure disorder

E. Client education

1. Provide verbal and written information about the etiology and treatment of epilepsy.

2. Discuss the importance of adherence to medication regimes, emphasizing that the maximum tolerated dose is one increment below the dose at which the patient experiences side effects (Alldredge, 2013).

3. Review the importance of lifestyle issues on seizure control: regular sleep–wake schedule, minimal or modest alcohol intake, maintaining hydration.

TABLE 55-3 Medication Treatment Strategies for Patients with Epilepsy

Establish an epilepsy syndrome diagnosis for each patient (Table 55-1).
Select medications appropriate for that epilepsy syndrome (Table 55-1).
Among the syndrome-appropriate medications, choose the agent best suited for the particular patient, based on patient and medication characteristics (Table 55-2).
Initiate and titrate the medication at doses, increments, and rates appropriate for that medication to enhance tolerability (Table 55-2).
Ascend the medication, regardless of serum levels, until complete seizure control is achieved, or until persistent, unacceptable side effects occur.
If satisfactory seizure control is not achieved, transition the patient to another agent appropriate for the epilepsy syndrome being treated. Attempt to arrive at antiepileptic drug monotherapy for each patient.
If trials with one or two agents fail to achieve acceptable results, refer the patient to an epilepsy specialist for consultation.

Modified with permission from "Management of seizures and epilepsy," 1998, *American Family Physician*. Copyright © 1998 American Academy of Family Physicians. All Rights Reserved; Modified from Marks, W. J., Jr., & Garcia, P. A. (1998). Seizures and epilepsy: Current management. *American Family Physician*, *57*(7), 1589–1600.

VI. Self-management resources

A. Epilepsy Foundation

An excellent resource for patient and families can be found at: www.epilepsy.com/. This site is sponsored by the Epilepsy Therapy Project and the Epilepsy Foundation. The individuals involved with this site are among the top epilepsy experts in the country. A wide variety of resources is available on diagnosis, treatment, clinical trials, and support for family and caregivers.

It is also a good resource for patients and families to identify local Epilepsy Foundation affiliates throughout the country. The local affiliates can help direct patients and families to local resources (advocacy, job training, support groups, etc).

The site has a function called "My Epilepsy Diary," which allows patients and families to enter seizures, medications, side effects, and healthcare appointments. It can be used to set alerts so that patients remember to take their medications at the proper times. The site also has a section for healthcare professionals, with more sophisticated information that tends to be highly accurate and carefully reviewed: http://professionals.epilepsy.com/homepage/index.html.

B. Seizure tracker

Seizure Tracker is a website that allows patients to enter data on medication dosages, seizure frequencies, use of rescue medications, and so forth and then share this information with healthcare providers of their choosing. https://www.seizuretracker.com/.

C. Citizens United for Research in Epilepsy (CURE)

CURE is an organization that promotes awareness and education of epilepsy and raises funds for research in epilepsy. www.cureepilepsy.org/.

REFERENCES

Alldredge, B. K. (2013). Seizure disorders. In Kimble, M., B. K. Alldredge, R. L. Corelli, M. E. Ernst, B. J. Guglielmo, P. A. Jacobson, W. A. Kradjan, & B. R. Williams (Eds.), *Koda-Kimble & Young's applied therapeutics: The clinical use of drugs.* (10th ed.). Baltimore: Wolters Kluwer Health/Lippincott Williams & Wilkins.

England, M. J., Liverman, C. T., Schultz, A. M., & Strawbridge, L. M. (2012). Epilepsy across the spectrum: Promoting health and understanding. A summary of the Institute of Medicine report. *Epilepsy & Behavior, 25,* 266–276.

Fisher, R., Acevedo, C., Arzimanoglou, A., Bogacz, J., Cross, H., Elger, C. E., et al. (2014). A practical clinical definition of epilepsy. *Epilepsia, 55*(4), 415–482.

Galanopoulou, A., Buckmaster, P. S., Staley, K., Moshé, S. L., Perucca, E., Engel J., Jr., et al. (2012). Identification of new epilepsy treatments: Issues in preclinical methodology. *Epilepsia, 53*(3), 571–582.

Hesdorffer, D., & Tomson, T. (2013). Sudden unexpected death in epilepsy. Potential role of antiepileptic drugs. *CNS Drugs, 27*(2), 113–119.

Lowenstein, D. H. (2008). Seizures and epilepsy. In A. S. Fauci, E. Braunwald, D. L. Kasper, S. L. Hauser, D. L. Longo, J. L. Jameson, et al. (Eds.), *Harrison's principles of internal medicine online* (17th ed.). New York: McGrawHill.

Marks, W. J., Jr., & Garcia, P. A. (1998). Management of seizures and epilepsy. *American Family Physician, 57*(7), 1589–1600.

Ramli, N., Rahmat, K., Lim, K. S., & Tan, C. T. (2015). Neuroimaging in refractory epilepsy. Current practice and evolving trends. *European Journal of Radiology, 84*(9), 1791–1800. doi:10.1016/j.ejrad.2015.03.024

GASTROESOPHAGEAL REFLUX DISEASE

Karen C. Bagatelos, Geraldine Collins-Bride, and Fran Dreier

CHAPTER **56**

I. Definition and overview

Gastroesophageal reflux disease (GERD) is defined as chronic symptoms or mucosal damage produced by the abnormal reflux of gastric acid into the esophagus, the oral cavity or the lung (Kahrilias, 2008). It is the most common gastrointestinal (GI) diagnosis recorded during outpatient clinic visits in the United States (Katz, Gerson, & Vela, 2013). GERD affects 19 million adults, accounting for 4,590,000 outpatient visits and 96,000 hospitalizations annually (Practice Parameters Committee of the American College of Gastroenterology, Wang, & Sampliner, 2008). Prevalence is estimated at 20–25% of adults (Practice Parameters Committee of the American College of Gastroenterology et al., 2008; Talley & Vakil, 2005). Studies show that 40% of adults in the United States report regular heartburn and regurgitation; 18% report it weekly. It is more common with increased age. It has become more prevalent in China, Japan, and other Asian countries because of the increasing adoption of a Western diet (Hauser, Oxentanko, & Sanchez, 2014).

A. Significance and complications

Recognizing and treating GERD is important, not only for symptomatic management, but also to avoid the complication of Barrett's esophagus and esophageal carcinoma (Kahrilias, 2008). Approximately 5.6% of the population in the United States has Barrett's esophagus (Spechler & Souza, 2014). Barrett's esophagus involves the replacement of normal squamous epithelium with columnar epithelium, which can occur when normal esophageal mucosa is exposed repeatedly to stomach acid. The columnar epithelium can transform into dysplasia, a precursor to cancer. The worldwide incidence of esophageal cancer is 65.8 cases per 1,000 patient-years in those with high-grade dysplasia. The risk with low-grade dysplasia is 16.98 cases per 1,000 patient-years compared to 5.98 cases without dysplasia (Hauser et al., 2014). The mortality rate is high with adenocarcinoma. Esophageal adenocarcinoma has increased in frequency by a factor of 7 in the United States in the past 4 decades (Spechler & Souza, 2014). Additional complications associated with GERD include esophagitis, esophageal ulceration, and esophageal strictures. Respiratory manifestations, such as chronic cough, shortness of breath, and exacerbation of asthma, are also commonly seen. *It is important to always consider the possibility of GERD in patients with respiratory symptoms* (Galmiche, Zerbib, & Des Varannes, 2008). Reflux of gastric acid can also cause sore throats and tooth decay. Antisecretory therapy and other treatment modalities for GERD produce a huge economic burden.

B. Pathophysiology and etiology of GERD

Several factors can contribute to the development of GERD. In normal individuals (i.e., those who do not have GERD), four mechanisms protect the esophageal epithelium from being damaged by reflux of gastric contents (Hauser et al., 2008).

1. A competent lower esophageal sphincter (LES), which acts as a barrier to reflux

2. Effective movement of contents through the esophagus

3. Secondary peristalsis, which sweeps refluxed material back into the stomach and closes the LES

4. The acid-neutralizing effect of swallowed saliva and mucous present in the upper GI (UGI) tract

    From a broad perspective, the final common path in the development of GERD is altered gastric motility or injury to the UGI tract. Esophageal dysmotility is associated with a great many illnesses, including rheumatologic and endocrine disorders. Altered gastric motility may be associated with a weak LES or transient LES relaxation, weak or disordered esophageal peristalsis, or delayed gastric emptying. GERD is sometimes the first symptom in young women with scleroderma, CREST syndrome, or mixed connective tissue disorders. Local esophageal damage can be caused by increased gastric acid secretion

TABLE 56-1 GERD Common Etiologies

Causative Factor	Clinical Examples
Motility disorders	Esophageal dysmotility caused by diminished peristalsis: rheumatologic and endocrine disorders, such as Sjögren syndrome, scleroderma, CREST syndrome, or mixed connective tissue disorders.
	Altered gastric motility including a weak lower esophageal sphincter or transient lower esophageal sphincter relaxation, weak or disordered esophageal peristalsis, and delayed gastric emptying seen with gastroparesis or gastric outlet obstruction.
Local damage	Increased gastric acid secretion or the retrograde passage of bile and pancreatic juices that cause damage to the esophageal mucosa.
Change in resistance to gastric acid	Factors that decrease the flow of acid and food through the upper gastrointestinal tract, such as reduced saliva (Sjögren syndrome, anticholinergic medications), increased hydrochloric acid (stress response or gastrinoma), or decreased mucosal blood flow (radiation therapy or ischemia).
Structural and physiologic changes	Associated with the following conditions: hiatal hernia, obstructive sleep apnea, weight gain, obesity, pregnancy, or wearing tight clothing.
Hormonal influences	Progesterone, cholecystokinin, secretin, and low gastrin.

or the retrograde passage of bile and pancreatic juice. Mucosal injury further decreases the rate of passage of the bolus of food through the UGI tract. Additional factors that decrease the flow of acid and food through the UGI tract include reduced saliva, increased hydrochloric acid, and decreased mucosal blood flow. Specific structural or physiologic conditions, such as a hiatal hernia or obstructive sleep apnea (Hauser et al., 2008), also decrease the rate of passage of food through the UGI tract. Motility is further affected by factors that increase abdominal pressure (pregnancy, weight gain, obesity, and tight clothing) and by hormonal influences (progesterone, cholecystokinin, secretin, and low gastrin). Hormonal influences can cause transient LES relaxation, excess acid production, and decreased UGI tract motility (**Table 56-1**).

II. **Database** (may include but is not limited to)

A. Subjective

1. Past medical history
   a. Peptic ulcer disease (associated with a hypersecretory state)
   b. Obesity (body mass index [BMI] > 29) causes increased pressure on the stomach and lower esophagus causing more acid to reflux. A recent weight gain, even in an individual of normal BMI, is also thought to have this effect (Katz et al., 2013).
   c. Gallbladder disease may cause symptoms similar to GERD
   d. Pregnancy can exacerbate reflux because of hormonal influences and increased pressure on the upper digestive tract
   e. Neurologic disease, such as a stroke or brain tumor, or any condition that affects neural pathways, including neurologic medications
   f. Diabetes can cause gastroparesis, which in turn causes increased reflux
   g. Collagen-vascular disease (scleroderma, mixed connective tissue disease, and systemic lupus erythematosis) can cause changes in the mucosa or the circulation in the UGI tract
   h. Recurrent pulmonary infections (possible aspiration) and asthma
   i. Cerebral palsy and other neurodevelopmental disabilities
   j. Medications: aspirin, nonsteroidal anti-inflammatory drugs, hormones, vitamins, adrenergics, and anticholinergics

2. Family history
   a. Peptic ulcer disease, GI cancer, gallbladder disease
   b. Diabetes, rheumatologic, and other endocrine disorders

3. Personal and social
   a. Current life stressors: stress can reduce the esophageal perception thresholds for pain (Mizyad, Fass, & Fass, 2009).
   b. Diet:
      i. Although it has been accepted in the past that alcohol, tobacco, caffeine (coffee, colas, and tea), spicy foods, fatty foods, acidic foods (tomatoes, oranges), carbonated beverages, mint, and chocolate can produce or worsen GERD, studies to date show conflicting evidence for the effect of these habits on the LES, and there are currently no published studies that document improvement in GERD symptoms or complications with cessation of these habits. Current guidelines call for individual patients with GERD to avoid those foods and habits that worsen their symptoms (Katz et al., 2013).
      ii. Large meals and late night eating are known provoking factors for GERD.
4. Review of systems
   a. Gastrointestinal
      i. Pain: the typical symptom is *heartburn*, a retrosternal burning sensation originating in the subxyphoid region and spreading upward into the chest occurring 30–60 minutes after meals. In severe episodes, there are esophageal spasms or noncardiac chest pain. The pain can radiate into the neck, shoulders, and back.
      ii. Dysphagia, episodes of choking (can present as coughing with eating)
      iii. Regurgitation of gastric contents into the mouth
      iv. Nausea and vomiting (can be seen with GERD, although not a common associated symptom)
      v. Aggravating factors for these symptoms
         a. Position (lying down, especially postprandial reclining; bending over and lifting heavy objects)
         b. Wearing tight clothing or belts
         c. Individual provoking factors (as noted previously, this may include tobacco, alcohol, caffeine, and certain foods)
   b. Ear, nose, and throat: chronic sore throat, early morning hoarseness
   c. Mouth: complaint of bad breath (halitosis)
   d. Cardiac: full cardiac review of systems is indicated
   e. Pulmonary: cough (especially nocturnal cough), wheezing (shortness of breath is not typically seen with GERD)

B. Objective

1. Physical examination
   a. General: appearance, development, nourishment; note tight clothing if present
   b. Weight, BMI
   c. Ear, nose, and throat: dentition changes, tooth decay, and pharyngeal erythema
   d. Cardiac examination: should be normal in a patient with GERD
   e. Chest examination: wheezing, adventitious sounds
   f. Abdominal examination: obesity, epigastric tenderness, distention, and tympanic bowel sounds
   g. Rectal examination: stool hemoccult

III. Assessment

A. Determine the diagnosis

GERD is most commonly diagnosed by history and presenting symptoms. The following diagnoses should be considered for all patients presenting with symptoms of GERD:

1. Cardiac disease or angina (should be excluded before beginning GI evaluation) (Katz et al., 2013)
2. Esophageal stricture or mass
3. Esophageal motility disorder
4. Esophageal spasm
5. *Helicobacter pylori* infection. In contrast to previous practice, screening for *H pylori* is not recommended in the diagnostic evaluation of GERD according to the 2013 practice guidelines of the American College of Gastroenterology (Katz et al., 2013).
6. Gastroparesis
7. Peptic ulcer disease
8. Zollinger-Ellison syndrome

B. Severity

Assess the severity of the disease, including duration of symptoms and risk for complications of untreated or poorly treated GERD. The diagnosis of GERD is currently subdivided into:

1. ERD (erosive disease)
2. NERD (nonerosive disease)

C. Significance and motivation

Assess the significance of the symptoms to the patient and explain the often chronic nature of this disorder. Determine the motivation and ability of the patient to follow through with the treatment plan that can involve significant modification of weight, habits, food choices, and timing of meals.

IV. Goals of clinical management

A. Screening

The American College of Gastroenterology recommends that patients with typical GERD symptoms of heartburn and/or regurgitation be managed pharmacologically. Patients with alarm symptoms or signs such as dysphagia or weight loss do require diagnostic studies such as esophago-gastroduodenoscopy (EGD). It has been reported that 50% of the patients who are screened with EGD have nonerosive gastroesophageal reflux (NERD) (Hauser et al., 2014).

B. Treatment

1. Medical management is designed to promote gastric emptying, augment the resting tone of the LES, and favorably alter the nature of refluxed material through nonpharmacologic and pharmacologic means.

2. Treatment aims to assist the patient in the management of GERD symptoms and enhance lifestyle modification to prevent recurrence of symptoms and disease.

C. Prevention of complications

These include the following: Barrett's esophagus, adenocarcinoma, esophagitis, dysphagia caused by esophageal strictures, narrowing or spasm, ulcers, persistent pain, and bleeding.

V. Plan

A. Screening

There are no screening tests available for the early detection or prevention of GERD. However, there are preventive measures that can be taken. These include maintaining normal body weight, reducing stress, and avoiding eating large fatty meals before bedtime.

B. Diagnostic tests

1. Laboratory tests: complete blood count, stool for occult blood. In unrelenting cases, check serum gastrin to evaluate for Zollinger-Ellison syndrome.

2. Electrocardiogram if chest pain is present. Perform or refer for additional cardiology diagnostic studies if angina is suspected.

3. UGI series: if dysphagia is present, consider UGI series to rule out a stricture or mass.

4. According to the 2013 Practice Guideline for the Diagnosis and Management of GERD (Katz et al., 2013), endoscopy is indicated in the following circumstances:

    a. Alarm signs or symptoms, such as persistent vomiting, hematemesis, evidence of GI blood loss, involuntary weight loss, progressive dysphagia, anemia, evidence of GI bleeding, chest pain proven to be of noncardiac etiology, or a mass, stricture, or ulcer found on imaging studies.

    b. Wheezing, orthopnea, or atypical respiratory symptoms

    c. Unrelenting symptoms despite therapy, or family history of esophageal cancer

    d. Patients who have reflux of many years' duration should receive an endoscopy to screen for Barrett's esophagus. If Barrett's esophagus is confirmed, then surveillance endoscopy should be done every 6 months to 3 years, depending on pathologic findings and the endoscopist's recommendations (Practice Parameters Committee of the American College of Gastroenterology et al., 2008). Caucasian men over 50 have the highest risk for Barrett's esophagus.

    e. Recurrent symptoms after antireflux surgery.

5. Special studies

    Additional evaluation includes tests to measure reflux and more precisely evaluate the motility of the esophagus and stomach (gastric emptying study, manometry with a 24-hour pH study, and endoscopy with biopsy). A gastric emptying study may reveal decreased gastric emptying, which can cause functional dyspepsia. A manometry with pH study can quantify the amount of reflux that a patient has in 24 hours and also measures the pressure in the upper and lower esophageal sphincters. These tests characterize GERD more precisely and also provide evidence for determining if the patient is an appropriate surgical candidate.

C. Management

Many patients with GERD respond to management with weight reduction, antacids or other medication, habit changes, elevation of the head of the bed, stress reduction, and other nonsurgical measures. For those who cannot be managed successfully with these measures but do respond to proton pump inhibitors (PPIs), and who do not want to take medication indefinitely, surgery is a viable option.

1. Nonpharmacologic measures

    a. Mechanical measures: raise the head of the bed 8–10 inches, and maintain an upright posture for a minimum of 30–60 minutes after eating.

    b. Dietary measures

        i. Do not eat within 3 hours of bedtime.

        ii. Avoid those foods that seem to aggravate symptoms.

    c. Smoking cessation should be considered

d. Weight loss when body mass index is greater than 29 or when there has been a recent weight gain

e. Stress management

2. Pharmacologic measures

Initial pharmacologic treatment of GERD is influenced by the frequency and severity of symptoms, and whether the patient is thought to have ERD (erosive reflux disease) or NERD (nonerosive reflux disease). Excellent documentation exists showing that PPIs are more effective and relieve symptoms more rapidly than H2 receptor antagonists (H2RAs), although those patients with ERD seem to have a higher rate of symptom relief.

a. *For mild symptoms*: patients with infrequent symptoms often respond well to antacids. Liquid preparations can be used, 15 mL (double-strength preparations) and 30 mL (single-strength preparations) 1 and 3 hours after meals and at bedtime until symptoms resolve.

b. *For mild to moderate symptoms in NERD*, H2RAs can be effective and are less expensive than PPIs. They work by blocking histamine-induced stimulation of gastric parietal cells. H2RAs are most effective when given as a divided dose twice daily.

Clinicians who use a "step-down approach" to the treatment of GERD often begin treatment with PPIs rather than with H2RAs. Clinicians who prefer a "step-up" approach begin with H2RAs.

c. For moderate to severe symptoms or for the suspicion or diagnosis of ERD, treatment of choice is a PPI. PPIs are potent inhibitors of gastric acid secretion, working by turning off the pumps in parietal cells. All PPIs seem to be equally effective. Selection of a particular PPI is often determined by insurance company formularies. There are many preparations on the market and the reader is encouraged to consult information for each agent. Most PPIs are given once daily, 30–60 minutes before the first meal of the day. Dosage can be increased to twice daily if needed or given at bedtime if nighttime symptoms are an issue. PPI treatment should achieve resolution of symptoms and complete healing of the esophagus in 8 weeks. If symptoms recur within 6 months, chronic therapy may be needed with either daily or twice-daily dosing of a PPI (**Table 56-2**). Patients who do have resolution of symptoms can continue taking PPIs or H2RAs on as needed basis. H2RAs can be added to PPIs to control nighttime symptoms, but it should be noted that H2RAs can exhibit waning effectiveness over time (tachyphylaxis) within a relatively short time.

See Table 56-2 for a list of side effects associated with GERD medications. Serious side effects can be associated with H2RAs, but these are rare. Although PPIs have a good safety profile, there can be side effects associated with their use. Because PPIs affect calcium metabolism, they should be used with caution in patients at high risk for hip fracture (Targownik & Leung, 2010). PPIs are also associated with an increased risk of *Clostridium difficile* and other enteric infections, and may be contraindicated in patients at high risk for these infections.

d. For patients with slow gastric emptying, consider using prokinetics/antiemetics:

i. Metoclopramide (Reglan®), 10 mg three to four times daily. This agent increases the rate of gastric and esophageal emptying by stimulating the smooth muscle of the intestine. The potential side effects of metoclopramide should be reviewed with the patient before initiating treatment. The most serious, although infrequent, side effects include tardive dyskinesia, agranulocytosis, supraventicular tachycardia, hyperaldosteronism, and neuroleptic malignant syndrome.

ii. Cisapride (Propulsid®), 10 mg four times daily before meals and at bedtime. Given its risk for potentially life-threatening arrhythmias, this agent is now only available for limited access protocol use by gastroenterologists. It is very effective in enhancing gastric emptying and generally has fewer side effects than metoclopramide.

iii. For nausea, one can use ondansetron (Zofran®) or promethazine (although the latter often produces drowsiness).

iv. Domperidone has been found to be effective but is not approved for GERD by the U.S. Food and Drug Administration.

e. For patients with gastroparesis who do not respond to medications, consider a referral to a tertiary medical center for a gastric stimulator.

3. Surgical options

The most common surgical procedure performed for GERD is the Nissen fundoplication. This surgery may be indicated in a small number of patients with severe reflux who do respond to PPIs but who may have reasons, such as drug side effects, for preferring surgical management. The patient must undergo detailed evaluation by a gastroenterologist before

TABLE 56-2 Commonly Used GERD Medications*

Medication Category with Examples	Initial Dose	Maintenance Dose	Precautions
Antacids			Use with caution in renal impairment. Many drug interactions, especially with higher doses (e.g., antipsychotics, anticonvulsants, and calcium channel blockers).
Aluminum hydroxide and magnesium hydroxide (Alamag OTC, Maalox®)	5–10 ml or 2–4 tablets 1–3 hours after meals and bedtimeHS	PRN according to symptoms	
Calcium carbonate and magnesium hydroxide (Mylanta® Gelcaps, Mylanta® Supreme, or Rolaids® Extra Strength)	Same as above	Same as above	Constipation is a frequent side effect
H2 receptor antagonists			Many adverse reactions including cardiac arrhythmias, reversible confusional states, and increased prolactin levels. Use with caution in renal impairment (creatinine clearance < 50). Monitor for vitamin B_{12} deficiency with long-term use.
Ranitidine (Zantac®)	150 mg twice daily or 300 mg daily (taken in the evening or at bedtime if single dose)	150 mg at bedtime	
Famotidine (Pepcid®)	20 mg twice daily, take second dose in the evening or at bedtime	20 mg at bedtime	
Nizatidine (Axid®)	150 mg twice daily or 300 mg daily (taken in the evening or at bedtime if single dose)	150 mg daily	
Proton pump inhibitors (PPIs)	Usually prescribed for 6–8 weeks for initial treatment		Check for drug interactions Good safety profile. Long-term safety use best studied with omeprazole, the first PPI on the market. Long-term use of PPIs: adjust to the lowest dose for symptom control (Kahrilias, Shaheen, & Vaezi, 2008). Take before breakfast. If twice daily dosing, take second dose before evening meal. No dose adjustment required for renal impairment
Omeprazole (Prilosec®)	20–40 mg daily	20–40 mg daily	Take 30 minutes before a meal.
Lansoprazole (Prevacid®)	15–30 mg daily	15–30 mg daily	Take 30 minutes before a meal.
Pantoprazole (Protonix®)	20–40 mg daily	20–40 mg daily	Take at least 1 hour before a meal.
Rabeprazole (AcipHex®)	20 mg daily	20 mg daily	
Esomeprazole (Nexium®)	40 mg daily	40 mg daily	

* Reflects suggested dosages for GERD. Dosages for erosive esophagitis and other esophageal disorders may vary.

surgery can be considered. Presurgical evaluation includes endoscopy, UGI series, and esophageal manometry with a 24-hour pH study.

The surgical treatment of choice for the obese patient is bariatric surgery.

D. Follow-up

1. Follow-up in approximately 4–6 weeks after initiating treatment or sooner if symptoms increase in severity. Assess adherence to treatment plan.

2. Gastroenterology consult if symptoms worsen or complications occur. If no response to treatment, consider EGD, UGI series, or Cine esophagram.

3. Assess for side effects of medications.

E. Patient education

1. Assist the patient and family to voice their concerns and develop coping strategies with respect to the disease process and its management.

2. Provide verbal and written information about the pathophysiology of GERD and its treatment. The National Institutes of Health has a very good handout that is available for distribution. See the website below.

3. Discuss what the patient can expect with diagnostic testing, including preparation and aftercare.

4. Explain the therapeutic benefit and side effects of any prescribed treatment.

5. Stress that follow-up is recommended in person or by telephone to monitor treatment response and make appropriate treatment regimen changes.

VI. Self-management resources

A. The National Institutes of Health

The National Institutes of Health has multiple brochures for patients. Refer to their website: http://digestive.niddk .nih.gov/ddiseases/pubs/gerd/.

B. The Mayo Clinic

The Mayo Clinic also has excellent resources: www .mayoclinic.com/health/gerd/DS00967.

REFERENCES

Galmiche, J. P., Zerbib, F., & Des Varannes, S. B. (2008). Review article: Respiratory manifestations of gastro-esophageal reflux disease. *Alimentary Pharmacology & Therapeutics, 27*(8), 449–464.

Hauser, S. C., Oxentanko, A. S., & Sanchez, W. (2014). *Mayo Clinic Gastroenterology and Hepatology Board Review.* Rochester, MN: Mayo Clinic Scientific Press.

Kahrilias, P. J. (2008). Gastroesophageal reflux disease. *New England Journal of Medicine, 359*(16), 1700–1707.

Kahrilias, P. J., Shaheen, N. J., & Vaezi, M. F. (2008). American Gastroenterological Association medical position statement on management of gastroesophageal reflux disease. *Gastroenterology, 135*(4), 1383–1391.

Katz, P. O., Gerson, L. B., & Vela, M. F. (2013). Guidelines for the diagnosis and management of gastroesophageal reflux disease. *American Journal of Gastroenterology, 108,* 308–328; doi: 10.1038/ajg.2012.444

Mizyad, I., Fass, S. S., & Fass, R. (2009). Gastro-oesophageal reflux disease and psychological comorbidity. *Alimentary Pharmacology & Therapeutics, 29*(4), 351–358.

Practice Parameters Committee of the American College of Gastroenterology, Wang, K. K., & Sampliner, R. (2008). Updated guidelines 2008 for the diagnosis, surveillance and therapy of Barrett's esophagus. *American Journal of Gastroenterology, 103,* 788–797.

Spechler, S. J., & Souza, R. F. (2014). Barrett's esophagus. *New England Journal of Medicine, 371,* 836–845.

Talley, N. J., & Vakil, N. (2005). Guidelines for the management of dyspepsia. *American Journal of Gastroenterology, 100,* 2324–2337.

Targownik, L. E., & Leung, S. L. (2010). Proton-pump inhibitor use is not associated with osteoporosis or accelerated bone mineral density loss. *Gastroenterology, 138*(3), 896–904.

GERIATRIC SYNDROMES

CHAPTER 57

Courtney Gordon

I. Introduction and general background

Geriatric syndromes are defined as common conditions seen in older adults that cannot be classified into a single disease but have a significant impact on well-being and quality of life. They are complex conditions more frequently seen among older adults that are multifactorial in etiology and require a multidisciplinary approach to management and treatment. The geriatric syndromes discussed in this chapter include many of the conditions commonly seen in primary care of older adults. Those syndromes are frailty, sensory impairment, falls, urinary incontinence, and delirium.

A. Frailty

1. Definition and overview

   Frailty is an increasingly recognized geriatric syndrome that has a tremendous impact on the older individual, their family, and society as a whole (Theou et al., 2011). Frailty is a condition made up of many different components. Presenting complaints commonly include decreased energy, poor appetite and inability to consume adequate nutrition, weight loss, weakness, and decreased physical activity. It is a chronic syndrome which is progressive in nature developing along a continuum of severity. Frailty is associated with a high risk for poor clinical outcomes due to inability to recover from stressors. These adverse clinical outcomes often include falls, functional impairment, loss of independence, and mortality. The main goal is prevention of frailty by maintaining muscle mass and activity level in older adults as well as adequate nutritional intake.

2. Prevalence

   Frailty tends to be more prevalent in the presence of any stressors to the body. Stressors in older adults can include factors such as infections, dehydration, new medications, depression, and any changes in living arrangements like moving or new caregivers, or recent hospitalization.

B. Sensory impairment

1. Definition and overview

   Both visual and hearing impairment greatly impact the quality of life for older adults. Other sensory impairments that are seen in advanced age include change of taste and smell. Along with sensory impairments comes social isolation, depression, anxiety, loss of independence, greater risk of falls, and functional decline.

   Visual impairment is defined as visual acuity less than 20/40. Blindness is defined as visual acuity less than 20/200 (Durso & Sullivan, 2013). There are many common eye conditions older adults are likely to develop as they age that result in worsening visual acuity. Those include but are not limited to cataracts, age-related macular degeneration, glaucoma, and diabetic retinopathy.

   Hearing impairment has a substantial negative impact on the way patients communicate. It has also been linked to increased incidence of cognitive deterioration, increased falls, and gait disorders. Presbycusis is defined as age-related hearing loss. There are many reasons why older adults suffer from hearing loss and it is important to recognize the different types of hearing loss. The most common type in older adults is sensorineural hearing loss. Other types of hearing loss are classified as conductive or mixed. Various infections can also cause hearing loss as well in older adults and some individuals may have an autoimmune inner ear disease that can contribute to hearing loss such as systemic lupus erythematous, Crohn's disease, and ulcerative colitis to name a few. Diabetes mellitus can affect the vasculature of the cochlea leading to hearing loss. Ototoxic medications like aminoglycoside antibiotics, antimalarial medications, platinum-based chemotherapy agents, loop diuretics, and nonsteroidal anti-inflammatory drugs can all worsen hearing loss. Acoustic neuroma, Meniere disease, trauma, and radiation can all also contribute to hearing loss in the older adult.

2. Prevalence

Both visual and hearing impairments increase in incident as people age. These impairments have a substantial impact on the quality of life of the older adult as well as the medical system. Chronic eye conditions are one of the most common reasons for office visits among those 65 years and older (Durso & Sullivan, 2013).

Hearing loss is one of the most common chronic conditions affecting people over the age of 65. The prevalence of hearing loss is 20–40% in adults aged 50 years or older and more than 80% for those aged 80 years or older (Chou, Dana, Bougatsos, Fleming, & Beil, 2011).

C. Falls

1. Definition and overview

Significant morbidity and mortality are associated with falls in older adults. The prognosis worsens in people with repetitive and frequent falls. Falls and gait disorders, like all geriatric syndromes, play an important role in the quality of life for older adults. Depression and confusion are often seen in patients who suffer from falls. Family members also begin thinking of placing their loved ones in a residential facility due to falls, gait disorders, and resultant risk of injury to themselves in the home. The fear of falling can also create stress to individuals and family. The fear of falling has been shown to increase overall fall risk. One of the major consequences of fear of falling is the restriction and avoidance of activities (Delbaere, Crombez, Vanderstraeten, Willems, & Cambier, 2004).

2. Prevalence

Falls are the most common event that in turn causes loss of independence in older adults. More than one-third of community-living adults older than 65 years fall each year. Approximately 10% of falls result in a major injury such as a fracture, soft tissue injury, or traumatic brain injury (Tinetti & Kumar, 2010). The incidence increases for those individuals over the age of 80 and those who reside in residential facilities.

D. Urinary incontinence

1. Definition and overview

Urinary incontinence is defined as any involuntary leakage or loss of urine. Urinary incontinence is a syndrome that can result from different medical conditions and the usage of certain medications.

Leading risk factors for urinary incontinence include female gender, cognitive impairment, abdominal surgery, obesity, impaired mobility, and increasing age. Incontinence has a substantial impact financially on the healthcare system as well as the individual's quality of life. An estimated 12 billion dollars is spent annually on incontinence supplies, medications, and caregiver time (Williams et al., 2014). The different types of urinary incontinence include functional incontinence, stress incontinence, urge incontinence, overflow incontinence, and mixed incontinence. Please refer to Chapter 25, Urinary Incontinence in Women, for more detailed information.

2. Prevalence

Urinary incontinence increases in incidence with age and is more common in women than men. Approximately 15–30% of healthy older adults experience some urinary leakage. The prevalence is nearly 50% among frail community dwellers and between 50% and 75% among institutionalized older adults (Williams et al., 2014). Incontinence often goes unreported by patients due to embarrassment and social stigma. Urinary incontinence, like falls, is one of the main reasons persons are moved out of their homes into residential nursing facilities. It has a great burden on caregivers and negatively affects quality of life. Family members have difficulty helping their loved ones with their toileting and as a result need more help. Urinary incontinence is associated with a 30% increase in functional decline, and a 2-fold increased risk of falls, depressive symptoms, and nursing home placement (Goode, Burgio, Richter, & Markland, 2010).

E. Delirium

1. Definition and overview

Like the previous syndromes, delirium is multifactorial and important to recognize in the geriatric population as individuals experiencing delirium are at an increased risk for poor clinical outcomes. Key features include an acute onset with a fluctuating course as well as waxing and waning of symptoms. Typically described as a transient syndrome some cases of delirium have been reported to last as long as a few weeks to months. Delirium often goes misdiagnosed as dementia especially in the acute care setting. It is important to remember most dementias typically present gradually and progressively over many months to years, unlike delirium, which occurs suddenly and changes often over the course of 24 hours. However, a major predisposing factor for the development of delirium is underlying cognitive impairment, so often older adults can have both delirium and dementia. Other predisposing factors for delirium include depression, coexisting medical conditions, drugs/medications, environmental changes, electrolyte disturbances, infection, injury, and change in functional status, poor appetite, and sensory impairment. Three different forms of delirium exist—hyperactive, hypoactive, and mixed. Hyperactive delirium is the individual who is very anxious and agitated, has difficulty sleeping, and can be aggressive with staff and caregivers. Hypoactive deliriums are often missed because the main symptoms are the patient is more lethargic and sleepy than their baseline. Mixed delirium is common and is a combination of the two (Wong, Holroyd-Leduc, Simel, & Straus, 2010).

2. Prevalence

Delirium is a common occurrence in older adults and is associated with high morbidity and mortality. Delirium is also associated with functional decline and immobility, which result in further complications of care. Delirium is the most common complication among hospitalized older adults (Witlox, Eurelings, de Jonghe, Kalisvaart, Eikelenboom, & van Gool, 2010). On admission to the hospital prevalence of delirium can range from 10% to 40% of older adults. Patients admitted to the ICU have an even higher incidence of 70–87% (Williams et al., 2014). The prevalence of delirium at the end of life is also reported to be quite high as well, upwards of 80–85% (Durso & Sullivan, 2013). Delirium complicates hospital stays for at least 20% of the 12.5 million patients 65 years of age or older who are hospitalized each year and increases hospital costs by $2,500 per patient, so that about $6.9 billion of Medicare hospital expenditures are attributable to delirium (Inouye, 2006).

II. Database

A. Subjective

1. Frailty

Subjective data are obtained from a detailed history from the patient if they are able to provide information as well as from any family members or caregivers who are present. Family members typically complain that their loved one is slowing down. The individual seems weaker or more tired than usual. Patients often complain of having no energy and feeling as if everything is a burden.

2. Sensory impairment

Patients with visual impairments will have various complaints. It is important to do a detailed history to decipher what requires attention from an ophthalmologist versus what can be handled in the outpatient setting. Questions to ask include: Do they now require reading glasses? Do they have associated pain? Is their vision blurred? What is the time frame for loss of vision?

Hearing loss data are often reported from family members and caregivers who find the patient is not hearing as well as normal. Hearing loss that is associated with age is gradual and spans many years. Common complaints from patients are not being able to hear well in large crowds; for example, when dining out they have difficulty engaging in conversations due to inability to hear well. Hearing loss is often considered by patients and family members as a normal part of aging and not something that can be fixed. Often this is not the case. As a clinician it is important to about ask the nature of the hearing loss, the timing (days, months, years), and any associated symptoms like ear pain, ringing, drainage, or dizziness. If they have already been examined and have hearing aids, are they wearing them appropriately? Do they know how to care for them?

3. Falls

During the detailed history it is important to ask if the patient has had any previous falls, balance issues, or worsening in vision recently. What medications is the person taking? Are they depressed or suffer from dizziness, and do they have any associated pain? These factors all contribute to the increased risk for falls. By targeting risk factors, interventions can be made to decrease incidence of falls.

4. Urinary incontinence

A thorough history of urinary incontinence must include gaining information from the patient, family member, or caregiver about frequency, duration, and severity of symptoms. Often an older adult is reluctant to discuss urinary incontinence due to embarrassment. Questions should also include: Do you ever leak urine when you cough or sneeze? Do you have problems making it to the bathroom in time? If yes, why do you have difficulty? Do you find yourself getting up frequently during the night to urinate?

5. Delirium

Clinical diagnosis is made after a detailed history, a cognitive assessment, and a physical and neurological exam. Knowing a patient's cognitive status at baseline is important to determine any fluctuations or subtle changes. Obtaining a detailed history from family members and caregivers is vital to ascertain any recent changes in mental status. It is important for clinicians to note the timing of the mental status change and the course thus far. Additionally, identify any preceding factors such as new medications, change in physical environment, or injury. It is important to diagnose delirium as it can be a medical emergency and improve with treatment quickly.

B. Objective: physical examination

1. Frailty
   a. Pertinent physical exam findings may include:
      i. Head, eyes, ears, nose, and throat (HEENT)—temporal wasting, dry mucous membranes
      ii. Cardiovascular—tachycardia or other arrhythmias
      iii. Weight loss and poorly fitting clothes
2. Sensory impairment
   a. Measure visual acuity using the Snellen chart.
   b. Examine whether the older adult's pupils respond to light.
   c. Assess visual fields via confrontation and extraocular motility.
   d. Examine the outer parts of the eye (lids, lashes, and brows)
   e. With an ophthalmoscope assess the lens for opacities; the optic disc for increased cupping or pallor, arteriovenous narrowing, nicking and/or copper and silver wiring; and the maculae for hemorrhages, exudates, and drusen.
   f. When assessing hearing it is imperative to examine with an otoscope and observe the ear canal as well as the tympanic membrane. Cerumen can occlude the ear canal resulting in significant hearing loss as well as discomfort and can be easily removed providing relief. When inspecting the ear canal look for any tumors, cysts, polyps, or foreign bodies that might impair hearing. It is important to look for any perforation of the tympanic membrane or significant thickening of the membrane, which can worsen hearing.
   g. When assessing hearing, clinicians can perform tuning fork tests with both the Weber and the Rinne to differentiate the type of hearing loss in the older adult.
3. Falls
   a. Examine footwear and clothing, which can impede safety.
   b. Obtain orthostatic vital signs.
   c. Assess cognitive status with a validated tool like the ones included in this chapter (see **Figures 57-1** and **57-2**).
   d. Check visual acuity (see previous section on sensory impairment).
   e. Pertinent physical exam findings can include:
      i. HEENT—Nystagmus and other ocular deficiencies contributing to the risk for falls. Ears impacted with cerumen contributing to dizziness and falls. Examine mouth to look for moist mucous membranes. Dry membranes are an indicator for dehydration, which can contribute to falls.
      ii. Cardiovascular—Assess for arrhythmias and other cardiac abnormalities that can cause syncope and falls. Assess both carotid arteries for bruits.
      iii. Musculoskeletal—Examine for strength and any movement disorders that can contribute to falls.
   f. There are several validated tests that measure balance and mobility in the older adult but are often not practical to perform in a busy clinic setting. The Timed Up and Go test and the functional reach test however are fairly easy to use and take relatively little time. (See **Table 57-1**).
4. Urinary incontinence
   a. Patients or their caregivers can complete a voiding or bladder diary, which the clinician can use to review episodes of incontinence regarding timing and frequency. Patients or their caregivers write down the time of urination, the amount, and any additional comments such as what they were doing, for example, coughing, sneezing, or sleeping.
   b. Physical exam is less useful for initial assessment of urinary incontinence than the detailed history (Goode et al., 2010). However, a thorough physical exam should include:
      i. Cardiovascular—A thorough cardiovascular assessment looking for signs of fluid overload associated with congestive heart failure, which can contribute to incontinence. Elevated jugular venous pressure, arrhythmias, increased edema to extremities, and shortness of breath.
      ii. Abdominal—Palpate the bladder for fullness and if there is any associated pain or tenderness. Examine the abdomen for any constipation, which can contribute to incontinence.
      iii. A rectal exam should be done in particular for men to assess for enlarged prostate, masses, or fecal impaction.

The Confusion Assessment Method Instrument:

1. *[Acute Onset]* Is there evidence of an acute change in mental status from the patient's beseline?
2A. *[Inattention]* Did the patient have difficulty focusing attention, for example, being easily distractible, or having difficulty keeping track of what was being said?
2B. *(If present or abnormal)* Did this behavior fluctuate during the interview, that is, tend to come and go or increase and decrease in severity?
3. *[Disorganized thinking]* Was the patient's thinking disorganized or incoherent, such as rambling or irrelevant conversation, unclear or illogical flow of ideas, or unpredictable switching from subject to subject?
4. *[Altered level of consciousness]* Overall, how would you rate this patient's level of consciousness? (Alert [normal]; Vigilant [hyperalert, overly sensitive to environmental stimuli, startled very easily], Lethargic [drowsy, easily aroused]; Stupor [difficult to arouse]; Coma; [unarousable]; Uncertain)
5. *[Disorientation]* Was the patient disoriented at any time during the interview, such as thinking that he or she was somewhere other than the hospital, using the wrong bed, or misjudging the time of day?
6. *[Memory impairment]* Did the patient demonstrate any memory problems during the interview, such as inability to remember events in the hospital or difficulty remembering instructions?
7. *[Perceptual disturbances]* Did the patient have any evidence of perceptual disturbances, for example, hallucinations, illusions or misinterpretations (such as thinking something was moving when it was not)?
8A. *[Psychomotor agitation]* At any time during the interview did the patient have an unusually increased level of motor activity such as restlessness, picking at bedclothes, tapping fingers or making frequent sudden changes of position?
8B. *[Psychomotor retardation]* At any time during the interview did the patient have an unusually decreased level of motor activity such as sluggishness, staring into space, staying in one position for a long time or moving very slowly?
9. *[Altered sleep-wake cycle]* Did the patient have evidence of disturbance of the sleep-wake cycle, such as excessive daytime sleepiness with insomnia at night?

The Confusion Assessment Method (CAM) Diagnostic Algorithm

Feature 1: *Acute Onset or Fluctuating Course*
This feature is usually obtained from a family member or nurse and is shown by positive responses to the following questions: Is there evidence of an acute change in mental status from the patient's baseline? Did the (abnormal) behavior fluctuate during the day, that is, tend to come and go, or increase and decrease in severity?

Feature 2: *Inattention*
This feature is shown by a positive response to the following question: Did the patient have difficulty focusing attention, for example, being easily distractible, or having difficulty keeping track of what was being said?

Feature 3: *Disorganized thinking*
This feature is shown by a positive response to the following question: Was the patient's thinking disorganized or incoherent, sach as rambling or irrelevant conversation, unclear or illogical flow of ideas, or unpredictable switching from subject to subject?

Feature 4: *Altered Level of consciousness*
This feature is shown by any answer other than "alert" to the following question: Overall, how would you rate this patient's level of consciousness? (alert [normal]), vigilant [hyperalert], lethargic [drowsy, easily aroused], stupor [difficult to arouse], or coma [unarousable])

The diagnosis of delirium by CAM requires the presence of features 1 and 2 and either 3 or 4.

FIGURE 57-1 Confusion Assessment Method (CAM)

Reproduced from Inouye, S., van Dyck, C., Alessi, C., Balkin, S., Siegal, A. & Horwitz, R. (1990). Clarifying confusion: The confusion assessment method. *Annals of Internal Medicine, 113*(12), 941–948.

MONTREAL COGNITIVE ASSESSMENT (MOCA)
Version 7.1 Original Version

NAME :
Education :
Sex :
Date of birth :
DATE :

VISUOSPATIAL / EXECUTIVE			POINTS

Copy cube

Draw CLOCK (Ten past eleven) (3 points)

[ ]   [ ]   [ ] Contour   [ ] Numbers   [ ] Hands   __/5

NAMING

[ ]   [ ]   [ ]   __/3

MEMORY	Read list of words, subject must repeat them. Do 2 trials, even if 1st trial is successful. Do a recall after 5 minutes.		FACE	VELVET	CHURCH	DAISY	RED	No points
		1st trial						
		2nd trial						

ATTENTION	Read list of digits (1 digit/ sec.).	Subject has to repeat them in the forward order [ ] 2 1 8 5 4	__/2
		Subject has to repeat them in the backward order [ ] 7 4 2	

Read list of letters. The subject must tap with his hand at each letter A. No points if ≥ 2 errors
[ ] FBACMNAAJKLBAFAKDEAAAJAMOFAAB   __/1

Serial 7 subtraction starting at 100   [ ] 93   [ ] 86   [ ] 79   [ ] 72   [ ] 65   __/3
4 or 5 correct subtractions: **3 pts**, 2 or 3 correct: **2 pts**, 1 correct: **1 pt**, 0 correct: **0 pt**

LANGUAGE	Repeat : I only know that John is the one to help today. [ ] The cat always hid under the couch when dogs were in the room. [ ]	__/2

Fluency / Name maximum number of words in one minute that begin with the letter F   [ ] ____ (N ≥ 11 words)   __/1

ABSTRACTION	Similarity between e.g. banana - orange = fruit [ ] train – bicycle [ ] watch - ruler	__/2

DELAYED RECALL	Has to recall words WITH NO CUE	FACE [ ]	VELVET [ ]	CHURCH [ ]	DAISY [ ]	RED [ ]	Points for UNCUED recall only	__/5
Optional	Category cue							
	Multiple choice cue							

ORIENTATION	[ ] Date [ ] Month [ ] Year [ ] Day [ ] Place [ ] City	__/6

© Z.Nasreddine MD   www.mocatest.org   Normal ≥ 26 / 30   TOTAL   __/30

Administered by: _____   Add 1 point if ≤ 12 yr edu

FIGURE 57-2 Montreal Cognitive Assessment (MOCA)

TABLE 57-1 Special Maneuvers

Timed Up and Go Test	Measure an older adult's strength and balance
The most frequently recommended screening test for mobility, takes less than 1 minute to administer	Patient should stand from a chair without using arms to push up
	Patient walks across the exam room and turns around
	Patient walks back to chair and sits down again without using arms
	Inability to do this test within 15 seconds indicates an increased fall risk
	Patient is also graded on a scale of 1 to 5 regarding muscle strength, balance, and gait abnormalities while performing test
Functional Reach Test	Performed with a leveled yardstick secured to the wall just above the patient's waist
	Patient being tested stands with shoulders perpendicular to the wall and he or she makes a fist and extends the arm as far forward as possible along the wall without losing balance or taking a step.
	Test should be done without shoes or socks
	The distance reached is measured using the yardstick
	Patient should accomplish 6 inches or greater
	Inability to do so is an indicator to pursue further testing and assessment for functional decline

Data from Tinetti, M. E., & Kumar, C. (2010). The patient who falls. "It's always a trade-off." *JAMA*, *303*(3), 258–266.

iv. For women, assess for prolapse or atrophy, which can contribute to incontinence, as well as any masses.

5. Delirium

a. Clinicians should use the Confusion Assessment Method (CAM) (see Figure 57-1), Minicog, MOCA (see Figure 57-2), or another validated tool to help determine cognitive status (Durso & Sullivan, 2013). These tests assess for cognitive changes, attention span, organization, and level of consciousness.

b. The CAM is simple to use and also comes in an ICU format for patient's admitted to intensive care units. It is easily administered at the bedside.

c. It is important to perform MOCA at routine follow-up visits in the outpatient setting to assess baseline cognitive functioning and therefore be able to identify any changes.

d. Pertinent physical exam findings may include:

i. Cardiovascular—Assess for cardiac arrhythmias such as atrial fibrillation, bradycardia, tachycardia, congestive heart failure (CHF) exacerbation, which could be the source of the delirium.

ii. Abdominal—Assess for distention, pain, and bowel sounds. Acute abdominal pain and constipation can cause delirium in the older adult.

iii. Neurological—Focus attention on mental status, which might show hyperalertness or lethargy. Assess mood, which can be agitated, anxious, more confused. Assess grip strength and motor skills to rule out stroke.

III. Assessment

A. Frailty

Using a comprehensive geriatric assessment allows clinicians to care for frail older adults. This allows clinicians to address the different components of frailty. A team-based approach including physicians, nurses, pharmacists, therapists, and dieticians has been shown to have positive effects when treating older adults. The focus of assessment in frailty is to eliminate or treat any underlying stressors that are contributing to frailty.

According to the American Geriatric Society a person must have three or more characteristics in order to be classified with frailty (Durso & Sullivan, 2013).

1. Weight loss—more than 10 lbs unintentionally in the past year

2. Exhaustion—sensation that everything takes an enormous effort to complete

3. Slowness—time to walk 15 feet

4. Low activity level—uses less than 270 kcal/week

5. Weakness—can calculate with grip strength measurement

A clinician should be able to recognize any precipitating causes of frailty and address these to promote functional improvement and decrease decline in status. Important to assess nutritional status, and note any impairments in their instrumental activities of daily living (IADLs) and activities of daily living (ADLs). ADLs are basic activities of daily living that persons do to function during the day: eating, bathing, toileting, transferring (walking), and continence. IADLs are things that are not considered to be necessary for fundamental functioning but do allow an individual to live independently in the community. IADLs include preparing meals, housework, managing medications, and taking medications.

B. Sensory impairment

It is important to recognize normal changes in the aging eye versus an acute or progressive visual problem. In all adults, presbyopia develops as a result of the lens becoming less flexible and losing the ability to accommodate. Older adults have the inability to focus their eyes on objects that are near. Most all older adults will require reading glasses in their lifetime in order to see objects that are near. Common ocular disorders to identify and/or to be suspicious of and refer to an ophthalmologist are dry eyes (keratoconjunctivitis sicca), cataracts, glaucoma, retinopathy, and macular degeneration.

Some predisposing factors of hearing impairment cannot be changed like genetic predisposition, sex, and aging of the cochlea. Other factors can be modified like removal of cerumen impaction, reduction of exposure to noise and ototoxic medications. Clinicians must be able to differentiate the different types of hearing loss in older adults.

C. Falls

Often falls are not a result of one single action but rather a culmination of events leading up to the fall. Independent risk for factors for falling in the older adult population include balance impairment, previous falls, decreased muscle strength, visual impairment, more than four medications or the use of a psychoactive medication, gait impairment, depression, dizziness, functional limitations, age greater than 80 years, female, low body mass index, urinary incontinence, cognitive impairment, arthritis, diabetes, and pain (Tinetti & Kumar, 2010).

D. Urinary incontinence

Once the cause and type of urinary incontinence the older adult is suffering from are identified, steps can be made to treat and correct contributing factors. Management of urinary incontinence should focus on the individual's goals and issues that are most problematic to the older adult.

E. Delirium

The diagnosis of delirium is primarily clinical and based on careful observation of key features. Key clinical features include acute onset and fluctuating course, inattention, disorganized thinking, altered level of consciousness, disorientation, memory impairment, perceptual disturbances, increased or decreased psychomotor activity, and disturbance of the sleep wake cycle (Wong et al., 2010).

A useful mnemonic to help identify reversible causes of delirium is listed in **Table 57-2**.

TABLE 57-2 Delirium Mnemonic

D Drugs	Any changes to prescription regimen. Any new medications, adjustments in dosage, and interactions with other medications and foods.
E Electrolyte disturbances	Dehydration, thyroid abnormalities, sodium and potassium deficiencies
L Lack of drugs	Withdrawal from medications, poor pain control due to inefficient prescribing and treatment, withdrawal from alcohol or other drugs
I Infection	Urinary tract and respiratory are the most commonly seen
R Reduced sensory input	Poor vision and inability to hear as well as changes in smell, taste, and touch
I Intracranial	Stroke, hemorrhage, brain injury, infectious process of the brain
U Urinary	Urinary retention, incontinence, and infection. Also includes fecal incontinence and impaction.
M Myocardial	Myocardial infarction, CHF, arrhythmias

Data from Geriatric Review Syllabus. (2013).

IV. Goals of clinical management

A. Screening

1. Thorough screening to determine geriatric syndrome

2. It is important to choose screening and diagnostic tools that are cost effective and patient appropriate

B. Treatment

1. Select a safe and effective treatment plan based on diagnosis of geriatric syndrome as well as patient's goals of care.

C. Patient adherence

1. Select an approach that maximizes patient adherence and continue to monitor patient adherence throughout treatment.

V. Plan

A. Frailty

1. Diagnostic studies (See **Table 57-3**)

2. Treatment/patient and caregiver education
   a. Prevention is key.
   b. Causes of frailty should be treated in order to prevent the human and economic burden associated with this syndrome (Theou et al., 2010).
   c. Immobility is often a precursor to worsening frailty so making sure the older adult remains physically active is important. Maintaining muscle mass and strength through routine exercises including stretching and weight resistance have been shown to be beneficial (Theou et al., 2010)
   d. Counseling patients and caregivers on adequate nutrition and caloric intake is important. Depending on the case, supplemental protein might be used.
   e. Counseling patients, family members, and caregivers on availability of community support systems. For example, meals on wheels or other home delivery food options.

B. Sensory impairment

1. Diagnostic studies are sometimes needed in the assessment and treatment of sensory impairments. When pursuing diagnostic studies it is important to review goals of care and what will be done with results of studies obtained. Occasionally a CT scan/MRI of the brain might be used if there is concern for a stroke or head injury contributing to impairment.

2. Treatment/patient and caregiver education
   a. By identifying the visual condition affecting the older adult, steps can be taken to fix the problem or allow the patient to accommodate to new visual changes. For example, dry eyes tend to be a common complaint in older adults, especially women. The use of nonprescription artificial tears can help alleviate dry eyes.
   b. Encourage patients to have an annual eye exam.
   c. Provide education regarding a safe visual environment in the home, meaning making sure there is adequate lighting. Older adults lose the ability to see well in dim light.
   d. Treatments for common conditions like cataracts, age-related macular degeneration, glaucoma, and diabetic neuropathy vary on the diagnosis so recognizing the condition can then allow you to guide treatment.
   e. Depending on the cause of the hearing loss some conditions can be helped with medical and or surgical intervention.
   f. To better assess hearing, refer to an audiologist for formal audiometric testing and assistance with obtaining hearing aids and other devices that can amplify hearing such as a pocket talkers if appropriate. There are many devices such as amplified telephones, visual alarm systems, and vibrating alarm clocks available to help older adults who suffer with hearing loss adjust to their living environment.
   g. Adaptive techniques, such as, teaching family members to speak directly in front of the patient and using low tones have been shown to be beneficial. Older adults lose the ability to hear high pitched tones.

C. Falls

1. Diagnostic studies (see Table 57-3)

2. Treatment/patient and caregiver education
   a. Fall prevention strategies are important. Working with families and institutions if the person is residing in a facility should be done to promote an environment that is safe and reduces risk of falls.
   b. Need to individualize treatment plans for patients based on cause of falls.
   c. Treat any modifiable risk factors that can contribute to falls, for example, correcting visual impairment and ensuring the older adult has appropriate footwear.
   d. Medication reduction and physical therapy have been shown to be helpful in reducing further falls (Cameron et al., 2010).

TABLE 57-3 Geriatric Syndromes and Labs/Imaging

Labs/Imaging to Obtain	Geriatric Syndrome	Rationale
Complete blood count	Frailty Falls Urinary incontinence Delirium	Assess for anemia and/or elevated white count, which could indicate an infectious process contributing to these particular geriatric syndromes
Serum electrolyte	Frailty Falls Urinary incontinence Delirium	Assess for hypo/hyperkalemia, hypo/hypernatremia, dehydration, which can contribute to these particular geriatric syndromes
Renal panel	Frailty Falls Urinary incontinence Delirium	Assess kidney functioning to determine if kidney injury, failure, or disease is contributing to these particular geriatric syndromes
Thyroid panel	Frailty Delirium	Assess for hyper/hypothyroidism. Hyperthyroidism can contribute to weight loss and frailty. Uncontrolled hyper/hypothyroidism can lead to delirium.
Urinalysis, urine culture	Frailty Falls Urinary incontinence Delirium	If concern for infectious process that is treatable and contributes often to frailty, falls, increased urinary incontinence, and delirium. Especially helpful in patients with dementia who cannot express symptoms of infection.
Albumin, prealbumin	Frailty	Indicator of protein intake and overall nutritional state
Serum glucose	Falls Delirium	Assess for hypoglycemia, which can lead to falls and delirium in the older adult
Vitamin B$_{12}$	Falls Delirium	Low levels are associated with proprioceptive problems contributing to falls and increased confusion resulting in delirium
Vitamin D	Falls	High risk for fractures from fall if level is low
Electrocardiogram	Falls Delirium	Evaluate for abnormal rhythm or cardiac pathology contributing to syncope resulting in a fall or delirium
Computerized tomography (CT) scan/ magnetic resonance imaging (MRI) brain	Sensory impairment Falls Delirium	If concern for stroke, bleed, or injury to the head, which can contribute to sensory impairment, falls, and/or delirium
Ultrasound of bladder	Urinary incontinence	To assess volume of urine inside the bladder. A postvoid residual is often done in the hospital setting to examine for urinary retention. This test is rarely needed in the ambulatory setting.
Renal ultrasound	Urinary incontinence	Evaluate for kidney disease and problems with the urinary tract
CT abdomen/pelvis	Urinary incontinence	Evaluate for obstructions, tumors, cysts
Arterial blood gas	Delirium	If concern for hypoxia, poor perfusion contributing to delirium
Toxicology	Falls Delirium	Assess for presence of illegal substances contributing to falls and delirium
Electroencephalogram	Sensory impairment Falls Delirium	If concern for seizure activity contributing to sensory impairment, falls, and/or delirium

e. Clinicians should work along with physical therapist colleagues to establish an exercise program for older adults.

f. Manage postural hypotension by titrating medications, optimizing fluid intake, and teaching behavioral strategies to reduce incidents.

g. Provide vitamin D supplement when appropriate to reduce risk of fractures from falls.

D. Urinary incontinence

1. Diagnostic studies (see Table 57-3)

2. Treatment/patient and caregiver education

   a. Initiate behavioral targeted therapies as well as medications or at times surgical intervention when appropriate based on type of urinary incontinence. Make referral to urology and/or urogynecology.

   b. It is also important to recognize medications that contribute to worsening of urinary incontinence and remove those from the patient if this can be done safely. Common medications include alpha-blockers, antipsychotics, loop diuretics, narcotics, and tricyclic antidepressants.

   c. Treat comorbid conditions contributing to urinary incontinence such as diabetes mellitus and dementia.

   d. Behavioral modifications include timed voiding, for example, having the patient empty the bladder every 2 hours, and pelvic muscle training, which are Kegel exercises to strengthen the pelvic floor and surrounding muscles.

   e. Medications can be used to treat some types of urinary incontinence. Anticholinergic drugs are the most commonly prescribed medications for incontinence and it is important to recognize the side effects of these medications in older adults, which can be quite problematic. Some of these side effects include confusion, constipation, dry eyes and mouth, and falls. Other agents often prescribed are antimuscarinics such as oxybutynin, tolterodine, trospium, and fesoterodine. Alpha-blockers and tricyclic antidepressants have also been used.

   f. Devices such as pessaries can be trialed in women who suffer from organ prolapse resulting in overflow incontinence. It is important to recognize pessaries do require some care from the individual so often they are not appropriate for older adults with cognitive impairment

   g. Several different surgical interventions can also be used if patient is deemed a surgical candidate. Appropriate referrals are needed to specialists. Please refer to Chapter 25, Urinary Incontinence in Women, for more detailed treatment regimens.

E. Delirium

1. Diagnostic studies (see Table 57-3)

2. Treatment/patient and caregiver education

   a. After accurate diagnosis of delirium, steps can be made to reduce complications and provide treatment.

   b. Important to identify and treat any reversible conditions contributing to delirium.

   c. Attempt to prevent further complications and decline by reducing medications where appropriate.

   d. Nonpharmacologic strategies include correcting any sensory impairment (see the section on sensory impairment for details), avoiding physical restraints including foley catheters that keep patients from being mobile, sleep hygiene, reorientation, and environment optimization.

   e. Pharmacologic strategies are useful for severe cases of delirium where the person's safety and well-being are at risk. Pharmacologic treatment strategies include the use of an antipsychotic such as Haldol, atypical antipsychotics such as risperidone, olanzapine, or quetiapine, a benzodiazepine such as lorazepam, and/or an antidepressant such as trazodone (Inouye, 2006). The same geriatric principles apply when prescribing these medications: starting low and going slow, meaning start with a low dose and titrate up slowly if needed.

   f. It is important to weigh goals of care for the individual being treated with invasiveness of procedure and tests.

VI. Online resources for clinicians, patients, and caregivers

A. *AARP (www.aarp.org)*

B. *Alzheimer's Association (www.alz.org)*

C. *American Geriatrics Society (www.americangeriatrics.org)*

D. *American Geriatrics Society Beers Criteria (http://geriatricscareonline.org/ProductAbstract /american-geriatrics-society-updated-beers -criteria-for-potentially-inappropriate-medication -use-in-older-adults/CL001)*

E. *Family Caregiver Alliance (www.caregiver.org)*

F. *Gerontological Advanced Practice Nurses Association (https://www.gapna.org)*

G. *John A. Hartford Foundation (www.jhartfound.org)*

H. *The Hartford Institute for Geriatric Nursing, College of Nursing, New York University (http:// consultgerirn.or/ or www.hartfordign.org)*

　1. The Hartford Institute Assessment Tools Try This (www.hartfordign.org/practice/try_this)

I. *The Hospital Elder Life Program (www. hospitalelderlifeprogram.org/about)*

J. *Medicare (www.medicare.gov)*

K. *National Institute on Aging (http://nia.nih.gov)*

L. *U.S. Preventive Services Task Force: Falls Prevention in Older Adults: Counseling and Preventive Medication (www .uspreventiveservicestaskforce.org/Page/Topic /recommendation-summary/falls-prevention -in-older-adults-counseling-and-preventive -medication)*

REFERENCES

Cameron, I. D., Murray, G. R., Gillespie, L. D., Robertson, M. C., Hill, K. D., Cumming, R. G., et al. (2010). Interventions for preventive falls in older people in nursing care facilities and hospitals. *Cochrane Database of Systematic Reviews, 1*.

Chou, R., Dana, T., Bougatsos, C., Fleming, C., & Beil, T. (2011). Screening adults aged 50 years or older for hearing loss: A review of the evidence for the U.S. Preventive Services Task Force. *Annals of Internal Medicine, 154*(5), 347–355.

Delbaere, K., Crombez, G., Vanderstraeten, G., Willems, T., & Cambier, D. (2004). Fear-related avoidance of activities, falls, and physical frailty. A prospective community-based cohort study. *Age and Ageing, 33*(4), 368–373.

Du Moulin, M. F., Hamers, J. P., Ambergen, A. W., Janssen, M. A., & Halfens, R. J. Prevalence of urinary incontinence among community-dwelling adults receiving home care. *Research in Nursing & Health, 31*(6), 604–612.

Durso, S., & Sullivan, G. (Eds.). (2013). *Geriatrics review syllabus: A core curriculum in geriatric medicine* (8th ed.). New York: American Geriatrics Society.

Goode, P. S., Burgio, K. L., Richter, H. E., & Markland, A. D. (2010). Incontinence in older women. *JAMA, 303*(21), 2172–2181.

Inouye, S. K. (2006). Delirium in older persons. *New England Journal of Medicine, 354*(11), 1157–1165.

Inouye, S., van Dyck, C., Alessi, C., Balkin, S., Siegal, A., & Horwitz, R. (1990). Clarifying confusion: The confusion assessment method. *Annals of Internal Medicine, 113*(12), 941–948.

Theou, O., Stathokostas, L., Roland, K. P., Jakobi, J. M., Patterson, C., Vandervoort, A. A., et al. (2011, April 4). The effectiveness of exercise interventions for the management of frailty: A systemic review. *Journal of Aging Research*, 1–19.

Tinetti, M. E., & Kumar, C. (2010). The patient who falls. "It's always a trade-off." *JAMA, 303*(3), 258–266.

Williams, B., Chang, A., Ahalt, C., Chen, H., Conant, R., Landefeld, S., et al. (Eds.). (2014). *Current diagnosis & treatment: geriatrics* (2nd ed.). New York: McGraw-Hill Education.

Witlox, J., Eurelings, L. S., de Jonghe, J. F. M., Kalisvaart, K. J., Eikelenboom, P., & van Gool, W. A. (2010). Delirium in elderly patients and the risk of postdischarge mortality, institutionalization, and dementia: A meta-analysis. *JAMA, 304*(4), 443–451.

Wong, C. L., Holroyd-Leduc, J., Simel, D. L., & Straus, S. E. (2010). Does this patient have delirium? Value of bedside instruments. *JAMA, 304*(7), 779–786.

HEART FAILURE

CHAPTER 58

Lisa Guertin and Barbara Boland

I. Introduction and general background

Heart failure is a common condition seen in the primary care setting. It is a clinical syndrome that can occur suddenly or over time and arises from cardiac derangements within the pericardium, myocardium, or endocardium, and/or structural abnormalities of the vessels or valves.

A. Definition and overview

Heart failure as defined by the American College of Cardiology and American Heart Association is a complex clinical syndrome that results from any structural or functional impairment of ventricular filling or ejection of the blood (Yancy et al., 2013). Heart failure is a clinical diagnosis based on the presentation of symptoms, which typically include dyspnea, fatigue, fluid retention, and exercise intolerance.

Heart failure can involve the left ventricle, right ventricle, or both ventricles. Left ventricular heart failure occurs when the left ventricle is unable to pump sufficiently to meet the body's demands. The myocardial muscle may be too weak and thin to eject the blood from the ventricle or the myocardial muscle may be too thick and stiff causing inadequate ventricular filling. Both forms of heart failure cause elevated left ventricular filling pressures.

The symptoms of left ventricular failure predominantly include dyspnea and fatigue. Dyspnea arises from pulmonary edema. Pulmonary edema occurs from the ineffective ejection of blood from the left ventricle, causing elevated left atrial pressures resulting in fluid back up in the lungs. Subsequently, the persistent increased pulmonary volume and pressure can begin to affect the right ventricle. Fatigue arises from the inability of the ventricles to eject enough blood to meet the needs of the body, causing decreased forward flow and ultimately decreased cardiac output. However, the symptom of fatigue occurs in both left and right ventricular failure. Signs of right ventricular failure, which include peripheral edema, ascites, and hepatic and splenic congestion, predominantly arise from systemic venous fluid congestion.

Two major clinical subsets of heart failure are systolic and diastolic. Systolic heart failure, often called heart failure with reduced ejection fraction or HFrEF, occurs when the heart loses its ability to contract normally. As systolic heart failure progresses the ventricle may become dilated. Reduced contractile function causes increased end systolic and end diastolic volumes, dilating the ventricle. This condition is called dilated cardiomyopathy (DCM). DCM is largely categorized into two etiologies: ischemic or nonischemic. Ischemic disease is the predominant cause of left ventricular systolic failure in the United States. There are multiple causes of nonischemic cardiomyopathy including but not limited to familial, alcohol induced, cardiotoxicity due to medications, infectious diseases, inflammatory diseases, rheumatologic disorders, thyroid disease, some muscular dystrophies, longstanding poorly controlled hypertension, and valvular heart disease.

Diastolic heart failure is abnormal filling of the left or right ventricle caused by impaired myocardial relaxation or stiffness of the heart muscle. Common causes of diastolic heart failure are chronic hypertension with left ventricular hypertrophy as well as restrictive, infiltrative, and hypertrophic cardiomyopathies. Fifty percent of patients with heart failure have a preserved ejection fraction (EF) (Yancy et al., 2013). Heart failure with preserved EF is now commonly referred to as HFpEF.

The New York Heart Association (NYHA) and American College of Cardiology Foundation/American Heart Association (ACCF/AHA) have complimentary classifications and staging for defining the functional status and severity of heart failure. NYHA classifications are (Criteria Committee of the American Heart Association, 1994):

1. Class I: no symptoms with or limitations in ordinary activities

2. Class II: slight, mild limitation of activity; the patient is comfortable at rest or with mild exertion

3. Class III: marked limitation of any activity; the patient is comfortable only at rest

4. Class IV: severe limitations; any physical activity causes discomfort and symptoms occur at rest

The ACCF/AHA staging of heart failure are (Yancy et al., 2013):

1. Stage A: Patients at high risk for developing heart failure but without structural heart disease or symptoms of heart failure.

2. Stage B: Structural heart disease but without signs or symptoms of heart failure.

3. Stage C: Structural heart disease with prior or current symptoms of heart failure.

4. Stage D: Refractory heart failure requiring specialized interventions.

B. Prevalence and incidence

The American Heart Association estimates 5.7 million Americans over the age of 20 have heart failure, occurring more frequently in men and in those over the age of 60 (Mozaffarian et al., 2015). The prevalence is expected to increase 46% by the year 2030, with 870,000 new cases diagnosed every year (Mozaffarian et al., 2015).

Multiple risk factors contribute to heart failure including but not limited to coronary disease, obesity, insulin resistance, inflammation and elevated inflammatory markers, men with hypertension, and cigarette exposure (Go et al., 2014). It is important to note 75% of heart failure cases have an antecedent of hypertension (Go et al., 2014). Although survival after a heart failure diagnosis has improved, mortality remains at 50% within 5 years of diagnosis (Go et al., 2014). According to the AHA and Centers for Disease Control and Prevention (CDC), the estimated annual cost of heart failure to the nation is between $30 billion and $32 billion (Mozaffarian et al., 2015; National Center for Chronic Disease Prevention and Health Promotion, 2013).

II. **Database** (may include but is not limited to)

A. Subjective

1. Past health history

   a. Medical history: hypertension, coronary artery disease (myocardial infarction [MI]), arrhythmia, valvular heart disease including aortic or pulmonic stenosis, mitral or tricuspid stenosis, or mitral or aortic regurgitation, congenital heart disease, obesity, peripheral vascular disease, diabetes, obstructive sleep apnea, hyperlipidemia, anemia, thyroid disease, peripartum myopathy, other hormonal disorders, systemic lupus erythematosus, scleroderma, sarcoidosis, amyloidosis, infectious diseases including HIV, Chagas disease, viral endocarditis and myocarditis, and malignancies requiring medications such as anthracycline, trastuzumab (Herceptin), high-dose cyclophosphamide, toxoids, mitomycin-C, 5-fluorouracil, and the interferons or other nonchemo cardiotoxic medications (Yancy et al., 2013).

   b. Surgical history: Cardiac surgeries, including valve replacements, myectomy, coronary artery bypass. Endovascular procedures such as stent placement, ethanol, or radiofrequency ablation.

   c. Medication history: Some categories of medications used in heart failure may have an adverse effect. For example, calcium channel blockers (harmful) and beta-blockers are negative inotropes. However, beta-blockers should not be excluded from the treatment regimen, as they remain part of the primary treatment for systolic heart failure. Antiarrhythmic medications and inotropes may be proarrhythmic. Thiazolidinediones and nonsteroidal anti-inflammatories can cause fluid retention. Other cardiotoxic medications are previously mentioned.

2. Family history: Atherosclerosis, MI, cerebrovascular accident (CVA), peripheral arterial disease, sudden cardiac death, arrhythmias, conduction disease (often requiring pacemakers or internal cardioverter defibrillators [ICDs]), heart failure, or cardiomyopathy

3. Occupational and educational history

   a. Exposures to chemicals or toxins

   b. Level of education

   c. Ability to work; days missed from work or school

4. Personal and social history

   a. Alcohol, cocaine, methamphetamine, and intravenous drug use

   b. Diet: Adherence to a heart-healthy and low-sodium diet.

   c. Exercise: Assess the distance able to ambulate without stopping due to fatigue or shortness of breath, the ability to climb stairs, and participation in routine exercise or sedentary lifestyle.

   d. Activities of daily living: Ability to perform routine tasks without fatigue or shortness of breath

   e. Culture and cultural practices

   f. Living situation

5. Review of symptoms

   a. Constitutional signs and symptoms: Recent hospitalizations, fever, chills, rigors, fatigue, weight gain or loss. Weight loss is concerning as it is a poor prognostic indicator of heart failure.

b. Respiratory: Dyspnea with or without exertion, shortness of breath, orthopnea, paroxysmal nocturnal dyspnea, and cough.

c. Cardiac: Chest pain, palpitations, edema, syncope, and presyncope.

d. Gastrointestinal: Anorexia, nausea, increasing abdominal girth, and abdominal discomfort.

e. Genitourinary: Sexual dysfunction, sexually transmitted disease exposure, and urination patterns.

f. Endocrine: Heat or cold intolerance

g. Neurologic: Lightheadedness, dizziness, frequent naps or inability to stay awake, decreased concentration, memory loss, and signs of transient ischemic attack (TIA) or CVA.

h. Psychiatric: Anxiety and/or depression.

B. Objective

1. Physical examination findings

   a. Height, weight, body mass index, body habitus, and general appearance

   b. Vital signs: orthostatic blood pressures

   c. Pulse: Assess strength and regularity throughout. Assess the character of the carotid upstroke

   d. Skin: Pallor, cyanosis, cool temperature

   e. Thyroid/neck: Goiter and/or bruits

   f. Lungs: Tachypnea, rales, wheezing, ability to speak full sentences

   g. Cardiac: Arrhythmia, elevated jugular venous pressure, additional heart sounds such as S3 gallop, S4, or murmur, laterally displaced point of maximum intensity (PMI), heaves, lifts, thrills, and edema (abdominal, peripheral, or sacral)

   h. Abdomen: Increased abdominal girth, abdominal tenderness, hepatomegaly and hepatojugular reflux lasting longer than 10 seconds with sustained abdominal pressure.

III. Assessment

A. Determine the diagnosis

Heart failure is a clinical diagnosis that is largely based on findings from the history and physical examination. Diagnostic testing is important and useful in confirming the diagnosis, the underlying etiology, and the severity of the disease.

1. Differential diagnosis

   a. Chronic obstructive pulmonary disease

   b. Asthma

   c. Pulmonary embolism

   d. Interstitial lung disease

   e. Pneumonia

   f. Sleep apnea

   g. Pulmonary artery hypertension

   h. Myocardial ischemia

   i. Valvular heart disease

   j. Atrial fibrillation or other arrhythmia

   k. Anemia or other blood dyscrasias

   l. Venous insufficiency or thrombosis

   m. Cirrhosis

   n. Gastrointestinal disorders

   o. Renal disease or failure

   p. Endocrine disorders such as thyroid disease

   q. Deconditioning

   r. Depression

   s. Obesity

   t. Adverse effects from medications

B. Severity

1. Assess the severity of the disease based on the NYHA classifications and/or ACCF/AHA heart failure staging.

C. Motivation and ability

1. Determine the patient's willingness and ability to adhere to a treatment plan.

IV. Goals of clinical management

A. Select and implement a treatment plan that appropriately manages heart failure in a beneficial and cost-effective manner.

B. Implement an appropriate treatment plan that enables patients' adherence.

C. Relieve symptoms.

D. Prevent/decrease admissions to an acute care facility.

E. Improve survival.

V. Plan

A. Diagnostic tests

1. Noninvasive testing

   a. General laboratory studies: Complete blood count (CBC), metabolic panel, calcium, magnesium, blood urea nitrogen, serum creatinine, liver function tests, fasting glucose, urinalysis, lipid panel, and thyroid-stimulating hormone.

b. Cardiac-specific laboratory studies: Natriuretic peptide: B-type natriuretic peptide (BNP) and N-terminal pro-B-type natriuretic peptide (NT pro-BNP) can be useful in patients with dyspnea and to assess severity of the disease (Yancy et al., 2013). It is important to consult the laboratory preforming the test to obtain their normal range of laboratory values. Additionally, there are multiple factors that may cause and elevated BNP and NT pro-BNP.

c. Electrocardiogram: Left ventricular hypertrophy, evidence of prior MI, arrhythmia, conduction problems, and axis deviation.

d. Chest radiograph: Cardiomegaly, pulmonary congestion.

e. Echocardiogram: Ventricular size, function, wall motion, atrial size, valvular function, and hemodynamic values.

f. Cardiovascular magnetic resonance may be appropriate for the initial evaluation of heart failure and may be helpful in assessing myocardial perfusion, viability, and fibrosis imaging (Patel et al., 2013).

2. Invasive testing

a. Hemodynamic monitoring with pulmonary artery catheter to guide treatment in patients who have respiratory distress and clinical evidence of impaired perfusion and intracardiac filling pressures cannot be determined from the clinical assessment (Yancy et al., 2013).

b. Coronary angiogram is recommended if the etiology of heart failure is concerning for ischemic heart disease and the patient is a candidate for revascularization (Patel et al., 2013).

c. Right heart catheterization may be useful in determining volume status, hemodynamic values, and intracardiac filling pressures to assess specific therapeutic questions (Yancy et al., 2013).

d. Endomyocardial biopsy (EMB) may be useful in diagnosis and management of acute onset unexplained cardiomyopathy that does not respond to the usual standard of practice. Furthermore, EMB plays a role in suspected infiltrative disease that presents either as unexplained hypertrophic cardiomyopathy or as restrictive disease (Bennett et al., 2013).

B. Management (includes treatment, consultation, referral, and follow-up care)

1. Acute heart failure: Immediate intervention of oxygen; arrange hospital admission. Depending on the severity, emergency response may be required and therefore admitted via the emergency department.

The patient may require ventilator support, intravenous diuretics, ultrafiltration, intravenous inotropes, vasopressors, vasodilators, or mechanical support (National Clinical Guideline Centre, 2014).

2. Chronic heart failure

a. Treatment is often performed in a progressive stepwise approach. A referral to cardiology should be initiated upon diagnosis (see **Figure 58-1**).

b. The focus of stage A heart failure management is on risk modification including hypertension control, diabetes control and lipid management to control atherosclerosis and obesity.

c. Stage B heart failure management includes stage A management plus intervention of structural heart disease. Special considerations should be given to patients with stage B heart failure patients with a history of MI and/or revascularization and structural heart disease.

d. The development of symptoms classifies patients as stage C. Stage C heart failure management is multifaceted and aims at reducing morbidity and mortality by self-care and pharmacologic strategies. ICD implantation may be appropriate for this group of patients for either primary or secondary prevention. Additionally, cardiac resynchronization therapy (CRT) may be indicated for a subset of patients.

e. Stage D heart failure patients are considered refractory and the disease progresses despite implementation of goal-directed therapy (strategies in stages A, B, and C). These patients may require intravenous inotropic support or other advanced therapies such as mechanical circulatory support or heart transplantation.

f. Lifestyle modification

   i. Smoking cessation

   ii. Alcohol cessation or restriction

   iii. Illicit drug use cessation

   iv. Exercise: Regular exercise 20–30 minutes three to five times per week. Referral to cardiac rehabilitation. Lack of improvement after a training program portends a poor prognosis (Tang & Francis, 2010).

   v. Diet: Sodium restriction in patients who are symptomatic. Less than 3 g/daily should be effective in symptom relief; 1.5 g/daily to aid in hypertension control in patients with stage A and B heart failure (Yancy et al., 2013).

   vi. Free water: Restrict daily intake to 1.5–2 L in patients with stage D heart failure and hyponatremia (Yancy et al., 2013).

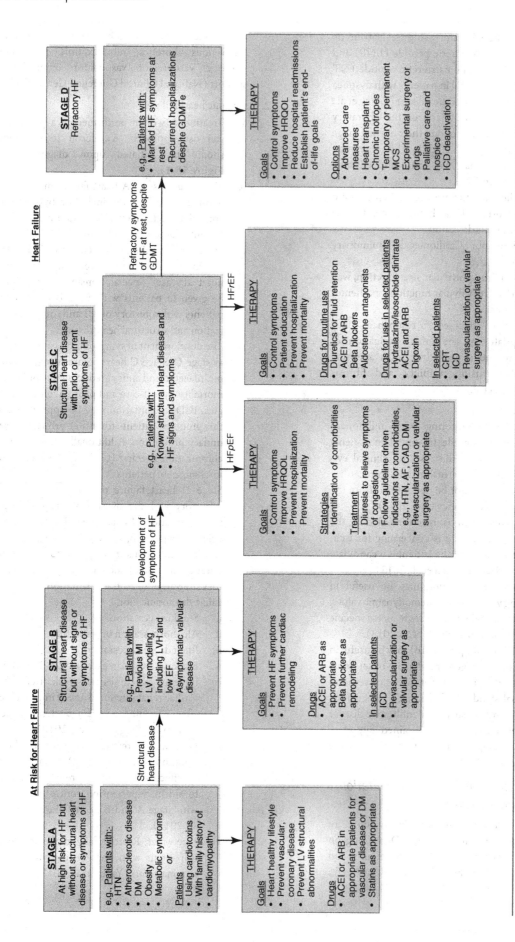

FIGURE 58-1 Heart Failure Risk

ACEI = angiotensin-converting enzyme inhibitor, CAD = coronary artery disease, DM = diabetes mellitus, GDMT = guideline-determined medical therapy. HRQOL= health-related quality of life, HTN = hypertension, MCS = mechanical circulatory support.

Reproduced from Yancy, C. W., Jessup, M., Bozkurt, B., Butler, J., Casey, D. E., Jr., Drazner, M. H., et al. (2013). 2013 ACCF/AHA guideline for the management of heart failure: A report of the American College of Cardiology Foundation/American Heart Association task force on practice guidelines. *Journal of the American College of Cardiology, 62*(16), e147–e239.

g. Weight and blood pressure monitoring: Document weight and blood pressure daily, at the same time every day; monitor trends. Provide parameters that indicate when the patient should contact the provider regarding weight gain, evidence of volume overload, and blood pressure.

h. Healthcare maintenance
  i. Annual flu vaccine
  ii. Pneumococcal vaccine
  iii. Medic alert information
  iv. Dental care

i. Treatment of other illnesses/conditions that may be causative or contributory to heart failure
  i. Diabetes (see Chapter 54, Diabetes Mellitus)
  ii. Hypertension (see Chapter 60, Hypertension)
  iii. Obesity (see Chapter 66, Obesity)
  iv. Sleep apnea
  v. Thyroid disorders (see Chapter 69, Thyroid Disorders)
  vi. Infection
  vii. Inflammation or inflammatory processes

j. Pharmacologic therapy for heart failure (systolic or diastolic), volume retention, heart rhythm and rate control, and hypertension. Start at a low dose and titrate up as patient tolerates until the maximum safe dosage allowable. See **Box 58-1** for medication approaches for systolic heart failure with low EF. Management for diastolic heart failure predominantly consists of controlling

---

BOX 58-1 *Medication Management for Systolic Heart Failure with Low Ejection Fraction (EF)*

1. Angiotensin-converting enzyme inhibitor (ACE-I) (see **Table 58-1**)
   a. Provides left ventricular remodeling and survival benefit. ACE-I can be replaced with an aldosterone receptor blocker (ARB) if unable to tolerate ACE-I, typically due to a dry, irritating cough. Monitor electrolytes and renal function closely after initiation of treatment and dosage adjustments.

2. Hydralazine in conjunction with a nitrate (see Table 58-1)
   a. Can be utilized if the patient is unable to tolerate both ACE and ARB; it can also be used as adjunctive therapy in NYHA class III–IV heart failure.

3. Beta-blockers (see Table 58-1)
   a. Can provide improvement in EF as well as anti-ischemic properties and reduce mortality.

4. Diuretic therapy (see **Table 58-2**)
   a. Indicated for patients to control volume retention.
   b. Monitor electrolytes and renal function closely after initiation of treatment and dosage adjustments.

5. Aldosterone antagonists (see Table 58-1 and 58-2)
   a. Recommended for patients with persistent symptoms with NYHA class II–IV heart failure and EF < 35%.
   b. Monitor electrolytes and renal function closely after initiation of treatment and dosage adjustments.

6. Digoxin
   a. Remains controversial in the patient population with systolic heart failure.
   b. Digoxin can be used in patients as adjunctive therapy if they remain symptomatic despite guideline directed management.
   c. Digoxin should be avoided in patients with sinus node or atrioventricular node conduction disease (Yancy et al., 2013).
   d. Monitor digoxin levels to ensure they remain in a therapeutic range and do not become toxic.

7. Amiodarone and dofetilide
   a. The only recommended antiarrhythmic medications to have neutral effects on mortality on patients with heart failure (Yancy et al., 2013).
   b. Prior to starting and after initiation of amiodarone, monitor thyroid-stimulating hormone.
   c. Monitor for signs of amiodarone induced pulmonary fibrosis, liver dysfunction, and thyroid toxicity.

8. Antithrombotics
   a. Use is based upon the CHA2DS2-VACs score for arrhythmia and dilated cardiomyopathy due to an increased risk of left ventricular thrombus (Yancy et al., 2013).
   b. Choose an appropriate, approved, and individualized antithrombotic agent for the patient.

(continues)

> **BOX 58-1 Medication Management for Systolic Heart Failure with Low Ejection Fraction (EF)** *(Continued)*
>
> 9. Harmful in NYHA class II–IV heart failure
>   a. Thiazolidinediones
>   b. Calcium channel blockers (CCB): The nondihydropyridine calcium channel blockers have negative inotropic properties and are considered harmful in patients with a low ejection fraction and therefore are not recommended. Amlodipine is the only CCB that may be considered in the management of hypertension or ischemic heart disease in patients with heart failure as it has neutral effects on morbidity and mortality (Yancy et al., 2013).
>   c. Nonsteroidal anti-inflammatory drugs (NSAIDs) and COX-2 inhibitors

TABLE 58-1 ACE Inhibitors

Drug	Initial Dose
ACE Inhibitors	
Captopril	6.25 mg three times daily
Enalapril	2.5 mg twice daily
Fosinopril	5–10 mg daily
Lisinopril	2.5–5 mg daily
Perindopril	2 mg daily
Quinapril	5 mg twice daily
Ramipril	1.25–2.5 mg daily
Trandolapril	1 mg daily
Angiotensin Receptor Blockers	
Candesartan	4–8 mg daily
Losartan	25–50 mg daily
Valsartan	20–40 mg twice daily
Aldosterone antagonists	
Spironolactone	12.5–25 mg daily
Eplerenone	25 mg daily
Beta-blockers	
Bisoprolol	1.25 mg daily
Carvedilol	3.125 mg twice daily
Carvedilol CR	10 mg daily
Metoprolol succinate extended-release	12.5–25 mg daily
Hydralazine and isosorbide dinitrate	
Fixed-dose combination	37.5 mg hydralazine/20 mg isosorbide dinitrate three times daily
Hydralazine and isosorbide dinitrate	Hydralazine 25–50 mg, three or four times daily and isosorbide dinitrate 20–30 mg three or four times daily

Adapted from Yancy, C. W., Jessup, M., Bozkurt, B., Butler, J., Casey, D. E., Jr., Drazner, M. H., et al. (2013). 2013 ACCF/AHA guideline for the management of heart failure: A report of the American College of Cardiology Foundation/American Heart Association task force on practice guidelines. *Journal of the American College of Cardiology, 62*(16), e147–e239.

TABLE 58-2 Loop Diuretics

Drug	Initial Dose
Loop diuretics	
Bumetanide	0.5–1 mg once or twice daily
Furosemide	20–40 mg once or twice daily
Torsemide	10–20 mg daily
Thiazide diuretics	
Chlorothiazide	250–500 mg once or twice daily
Chlorthalidone	12.5–25 mg daily
Hydrochlorothiazide	25 mg once or twice daily
Indapamide	2.5 mg daily
Metolazone	2.5 mg daily
Aldosterone antagonists (potassium-sparing diuretics)	
Amiloride	5 mg daily
Spironolactone	12.5–25 mg daily
Triamterene	50–75 mg twice daily
Sequential nephron blockade	
Metolazone	2.5–10 mg daily + loop diuretic
Hydrochlorothiazide	25–100 mg once or twice daily + loop diuretic
Chlorothiazide (IV)	500–1,000 mg daily + loop diuretic

Adapted from Yancy, C. W., Jessup, M., Bozkurt, B., Butler, J., Casey, D. E., Jr., Drazner, M. H., et al. (2013). 2013 ACCF/AHA guideline for the management of heart failure: A report of the American College of Cardiology Foundation/American Heart Association task force on practice guidelines. *Journal of the American College of Cardiology, 62*(16), e147–e239.

hypertension (see Chapter 60, Hypertension, for the related guidelines) and myocardial ischemia as well as symptom management with the judicious use of diuretics.

k. ICD device therapy is recommended as primary prevention for patients with DCM or ischemic heart disease; with an EF < 35% and NYHA class II or higher heart failure or with an EF < 30% and NYHA class I heart failure; or who are on guideline-directed therapy and are at risk of sudden cardiac death (McMurray et al., 2012). CRT is recommended for patients with EF < 35% after 3 months of optimal medical therapy, in sinus rhythm with a QRS duration of 150 ms or greater, or with left bundle branch (LBBB) morphology (Yancy et al., 2013).

l. End-of-life and palliative care
   i. Consider for patients who have advanced persistent symptoms at rest despite pharmacologic therapy
   ii. Recurrent heart failure hospitalizations
   iii. Poor quality of life, including little or no ability to conduct activities of daily living
   iv. Need for continuous intravenous inotropic support
   v. Further advanced heart failure therapy is not clinically indicated or is unwanted
   vi. Consider hospice referral
   vii. Advanced directives and durable power of attorney should be in place

m. Appropriate follow-up for interventions implemented or anticipated implementation.

n. Collaborate with prescribing providers regarding the ongoing treatment plan as well as elimination of the medications or treatments that cause or exacerbate heart failure.

C. Client education and support

1. The patient must be able to adhere to the treatment plan and have adequate resources to comply effectively with the regimen. Instituting the plan may take time. The patient and patient's support must have an understanding of the treatment regimen, disease progression and potential complications, which will require ongoing education. Anticipate barriers to the treatment plan as this may prevent future complications.

2. It is also important to provide both verbal and written information to the patient and his or her support system. This information should include but is not limited to heart failure education, symptoms, prognosis, complications, and disease management. The patient should be referred to social services in order to ensure that a full spectrum of resources is available. Social services are useful in providing emotional support for both the patient and support system to improve coping skills and provide any additional financial resources.

VI. Self-management resources and tools

A. Patient education

1. American Heart Association (www.heart.org /HEARTORG/Conditions/HeartFailure/Heart -Failure_UCM_002019_SubHomePage.jsp). The American Heart Association has print and online education materials and online videos. Websites are available in Spanish, Chinese, Vietnamese, and English.

2. Centers for Disease Control and Prevention (www. cdc.gov/heartdisease/materials_for_patients.htm).

3. Medline Plus from the National Library of Medicine and National Institutes of Health (www.nlm.nih.gov /medlineplus/heartfailure.html). Provides an interactive tutorial in English and Spanish and extensive resources for aspects of the disease.

4. Heart Failure Matters (www.heartfailurematters .org/en_GB). This is an interactive, multilingual, educational website containing animations, videos, and tools for patients with heart failure. It is available in English, French, German, and Spanish. It has a family and caregiver section and links to a variety of other related websites.

5. HeartFailure.org (www.heartfailure.org/). Provides online education as well as additional links to other resources.

6. MegaHeart.com (http://megaheart.com/). Provides recipes and dietary support and recommendations.

B. Community support groups

1. The American Heart Association offers a variety of community events and support groups for individuals with heart disease.

2. Mended Hearts (www.mendedhearts.org/) is an organization for individuals with heart disease. Patients must pay to join. They have group meetings, hospital visiting programs, an annual convention, educational resources, and various events. Patients can join a local chapter.

REFERENCES

Bennett, M. K., Gilotra, N. A., Harrington, C., Rao, S., Dunn, J. M., Freitag, T. B., et al. (2013). Evaluation of the role of endomyocardial biopsy in 851 patients with unexplained heart failure from 2000-2009. *Circulation. Heart Failure, 6*(4), 676–684.

Criteria Committee of the American Heart Association. (1994). *Nomenclature and criteria for diagnosis of diseases of the heart and great vessels* (9th ed.). Boston, MA: Little Brown.

Go, A. S., Mozaffarian, D., Roger, V. L., Benjamin, E. J., Berry, J. D., Blaha, M. J., et al. (2014). Heart disease and stroke statistics—2014 update: A report from the American Heart Association. *Circulation, 129*(3), e28–e292.

McMurray, J. J., Adamopoulos, S., Anker, S. D., Auricchio, A., Bohm, M., Dickstein, K., et al. (2012). ESC guidelines for the diagnosis and treatment of acute and chronic heart failure 2012: The task force for the diagnosis and treatment of acute and chronic heart failure 2012 of the European Society of Cardiology. Developed in collaboration with the Heart Failure Association (HFA) of the ESC. *European Heart Journal, 33*(14), 1787–1847.

Mozaffarian, D., Benjamin, E. J., Go, A. S., Arnett, D. K., Blaha, M. J., Cushman, M., et al. (2015). Heart disease and stroke statistics—2015 update: A report from the American Heart Association. *Circulation, 131*(4), e29–e322.

National Center for Chronic Disease Prevention and Health Promotion, Division for Heart Disease and Stroke Prevention. (2013). *Heart failure fact sheet.* Retrieved from www.cdc.gov/DHDSP/data_statistics/fact _sheets/fs_heart_failure.htm

National Clinical Guideline Centre (UK). (2014). Acute heat failure: diagnosis and management. Retrieved at http://www.nice.org.uk /guidance/cg187

Patel, M. R., White, R. D., Abbara, S., Bluemke, D. A., Herfkens, R. J., Picard, M., et al. (2013). 2013 ACCF/ACR/ASE/ASNC/SCCT/ SCMR appropriate utilization of cardiovascular imaging in heart failure: A joint report of the American College of Radiology appropriateness criteria committee and the American College of Cardiology Foundation appropriate use criteria task force. *Journal of the American College of Cardiology, 61*(21), 2207–2231.

Tang, W. H. W., & Francis, G. S. (2010). The year in heart failure. *Journal of the American College of Cardiology, 55*(7), 688.

Yancy, C. W., Jessup, M., Bozkurt, B., Butler, J., Casey, D. E., Jr., Drazner, M. H., et al. (2013). 2013 ACCF/AHA guideline for the management of heart failure: A report of the American College of Cardiology Foundation/American Heart Association task force on practice guidelines. *Journal of the American College of Cardiology, 62*(16), e147–e239.

HERPES SIMPLEX INFECTIONS

Hattie C. Grundland and Geraldine Collins-Bride

I. Introduction and general background

Herpes simplex is a DNA virus belonging to the herpes virus group. The virus causes a recurring vesicular eruption to the skin or mucus membrane surfaces that have a prior contact exposure. Similar to other herpes viruses, after initial infection, a latent state is established that can be followed by reactivation of the virus and recurrent local disease. Herpes simplex virus (HSV) infection is lifelong. The course of disease, however, varies among individuals from asymptomatic to recurrent clinical presentations. Management of genital HSV should address the chronic nature of the disease rather than focusing solely on treatment of acute episodes of genital lesions (Centers for Disease Control and Prevention [CDC], 2015).

A. Types of HSV

1. HSV-1

   HSV-1 is responsible for most of the infections in the face and upper body. Oral and perioral lesions, often referred to by the public as "cold sores" or "fever blisters," are common presentations. HSV-1 can infect mucus membranes or abraded skin at any site including the eye, the genitals, and nongenital skin. Serious manifestations of HSV disease, such as encephalitis and meningitis, are rare in the immunocompetent patient. HSV is a common infection worldwide. Each year in the United States, there are approximately 500,000 primary infections (Scott, Coulter, & Lamey, 1997). HSV-1 is commonly transmitted in childhood with 90% of individuals seropositive for HSV-1 by the fourth decade of life (Buddingh, Schrum, & Lanier, 1953; Corey, 1986).

2. HSV-2

   HSV-2 is responsible for most genital skin infections. Most cases of recurrent genital herpes are caused by HSV-2, although seroprevalence trends show that the percentage of genital herpes caused by HSV-1

is increasing (Langenberg, Corey, Ashley, Leong, & Straus, 1999; Xu et al., 2006). A total of 20–25% of the adult population has serologic evidence of HSV-2 infection (Fleming et al., 1997). Subclinical viral shedding is common in the first few years after the primary HSV infection and then becomes less frequent—from 25% of days in the first year after infection to 4% of days in later years. The majority of genital infections are acquired during contact with persons unaware that they have the infection and who are asymptomatic when transmission occurs. In addition, individuals may not attribute symptoms such as vulvar rashes, irritation, or fissures with genital herpes ulcers. Thus, subclinical viral shedding and unrecognized mild symptoms are key factors in both horizontal (to a partner) and vertical (mother to newborn) transmission (Schillinger et al., 2008).

HSV-2 infection is an important risk factor for both HIV acquisition (Todd et al., 2006) and transmission. Persons with dual HIV and HSV infections are more likely to shed both viruses from open herpes ulcers caused by HSV-2, offering an explanation for the increased risk of HIV transmission from individuals with HSV-2 infections (Schacker et al., 1998). Conversely, the likelihood of horizontal acquisition of HIV infection significantly increases from twofold to three- or fourfold in persons with HSV infection, as a result of open herpes lesions coming into contact with the bodily fluids of an HIV infected partner (Freeman et al., 2006).

Neonatal infection with HSV is associated with high neonatal morbidity and mortality. The risk for transmission to the neonate from an infected mother is high (30–50%) among women who acquire genital herpes near the time of delivery and low (< 1%) among women with prenatal histories of recurrent herpes or who acquire genital HSV during the first half of pregnancy (CDC, 2015). Most pregnant women with a history of recurrent genital herpes can deliver their infants vaginally with a risk of neonatal transmission of less than 1% (Prober et al., 1987). According to the 2015 CDC sexually transmitted disease treatment guidelines, women without known genital herpes should be counseled to abstain from vaginal intercourse during the third trimester with partners known or suspected of having genital herpes. In addition, pregnant women without known orolabial herpes should be advised to abstain from receptive oral sex during the third trimester with partners known or suspected to have orolabial herpes. In women with active genital lesions at the time of delivery, a cesarean section delivery is recommended.

There is limited evidence that the use of routine serologic screening for HSV-2 or prophylactic antiviral therapy given in the third trimester in women with a history of recurrent HSV decreases neonatal herpes infection, and therefore neither intervention is recommended (CDC, 2015; U.S. Preventive Services Task Force, 2014). However, suppressive acyclovir treatment late in pregnancy reduces the frequency of cesarean delivery among women who have recurrent genital herpes by diminishing the frequency of recurrences at term (Scott et al., 2002; Sheffield, Hollier, Hill, Stuart, & Wendel, 2003). Treatment may not protect against transmission to neonates in all cases (Pinninti et al., 2012).

B. Clinical presentations: primary, nonprimary first-episode, and recurrent HSV

1. Primary infection

   This is the first clinical episode of genital herpes in an individual *without antibodies* to HSV-1 or HSV-2. Primary infection can be severe with painful genital ulcers and systemic symptoms, such as fever, myalgias, malaise, and tender inguinal lymphadenopathy. Lesions classically appear as vesicles or pustules that open in 12–24 hours to form shallow ulcers. Symptoms usually occur within a few weeks after infection and resolve within 2 weeks (**Figure 59-1**). Complications of HSV infection are more likely in primary infection and can include aseptic meningitis, sacral autonomic nervous system dysfunction, and disseminated lesions (Corey, Adams, Brown, & Holmes, 1983).

2. Nonprimary first-episode infection

   This is the first clinical episode of herpes in an individual *with serologic evidence of prior infection* with either HSV-1 or HSV-2. The clinical presentation usually is less severe compared to primary infection with fewer local lesions, mild to no systemic symptoms, and shorter duration of symptoms (Corey et al., 1983; Kimberlin & Rouse, 2004).

3. Recurrent infection

   Recurrent clinical episodes of herpes typically are less severe than primary and nonprimary first

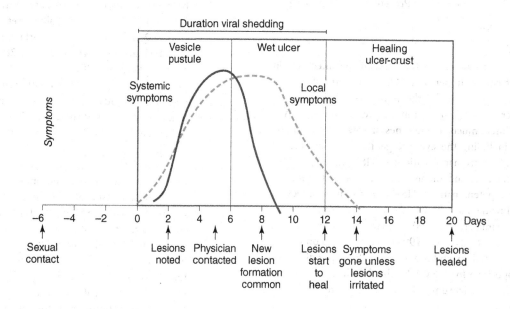

FIGURE 59-1 Clinical Course of Primary Genital Herpes Simplex Virus Infection

Reproduced from Corey, L., Adams, H. G., Brown, Z. A., & Holmes, K. K. (1983). Genital herpes simplex virus infections: Clinical manifestations, course, and complications. *Annals of Internal Medicine*, 98(6), 958–972. Reprinted with permission.

episodes. Systemic symptoms are uncommon. Time of healing of local ulcers and duration of viral shedding is shorter (Wald, Zeh, Selke, Ashley, & Corey, 1995). Triggers that may cause recurrent disease include acute illness, stress, sunlight, fatigue, menstrual periods, and unknown factors. Fifty percent of patients with recurrent episodes experience prodromal symptoms, such as sensitivity to touch (hyperesthesia), local tingling or itching, and peripheral nerve pain (Kimberlin & Rouse, 2004). A smaller number of patients develop frequent recurrence of HSV outbreaks that can cause both physical and emotional distress. For individuals who experience six or more outbreaks yearly, suppressive antiviral therapy should be offered (CDC, 2015). Although the medical complications from recurrent infection are uncommon, the psychosocial and psychosexual impact can cause significant distress for patients.

4. Asymptomatic infection

In asymptomatic infections, an individual has serum antibodies yet there is no history of clinical outbreaks. Unrecognized mild symptoms of HSV-2 are common, however, and may account for nearly two-thirds of individuals with what appears to be asymptomatic infections (CDC, 2015).

II. Database

A. Subjective

1. Past medical history and situational factors (may include but are not limited to)
   a. History of similar ulcer eruption (i.e., location of lesion and duration of the outbreaks). Note results of culture if done previously.
   b. History of contact exposure to individual with known HSV infection
   c. History of stimulus known to trigger eruption: sunlight, menses, fever, other illnesses, stress, and increased sexual activity
   d. History of rash, eczema, and erythema multiforme
   e. History of immunocompromise: HIV/AIDS, leukemia, lymphoma, other malignancies, autoimmune diseases, and posttransplant patients
   f. History of sexual practices, including oral–genital contact
   g. Currently pregnant
2. Occupational history
   a. Exposure history
   b. Type of profession (e.g., healthcare worker and dentist [herpetic whitlow])
   c. Contacts and personal protection

3. Symptomatology
   a. Fever, headache, malaise, myalgias, and tender lymph nodes
   b. Burning pain, tingling, hyperesthesia, or itching of involved skin and mucous membranes defines the prodromal symptoms of recurrent infection preceding outbreak of lesions by a few hours to up to 2 days.
   c. Depending on the site of infection
      i. Genital lesions: dysuria, urinary retention, sacral or genital paresthesias, rectal tenesmus, and constipation
      ii. Oral lesions: facial paresthesias, mouth pain (gingivostomatitis), difficulty eating, and visual disturbances or pain
   d. No symptoms

B. Objective

1. Vital signs: fever infrequent, most common in primary infection or with secondary complications, such as aseptic meningitis

2. Skin: tender, single, or clustered vesicles, pustules, or ulcers on a clean erythematous base. Ulcers may appear crusted over in the period before resolution. Lesions most frequently occur in or around the mouth, on the vulva, on penile glans or shaft, or perianally. May occur on distal fingers (herpetic whitlow), especially of healthcare workers.

3. Eye: unilateral conjunctivitis, blepharitis with vesicles on the lid margin, keratitis with dendritic lesions, or with punctuate opacities on ophthalmic examination

4. Mouth: small ulcers located on the soft palate, buccal mucosa, tongue, or floor of the mouth

5. Lymph: may have tender, nonfluctuant regional lymphadenopathy, especially in primary outbreaks.

6. Genitourinary: may see urethral, vaginal, or rectal discharge depending on severity of involvement. If rectal involvement, on anoscopy may see either ulcerations (not distinct lesions) and/or swollen inflamed mucosa.

III. Assessment

A. Determine the diagnosis

1. Primary
2. Nonprimary first episode
3. Recurrent
4. Asymptomatic
5. Other conditions that may explain the patient's presentation:

a. Infectious genital ulcer diseases: syphilis, chancroid, lymphogranuloma venereum, or granuloma inguinale
b. Noninfectious genital ulcers: Behçet syndrome, Crohn's disease, or fixed drug eruption
c. Mucopurulent cervical discharge: chlamydia, gonorrhea, or mycoplasmas
d. Vulvar rashes: allergic contact dermatitis (especially poison oak or poison ivy vulvitis), impetigo, psoriasis
e. Orolabial ulcers: aphthous stomatitis
f. Herpes zoster
g. Other etiologies of proctitis

B. Severity

Assess the severity of the infection including diagnosis of complications:

1. Urine retention resulting from bladder neck spasm
2. Proctitis, particularly in men who have sex with men (Klausner, Kohn, & Kent, 2003)
3. Constipation
4. Difficulty eating solid foods
5. Secondary bacterial infections caused by streptococci or staphylococci
6. Erythema multiforme
7. Herpes keratitis
8. Disseminated herpes
9. Aseptic meningitis
10. Neonatal herpes
11. Emotional stress and psychological morbidity especially seen with recurrent genital HSV

IV. Goals of clinical management

A. Choose a cost-effective approach for diagnosing HSV infection

B. Select a treatment plan that addresses the patient's symptom severity, frequency of recurrence, transmission risk to uninfected partner, and cost

C. Select an approach that maximizes patient adherence

D. Provide an education plan that empowers patients to cope with a chronic, recurrent sexually transmitted disease through self-management resources

V. Plan

A. Screening

The American Academy of Family Physicians and the U.S. Preventive Services Task Force (USPSTF) recommend against routine serologic screening for the general population and for pregnant women to prevent neonatal HSV infections. Counseling around the risks and benefits of serologic screening should be discussed and offered to select groups of patients including patients who may have HSV-infected sex partners and HIV-positive patients (American Academy of Family Physicians, 2009; USPSTF, 2014). HSV serologic testing should be considered for persons presenting for evaluation of sexually transmitted infections (STIs), especially for those persons with multiple sex partners; persons with HIV infection; and men who have sex with men (MSM) at increased risk for HIV acquisition (CDC, 2015).

B. Diagnostic tests

1. HSV viral culture if active lesions are present.
   The gold standard for diagnosis of HSV if an active lesion is present. Viral culture is highly specific (> 99%) but sensitivity depends on the stage of the lesion. Sensitivity is highest (90%) when lesion vesicles are unroofed and the base of an ulcer can be sampled. As lesions start to heal, the culture sensitivity decreases rapidly (sensitivity at ulcer stage = 70% and crust stage = 30%) (Corey et al., 1983). Determination of the HSV-type of infection predicts recurrence risk (50% with HSV-2, 10% with HSV-1) but otherwise is not necessary or helpful.

2. HSV polymerase chain reaction (PCR).
   PCR is highly sensitive but at significantly increased cost. PCR is now approved by the Food and Drug Administration for testing of anogenital specimens but cost prohibits this method of testing in the majority of clinical settings. PCR should be used to detect HSV in spinal fluid in cases where central nervous system infection is suspected.

3. Cytology (Pap or Tzanck).
   Is no longer recommended due to low sensitivity and specificity.

4. Type-specific herpes virus serology.
   Antibodies to HSV-1 and HSV-2 can be detected anywhere from 3 weeks to 3 months after infection and remain indefinitely. Testing may be clinically useful in the following cases:
   a. To rule out HSV diagnosis if the serology is negative at least 6 weeks after the onset of the outbreak

b. To determine primary herpes infection if patient is seronegative during initial symptoms then converts to seropositive after 6 weeks from the onset of the outbreak

c. In asymptomatic patients who have a sex partner with genital herpes

d. For patients at increased risk for STIs (i.e., multiple sex partners, HIV infection, and among MSM at increased risk for HIV acquisition) who request comprehensive STI screening (CDC, 2015)

5. Diagnostic tests as necessary to rule out etiologies other than HSV infection include syphilis serology to rule out primary or secondary syphilis.

6. HIV screening should be offered to all patients.

C. Management

1. Preventive

a. Avoid contact with persons with a known or suspected active herpes lesion

b. Use of condoms, gloves, or other barrier methods

c. Avoid or decrease exposure to known recurrence triggers

d. Antiviral medications used to treat or suppress recurrent outbreaks or prophylactic therapy of an infected person to prevent horizontal transmission to an uninfected partner (**Table 59-1**)

2. Symptomatic

a. Sitz bath or cool compresses

b. Topical anesthetic or viscous lidocaine as needed

TABLE 59-1 Drug Treatment of Herpes Simplex Infections

HSV Treatment Type	Drug	Dosage	Notes
Oral HSV primary	Acyclovir*	200 mg orally five times daily or 400 mg orally three times daily for 7–10 days	Begin treatment early in infection
Oral HSV Episodic treatment for recurrent symptoms	Acyclovir	200 mg orally five times daily for 10 days	Treatment for recurrent oral herpes offers mild benefit. Topical antiviral medications are not recommended due to limited clinical benefit (i.e., docosanol 10%, penciclovir 1%, acyclovir 5%).
Genital HSV primary	Acyclovir or Famciclovir or Valacyclovir	400 mg orally three times a day for 7–10 days or 200 mg orally five times a day for 7–10 days 250 mg orally three times a day for 7–10 days 1 g orally twice a day for 7–10 days	Extending treatment is an option if healing is incomplete after 10 days of therapy
Genital HSV Episodic therapy for recurrent symptoms	Acyclovir or Famciclovir or Valacyclovir	400 mg orally three times a day for 5 days or 800 mg orally twice a day for 5 days or 800 mg orally three times a day for 2 days 125 mg orally twice daily for 5 days or 1,000 mg orally twice daily for 1 day or 500 mg once, followed by 250 mg twice daily for 2 days 500 mg orally twice a day for 3 days or 1 g orally once a day for 5 days	Begin treatment at first sign of infection; an option for patients with mild or infrequent recurrent symptoms (< 6 outbreaks per year) Immuncocompromised patients can have longer duration and more severe symptoms. Consider increasing the doses of antiviral drugs to improve clinical healing in immunocompromised patients

(continues)

TABLE 59-1 Drug Treatment of Herpes Simplex Infections *(Continued)*

HSV Treatment Type	Drug	Dosage	Notes
Genital HSV Suppressive therapy	Acyclovir or	400 mg orally twice a day	An option for patients with more frequent or severe symptoms (> 6 outbreaks per year)
	Famciclovir or	250 mg orally twice a day	Shown to decrease transmission in discordant couples with HSV-2
	Valacyclovir	500 mg orally once a day or 1 g orally once a day (for episodes ≥ 10 per year)	Patients and their partners should be counseled that suppressive therapy reduces but does not eradicate viral shedding.
HSV treatment in patients with HIV			For guidelines on HSV treatment in people with HIV, see Chapter 66, Primary Care of HIV-Infected Adults*

*Intravenous acyclovir therapy should be provided for patients who have severe primary HSV disease or complications that necessitate hospitalization (e.g., disseminated infection, pneumonitis, or hepatitis) or central nervous system complications (e.g., meningitis or encephalitis). The recommended regimen is acyclovir, 5–10 mg/kg body weight intravenously every 8 hours for 2–7 days or until clinical improvement is observed, followed by oral antiviral therapy to complete at least 10 days of total therapy.

Data from Centers for Disease Control and Prevention. (2015). *2015 sexually transmitted diseases: Treatment guidelines.* Retrieved from http://www.cdc.gov/std/tg2015/herpes.htm.

c. Anticonstipating diet or stool softeners as needed

d. Nonsteroidal anti-inflammatory medications to reduce pain

e. Antiviral medications for primary or recurrent outbreaks (Table 59-1)

3. Criteria for consultation or specialty referral

a. Generalized involvement

b. Any complications present

c. Pregnancy

4. Follow-up

a. As medically indicated for patients with primary herpes, depending on the severity of the infection

b. Not medically necessary for follow-up with infrequent recurrent outbreaks, although some patients may require follow-up visits to focus on counseling and education

c. Patients on suppressive therapy should be reevaluated every 12 months

D. Patient education

1. Goal: Educate on the clinical course of the disease, emphasizing risk factors for HSV transmission. Address concerns and feelings to help patients cope with herpes as a chronic disease. Recommended counseling topics listed in the 2015 CDC STD Treatment Guidelines can be found in **Figure 59-2.**

FIGURE 59-2 Genital HSV Counseling Topics

The following topics should be discussed when counseling persons with genital HSV infection:

- the natural history of the disease, with emphasis on the potential for recurrent episodes, asymptomatic viral shedding, and the attendant risks of sexual transmission
- the effectiveness of suppressive therapy for persons experiencing a first episode of genital herpes in preventing symptomatic recurrent episodes
- use of episodic therapy to shorten the duration of recurrent episodes
- importance of informing current sex partners about genital herpes and informing future partners before initiating a sexual relationship

FIGURE 59-2 Genital HSV Counseling Topics *(Continued)*

- potential for sexual transmission of HSV to occur during asymptomatic periods (asymptomatic viral shedding is more frequent in genital HSV-2 infection than genital HSV-1 infection and is most frequent during the first 12 months after acquiring HSV-2)

- importance of abstaining from sexual activity with uninfected partners when lesions or prodromal symptoms are present

- effectiveness of daily use of valacyclovir in reducing risk for transmission of HSV-2, and the lack of effectiveness of episodic or suppressive therapy in persons with HIV and HSV infection in reducing risk for transmission to partners who might be at risk for HSV-2 acquisition

- effectiveness of male latex condoms, which when used consistently and correctly can reduce (but not eliminate) the risk for genital herpes transmission (Martin et al.,2009)

- HSV infection in the absence of symptoms (type-specific serologic testing of the asymptomatic partners of persons with genital herpes is recommended to determine whether such partners are already HSV seropositive or whether risk for acquiring HSV exists)

- risk for neonatal HSV infection

- increased risk for HIV acquisition among HSV-2 seropositive persons who are exposed to HIV (suppressive antiviral therapy does not reduce the increased risk for HIV acquisition associated with HSV-2 infection) (Baeten et al., 2012)

Asymptomatic persons who receive a diagnosis of HSV-2 infection by type-specific serologic testing should receive the same counseling messages as persons with symptomatic infection. In addition, such persons should be educated about the clinical manifestations of genital herpes.

Pregnant women and women of childbearing age who have genital herpes should inform the providers who care for them during pregnancy and those who will care for their newborn infant about their infection.

Reproduced from Centers for Disease Control and Prevention. (2015). *2015 sexually transmitted diseases: Treatment guidelines.* Retrieved from http://www.cdc.gov/std/tg2015/herpes.htm.

VI. Self–management resources and tools

A. Patient education

1. Basic fact sheet address frequently asked questions by patients about HSV infection can be printed from the Centers for Disease Control and Prevention: www.cdc.gov/std/herpes/stdfact-herpes.htm.

2. Herpes Resource Center
   American Sexual Health Association (1-800-230-6039; http://ashastd.org)

3. National Institute of Allergy and Infectious Disease (http://niaid.nih.gov)

B. Community support groups

1. The Herpes Resource Center has an affiliated network of local support (HELP) group for people concerned about herpes simplex virus. The network of support groups can be accessed on the American Sexual Health Association website (http://ashastd.org).

REFERENCES

American Academy of Family Physicians. (2009). *Summary of AAFP recommendations for clinical preventive services.* Retrieved from http://www.aafp.org/online/en/home/clinical/clinicalrecs.html.

Baeten, J. M., Donnell, D., Ndase, P., Mugo, N. R., Campbell, J. D., Wangisi, J., et al. (2012). Antiretroviral prophylaxis for HIV prevention in heterosexual men and women. *New England Journal of Medicine, 367,* 399–410.

Buddingh, G. J., Schrum, D. I., & Lanier, J. C. (1953). Studies of the natural history of herpes simplex infections. *Pediatrics, 11*(6), 595–610.

Centers for Disease Control and Prevention. (2015). *2015 sexually transmitted diseases: Treatment Guidelines.* Retrieved from www.cdc.gov/std/tg2015/herpes.htm/.

Corey, L. (1986). Genital herpes. In A. Nahmias & B. Roizman (Eds.), *The herpes viruses* (pp. 1–35). New York: Plenum Press.

Corey, L., Adams, H. G., Brown, Z. A., & Holmes, K. K. (1983). Genital herpes simplex virus infections: Clinical manifestations, course and complications. *Annals of Internal Medicine, 98*(6), 958–972.

Fleming, D. T., McQuillan, G. M., Johnson, R. E., Nahmias, A. J., Aral, S. O., Lee, F. K., et al. (1997). Herpes simplex virus type 2 in the United States, 1976 to 1994. *New England Journal of Medicine, 337*(16), 1105–1111.

Freeman, E. E., Weiss, H. A., Glynn, J. R., Cross, P. L., Whitworth, J. A., & Hayes, R. J. (2006). Herpes simplex virus 2 increases HIV acquisition in men and women: A systematic review and meta-analysis of longitudinal studies. *AIDS, 20*, 73–83.

Kimberlin, D. W., & Rouse, D. J. (2004). Clinical practice. Genital herpes. *New England Journal of Medicine, 350*(19), 1970–1977.

Klausner, J. D., Kohn, R., & Kent, C. (2003). Etiology of clinical proctitis among men who have sex with men. *Clinical Infectious Disease, 38*(2), 300–302.

Langenberg, A. G., Corey, L., Ashley, R. L., Leong, W. P., & Straus, S. E. (1999). A prospective study of new infections with herpes simplex virus type 1 and type 2. Chiron HSV Vaccine Study Group. *New England Journal of Medicine, 341*(19), 1432–1438.

Martin, E. T., Krantz, E., Gottlieb, S. L., Magaret, A. S., Langenberg, A., Stanberry, L., et al. (2009). A pooled analysis of the effect of condoms in preventing HSV-2 acquisition. *Archives of Internal Medicine, 169*, 1233–1240.

Pinninti, S. G., Angara, R., Feja, K. N., Kimberlin, D. W., Leach, C. T., Conrad, D. A., et al. (2012). Neonatal herpes disease following maternal antenatal antiviral suppressive therapy: a multicenter case series. *Journal of Pediatrics, 161*, 134–138.

Prober, C. G., Sullender, W. M., Yasukawa, L. L., Au, D. S., Yeager, A. S., & Arvin, A. M. (1987). Low risk of herpes simplex virus infections in neonates exposed to the virus at the time of vaginal delivery to mothers with recurrent genital herpes simplex virus infections. *New England Journal of Medicine, 316*, 240–244.

Schacker, T., Ryncarz, A. J., Goddard, J., Diem, K., Shaughnessy, M., & Corey, L. (1998). Frequent recovery of HIV-1 from genital herpes simplex virus lesions in HIV-1-infected men. *JAMA, 280*(1), 61–66.

Schillinger, J. A., McKinney, C. M., Garg, R., Gwynn, R. C., White, K., Lee, F., et al. (2008). Seroprevalence of herpes simplex virus type 2 and characteristics associated with undiagnosed infection. *Sexually Transmitted Disease, 35*(6), 599–606.

Scott, D. A., Coulter, W. A., & Lamey, P. J. (1997). Oral shedding of herpes simplex virus type 1: A review. *Journal of Oral Pathology Medicine, 26*(10), 441–447.

Scott, L. L., Hollier, L. M., McIntire, D., Sanchez, P. J., Jackson, G. L., & Wendel, G. D., Jr. (2002). Acyclovir suppression to prevent recurrent genital herpes at delivery. *Infectious Diseases in Obstetrics and Gynecology, 10*, 71–77.

Sheffield, J. S., Hollier, L. M., Hill, J. B., Stuart, G. S., & Wendel, G. D. (2003). Acyclovir prophylaxis to prevent herpes simplex virus recurrence at delivery: A systematic review. *Obstetrics & Gynecology, 102*, 1396–1403.

Todd, J., Grosskurth, H., Changalucha, J., Obasi, A., Mosha, F., & Balira, R. (2006). Risk factors influencing HIV infection incidence in a rural African population: A nested case-control study. *Journal of Infectious Disease, 193*(3), 458–466.

U.S. Preventive Services Task Force. (2014). *Guide to clinical preventive services.* Retrieved from http://www.ahrq.gov/clinic/pocketgd1011/gcp10s1.htm.

Wald, A., Zeh, J., Selke, S., Ashley, R. L., & Corey, L. (1995). Virologic characteristics of subclinical and symptomatic genital herpes infections. *New England Journal of Medicine, 333*(12), 770–775.

Xu, F., Sternberg, M. R., Kottiri, B. J., McQuillan, G. M., Lee, F. K., & Nahmias, A. J. (2006). Trends in herpes simplex virus type 1 and type 2 seroprevalence in the United States. *JAMA, 296*(8), 964–973.

HYPERTENSION

Judith Sweet and Steve Protzel

I. Introduction and definition

Hypertension is one of the most common conditions seen in primary care and is also considered one of the most significant preventable causes of disease and death, primarily because of its association with heart disease, stroke, and renal failure (James et al., 2014). Most patients with hypertension have additional risk factors, including dyslipidemias, glucose intolerance or diabetes, a family history of early cardiovascular events, obesity, and/or cigarette smoking (Weber et al., 2014). Unfortunately, successful treatment of hypertension has been poor overall, and in some communities, fewer than 50% of all hypertensive patients have adequately controlled blood pressure (Weber et al., 2014).

A. Prevalence

The National Health and Nutrition Examination Survey (NHANES) (Nwankwo, Yoon, Bury, & Gu, 2013) reported the prevalence of hypertension (HTN) in 2011–2012 among U.S. adults aged 18 and over was approximately 30% with similar distribution across races and sexes. The prevalence does increase with age and is highest among older adults and is highest among non-Hispanic black adults at 42%.

The World Health Organization (WHO, 2013) considers HTN to be the main attributable risk factor for death worldwide. According to a 2013 WHO report, HTN is responsible for at least 45% of worldwide deaths due to heart disease and over 50% of deaths due to stroke. The number of adults with a diagnosis of HTN rose from 60 million in 1980 to over a billion in 2008. The prevalence of hypertension is greatest in middle- and low-income countries with larger populations and poorer access to health care (WHO, 2013).

B. Definition

Hypertension is an elevation in arterial blood pressure (BP) confirmed when the average of two or more (seated) readings done at two or more office visits is greater than 140 systolic or 90 diastolic.

Hypertension is a continuous and independent risk factor for cardiovascular disease, and the presence of additional risk factors (elevated total cholesterol, high-density lipoprotein cholesterol < 35, smoking, diabetes, and left ventricular hypertrophy as the most significant) compounds the risk from HTN. Elevated systolic BP (SBP) and diastolic BP (DBP) are each considered important risk factors.

Diastolic HTN is a stronger cardiovascular risk factor and more common before the age of 50 than systolic HTN. However, systolic HTN is more common after the age of 50 than diastolic HTN. Diastolic BP may actually decrease whereas systolic blood pressure increases with aging. This is most likely due to the progressive stiffening of the arterial circulation that occurs with aging (Weber et al., 2014).

C. Classification and Treatment Goal Recommendations

In 2004, the seventh report of the Joint National Committee on Prevention, Detection, Evaluation, and Treatment of High Blood Pressure (JNC 7) categorized BP as follows: (1) normal, (2) pre-HTN, (3) HTN stage 1, and (4) HTN stage 2 (**Table 60-1**). The designation of "pre-HTN" is meant to identify those individuals at high risk of developing frank HTN who may benefit from adapting lifestyle modifications that either lower BP or slow the rate of progression (JNC 7, 2004). This stage should not be viewed as a disease category, but rather as a warning and an incentive for care providers to strongly counsel these individuals regarding lifestyle modifications. These individuals are not candidates for medication treatment unless they also have diabetes or kidney disease (U.S. Department of Health and Human Services [USDHHS], 2004).

The eighth JNC report in 2014 specifically focused on evidence to support the need to initiate antihypertensive pharmacologic therapy at specific BP thresholds (see Table 60-1) and whether there is evidence to support adjusting pharmacologic treatment to specified BP goals (James et al., 2014). The panel members also changed general recommendations on how aggressively to treat older adults (over age 60) based on their extensive

TABLE 60-1 A Comparison Between JNC-7 and JNC-8 Blood Pressure (BP) Definitions

JNC-7 defines by BP classification			JNC-8 defines by BP treatment threshold		
BP Classification	Systolic BP mm Hg	Diastolic BP mm Hg	Population	Systolic BP mm Hg Treatment Threshold	Diastolic BP mm Hg Treatment Threshold
Normal	< 120	and < 80	General population aged ≥ 60 years	≥ 150	≥ 90
Prehypertension	120–139	or 80–89	General population 18–60 years	≥ 140	≥ 90
Stage 1 hypertension	140–159	or 90–99	In the population aged ≥18 years with chronic kidney disease	≥ 140	≥ 90
Stage 2 hypertension	≥ 160	or ≥100	In the population aged ≥18 years with diabetes	≥ 140	≥ 90

Data from James, P. A., Oparil, S., Carter, B. L., Cushman, W. C., Dennison-Himmelfarb, C., Handler, J., et al. (2014). 2014 evidence-based guidelines for the management of high blood pressure in adults: Report from the panel members appointed to the Eighth Joint National Committee (JNC 8). *JAMA, 311*(5), 507–520. doi: 10.1001/jama.2013.284427.

review of the evidence accumulated since JNC 7 in 2004 (James et al., 2014). However, there was disagreement among members of the JNC 8 and overall controversy among experts about the recommendations made for older adults, specifically from the American Society of Hypertension (ASH) and the International Society for Hypertension (ISH) (Ram, 2014).

The following recommendations were made by JNC 8 panel members regarding when to initiate pharmacologic treatment (James et al., 2014):

1. In the general population ≥ age 60, initiate medication treatment at SBP ≥ 150 mm Hg or DBP ≥ 90 mm Hg and treat to a goal of SBP < 150 and DBP < 90.
   a. (corollary to #1): If pharmacologic treatment for persons ≥ 60 years old lowers BP to less than 150/90 and the treatment is well tolerated without adverse effects, the treatment does not need to be adjusted.
2. In the general population < 60, begin medication at DBP ≥ 90 and treat to a goal < 90.
3. In the general population < 60, begin medication to lower BP at SBP ≥ 140 with a goal of SBP < 140.
4. In the population ≥ 18 years old with diabetes, initiate medication at SBP ≥ 140 or DBP ≥ 90 and treat to a goal of SBP < 140 and/or DBP < 90.
5. In the population > 18 with chronic kidney disease (CKD), begin pharmacologic therapy at SBP ≥ 140 or DBP ≥ 90 and treat to a goal of SBP < 140 and/or DBP < 90.

6. The ASH/ISH guidelines differ from these recommendations in recommending treating all adults 18–79 at a BP ≥ 140/90. For adults age ≥ 80 years old, the ASH/ISH guidelines recommend that treatment should start at BP of ≥ 150/90 or ≥ 140/90 if diabetic or with renal disease, respectively.

II. Database (may include but is not limited to)

A. Subjective

1. Most patients are asymptomatic.
   a. Although most patients are asymptomatic, some may experience headaches, dizziness, blurred vision, tinnitus, chest pain, shortness of breath, nausea, vomiting, extremity swelling, or anxiety, which may be unrelated to actual elevated blood pressure or be caused by end-organ damage.
2. The following symptoms suggest secondary causes for HTN.
   a. Muscle cramps, polyuria, weakness, and excessive thirst: primary aldosteronism (rare)
   b. Headache, pallor, palpitations, sweating, and flushing: pheochromocytoma (very rare)
   c. Hirsutism, easy bruising, and symptoms of diabetes mellitus: Cushing's syndrome (rare)
   d. Severe chest pain radiating to back: aortic dissection or aneurysm (common)

e. Claudication: coarctation of aorta (rare to be found late in life)

f. Snoring and daytime fatigue: sleep apnea (common)

g. Palpitations, insomnia, anxiety, and weight loss: hyperthyroidism (common) (see Chapter 66 on thyroid disorders for details)

3. Symptoms suggestive of target organ damage

a. Exertional chest pain, shortness of breath, orthopnea, peripheral edema, and paroxysmal nocturnal dyspnea: coronary artery disease or heart failure

b. Fatigue, pruritus, or peripheral edema: renal failure

c. Syncopal episodes or dizziness, memory loss, motor weakness, speech difficulties, or other focal neurologic findings: cerebrovascular disease

d. Claudication and sudden loss of vision: peripheral arterial disease

4. Past health history

a. History and work-up of HTN (When was patient first told he or she has high BP?); course of treatment and complications including medications tried and failed or with adverse effects.

b. Diabetes, lipid abnormalities, gout, cardiovascular and cerebrovascular disease, and renal disease.

c. Use of prescribed or over-the-counter drugs and street drugs that may influence BP or interfere with the effectiveness of an antihypertensive drug (e.g., hormonal contraceptives, steroids, nonsteroidal anti-inflammatory drugs, alcohol, cocaine, amphetamines, appetite suppressants or other "diet" supplements, tricyclic antidepressants, monoamine oxidase inhibitors, or decongestants [pseudoephedrine and phenylpropanolomines or analogues]) (**Table 60-2**).

d. Dietary supplement use including products containing "herbal ecstasy," ma huang/ephedra, ergot-containing products, and St. John's wort.

e. If overweight, note history of weight gain.

5. Family history: history of HTN, stroke, sudden cardiac death, diabetes, heart failure, renal disease, or other cardiovascular disease.

6. Personal and social history: habits

a. Alcohol use: chronic use and withdrawal elevates BP

b. Recreational or street drug use, especially cocaine, crack, and amphetamines; anabolic steroids; recent withdrawal from narcotics

c. Diet: includes sodium intake, use of canned or prepared foods, vegetable and fruit intake, fat and cholesterol intake

d. Exercise: type, frequency, and level of exercise

e. Tobacco use: not a cause of HTN but is an additional risk factor for cardiovascular disease, and withdrawal may be associated with elevated BP

f. Ethnic or racial background

g. May affect responsiveness to certain medications (see pharmacologic treatment section V. B.)

h. Other factors influencing BP control

i. Emotional stress including social support system (if any), family and living situation, employment and working situation and stress, ability to obtain and pay for healthcare services, and educational level and literacy (may affect understanding of treatment recommendations, and/or ability to read patient handouts)

B. Objective

1. Physical examination

a. Vital signs including BP should be taken after the patient has been sitting quietly for at least 5 minutes with arm resting on a flat surface and feet on the floor. Additionally, the patient should not have used caffeine, tobacco, or alcohol and nor exercised for at least 30 minutes before the BP measurement. The initial evaluation should include a BP measurement in both arms. At least two measurements should be obtained with the average of the two recorded. Periodic standing BP measurements are recommended for those at risk for postural BP changes or with such symptoms and when adding or changing medications. The preferred method of BP measurement is the auscultatory (not digital) method. A proper sized cuff is essential; the cuff bladder should encircle at least 80% of the arm to assure an accurate BP reading (USDHHS, 2004).

b. Complete a fundoscopic evaluation for arteriovenous nicking, arteriolar narrowing, papilloedema, hemorrhages, or exudates.

c. Assess neck for carotid bruits, distended veins, and enlarged thyroid.

d. Evaluate the heart for precordial heave, thrills, rate, murmurs, or other extra sounds, such as S3 and S4.

e. Auscultate the lungs for adventitious sounds (e.g., crackles and wheezing).

f. Evaluate the abdomen for bruits, enlarged kidneys, or striae.

g. Assess the extremities for diminished or absent peripheral arterial pulses, edema, or femoral artery bruits.

h. Neurologic assessment as baseline and for evaluation of abnormal sensory, motor, and cognitive findings suggestive of target organ damage.

TABLE 60-2 Common Substances Associated with Hypertension in Humans

Prescription Drugs	Street Drugs and Other "Natural Products"	Food Substances	Chemical Elements and Other Industrial Chemicals
Cortisone and other steroids: (both corticosteroids and mineralosteroids), adrenocorticotropic hormone (ACTH)	Cocaine and cocaine withdrawal	Sodium chloride	Lead
Estrogens (usually just oral contraceptive agents with high estrogenic activity)	Ma huang, "herbal ecstasy," and other phenyl propanolamine analogues	Ethanol	Mercury
Nonsteroidal anti-inflammatory drugs	Nicotine and withdrawal	Licorice	Thallium and other heavy metals
Phenylpropanolamines and analogues	Anabolic steroids	Tyramine-containing foods (with monoamine oxidase inhibitors)	Lithium salts, especially the chloride
Cyclosporine and tacrolimus	Narcotic withdrawal	Caffeine	
Erythropoietin	Methylphenidate		
Sibutramine	Phencyclidine		
Ketamine	Ketamine		
Desflurane	Ergotamine and other ergot-containing herbal preparations		
Carbamazepine	St. John's wort		
Bromocriptine			
Metoclopramide			
Antidepressants (especially venlafaxine)			
Buspirone			
Clonidine (abrupt withdrawal) with or without the simultaneous initiation of beta-adrenergic blocking agents			
Pheochromocytoma: beta-adrenergic blocking agent without alpha-blocker first; glucagon			
Clozapine			
Weight loss drugs			

Modified from U.S. Department of Health and Human Services. (2004). *Seventh report of the Joint National Committee on Prevention, Detection, Evaluation, and Treatment of High Blood Pressure (JNC 7)* (NIH Publication no. 0405230) (p. 59). Washington, DC: National Institutes of Health, National Heart, Lung, and Blood Institute, National High Blood Pressure Education Program, U.S. Department of Health and Human Services. Retrieved from http://www.nhlbi.nih.gov/guidelines/hypertension/jnc7full.htm.

2. Diagnostic tests
   a. Laboratory: urinalysis (for proteinuria or hematuria suggesting end-organ damage or secondary HTN), fasting blood glucose or hemoglobin A1C (for hyperglycemia suggesting diabetes), hematocrit (for anemia suggesting other disease or polycythemia), serum potassium (may affect medication choice and/or suggest etiology or -organ damage), creatinine and estimated glomerular filtration rate (may affect medication choice or suggest end-organ damage or secondary HTN), calcium (may be associated with renal disease and thyroid disease), thyroid-stimulating hormone (TSH) and free L-thyroxine (FT4) (for hyperthyroidism), and fasting lipid profile (as is associated risk factor)
   b. Twelve-lead electrocardiogram (as baseline and/or for evidence of arrhythmias, conduction defects, ischemia and/or infarct, and/or left ventricular hypertrophy)

TABLE 60-3 Screening Tests for Identifiable Causes of Hypertension

Diagnosis	Diagnostic Test
Chronic kidney disease	Estimated glomerular filtration rate
Coarctation of the aorta	Computerized tomography angiography
Cushing's syndrome and other glucocorticoid excess states including chronic steroid therapy	History; dexamethasone suppression test
Drug induced or related	History and drug screening
Pheochromocytoma	24-Hour metanephrine and normetanephrine
Primary aldosteronism and other mineralocorticoid excess states	24-Hour urinary aldosterone level or specific measurements of other mineralocorticoids
Renovascular hypertension	Doppler flow study; magnetic resonance angiography
Sleep apnea	Sleep study with O_2 saturation
Thyroid or parathyroid disease	Thyroid-stimulating hormone, serum parathyroid hormone

Reproduced from U.S. Department of Health and Human Services. (2004). *Seventh report of the Joint National Committee on Prevention, Detection, Evaluation, and Treatment of High Blood Pressure (JNC 7)* (NIH Publication no. 0405230). Washington, DC: National Institutes of Health, National Heart, Lung, and Blood Institute, National High Blood Pressure Education Program, U.S. Department of Health and Human Services. Retrieved from http://www.nhlbi.nih.gov/guidelines/hypertension/jnc7full.htm.

   c. If secondary HTN is suspected based on the patient's presentation, other tests should be included (**Table 60-3**)

III. Assessment

   A. *Determine the diagnosis (see Table 60-1)*

   B. *Severity*
   1. Assess severity based on level of BP and presence or absence of other risk factors or other compelling diseases.
      a. Hypertensive emergencies are characterized by severe elevations in BP (> 180/120 mm Hg) and complicated by evidence of impending or progressive target organ dysfunction. They require immediate BP reduction (not necessarily to normal) to prevent or limit target organ damage (e.g., intracerebral hemorrhage or acute myocardial infarction).
      b. Hypertensive urgencies are those situations associated with severe elevations in BP without progressive target organ dysfunction (USDHHS, 2004).

   C. *Significance and patient's motivation and ability*
      Assess the significance of this diagnosis to the patient and to significant others. Additionally, assess patient's understanding of the disorder and willingness and ability to follow a treatment plan, including lifestyle modifications. This assessment should be made on an ongoing basis throughout follow-up visits.

IV. Goals of clinical management

   A. *Public health goal*
      Reduce the cardiovascular and renal morbidity and mortality.

   B. *Individual's goal related to self-management and patient adherence*
      Choose a plan including medications, lifestyle modifications, and follow-up that is tailored to the patient.

   C. *BP goal (see section I, C for BP goals for different groups of affected individuals)*

V. Plan and management
(see **Figure 60-1**)

   A. *Lifestyle modification*
      This is the first step in counseling and treating patients with pre-HTN and stage 1 HTN and is an essential component

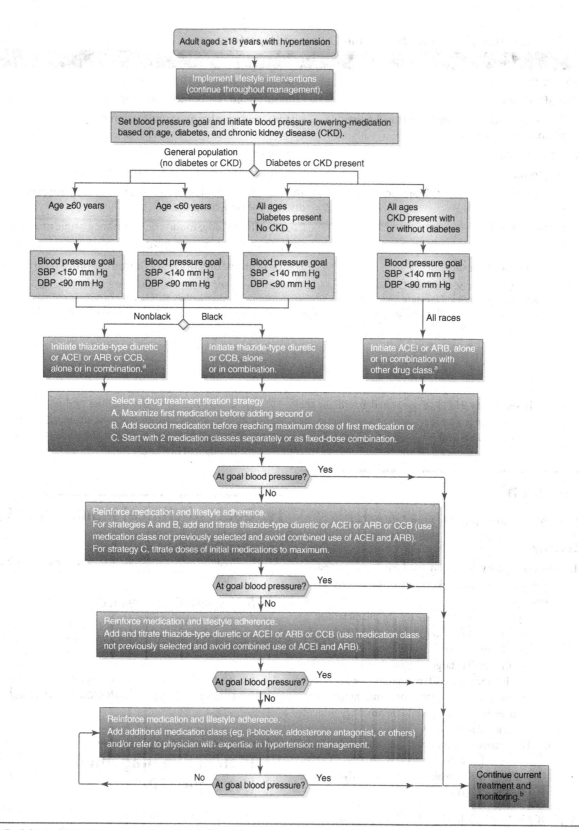

FIGURE 60-1 2014 Hypertension Guideline Management Algorithm

Reproduced from James, P. A., Oparil, S., Carter, B. L., Cushman, W. C., Dennison-Himmelfarb, C., Handler, J., et al. (2014). 2014 evidence-based guidelines for the management of high blood pressure in adults: Report from the panel members appointed to the Eighth Joint National Committee (JNC 8). *JAMA, 311*(5), 516. doi: 10.1001/jama.2013.284427.

of treatment for stage 2 HTN. In patients with prehypertension or mild stage 1 HTN, lifestyle modifications may be definitive therapy, and in others they may reduce the number and doses of antihypertensives required to reach goal BP and decrease risk of or delay progression to end-organ damage.

1. Weight
   a. Weight loss of as little as 10 lb (4.5 kg) reduces BP or prevents HTN in many overweight individuals (USDHHS, 2004).

2. Diet
   a. There is strong evidence that consuming a diet that emphasizes vegetables, fruits, whole grains, low-fat dairy, poultry, fish, legumes, nontropical vegetable oils, and nuts and limits intake of sweets, sugar-sweetened beverages, and red meats can benefit BP lowering (Eckel et al., 2013). The DASH (Dietary Approaches to Stop Hypertension) diet or the American Heart Association diet are diets consistent with these recommendations and generally recommended (American Heart Association [AHA], 2014; Heller, 2015).
   b. Strong evidence also exists for consuming no more than 2,400 mg of sodium daily, and reducing further to 1,500 mg/day is associated with greater BP reduction. Even reducing sodium intake by at least 100 mg a day, though not ideal, can lower BP (Eckel et al., 2013)

3. Alcohol
   Alcohol intake should be limited to 1 oz or less daily of ethanol (two drinks in men) and no more than 0.5 oz (AHA, 2014).

4. Exercise
   Regular aerobic activity often lowers BP in adults. Three to four sessions a week of approximately 40 minutes each involving moderate to vigorous intensity exercise are recommended (Eckel et al., 2013).

5. Tobacco abstinence
   For overall cardiovascular risk reduction, smoking cessation is essential and should be a major focus of counseling for providers.

6. Other lifestyle modifications or alternative treatments
   Numerous other modalities and lifestyle treatments have been tried and studied over the past several decades, but in general the research done on these strategies is less rigorous, or lacking in statistical power, to make strong recommendations (Eckel et al., 2013).
   However, several modalities have moderately good evidence to support recommending to patients with pre-HTN as a trial therapy and to any patient with HTN as an adjuvant therapy: (1) transcendental meditation and possibly other meditation techniques (the latter less studied) and (2) biofeedback, device-guided breathing (such as the RESPeRATE, which is approved by the Food and Drug Administration as an over-the-counter product for stress reduction and adjunct to treating HTN; USDHHS, 2002). Other alternative approaches that have been used successfully but have not been adequately researched include acupuncture (including electroacupuncture), cognitive behavioral techniques for stress reduction, progressive muscle relaxation, and yoga (Eckel et al., 2013).

B. **Pharmacologic treatment (Table 60-4)**
Reducing elevated BP with medications has been shown in numerous studies to decrease the incidence of cardiovascular mortality and morbidity.

1. Factors to be considered in the selection of therapy
   a. Cost of medication
   b. Metabolic and subjective side effects
   c. Potential drug–drug interactions
   d. Concomitant diseases that may be beneficially or adversely affected by the antihypertensive agent chosen
   e. Ethnicity and race: There is a great variance in HTN-related morbidity and mortality among various ethnic groups in the United States, because of many factors including physiologic differences in response to some drugs; socioeconomic conditions; access to healthcare services; attitudes and beliefs related to health information; and differences in lifestyle practices, such as diet (USDHHS, 2004).
      i. African Americans may respond to a low-sodium diet and diuretics with greater BP reductions than other demographic subgroups (James et al., 2014) Also, the JNC 8 panel recommends using a calcium channel blocker (CCB) rather than an angiotensin converting enzyme inhibitor (ACEI) initially in Blacks because of increased stroke risk in Blacks started initially on an ACEI in one large randomized control trial (The ALLHAT Officers and Coordinators for the ALLHAT Collaborative Research Group, 2002).
      ii. Mexican Americans and Native Americans tend to have lower control rates of HTN than non-Hispanic whites and African Americans (USDHHS, 2004), which may mean closer attention to dietary sodium intake and/or greater need for use of medications from two or more classes.

TABLE 60-4 Commonly Used Antihypertensive Medications*

Class of Drug	Drug Name	Usual Dose Range (mg/day)	Usual Daily Frequency	Mechanism	Comments
Thiazide diuretics	Chlorthalidone	12.5–25	1	Decreased plasma volume and extracellular fluid volume, decreased cardiac output initially, followed by decreased total peripheral resistance with normalization of cardiac output. Long-term effects include slight decreases in extracellular fluid volume.	For thiazide and loop diuretics, lower doses and dietary counseling should be used to avoid metabolic changes (e.g., potassium, sodium losses).
	Chlorothiazide	125–500	1–2		
	Hydrochlorathiazide	12.5–50	1		Check electrolytes 1–2 weeks after initiating these medications.
	Indapamide	1.25–2.5	1		
	Polythiazide	2–4	1		
	Metolazone (Zaroxolyn)	2.5–5.0	1		
Loop diuretics	Bumetanide	0.5–2	2	See thiazides.	Higher doses may be needed for patients with renal impairment or congestive heart failure.
	Ethacrynic acid	50–100	1–2		Ethacrynic acid is the only alternative for patients with allergy to thiazide and sulfur-containing diuretics.
	Furosemide	10–80	2		
	Torsemide	2.5–10	1		
β-Blockers	Atenolol	25–100	1	Decreased cardiac output and increased total peripheral resistance; decreased plasma renin activity; atenolol, betaxolol, bisoprolol, and metroprolol are cardioselective.	Selective agents also inhibit in higher doses (e.g., all may aggravate asthma).
	Betaxolol	5–20	1		
	Bisoprolol	2.5–10	1		
	Metoprolol	50–200	1–2		
	Metoprolol extended release	25–100	1		
	Nadolol	40–120	1		
	Propranolol	40–160	2		
	Propranolol long-acting	60–180	1		
		10–40	2		
β-Blockers with intrinsic sympathomimetic activity	Acebutolol	200–800	2	See β-blockers	Use intrinsic sympathomimetic activity agents for those with bradycardia who must receive β-blockers.
	Penbutolol	10–40	1	Acebutolol is cardioselective.	
	Pindolol	10–40	2		

Class	Drug	Dosage range	Frequency	Mechanism of action	Comments
Angiotensin-converting enzyme inhibitors (ACEIs)	Benzapril	10–40	1	Block formation of angiotensin II by cleaving angiotensin I thereafter promoting vasodilation and reducing the circulation of aldosterone that results in decreased sodium and water retention. They also increase bradykinin and vasodilatory prostaglandins.	Diuretic doses should be reduced or discontinued before starting angiotensin-converting enzyme inhibitors whenever possible to prevent excessive hypotension. May cause hyperkalemia in patients with renal impairment or in those receiving potassium-sparing agents. Can cause acute renal failure in patients with severe bilateral renal artery stenosis or severe stenosis in artery in a solitary kidney.
	Captopril	25–100	2		
	Enalapril	5–20	1–2		
	Fosinopril	10–40	1		
	Lisinopril	10–40	1		
	Moexipril	7.5–30	1		
	Perindopril	4–8	1		
	Quinapril	10–80	1		
	Ramipril	2.5–2.0	1		
	Trandolapril	1–4	1		
Angiotensin II receptor blockers	Candesartan	8–32	1	Blocks the angiotensin II receptor thus inhibiting the action of angiotensin II as noted previously. Bradykinin levels are not altered so there is lower incidence of an associated dry cough than with angiotensin-converting enzyme inhibitors.	See angiotensin-converting enzyme inhibitors.
	Eprosartan	400–800	1–2		
	Irbesartan	150–300	1		
	Losartan	25–100	1–2		
	Olmesartan	20–40	1		
	Telmisartan	20–80	1		
	Valsartan	80–320	1–2		
Calcium channel blockers	Amlodipine	2.5–10	1	Block inward movement of calcium ion across cell membranes and cause smooth muscle relaxation.	Dihydropyridines—more potent peripheral vasodilators than other calcium channel blockers and, as such, may cause more dizziness, headache, flushing, peripheral edema, and tachycardia. All can reduce sinus rate and produce heart block, especially in combination with other antihypertensives.
	Diltiazem (Sutters, 2015)				
	*Cardizem SR®	180–360	1		
	*Cardizem CD®	180–360	1		
	*Dilacor XR®	180–480	1		
	*Tiazac SA®	180–540	1		
	Felodipine	2.5–2.0	1		
	Isradipine	2.5–5	2		
	Nicardipine	20–40	2		
	Nicardipine SR	30–60	2		
	Nifedipine XL	30–120	2		
	Nisoldipine	17–34	1		
	Verapamil (long acting and sustained release) (Sutters, 2015)	180–480	1–2		

*"In some patients treated once daily, the antihypertensive effect may diminish toward the end of the dosing interval (trough effect). Blood pressure (BP) should be measured just prior to dosing to determine if satisfactory BP control is obtained" (USDHHS, 2004, p. 11).

Data from James, P. A., Oparil, S., Carter, B. L., Cushman, W. C., Dennison-Himmelfarb, C., Handler, J., et al. (2014). 2014 evidence-based guidelines for the management of high blood pressure in adults: Report from the panel members appointed to the Eighth Joint National Committee (JNC 8). *JAMA, 311*(5), 507–520. doi: 10.1001/jama.2013.284427; Sutters, M. (2015). Chapter 11: Systemic hypertension. In M. A. Papadakis, S. McPhee, & M. W. Rabow (Eds.), *Current medical diagnosis and treatment* (54th ed.). New York: McGraw-Hill Education.

iii. African Americans and Asians have a three to four times higher risk of developing angioedema and more cough associated with the use of angiotensin-converting enzyme inhibitors than whites (USDHHS7, 2004).

2. General treatment guidelines.

a. Consider first of all that most patients will require more than one drug to achieve good BP control (Weber et al., 2014).

b. In the general non-Black population, including those with diabetes, initial pharmacologic treatment should include a thiazide-type diuretic, CCB, ACEI, or angiotensin receptor blocker (ARB) (James et al., 2014)

c. In the general Black population, including those with diabetes, initial pharmacologic antihypertensive treatment should include a thiazide-type diuretic or CCB (James et al., 2014)

d. If goal BP is not reached within a month of treatment, add another agent from (a) or (b). Continue to assess BP regularly and adjust treatment regimen to desired BP goal.

e. If goal BP is not reached with two drugs, add a third from this list (CCB, ACEI, ARB, or thiazide diuretic). Note: Do not use an ACEI and ARB in same patient.

f. If goal BP is not reached with titration of drugs from this list due to a contraindication or the need to use more than three drugs, other antihypertensive medications (from other classes) may be used.

g. Consider referral to a hypertensive specialist if goal BP is not reached using four medications and after a careful review of patient's compliance with medication and lifestyle modifications. (James et al., 2014)

h. Simplify the regimen to once daily dosing if possible for greater adherence.

i. In some patients on once-daily dosing, there may be a trough effect: waning of effectiveness of medications at the end of dosing interval. Therefore, it is best to measure the BP just before the next dose to determine the need for dosage adjustment (USDHHS, 2004).

j. In stage 2 HTN, consider starting therapy with two drugs, either as separate prescriptions or in fixed-dose combinations, because this increases the likelihood of reaching BP goal more promptly than with one agent (USDHHS, 2004).

C. Patient education

It is essential that this be done in the language in which the patient is fluent (oral and written) and at a reading level appropriate to patient's education. When in doubt, aim at a sixth grade or lower level of reading.

1. Provide oral and written information on cardiovascular risk factors associated with HTN and long-term prognosis of HTN if untreated.

2. Elicit the patient's concerns regarding the diagnosis, including his or her acceptance of the diagnosis.

3. Provide the patient with a written copy of his or her BP reading at each visit. If possible provide a wallet card that contains multiple readings.

4. Come to a mutual agreement with the patient on BP goal.

5. Provide specific, preferably written, information on lifestyle modifications that you are recommending for this patient.

6. Be sure to underscore the importance of the need to continue treatment, most likely for their lifetime. Emphasize "control does not mean cure" (USDHHS, 2004, p. 62)

7. Explain that most individuals with HTN are usually asymptomatic, so the patient will not usually be able to tell if the BP is elevated or not based on his or her symptoms.

8. Have the patient repeat his or her understanding of treatment regimen before the end of the visit.

9. Include in the patient education cautions regarding use of cold preparations and over-the-counter analgesics (e.g., pseudoephedrine, nonsteroidal anti-inflammatory drugs, respectively).

10. Encourage the use of validated home BP-monitoring devices for interested and able patients, especially those with refractory HTN.

D. Follow-up and monitoring

1. If treating initially with lifestyle modifications alone, have the patient follow up in 3 months to assess both effectiveness on BP and the patient's ability to carry through lifestyle changes.

2. After initiating antihypertensive drug therapy, have the patient return in 1 month for a BP check and review of adverse or other effects of medications.

3. Continue follow-up visits at 1- to 3-month intervals until BP goal is achieved.

4. If stage 2 HTN or with the presence of other comorbid conditions, such as diabetes or chronic kidney disease, more frequent visits may be warranted.

5. Once the BP is stable, schedule visits at 3- to 6-month intervals.

6. Laboratory follow-up
   a. Check serum electrolytes 2–4 weeks after starting a diuretic.
   b. Check serum potassium and creatinine 2–4 weeks after starting an angiotensin-converting enzyme inhibitor.
   c. Check serum electrolytes and creatinine at least annually for all patients on antihypertensive medications.

7. Have the patient bring in all medications to each follow-up visit.

8. Failure to reach target BP goal
   a. Consider nonadherence to medication or lifestyle recommendations, including excessive sodium intake or increased alcohol intake.
   b. Consider use of over-the-counter medications or street drugs.
   c. Evaluate for high levels of stress or psychiatric conditions that can affect BP, such as anxiety disorders and panic disorder.
   d. Reconsider secondary causes for HTN.
   e. Always maintain an attitude of empathetic concern and genuine interest in developing the best possible, workable plan for the patient, as a partner in treatment.

REFERENCES

American Heart Association (2014). .*The American Heart Association's diet and lifestyle recommendations*. Retrieved from www.heart.org/HEARTORG/GettingHealthy/NutritionCenter/HealthyEating/The-American-Heart-Associations-Diet-and-Lifestyle-Recommendations_UCM_305855_Article.jsp.

Eckel, R. H., Jakicic, J. M., Ard, J. D., de Jesus, J. M., Houston Miller, N., Hubbard, V. S., et al. (2013). 2013 AHA/ACC guideline on lifestyle management to reduce cardiovascular risk: A report of the American College of Cardiology/American Heart Association Task Force on Practice Guidelines. *Circulation, 129*(25, Suppl. 2), S76–S99. doi:10.1161/01.cir.0000437740.48606.d1.

Heller, M. (2015). *The DASH diet eating plan*. Retrieved from http://dashdiet.org/default.asp.

James, P. A., Oparil, S., Carter, B. L., Cushman, W. C., Dennison-Himmelfarb, C., Handler, J., et al. (2014). 2014 evidence-based guidelines for the management of high blood pressure in adults: Report from the panel members appointed to the Eighth Joint National Committee (JNC 8). *JAMA, 311*(5), 507–520. doi: 10.1001/jama.2013.284427.

Nwanko, T., Yoon, S. S., Bury, V., & Gu, Q. (2013) *Hypertension among adults in the United States: National Health and Nutrition Examination Survey, 2011–2012* (NCHS data brief, no. 133). Hyattsville, MD: Centers for Disease Control and Prevention, National Center for Health Statistics. Retrieved from www.cdc.gov/nchs/data/databriefs/db133.htm. Ram, C. V. (2014). Hypertension guidelines in need of guidance. *Journal of Clinical Hypertension, 16*(4), 251–254. doi: 10.1111/jch.12306.

Sutters, M. (2015). Chapter 11: Systemic hypertension. In M. A., Papadakis, S., McPhee, & M. W., Rabow (Eds.), *Current medical diagnosis and treatment* (54th ed.). New York: McGraw-Hill Education.

The ALLHAT Officers and Coordinators for the ALLHAT Collaborative Research Group. (2002). Major outcomes in high-risk hypertensive patients randomized to angiotensin-converting enzyme inhibitor or calcium channel blocker vs diuretic: The Antihypertensive and Lipid-Lowering Treatment to Prevent Heart Attack Trial (ALLHAT). *The Journal of the American Medical Association, 288* (23), 2981–2997.

U.S. Department of Health and Human Services, U.S. Food and Drug Administration. (2002). Summary for The Intercure Ltd. RESPeRATE. Retrieved from http://www.accessdata.fda.gov/cdrh_docs/pdf2/k020399.pdf.

U.S. Department of Health and Human Services. (2004). *Seventh report of the Joint National Committee on Prevention, Detection, Evaluation, and Treatment of High Blood Pressure (JNC 7)* (NIH Publication no. 0405230). Washington, DC: National Institutes of Health, National Heart, Lung, and Blood Institute, National High Blood Pressure Education Program, U.S. Department of Health and Human Services. Retrieved from http://www.nhlbi.nih.gov/guidelines/hypertension/jnc7full.htm.

Weber, M. A., Schriffin, E. L., White, W. B., Mann, S., Lindholm, L. H., Kenerson, J. G., et al. (2014). Clinical practice guidelines for the management of hypertension in the community: A statement by the American Society of Hypertension and the International Society of Hypertension. *Journal of Clinical Hypertension, 16*(1), 14–26. doi: 10.1111/jch.12237

World Health Organization. (2013). A global brief on hypertension: Silent killer, global public health crisis (Document no. WHO/DCO/WHD/2013.2). Retrieved from www.who.int/cardiovascular_diseases/publications/global_brief_hypertension/en/.

INTIMATE PARTNER VIOLENCE (DOMESTIC VIOLENCE)

Rosalind De Lisser, Deborah Johnson, JoAnne Saxe, and Cecily Reeves

CHAPTER 61

I. Introduction and general background

Intimate partner violence (IPV) is a serious, preventable public health problem that affects millions of Americans (Centers for Disease Control and Prevention [CDC], 2015b). In the United States, IPV is also commonly referred to as domestic violence, and can occur among heterosexual or same sex partners, either current or former, and does not require sexual intimacy, legal ties, or even cohabitation (CDC, 2015b). The term IPV also encompasses dating violence, defined as violence committed by a person who is or has been in a social relationship of a romantic or intimate nature with the victim (U.S. Department of Health & Human Services, 2009). IPV involves a "pattern of abusive behavior" with the intention to intimidate, control, and instill fear in the victim (U.S. Department of Justice [USDOJ], 2015). Victims, survivors who withstand the violence, can be male or female, educated or illiterate, able bodied or disabled, wealthy or poor, and any age (National Center for Victims of Crime, 2008a). They can be of any racial, ethnic, or cultural background, of any sexual orientation, and of any immigration/citizenship status; in fact, disclosure of IPV is often complicated for individuals who experience oppression or have fear of authority.

According to the 2009 California Penal Code Handbook (Section 1M.6, 137W, 242, 243, 273.5), acts of partner abuse include those that intentionally or recklessly cause, or attempt to cause, bodily injury or that place another person in reasonable apprehension of imminent serious bodily injury. IPV is considered by many as a prelude to murder (Ferguson, 2007; Strack & Gwinn, 2011). For this reason, clinicians play an important role in identifying indications of abuse as well as risk factors that indicate that the abuse will reoccur or heighten.

A. Definition and overview

The U.S. Department of Justice (2015) defines IPV in terms of the following five categories:

1. *Physical abuse* is defined as acts of hitting, slapping, shoving, grabbing, biting, etc. and also includes denying a partner medical care or forcing alcohol or drugs upon him or her.

2. *Sexual abuse* is coercing or attempting to coerce any sexual contact or behavior without consent, marital rape, forcing sex after physical violence, treating one in a sexually demeaning manner, and birth-control sabotage.

3. *Emotional abuse* involves undermining an individual's sense of self-worth, name calling, diminishing one's abilities, or damaging one's relationship with his/her children.

4. *Economic abuse* is defined as making or attempting to make an individual financially dependent by controlling or withholding one's access to money or forbidding attendance at school or employment.

5. *Psychological abuse* is different from emotional abuse as it involves causing fear by intimidation through threats to harm self, partner, children, or other individuals/pets/property involved in the victim's life. It also involves forcing isolation from one's community or threatening the victim's immigration status or custody of his/her children.

These categories of IPV are not mutually exclusive; they often present together as a complex ongoing pattern of abuse. Although all states have legislation that defines IPV, those definitions vary across states. IPV constitutes the willful intimidation, assault, battery, sexual assault, or other abusive behavior perpetrated by one family member, household member, or intimate partner against another (National Center for Victims of Crime, 2008a). In most state laws addressing IPV, the relationship necessary for a charge of domestic assault or abuse generally includes a spouse, former spouse, persons currently residing together or those that have within the previous year, or persons who share a common child. In addition, as of 2007, most states provide some level of statutory protection for victims of dating violence (National Center for Victims of Crime, 2008a).

B. Prevalence and incidence

In 2010 the Centers for Disease Control and Prevention's National Center for Injury Prevention and Control, in collaboration with the National Institutes of Justice and the Department of Defense, developed a telephone survey, the National Intimate Partner and Sexual Violence Survey (NISVS). The NISVS began collecting ongoing population-based surveillance data, generating accurate and reliable incidence and prevalence estimates for intimate partner violence, sexual violence, dating violence, and stalking victimization (CDC, 2015a). The first report, released in 2014, stated that 20 people per minute are victims of physical violence by an intimate partner in the United States. The National Intimate Partner and Sexual Violence Survey data are summarized next.

1. Sexual Violence by Any Perpetrator

   One in 5 women or 18.3% of all women in the United States and 1 in 71 men or 1.4% of all men in the United States have been raped at some time in their lives. This includes full and attempted forced penetration and drug/alcohol facilitated violations.

2. Stalking Victimization by Any Perpetrator

   One in 6 women or 16.6% and 1 in 19 men or 5.2% report stalking victimization in the United States.

Stalking victimization results in victims feeling fearful that they or someone close to them will be harmed or killed by the stalker; 66% of female victims of stalking were stalked by a current or former partner, and 41% of male victims were stalked by a partner.

3. Violence by an Intimate Partner

   One in 3 women (35.6%) and 1 in 4 men (28.5%) in the United States have experienced rape or violence and/or stalking by their intimate partner during their lifetime. Of those victims 1 in 4 women (24.3%) and 1 in 7 men (13.8%) have experienced severe violence, characterized by being hit by a fist or other object, beaten, or slammed against something hard. The survey also reports that half of all men and women have experienced psychological aggression. Of all victims of intimate partner violence, 69% of females and 53% of males experienced the first episode before the age of 25.

4. Violence by an Intimate Partner Experienced by Race/Ethnicity (**Table 61-1**)

C. Consequences

Although the severity of IPV can vary, the type of IPV that is repetitive and prolonged has been most closely associated with negative health sequelae (Humphreys &

TABLE 61-1 National Intimate Partner and Sexual Violence Survey: Victimization by Race/Ethnicity

Race/Ethnicity	U.S. Total	Black Non-Hispanic	White Non-Hispanic	Hispanic	American Indian or Alaska Native	Multiracial Non-Hispanic	Asian/Pacific Islander
Event	% per total U.S. population						
Intimate Partner Violence (IPV), lifetime: WOMEN	31.5%	41.2%	30.5%	29.7%	51.7%	51.3%	15.3%
IPV, lifetime: MEN	27.5%	36.3%	26.6%	27.1%	43.0%	39.3%	11.5%
IPV Rape Victimization during lifetime: WOMEN	8.8%	8.8%	9.6%	6.2%	*	11.4%	*
IPV Rape Victimization during lifetime: MEN	0.5%	*	*	*	*	*	*
IPV Sexual Violence other than rape: WOMEN	15.8%	17.4%	17.1%	9.9%	*	26.8%	*
IPV Sexual Violence other than rape: MEN	9.5%	24.4%	22.2%	26.6%	24.5%	39.5%	15.8%
IPV Stalking Victimization, lifetime: WOMEN	**	9.5%	9.9%	6.8%	*	13.3%	*
IPV Stalking Victimization, lifetime: MEN	**	*	1.7%	*	*	*	*

* No data as not statistically reliable due to small case count.

** Data not available.

Data from Breiding, M. J., Smith, S. G., Basile, K. C., et al. (2014). Prevalence and Characteristics of Sexual Violence, Stalking, and Intimate Partner Violence Victimization—National Intimate Partner and Sexual Violence Survey, United States, 2011. *MMWR, 63*(SS08), 1–18. Retrieved from http://www.cdc.gov/mmwr/preview/mmwrhtml/ss6308a1.htm#Table1

Campbell, 2010). This violence results in nearly 2 million injuries and nearly 1,300 deaths. Of the IPV injuries, more than 555,000 require attention by a healthcare provider, and more than 145,000 are serious enough to warrant hospitalization for 1 or more nights. In 2008, nearly 45% of female homicide victims were killed by intimate partners (Bureau of Justice Statistics, 2009b). Of note, IPV is the leading cause of premature death from homicide and injury among African American women between the ages of 15 and 24 years (Rennison & Welchans, 2002). As noted in the NISVS, 24.3% of women and 13.8% of men in the United States have been a victim of *severe* physical violence and nearly 15% of women and 4% of men have been injured as a result (Breiding et al., 2014). Research suggests that the risk of suffering from six or more chronic physical symptoms increases with the number of forms of violence experienced, even when the last episode was over 30 years ago (Nicolaidis, Curry, McFarland, & Gerrity, 2004). IPV costs in the United States are estimated at $12.6 billion on an annual basis, 0.1% of the gross domestic product (Waters et al., 2004). IPV also results in more than 18.5 million mental healthcare visits each year and 13.6 million days of lost productivity from paid work and household chores among IPV survivors and the value of IPV murder victims' expected lifetime earnings (National Center for Injury Prevention and Control, 2003).

In addition to the injuries inflicted during violent episodes, physical and psychological abuses are linked to a number of adverse health effects. These include arthritis; chronic neck or back pain; migraine or other types of headache; sexually transmitted infections (including HIV); chronic pelvic pain; peptic ulcers; irritable bowel syndrome; and frequent indigestion, diarrhea, or constipation (Coker, Smith, Bethea, King, & McKeown, 2000). Psychological consequences include posttraumatic stress disorder, depression, substance abuse, and suicidal behaviors (Ellsberg, Jansen, Heise, Watts, & Garcia-Moreno,

2008). Six percent of all pregnant women are battered. Pregnancy complications, including low weight gain, anemia, infections, and first- and second-trimester bleeding, are significantly higher for abused women, as are maternal rates of depression, suicide attempts, and substance abuse (Parker, McFarlane, & Soeken, 1994).

Health behaviors are also significantly affected by IPV and research demonstrates that the more severe the violence the more impaired the health behaviors become, including engaging in high-risk sexual behavior, using harmful substances, and unhealthy diet-related behaviors, all resulting in overuse of the health services (Heise & Garcia-Moreno, 2002).

D. Risk factors

Factors that should heighten the clinician's index of suspicion regarding the possibility of IPV include medical records indicating repeated visits or previous injuries, a history of IPV or a history with inconsistent descriptions of injuries, and a past history of suicide attempts. Vague and nonspecific responses to questions with a history of anxiety, depression, sleeplessness, fatigue, or chronic somatic complaints may indicate intrafamilial crisis. Abuse is a frequent precipitant of suicide attempts, and those who attempt suicide are likely to have a history of IPV (Ellsberg et al., 2008).

E. Special populations

Special populations at increased risk of IPV include poor or homeless individuals; teenagers; pregnant or immigrant women; those with chronic illnesses (HIV) or disabilities; lesbian, gay, bisexual, and transgender individuals; and the elderly. Risks to note in these special populations and additional resources are highlighted in (**Table 61-2**). Clinicians should be aware of agencies or resources in the area that do focused work with these special populations. Clinicians should seek out additional information and culturally competent training to provide best practice care to these individuals.

TABLE 61-2 Special IPV Risk Populations

Risk	Data	Sources
Chronic illness (HIV)	The IPV risk for women with HIV may be as high as 67%, a rate three to four times greater than among HIV-negative women.	Brief, Vielhauer, & Keane, 2006; Cobb, 2008; Gielen et al., 2007
	HIV-positive women seem to experience IPV at rates comparable to HIV-negative women from the same underlying populations; however, their abuse seems to be more frequent and more severe.	
Individuals with disabilities	Those with disabilities and deaf women have an increased risk of both typical and unique forms of violence. The greater the degree of cognitive impairment, the greater the risk for victimization and abuse.	Barrett, O'Day, Roche, & Carlson, 2009; Curry, Powers, Oschwald, & Saxton, 2004

TABLE 61-2 Special IPV Risk Populations *(Continued)*

Risk	Data	Sources
Immigrant women	More difficult for these women to seek or obtain help because of abusive partners using immigration status against her, threatening deportation. Language barriers, isolation, and a lack of familiarity with the United States social services system and legal rights. Fear that if she reports violence she will be treated with insensitivity, hostility, or discrimination by authorities. Low level of awareness about IPV among immigrants or refugees. Not seen as a problem in their community. May be recognized, but only as a family or private issue. Community members may condone IPV or do not consider various abusive or controlling acts to be IPV.	Kulwicki & Miller, 1999; Moracco, Hilton, Hodges, & Frasier, 2005; Murdaugh, Hunt, Sowell, & Santana, 2004; Runner, Yoshihama, & Novick, 2009; Shiu-Thornton, Senturia, & Sullivan, 2005; Yoshihama, 2008
Lesbian, gay, bisexual, or transgender individuals	Lifetime prevalence of IPV for women: Lesbian 43.8%, bisexual 61.1%, heterosexual 35.0%. Lifetime prevalence of IPV for men: Gay 26.0%, bisexual 37.3%, heterosexual 29.0%. Transgender: estimated 50% of transgender individuals report lifetime sexual violence Lesbian, gay, bisexual, or transgender individuals who are incarcerated are sexually assaulted at a rate 15 times higher than that of the general inmate population.	FORGE, 2012; Walters, Chen, & Breiding, 2013
Poor or homeless	IPV is the primary cause of family homelessness in 28% of cities surveyed across the United States, and 15% of homeless persons were victims of IPV. Between 25% and 50% of homeless families have lost their homes as a result of intimate partner abuse. Homelessness and poverty *significantly* increase a child's exposure to parental IPV. Women living in disadvantaged neighborhoods are more than twice as likely to be the victims of IPV as women in more affluent neighborhoods.	U.S. Conference of Mayors, 2008; Institute for Children and Poverty, 2010
Pregnant women	IPV in women of childbearing age may include reproductive coercion, sabotaged contraception, and forced pregnancy continuation or abortion, and may lead to gynecological disorders, pregnancy complications, unintended pregnancy, and sexually transmitted infections, including human immunodeficiency virus (HIV). Other adverse outcomes correlating with IPV include poor pregnancy weight gain, infection, anemia, tobacco use, stillbirth, pelvic fracture, placental abruption, fetal injury, preterm delivery, and low birth weight. The severity of violence may escalate during pregnancy or the postpartum period, and homicide has been reported as a leading cause of maternal mortality, with the majority perpetrated by a current or former intimate partner. Abused women were twice as likely to begin prenatal care during the third trimester and more likely to abuse substances before and during pregnancy.	Bureau of Justice Statistics, 2009a; Cha & Masho, 2014; Chamberlain, &. Levenson, 2013; Cheng & Horon, 2010; Madkour, Xie, & Harville, 2014; Silverman et al., 2011; World Health Organization, 2013

(continues)

TABLE 61-2 Special IPV Risk Populations *(Continued)*

Risk	Data	Sources
Teenagers	The 2013 Youth Risk Behavior Surveillance reports a prevalence of physical dating violence between 13% (female) and 7.4% (male) among youth in grades 9 through 12. The prevalence of youth reporting sexual dating violence was 14.4% (female) and 6.2% (male).	CDC, 2014b; Foshee, Reyes, Gottfredson, Chang, & Ennett, 2013; Keenan-Miller, Hammen, & Brennan, 2007; Miller et al., 2013; Silverman et al., 2011; Stöckl, March, Pallitto, & Garcia-Moreno, 2014; Vagi, Rothman, Latzman, Tharp Hall, & Breiding, 2013
	Among adult victims of rape, physical violence, and/or stalking by an intimate partner, 22% of females and 15% of males report their first experience of partner violence occurred between 11 and 17 years of age.	
	When youth responses were evaluated based on reported race, Hispanic females (13.6/12.9%) followed by white females (12.9/14.6%) and black males (8.2/8.9%) followed by Hispanic males (7.0/6.7%) reported the highest incidence of both physical and sexual dating violence, respectively.	
	Numerous risk factors have been correlated with adolescent dating violence, ranging from individual (substance use, depression, anxiety, age/gender, race/ethnicity, personal violence history, acceptance of violent behavior) to relationship level (aversive family communication, harsh parenting, hostile friendships, low parental monitoring). Protective factors include high empathy, high grade point average, high verbal IQ, positive relationship with mother, and attachment to school. Detrimental consequences may include increased alcohol, cigarette, and marijuana use; increased internalizing; and decreased number of close friends.	

F. Screening

The U.S. Preventive Services Task Force (USPSTF) now recommends IPV screening and has found benefits of detection and early intervention to reduce violence and improve health outcomes in women of childbearing age (Moyer, 2013). The USPSTF, however, has determined that current evidence is insufficient to assess the balance between the benefits and harms of screening for IPV in elderly or vulnerable adult populations (USPSTF, 2013). There are no current recommendations regarding screening men for IPV.

II. **The focused IPV assessment and database** (may include but is not limited to)

A. Subjective

Although many individuals may not bring up the subject of abuse on their own, many will discuss it in a private, confidential setting when asked simple, direct, nonjudgmental questions. See **Table 61-3** for approaches to phrasing questions. A variety of tools can be used to accurately measure victimization and offer the clinician specific scales in the areas of physical, sexual, psychological, and emotional victimization and stalking

to guide their inquiries (Basile, Hertz, & Back, 2007; Thompson, Basile, Hertz, & Sitterle, 2006).

1. When IPV is identified:

a. It is important to determine the identity of the person allegedly inflicting the injuries and document the circumstances surrounding the event, any past history of abuse, the nature of the injuries, and use of any threats or weapons. Whenever possible, use the patient's exact words and quotation marks.

b. Additional history related to other health-risk behaviors (e.g., alcohol or drug use, tobacco) and chronic conditions, such as sleep problems, depression, and eating disorders, should be elicited. These conditions, along with currently being the victim of IPV, are predictors of the women's physical and psychological health (Svavarsdottir & Orlygsdottir, 2009).

B. Objective

Perform a complete head-to-toe examination or focused evaluation as indicated by history or report of injuries. Document the character and extent of all physical injuries, including areas of pain and tenderness, even if there is as yet no obvious bruising or injury. It is recommended to use photos or drawings whenever possible.

Additional components of the physical examination are listed in **Table 61-4**.

TABLE 61-3 Screening History Questions

USPSTF recommends use of a screening scale with women of reproductive age, elderly, and vulnerable. Those with the highest levels of sensitivity and specificity for identifying IPV are Hurt, Insult, Threaten, Scream (HITS; English and Spanish versions); Ongoing Abuse Screen/Ongoing Violence Assessment Tool (OAS/OVAT); Slapped, Threatened, and Throw (STaT); Humiliation, Afraid, Rape, Kick (HARK); Modified Childhood Trauma Questionnaire–Short Form (CTQ-SF); and Woman Abuse Screen Tool (WAST) (Rabin, Jennings, Campbell, & Bair-Merritt, 2009).

HITS

How often does your partner: (1) Physically hurt you? (2) Insult you or talk down to you? (3) Threaten you with harm? (4) Scream or curse at you?

WAST

(1) In general, how would you describe your relationship—a lot of tension, some tension, no tension? (2) Do you and your partner work out arguments with great difficulty, some difficulty, or no difficulty? (#3–#7 response options: often, sometimes, never) (3) Do arguments ever result in you feeling down or bad about yourself? (4) Do arguments ever result in hitting, kicking, or pushing? (5) Do you ever feel frightened by what your partner says or does? (6) Has your partner ever abused you physically? (7) Has your partner ever abused you emotionally? (8) Has your partner ever abused you sexually?

For women of reproductive age, select a scale for physical/sexual, psychological–emotional, stalking screening based on evidence of sensitivity and specificity for identifying IPV as well as utility within the clinical setting. The clinician must remain alert to clinical clues of IPV, abuse, and neglect of all populations, inclusive of elderly and vulnerable adults, males, and prepubescent females and assess further when indicated on clinical grounds.

Phrasing the Interview Questions

1. Begin with a framing statement such as "We've started talking to all of our patients about safe and healthy relationships because it can have such a large impact on your health" (Chamberlain & Levenson, 2013).

2. Advise patient of the limits of confidentiality, based on state mandates. For example, "Before we get started, I want you to know that everything here is confidential, meaning that I won't discuss what is said unless you tell me that… (insert the laws in your state about what is necessary to disclose)."

3. Sample questions:

Phrasing Questions: The Use of One of the Victimization Scales for Physical–Sexual, Psychological–Emotional, Stalking.

1. "Are you in a relationship in which you have been physically hurt or threatened by your partner? Have you ever been in such a relationship?"

2. "Has your partner ever destroyed things that you cared about? Ever threatened or abused your children? Ever forced you to have sex when you didn't want to?"

3. "What happens when you and your partner disagree or fight? Do you ever feel afraid of your partner?"

4. "Has your partner ever prevented you from leaving the house, seeking friends, getting a job, or continuing your education?"

5. "If your partner uses alcohol or drugs, is s/he ever physically or verbally abusive to you when using?"

6. "Do you have guns or other weapons in your home? If so, has your partner ever threatened to use them?"

TABLE 61-4 Physical Examination

Components of the Physical Examination

Assess general appearance: Level of distress

Vital signs

Other physical examination data:

1. Look carefully for multiple abrasions and contusions to different anatomic sites and multiple injuries in various stages of healing.

2. Most accidents involve the extremities, whereas IPV injuries often involve the face, neck, chest, breasts, abdomen, genitalia, or anus.

Mental status examination: Evaluate mood, orientation, thought processes, and judgment.

III. Assessment

Evaluate the extent of any injuries and the need for immediate medical intervention. See **Table 61-5** for additional components of the assessment. Assess the need for mandatory reporting as cited in the respective state's penal codes (Durborow, Lizdas, O'Flaherty, & Marjavi, 2010). Legal requirement of health professionals to report suspected adult abuse to law enforcement is currently implemented in 16 states and remains a controversial issue. Victims report greater access to legal protection without the responsibility to report abuse themselves, a reduced sense of aloneness and guilt, teaching partners the seriousness of abuse, documentation of the incident and potentially positive interaction with police. However, concerns such as the risk of retaliation, fear of lost custody of their children, anxiety induced by required interactions with a social worker or other government authorities, being victimized by the health system, financial responsibility for the intimate partner violence report, as well as loss of autonomy and confidentiality are reportedly more significant than the benefits (World Health Organization, 2013). Although mandatory reporting is thought by some

TABLE 61-5 Assessment

Components of the Assessment

Determine the diagnosis (not mutually exclusive).

1. History of prior IPV.
2. Recent IPV without observable injury.
3. Current history of IPV with observable injury.
    a. Report as required by state regulations.

Determine the ICD (International Classification of Diseases) codes for IPV, which are divided into four categories (Rudman, 2000).

1. Adult maltreatment and abuse (995-81).
2. The primary diagnosis (underlying reason for admittance).
3. Modifier codes that provide details (E-codes).
4. History codes that provide information on previous incidents (V-codes).

With ICD-10 implementation, code 995 will be replaced with T74 (confirmed) and T76 (suspected) and the coding will include:

    a. Suspected or Confirmed
    b. Encounter type (Initial encounter, Subsequent encounter, Sequela encounter) (Bryant, 2014)

Assess for suicidal or homicidal ideation.

Evaluate the safety of the patient and family members and children.

Identify any immediate risk and need for emergency housing, legal, or social service consultations.

Assess social support systems.

Determine ongoing risk of IPV.

Physical abuse ranking scale. More than five affirmatives indicate high danger (Wadman & Foral, 2007).

1. Throwing things, punching the wall—lower risk
2. Pushing, shoving, grabbing, throwing things
3. Slapping with an open hand
4. Kicking, biting
5. Hitting with closed fists
6. Attempted strangulation
7. Beating up, pinning to the wall or floor, repeated
8. Threatening with a weapon
9. Assault with a weapon—higher risk

authorities to help the victim and perpetrator to receive treatment, many health professionals are concerned that victims may be discouraged from disclosing information based on compromised provider–patient confidentiality and individual autonomy. Other concerns include the expense in time and resources and the risk of retaliation or escalation in partner violence in the event of unsuccessful prosecutions (American College of Emergency Physicians, 2014; Feder, Wathen, & MacMillan, 2013).

Whether or not forensic requirements of the criminal justice system require mandated reporting, appropriate management of the sexually assaulted patient is built upon therapeutic communication and requires the clinician to address the medical and emotional needs of the patient within the context of patient-centered care. Providers must be informed of the laws governing mandated reporting in their regions. A summary of the *Professions Mandated to Report* can be found at www.ncsl.org/research/human-services/child-abuse-and-neglect-reporting-statutes.aspx#1 (Child Welfare Information Gateway, 2014).

IV. Goals of clinical management

The goals in managing victims of IPV include consistent screening through thoughtful inquiry in a safe and confidential environment, identifying immediate injury and safety risks, appropriate reporting and referral, and the provision of information and support. Being aware of immigration concerns and cultural or ethnic differences is an important element in patient care. One of the earliest efforts to systematically address IPV in the clinical environment was the development of RADAR, which remains commonly used in practice. RADAR summarizes action steps that the clinician can use to increase comfort and ability recognize and treat victims of IPV (Harwell et al., 1998)

- **R**emember to routinely inquire about partner violence
- **A**sk directly about violence (see questions in Table 61-3), always in a private area
- **D**ocument findings of suspected or reported partner violence in the patient's chart
- **A**ssess patient safety (lethality or abuse scales)
- **R**espond, review patient options, and refer (Institute for Safe Families, 2002).

V. Plan

A. Diagnostic testing

Obtain radiographs, computed tomography, or magnetic resonance imaging based on the extent of injury.

B. Management (includes treatment, consultation, referral, and follow-up care)

Interventions designed to decrease health-risk behaviors, treat chronic health conditions or illnesses, and offer best practice first response to women who are victims of IPV can be offered to reduce the short- and long-term effects of violence on their physical and psychological health (Svavarsdottir & Orlygsdottir, 2009).

Patient management includes treatment, consultation, referral, and follow-up care. In the event there is a history of recent sexual assault (within 72 hours), it is important to refer the patient to the sexual assault response team or emergency department. In most instances law enforcement involvement is necessary to authorize a forensic examination and a report is filed both via telecommunications and in writing to the respective authorities. The clinician will follow the reporting guidelines as cited in the respective state's penal codes.

C. Client/patient education

Priority educational areas include the nature of IPV and the identification of emergency strategies. A personalized safety plan for patients can be found at www.domesticviolence.org/personalized-safety-plan/

VI. Self-management resources and tools

A. Educational resources and support

1. The clinician should be prepared to provide patient education brochures or frequently asked questions documents and to direct the patient to appropriate community agencies and support groups for victims of domestic violence (e.g., local shelters), statewide coalitions and helplines (e.g., Jane Doe in Massachusetts, APIADV in San Francisco, CA), and national resources, such as the National Domestic Violence Hotline (1-800-799-SAFE, 1-800-799-7233, or www.thehotline.org), National Dating Abuse Helpline and Love Is Respect (1-866-331-9474, text 77054, or www.loveisrespect.org), or the National Sexual Assault Hotline (1-800-656-HOPE or 1-800-656-4673).

B. Resources for reducing stigma and increasing awareness of domestic violence

1. Resources for reducing stigma and increasing awareness of domestic violence can be found at www.nomore.org. Social media and campaign efforts may be appropriate for use within the clinic setting and to promote open disclosure with anticipatory guidance.

C. Other services and resources

1. National Sexual Violence Resource Center (www.nsvrc.org)

2. National Center for Victims of Crime's Stalking Resource Center (www.victimsofcrime.org/our-programs/stalking-resource-center)

3. National Coalition of Anti-Violence Programs (www.avp.org/about-avp/coalitions-a-collaborations/82-national-coalition-of-anti-violence-programs)

4. National Online Resource Center on Violence Against Women (www.vawnet.org/)

5. Rape, Abuse, and Incest National Network (www.rainn.org), hotline at 1-800-656-HOPE

REFERENCES

American College of Emergency Physicians. (2014). *Domestic family violence.* Retrieved from www.acep.org/Clinical—Practice-Management/Domestic-Family-Violence/.

Barrett, K. A., O'Day, B., Roche, A., & Carlson, B. L. (2009). Intimate partner violence, health status, and healthcare access among women with disabilities. *Women's Health Issues, 19*(2), 94–100.

Basile, K. C., Hertz, M. F., & Back, S. E. (2007). *Intimate partner violence and sexual violence victimization assessment instruments for use in healthcare settings* (Ver. 1). Atlanta, GA: Centers for Disease Control and Prevention, National Center for Injury Prevention and Control.

Black, M. C., & Breiding, M. J. (2008). Adverse health conditions and health risk behaviors associated with intimate partner violence—United States, 2005. *Morbidity and Mortality Weekly Report, 57*, 113–118.

Black, M. C., Basile, K. C., Breiding, M. J., Smith, S. G., Walters, M. L., & Merrick, M. T. (2011). *The National Intimate Partner and Sexual Violence Survey (NISVS): 2010 summary report.* Atlanta, GA: National Center for Injury Prevention and Control, Centers for Disease Control and Prevention.

Breiding, M. J., Smith, S. G., Basile, K. C., Walters, M. L., Chen, J., & Merrick, M. T. (2014). Prevalence and characteristics of sexual violence, stalking, and intimate partner violence victimization—National Intimate Partner and Sexual Violence Survey, United States, 2011. *MMWR Surveillance Summaries, 63*(SS08), 1–18.

Brief, D., Vielhauer, M., & Keane, T. (2006). University of California, San Francisco, AIDS Health Project. The interface of HIV, trauma, and posttraumatic stress disorder. *Focus, 21*(4), 1–4.

Bryant, G. (2014). ICD-10 Brings Value to Injury Data Like Domestic Violence. ICD-10 Monitor. Accessed at http://icd10monitor.com/enews/item/1271-icd-10-brings-value-to-injury-data-like-domestic-violence Bureau of Justice Statistics. (2009a). *Domestic violence and sexual assault data resource center.* Retrieved from www.jrsa.org/dvsa-drc/dv-data.shtml

Bureau of Justice Statistics (2009b). *Intimate homicide.* Retrieved from www.bjs.gov/content/pub/pdf/htus8008.pdf.

California Penal Code Handbook 2009. (2008). San Francisco: Matthew Bender & Company LexisNexis.

Centers for Disease Control and Prevention. (2014a). *Understanding teen dating violence.* Retrieved from www.cdc.gov/violenceprevention/intimatepartnerviolence/teen_dating_violence.html.

Centers for Disease Control and Prevention. (2014b). Youth risk behavior surveillance, United States, 2013. *MMWR Surveillance Summaries, 63*(4), 1–168. Retrieved from www.cdc.gov/mmwr/pdf/ss/ss6304.pdf.

Centers for Disease Control and Prevention. (2015a). *The National Intimate Partner and Sexual Violence Survey.* Retrieved from www.cdc.gov/violenceprevention/nisvs/index.html.

Centers for Disease Control and Prevention. (2015b). Intimate Partner Violence Surveillance: Uniform Definitions and Recommended Data Elements. Retrieved from www.cdc.gov/violenceprevention/pdf/intimatepartnerviolence.pdf

Cha, S., & Masho, S. (2014). Intimate partner violence and utilization of prenatal care in the United States. *Journal of Interpersonal Violence, 29*(5), 911–927.

Chamberlain, L., & Levenson, R. (2010). *Reproductive health and partner violence guidelines: An integrated response to intimate partner violence and reproductive coercion.* San Francisco, CA: Family Violence Prevention Fund. Retrieved from www.futureswithoutviolence.org/userfiles/file/HealthCare/Repro_Guide.pdf.

Chamberlain, L., & Levenson, R. (2013). *Addressing intimate partner violence reproductive and sexual coercion: A guide for obstetric, gynecologic, reproductive healthcare settings* (3rd ed.). San Francisco, CA: Futures Without Violence; Washington, DC: American College of Obstetricians and Gynecologists.

Cheng, D., & Horon, I. (2010). Intimate-partner homicide among pregnant and postpartum women. *Obstetrics and Gynecology, 115*(6), 1181–1186.

Child Welfare Information Gateway. (2014). Mandatory reporters of child abuse and neglect. Washington, DC: U.S. Department of Health and Human Services, Children's Bureau. Retrieved from www.ncsl.org/research/human-services/child-abuse-and-neglect-reporting-statutes.aspx#1.

Cobb, A. J. (2008, August 25–28). *The intersection: HIV/AIDS and intimate partner violence.* Paper presented at the Ryan White All-Grantee Meeting, Washington, DC.

Coker, A., Smith, P., Bethea, L., King, M., & McKeown, R. (2000). Physical health consequences of physical and psychological intimate partner violence. *Archives of Family Medicine, 9*, 451–457.

Curry, M. A., Powers, L. E., Oschwald, M., & Saxton, M. (2004). Development and testing of an abuse screening tool for women with disabilities. *Journal of Aggression, Maltreatment and Trauma, 8*(4), 123–141.

Durborow, N., Lizdas, K., O'Flaherty, A., Marjavi, A. (2010). Compendium of state statutes and policies on domestic violence and health care. San Francisco, CA: Family Violence Prevention Fund. Retrieved from www.postandcourier.com/tilldeath/assets/d1-38.pdf.

Ellsberg, M., Jansen, H. A., Heise, L., Watts, C. H., & Garcia-Moreno, C. (2008). Intimate partner violence and women's physical and mental health in the WHO multi-country study on women's health and domestic violence: An observational study. *Lancet, 371*(9619), 1165–1172.

Feder, G., Wathen, N., & MacMillan, H. (2013). An evidence-based response to intimate partner violence: WHO guidelines. *JAMA, 31*(5), 479–480.

Ferguson, E. E. (2007). Domestic violence by another name: Crimes of passion in fin-de-siècle Paris. *Journal of Women's History, 19*(4), 12–34.

FORGE. (2012). Transgender rates of violence. Retrieved from http://forge-forward.org/wp-content/docs/FAQ-10-2012-rates-of-violence.pdf.

Foshee, V., Reyes, H., Gottfredson, N., Chang, L., & Ennett, S. (2013). A longitudinal examination of psychological, behavioral, academic, and relationship consequences of dating abuse victimization among a primarily rural sample of adolescents. *Journal of Adolescent Health, 53*(6): 723–729.

Gielen, A. C., Ghandour, R. M., Burke, J. G., Mahoney, P., McDonnell, K. A., & O'Campo, P. (2007). HIV/AIDS and intimate partner violence: Intersecting women's health issues in the United States. *Trauma, Violence, & Abuse, 8*(2), 178–198.

Harwell, T. S., Casten, R. J., Armstrong, K. A., Dempsey, S., Coons, H. L., & Davis, M. (1998) Results of a domestic violence training program offered to the staff of urban community health centers. *American Journal of Preventive Medicine, 15*(3), 235-242.

Heise, L., & Garcia-Moreno, C. (2002). Violence by intimate partners. In E. E. Krug, L. L. Dahlberg, J. A. Mercy, A. B. Zwi, & R. Lozano (Eds.), *World report on violence and health* (pp. 87–121). Geneva, Switzerland: World Health Organization.

Humphreys, J., & Campbell, J. C. (Eds.). (2010). *Family violence and nursing practice* (2nd ed.). Philadelphia, PA: Lippincott Williams & Wilkins.

Institute for Children and Poverty. (2010). *Exposure to intimate partner violence among poor children experiencing homelessness or residential instability* (Research Brief). New York: Author. Retrieved from www.icphusa.org/PDF/reports/ICP_ResearchBrief_ExposureToIntimate PartnerViolenceAmongPoorChildren.pdf.

Institute for Safe Families. (2002). RADAR pocket cards. Retrieved from www.instituteforsafefamilies.org/materials/health-care.

Keenan-Miller, D., Hammen, C., & Brennan, P. (2007). Adolescent psychosocial risk factors for severe intimate partner violence in young adulthood. *Journal of Consulting and Clinical Psychology, 75*(3), 456–463.

Kulwiki, A. D., & Miller J. (1999). Domestic violence in the Arab American population: Transforming environmental conditions through community education. *Issues in Mental Health Nursing, 20*(3), 199–215.

Madkour, A. S., Xie, Y., & Harville, E. W., (2014). Pre-pregnancy dating violence and birth outcomes among adolescent mothers in a national sample. *Journal of Interpersonal Violence, 29*(10), 1894–1913. Retrieved from http://jiv.sagepub.com/content/29/10/1894.full.pdf+html

Miller, E., Tancredi, D., McCauley, H., Decker, M., Virata, C., Anderson, H., et al. (2013). One-year follow-up of a coach-delivered dating violence prevention program: A cluster randomized controlled trial. *American Journal of Preventive Medicine, 45*, 108–112.

Moracco, K. E., Hilton, A., Hodges, K. G., & Frasier, P. Y. (2005). Knowledge and attitudes about intimate partner violence among immigrant Latinos in rural North Carolina. *Violence Against Women, 11*, 337–352.

Moyer, V. A. (2013) Screening for intimate partner violence and abuse of elderly and vulnerable adults: U.S. Preventive Services Task Force recommendation statement. *Annals of Internal Medicine, 158*(6), 478–486.

Murdaugh, C., Hunt, S., Sowell, R., & Santana, I. (2004). Domestic violence in Hispanics in the southeastern United States: A survey and needs analysis. *Journal of Family Violence, 19*, 107–116.

National Center for Injury Prevention and Control. (2003). *Costs of intimate partner violence against women in the United States.* Atlanta, GA: Centers for Disease Control and Prevention. Retrieved from www.cdc.gov/violenceprevention/pdf/IPVBook-a.pdf.

National Center for Victims of Crime. (2008a). Victims Rights. Retrieved from www.victimsofcrime.org/help-for-crime-victims/get-help-bulletins -for-crime-victims/victims'-rights.

Nicolaidis, C., Curry, M., McFarland, B., & Gerrity, M. (2004). Violence, mental health and physical symptoms in an academic internal medicine practice. *Journal of General Internal Medicine, 19*(8), 819–827.

Parker, B., McFarlane, J., & Soeken, K. (1994). Abuse during pregnancy: Effects on maternal complications and infant birth weight in adult and teen women. *Obstetrics & Gynecology, 841*, 323–328.

Rabin, R., Jennings, J., Campbell, J., & Bair-Merritt, M. H. (2009). Intimate partner violence screening tools: A systematic review. *American Journal of Preventive Medicine, 36*(5), 439–445.

Rennison, C. M., & Welchans, S. (2002). *Intimate partner violence* (Bureau of Justice Statistics Special Report NCJ 178247). Washington, DC: U.S. Department of Justice, Bureau of Justice Statistics.

Rudman, W. J. (2000). *Coding and documentation of domestic violence.* San Francisco, CA: Family Violence Prevention Fund. Retrieved from www .futureswithoutviolence.org/userfiles/file/HealthCare/codingpaper .pdf.

Runner, M., Yoshihama, M., & Novick, S. (2009). *Intimate partner violence in immigrant and refugee communities: Challenges, promising practices and recommendations.* San Francisco, CA: Family Violence Prevention Fund. Retrieved from https://www.futureswithoutviolence.org/userfiles /file/ImmigrantWomen/IPV_Report_March_2009.pdf.

Shiu-Thornton, S., Senturia, K., & Sullivan, M. (2005). Like a bird in a cage: Vietnamese women survivors talk about domestic violence. *Journal of Interpersonal Violence, 20*, 959–976.

Silverman, J. G., McCauley, H. L., Decker, M. R., Miller, E., Reed, E., & Raj, A. (2011). Coercive forms of sexual risk and associated violence perpetrated by male partners of female adolescents. *Perspectives on Sexual and Reproductive Health, 43*(1), 60–65. doi: 10.1363/4306011.

Stöckl, H., March, L., Pallitto, C., & Garcia-Moreno, C. (2014). Intimate partner violence among adolescents and young women: Prevalence and associated factors in nine countries: A cross-sectional study. *BioMedCentral (BMC) Public Health, 14*, 751. Retrieved from www .biomedcentral.com/1471-2458/14/751.

Strack, G. B., & Gwinn, C. (2011). On the edge of homicide: Strangulation as a prelude. *Criminal Justice, 26*(3), 32–36.

Svavarsdottir, E. K., & Orlygsdottir, B. (2009). Intimate partner abuse factors associated with women's health: A general population study. *Journal of Advanced Nursing, 65*(7), 1452–1462.

Thompson, M. P., Basile, K. C., Hertz, M. F., & Sitterle, D. (2006). *Measuring intimate partner violence victimization and perpetration: A compendium of assessment tools.* Atlanta, GA: Centers for Disease Control and Prevention. Retrieved from http://stacks.cdc.gov/view/cdc/11402.

U.S. Conference of Mayors. (2008). *Hunger and Homeless Survey: A status report on hunger and homelessness in America's cities: A 25-city survey.* Washington, DC: Author.

U.S. Department of Health and Human Services, National Women's Health Information Center. (2009). *Violence against women: Dating violence.* Retrieved from www.womenshealth.gov/violence-against-women/types -of-violence/dating-violence.html.

U.S. Department of Justice. (2015). *Domestic violence.* Retrieved from www .justice.gov/ovw/domestic-violence.

U.S. Preventive Services Task Force. (2013). *Final recommendation statement: Intimate partner violence and abuse of elderly and vulnerable adults.* Retrieved from www.uspreventiveservicestaskforce.org/Page /Document/RecommendationStatementFinal/intimate-partner -violence-and-abuse-of-elderly-and-vulnerable-adults-screening.

Vagi, K., Rothman, E., Latzman, N., Tharp A., Hall, D., & Breiding, M. (2013). Beyond correlates: A review of risk and protective factors for adolescent dating violence perpetration. *Journal of Youth and Adolescence, 42*(4), 633–649.

Wadman, M. C., & Foral, J. (2007). *Domestic violence, determining risk.* Emedicinehealth. Retrieved from www.emedicinehealth.com/domestic _violence/page7_em.htm.

Walters, M. L., Chen, J., & Breiding, M. J. (2013). *The National Intimate Partner and Sexual Violence Survey (NISVS): 2010 findings on victimization by sexual orientation.* Atlanta, GA: National Center for Injury Prevention and Control, Centers for Disease Control and Prevention. Retrieved from www.cdc.gov/violenceprevention/pdf/nisvs_sofindings.pdf.

Waters, H., Hyder, A., Rajkotia, Y., Basu, S., Rehwinkel, J. A., & Butchart, A. (2004). *The economic dimensions of interpersonal violence.* Geneva, Switzerland: Department of Injuries and Violence Prevention, World Health Organization.

World Health Organization. (2013). *Responding to intimate partner violence and sexual violence against women: WHO clinical and policy guidelines.* Geneva, Switzerland: Author. Retrieved from http://apps .who.int/iris/bitstream/10665/85240/1/9789241548595_eng .pdf?ua=1.

Yoshihama, M. (2008). Literature on intimate partner violence in immigrant and refugee communities: Review and recommendations. In *Intimate partner violence in immigrant and refugee communities: Challenges, promising practices and recommendations.* A report by the Family Violence Prevention Fund (pp. 34–64). Princeton, NJ: Robert Wood Johnson Foundation. Retrieved from https://www .futureswithoutviolence.org/userfiles/file/ImmigrantWomen/IPV _Report_March_2009.pdf.

IRRITABLE BOWEL SYNDROME

Karen C. Bagatelos, Geraldine Collins-Bride, and Fran Dreier

CHAPTER **62**

I. Introduction and general background

Irritable bowel syndrome (IBS) is a "functional bowel disorder," a disorder of intestinal motility and visceral sensory perception. There are no structural or biochemical causes associated with IBS. Although often associated primarily with the lower intestinal tract, the signs and symptoms of IBS can be found along the entire gastrointestinal tract.

The main symptoms of IBS are abdominal pain and discomfort associated with a change in the consistency or frequency of stool and relief of the pain with defecation (Ringel, Sperber, & Drossman, 2001). This constellation of symptoms led to the development of the Rome Criteria, which was done in conjunction with the World College of Gastroenterology in Rome, Italy, in 1998 (Rome I), again in 1999 (Rome II), and subsequently in 2006 (Rome III). The Rome criteria are used to aid in the diagnosis of IBS.

The following is a list of the Rome III criteria for IBS diagnosis: recurrent abdominal pain or discomfort at least 3 days per month in the last 3 months associated with two of the following features:

- Improvement with defecation,
- Onset associated with change in frequency of stool, and
- Onset associated with a change in the form of stools (Drossman, 2006).

Other features that are included in the diagnosis are:

- Abnormal stool frequency (more than three bowel movements per day or less than three per week),
- Abnormal stool form, abnormal stool passage, passage of mucus, and abdominal bloating or distention (Drossman, Camilleri, Mayer, & Whitehead, 2002), and
- Exacerbation triggered by stressful life events.

Diagnosis can be made if all other diagnoses, structural or metabolic, have been eliminated. One must keep in mind that symptom expression differs among patients and may be any combination of these factors.

A. Epidemiology

1. Prevalence

   The prevalence of IBS is 1–2 in 10 or 10–20% of the population. Studies have also shown a prevalence of 8–22 per 100 adults (Ringel et al., 2001). These numbers are difficult to assess because in many patients symptoms resolve and/or medical attention and treatment are not sought. Approximately 10–20% of patients with IBS actually seek care (Lehrer & Lichenstein, 2009).

2. Impact

   The costs of healthcare use and absenteeism from work are substantial. It is estimated that approximately $8 billion is spent per year in the United States on the care of patients with IBS (Hauser, Pardi, & Poterucha, 2008). Annually, IBS accounts for 3.5 million physician visits, 2.2 million prescriptions, and 35,000 hospitalizations annually (Hauser, Oxentenko, & Sanchez, 2014).

3. Risk factors

   Female gender confers greater risk with a ratio of 2:1. These numbers may be somewhat inflated because females seek medical care more frequently than males; thus the number of men with IBS may not be accurately reported. The prevalence of IBS decreases with age; however, there have been rare cases of new-onset IBS in the elderly. There are no consistent racial or ethnic differences in individuals with and without IBS (Hauser et al., 2008). Although IBS seems to have a "familial component," a confirmed genetic risk has not been clearly established.

   IBS has been associated with psychiatric illness and can also be exacerbated by stress, anxiety, and depression. Studies have shown that physical and sexual abuse may have a role in the development of IBS (Lehrer & Lichenstein, 2009). In some cases, the onset of symptoms can occur after acute inflammatory conditions of the gastrointestinal tract, such as postinfectious IBS. Food sensitivities and allergies may also have a role, although formal food allergy testing is generally not recommended.

B. Pathophysiology

The etiology of IBS is not completely understood. There are many possible mechanisms and causative factors. In some patients, IBS seems to be associated with visceral hypersensitivity as demonstrated by balloon distention studies (Yuan et al., 2003). These studies have shown that IBS patients have lower thresholds for pain. Balloon inflation in the sigmoid colon causes increased pain in IBS patients as opposed to normal controls (Horwitz & Fisher, 2001). Patients with IBS can have hypersensitivity throughout the entire digestive tract.

IBS is also associated with altered bowel motility. Signals from the central nervous system are either exaggerated or diminished, which causes an increase or decrease in bowel motility (Horwitz & Fisher, 2001), thus explaining why some patients have diarrhea-predominant and others have constipation-predominant IBS. It has been postulated that serotonin or other neurotransmitters can play a role. There can be underexpression or overexpression of some neurotransmitters or increased amounts of receptors in the central and enteric (intestinal) nervous system transmitting signals at abnormal rates. This etiology remains under investigation.

The possible role of bacterial overgrowth and inflammation is also being investigated. Bacterial overgrowth may be the primary cause of IBS symptomatology in some patients as some individuals improve significantly with antibiotic treatment. In some patients, the flora of the digestive tract becomes imbalanced, with "bad" bacteria overcoming "good" bacteria. Psychosocial factors, such as stress and anxiety, and dietary factors can also play a role in the expression of this syndrome (Drossman et al., 2002).

II. Database (may include but is not limited to)

A. Subjective findings

1. Past medical history
   a. Multiple abdominal surgeries: can cause adhesions
   b. Surgery that has damaged the vagus nerve: any upper abdominal surgery, in particular gastric and esophageal surgeries, can cause diarrhea (Ukleja, Woodward, & Achem, 2002)
   c. Psychiatric illness, including trauma and abuse
   d. Substance abuse (including laxatives)
   e. Thyroid disease
   f. Food sensitivities, especially lactose intolerance
   g. Carcinoid syndrome: causes profound diarrhea
   h. Gastroesophageal reflux disease: frequently seen in patients with slow overall motility
   i. Medications prone to altering gastrointestinal motility, such as opiates, stimulants, or laxatives

2. Family history: IBS, inflammatory bowel disease, colon cancer, diabetes, and thyroid disease

3. Psychosocial history
   a. Habits: alcohol, tobacco, or illicit drug use
   b. Situational stressors, coping mechanisms, and social support systems
   c. Exercise and physical activity: sedentary lifestyle is commonly seen in patients with constipation and other bowel motility disorders
   d. Diet history: note typical diet, foods that trigger symptoms, amount of water and caffeine intake, use of artificial sweeteners (sorbitol, saccharin, or NutraSweet), chewing gum, and fiber intake

4. Review of systems
   a. Fever, chills, weight gain or loss, and fatigue
   b. Changes in skin, hair, nails, and other symptoms suggestive of thyroid disease
   c. Lower abdominal pain relieved with defecation, particularly in the left lower quadrant
   d. Constipation, diarrhea, or alternating diarrhea and constipation
   e. Bloating (upper and lower intestinal tract) and gas
   f. Frequency of stools and presence of mucus or blood in the stool (*patients with IBS typically do not have blood in the stool*)
   g. Anxiety, depression, other psychiatric symptoms
   h. Nausea, vomiting, dyspepsia, and other upper gastrointestinal symptoms

B. Objective findings

1. Physical examination: a full physical examination is recommended with particular attention to:
   a. Vital signs (note any orthostatic changes), weight, and body mass index
   b. Thyroid examination
   c. Abdominal examination noting bowel sounds, any masses, and tenderness (especially in the left lower quadrant)
   d. Pelvic examination noting any uterine or adnexal enlargement
   e. Mental status examination noting appearance, behavior, mood, affect, and thought content

III. Assessment

A. Determine the diagnosis

IBS is a diagnosis of exclusion. That being said, many patients with IBS undergo expensive and unnecessary testing and continue to pursue diagnostic work-ups in search of the answer to "what is wrong with me?" The diagnostic and management approaches to patients with IBS rest with careful history and physical examination skills in additional to building a strong therapeutic alliance with the patient to help understand the underlying disorder and symptom-based treatment. The following diagnoses should be considered for all patients presenting with suspected IBS.

1. Bacterial infections
2. Colon cancer
3. Diverticulosis and diverticulitis
4. Eating disorders
5. Adhesions
6. Fecal incontinence
7. In females: ovarian tumors, endometriosis, and adnexal cysts
8. Inflammatory bowel disease
9. Atypical colitis, microscopic colitis, lymphocytic colitis, or eosinophilic gastroenteritis
10. Thyroid disease, diabetes, and other endocrine disorders
11. Celiac disease
12. Depression, anxiety, and other mental health disorders
13. Pelvic floor dysfunction caused by pelvic floor damage
14. Arteriovenous malformations with bleeding
15. Large polypoid mass (can cause constipation) or a malignant tumor
16. Trauma to the rectum
17. Carcinoid syndrome

B. Severity

Assess the severity of the disease.

C. Significance

Assess the significance of the symptoms and chronic nature of the disorder to the patient and significant others.

IV. Goals of clinical management

A. Assist the patient with medications, stress management, and psychosocial support.

B. Prevent pain by performing adequate pain assessments and referring to pain management for assistance if needed.

C. Assist the patient to achieve optimal level of functioning with daily activities and quality of life while living with a chronic, often relapsing disorder.

V. Plan

A. Screening

There are no screening tests available for early detection or prevention of IBS.

B. Diagnostic studies

Based on symptoms and history

1. Diet diary. The diet diary is an essential initial diagnostic tool for IBS management. The diary helps both the patient and the clinician to make associations between symptoms and foods. It also engages the patient in a meaningful way as a partner in both the diagnostic and treatment processes. The diary should note time of meals and snacks, type and quantity of foods eaten, and associated gastrointestinal symptoms before or after food consumption, noting the time frame of symptom development.

2. For recommended first- and second-line symptom-based diagnostic testing see **Tables 62-1** and **62-2**.

3. *Alarm symptoms* warranting a gastroenterology referral include:
   a. Unrelenting symptoms despite treatment
   b. Rectal bleeding, abnormal stool studies
   c. Unexplained anemia
   d. Anorexia
   e. Blood in the stool
   f. Severe unrelenting diarrhea or constipation
   g. Nocturnal symptoms
   h. Onset in patients older than 50 years
   i. Palpable abdominal or rectal mass (Kolfenbach, 2007; World Gastroenterology Organization, 2009). These symptoms are particularly worrisome if the patient has a family history of inflammatory bowel disease, celiac sprue, or colorectal cancer.

C. Management

The mainstay of any treatment regimen for patients with suspected or confirmed IBS is first and foremost to build a therapeutic alliance with the patient. The underpinnings of this alliance include careful listening, validation of symptoms, and compassion for the distress that

TABLE 62-1 Initial Symptom-Based Diagnostic Work-Up for Irritable Bowel Syndrome

Diarrhea-Predominant Symptoms	Constipation-Predominant Symptoms	Upper Gastrointestinal-Predominant Symptoms
Stool sample: culture and sensitivity, ova and parasites, and *Clostridium difficile* • To rule out bacterial and parasitic infections	Complete blood count with differential • To look for evidence of anemia seen with malignancies, inflammatory bowel disease (IBD), and other systemic disease • To look for leukocytosis seen with IBD and infections	Upper gastrointestinal series with a small bowel follow-through • To rule out structural abnormality or adhesions; also to evaluate transit time with constipation and diarrhea
Stool sample for *Giardia* • To rule out *Giardia lamblia* infection. Increased risk in individuals with immunocompromise and those with a recent travel history	Thyroid-stimulating hormone • To rule out hypothyroid disorders	Abdominal sonogram • To rule out gallstones
Stool sample for fecal occult blood • To rule out malignancy, IBD, and other systemic causes of intestinal bleeding	Plain abdominal film (also called a "flat plate of the abdomen") • To look for a bowel obstruction or ileus, adhesions, and pseudo-obstruction	Serum liver function tests • To evaluate liver health and rule out hepatitis, cirrhosis, and other liver diseases
Stool sample for fecal fat/pancreatic elastase • Seen with malabsorption and pancreatic insufficiency	Stool sample for fecal occult blood • To rule out malignancy, IBD, and other systemic causes of intestinal bleeding	Serum lipase and amylase • To rule out pancreatitis
Complete blood count with differential • To look for evidence of anemia seen with malignancies, IBD, and other systemic disease • To look for leukocytosis seen with IBD and infections	Serum potassium and calcium • To rule out hypokalemia and hypercalcemia, both associated with constipation	
Erythrocyte sedimentation rate • Nonspecific marker of IBD and malignancy		
Fasting blood sugar • To rule out diabetes mellitus, which can present with diarrhea because of diabetic gastroenteropathy		
Thyroid-stimulating hormone • To rule out hyperthyroid disorders		
Electrolytes (depending on severity of symptoms) • To look for electrolyte disturbances seen with severe diarrhea and malabsorption		

Data from American College of Gastroenterology Task Force on Irritable Bowel Syndrome. (2009); World Gastroenterology Organization Global Guideline. (2009). *Irritable bowel syndrome: A global perspective*, 1–20.

TABLE 62-2 Second-Line Symptom-Based Diagnostic Work-Up for Irritable Bowel Syndrome

Diarrhea-Predominant Symptoms	Constipation-Predominant Symptoms	Upper Gastrointestinal-Predominant Symptoms
Celiac serologies (tissue transglutaminase IgA most sensitive) • To rule out celiac sprue disease	Colonoscopy or flexible sigmoidoscopy with a barium enema • To rule out mucosal (atypical colitis) or structural abnormalities	Endoscopy • To rule out celiac disease, gastric or duodenal ulcer, and gastroesophageal reflux disease with esophageal spasm
Repeat stool sample for ova and parasites and *Clostridium difficile* • To rule out a recurrent bacterial infection or *C. difficile*, commonly seen with recent history of antibiotic use	Abdominal and pelvic computerized tomography scan • To rule out cancer and other pathologic conditions	
Allergy testing (controversial) • To look for food allergies		
Endoscopy • To rule out celiac disease by taking small bowel biopsies looking for villous blunting with diarrhea, bloating, and pain		

Data from American College of Gastroenterology Task Force on Irritable Bowel Syndrome. (2009); World Gastroenterology Organization Global Guideline. (2009). *Irritable bowel syndrome: A global perspective*, 1–20.

symptoms may cause for the patient. Such an alliance provides a platform for working with the patient through the symptom-based diagnostic and treatment process.

There are few studies that offer convincing evidence of effectiveness in curing the IBS symptom complex (Akehurst & Kaltenthaler, 2001). Current treatment guidelines focus on symptom-based treatment management (World Gastroenterology Organization, 2009).

1. For diarrhea-predominant symptoms:
   a. Diet
      All patients should try a *low FODMAP diet*. FODMAPs (fermentable oligo-, di- and monosaccharides and polyols) are short-chain sugars that are poorly absorbed by the small intestine. Studies show that a low FODMAP diet may help reduce symptoms of gas, bloating, diarrhea, and abdominal discomfort (Halmos, Power, Shepherd, Gibson, & Muir, 2014; Shepherd, Lomer, & Gibson, 2013). Limit the high FODMAP foods: gas-producing vegetables, such as onions, garlic, beans, broccoli, cabbage, Brussels sprouts, asparagus, and cauliflower. Other dietary restrictions include limiting dairy products, carbonated beverages, caffeine, alcohol, red meats, artificial fats, sugars such as honey, high-fructose

corn syrup, and artificial sweeteners (sorbitol-containing products).

It can be overwhelming to restrict all of these foods and substances at once. Often, selecting 1–2 food groups to eliminate and monitoring the effect is a reasonable approach to begin the dietary modification process. Referral to a nutritionist may also be helpful.

   b. *Concentrated fiber* to help form stools (i.e., ½–1 tablespoon daily working up to 1 heaping tablespoon of psyllium fiber or other similar fiber in 4 ounces of water one to three times per day, depending on symptoms and symptom response). Patients should try insoluble fiber, incorporated into their diet, such as whole grain foods, fresh fruits, fresh vegetables, wheat bran, and beans. Insoluble fiber absorbs water from the intestinal tract and helps to decrease diarrhea.
   c. Loperamide, 4 mg orally two to four times daily, as needed to reduce stool frequency.
   d. Empiric antibiotic trial (see options that follow) followed by a probiotic to treat bacterial overgrowth and repopulate the intestines with beneficial flora. Probiotics have been found to be beneficial in some patients. A systematic review from the American College of Gastroenterology

Task Force (2009) on the treatment of IBS concluded that *Lactobacillus* alone does not seem to be effective in single-organism studies and combinations of probiotic studies. However, *Bifidobacterium* does demonstrate some efficacy. Future studies are needed to determine the efficacy of specific strains of probiotics in the treatment of IBS (Aragon, Graham, Borum, & Doman, 2010). With further study, it may be possible to target symptoms with specific strains of bacteria that facilitate better targeting of treatment and enhanced efficacy (Spiller, 2008). At this time, it is not possible to make recommendations as to a specific brand or bacterial strain because no documented studies exist. There is also no standardization of these products.

One of the following oral antibiotics regimens may be used:

i. Rifaximin, 400 mg three times daily for 7 days

ii. Levofloxacin, 500 mg daily for 7 days

iii. Ciprofloxacin, 500 mg twice daily for 7 days

iv. Metronidazole, 500 mg three times daily for 7 days

2. For constipation-predominant symptoms:

a. High-fiber diet with the addition of dietary fiber, psyllium, or Benefiber® (i.e., 1 heaping tablespoon in 8 oz of fluids one to two times taken by mouth per day with plenty of water). Also, add insoluble fiber (see list mentioned previously). Insoluble fiber helps the stool absorb water to facilitate passage and prevent constipation.

b. Laxatives

i. Polyethylene glycol (Miralax®), 18 g mixed in 8 oz of liquid one to two times per day, is very effective for constipation but patients may continue to experience bloating and abdominal pain

ii. Bisacodyl (Dulcolax®): 5-to 15-mg tablets as a single dose; may take up to 30 mg if complete bowel evacuation is needed; 10 mg suppository as a single daily dose prn

iii. Senna or Cascara tablets should be avoided long term due to the increased risk of melanosis coli (dark pigment deposits in the lining of the large intestine), which can worsen constipation.

c. Empiric antibiotic treatment followed by a probiotic therapy as mentioned previously

d. Chloride channel activator that acts to increase intestinal fluid secretion and intestinal motility:

i. Lubiprostone (Amitiza®), 8 mcg orally twice daily, for women age 18 and older

ii. Linaclotide (Linzess®), 290 mcg by mouth daily. Long-term safety profile is unknown. *Consultation with gastrointestinal specialist is recommended.*

e. Increase oral fluids: water is best, followed by low-sugar-content fluids.

f. Physical activity: assist the patient in developing a regular daily exercise and activity plan. Physical activity has been shown to promote healthier bowel motility and overall better mental and physical health.

3. For abdominal pain–predominant IBS:

a. Antispasmodic agents

i. Dicyclomine (Bentyl®), 20 mg orally four times per day prn. Can titrate up to a maximum of 160 mg per day.

ii. Hyoscyamine, 0.125–0.25 mg orally three-four times daily prn pain. Take before food. Maximum dosage is 1.5 mg in 24 hours. Because of anticholinergic properties, use these medications with caution in the geriatric population

b. Low-dose tricyclic antidepressants (help to reduce visceral sensation): amitriptyline 25 mg orally at bedtime, may titrate up to 100 mg at bedtime

c. Serotonin reuptake inhibitor or other antidepressant if depression is suspected.

d. Pain management: suggest nonpharmacologic measures first, such as relaxation, acupuncture, and meditation. Avoid the use of narcotic analgesics because of their addiction potential. See Chapter 50 on chronic pain management for further suggestions.

4. For alternating diarrhea and constipation:

a. High-fiber diet (insoluble fiber) examples include whole grain foods; fresh fruits; fresh vegetables; wheat bran; beans; or a fiber supplement, such as psyllium husk, methylcellulose (Citrucel®), or Benefiber. The dose for constipation is 1 tablespoon in 8 oz of fluid taken orally one to two times per day. The dose for diarrhea is 1 tablespoon in 4 oz of water taken orally one to three times per day.

b. Antidiarrheal medications during diarrhea phase (loperamide 4 mg orally two–three times daily) and laxative during constipation phase (polyethylene glycol, 18 g in 8 oz of liquid taken orally each day).

c. Empiric antibiotic followed by a probiotic.

5. For abdominal bloating–predominant symptoms

a. Empiric antibiotic followed by a probiotic.

TABLE 62-3 Diet Strategies for the Management of Constipation and Diarrhea: Avoid the following FoodS

Constipation	Diarrhea
Prepared protein-laden foods: cooked, fried, baked, steamed, or canned	Caffeine: found in coffee, tea, cola, and chocolate
Wheat products: bread, pasta, cookies, pastries, and so forth	Nicotine from cigarettes, chewing tobacco, and nicotine replacement products
Supplementary iron	Gas-producing foods, such as beans, broccoli, cabbage, and apples
Dairy products: all dairy	Dairy products that contain lactose
Supplementary calcium	High-sugar foods, such as juices, soda, candy, cookies, and other packaged sweets
All processed foods	Foods high in fat, such as bacon, sausage, butter, oils, and deep fried foods
	Sorbitol and xylitol, and other artificial sweeteners

Data from American College of Gastroenterology Task Force on Irritable Bowel Syndrome. (2009); Halmos, E., Power, V., Shepherd, S., et al. (2014). A diet low in FODMAPs reduces symptoms of irritable bowel syndrome. *Gastroenterology*, 146–167.

    b. Food diary to identify and eliminate any aggravating foods.

    c. Diet: avoid cruciferous vegetables (cauliflower, broccoli, cabbage, and so forth) and dairy products (**Table 62-3**).

    d. Incorporate stress management strategies; if needed, refer for mental health treatment. In the event of refractory pain, a referral to gastroenterology is warranted.

D. Follow-up

Reevaluate the patient in 3–6 weeks after initial treatment program and evaluation are done. If symptoms persist, consider changing treatment regimen or obtaining further diagnostic testing as indicated based on predominant symptoms. The following are recommendations for further testing after the initial evaluation, which are often done by a gastroenterologist

1. Refractory constipation: evaluate colonic transit time, pelvic floor function, and adhesions by considering the following additional tests:

    a. Colonic transit test

    b. Anorectal manometry

    c. Rectal sensation testing and emptying study

2. Refractory diarrhea: evaluate for bacterial overgrowth, laxative abuse, atypical colitis, carcinoid syndrome, and increased colonic transit.

    a. Stool chemistry for surreptitious laxative abuse

    b. Duodenal aspirate for bacterial overgrowth

    c. Colonic biopsies for microscopic or collagenous colitis

    d. Urinary 5-hydroxy indolacetic acid for carcinoid syndrome

    e. Small bowel transit study for increased transit

3. Pain: evaluate small or large intestine for obstruction, intermediate obstruction, cancer, or adhesions.

    a. Plain abdominal radiograph for obstruction and intermediate obstruction

    b. CT scan of the abdomen for cancer and obstruction

    c. CT enterography for cancer, obstruction, and colitis

    d. Upper gastrointestinal series with a small bowel follow-through for adhesions; can also evaluate transit time

E. Client education

1. Assist the patient and family in verbalizing their concerns and coping strategies with respect to the disease process and management.

2. Provide verbal and written information about the pathophysiology of IBS and treatment.

3. Discuss what the patient can expect with diagnostic testing, preparation, and after-care.

4. Explain the therapeutic benefits and side effects of any prescribed treatment.

5. Reassure the patient that assistance is available when needed.

6. Emphasize the importance of stress management and good mental health in coping with this disorder

VI. Self-management eResources

A. The National Institutes of Health has multiple brochures for IBS patients
(http://digestive.niddk.nih.gov/ddiseases/pubs/ibs/)

B. Irritable Bowel Syndrome Association
(www.ibsgroup.org/ibsassociation)

C. IBS FODMAP Dieting Guide
(www.ibsdiets.org/fodmap-diet/fodmap-food-list/)

REFERENCES

Akehurst, R., & Kaltenthaler, E. (2001). Treatment of irritable bowel syndrome: A review of randomized controlled trials. *Gut, 48,* 272–282.

American College of Gastroenterology Task Force on Irritable Bowel Syndrome. (2009). An evidence-based systematic review on the management of irritable bowel syndrome. *American Journal of Gastroenterology, 104*(Suppl. 1), S1–S35.

Aragon, G., Graham, D. B., Borum, M., & Doman, D. B. (2010). Probiotic therapy for irritable bowel syndrome. *Gastroenterology and Hepatology, 6*(1), 39–44.

Drossman, D. A. (2006). The functional GI disorders and the Rome III process. *Gastroenterology, 130*(5), 1377–1390.

Drossman, D. A., Camilleri, M., Mayer, E. A., & Whitehead, W. E. (2002). AGA technical review on irritable bowel syndrome. *Gastroenterology, 123*(6), 2108–2131.

Halmos, E., Power, V., Shepherd, S., Gibson, P. R., & Muir, J. G. (2014). A diet low in FODMAPs reduces symptoms of irritable bowel syndrome. *Gastroenterology, 146*(1), 67–75.

Hauser, S. C., Pardi, D. S., & Poterucha, J. J. (2008). *Mayo Clinic gastroenterology and hepatology board review* (3rd ed.). Rochester, MN: Mayo Clinic Scientific Press.

Hauser, S. C., Oxentenko, A. S., & Sanchez, W. (2014). *Mayo Clinic gastroenterology and hepatology board review* (4th ed.). Rochester, MN: Mayo Clinic Scientific Press.

Horwitz, B. J., & Fisher, R. S. (2001). The irritable bowel syndrome. *New England Journal of Medicine, 344,* 1846–1850.

Kolfenbach, L. (2007). The pathophysiology, diagnosis, and treatment of IBS. *Journal of the American Academy of Physician Assistants, 20*(1), 16–20.

Lehrer, J. K., & Lichenstein, G. R. (2009). *Irritable bowel syndrome.* Retrieved from http://emedicine.medscape.com/article/180389-overview.

Ringel, Y., Sperber, A. D., & Drossman, D. A. (2001). Irritable bowel syndrome. *Annual Review of Medicine, 52,* 319–338.

Shepherd, S., Lomer, M., & Gibson, P. (2013). Short-chain carbohydrates and functional gastrointestinal disorders. *American Journal of Gastroenterology, 108*(5), 707–717.

Spiller, R. (2008). Review article: Probiotics and prebiotics in irritable bowel syndrome. *Alimentary Pharmacologic Therapy, 28*(4), 385–396.

Ukleja, A., Woodward, T. A., & Achem, S. R. (2002). Vagus nerve injury with severe diarrhea after laparoscopic antireflux surgery. *Digestive Diseases and Sciences, 47*(7), 1590–1593.

World Gastroenterology Organization. (2009). *Irritable bowel syndrome: A global perspective.* Milwaukee, WI: Author. Retrieved from www.worldgastroenterology.org/guidelines/global-guidelines/irritable-bowel-syndrome-ibs/irritable-bowel-syndrome-ibs-english.

Yuan, Y. Z., Tao, R. J., Xu, B., Sun, J., Chen, K. M., Miao, F., et al. (2003). Functional brain imaging in irritable bowel syndrome with rectal balloon-distention by using fMRI. *World Journal of Gastroenterology, 9*(6), 1356–1360.

LIPID DISORDERS

CHAPTER 63

Caitlin Garvey

I. Introduction and general background

Cardiovascular disease (CVD) is the leading cause of death in the United States (Kochanek, Xu, Murphy, Miniño, & Kung, 2011). Many studies have demonstrated the relationship between serum cholesterol levels, particularly low-density lipoprotein (LDL-c) levels, with atherosclerosis and coronary vessel disease. For this reason, the identification and management of lipid disorders is of great significance in mitigating cardiovascular risk.

Lipid metabolism involves several types of lipoproteins responsible for transporting cholesterol and triglycerides within endogenous and exogenous pathways for lipid synthesis and delivery, as well as reverse cholesterol transport. This physiology is not discussed in detail here; however, it is important to highlight that that different lipoproteins fulfill different roles.

LDL's primary role is carrying cholesterol to extrahepatic cells, and its excess can result in atherogenesis. High-density lipoprotein (HDL) transports cholesterol from extrahepatic cells to the liver; it is antiatherogenic and higher levels of HDL are associated with lower cardiovascular risk. It is also important to remember that these pathways rely on normal functioning of the liver and the intestine, from where dietary cholesterol and triglycerides are absorbed.

A. Definition and overview

Lipid disorders are defined by elevations in serum lipids (cholesterol, phospholipids, or triglycerides). The phospholipids include LDL, HDL, very-low-density lipoproteins (VLDL), intermediate-density lipoproteins (IDL), and chylomicrons.

Lipid disorders fall into two main categories: (1) primary (genetic or inherited) disorders of lipid metabolism, and (2) lipid disorders that are secondary to other diseases (Durrington, 2003; Vodnala, Rubenfire, & Brook, 2012). For many patients, the causes of lipid disorders may be multifactorial with primary and secondary etiologies at play.

B. Prevalence

An estimated 43.4% of Americans have total cholesterol levels ≥ 200 mg/dL and an estimated 31.1% have LDL cholesterol levels ≥ 130 mg/dL (Centers for Disease Control and Prevention [CDC], 2011). Low-income adults and Mexican Americans are disproportionately affected by hyperlipidemia.

C. Diagnostic classifications

1. Inherited disorders of LDL-metabolism

    a. Definition and overview: Primary or genetic disorders of lipid metabolism are less common than other types of dyslipidemia, but they are often responsible for the most severe dyslipidemias. These disorders may be monogenic or polygenic. They may result in elevated LDL-c with normal triglyceride levels or elevated triglycerides in isolation (see section C. 2., Hypertriglyceridemia). Most are rare outside of certain specific demographic groups.

    Primary disorders resulting in elevated LDL-c and normal triglycerides:

    i. Familial hypercholesteremia
    ii. Familial defective ApoB-100
    iii. Autosomal dominant hypercholesterolemia due to mutations in PCSK9
    iv. Autosomal recessive hypercholesterolemia
    v. Sitosterolemia
    vi. Polygenic hypercholesterolemia
    vii. Elevated plasma levels of lipoprotein(a)

2. Hypertriglyceridemia

    a. Hypertriglyceridemia is generally believed to be an independent risk factor for cardiovascular disease, but the amount of excess risk is small. Elevated levels of triglycerides are also associated with lower levels of HDL due to the physiology of metabolic pathways.

    b. May be primary, secondary, or multifactorial.

613

c. Primary lipid disorders causing elevated triglycerides and normal LDL
   i. Familial chylomicronemia
   ii. ApoA-V deficiency
   iii. GPIHBP1 deficiency
   iv. Hepatic lipase deficiency
   v. Familial dysbetalipoproteinemia
   vi. Familial hypertriglyceridemia: autosomal dominant disorder and causes moderately elevated triglyceride levels
   vii. Familial combined hyperlipidemia

d. Secondary causes include obesity, type 2 diabetes with poor glycemic control, nephrotic syndrome, hypothyroidism, and pregnancy. Associated medications include tamoxifen, beta-blockers, immunosuppressives, HIV antiretrovirals, and retinoids.

e. Very high levels of triglycerides are associated with pancreatitis. In patients with hypertriglyceridemia, additional factors associated with pancreatitis include poorly controlled diabetes, excessive alcohol use, and drug- or diet-induced hypertriglyceridemia.

3. Secondary disorders of lipoprotein metabolism
   a. Type 2 diabetes is one of the most important secondary causes of hyperlipidemia in primary care.
   b. Other secondary causes include:
      i. Excessive alcohol use
      ii. Hypothyroidism
      iii. Obesity
      iv. Pregnancy
      v. Cholestatic liver disease
      vi. Nephrotic syndrome
      vii. Immunoglobulin excess
      viii. Tobacco use (smoking)
      ix. Medications: oral estrogens, steroid hormones, protease inhibitors, and some atypical antipsychotics

D. Treatment of hypercholesteremia for secondary prevention

1. This includes treatment for patients with known coronary heart disease (CHD), cerebrovascular disease, or peripheral artery disease (PAD)

E. Treatment of hypercholesteremia for primary prevention

1. Because the risk of cardiovascular disease (CVD) related events is smaller for those without known CVD, the absolute benefit of lipid-lowering therapy is smaller in primary prevention.

II. Database

A. Subjective

1. Past health history
   a. CVD (coronary artery disease [CAD]/coronary heart disease [CHD], myocardial infarction [MI], angina, coronary revascularization, peripheral vascular disease, abdominal aortic aneurysm)
      i. Premature CAD should raise suspicion for primary lipid disorders
   b. Hypertension
   c. Cerebrovascular disease
   d. Excessive alcohol use
   e. Hypothyroidism
   f. Obesity
   g. Pregnancy
   h. Cholestatic liver disease
   i. Nephrotic syndrome
   j. Immunoglobulin excess
   k. Pancreatitis
   l. Diabetes mellitus

2. Medications
   a. Medications that can promote hyperlipidemia: oral estrogens, steroid hormones, protease inhibitors, and some atypical antipsychotics
   b. Medications that can promote hypertriglyceridemia: tamoxifen, immunosuppressives, HIV antiretrovirals, and retinoids

3. Family history
   a. First-degree relative(s) with dyslipidemia
   b. First-degree relative with premature CHD (e.g., before age 55 in men and 65 in women)

4. Personal-social history: health-related behaviors
   a. High dietary saturated fat and cholesterol intake (total cholesterol and LDL)
   b. Excess total calorie intake
   c. Sedentary lifestyle
   d. Tobacco use (current and former)
   e. Excess alcohol use

B. Objective

1. Physical exam
   a. Most cases will lack physical exam findings, yet some findings may include:
      i. Tendon xanthomas (may be seen in primary/severe hyperlipidemias)
      ii. Xanthelasmas (may be seen in primary/severe hyperlipidemias)

      iii. Physical exam may reveal evidence of secondary causes (e.g., findings consistent with diabetes mellitus) or pancreatitis

  b. Diagnostic tests

      i. Lipid panel reference ranges (adults)

        a. Total cholesterol: 125–200 mg/dL

        b. LDL: < 130 mg/dL

        c. HDL: ≥ 40 mg/dL

        d. Triglycerides: ≤ 150 mg/dL

        e. Very high triglycerides: ≥ 500 mg/dL

      ii. Risk calculators

        a. Pooled Cohort Equation (Stone et al., 2014)

        b. Framingham (D'Agostino et al., 2008)

III. Assessment

A. Determining diagnosis

1. Hyperlipidemia (pure, mixed, or unspecified)

2. Hypertriglyceridemia

3. Secondary causes of lipid disorders (e.g., type 2 diabetes with diabetic hyperlipidemia or hyperlipidemia due to steroid)

B. Severity

1. Assess severity of the disease with a need to treat based on history, physical, diagnostics, and calculated risk estimates using risk calculator

C. Significance

1. Assess significance to patient

2. Consider significance to caregivers and family

D. Motivation

1. Assess patient's preferences and willingness to adhere to recommended treatment plan

IV. Goals of clinical management

A. Screening

1. Use cost-effective and evidence-based tools to identify patients at elevated risk for CVD events

B. Treatment

1. Reduce risk of CVD event

C. Patient adherence

1. Develop plan that fits patient preferences and ability to adhere to treatment

V. Plan

A. Screening

1. U.S. Preventive Services Task Force (USPSTF) strongly recommends screening for lipid disorders in:

  a. Men ≥ 35 years old (Grade A)

  b. Women ≥ 45 years old at elevated risk for coronary heart disease (CHD) (Grade A)

  c. Men 20–35 years old at elevated risk for CHD (Grade B)

  d. Women 20–45 years old at elevated risk for CHD (Grade B)

  e. Risk factors for CHD: diabetes, previous history of CHD or noncoronary atherosclerosis, family history of cardiovascular disease before the age of 55 in first-degree male relatives or age 65 in first-degree female relatives, tobacco use, hypertension, and obesity.

Grade	Definition
A	The USPSTF recommends the service. There is high certainty that the net benefit is substantial.
B	The USPSTF recommends the service. There is high certainty that the net benefit is moderate or there is moderate certainty that the net benefit is moderate to substantial.
C	The USPSTF recommends selectively offering or providing this service to individual patients based on professional judgment and patient preferences. There is at least moderate certainty that the net benefit is small.

Modified from U.S. Preventive Services Task Force. (2008). *Lipid disorders in adults (cholesterol, dyslipidemia): Screening.* Retrieved from http://www.uspreventiveservicestaskforce.org/Page/Document/UpdateSummaryFinal/lipid-disorders-in-adults-cholesterol-dyslipidemia-screening.

2. U.S. Preventive Services Task Force does not make recommendations for or against routine screening regarding screening for men 20–35 years old and women who are not at increased risk for CHD (Grade C).

3. Note USPSTF Grade Definitions (U.S. Preventive Services Task Force, 2008)

B. Diagnostics

1. Evaluate for primary causes

   a. Hypertriglyceridemia: suspect primary cause if fasting plasma triglycerides > 1,000 mg/dL

   b. Elevated LDL-c: if levels greater than 95th percentile, suspect primary hyperlipidemia

   c. Molecular studies: rarely indicated given diagnosis is usually clinical and differentiation between specific types of primary hyperlipidemias rarely informs management

   d. Evaluate for secondary causes

      i. Diabetes: fasting glucose and/or glycohemoglobin

      ii. Excessive alcohol use: Alcohol Use Disorders Identification Test (AUDIT-c) (Bush, Kivlahan, McDonell, Fihn, & Bradley, 1998)

      iii. Hypothyroidism: thyroid-stimulating hormone (TSH)

      iv. Nephrotic syndrome and chronic renal insufficiency: urine protein and serum creatinine

      v. Hepatitis and cholestasis: liver function tests

      vi. Drugs: careful medication reconciliation

   e. Patient monitoring

      i. Lipid panels every 6–12 months to ensure adherence and efficacy of therapy

C. Management

1. Before initiating therapy for any type of lipid disorder, evaluate and treat for hypothyroidism, nephrotic syndrome, and obstructive liver disease

2. Even for patients with suspected or known primary hyperlipidemias, management should always involve evaluation and treatment of secondary causes

3. Inherited disorders of LDL-c metabolism

   a. Statins and a second therapy (usually absorption inhibitor and/or bile acid sequestrant) are generally required at minimum. In some cases, particularly for patients with homozygous familial hypercholesterolemia, additional agents are required.

   b. Apheresis, a method for removing LDL from the blood, can also be used when pharmacologic therapy is not enough.

4. Hypertriglyceridemia

   a. Lifestyle: weight management with aerobic exercise and dietary portion control, low-fat diet with avoidance of high-carbohydrate, high-glycemic, and high-fructose foods. Particularly important for patients with very high triglycerides to avoid "refeeding" or binging, which can precipitate pancreatitis.

   b. Pharmacologic management directed at lowering CVD risk: There are limited data to guide who is treated for hypertriglyceridemia and what medication to select. Cardiovascular risk reduction can be achieved with statins and given this is the primary goal of all lipid-lowering therapy, they are considered first line even though they are not particularly effective in lowering serum triglyceride levels.

   c. Pharmacologic management directed at lowering triglycerides: gemfibrozil, fenofibrate, nicotinic acid, fish oil

5. Treatment of hypercholesteremia for secondary prevention

   a. Diet and lifestyle interventions are first line.

   b. American Heart Association diet (American Heart Association, 2014a)

      i. Low saturated fat

      ii. Aerobic exercise

      iii. Healthy weight

   c. Pharmacologic management: American College of Cardiology (ACC) and American Heart Association (AHA) cholesterol treatment guidelines (Stone et al., 2014)

      i. Compared to previous guidelines, ACC/AHA 2013 guidelines focus on statin therapy tailored for cardiovascular risk as assessed by their newly developed Pooled Cohort Equation. These guidelines deemphasize previously relied upon LDL targets and nonstatin therapy.

      ii. Statin therapy (see **Table 63-1**)

         a. Check baseline liver enzymes and TSH prior to initiating statin therapy

         b. Nonstatin therapy is not currently recommended as first-line pharmacologic management. Nonstatin agents may be used if statin therapy is contraindicated or not tolerated (see **Table 63-2**, Lipid-Lowering Agents).

         c. Nonstatin agents do not add additional benefit when used in conjunction with statins

      iii. Engage in evidence-based treatment of underlying disease contributing to disordered lipid metabolism, such as diabetes.

TABLE 63-1 Summary of Statin Therapy

Statin Classification	Indication	Therapy
High Intensity	• Patients age ≤ 75 with clinical ASCVD* • Patients with type 1 or 2 diabetes between 40 and 75 years of age and estimated 10-year risk ≥ 7.5%[†‡] • Patients with LDL-c ≥ 190 mg/dL	• Expected to lower LDL-c ≥ 50% • Atorvastatin 40–80 mg, Rosuvastatin 20–40 mg
Moderate Intensity	• Patients age > 75 with clinical ASCVD • Patients with type 1 or 2 diabetes between 40 and 75 years of age and estimated 10-year risk < 7.5% • Patients between 40 and 75 year of age with an LDL between 70 and 189 mg/dL and estimated 10-year risk ≥ 7.5% • Patients who are recommended, but cannot tolerate high-intensity statin therapy	• Expected to lower LDL-c 30–49% • Atorvastatin 10–20 mg, Rosuvastatin 5–10 mg, Simvastatin 20–40 mg, Pravastatin 40–80 mg, Lovastatin 40 mg, Fluvastatin XL 80 mg, Fluvastatin 40 mg bid, Pitavastatin 2–4 mg
Low Intensity	• Not recommended in AHA/ACC 2013 guidelines • May be considered in patients who are recommended, but cannot tolerate, high- or moderate-intensity statin therapy	• Expected to lower LDL-c < 30% • Simvastatin 10 mg, Pravastatin 10–20 mg, Lovastatin 20 mg, Fluvastatin 20–40 mg, Pitavastatin 1 mg

*Clinical atherosclerotic cardiovascular disease (ASCVD) includes patients with history of acute coronary syndrome, myocardial infarction, angina, coronary revascularization, stroke, transient ischemic attack, or peripheral artery disease.

[†]Pooled Cohort Equation can be used to estimate 10-year risk. This equation incorporates age, sex, race, total cholesterol, HDL cholesterol, systolic blood pressure, antihypertensive therapy, diabetes diagnosis, and tobacco use.

[‡]There is limited data for adults under age 40. If the adult under age 40 has diabetes and estimated 10-year risk ≥ 7.5%, it is reasonable to consider statin therapy

Adapted from Stone, N. J., Robinson, J. G., Lichtenstein, A. H., Merz, C. N. B., Blum, C. B., Eckel, R. H., et al. (2014). 2013 ACC/AHA guideline on the treatment of blood cholesterol to reduce atherosclerotic cardiovascular risk in adults: a report of the American College of Cardiology/ American Heart Association Task Force on Practice Guidelines. *Circulation, 129*(25 Suppl. 2), S1–45.

TABLE 63-2 Lipid-Lowering Agents

Class	Notes
Statin (HMG-CoA reductase inhibitors)	Block the enzyme required for a rate-limiting step in the synthesis of cholesterol. This is the only class of lipid-lowering medication shown to reduce mortality and is the only class advised by 2013 AHA/ACC guidelines. Statins lower LDL, lower triglycerides, and modestly raise HDL. Adverse effects include, but are not limited to, hepatotoxicity, myopathy, and increased risk for diabetes.
Fibrates	Includes gemfibrozil and fenofibrate. Works by inhibiting the secretion of VLDL (which transports endogenous triglycerides and cholesterol). Generally used to lower triglycerides, given limited efficacy in lowering LDL. Side effects include dyspepsia, gallstones, and myopathy.
Absorption Inhibitors	Includes ezetimibe. Works by blocking intestinal absorption of cholesterol. Effective in lowering LDL-c, particularly when used in combination with statin. Does not significantly affect triglycerides or HDL-c.
Bile acid sequestrants	Includes cholestyramine and colestipol. Works by reducing bile acid reabsorption from the intestine causing the liver to use available cholesterol for increased bile acid synthesis. Most common side effects are gastrointestinal related (bloating, constipation).
Nicotinic acid (niacin)	Reduces LDL-c and triglycerides. Can cause flushing and increased blood glucose levels.

   d. Treatment of hypercholesteremia for primary prevention
      i.   Diet and lifestyle
      ii. If treatment is pursued, consider moderate- or high-intensity statin
      iii. Nonstatin lipid-lowering medication is not recommended in primary prevention
6. Interprofessional team use and referral
   a. Endocrine: Consider for refractory hyperlipidemia or difficult to treat hyperlipidemias related to diabetes, obesity, or thyroid disease.
   b. Nutrition: For overweight patients, weight loss through diet and physical activity
   c. Tobacco cessation: The importance of tobacco cessation in reducing cardiovascular risk cannot be understated. For patients who use tobacco, motivational interviewing, nicotine replacement, pharmacologic therapy, and group support should be considered and offered as appropriate at each encounter.

VI. Self-management resources and tools

A. Patient education

1. Inform the patient and/or caregiver that hyperlipidemia, especially elevated triglycerides, is associated with alcohol misuse and poor diet. Low HDL is associated with sedentary lifestyle, obesity, and smoking.

B. Online resources

1. American Heart Association's Heart360 (American Heart Association, 2014b)

2. National Heart, Lung, and Blood Institute's heart and vascular disease patient information online publications (National Heart, Lung, and Blood Institute, 2014)

REFERENCES

American Heart Association. (2014a). *The American Heart Association's diet and lifestyle recommendations*. Retrieved from http://www.heart.org/HEARTORG/GettingHealthy/NutritionCenter/HealthyEating/The-American-Heart-Associations-Diet-and-Lifestyle-Recommendations_UCM_305855_Article.jsp.

American Heart Association. (2014b). *Heart360*. Retrieved from https://www.heart360.org/Default.aspx?cid=9ea5cba5ffa4c87aab69dcac799a03de.

Bush, K., Kivlahan, D. R., McDonell, M. B., Fihn, S. D., & Bradley, K. A. (1998). The AUDIT alcohol consumption questions (AUDIT-C): An effective brief screening test for problem drinking. Ambulatory care quality improvement project (ACQUIP). *Archives of Internal Medicine, 158*(16), 1789–1795.

Centers for Disease Control and Prevention. (2011). Vital signs: Prevalence, treatment, and control of high levels of low-density lipoprotein cholesterol. United States, 1999–2002 and 2005–2008. *MMWR, 60*(4), 109–114.

D'Agostino, R. B., Sr., Vasan, R. S., Pencina, M. J., Wolf, P. A., Cobain, M., Massaro, J. M., et al. (2008). General cardiovascular risk profile for use in primary care: The Framingham heart study. *Circulation, 117*(6), 743–753.

Durrington, P., (2003). Dyslipidaemia. *Lancet, 362*(9385), 717–731. doi: 10.1016/S0140-6736(03)14234-1.

Kochanek, K. D., Xu, J. Q., Murphy, S. L., Miniño, A. M., & Kung, H. C. (2011). Deaths: Final data for 2009. *National Vital Statistics Reports, Vol. 60, No. 3*. Hyattsville, MD: Centers for Disease Control and Prevention, National Center for Health Statistics.

National Heart, Lung, and Blood Institute. (2014). *Heart & vascular diseases*. Retrieved from http://www.nhlbi.nih.gov/health/resources/heart.

Stone, N. J., Robinson, J. G., Lichtenstein, A. H., Merz, C. N. B., Blum, C. B., Eckel, R. H., et al. (2014). 2013 ACC/AHA guideline on the treatment of blood cholesterol to reduce atherosclerotic cardiovascular risk in adults: A report of the American College of Cardiology/American Heart Association Task Force on Practice Guidelines. *Circulation, 129*(25, Suppl. 2), S1–S45.

U.S. Preventive Services Task Force. (2008). *Lipid disorders in adults (cholesterol, dyslipidemia): Screening*. Retrieved from http://www.uspreventiveservicestaskforce.org/Page/Topic/recommendation-summary/lipid-disorders-in-adults-cholesterol-dyslipidemia-screening.

Vodnala, D., Rubenfire, M., & Brook, R., (2012). Secondary causes of dyslipidemia. *American Journal of Cardiology, 110*(6), 823–825. doi:10.1016/j.amjcard.2012.04.062.

LOW BACK PAIN

CHAPTER 64

H. Kate Lawlor

I. Introduction/general background

The lumbosacral spine is the fulcrum of the body. Its skeletal structure, muscles, and ligaments bear the stressors of bending over, straightening up, lifting, carrying, and supporting the body's weight. So it is not surprising that up to 60% of the U.S. population will experience low back pain (LBP) at some time during their adult life (van Tulder, Koes, & Bombardier, 2002). After upper respiratory infections, back pain is the next most common reason to seek nonemergency care (Atlas & Deyo, 2001). The differential diagnosis for LBP is lengthy, and a precise diagnosis cannot be made in more than 80% of cases (Chou et al., 2007); yet 80% of episodes of LBP in a primary care setting will spontaneously improve in 1–2 weeks, and 90% resolve within 6 weeks. The diagnostic challenge is to identify those patients who require a more extensive or urgent evaluation at their initial presentation (Papadakis & McPhee, 2015).

The differential diagnosis for LBP includes both muscular and focal spine disorders (i.e., disc herniation, spinal fracture, and stenosis of the spinal canal), regional nonspinal disorders (i.e., pelvic inflammatory disease, aortic aneurysm, and kidney stones), and systemic diseases (such as ankylosing spondylitis and metastatic cancer). Even if anatomic defects like narrowed disk space or the vertebral osteophytes of degenerative arthritis are found on x-rays, causality cannot be absolutely assumed, because these defects are also common in asymptomatic patients and increase in frequency with age (Ehrlich, 2003). In fact, more than one-third of asymptomatic individuals older than age 60 will have evidence of disc herniation or spinal stenosis on specialized imaging (Ehrlich, 2003).

Table 64-1 lists the potential causes of LBP grouped by category. The most common causes are pain due to mechanical or degenerative processes. The most frequent sources of pain in these categories are lumbar-sacral strain and symptomatic herniated disc (Chou et al., 2007). The obligation for the clinician is to promptly identify those other patients whose pain may be due to urgent causes ("red flags"), such as (in order of frequency) ankylosing spondylitis, cord compression, a compression fracture, cancer, or cauda equine syndrome (see description in the following section) (Chou et al., 2007).

These guidelines review the history and physical exam (PE) necessary to differentiate mechanical or degenerative LBP from more urgent causes. The treatment and patient education for causes of LBP that are appropriately managed by primary care providers are emphasized. For most patients, the history and physical exam is sufficient to exclude the "red flags" that suggest more serious disorders (**Table 64-2**) (Ehrlich, 2003).

II. Database (may include but is not limited to)

A. Subjective

1. History of present illness
   a. Onset and duration (intermittent vs. constant)
   b. Circumstances when first occurred (trauma? work related?)
   c. Location and radiation of pain: Atypical location such as midback is more common in cancer. Pain that is localized in the midbuttock may not be a spinal problem. The less frequently occurring piriformis syndrome (PS) is due to inflammation or spasm of the piriformis muscle that follows overuse or athletic injury. Because the muscle overlies the sciatic nerve, irritation of the piriformis muscle can cause the same sciatic nerve entrapment symptoms (see Section 7) as lumbosacral disorders. Thus, it is often difficult to differentiate.
   d. Quality and severity of pain: use specific descriptors and pain severity scale.
   e. Progression of symptoms over time: Symptoms lasting > 3 months represent "chronic" LBP.

TABLE 64-1 Most Common Causes of Low Back Pain

I. Mechanical (74%)
    A. Poor back or core abdominal muscle tone (may be secondary to obesity, pregnancy, or deconditioning)
    B. Chronic postural or lumbar-sacral strain

II. Structural/Degenerative (17%)
    A. Degenerative joint disease (osteoarthritis, degenerative disc disease, facet process) (10%)
    B. Sacroiliitis
    C. Scoliosis, kyphosis
    D. Disc protrusion or herniation (4%)
    E. Spinal stenosis (narrowing of spinal canal) (3%)
    F. Osteoporosis
    G. Piriformis syndrome
    H. Cauda equina syndrome (characterized by lower extremity weakness and sensory loss, saddle anesthesia/fecal incontinence, urinary retention or incontinence)

III. Trauma (6%)
    A. Fall
    B. Work-related injury
    C. Compression fracture due to fall, osteoporosis, or chronic steroid use (4%)
    D. Subluxation of facet joint (spondylolisthesis) (2%)

IV. Inflammatory Diseases (0.3%)
    A. Ankylosing spondylitis (or other spondyloarthropathies)
    B. Rheumatoid arthritis

V. Infection (0.03%)
    A. Osteomyelitis
    B. Urinary tract infection (from indwelling catheter)
    C. Tuberculosis
    D. IV drug abuse

VI. Cancer (0.7%)
    A. Multiple myeloma
    B. Metastatic cancer of prostate, breast, and lung
    C. Spinal cord tumors

VII. Visceral Disease (2%)
    A. Dissecting abdominal aneurysm (usually history of hypertension)
    B. Renal disease
    C. Pelvic disease

VIII. Psychogenic
    A. Tension/stress related
    B. Malingering (more often in setting of worker's compensation claim)

Data from Atlas, S., & Deyo, R. (2001). Evaluating and managing acute low back pain in the primary care setting. *Journal of General Internal Medicine, 16,* 120–131.

TABLE 64-2 History and Physical Examination Findings Associated with Increased Likelihood of Serious Spine Condition ("red flags")

Disorder	History	Physical Exam/Studies for Diagnosis
All	• Failure to improve > 6 weeks • No relief with bed rest	
Cancer	• Age > 50 yrs • Previous history of cancer (esp. multiple myeloma) • Unexplained weight loss of > 10 lbs in 6 months • Failure to improve after 1 month; worse at night • No relief with bedrest	• Lymphadenopathy • Plain lumbar-sacral (LS) spine films • Magnetic resonance imagining (MRI) • Elevated erythrocyte sedimentation rate (ESR)
Fracture	• Age > 50 yrs; especially > 70 yrs • Weight < 57 kg • History of cancer (causes lytic metastases) • History of smoking (increased risk of osteoporosis) • History of significant trauma (fall from height, motor vehicle accident, or direct blow) • History of osteoporosis • Long-term steroid use (causes decreased bone density) • Substance abuse (increased risk of falls; alcohol use)	• Vertebral point tenderness • Plain LS spine film
Bone Infection	• Fever, chills • Pain increased at rest • Recent skin or genital-urinary infection (history of indwelling catheter) • Recreational injection drug use • Immunosuppression	• Fever > 100°F • Tenderness over a spinous process • MRI • Elevated ESR, positive C-reactive protein, elevated white blood count
Ankylosing Spondylitis	• Male > female; < 45 years old • Positive family history of irritable bowel disease (IBD), ankylosing spondylitis • Pain > 3 mos; especially buttock pain • Pain in latter part of night; morning stiffness • Pain improved with exercise • May be associated with IBD, psoriasis, uveitis, plantar fasciitis, or Achilles tendinitis	• May be decreased chest expansion • Decreased spinal flexibility in sideways, frontal, and backward motions • May be sacroiliac (SI) joint tenderness • May be radiologic evidence of sacroiliitis on anteroposterior pelvic plain films • Elevated ESR, positive C-reactive protein • 90% + histocompatibility complex (HLA)-B27
Cauda Equina Syndrome	• Urinary retention or incontinence • Bowel incontinence • Progressive leg/foot weakness • Sensory loss in lower extremity(ies)	• Saddle anesthesia • Diminished anal sphincter tone • Severe unilateral or bilateral leg/foot weakness • Bladder distension • MRI

Data from Atlas, S., & Deyo, R. (2001). Evaluating and managing acute low back pain in the primary care setting. *Journal of General Internal Medicine, 16,* 120–131; Chou, R., Qaseem, A., Snow, V., Casey, D., Cross, J. T. Jr., Shekelle, P., . . . American Pain Society Low Back Pain Guidelines Panel. (2007). Diagnosis and treatment of low back pain: A joint clinical practice guideline from the American College of Physicians and the American Pain Society. *Annals of Internal Medicine, 147*(7), 478–491.

f. Aggravating and alleviating factors

g. Worse with bending, lifting, prolonged standing, or sitting (most common with mechanical back pain)

h. Worse in AM: if pain less than 30 minutes after waking or shifting positions, suggests degenerative changes of vertebrae.

i. Relief with activity; worse with rest (typical of ankylosing spondylitis)

j. Relief with sitting or bending forward (suggestive of spinal stenosis)

k. Worse with cough, bowel movement, or sneezing (suggests disc pathology)

l. Complaints of urinary retention or incontinence from loss of sphincter function, bilateral motor weakness of lower extremities, and decrease in sensation over buttocks or perineum ("saddle anesthesia") suggest cauda equina syndrome—usually due to massive, centrally herniated disc causing compression of nerve roots of lower cord segments.

m. Interventions attempted to relieve pain and results

i. Medications: (aspirin [ASA], nonsteroidal anti-inflammatory drugs [NSAIDS], acetaminophen [Tylenol], and opioids)

ii. Herbal products

iii. Chiropractic care

iv. Physical therapy

v. Massage

vi. Acupuncture

vii. Heat/cold application

n. Associated signs and symptoms

i. Constitutional symptoms: fever, malaise, fatigue, weight loss (each suggests a more serious concern: osteomyelitis, abscess, or cancer)

ii. Ocular: painful, inflamed, or gritty eye (uveitis is associated with ankylosing spondylitis)

iii. Neurologic

a. Sciatica: burning pain that radiates down the posterior or lateral aspect of one or both legs past the knee—95% sensitive for nerve root irritation (Atlas & Deyo, 2001). Sciatica occurs with herniated disc, spinal stenosis, and piriformis syndrome. Other neurologic abnormalities and location of pain found in setting of sciatica help to identify which nerves are affected. See **Table 64-3**.

b. Sharp back pain when coughs or sneezes (indicative of disc compression)

c. Leg pain with standing or walking (neurogenic claudication); relief with sitting (suggests spinal stenosis)

d. Leg or foot weakness; gait disturbance; urinary retention or urinary incontinence; bowel incontinence (these

TABLE 64-3 Specific Nerve Root Impingements Associated with Particular Physical Examination Findings

Strength	Unilateral Altered Sensation	Reflex	Nerve Root
Iliapsoas: have the patient seated with legs dangling over the edge of the examination table. Then stabilize the pelvis by placing your hand over the iliac crest while the patient actively raises the thigh from the table. Second, place your other hand over the distal femoral portion of the knee, and ask the patient to attempt to raise the thigh further from the table while you resist this motion. Compare resistance results testing on the other, uninvolved side (Hoppenfeld, 1976, p. 250).	Anterior thigh/groin	—	L2
Quadriceps: squatting then rising, or strengthening a bent knee against resistance while seated	Anterolateral thigh	Patellar	L3
Quadriceps; ankle dorsiflexion (heel walking)	Medial ankle/foot	Patellar	L4
First toe dorsiflexion	Dorsum of foot	—	L5
Ankle plantar flexion (toe walking)	Lateral plantar foot	Achilles	S1

Note: Over 95% of herniated discs involve the L4-5 or L5–S1 interspaces (Chou et al., 2007).

Data from Atlas, S., & Deyo, R. (2001). Evaluating and managing acute low back pain in the primary care setting. *Journal of General Internal Medicine, 16*, 120–131; Hoppenfeld, S. (1976). *Physical exam of the spine and the extremities.* East Norwalk, CT: Appleton-Century-Crofts/Prentice-Hall.

symptoms in the aggregate suggest cauda equina syndrome resulting from cord compression, a surgical emergency)

    iv. Abdominal: pain or diarrhea (inflammatory bowel disease can be associated with ankylosing spondylitis)

    v. Genitourinary: dysuria, urinary frequency or urgency, recent indwelling catheter use (suggests urinary tract infection, pyelonephritis may present with flank pain and fever). Vaginal discharge, pelvic pain (suggests pelvic infection)

    vi. Vascular: chest pain or throbbing abdominal pain (LBP with these symptoms may signal an abdominal aortic aneurysm)

    vii. Skin: history of psoriasis (associated with ankylosing spondylitis) or recent skin infection (may cause spinal infection)

    viii. Psychologic: recent sleep disturbances, depressed or anxious mood, diminished participation in social activities (may signal depression)

  o. Patient's concern/theory about of source of symptoms

2. Past health history

  a. Prior spinal diagnoses, fractures or surgery, history of current or previous cancers

  b. Previous radiologic or imaging studies of spine. Prior bone density testing.

  c. Medications

    i. Used for back pain (especially opiates: dosage and frequency)

    ii. Prescription (steroid use can be risk factor for osteoporosis and compression fractures)

    iii. Over the counter

    iv. Herbal/alternative

3. Family history

  a. Disc disease

  b. Osteoporosis

  c. Rheumatoid arthritis, ankylosing spondylitis

  d. Vascular disease

  e. Scoliosis

4. Occupational

  a. Physical requirements of job

  b. How many hours worked per week

  c. Number of hours spent in prolonged sitting (risk factor for piriformis syndrome and deconditioning)

  d. Recent job injury

  e. Prior ergonomic assessments performed and results

  f. Current worker's compensation claim or permanent disability

  g. Job satisfaction

5. Personal/social (factors that may predict poorer or delayed resolution)

  a. Other pending litigation: occupational or trauma

  b. Impact of pain on activities of daily living (ADLs) or current relationships

  c. History of depression

  d. Outstanding disability claims

  e. Previous worker's comp claims

  f. Habits

    i. Smoking (risk factor for osteoporosis)

    ii. Injectable drug use (risk factor for spinal infection)

    iii. Alcohol use (be alert to increased use for self-medicating pain)

    iv. Recreational drug use

B. Objective: physical exam

Patient should be undressed. Exam should include but is not limited to:

1. Height (loss of height suggests kyphosis, compression fracture)

2. Weight (unexplained weight loss may suggest cancer; low body weight is risk factor for osteoporosis; obesity is risk factor for osteoarthritis)

3. Age (> 50 yrs at greater risk for cancer; > 75 yrs at greater risk for osteoporosis)

4. Gender (males at greater risk for ankylosing spondylitis; females > 30 yrs are largest population for PS).

5. Vital signs, including temperature (fever > 100°F suggests infection)

6. Spine (performed with patient unclothed in gown and underwear)

In the absence of a history suggestive of a serious condition, systemic disease, and/or illness not localized to the back region (see Table 64-1), a focused spine and neurologic exam as described next should be an adequate screening exam to rule out serious or urgent causes of LBP, unless any red flags (see Table 64-2) are identified (Ehrlich, 2003).

  a. Inspection: look for changes in normal spine curvature that may occur if muscle spasm, scoliosis, hyperkyphosis, or ankylosing spondylitis

  b. Standing: assess symmetry and posture

  c. Palpation: assess for bone tenderness versus muscle spasm. With patient forward flexed, assess for lateral curvature and rotation of the spine; may suggest scoliosis. Exclusively lateral curve could signal hyperkyphosis. Palpate the area over the piriformis muscle at the sciatic notch if the patient complains of buttock pain. Eliciting tenderness with deep palpation suggests that the source of the patient's pain may be PS, not lumbar-sacral disorders.

d. Range of motion: assess flexibility as well as complaints of pain. Ask which movement causes the most pain. (Flexion causes increased pressure on the disc; extension narrows the diameter of the spinal canal [spinal stenosis]; lateral bending causes increased pain if disc is herniated.)

e. Gait; check heel and toe walking separately (heel walk involves the anterior tibialis and L4 innervation; toe walk uses the gastrocnemius and S1 innervation)

f. Measure leg length. (Difference of > 2 cm causes significant postural alteration that can result in LBP.)

7. Focused neurologic exam

a. Straight leg raises (SLR): screen for nerve root irritation, most commonly due to a herniated disc in the L5 or S1 nerve roots. While patient is supine, the affected leg should be elevated by the clinician with the ankle dorsiflexed and the knee fully extended. A (+) response ("sciatica") reproduces sharp or burning pain when the limb is raised to 30–70 degrees. This occurs in the setting of disc herniation or degenerative conditions causing neural foraminal stenosis, and less often, PS. The earlier the onset of pain during the test and the greater the severity, the more specific is the result. The SLR test is 64–98% sensitive, but less specific (11–61%) for lumbosacral disc herniation (McGee, 2007). Additionally, sciatic symptoms that occur down the opposite leg during testing usually indicate a large disc herniation (Papadakis & McPhee, 2015). Sciatica due to spinal stenosis is more common in older patients, and pain is often bilateral (see Table 64-3 for exam findings associated with impingement of specific nerve roots). Pain that is limited to the back or the hip during the SLR is considered a (−) test. A (−) test argues against disc herniation of the L4–S1 area. If (+) SLR or a red flag is present, the clinician needs to proceed with more detailed neurologic exam of the lower extremities as described in Section 8.

Much less L4 and minimal L2 or L3 disc movement occurs during the SLR test, so that it is less useful in detecting disc herniation above L4. Flexing the knee with the patient in a prone position may reproduce the back and anterior thigh pain of upper lumbar disc herniation (Goroll & Mulley, 2014).

8. Expanded neurologic exam

a. Comparative muscle strength testing of upper and lower extremities: knee, great toe, and ankle dorsiflexion

b. Dermatomal sensation testing of lower extremities and feet

c. Reflex testing of patellae and Achilles tendon and Babinski

d. Measure muscle mass of thighs and calves: difference of > 2 cm may indicate neurologic involvement of limb with smaller muscle mass.

e. If complaints and exam findings are consistent with cauda equine syndrome (severe unilateral or bilateral leg weakness, urinary retention/distended bladder, or fecal incontinence), check for saddle anesthesia and diminished anal sphincter tone.

9. Systemic exam

a. Eye exam: if c/o eye pain or irritation. Anterior uveitis can be associated with ankylosing spondylitis.

b. Pulmonary exam (chest expansion decreased in ankylosing spondylitis)

c. Cardiac exam: note evidence of aortic valve incompetence (can occur in ankylosing spondylitis) including testing for aortic bruits to assess if aortic aneurysm is suspected as the source of LBP.

d. Urinary exam: assess for distended bladder (saddle anesthesia and/or diminished anal sphincter tone with fecal incontinence and urinary retention suggests cauda equina syndrome, a surgical emergency)

e. Genitourinary exam: note any pelvic tenderness or masses, or cervical motion tenderness or discharge (suggests pelvic inflammatory disease in females); urethral discharge or dysuria (can be associated with ankylosing spondylitis); prostate enlargement, tenderness, or masses (can signal infection or prostate cancer).

f. Abdominal exam: pulsatile mass near umbilicus suggests an aortic aneurysm

g. Rectal exam: check for saddle anesthesia of the perineum or diminished anal sphincter tone if suspicion of cauda equine syndrome

C. Diagnostic tests (may include, but not limited to)

1. Radiographs: basic x-ray findings are poorly correlated with specific symptoms and are not sensitive for important abnormalities (Chou et al., 2007). In addition, in several studies of asymptomatic

individuals, disc degeneration was a common finding that increased with age (Atlas & Deyo, 2001). Therefore, plain x-rays of the spine have a very low sensitivity and specificity in the majority of cases, and should not be obtained for patients with nonspecific low back pain unless pain has persisted for > 6 weeks.

a. Only consider plain radiograph of the lumbosacral spine when:

    i. There are red flags in the patient's history or physical exam (see Table 64-2).

    ii. If back pain is primarily in the high lumbar or thoracic regions (pain here is suggestive of a compression fracture or metastatic tumor)

    iii. If the patient has not improved after a 6-week course of conservative therapy.

b. Consider pelvic radiograph to look for sacroiliitis if suspicion of ankylosing spondylitis based on patient's history or exam (Chou et al., 2007).

c. Consider chest x-ray if findings suggestive of abdominal aortic aneurysm.

d. Advanced radiographic studies (computerized tomography [CT], magnetic resonance imaging [MRI]) are appropriate to consider in the situations below:

    i. If severe or progressive neurologic deficits

    ii. If suspicion of infection, tumor, or cauda equina syndrome, urgent study is warranted

    iii. If sciatic symptoms suggest disc herniation or spinal stenosis

        a. Treat with course of conservative care first (see Plan, Section IV A), which may be sufficient (Atlas & Deyo, 2001).

        b. If surgery is likely to be needed for unimproved symptoms of disc herniation or spinal stenosis, consider referral to orthopedic or neurosurgical specialist *before* advanced studies are ordered, as they may have a particular preferred test.

e. Despite frequent patient requests for imaging, its utility is largely limited to situations in which an interventional procedure is likely. Again, to emphasize this important point: in 22–26% of asymptomatic adults, disc herniations are seen on MRI. Asymptomatic patients over age 60 have up to 21% incidence of spinal stenosis (Jarvik, 2002; Weinstein et al., 2006). Patient education is important to explain the risk of unnecessary radiation and to underscore the frequency of false-positive results.

2. Routine blood and urine testing is unnecessary. Select tests may be helpful if particular pathology is suspected:

a. Erythrocyte sedimentation rate (ESR): if question of malignancy, ankylosing spondylitis, or consideration of infection

b. Complete blood count (CBC): may be used as screening test for neoplasms, infections, or inflammatory processes

c. Prostate-specific antigen (PSA): if suspicion of metastatic prostate cancer

d. Urinalysis: if question of urinary tract disease

e. C-reactive protein: as screen for vertebral infection or ankylosing spondylitis

f. HLA-B27: as screen for ankylosing spondylitis (rate of reliability as a screen differs markedly among ethnic populations; strongest association with ankylosing spondylitis is in caucasians) (Khan, 2002).

g. Serum calcium and vitamin D level if concern of osteoporosis

h. Alkaline phosphatase

3. Electromyography and nerve conduction studies should be reserved for use by specialists in recalcitrant or complex cases.

III. Assessment

More than 85% of cases of acute LBP presenting to a primary provider *cannot* reliably be attributed to a specific disease or spinal abnormality (Chou et al., 2007) but will recover within 6 weeks of conservative therapy as described in the Plan, section IV (Papadakis & McPhee, 2015).

A. *Determine if evidence of nerve impingement due to disc herniation or spinal stenosis (Tables 64-2 and 64-3).*

B. *Determine if presence of red flags suggests more serious pathology (cancer, infection, inflammatory condition, fracture; see Table 64-2).*

C. *If no "red flags" are present, even if there is evidence of simple nerve impingement (i.e., sciatica but no evidence of cauda equina), treat as mechanical musculoskeletal back pain **or** PS, if presentation suggests it, and follow Plan outlined in section IV.*

D. *Determine if medical-legal issues concerning possible worker's compensation or disability claim are present. If medical-legal issues, refer to a specialist.*

IV. Plan

A. Acute low back pain (acute: < 2–6 weeks; may include sciatica, but no red flags)

1. Physical measures: in a synthesis of 17 randomized controlled trials of nonpharmacologic therapies for LBP (Chou & Huffman, 2007b), only the following interventions showed evidence of efficacy:

   a. Bed rest (BR) only if sciatic or muscle symptoms make walking/sitting difficult. Limit use of BR for only severe pain; bed rest for > 48 hours is not only of no value, it contributes to counterproductive deconditioning (Ehrlich, 2003).

   b. Patient contact should be made at 1 week, 2–4 weeks, and 6 weeks to assess expected improvement in pain. Any worsening of pain or new/worsening of neurologic losses should be evaluated promptly.

   c. Avoid prolonged sitting or standing; get up at regular intervals (every 30 minutes) to walk and stretch the paraspinal muscles.

   d. Activity modification as warranted by pain level/location. Avoid heavy lifting, extreme spinal flexion.

   e. Local application of moist heat or cold may offer relief.

   f. If suspicion of PS, referral to physical therapist for training in stretching and strengthening of hip abductors, external rotators, and extensors.

   g. Spinal manipulation and gentle massage by physical therapist (PT) or osteopathic doctor (DO) may be helpful in producing short-term improvements in pain. Patients should not undergo spinal manipulation if they have radicular symptoms or do back exercises not specifically designed for them as symptoms may be aggravated.

   h. Other nonpharmacologic therapies like acupuncture, back schools, low-level laser, lumbar supports, traction, transcutaneous electrical nerve stimulation (TENS) units, and ultrasonography lack reliable evidence of effectiveness in managing acute LBP. There have been no studies that evaluate the effect of different mattresses or pillows on pain intensity.

2. Medications. In a review of 51 randomized, controlled trials for the treatment of LBP from the Cochrane Central Registry of Controlled Trials (Chou & Huffman, 2007a):

   a. NSAIDS were superior to placebo for global improvement of back pain with or without sciatica. No one agent was found to be superior to any other drug in the same class.

   b. Acetaminophen at dosages up to 4 g/day produced relief equivalent to NSAIDS for patients who could not tolerate NSAIDS.

   c. There was insufficient evidence to judge the independent benefit of ASA.

   d. Opioid analgesics offered moderate benefits in relieving pain not controlled by NSAIDS or acetaminophen. Their use should be limited to < 1 week and reserved for patients whose pain cannot be controlled by agents like NSAIDs or acetaminophen or who should not take these medications for other medical reasons.

   e. Muscle relaxants (e.g., diazepam, tizanidine, cyclobenzaprine, baclofen): use for < 2 weeks; reserved for patients whose pain cannot be controlled alone by NSAIDs or acetaminophen because of *true* muscle spasm. Most effective when combined with NSAID or acetaminophen.

   f. The decision to prescribe antidepressants, antiepileptic drugs, or epidural steroid injections for patients with sciatica should be left to a specialist. However, they were not shown to offer any independent, sustained pain relief.

3. For *Return to Work Guidelines*, see the *AHRQ Official Disability Guidelines* at http://www.guideline.gov/content.aspx?id=47586. Modify as directed if sciatic symptoms still present.

4. File a "Physician's First Report of Injury" if symptoms are due to a work-related injury.

B. Subacute low back pain (1–3 months)

1. Physical measures (Chou & Huffman, 2007a)

   a. Intermittent bed rest (of no more than 48 hours at a time) only if radicular symptoms persist

   b. Modify activity as needed to control symptoms

   c. Low-stress aerobic exercise (walking, swimming) as tolerated; avoid heavy lifting, prolonged sitting and standing

   d. Refer workers with LBP beyond 6 weeks to a comprehensive return-to-work rehabilitation program. Effective programs are multidisciplinary and involve case management, education about keeping active, behavioral treatment, and participation in an exercise program.

   e. Exercise training by PT or DO for improvements in posture, core stability training, physical conditioning, and activity modification to decrease physical strain are keys for ongoing management (Papadakis & McPhee, 2015). Current guidelines contraindicate spinal manipulation in people with severe or progressive neurologic deficits.

f. There is insufficient evidence to recommend for or against any *specific* type of exercise program or its frequency.

g. Local heat/cold if provides relief

h. There is insufficient evidence to recommend for or against acupuncture, massage therapy, herbal medicine, yoga, laser therapy, and diathermy.

i. Lumbar corsets ("back belts"), traction, TENS unit use, systemic steroids, and ultrasonography have failed to demonstrate benefit in numerous controlled trials.

2. Medications (Chou & Huffman, 2007b)

a. Nonnarcotic analgesics only (e.g., acetaminophen, NSAIDs) unless contraindicated. Again, no single NSAID is superior to any other in controlling pain and symptoms.

b. Short-term use of benzodiazepines may offer some benefit if skeletal muscle spasm persists; other skeletal muscle relaxants did not demonstrate benefits in controlled trials (Chou & Huffman, 2007b).

c. Opioids should be avoided because of risk of dependency or abuse, unless brief course (1–2 weeks) needed for severe pain

d. Consider course of tricyclic antidepressants (e.g., amitriptyline) if radicular pain is present. (When used for nerve pain, start at 10 mg at bedtime, then increase to 25 mg after 1 week, then up to 50 mg as maintenance dose). This is a subtherapeutic dose for depression. Caution with use in patients with history of bipolar affective disorder, mood swings, glaucoma, or history of palpitations.

3. Conditioning (after initial pain has subsided)

a. Biofeedback

b. "Back school"

c. Conditioning training by PT, DO, or other health professional to improve core muscle strength. More rigorous conditioning regimens are associated with the best outcomes (Chou et al., 2007).

d. Ergonomic evaluation of the workplace if symptoms suggest aggravation by work activities.

4. Referral for specialty evaluation (Atlas & Deyo, 2001)

a. Refer to a specialist for consideration of epidural steroid injections if sciatic pain (suggesting disc herniation) remains incapacitating during the latter 6 weeks of conservative therapy. Typically, two injections will be given 3–4 weeks apart. Pain relief will be short term (averaging 3–6 weeks) but may help patient to manage during period between "end" of conservative therapy and point of surgical decision making.

b. Refer for surgical evaluation if patient with sciatica has not improved after 4–12 weeks of conservative therapy, and/or imaging with CT or MRI shows lesion in an area that corresponds to symptoms.

c. Refer for diagnostic/specialty evaluation if new red flag symptoms appear while patient is being treated with conservative therapy.

d. Refer for evaluation by specialist if symptoms caused by a workplace injury or the patient plans to file a disability claim.

5. For *Return to Work Guidelines* see the *AHRQ Official Disability Guidelines* at http://www.guideline.gov/content.aspx?id=47586. Modify as directed if sciatic symptoms still present.

6. Patient education (see sample patient education handout in **Figure 64-1**).

a. Provide written information that includes all the teaching points detailed in requirements described in management of acute episode of LBP

7. Career counseling: consider referral for vocational evaluation if patient's work repeatedly produces back pain despite conditioning, and patient is not amenable to surgical correction.

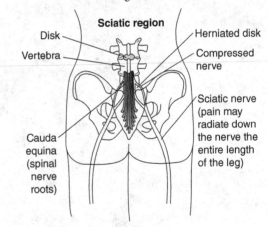

FIGURE 64-1 Sample Patient Education (To accompany the patient education material noted on pages 628-631.)

FIGURE 64-1 Sample Patient Education (Continued)

What Is Back Pain?

Fast Facts: An Easy-to-Read Series of Publications for the Public

Back pain can range from a dull, constant ache to a sudden, sharp pain that makes it hard to move. It can start quickly if you fall or lift something too heavy, or it can get worse slowly.

Who Gets Back Pain?

Anyone can have back pain, but some things that increase your risk are:

- Getting older. Back pain is more common the older you get. You may first have back pain when you are 30 to 40 years old.
- Poor physical fitness. Back pain is more common in people who are not fit.
- Being overweight. A diet high in calories and fat can make you gain weight. Too much weight can stress the back and cause pain.
- Heredity. Some causes of back pain, such as ankylosing spondylitis, a form of arthritis that affects the spine, can have a genetic component.
- Other diseases. Some types of arthritis and cancer can cause back pain.
- Your job. If you have to lift, push, or pull while twisting your spine, you may get back pain. If you work at a desk all day and do not sit up straight, you may also get back pain.
- Smoking. Your body may not be able to get enough nutrients to the disks in your back if you smoke. Smoker's cough may also cause back pain. People who smoke are slow to heal, so back pain may last longer.

Another factor is race. For example, black women are two to three times more likely than white women to have part of the lower spine slip out of place.

What Are the Causes of Back Pain?

There are many causes of back pain. Mechanical problems with the back itself can cause pain. Examples are:

- Disk breakdown
- Spasms
- Tense muscles
- Ruptured disks

Injuries from sprains, fractures, accidents, and falls can result in back pain.

Back pain can also occur with some conditions and diseases, such as:

- Scoliosis
- Spondylolisthesis
- Arthritis
- Spinal stenosis
- Pregnancy
- Kidney stones
- Infections
- Endometriosis
- Fibromyalgia

Other possible causes of back pain are infections, tumors, or stress.

Can Back Pain Be Prevented?

The best things you can do to prevent back pain are:

- Exercise often and keep your back muscles strong.
- Maintain a healthy weight or lose weight if you weigh too much. To have strong bones, you need to get enough calcium and vitamin D every day.

FIGURE 64-1 *Sample Patient Education* (Continued)

- Try to stand up straight and avoid heavy lifting when you can. If you do lift something heavy, bend your legs and keep your back straight.

When Should I See a Healthcare Provider for Pain?

You should see a healthcare provider if you have:

- Numbness or tingling
- Severe pain that does not improve with rest
- Pain after a fall or an injury
- Pain plus any of these problems:
  - Trouble urinating
  - Weakness
  - Numbness in your legs
  - Fever
  - Weight loss when not on a diet.

How Is Back Pain Diagnosed?

To diagnose back pain, your healthcare provider will take your medical history and do a physical exam. Your healthcare provider may order other tests, such as:

- X-rays
- Magnetic resonance imaging (MRI)
- Computerized tomography (CT) scan
- Blood tests

Medical tests may not show the cause of your back pain. Many times, the cause of back pain is never known. Back pain can get better even if you do not know the cause.

What Is the Difference Between Acute and Chronic Pain?

Acute pain starts quickly and lasts less than 6 weeks. It is the most common type of back pain. Acute pain may be caused by things like falling, being tackled in football, or lifting something heavy. Chronic pain lasts for more than 3 months and is much less common than acute pain.

How Is Back Pain Treated?

Treatment for back pain depends on what kind of pain you have. Acute back pain usually gets better without any treatment, but you may want to take acetaminophen, aspirin, or ibuprofen to help ease the pain. Exercise and surgery are not usually used to treat acute back pain.

Following are some types of treatments for chronic back pain.

Hot or Cold Packs (or Both)

Hot or cold packs can soothe sore, stiff backs. Heat reduces muscle spasms and pain. Cold helps reduce swelling and numbs deep pain. Using hot or cold packs may relieve pain, but this treatment does not fix the cause of chronic back pain.

Exercise

Proper exercise can help ease chronic pain but should not be used for acute back pain. Your healthcare provider or physical therapist can tell you the best types of exercise to do.

Medications

The following are the main types of medications used for back pain:

- Analgesic medications are over-the-counter drugs such as acetaminophen and aspirin or prescription pain medications.

(continues)

FIGURE 64-1 *Sample Patient Education* *(Continued)*

- Topical analgesics are creams, ointments, and salves rubbed onto the skin over the site of pain.
- Nonsteroidal anti-inflammatory drugs (NSAIDs) are drugs that reduce both pain and swelling. NSAIDs include over-the-counter drugs such as ibuprofen, ketoprofen, and naproxen sodium. Your healthcare provider may prescribe stronger NSAIDs.
- Muscle relaxants and some antidepressants may be prescribed for some types of chronic back pain, but these do not work for every type of back pain.

Behavior Changes

You can learn to lift, push, and pull with less stress on your back. Changing how you exercise, relax, and sleep can help lessen back pain. Eating a healthy diet and not smoking also help.

Injections

Your healthcare provider may suggest steroid or numbing shots to lessen your pain.

Complementary and Alternative Medical Treatments

When back pain becomes chronic or when other treatments do not relieve it, some people try complementary and alternative treatments. The most common of these treatments are:

- Manipulation. Professionals use their hands to adjust or massage the spine or nearby tissues.
- Transcutaneous electrical nerve stimulation (TENS). A small box over the painful area sends mild electrical pulses to nerves. *Studies have shown that TENS treatments are not always effective for reducing pain.*
- Acupuncture. This Chinese practice uses thin needles to relieve pain and restore health. Acupuncture may be effective when used as a part of a comprehensive treatment plan for low back pain.
- Acupressure. A therapist applies pressure to certain places in the body to relieve pain. *Acupressure has not been well studied for back pain.*

Surgery

Most people with chronic back pain do not need surgery. It is usually used for chronic back pain if other treatments do not work. You may need surgery if you have:

- Herniated disk. When one or more of the disks that cushion the bones of the spine are damaged, the jelly-like center of the disk leaks, causing pain.
- Spinal stenosis. This condition causes the spinal canal to become narrow.
- Spondylolisthesis. This occurs when one or more bones of the spine slip out of place.
- Vertebral fractures. A fracture can be caused by a blow to the spine or by crumbling of the bone due to osteoporosis.
- Degenerative disk disease. As people age, some have disks that break down and cause severe pain.

Rarely, when back pain is caused by a tumor, an infection, or a nerve root problem called cauda equina syndrome, surgery is needed right away to ease the pain and prevent more problems.

What Kind of Research Is Being Done?

Highlights of recent research include:

- Cost and effectiveness comparisons of surgical versus nonsurgical treatments for various types of back pain
- Factors that go into patients' decisions about whether or not to have surgery for herniated disks
- National statistics on back pain costs
- Socioeconomic factors that relate to back pain costs and treatment.

Goals of current research are to:

- Understand the many factors that can cause back pain
- Identify ways to prevent back pain
- Improve surgical and nonsurgical treatments for back pain
- Prevent disability in people who suffer from back pain.

FIGURE 64-1 Sample Patient Education (Continued)

For More Information About Back Pain and Other Related Conditions:

National Institute of Arthritis and Musculoskeletal and Skin Diseases (NIAMS)

Information Clearinghouse

National Institutes of Health

Website: http://www.niams.nih.gov

The information in this publication was summarized in easy-to-read format from information in a more detailed NIAMS publication. To order Back Pain: Handout on Health full-text version, please contact NIAMS using the contact information above. To view the complete text or to order online, visit http://www.niams.nih.gov.

Reproduced from National Institute of Arthritis and Musculoskeletal and Skin Diseases (NIAMS). (2015). *Handout on Health: Back Pain.* (NIH Publication No. 15-5282). Retrieved from http://www.niams.nih.gov/Health_Info/Back_Pain/default.asp#Fig1.

C. Recurrent or chronic low back pain (> 3 months)

1. Appropriate to do radiologic and/or imaging studies, and/or blood tests if not resolved yet, especially if pain arose from work setting

2. Refer to specialist for further evaluation/management if neurologic losses remain present despite compliance with conservative therapy, especially if pain is work-related or disability claim filed

3. Physical measures (Chou et al., 2007)
   a. Modify activity to control symptoms; avoid heavy lifting, prolonged sitting/standing
   b. Low-stress aerobic exercise
   c. Massage
   d. Yoga as long as no radicular (sciatic) symptoms
   e. Manipulation by PT or DO may be helpful as long as no sciatic symptoms present
   f. Acupuncture may offer additive short-term pain relief
   g. Patient-specific exercises and activities per PT or DO to improve core muscle strength and posture may reduce the likelihood of recurrence.
   h. Exercising in warm water can be effective analgesic. Do not do any exercises that increase the pain.
   i. Encourage return to work and ADLs as tolerated
   j. A regular program of daily walking and low-stress aerobic activities once pain has resolved helps develop core muscle support

4. Medications (Chou & Huffman, 2007b)
   a. Nonnarcotic analgesics only (acetaminophen or NSAIDs)

   b. Consider a course of low-dose tricyclic antidepressant if it has not been tried for back pain [see details under Subacute LBP: Section B2(b)].

5. Refer to pain management specialist or physiatrist who specializes in the spine if insufficient relief with above measures and no evidence of structural disorder or discogenic cause of pain on imaging.

6. There is strong evidence that several psychosocial factors correlate with the development of chronic back pain. Because strategies aimed at addressing these risk factors have not been individually evaluated, it is reasonable to refer the patient to a mental health professional trained in cognitive behavioral therapy.

7. Conditioning: can use if not previously attempted, or if had good relief with prior use
   a. Biofeedback
   b. "Back school": interdisciplinary rehabilitation most effective when presented at patient's worksite if involves a work-related injury (Chou & Huffman, 2007a)
   c. Conditioning training by PT or DO
   d. Ergonomic evaluation of workplace if symptoms suggest aggravation by work activities and evaluation not already conducted

8. Patient education (see sample in Figure 64-1)

D. Follow-up care to prevent recurrence after symptoms have improved

Because relapses in back pain are common—approaching 75% (Goroll & Mulley, 2014)—and the societal burden of chronic pain is large, strategies to prevent acute back pain from becoming chronic have been investigated.

The U.S. Preventive Services Task Force (USPSTF, 2007) and Agency for Healthcare Research and Quality (AHRQ, 2001) have synthesized the evidence on prevention:

1. Both reports emphasized the importance of clinician education and support in explaining the usually benign course of LBP, even though symptoms may persist for more than 1 month. Written materials reinforcing the clinician's message are useful to provide as a supplement (see Resources at end of chapter).

2. Although both analyses determined that it is important to resume physical activity quickly after the acute pain has resolved, both concluded that there is insufficient evidence to recommend for or against the routine use of *specific* exercise interventions to prevent back pain.

3. Consider encouraging the patient to attend a community-based exercise program or gym program to support performance of exercises and obtain benefit of peer support in strengthening core musculature, reducing likelihood of recurrence.

4. Other nonpharmacologic interventions listed in Plan section IV A *1* (h) were not found to offer additional benefit or relief.

5. It has not been verified that a reduction in risk factors (i.e., obesity and smoking) will prevent the recurrence of back pain, although it intuitively seems a reasonable expectation.

6. The physical measures listed in C3 earlier in the Plan for Chronic LBP have not been validated as either preventing or not preventing recurring episodes of LBP.

7. The earlier agents that have been recommended to avoid, still apply in preventing recurrences of LBP.

8. Consult or refer for evaluation by an orthopedic spine surgeon or neurosurgeon if:
   a. Symptoms consistent with cauda equina syndrome
   b. Lower limb weakness or sensory losses
   c. Progressive neurologic deficit
   d. Presence of red flags (symptoms suggestive of cancer, bone infection, or ankylosing spondylitis require referral to other appropriate specialists)
   e. Severe spinal deformity
   f. Abnormal findings on CT or MRI
   g. Failure to secure relief of symptoms, or worsening of symptoms *after 6 weeks* of conservative measures described previously.

   Because the vast majority of cases of uncomplicated LBP resolve within 6 weeks, even if there is evidence of nerve root irritation, a major question exists: when are the risk and cost of spinal surgery clinically warranted and cost-effective in these types of cases?

   In a widely referenced study that followed 2,427 patients for 4 years (2000–2005), the cost effectiveness of surgery vs. nonoperative care was evaluated for the diagnoses of either disc herniation, degenerative spondylolisthesis, or spinal stenosis (Spine Patient Outcomes Research Trial; Tosteson et al., 2011). For each diagnosis, cost per quality-adjusted life-year (QALY) was calculated to determine whether surgery or nonsurgical care was more cost effective as measured by patient-reported actual financial cost of medical care as well as satisfaction with quality of life for each image-confirmed diagnosis. After 4 years of a projected 9-year data collection, it appears that the cost of the surgery at the outset of the study was significantly eclipsed by the continuing costs sustained by the nonoperative patient population, predominantly due to their productivity losses. Although total costs after 4 years remained higher for the surgically treated group, this difference was most minimal in patients with disc herniation ($6,994). This patient group noted a large improvement in their sciatic symptoms and an improved quality of life following surgery. The cost difference was highest for those with degenerative spondylolisthesis ($22,127). In patients with spinal stenosis, the higher cost in surgical patients compared with nonoperable care after 4 years was $13,127. These data support an argument that surgery is a cost-effective option for those patients who have a positive impression of the benefit of undergoing surgery for relief of protracted disc herniation symptoms after a prolonged period of continuing symptoms despite compliance with conservative therapy and do not have red flags.

   However, it is important to note that patients who were reluctant to have surgery also recovered with nonoperative conservative treatment as long as they considered the pain as "tolerable," and they did not have evidence of neurologic defects. Importantly, delaying or avoiding surgery did not cause additional neurologic injury or damage.

9. Patient education (see sample in Figure 64-1)
   a. Provide written information that reinforces the clinician's information and includes:
      i. Most common cause of symptoms
      ii. Difference in symptoms caused by musculoskeletal strain vs. nerve root impingement
      iii. Reassurance that testing rarely helpful initially, and spontaneous resolution is most common
      iv. Physical recommendations

v. Analgesic recommendations

vi. Exercise/activity precautions

vii. Call/see provider if

a. No improvement after 2 weeks of sciatic symptoms

b. No improvement after 6 weeks of nonspecific LBP

c. Symptoms progress in severity

d. Red flags occur

viii. Conditioning/prevention recommendations once acute phase subsides

V. Self-management resources and tools

See **Table 64-4** for additional resources.

TABLE 64-4 Web-Based Patient Education Materials

The Internet has volumes of information available on the causes, evaluation, and treatment of low back pain. The following are suggested because the vocabulary is appropriate for a lay audience, they do not focus exclusively on surgical remedies, and they are not overly long. *This list is not exclusive*; other websites may be found to be valuable as well.

American Academy of Rheumatology. (2008). *Back pain.* Retrieved from http://www.rheumatology .org/I-Am-A/Patient-Caregiver/Diseases-Conditions /Living-Well-with-Rheumatic-Disease/Back-Pain.

American Association of Neurological Surgeons. (2005). *Cauda equina syndrome.* Retrieved from http://www .aans.org/Patient%20Information/Conditions%20and%20 Treatments/Cauda%20Equina%20Syndrome.aspx.

Annals of Internal Medicine. (2009). *Low back pain.* Retrieved from http://www.medicinenet.com/low_back _pain/page4.htm.

Family Doctor. (2009). *An overview of low back pain.* Retrieved from http://familydoctor.org/familydoctor/en /diseases-conditions/low-back-pain.html.

National Institutes of Health. (2009). *Low back pain fact sheet.* Retrieved from http://www.ninds.nih.gov/disorders /backpain/detail_backpain.

National Institute of Neurologic Disorders and Stroke (NIH). (2003). *Low back pain fact sheet.* Retrieved from http://www.ninds.nih.gov/disorders/backpain/detail _backpain.WebMD. (2008). *Overview of low back pain.* Retrieved from http://www.webmd.com/back-pain/tc /low-back-pain-treatment-overview.

REFERENCES

Atlas, S., & Deyo, R. (2001). Evaluating and managing acute low back pain in the primary care setting. *Journal of General Internal Medicine, 16,* 120–131.

Agency for Healthcare Research and Quality. (2001). Guideline for the evidence-informed primary care management of low back pain. Retrieved from http://www.guideline.gov/content.aspx?id=37954.

Chou, R., & Huffman, L. (2007a). Medications for acute and chronic low back pain: A review of the evidence for an American Pain Society/ American College of Physicians Clinical Practice Guideline. *Annals of Internal Medicine, 147*(7), 505–514.

Chou, R., & Huffman, L. (2007b). Nonpharmacologic therapies for acute and chronic low back pain: A review of the evidence for an American Pain Society/American College of Physicians Clinical Practice Guideline. *Annals of Internal Medicine, 147*(7), 492–504.

Chou, R., Quaseem, A., Snow, V., Casey, D., Cross, J. T., Jr., Shekelle, P., et al. (2007). Diagnosis and treatment of low back pain: A joint clinical practice guideline from the American College of Physicians and the American Pain Society. *Annals of Internal Medicine, 147*(7), 478–491.

Ehrlich, G. (2003). Back pain. *Journal of Rheumatology, 30*(67), 26–31.

Goroll, A. H., & Mulley, A. (2014). *Primary care medicine* (7th ed.). Philadelphia: Wolters Kluwer Health.

Hoppenfeld, S. (1976). *Physical exam of the spine and the extremities.* East Norwalk, CT: Appleton-Century-Crofts/Prentice-Hall.

Jarvik, J. G., & Deyo, R. (2002). Diagnostic evaluation of low back pain with emphasis on imaging. *Annals of Internal Medicine, 137,* 586–597.

Khan, M. A. (2002). Update on spondyloarthropathies. *Annals of Internal Medicine, 136*(12), 896–907.

McGee, S. (2007). The leg. In *Evidence based physical diagnosis* (2nd ed.). St. Louis, MO: Saunders Elsevier.

Papadakis, M., & McPhee, S. (Eds.). (2015). Low back pain. In *Current medical diagnosis and treatment* (54th ed.). New York: McGraw-Hill Education.

Tosteson, A., Tosteson, T., Lurie, J., Abdu, W., Herkowitz, H., Andersson, G., et al. (2011). Comparative effectiveness evidence from the spine patient outcomes research trial. *Spine, 16*(24), 2061–2068.

van Tulder, M., Koes, B., & Bombardier, C. (2002). Low back pain. *Best Practice and Research. Clinical Rheumatology, 16,* 761–765.

Weinstein, J., Lurie, J. D., Tosteson, T. D., Skinner, J. S., Hanscom, B., et al. (2006). Surgical vs. non-operative treatment for lumbar disk herniation. *JAMA, 296*(20), 2441–2450.

OBESITY

Sherri Borden, David Besio, and
Geraldine Collins-Bride

CHAPTER 65

I. Introduction and general background

Obesity is a major public health concern in the United States. According to the 2011–2012 National Health and Nutrition Examination Survey (NHANES), obesity prevalence in adults has remained relatively constant at an overall rate of 35.7% with 33.1% of adults in the overweight category. There was an increase in obesity noted in older adults (particularly women) age 60 and older (Ogden, Carroll, Kit, & Flegal, 2014).

Obesity trends are more prevalent in minority groups, lower socioeconomic groups, and less educated individuals and contribute to a number of significant chronic healthcare issues. In addition, an overweight and obese population contributes to substantial economic costs, estimated at $190.2 billion annually (Institute of Medicine [IOM], 2012).

Clinically, overweight is defined as a body mass index (BMI) of 25–29.9 kg/m² and obesity as greater than or equal to 30 kg/m². Overweight and obesity for those 18 years and older substantially increase the risks of morbidity for hypertension (HTN), dyslipidemia, type 2 diabetes, coronary artery disease, stroke, gallbladder disease, osteoarthritis, sleep apnea, and respiratory problems. Additional health risks include higher rates of endometrial, breast, prostate, and colon cancer. Overweight individuals also endure social stigmatization and discrimination (Centers for Disease Control and Prevention [CDC], 2009a, 2009c; IOM, 2012).

The goal of Healthy People 2010 was to promote health and reduce chronic disease associated with diet and weight by reducing the number of adults 20 years or older with a BMI over 30 to 15% of the population. The Healthy People 2020 objectives, discussed next, have been expanded and modified to include changes in state policies, expectations for primary care visits, and nutrition and weight management counseling for individuals older than age 2. Although the goals are ambitious, weight-related diseases are a major preventable cause of death, pose an important public health challenge, and should not be overlooked (IOM, 2012; U.S. Department of Health and Human Services, 2000).

A. Healthy People 2020, summarized (U.S. Department of Health and Human Services, 2009)

1. Objectives retained from 2010
   a. Increase the proportion of adults who are at a healthy weight.
   b. Reduce the proportion of adults who are obese.
2. Objective retained but modified
   a. Reduce the number of children and adolescents who are obese.
   b. For individuals age 2 and older: increase the consumption of fruits, vegetables, whole grains, and calcium. Reduce the consumption of saturated fat and sodium.
   c. Increase the number of healthcare visits that include counseling or education for weight management.
   d. Eliminate very low food security among children in U.S. households.
3. Objectives new to Healthy People 2020
   a. Prevent inappropriate weight gain in youth and adults.
   b. Increase the number of primary care providers who regularly calculate the BMI of their patients.
   c. Reduce the consumption of calories from solid fats and sugars, increase the number of states with food standards for children, and increase the percentage of schools that offer nutritious food and beverages outside of school meals.
   d. Changes in state-level policies for food outlets.
4. Measuring overweight and obesity: BMI provides a reasonable indicator for body adiposity and weight categories that may lead to significant health problems. BMI categories as defined by the National Institutes of Health include:
   a. 18.5–24.9 kg/m² (normal)
   b. 25–29.9 kg/m² (overweight)
   c. 30–34.9 kg/m² (Class I obesity)

d. 35–39.9 kg/m² (Class II obesity)

e. Greater than or equal to 40 kg/m² (Class III obesity)

B. Causes of obesity in adults

1. The most common causes of obesity are the result of energy imbalances with excessive caloric intake from food, beverages, or alcohol and insufficient physical activity and/or sedentary lifestyle. Both genetic influences (in particular genes that affect the leptin receptor) and environmental influences are thought to play a significant role (Baron, 2015).

2. The following medical problems may also contribute to the etiology of obesity:

   a. Hypothyroidism

   b. Cushing syndrome

   c. Hypogonadism

   d. Hypothalamic injuries

   e. Polycystic ovary (Stein-Leventhal syndrome)

   f. Pseudo-hypoparathyroidism

   g. Insulinoma

   h. Medications may also contribute to overweight and obesity: corticosteroids; progesterone; anticonvulsants and psychotropic medications, in particular atypical antipsychotics, such as clozaril and olanzapine; insulin; and select oral hypoglycemic agents

3. Consequences of obesity: as weight increases to the categories of overweight and obesity, risks for chronic health problems increase. These health problems include:

   a. Coronary artery disease

   b. Type 2 diabetes

   c. Cancers (endometrial, breast, and colon)

   d. HTN

   e. Dyslipidemia

   f. Stroke

   g. Liver and gallbladder disease

   h. Sleep apnea and respiratory problems

   i. Osteoarthritis

   j. Gynecological problems (abnormal menses and fertility problems)

   k. Metabolic syndrome (Kanaya, 2010). Also known as syndrome X, insulin resistance syndrome, and the dysmetabolic syndrome, metabolic syndrome is a group of risk factors that confers higher risk for stroke, coronary artery disease, and type 2 diabetes. The syndrome includes three or more of the following criteria:

      i. Waist circumference according to population-specific criteria :

         a. White, European: men ≥ 102 cm, women ≥ 88 cm

         b. Asian: men ≥ 90 cm, women ≥ 80 cm

         c. Middle East, Mediterranean: men ≥ 94 cm, women ≥ 80 cm

         d. Sub-Saharan African: men ≥ 94 cm, women ≥ 80 cm

         e. Central and South American: men ≥ 90 cm, women ≥ 80 cm

      ii. High-density lipoprotein (HDL): men < 40, women < 50 or niacin or fibrate use

      iii. Triglycerides: ≥ 150 mg/dL, or niacin or fibrate use

      iv. Blood pressure ≥ 130/85 or taking blood pressure medications

      v. Fasting glucose ≥ 100 mg/dL or using diabetes medications

C. Obesity in children and adolescents

Child and adolescent obesity continues to have a high prevalence in the United States. Obesity is a serious health issue for children and adolescents for numerous reasons including risk of obesity in adolescence and adulthood; increased risk for cardiovascular disease (CVD), such as high blood pressure, high cholesterol, and type 2 diabetes (Whitaker, Wright, Pepe, Seidel, & Dietz, 1997); and alterations in body image with subsequent social stigmatization. In a meta-analysis of the association between BMI and health-related quality of life (HRQoL) among children and adolescents, Ul-Haq, Mackay, Fenwick, & Pell (2013) found that as BMI increased, HRQoL decreased from normal weight through overweight and obesity. In addition, obese children and adolescents have decreased HRQoL. For more discussion, see Chapter 16 on childhood obesity.

D. Obesity in individuals with mental illness

As in other populations, individuals with mental illness who are overweight or obese are at increased risk for developing chronic diseases, such as CVD and type 2 diabetes. Excessive weight gain is not always addressed by clinicians such as psychiatrists, primary care physicians, and advanced practice nurses, who feel poorly equipped to deal with this problem and fear patient treatment noncompliance or psychiatric symptom decompensation.

There are no clear interventions to prevent and treat overweight and obesity in this population. Individuals with mental illness who gain more than 11 lbs in adulthood have approximately twice the rate of type 2 diabetes (Boyd, 2002). Excessive weight gain and obesity is two to three times more prevalent than in the general population (Aquila, 2002). This increased occurrence has been strongly associated with several important factors including diet, exercise, environmental factors, and psychotropic medications. Individuals with mental illness tend to eat a diet higher in saturated fat and calories; consume greater amounts of high-carbohydrate beverages; and eat a diet lower in fiber, fresh fruits, and vegetables. They also tend to exercise less, living a more sedentary lifestyle as a result of institutionalization and other factors (Greenberg, Chan, & Blackburn, 1999).

Weight gain has also been reported during treatment with many medications, such as conventional antipsychotic agents, phenothiazines, and thioxanthenes, and was reported in novel antipsychotic agents, such as clozapine, risperidone, and olanzapine (Basson et al., 2001). Although novel antipsychotic medications improve psychiatric outcomes, estimates for associated weight gain range from virtually zero weight gain, as seen in ziprasidone, to an average gain of 4–4.5 kg after 10 weeks of treatment with both olanzapine and clozapine, to nearly 12 kg at 1 year with olanzapine (Allison et al., 1999; Fontaine et al., 2001). The variability of novel antipsychotic weight gain experienced by patients suggests that several factors are involved. Weight gain is often rapid in the first few weeks of treatment and then reaches a plateau. Weight gain with novel antipsychotic treatment has been correlated with an excessive appetite, thought to be directly related to the atypical antipsychotics affinity for histamine H1 receptors of blockade of the hypothalamic sites regulating satiety (Rummel-Kluge et al., 2010).

Although lifestyle intervention is an important component in preventing and managing weight gain related to the second-generation antipsychotics (SGA), some studies have examined the off-label use of metformin in the management of SGA-induced weight gain. Metformin, an antidiabetic agent used mostly in type 2 diabetes, has also been used in patients with polycystic ovarian syndrome to induce ovulation. Because metformin is associated with some weight reduction in diabetic patients and is relatively well tolerated, several studies have aimed to determine the effect of metformin treatment on SGA-induced weight gain. In a systematic review and meta-analysis by Bjorkhem-Bergman, Asplund, & Lindh (2010), the authors found that those on metformin had significant weight reduction, especially those who had gained weight on antipsychotic agents. Although there are still no current recommendations for the routine use of metformin in those prescribed SGA, a more recent systematic review conducted by Newall et al. (2012) concluded that if weight gain occurs despite lifestyle intervention, metformin should be considered as an adjunct therapy. Although the authors reported limitations in the primary research available, they concluded that metformin may be more useful in younger people and those with shorter SGA treatment duration. They recommend starting metformin in those who have gained greater than 10% of their body weight despite lifestyle interventions (Newall et al., 2012).

II. Database

A. Subjective

1. Developmental patterns and past medical history
   a. Infant and childhood obesity: no correlation found in infancy; however, there seem to be links to intrauterine imprinting (Bray & Champagne, 2005). Obesity beginning at age range of 5–6 years has a documented correlation to adult obesity secondary to genetic and environmental factors, such as overfeeding, poor food choices, and sedentary lifestyle.
   b. Adolescent obesity: adolescents with obesity are at an increased risk of CVD, type 2 diabetes, and respiratory and sleep problems. According to the American Academy of Child and Adolescent Psychiatry (2006), adolescent obesity is also associated with lower self-esteem, depression, anxiety, and obsessive–compulsive disorder.
   c. Obesity of early adulthood (postpartum)
   d. Middle-age obesity: decrease in metabolic rate, decrease in activity level, increase in body weight increases the risk of developing CVD and type 2 diabetes.
   e. Past medical history of obesity-related medical problems: arthritis, gallbladder disease, HTN, CVD, diabetes, depression, and obstructive sleep apnea.

2. Family history: note history of obesity; CVD; HTN; genetic syndromes; and thyroid, diabetes, and other endocrine disorders

3. Dietary history
   a. 24-hour recall of current usual intake: type and quantity of food, meal times, and variability of intake
   b. Intake of high caloric foods: sugar, fats, and beverages (alcohol, soda, and fruit juices)
   c. Meal preparation: cooking techniques and use of fats and oils
   d. Emotional and behavioral cues to eating
      i. Internal and emotional reaction to self or others, and sabotaging thoughts, such as "I deserve a treat"
      ii. External sight or smell of food; associations of food with time, place, or activity; and celebration or parties
   e. Availability: cost and quality of food, cooking facilities, and food insecurity
   f. Cultural orientation to food and weight

4. Exercise and activity: note type and amount of daily activity, including assets and barriers to

exercise (affordability, access, level of priority, and seasonality)

5. Self-image, self-esteem, and self-confidence: effect on relationships, jobs, and daily life

6. Motivation and interest in weight control

7. Weight loss and dieting history, including use of over-the-counter (OTC) medications, supplements, and herbal treatments; diuretics and laxatives; diet pills; and prescription drugs. Note history of binge and purge behavior or self-starvation

8. Review of systems: in general, the mild to moderately obese individual is asymptomatic. In cases of class III obesity (BMI ≥ 40), the following symptoms can be manifestations of mechanical difficulties or medical consequences:

   a. Easy fatigability and dyspnea on exertion

   b. Somnolence

   c. Malaise and weakness

   d. Abdominal bloating and dyspepsia

   e. Ankle swelling

   f. Joint pains, especially weight-bearing joints: low back, hips, knees, and ankles

   g. Skin rashes: acne and chronic candidiasis in skin folds

   h. Menstrual irregularities

   i. Symptoms of depression

   j. To rule out endocrine disorders, consider the following history

      i. Lethargy, ankle swelling, somnolence, heat or cold intolerance, hair loss, dry skin, constipation and menstrual irregularities: *consider hypothyroidism.*

      ii. Acne, increase in hair growth, change in facial appearance, easy bruising, and skin rashes: *consider Cushing syndrome.*

      iii. Delayed puberty, decreased or absent libido: *consider hypogonadism.*

      iv. Amenorrhea or menstrual irregularities and hirsutism: *consider polycystic ovary syndrome.*

      v. Arthralgias, muscle cramps, weakness, numbness or tingling, seizures, and emotional lability: *consider pseudo-hypoparathyroidism.*

B. Objective

1. Physical examination

   a. Most individuals who are obese require general observation; height, weight, and BMI measurement; and a complete set of vital signs. However, a complete physical examination is generally preferred to rule out secondary causes and evidence of obesity-related health risks. The examination should focus in particular on the thyroid, cardiovascular, pulmonary, musculoskeletal, and neurologic examination in all patients.

   b. Measuring abdominal circumference helps assess distribution of fat. Waist circumference provides a clinically acceptable measurement of abdominal fat before and during weight loss. Waist circumference in men should be less than 102 cm (40 in) and in women less than 88 cm (35 in). Cutoffs can be used to identify increased relative risk for the development of obesity-associated risk factors in most adults with a BMI from 25–34.9. Waist circumference is measured by placing the measuring tape at the most superior point of the hip bone, keeping it horizontal, and taking the reading at the point of exhalation.

   c. The following complexes of physical signs may provide clues to underlying endocrine disorders:

      i. Cool, dry skin; hoarse voice and facial edema; thick tongue; delayed or absent deep tendon reflexes: *consider hypothyroidism.*

      ii. Round, "moon face"; hirsutism; truncal obesity; purple striae; ecchymosis: *consider Cushing syndrome.*

      iii. Small stature, lack of secondary sex characteristics, poor muscular development: *consider hypogonadism.*

      iv. Short, stocky stature; round face; intellectual disability; joint deformities; cataracts; papilledema: *consider pseudo-hypoparathyroidism*

2. Diagnostic testing: depends on the severity of obesity, potential for secondary cause, and evaluation of obesity-related health risks. Consider the following tests:

   a. *Electrolytes, fasting glucose, blood urea nitrogen, and creatinine

   b. *Thyroid-stimulating hormone (T4 if on thyroid medication)

   c. *Fasting low-density lipoprotein (LDL) and HDL cholesterol and serum triglycerides

   d. Pulmonary function tests and arterial blood gas

   e. Steroid studies: cortisol level and dexamethasone suppression test

   f. Hemoglobin A_{1C}

   g. Growth hormones

   h. Testosterone

   i. Follicle-stimulating hormone, luteinizing hormone, and prolactin levels

   *Most commonly ordered as initial screening tests

III. Assessment

A. *Determine the diagnosis*

Distinguish between secondary and primary obesity. Rule out endocrine disorders as described previously.

B. *Severity*

Assess the severity of obesity, including current and future health risks.

C. *Significance*

Assess the significance of obesity to the patient and significant others including impact on daily functioning, work, relationships, and self-esteem.

D. *Motivation and ability:*

1. Assess the motivation of the patient, including reasons for weight reduction, previous history of weight loss, understanding of the causes of obesity, ability to engage in action plan, and financial considerations.

2. Assess stage of change (Prochaska & DiClemente, 1982) to help identify possible interventions and develop patient-specific process goals and cognitive and behavioral therapy strategies (Fabricatore, 2007).

   a. Precontemplation: provide weight and health education and explain health benefits of exercise.

   b. Contemplation
      i. Identify and list advantages and disadvantages of weight loss (Brownell, 2000)
      ii. Make a list of potential exercises and activities

   c. Preparation
      i. Positive goal setting (specific, measurable, attainable, reasonable, and time limited)
      ii. Environmental control: stocking the refrigerator with fresh vegetables and fruits, removing easy access to sweets and treats, eating slowly without distractions, using smaller plates and bowls, shopping from a list, menu planning, buying prepackaged healthy calorie-controlled meals to eat as "Plan B," identifying possible alternative exercises, and monitoring such as checking weekly or biweekly weights at home, keeping a food record and exercise log
      iii. Identify potential diet intervention (**Figures 65-1** and **65-2**)

   d. Action: implement goals of dietary and lifestyle change; reevaluate goals regularly to encourage additional progress.

   e. Maintenance: develop coping strategies for diet and exercise lapses.

   f. Relapse: encourage patient regarding positive accomplishments, reevaluate advantages and disadvantages, and reinitiate preparation strategies.

IV. Goals of clinical management

A. *Risk reduction*

Being overweight or obese clearly increases morbidity and mortality, and strong evidence suggests that weight loss reduces risk factors for CVD and diabetes. Weight loss reduces blood pressure in both overweight hypertensive and nonhypertensive individuals, lowers serum triglycerides, increases HDL cholesterol, and generally produces reductions in LDL and total serum cholesterol. Additionally, modest weight loss of 5–10% reduces blood glucose levels and HbA_{1C} in some patients with type 2 diabetes (National Heart, Lung, and Blood Institute [NHLBI], 1998).

B. *Prevention of obesity*

Although the physical consequences of obesity are a significant problem, the impact on self-esteem and body image is also an important factor to consider. Physical health is closely linked to mental health and physical problems may negatively affect a patient's body image. Clinicians can play an integral role in helping a patient understand the health risks associated with obesity. Therefore, one of the primary goals should be to initiate healthcare maintenance measures early to prevent or intervene in weight gain. It is important to take into account a variety of factors when choosing treatment plans to provide comprehensive holistic care including the patient's personal, cultural, and family history; knowledge of the development of chronic health conditions; and impact of overweight and obesity on body image. According to the IOM 2012 report, *Accelerating Progress in Obesity Prevention*, the following goals were recommended:

- Make physical activity an integral part of life
- Create food and beverage environments that ensure healthy food and beverage options are the routine, easy choice
- Transform messages about physical activity and nutrition
- Expand the roles of healthcare providers, insurers, and employers
- Make schools a national focal point

To date, there is an explosion of healthy nutrition and regular physical activity messages in the media, along with farmers' markets, food labeling, and more "healthier food choices" even in the fast food industry. One of the biggest challenges facing providers and patients is the cost and access to healthier foods and physical activities for those patients with limited means.

FIGURE 65-1 One-Week Food Record

	Day 1	Calories	Day 2	Calories	Day 3	Calories	Day 4	Calories
Breakfast								
Time								
Place								
Hunger level*								
Lunch								
Time								
Place								
Hunger level*								
Dinner								
Time								
Place								
Hunger level*								
Snack (please note all snacks)								
Exercise								

(continues)

FIGURE 65-1 One-Week Food Record (Continued)

	Day 5	Calories	Day 6	Calories	Day 7	Calories	To Document Intake:
Breakfast							Record everything you eat or drink during the day (as soon as possible after intake). List the food and amount eaten and calories to the best of your ability.
							For example:
Time							2 slices w/w Light bread 120
Place							8 oz nonfat milk 90
Hunger level							1 hard-boiled egg 80
Lunch							Total 335
Time							**Goal 1:**
Place							
Hunger level							
Dinner							
							Goal 2:
Time							
Place							
Hunger level							
Snack (please note all snacks)							
Exercise							**Feelings/Comments/Concerns**

* Hunger Level:1 = Starving 10 = Stuffed

Produced by UCSF Nutrition and Food Services. Used with permission by UCSF Medical Center.

FIGURE 65-2 *Wellness Agreement*

A goal should be realistic and measurable based on baseline patterns

Current diet recall indicates that patient has vegetables 3 times/week

- Unrealistic goal: I will eat lots of vegetables every day
- More realistic goal: I will eat a serving of vegetables at dinner 6 nights this week
- Work towards bigger goals over time

Reward yourself for accomplishing your goal. Examples: take a bubble bath, rent a favorite movie, get a massage, sleep in late, or just pat yourself on the back!

- ❑ Create no more than 3 goals per week
- ❑ Check in with a supportive friend, family member, or health professional to help keep you on track. A check-in can be by phone, text or e-mail—taking advantage of current technologies

	Goal	Reward
Food		
Exercise		
Stress Management		

I will focus on these wellness goals for the week.

_____ Signature _____ Date

Produced by UCSF Nutrition and Food Services. Used with permission by UCSF Medical Center.

V. Plan

A. Management

Treatment requires a fundamental change in lifestyle. Weight loss depends on adherence to an agreement outlining lifestyle changes that factor in individual motivation, support systems, and underlying medical or psychological conditions. The management plan should consist of the following considerations:

1. Treat the underlying cause, if secondary obesity.

2. Establish a patient agreement: determine short- and long-range goals and outcomes, using healthy body weight range based on BMI, patient's desired weight, and practitioner's assessment of desired weight.

3. Meal plans: although in the short-term lower carbohydrate meal plans seem to result in weight loss without adverse health consequences (Baron, 2015; Gardner et al., 2007), using a variety of dietary interventions (including low-calorie meal replacements) is reasonable because there does not seem to be an advantage of one macronutrient distribution versus another (Sacks et al., 2009; Vesely & DeMattia, 2014). Induce a 500- to 1,000-calorie deficit to promote 1- to 2-lb weight loss per week resulting in approximately an 8–10% total weight loss outcome. Refer to a weight management group with comprehensive lifestyle interventions focusing on meal plans, lifestyle, and behavior therapy provided by team of professionals, which may include nutritionist, behaviorist, exercise specialists, and trained practitioners (Millen, Wolongevicz, Nonas, & Lichtenstein, 2014) (**Figure 65-3**).

4. Physical activity: discuss the health benefits of physical activity, even if weight loss is not accomplished. Assist the individual in developing an activity regimen, setting reasonable short-term goals to increase to a long-term goal of six times per week for 60 minutes per session. According to the National Weight Control Registry only 9% of participants in the registry reported keeping weight off *without* engaging in some physical activity. Walking seemed to be the most popular form of physical activity. Half of the participants also combined walking with another form of planned exercise, such as aerobics, bicycling, or swimming (Hill & Wing, 2003).

5. Medications: OTC appetite suppressants are not helpful with long-term management of obesity. Although they do reduce appetite, tolerance and dependence are potentially dangerous side effects.
   a. Pharmacologic therapy
      i. Sibutramine: an appetite suppressant that has been used for long-term use, up to 1 year, and seems to enhance weight loss modestly when used with diet and lifestyle changes. It also may help promote weight control. However, in 2010, the U.S. Food and Drug Administration (FDA) removed sibutramine from the market because of clinical trial data indicating an increased risk of cardiovascular adverse events, including heart attack and stroke, in the studied population (Food and Drug Administration, 2010a).
      ii. Orlistat: a gastric lipase inhibitor, which reduces fat absorption by approximately 30%, is also approved for longer term use, up to 1 year, and results in modest additional weight loss with diet and lifestyle change (Fabricatore & Wadden, 2003). The recommended dose is 120 mg three times daily. It is currently sold in lower doses (60 mg) OTC as Alli®. Typical side effects from Orlistat are primarily gastrointestinal including flatus, abdominal cramping, fecal incontinence, and oily fecal staining. Absorption of fat soluble vitamins may be reduced with Orlistat use. Patients with a history of kidney stones should not be prescribed this medication. There have been rare reports of severe liver injury, including liver failure in patients taking Orlistat (FDA, 2010b). Clinicians should educate all patients taking Orlistat about the signs and symptoms of liver disease (FDA, 2010b).
      iii. Phentermine: the most commonly prescribed appetite suppressant because of low cost, phentermine is approved for only short-term use ($\leq$ 12 weeks) due to potential for abuse. Side effects include increased blood pressure (Millen et al., 2014; Sacks et al., 2005).
      iv. Phentermine/topiramate (Qsymia®): approved for use in 2012, the drug increases metabolism and satiety for patients with BMIs over 30 kg/m² or greater and 27 kg/m² with at least one weight-related medical comorbidity. As with other weight loss drugs, it is to be used in conjunction with low-calorie diets and increased activity and can result in weight loss on average of approximately 10%. Significant side effects include birth defects if taken during pregnancy, increased heart rate, vision problems, and potential suicidal thoughts or actions.

FIGURE 65-3 *Instructions for Use of the Plate Method*

STEP 1: Fill Half (1/2) of Your Plate with Nonstarchy Vegetables.

❏ Nonstarchy vegetables are low in calories, low in carbohydrate, and high in fiber. This means nonstarchy vegetables can help you feel full and more satisfied with your meal but not lead to weight gain and high blood sugar.

❏ Aim for 1 to 2 cups of any vegetable (EXCEPT starchy vegetables listed in Step 3).

❏ Vegetables can be raw or cooked.

STEP 2: Limit Protein to a Quarter (1/4) of Your Plate.

❏ Choose lean meat, poultry, or fish. Your portion should not be bigger than the palm of your hand. Try 1 to 2 whole eggs or just the egg whites for lower cholesterol.

❏ Choose tofu, nuts, or seeds. Aim for about 2 tablespoons of nuts and seeds or 1/2 cup of tofu.

STEP 3: Limit Starch to a Quarter (1/4) of Your Plate.

❏ Starch is a source of carbohydrate. Carbohydrate turns into an important fuel, called glucose, and limiting the portion size of starch helps control body weight and blood sugar.

❏ Choose a bun, tortilla, bread, bagel, rice, grains, cereal, pasta, or a starchy vegetable.

- If you choose bread, limit to 2 slices or 1/2 bagel.
- If you choose a hamburger/hotdog bun, limit to 1 bun.
- If you choose a tortilla, limit to 2 small tortillas or 1 large tortilla.
- If you choose rice, grains, pasta, cereal, or a starchy vegetable, limit the portion to no more than 1 cup—this is about the size of a woman's fist. Starchy vegetables include beans, potatoes, corn, yams, peas, and winter squash.

❏ Choose most of your starches from whole grains, such as whole wheat bread or tortillas, brown rice, whole wheat pasta, whole grain and bran cereals, or beans.

STEP 4: If Desired, Add 1 Portion of Fruit or Milk to Your Meal.

❏ Fruit, milk, and yogurt are also sources of carbohydrate. To best control body weight and blood sugar, limit yourself to either fruit or milk at your meal. You may choose to save the fruit or milk as a snack.

❏ Because high carbohydrate liquids can quickly raise blood sugar, avoid drinking fruit juice.

❏ Examples of fruit portion sizes are:

- 1 small apple, orange, peach, pear, banana, or nectarine (or half of a larger fruit)
- 3/4 cup fresh pineapple chunks, blueberries, or blackberries
- 17 grapes
- 1 and 1/4 cups strawberries or watermelon
- 1 cup cantaloupe, honeydew, or papaya

❏ Choose low fat or nonfat dairy products for heart health and weight control.

❏ Examples of milk and yogurt portion sizes are:

- 1 cup (8 ounces) of nonfat, 1%, or soy milk
- 2/3 to 1 cup plain nonfat or aspartame-sweetened fruit yogurt

STEP 5: Limit Added Fats.

❏ Avoid adding fats to your foods like butter, margarine, shortening, mayonnaise, gravies, cream sauces, salad dressing, and sour cream. Instead, season foods with herbs and spices.

❏ Cook using low fat methods such as baking, steaming, broiling, or grilling. Avoid frying foods.

(continues)

Plate method
For healthy meal planning

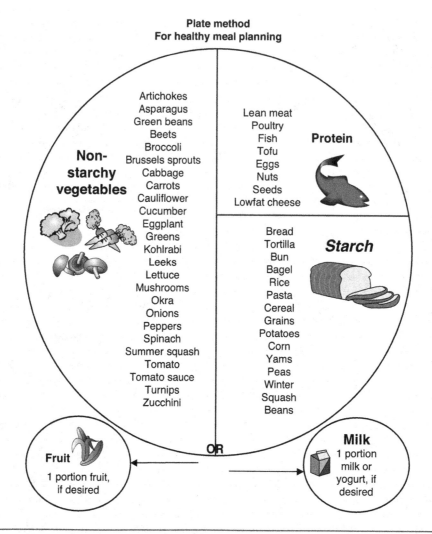

FIGURE 65-3 Instructions for Use of the Plate Method *(Continued)*
Produced by UCSF Nutrition and Food Services. Used with permission by UCSF Medical Center.

v. Lorcaserin (Belviq®): selective serotonin 2C receptor agonist. Approved for use for weight loss in 2012, the drug binds to receptors that regulate appetite. Weight loss results are slightly less than phentermine/topiramate when used in conjunction with diet and lifestyle modifications but with fewer side effects (Verpeut & Bello, 2014). Most common adverse events include headache, nausea, and dizziness (Fidler et al., 2011). Other side effects may include hallucinations, valvulopathy, and changes in attention and memory.

vi. Liraglutide (Saxenda®): a glucagon-like peptide-1 (GLP-1) receptor agonist, approved by the FDA in December 2014 for chronic weight management of adults who are overweight or obese and have at least one comorbidity such as hypertension, diabetes, or dyslipidemia. Saxenda®, administered as a once daily subcutaneous injection, has the same active ingredient as Victoza® (liraglutide), a medication used to treat type 2 diabetes, but in different doses—1.8 mg (Victoza®) versus 3 mg (Saxenda®). Three clinical trials were conducted for the safety and effectiveness of Saxenda® with 4,800 obese and overweight patients plus diet and exercise. In one study 62% of patients lost 5% or more of their baseline body weight versus 34% of placebo. In a second study that included patients with type 2 diabetes, 49% lost 5% or more of their baseline body weight verses 16% of placebo. The most common side effects of Saxenda® include nausea, vomiting, diarrhea, headache, and constipation. The medication should be discontinued if an individual does not lose 4% of their baseline body weight in the first 16 weeks, as the medication is unlikely to be effective. It carries a black box warning for thyroid C-cell tumor risk. As a condition of FDA approval, additional postmarketing studies must include evaluation for safety, effectiveness, and dosing in pediatric patients, assessment of growth, sexual maturation, and central nervous system development in mice, as well as medullary thyroid carcinoma case registry of at least 15 years and evaluation of potential increases in breast cancer (FDA, 2014).

b. Psychotropic medications, such as bupropion, fluoxetine, and sertraline, also have a short-term anorexic effect and can be helpful in treatment of individuals with coexisting depression. However, these medications are not approved for weight loss by the U.S. Food and Drug Administration (Sacks et al., 2005).

c. Investigational products (Nkansah, 2010)

   i. Bupropion/zonisamide (Empatic®): increases metabolism and suppresses appetite.

   ii. Bupropion/naltrexone (Contrave®): increases metabolism and counteracts body "starvation effect." Bupropion is a norepinephrine/dopamine reuptake inhibitor used to treat depression and smoking cessation and naltrexone is an opioid antagonist used in the treatment of opioid and alcohol dependency. In trials, it appears to have greater weight loss associated with its use than Orlistat or lorcarserin, although less than phentermine/topiramate but with less severe side effects (Verpeut & Bello, 2014).

6. Support groups, including family, friends, work-site support, and structured programs.

7. Cognitive–behavioral therapy for lifestyle modification can be a beneficial addition to a weight loss program.

B. Follow-up

Follow-up is a critical aspect of success in a weight management program, either individual or group based, with frequent visits in the beginning, then negotiated with the patient and their support system. Follow-up should include the following:

1. Reinforcement of successes and review of difficulties and barriers to change

2. Reevaluation of motivation and degree of adherence

3. Reevaluation of the individual agreement or contract

C. Bariatric surgery

This type of treatment is known to be the most effective and intensive treatment for morbid obesity, with improvement in medical comorbidities, such as HTN, diabetes mellitus, dyslipidemia, sleep apnea, and gastroesophageal reflux disease (in Roux-en-Y gastric bypass [RYGBP]). It is recommended for those who meet the surgical criteria and who have not been able to lose weight despite repeated attempts or maintain weight loss with diet and exercise (Sacks et al., 2005). Surgery may be appropriate for those who meet the medical screening criteria: BMI of greater than or equal to 40 or a BMI of 35–39.9 with serious health-related problems, such as diabetes or high blood pressure.

For patients considering weight loss surgery, the practitioner should perform a complete physical and thorough examination of the thyroid as part of the pretreatment evaluation. During this assessment, practitioners should focus on assessing the causes and complications of obesity, including family history of polycystic ovarian disease, hypothyroidism, and medications. The practitioner should screen for existing complications, such as type 2 diabetes, HTN, hyperlipidemia, atherosclerotic CVD, gallbladder disease, gout, cancers, osteoarthritis of the lower extremities, and sleep apnea. Baseline and diagnostic assessments should include electrolytes, liver function tests, complete blood count, total cholesterol, HDL and LDL cholesterol, triglycerides, thyroid function tests, and an electrocardiogram if a recent one is not available (NHLBI, 1998).

1. Other considerations

   a. Medical conditions that are contraindicated for bariatric surgery include end-stage lung disease, unstable CVD, multiorgan failure, and gastric varices.

   b. Psychiatric conditions with contraindications for weight loss surgery include current substance use, current heavy alcohol intake, active schizophrenia, severe intellectual disability, lack of knowledge regarding surgeries, and medical nonadherence (Bauchowitz et al., 2005).

2. Types of bariatric surgeries

   a. Roux-en-Y gastric bypass is the most popular procedure in the United States (Baron, 2015). Performed both open and laparoscopically, RYGBP is restrictive and malabsorptive in nature. It provides changes in physiology that seem to affect and reset energy equilibrium.

There is strong evidence to suggest that secretion of gastrointestinal hormones, such as grehlin, peptide tyrosine-tyrosine (PYY), and glucagon-like peptide-1, are altered by RYGBP helping to promote weight loss (Beckman, Beckman, & Earthman, 2010). Additionally, other factors such as increased bile acid concentration and altered gut microbiota may contribute to the effects on weight loss from RYGBP (Lutz & Bueter, 2014). Excess body weight loss is anticipated to be approximately 60–70%.

b. Adjustable gastric banding is primarily restrictive in nature. Placement of a foreign body-band around the upper portion of the stomach creates a small stomach pouch. Based on weight loss and tolerance, this is then adjusted with "fills" to decrease the flow rate of food into the larger portion of stomach to provide a longer feeling of fullness. Anticipated excess body weight loss is approximately 50%. Recent long-term studies in Europe, however, have shown that complications (such as band erosion and hiatal hernia) and lack of maintained weight loss have led to large numbers of patients having the band removed or converted to RYGBP; one study performed in a Dutch center found that after ~ 14 years over half the patients fell into this category (Aarts et al., 2014).

c. The biliopancreatic diversion with duodenal switch is primarily malabsorptive. Although expected excess body weight loss is anticipated at approximately 70%, the higher rates of severe side effects, such as diarrhea and nutritional deficiencies, make this surgery less frequently performed (Buchwald, 2005).

d. Vertical sleeve gastrectomy is restrictive with the amount of weight loss similar to RYGBP. It is usually performed laparoscopically and limits the volume of food in the stomach by creating a small pouch slightly larger than that created by the lap band procedure. The procedure keeps the pylorus intact and removes the remainder of the stomach. One specific problem, which is unique to sleeve gastrectomy, is an increase in gastroesophageal reflux disease (GERD) symptoms after surgery leading to increased treatment and use of proton pump inhibitors (Sheppard, Sadowski, de Gara, Karmali, & Birch, 2014). Although weight loss appears to be similar among RYGB and sleeve gastrectomy, sleeve gastrectomy does not appear to be effective in resolving diabetes mellitus as well as RYGB. Studies indicate that RYGB is more effective at improving insulin sensitivity and beta-cell function than is sleeve gastrectomy (Kashyap et al., 2013).

3. Preoperative and postoperative care
   a. Diet and lifestyle modifications need to be reinforced.
   b. Medications must be evaluated at the time of surgery. With rapid weight loss, diabetes and antihypertensive medications need to be reduced or eliminated as needed (Pi-Sunyer & Nonas, 2004).
   c. All time-released medications (for RYGBP) and nonsteroidal anti-inflammatory drugs need to be evaluated for appropriateness. Ursodiol® is typically used to prevent bile sludge and stones, so patients who have an intact gallbladder are started on Ursodiol®.
   d. Discussion with the surgeon should include medication evaluation for change in delivery (e.g., crushed, liquid, or quartered).
   e. Referral should be made to a registered dietitian experienced with bariatric surgical patients for evaluation of diet and multivitamin and mineral requirement needs.
   f. In addition to surgical complications, multiple early complications need to be monitored for including dehydration, dumping syndrome, nausea and vomiting, and lactose intolerance. Late complications, depending on the type of surgery, may include a variety of vitamin and mineral deficiencies (thiamine, folate, vitamin D, vitamin B_{12}, calcium, and iron and other fat-soluble vitamins for biliopancreatic diversion with duodenal switch); gallstones; weight regain; and other surgical complications.

D. Patient and family education

Patient education and instruction should revolve around the following issues and topics:

1. Multifactorial etiology of obesity and associated health risks
2. Meal plan and nutrition counseling with provision of specific caloric and portion information, including sample menus
3. Importance of exercise and physical activity scheduled into daily routine
4. Family involvement and participation and support
5. Patient expectation geared to slow weight loss over months

VI. Self-management resources

A. For online and smart phone food record keeping to increase patients' awareness of their eating

1. www.fitday.com
2. www.myfitnesspal.com

B. For healthy nutrition and weight loss diets

1. American Heart Association, www.heart.org, for healthy recipes, heart healthy tips, and risk calculators for heart disease
2. U.S. Department of Agriculture: www.choosemyplate.gov. This site has resources on the plate method, weight management and calorie counting, physical activity, healthy eating tips, and other nutrition information including printable materials for education.

C. For physical activity and exercise resources

1. Let's Move!: www.letsmove.gov/
2. American College of Sports Medicine: www.acsm.org
3. American Heart Association: www.heart.org/
4. Active at Any Size: http://win.niddk.nih.gov/publications/active.htm#activeat
5. There are also smart phone apps for measuring activity including step counting and GPS devices that appear be helpful in increasing awareness of activity (Morrison et al., 2014).

REFERENCES

Aarts, E. O., Dogan, K., Koehestanie, P., Aufenacker, T. J., Janssen, I. M., & Berends, F.J. (2014). Long-term results after laparoscopic adjustable gastric banding: A mean fourteen year follow-up study. *Surgery for Obesity Related Diseases, 10*(4), 633–640.

Allison, D. B., Mentor, J. L., Heo, M., Chandler, L. P., Cappelleri, J. C., Infante, M. C., et al. (1999). Antipsychotic-induced weight gain: A comprehensive research synthesis. *American Journal of Psychiatry, 156*(11), 1686–1696.

American Academy of Child and Adolescent Psychiatry. (2006). *Facts for families: Obesity in children and teens. No. 79, updated May 2008.* Retrieved from http://www.aacap.org/AACAP/Families_and_Youth/Facts_for_Families/FFF-Guide/Obesity-In-Children-And-Teens-079.aspx.

Aquila, R. (2002). Management of weight gain in patients with schizophrenia. *Journal of Clinical Psychiatry, 63*(Suppl. 4), 33–36.

Baron, R. (2015). Nutritional disorders. In M. Papadakis & S. McPhee (Eds.), *2015 current medical diagnosis & treatment* (pp. 1246–1249). New York: McGraw-Hill.

Basson, B. R., Kinon, B. J., Taylor, C. C., Szymanski, K. A., Gilmore, J. A., & Tollefson, G. D. (2001). Factors influencing acute weight change in patients with schizophrenia treated with olanzapine, haloperidol, or risperidone. *Journal of Clinical Psychiatry, 62*, 231–238.

Bauchowitz, A. U., Gonder-Frederick, L. A., Olbrisch, M. E., Azarbad, L., Ryee, M. Y., Woodson, M., et al. (2005). Psychosocial evaluation of bariatric surgery candidates: A survey of present practices. *Psychosomatic Medicine, 67*(5), 825–832.

Beckman, L. M., Beckman, T. R., & Earthman, C. P. (2010). Changes in gastrointestinal hormones and leptin after Roux-en-Y gastric bypass procedure: A review. *Journal of the American Dietetic Association, 110,* 571–584.

Bjorkhem-Bergman, L., Asplund, A. B, & Lindh, J. D. (2010). Metformin for weight reduction in non-diabetic patients on antipsychotic drugs: A systemic review and meta-analysis. *Journal of Psychopharmacology, 25*(3), 299–305.

Boyd, M. A. (2002). Atypical antipsychotics: Impact on overall health and quality of life. *Journal of the American Psychiatric Nurses Association, 8*(4), 9–17.

Bray, G. A., & Champagne, C. M. (2005). Beyond energy balance: There is more to obesity than kilocalories. *Journal of the American Dietetic Association, 105,* S17–S23.

Brownell, K. D. (2000). *The LEARN Program for weight management 2000.* Dallas, TX: American Health Publishing Company.

Buchwald, H. (2005). Consensus conference statement bariatric surgery for morbid obesity: Health implication for patients, health professionals and third-party payers. *Journal of American College Surgery, 200,* 593–604.

Centers for Disease Control and Prevention. (2009a). Defining overweight and obesity. Retrieved from http://www.cdc.gov/obesity/defining.html.

Centers for Disease Control and Prevention. (2009b). Obesity prevalence among low-income preschool-aged children—United States, 1998–2008. *Morbidity and Mortality Weekly Review, 58*(28), 769–773. Retrieved from www.cdc.gov/mmwr/preview/mmwrhtml/mm5828a1.htm.

Centers for Disease Control and Prevention. (2009c). Overweight and obesity: Health consequences. Retrieved from www.cdc.gov/obesity/causes/health.html.

Centers for Disease Control and Prevention. (2013). Obesity—United States, 1999–2010. Retrieved from www.cdc.gov/mmwr/preview/mmwrhtml/su6203a20.htm.

Fabricatore, A. N. (2007). Behavior therapy and cognitive-behavioral therapy of obesity: Is there a difference? *Journal of the American Dietetic Association, 107,* 92–99.

Fabricatore, A. N., & Wadden, T. A. (2003). Treatment of obesity: An overview. *Clinical Diabetes, 21*(2), 67–72.

Fidler, M. C., Sanchez, M., Raether, B., Weissman, N. J., Smith, S. R., Shanahan, W., et al. (2011). A one-year randomized trial of lorcaserin for weight loss in obese and overweight adults: The BLOSSOM trial. *Journal of Clinical Endocrinology Metabolism, 10,* 3067–3077.

Fontaine, K. R., Heo, M., Harrigan, E. P., Shear, C. L., Lakshminarayanon, M., Casey, D. E., et al. (2001). Estimating the consequences of antipsychotic induced weight gain on health and mortality rates. *Psychiatry Research, 101,* 277–288.

Food and Drug Administration. (2010a). FDA drug safety communication: FDA recommends against the continued use of Meridia (sibutramine). Retrieved from www.fda.gov/Drugs/DrugSafety/ucm228746.

Food and Drug Administration. (2010b). Postmarket drug safety information for patients and providers. Retrieved from www.fda.gov/drugs/drugsafety/postmarketdrugsafetyinformationforpatientsandproviders/default.htm.

Food and Drug Administration. (2014). FDA approves weight-management drug Saxenda. Retrieved from www.fda.gov/NewsEvents/Newsroom/PressAnnouncements/ucm427913.htm.

Gardner, C. D., Kiazand, A., Alhassan, S., Kim, S., Stafford, R. S., Balise, R. R., et al. (2007). Comparison of the Atkins, Zone, Ornish and LEARN diets for change in weight and related risk factors among overweight premenopausal women. The A to Z Weight Loss Study: A randomized trial. *JAMA, 297*, 969–977.

Greenberg, I., Chan, S., & Blackburn, G. L. (1999). Nonpharmacologic and pharmacologic management of weight gain. *Journal of Clinical Psychiatry, 60*(Suppl. 21), 31–36.

Hill, J., & Wing, R. (2003). The National Weight Control Registry. *The Permanente Journal, 7*(3), 34–37.

Institute of Medicine. (2012). *Accelerating progress in obesity prevention: Solving the weight of the nation* Washington, DC: National Academies Press. http://iom.edu/reports/2012/accelerating-progress-in-obesity-prevention.aspx.

Kanaya, A. (2010, February 26). *Obesity, metabolic syndrome, and diabetes: Making the connections.* Presented at the Obesity Summit 2010, University of California, San Francisco, California.

Kashyap, S., Bhatt, D., Wolski, K., Wtanabe, R., Abdul-Ghani, M., Abood, B., et al. (2013). Metabolic effects of bariatric surgery in patients with moderate obesity and type 2 diabetes: Analyses of a randomized control trial comparing surgery with intensive medical treatment. *Diabetes Care, 36*(8), 2175–2182.

Lutz, T., & Bueter, M. (2014). The physiology underlying Roux-en-Y gastric bypass—A status report. Abstract. *American Journal of Physiology, Regulatory, Integrative and Comparative Physiology, 307*(11), R1275–R1291.

Millen, B., Wolongevicz, D., Nonas, C., & Lichtenstein, A. (2014). American Heart Association/American College of Cardiology/The Obesity Society Guidelines for the Management of Overweight and Obesity in Adults: Implications and new opportunities for registered dietitian nutritionists. *Journal of the Academy of Nutrition and Dietetics, 114*(11), 1730–1735.

Morrison, L. G., Hargood, C., Lin, S. X., Dennison, L., Joseph, J., Hughes, S., et al. (2014). Understanding usage of a hybrid website and smartphone app for weight management: A mixed-methods study. Abstract. *Journal of Medical Internet Research, 16*(10).

National Heart, Lung and Blood Institute. (1998). *The clinical guidelines on the identification, evaluations, and treatment of overweight and obesity in adult: The Evidence Report.* Retrieved from www.nhlbi.nih.gov/files/docs/guidelines/ob_gdlns.pdf.

Newall, H., Myles, N., Ward, P. B., Samaras, K., Shiers, D., & Curtis, J. (2012). Efficacy of metformin for prevention of weight gain in psychiatric populations: A review. *International Clinical Psychopharmacology, 27*, 69–75.

Nkansah, N. (2010, February 26). *Medications for obesity: Why no magic bullets?* Presented at the Obesity Summit 2010, University of California, San Francisco, California.

Ogden, C. L., Carroll, M. D., Kit, B. K., & Flegal, K. M. (2014). Prevalence of childhood and adult obesity in the United States 2011-2012. *JAMA, 311*(8), 806–814.

Pi-Sunyer, F., & Nonas, C. (2004). Clinical monitoring. In G. D. Foster & C. A. Nonas (Eds.), *Managing obesity: A clinical guide* (Chapter 3, pp. 43–64). Chicago, IL: American Dietetic Association.

Prochaska, J., & DiClemente, C. C. (1982). Transtheoretical approach: Toward a more integrative model of change. *Psychotherapy: Theory, Research and Practice, 20*, 161.

Rummel-Kluge, C., Komossa, K., Schwarz, S., Hunger, H., Schmid, F., Lobos, C. A., et al. (2010). Head-to-head comparisons of metabolic side effects of second generation antipsychotics in the treatment of schizophrenia: A systematic review and meta-analysis. *Schizophrenia Research, 123*, 225–233.

Sacks, F. M., Bray, G. A., Carey, V. J., Smith, S. R., Ryan, D. H., Anton, S. D, et al. & Clinical Efficacy Assessment Subcommittee of the American College of Physicians. (2005). Pharmacologic and surgical management of obesity in primary care: A clinical practice guideline from the American College of Physicians. *Annals of Internal Medicine, 142*(7), 525–531.

Sheppard C. E., Sadowski, D. C., de Gara, C. J., Karmali, S., & Birch, D. W. (2014, November 20). Rates of reflux before and after laparoscopic sleeve gastrectomy for severe obesity. Abstract. *Obesity Surgery.* doi: 10.1007/s11695-014-1480-y.

Ul-Haq, Z., Mackay, D. F., Fenwick, E., & Pell, J. P. (2013). Meta-analysis of the association between body mass index and health-related quality of life among children and adolescents. Assessed using the pediatric quality of life inventory index. *Journal of Pediatrics, 162*, 280–286.

U.S. Department of Health and Human Services. (2000). *Healthy People 2010.* Objectives. Retrieved from www.healthypeople.gov/2010/?visit=1.

U.S. Department of Health and Human Services. (2009). *Healthy People 2020 proposed objectives.* Retrieved from www.healthypeople.gov/2020/topics-objectives/topic/nutrition-and-weight-status

Verpeut, J. L., & Bello, N. T. (2014). Drug safety evaluation of naltrexone/buproprion for the treatment of obesity. *Expert Opinion Drug Safety, 13*(6), 831–841.

Vesely, J. M., & DeMattia, L. G. (2014). Obesity: Dietary and lifestyle management. *FP Essentials, 425*, 11–15.

Whitaker, R. C., Wright, J. A., Pepe, M. S., Seidel, K. D., & Dietz, W. H. (1997). Predicting obesity in young adulthood from childhood and parental obesity. *New England Journal of Medicine, 337*, 869–873.

CHAPTER

66

PRIMARY CARE OF HIV-INFECTED ADULTS

Suzan Stringari-Murray and
Christopher Berryhill Fox

I. Introduction and general background

Since the first cases of acquired immunodeficiency syndrome (AIDS) were diagnosed in 1981, there have been significant scientific advances in the understanding of the biology, natural history, and clinical management of human immunodeficiency virus (HIV) infection. Far from the bleak years of the early epidemic, HIV infection is now a manageable chronic condition. Both the U.S. Department of Health and Human Services (USDHHS; 2015a) and the Infectious Diseases Society of America (IDSA) publish evidence-based guidelines identifying best practices in the clinical management of HIV/AIDS (Aberg et al., 2013).

This chapter reviews and summarizes current DHHS and IDSA guidelines for those advanced practice nurses who do not have expertise in HIV/AIDS but who may be providing primary care for people living with HIV/AIDS (PLWH). The chapter also includes information on HIV screening and testing, because diagnosing new HIV infections is the first step in the HIV/AIDS care continuum, a model for evaluating the U.S. epidemic that has emerged in recent years (USDHHS, 2013). In addition to HIV screening and testing, clinicians who are generalists can provide primary care to PLWH, offer HIV-specific healthcare maintenance and disease prevention, and initiate or follow antiretroviral therapy (ART) in consultation with HIV experts.

A. Epidemiology

HIV is the virus that causes AIDS. There are two types of HIV: HIV-1 and HIV-2. HIV-1 is the most prevalent globally and, without treatment, typically progresses to death within 8–10 years. HIV-2 occurs mostly in West Africa and has a slower clinical progression (Maartens, Celum, & Lewin, 2014). This chapter focuses exclusively on HIV-1, and use of the term HIV should be understood as referring to HIV-1.

HIV is transmitted through certain bodily fluids: semen, preseminal fluids (or preejaculate), rectal secretions, vaginal secretions, blood, and breast milk. Transmission occurs when an infected fluid enters the body of an HIV-uninfected person via a mucous membrane (particularly the rectal or vaginal mucosa) or the bloodstream. Vertical transmission, now rare in the United States, can occur during pregnancy, labor, delivery, or breastfeeding. Nonvertical HIV exposures that carry the highest risk for transmission are parenteral (blood transfusion, needle sharing during injection drug use, and percutaneous such as needle stick) and sexual (specifically anal and penile-vaginal sex) (Patel et al., 2014). Oral sex carries low risk of HIV transmission, and exposures through biting, spitting, throwing bodily fluids, and sharing sex toys have negligible risk (Centers for Disease Control and Prevention, 2014b; Patel et al., 2014; Pretty, Anderson, & Sweet, 1999).

AIDS represents the advanced stages of HIV infection and is characterized by the progressive depletion of CD4 T lymphocytes, resulting in life-threatening HIV-related opportunistic infections (OI) and certain malignancies. For the purpose of disease surveillance, the Centers for Disease Control and Prevention (CDC) developed a case definition for AIDS that has been revised several times to reflect advances in testing, diagnosis, and treatment of HIV. The current case definition of AIDS includes all HIV-infected people with CD4 counts ≤ 200 cells/mm^3 or diagnosis of certain AIDS-defining illnesses (**Table 66-1**) (CDC, 2014d).

The CDC has been tracking AIDS since 1981, when the first cases of a fatal pneumonia called *Pneumocystis carinii* (later renamed *P. jiroveci*) appeared in young, otherwise healthy gay men. Based on these data, there was an estimated cumulative total of over 1.1 million cases of AIDS in the United States at the end of 2012 (CDC, 2014a). By 2011, there was an estimated cumulative total of 648,459 deaths from AIDS in the United States (CDC, 2014a).

In addition to surveillance of AIDS cases, the CDC has fully established an HIV incidence surveillance system to effectively track trends in new HIV infections. As of 2008, confidential names-based reporting systems have been

TABLE 66-1 AIDS-Defining Illnesses in Adolescents and Adults

Candidiasis of bronchi, trachea, or lungs

Candidiasis of esophagus

Cervical cancer, invasive

Coccidioidomycosis, disseminated or extrapulmonary

Cryptococcosis, extrapulmonary

Cryptosporidiosis, chronic intestinal (> 1 month's duration)

Cytomegalovirus disease (other than liver, spleen, or nodes), onset at age > 1 month

Cytomegalovirus retinitis (with loss of vision)

Encephalopathy attributed to HIV

Herpes simplex: chronic ulcers (> 1 month's duration) or bronchitis, pneumonitis, or esophagitis

Histoplasmosis, disseminated or extrapulmonary

Isosporiasis, chronic intestinal (> 1 month's duration)

Kaposi sarcoma

Lymphoma, Burkitt (or equivalent term)

Lymphoma, immunoblastic (or equivalent term)

Lymphoma, primary, of brain

Mycobacterium avium complex or *Mycobacterium kansasii*, disseminated or extrapulmonary

Mycobacterium tuberculosis of any site, pulmonary, disseminated, or extrapulmonary

Mycobacterium, other species or unidentified species, disseminated or extrapulmonary

Pneumocystis jirovecii (previously known as *Pneumocystis carinii*) pneumonia

Pneumonia, recurrent

Progressive multifocal leukoencephalopathy

Salmonella septicemia, recurrent

Toxoplasmosis of brain

Wasting syndrome attributed to HIV

Modified from Centers for Disease Control and Prevention. (2014). Revised surveillance case definition for HIV infection—United States, 2014. *MMWR, 63*(3), 1–10. Retrieved from http://www.cdc.gov/mmwr/pdf/rr/rr6303.pdf.

implemented in all 50 states, the District of Columbia, and six U.S. dependent areas (American Samoa, Guam, the Northern Mariana Islands, Puerto Rico, the Republic of Palau, and the U.S. Virgin Islands) (CDC, 2014a).

The CDC (2014d) estimates that as of 2011 (the last year for which data are available), there were 1.2 million PLWH age 13 years or older in the United States. In 2012, there was an estimated incidence of 47,989 new HIV infections, with an incidence rate of 15.3 per 100,000 (CDC, 2014a).

HIV disproportionately affects gay, bisexual, and other men who have sex with men (MSM) in the United States. Although less than 4% of the male population is MSM, this group accounted for 57% of all diagnosed HIV/AIDS cases in 2011 (CDC, 2015c; Purcell et al., 2012).

In 2011, women represented one-quarter of all diagnosed HIV infections in the United States. Heterosexual activity accounted for 84% of new transmissions in this group (CDC, 2014a).

In recent years, new attention has been directed toward older adults living with HIV/AIDS in the United States., with 15% of PLWH now age 55 or older (CDC, 2013a). The graying of the HIV/AIDS epidemic in the United States is attributed to increased survival from ART, as well as infection with HIV later in life. Older adults may be unaware of their HIV risk or never offered testing by a healthcare provider. Compared to their younger counterparts, older adults are more likely to discover their new HIV infections late in disease progression (CDC, 2013a).

Although there are few data describing transgender populations, current evidence suggests that this group is at high risk for HIV, especially among male to female or transgender women (CDC, 2013b). In particular, transgender women who are sex workers, both in the United States and globally, have a high prevalence of HIV infection. Data describing HIV incidence, prevalence, or risk among female-to-male or transgender men are severely lacking.

There are significant racial and ethnic disparities in HIV/AIDS incidence, prevalence, and survival in the United States, particularly among African Americans, who are the group most affected by HIV/AIDS (CDC, 2015b). African Americans comprise 12% of the U.S. population but accounted for 47% of all new HIV diagnoses in 2012 (CDC, 2015b). New HIV infections are increasing fastest in young African American MSM (ages 13–24), who had nearly twice the new infections as young white or Hispanic MSM in 2010 (CDC, 2015b). African American women have the highest incidence of non-MSM new HIV infections in the United States, with an incidence rate 20 times that of white women and 5 times that of Hispanic women (CDC, 2015b). African Americans also had the highest HIV death rate in 2010 at 11.6 per 100,000—a dramatic contrast from the death rates of whites (1.1 per 100,000) and Hispanics (2.8 per 100,000) (National Center for Health Statistics, 2014).

Historically, most PLWH have been clustered in major metropolitan areas in three states: California, New York, and Florida. Now urban and rural areas in the South, as well as the District of Columbia, have emerged as a locus of HIV/AIDS. The District of Columbia has the highest estimated prevalence rate of HIV in the United States and dependent areas at 2,721.6 per 100,000 compared to 342.1 per 100,000 overall (CDC, 2014a).

Globally, there have been 78 million people infected with HIV since the start of the epidemic, resulting in 39 million deaths (United Nations Joint Programme on HIV/AIDS [UNAIDS], 2014). As of 2013, UNAIDS estimates that there were a total of 35 million PLWH globally, with the majority (70%) of cases in Sub-Saharan Africa. Heterosexual sex is the main mode of transmission in this region. Among countries, South Africa continues to carry the greatest HIV/AIDS burden, with 18% of global infections (UNAIDS, 2014).

Deaths from AIDS-related causes peaked globally in 2005 and have now fallen 35% with advances in prevention and treatment, as well as increased access to ART. Even so, in 2013, only 37% of PLWH globally had access to ART (UNAIDS, 2014).

New HIV infections around the globe have decreased 38% since 2001 (UNAIDS, 2014). In 2013, there were 2.1 million new HIV infections, compared to 3.4 million in 2001. Despite this downward trend, certain groups remain highly vulnerable to new HIV infections, including adolescent and young women, MSM, transgender people, sex workers, intravenous drug users (IVDUs), and incarcerated individuals (UNAIDS, 2014).

B. Pathogenesis and natural history of HIV infection

Transmission of HIV is followed within days to weeks by a nonspecific viral syndrome or seroconversion illness characterized by fever, generalized maculopapular rash, lymphadenopathy, and pharyngitis. Approximately 40–90% of patients acutely infected with HIV will experience this nonspecific and self-limiting viral syndrome (Panel on Antiretroviral Guidelines for Adults and Adolescents [PAGAA], 2015a). The period of acute HIV infection is characterized by an initial burst of viremia. Recent infection is the phase up to six months after infection when HIV-specific antibodies are detectable. Individuals with acute HIV have high levels of replicating virus, and transmission of HIV to an uninfected partner(s) is more likely during this phase of infection. Following transmission, HIV disseminates throughout the body infecting CD4 T-helper lymphocytes, a main target of the virus. HIV enters the host cell by attaching and binding to coreceptors on the surface of the cell (CCR5 and CXCR4). Once in the cell cytoplasm, viral enzymes reverse transcribe viral RNA into viral DNA. Viral DNA enters the cell nucleus and integrates into the host cell genome. Once integrated into the host cell genome, HIV persists as a latent reservoir of virus despite fully suppressive ART (Hare, 2009).

Research on the immunopathogenesis of HIV has resulted in an improved understanding of how HIV causes AIDS. An active site of HIV replication is the lamina propria of the gut wall, which is rich in lymphoid tissue and contains large numbers of CCR5 expressing CD4 T-helper lymphocytes. During acute HIV, gut-associated lymphoid tissue (GALT) is rapidly infected and destroyed, leading to local inflammation and increased gut permeability. It is hypothesized that leakage of microbes or "microbial translocation" from the gut results in a state of chronic immune system activation and inflammation (Douek, Picker, & Koup, 2003). Chronic immune system activation helps to sustain HIV replication through the continuous production of HIV-infected activated CD4 cells, which produce HIV and perpetuate a continuous cycle of viral replication. High levels of virus in the blood (viral load) are associated with more rapid destruction of CD4 lymphocytes and more rapid clinical progression. If HIV infection goes unrecognized, over a period of months to years (on average, 8–10 years) progressive depletion of CD4 lymphocytes leads to immune system failure and death from HIV, usually as a result of AIDS-related illnesses (**Figure 66-1**). Once HIV infection is established, chronic inflammation and immune activation persist even in patients on ART who have undetectable viral loads.

Currently recommended ART regimens are potent and effective in suppressing HIV replication but cannot eradicate HIV in host cells. Effective HIV treatment requires lifelong therapy and adherence to ART. Incomplete or intermittent adherence to ART can result in the failure to

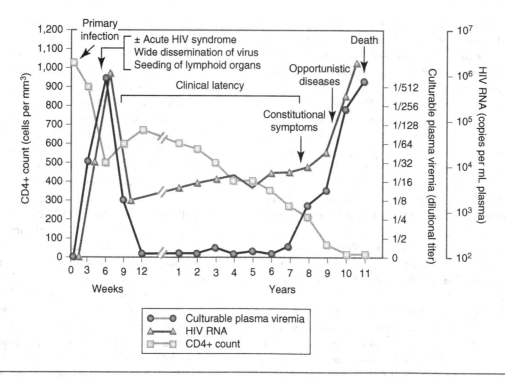

FIGURE 66-1 Typical Course of HIV Infection

During the period following primary infection, HIV disseminates widely in the body; an abrupt decrease in CD4+ T cells in the peripheral circulation is often seen. An immune response to HIV ensues, with a decrease in detectable viremia. A period of clinical latency follows, during which CD4+ T cell counts continue to decrease, until they fall to a critical level below which there is a substantial risk of opportunistic infections. (Adapted from Pantaleo et al., 1993.)

Reproduced from National Institute of Allergy and Infectious Diseases. (2010). *The relationship between the human immunodeficiency virus and the acquired immunodeficiency syndrome*. Retrieved from http://www.niaid.nih.gov /topics/hivaids/understanding/howhivcausesaids/pages/relationshiphivaids.aspx

fully suppress HIV replication and lead to the development of HIV–drug resistant virus.

Significant improvements have occurred in the potency, tolerability, and frequency of dosing for ART regimens. Recommended regimens for initial treatment of HIV consist of a combination of three or more drugs. Several of these combinations are now available as daily single tablet regimens (STR), which simplify therapy and support adherence by reducing pill burden (PAGAA, 2015a).

Historically, the initiation of ART has been guided by CD4 T lymphocyte counts. Current evidence-based guidelines recommend ART for all regardless of the pretreatment CD4 T lymphocyte count (**Table 66-2**). This recommendation is based on evidence from randomized controlled trials and observational studies that show a reduction in mortality for both AIDS-defining illnesses and non-AIDS-defining illnesses (e.g., cardiovascular, liver, or kidney disease) in individuals who are started on ART at higher pretreatment CD4 cell counts (PAGAA, 2015a).

C. HIV primary care and the HIV care continuum

HIV is now considered a chronic primary care disease. The HIV Care Continuum identifies a series of steps to fully engage and retain patients in primary care. Current estimates of HIV/AIDS care in the United States indicate that of those individuals who know they are HIV infected, only 37% are on ART, and of those individuals who are on ART, only 30% are virally suppressed (**Figure 66-2**). Nurse Practitioners (NPs) play an essential role in improving health outcomes of PLWH along all steps of the HIV Care Continuum (CDC, 2014e). The most significant impact for reducing HIV infections is achieved by providing HIV testing as a routine part of care in all medical settings and immediately linking patients diagnosed with HIV to medical care. Once patients are engaged in care, rapid initiation of ART and viral load suppression improves individual health outcomes and prevents further transmission of HIV.

Treatment with ART has significantly reduced deaths due to AIDS-defining illnesses (Table 66-1). Chronic conditions such as cardiovascular disease (CVD),

TABLE 66-2 Initiating Antiretroviral Therapy in Treatment-Naïve Adults and Adolescents

Antiretroviral therapy (ART) is recommended for all HIV-infected individuals to reduce the risk of disease progression.

- ART is recommended for all (CD4) cell counts: CD4 count < 350 cells/mm³ (AI); CD4 count 350 to 500 cells/mm³ (AII); CD4 count > 500 cells/mm³ (BIII).

- ART is also recommended for HIV-infected individuals to prevent transmission of HIV. The strength of and evidence for this recommendation vary by transmission risks: perinatal transmission (AI); heterosexual transmission (AI); other transmission risk groups (AIII).

- Patients starting ART should be willing and able to commit to treatment and understand the benefits and risks of therapy and the importance of adherence (AIII). Patients may choose to postpone therapy, and providers, on a case-by-case basis, may elect to defer therapy on the basis of clinical and/or psychosocial factors.

Rating of Recommendations: A = Strong; B = Moderate; C = Optional Rating of Evidence: I = Data from randomized controlled trials; II = Data from well-designed nonrandomized trials or observational cohort studies with long-term clinical outcomes; III = Expert opinion

Data from U.S. Department of Health and Human Services, Panel on Antiretroviral Guidelines for Adults and Adolescents. (May 1, 2014). *Guidelines for the use of antiretroviral agents in HIV-1-infected adults and adolescents*, p. E-1. Retrieved from https://aidsinfo.nih.gov/guidelines.

non-AIDS-defining malignancies, diabetes, chronic obstructive pulmonary disease, osteoporosis, thromboembolic disease, liver disease, renal disease, and neurocognitive dysfunction are increasingly the most common causes of morbidity and mortality in PLWH (Antiretroviral Therapy Cohort Collaborative, 2008; Strategies for Management of Antiretroviral Therapy [SMART] Study Group et al., 2006). HIV care now consists of more than

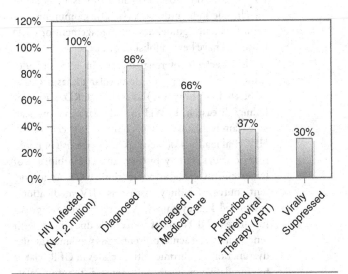

FIGURE 66-2 HIV/AIDS Care Continuum in the United States, 2011

Modified from Centers for Disease Control and Prevention. (2014). Vital signs: HIV diagnosis, care, and treatment among persons living with HIV—United States, 2011. *Morbidity and Mortality Weekly Report, 63*(47), 1113–1117. Retrieved from http://www.cdc.gov/mmwr/preview/mmwrhtml/mm6347a5.htm.

initiating and managing ART. Improved survival for PLWH has increased the prevalence of older adults (age > 50 years) living with HIV who have multiple chronic conditions complicated by HIV and HIV treatment. Improvements in life expectancy of PLWH beyond those that can be achieved with the use of ART will depend on optimal management of their multiple comorbidities.

Most evidence-based guidelines for chronic diseases do not address the impact of HIV in the management of chronic diseases. To address this gap in recommendations the HIV Medicine Association (AAHIVM) of the Infectious Disease Society of America (IDSA) has developed guidelines for managing comorbid conditions commonly seen in PLWH (see Resources). The following is a summary of some of these recommendations.

1. HIV, CVD, and dyslipidemias: Despite effective ART, PLWH have an increased risk of CVD and myocardial infarction (MI) when compared to the general population. In a retrospective study of an HIV-infected urban population, sudden cardiac death occurred at a rate four time higher in HIV-infected compared to non-HIV-infected subjects (Tseng et al., 2012). Underlying mechanisms proposed for this observed increased risk of MI include chronic immune activation and inflammation, ART-related side effects, and a greater prevalence of cardiovascular risk factors. Observational cohort studies of PLWH have documented past or current smoking in > 50% of study subjects as well as high rates of dyslipidemias (Friis-Møller et al., 2003). Nationally representative surveys of adults with HIV have shown that smoking prevalence is two times higher than in the general U.S. population (Mdodo et al., 2015).

   Strategies to address increased risk for CVD have included changing ART regimens associated with dyslipidemias and body fat redistribution syndromes and an increased emphasis on managing traditional risk factors such as smoking, abnormal lipids, and hypertension. Abacavir, a component of some ART regimens, has been associated with an increased risk of CVD. Studies supporting this association are conflicting and consensus on avoidance of abacavir in individuals at risk for MI has not been reached. Current ART treatment recommendations provide clinicians with guidance regarding regimen characteristics and consideration of specific clinical scenarios for the selection of initial ART regimens (PAGAA, 2015a).

Lipid management guidelines published in 2013 by the American Cardiology Association/American Heart Association (ACA/AHA) have been shown to underestimate the need for statin therapy in PLWH who have CT evidence of coronary plaque, suggesting that population-based guidelines may be inadequate for PLWH (Zanni et al., 2014). Despite evidence suggesting that CV disease risk is underestimated, current recommendations for lipid management in the general population apply to PLWH. Use of lovastatin and simvastatin are contraindicated in patients on protease inhibitor containing ART regimens due to significant drug-drug interactions. Medications should be reviewed for known or potential interactions between ART and commonly prescribed statins, antihypertensives, anticoagulants, and antiplatelet medications (PAGAA, 2015a).

2. HIV and diabetes mellitus (DM): The prevalence of DM in PLWH has been noted to range between 4–14% (Brown et al., 2005; Friis-Møller et al., 2003). First-generation protease inhibitors (indinavir) have been shown to impair glucose metabolism, and older NRTIs (stavudine) are associated with lipoatrophy and lead to development of DM. PLWH also have a higher prevalence of conditions associated with DM such as chronic HCV and ART-related fat redistribution syndromes. Important clinical management differences for PLWH who are diagnosed with DM include drug–drug interactions between metformin and dolutegravir (PAGAA, 2015a) and HbA1c discordance with fasting plasma glucose (FPG) levels. Some experts recommend use of FPG to screen for DM and suggest that lower target goals for HbA1c may be needed (Monroe, Gelsby, & Brown, 2015). At this time, treatment goals, lifestyle modification, and clinical management of DM are the same as for the general population.

3. HIV and malignancies: There are three AIDS-defining cancers: Kaposi sarcoma (KS) caused by human herpes virus-8, Non-Hodgkin's lymphoma,

and cervical cancer (Table 66-1). In addition to AIDS-defining cancers PLWH also have an increased risk of non-AIDS-defining cancers that are virally mediated or related to specific health behaviors: lung cancer (tobacco), liver cancer (HBV, HCV, and alcohol abuse), and anal cancer (HPV). Cervical cancer screening in women with HIV differs from the current U.S. Preventive Services Task Force (USPSTF) recommendations for initiation of screening, frequency of screening, and management of abnormal Pap smears (**Table 66-3**).

The incidence of breast, colon, and prostate cancer is similar to the general population. Significant declines in the incidence and prevalence of KS and primary CNS lymphoma have occurred in with widespread use of ART. The incidence of cervical cancer has not changed with the introduction of ART, however, the incidence of anal cancer has increased in both men and women. National multicenter studies are ongoing to determine cancer rates in PLWH to guide future policy on the impact of HIV infection on cancer risk and cancer related morbidity and mortality (U.S. National Institutes of Health, National Cancer Institute, n.d.). Cancer is a disease of aging. As PLWH grow older and reach their normal life expectancy, providers will likely see more cancer diagnoses in HIV-treated populations.

4. HIV and renal disease: HIV infection is a risk factor for chronic kidney disease (CKD). Comprehensive clinical practice guidelines for management of CKD in PLWH have been published (Lucas et al., 2014).

The spectrum of renal disease in HIV includes acute kidney injury and glomerular diseases (HIV-associated nephropathy) as well as CKD. Risks for kidney disease in PLWH include African American race, family history, CD4 count < 200 cells/mm³, HIV viral load > 4,000 copies/mL, past use of nephrotoxic drugs, family history, and comorbidities of hypertension, diabetes, and chronic HCV. An important source of kidney disease is HIV medication–associated kidney injury, with tenofovir disoproxil fumarate (TDF) of most concern. Kidney injury with tenofovir can be acute, presenting as proximal tubular dysfunction, or chronic with declines in GFR related to cumulative exposure to tenofovir. Tenofovir alafenamide, (TAF) an oral prodrug of tenofovir, is now approved as a component of a fixed-dose combination tablet for initial treatment of HIV. The potential for adverse kidney and bone effects is less with TAF than with TDF. Cobicistat, a pharmacokinetic booster found in some ART regimens, is approved for use in patients with a creatinine clearance (CrCl) of > 70 mL/min. Recommendations for dosing of

TABLE 66-3 Healthcare Maintenance and Disease Screening

Test	Frequency	Comments
Mycobacterium tuberculosis (MTB) skin test (TST) and interferon-γ release assay (IGRA)	Screen at entry into care and annually regardless of CD4 count	• PLWH who have latent tuberculosis infection (LTBI) have a 3–16% annual risk of active MTB • Routine use of both TST and IGRA is not recommended. • TST: Criteria for a positive skin test ≥ 5 mm induration at 48–72 hours. • IGRA: Has advantages over TST for TB screening in adults with HIV, including single patient visit to conduct test; results available in 24 hours; does not cross-react in patients who have been previously vaccinated with BCG; and has higher specificity (92–97%) compared to TST. Disadvantages include cost and limited data on PLWH. • Rescreen if CD4 increases to 200/mm^3 and previous TB screening was negative.
Cytomegalovirus-CMV IgG	At entry into care	• Screen in patients where likelihood of cytomegalovirus seropositivity is low (higher CMV seropositive prevalence in MSM and IDU).
Herpes simplex virus (HSV-2)	At entry into care	• Prevention of acquisition of HSV is recommended. Disclosure of HSV-2 in heterosexual HSV-2-discordant couples has been associated with reduced risk of transmission of HSV-2. • PLWH who are seronegative for HSV-2 should ask their sexual partners to be screened for HSV-2 (BII).
Neisseria gonorrhoeae (GC) and *Chlamydia trachomatis* (CT) *Trichomonas vaginalis*	At entry into care regardless of symptoms and when clinically indicated (multiple partners, reported high-risk behaviors, recurrent STDs) Women < age 25 and/or high-risk men and women who test positive for GC, CT, and trichomoniasis	• Nucleic acid amplification tests (NAAT) are sensitive and preferred for both genital and extragenital sampling. • Sexually active MSM, particularly ≤ 25 yrs, have a high burden of disease for CT and GC. NAATs are not approved by the Food and Drug Administration for testing rectal and oropharyngeal sites yet are sensitive and specific compared to culture. Check local health departments for guidance in using these tests. • Sexual partners should be referred for evaluation, testing, and presumptive treatment if they had sexual contact with the partner during the 60 days preceding the patient's onset of symptoms or chlamydia diagnosis (Centers for Disease Control and Prevention, 2015d) • Increased risk of HIV transmission and pelvic inflammatory disease in untreated trichomoniasis • Reinfection rates of STDs are high and repeat of all positive tests at 3 months following treatment is recommended

(continues)

TABLE 66-3 Healthcare Maintenance and Disease Screening *(Continued)*

Test	Frequency	Comments
Syphilis-Venereal Disease Research Laboratory (VDRL) or Rapid plasma reagin (RPR)	At entry into care and annually. More frequent screening (q 3–6 months) for those with multiple partners, sex without condoms, and partner recently treated for STDs	• Nontreponemal tests are sensitive and specific in PLWH. Some labs may use enzyme immunoassays (EIA) in syphilis testing algorithms followed by a reflex-quantitative, nontreponemal test if the EIA is positive. • Screening for other STDs (GC and CT) at anatomic sites of exposure should be done when screening or treating syphilis
Dilated retinal examination	CD4 < 100 annually and when clinically indicated	• Screen for HIV-related retinopathy and asymptomatic cytomegalovirus retinitis.
Chest radiograph	Baseline	• If positive TB screening test and history and exam suggestive of preexisting lung disease
Serum testosterone level	Men Morning specimen	• In males with fatigue, weight loss, and erectile dysfunction
Anal cancer screening	Men and women. At entry and annually based on risk	• Incidence of anal cancer is increasing in PLWH due to improved length of survival and reduced rates of HPV clearance in PLWH despite ART. Although there are no national guidelines for anal cancer screening, some experts recommend screening (CIII). • If resources for referral of abnormal anal cytology are not available, screening is optional (CIII).
Cervical cancer screening	*≤ 30 yrs old:* Screen at time of initial diagnosis. If normal, repeat in 12 months (BII). If 3 consecutive normal pap smears, repeat every 3 years. *≥ 30 years old:* Pap testing only: At baseline, and every 12 months (BII). If results of the 3 consecutive Pap tests are normal, recommend follow-up Pap tests every 3 years (BII) See Chapter 20, Screening for Intraepithelial Neoplasia and Cancer of the Lower Genital Tract, for details.	• Women with HIV have a higher prevalence of HPV infection and increased incidence of cervical cancer compared to women who are not HIV infected. • Begin screening at onset of sexual activity regardless of mode of transmission (e.g., sexual, perinatal exposure) but no later then 21 yrs old. • Co-testing with HPV is not recommended for HIV-infected women < 30 yrs old. • See Chapter 20, Screening for Intraepithelial Neoplasia and Cancer of the Lower Genital Tract, for additional details.
Breast, prostate, colon, and lung		• Cancer screening guidelines for general population apply to PLWH
Bone mineral density screen	Perform baseline exam in postmenopausal women and men age > 50 yrs.	• PLWH have increased prevalence of osteopenia and osteoporosis and increased risk of fragility fractures compared to general population

Rating of Recommendations: A = Strong; B = Moderate; C = Optional Rating of Evidence: I = Data from randomized controlled trials; II = Data from well-designed nonrandomized trials or observational cohort studies with long-term clinical outcomes; III = Expert opinion" as noted in table 66-2

Data from Centers for Disease Control and Prevention. (2010, June 25). Updated guidelines for using interferon gamma release assays to detect *Mycobacterium tuberculosis* infection in the United States, 2010. *MMWR Recommendations and Reports, 59*(RR05), 1–25. Retrieved from www.cdc .gov/mmwr/preview/mmwrhtml/rr5905a1.htm?s_cid=rr5905a1_e; Centers for Disease Control and Prevention. (2015). *Sexually transmitted disease treatment guidelines, 2015. MMWR Recommendations and Reports, 64*(RR3), 1–137. Retrieved from www.cdc.gov/mmwr/preview/mmwrhtml /rr6403a1.htm; Panel on Opportunistic Infections in HIV-Infected Adults and Adolescents. (2013). *Guidelines for the prevention and treatment of opportunistic infections in HIV-infected adults and adolescents: recommendations from the Centers for Disease Control and Prevention, the National Institutes of Health, and the HIV Medicine Association of the Infectious Diseases Society of America.* Retrieved from http://aidsinfo.nih.gov /contentfiles/lvguidelines/adult_oi.pdf.

ART regimens in patients with renal and/or hepatic disease can be found in the treatment guidelines (PAGAA, 2015a).

5. HIV and bone disease: Low bone mineral density (BMD) is highly prevalent in PLWH (~15%), with a 3.7-fold increase compared with age-matched controls, and rates of bone fracture for PLWH are higher than the general population (Young et al., 2011). The causes of low BMD are multifactorial and include traditional risks as well as HIV-specific risk factors such as chronic inflammation, ART-associated bone loss, and HIV/HCV confection. Following the initiation of ART, a 2–6% decrease in BMD occurs over the first 2 years of therapy (McComsey et al., 2010). All ART regimens have been implicated in bone loss with tenofovir having the strongest association with an acute decrease in BMD compared to other NRTIs (Rothman & Bessesen, 2012).

6. HIV and chronic HBV and HCV: Chronic viral hepatitis is more prevalent in PLWH due to similar routes of transmission (sexual transmission and IDU). Coinfection with chronic HBV or HCV results in a more rapid progression to fibrosis and cirrhosis and an increased risk of hepatocellular carcinoma (HCC). Both HBV and HCV may complicate the treatment of HIV due to hepatotoxicity associated with ART.

HIV/HBV coinfected patients have higher levels of HBV viremia and a lower likelihood of clearing their infection following acute HBV infection. All HIV-infected patients without evidence of immunity to HBV should be vaccinated with HBV vaccine (**Table 66-4**).

There are three antiretroviral drugs from the NRTI class with activity against HBV: lamivudine, emtricitabine, and tenofovir. Some are available alone or in a fixed-dose combination. HBV and HIV must be treated concurrently with ART that is active against both infections. For example, the fixed-dose combination of abacavir/lamivudine is a recommended regimen for treating HIV when combined with dolutegravir, but is inadequate for effectively treating HBV (PAGAA, 2015a). Treating HBV with tenofovir only in an HIV-infected patient would be inadequate treatment for HIV and lead to HIV drug resistance. Return to immune competence with increases in CD4 lymphocyte counts occurs after initiation of ART and can lead to reactivation of HBV-related liver disease. Liver transaminases must be followed more closely when initiating ART in HIV/HBV coinfected patients (Panel on Opportunistic Infections in HIV-Infected Adults and Adolescents, 2013).

HIV/HCV: The management of HCV is rapidly evolving, and several newer oral agents have been approved for treatment. Studies of HCV direct-acting antiviral agents (DAA) have shown that these drugs are safe and effective in HIV/HCV coinfection. PLWH who have chronic HCV have been categorized as high priority patients for treatment with these agents. (See Chapter 51, Chronic Viral Hepatitis.) Recommendations for concomitant use of HCV DAAs and drug interactions with ART are provided in current guidelines (PAGAA, 2015b).

II. HIV screening and testing

A. Rationale

Fourteen percent of Americans with HIV do not know that they are infected (CDC, 2014a), which has led the USDHHS (2014) to identify increasing awareness of HIV serostatus as a Leading Health Indicator in Healthy People 2020. Increased HIV serostatus awareness is also a goal of the National HIV/AIDS Strategy (White House Office of National AIDS Policy, 2010).

Early detection of HIV infection benefits patients by creating an opportunity to initiate ART, thereby preventing further immune destruction with its resulting morbidity and mortality. Knowledge of HIV serostatus also has major public health implications: Individuals with HIV who do not know their serostatus are the source of approximately 54% of new HIV transmissions (Marks, Crepaz, & Janssen, 2006). A person with unsuppressed virus is significantly more likely to transmit virus to a sexual or needle-sharing partner. Individuals with acute HIV infection may have very high levels of HIV. Individuals may also unknowingly facilitate viral transmission by participating in high-risk behaviors that would otherwise avoid if they were aware of their HIV serostatus.

In a nationwide survey of Americans, the top reasons that individuals gave for never receiving an HIV test were lack of perceived risk (#1) and testing had never been recommended by a doctor (#2) (Henry J. Kaiser Family Foundation, 2009). Therefore, it is incumbent upon clinicians to discuss HIV risk with patients and offer routine testing.

B. Guidelines

1. National recommendations
   a. The CDC (2006) recommends screening all patients ages 13–64 years, except in settings of low undiagnosed HIV prevalence (defined as < 0.1%, or less than 1 in every 1,000 HIV tests is positive).

TABLE 66-4 Immunizations for HIV-Infected Adults

All PLWH should be immunized according to CDC vaccine schedules for adults and adolescents. In general, the immune response to vaccines in PLWH is not as robust compared to HIV noninfected populations. Some clinicians may defer vaccines if an increase in CD4 T lymphocyte count to ≥ 200 mm³ is anticipated as a result of initiating ART. Some vaccines should not be deferred regardless of CD4 cell count.

Vaccines that are contraindicated in PLWH.

- Live attenuated intranasal influenza (LAIV-Flumist)
- Oral polio virus (OPV)
- Smallpox
- Typhoid oral vaccine (Ty21a)
- Bacillus Calmette-Guerin (BCG)

*Close contacts of persons with HIV should receive all age-appropriate vaccines, with the exception of live OPV and smallpox vaccine

Live vaccines that can be administered when CD4 counts are > 200 mm³.

Measles/Mumps/Rubella (MMR): Vaccine schedule and dosing are the same as for the general population.	• Persons with HIV infection are at increased risk for severe complications if infected with measles. • Newly diagnosed adults without acceptable evidence of measles immunity should receive mumps-measles-rubella vaccine unless they have evidence of severe immunosuppression (CD4 ≤ 200 mm³). If necessary separate components of vaccine can be given.
Varicella: Vaccine schedule and dosing are the same as for the general population	• People born before 1980 do not need to receive this vaccine. • No studies have evaluated the vaccine in HIV-infected adolescents or adults. Varicella vaccination may be considered in HIV-seropositive/VZV seronegative persons ≥ 8 years old with CD4 counts ≥ 200 cells/mm³. • Do not administer during pregnancy.
Varicella Zoster (VZV): Vaccine schedule and dosing are the same as for the general population	• Safety and efficacy in PLWH is unknown. Consider in patients 60 years of age with a CD4 > 200 mm³. • Serologic testing of prior exposure not required. • If susceptible to VZV avoid exposure to individuals with varicella. • Household contacts should be vaccinated to prevent transmission of varicella to PLWH. • If a known or suspected VZV exposure occurs post exposure prophylaxis is recommended with Varicella Zoster Immune Globulin (VZIG).
Yellow fever: Vaccine schedule and dosing are the same as for the general population	• Safe in patients without severe immunosuppression (CD4 > 200) • Less immunogenic in PLWH • Use with caution in persons on ART regimens containing CCR5 Inhibitors due to hypothetical concern regarding increased severity of vaccine-associated adverse events (Roukens, Visser, & Kroon, 2009).

Vaccines that can be administered at any CD4 cell count.

Inactivated, recombinant, subunit, polysaccharide, and conjugate vaccines and toxoids are safe and can be administered to all HIV-infected patients.

Inactivated Influenza A & B virus infection- Inactivated Influenza: Vaccine schedule and dosing are the same as for the general population	• Indicated for all adolescent and adult PLWH regardless of age or comorbid conditions
Hepatitis A: Vaccine schedule and dosing are the same as for the general population	• Immunize all nonimmune men who have sex with men (MSM) and those with increased risk of acquiring hepatitis A virus or at risk of experiencing severe illness if acutely infected with hepatitis A virus (HAV): chronic hepatitis B virus (HBV) or hepatitis C virus (HCV), injection drug use (IDU), hemophiliacs, and travel to high-risk areas.

TABLE 66-4 Immunizations for HIV-Infected Adults *(Continued)*

Hepatitis B: Vaccination schedule and dosing differ from general population. Engerix-B® 20 mcg/mL or Recombivax HB® 10 mcg/mL at 0, 1, and 6 months (AII), Or Engerix-B® 40 mcg/mL or Recombivax HB® 20 mcg/mL) at 0,1,2 and 6 months **(BI)** or Combined HAV and HBV vaccine (Twinrix®) as a 3-dose series at 0, 1, and 6 months or as a 4-dose series at 0, 7, 21 to 30, and 12 months) (AII) *Alternative Vaccine Dose for Non-Responders:* HBV vaccine IM (Engerix-B® 40 mcg/mL or Recombivax HB® 20 mcg/mL) at 0,1,2 and 6 months **(BI)**,	• Prevaccination screening includes anti-HBs, HBsAg, and anti-HBc • Presence of anti-HBs > 10 international units/mL (IU/mL) indicates immunity. • Vaccinate all patients without immunity to HBV. • Vaccinate patients with isolated anti-HBc (no detected anti-HBs or HBsAg) • Early vaccination is recommended before CD4 count falls below 350 cells/mm³. However, in a patient with low baseline CD4 cell count, vaccination should not be deferred until CD4 reaches > 350 cells/mm³. • Anti-HBs should be obtained 1 month after completion of the vaccine series. • Anti-HBs < 10 IU/mL at 1month is considered a nonresponder. (BIII) • For vaccine nonresponders revaccinate with second vaccine series (BIII) or for patients with low CD4 at time of first series, defer repeating series while awaiting a rise in CD4 count to ≥ 350 cells/mm³. (C-III)
Hemophilus influenzae type B (Hib)	• No longer indicated due to low risk of disease in HIV infected
Human papillomavirus (HPV): Vaccine schedule and dosing are the same as for the general population.	• Cervical and anal intraepithelial neoplasia rates are significantly higher in HIV infected than general population. • HPV vaccine is safe and immunogenic in HIV infected and the potential benefit is high. • Catch-up immunizations are recommended for girls age 13–26 yrs. (do not administer during pregnancy) and for males age 13–26 yrs.
Meningococcal: Vaccine schedule and dosing are the same as for the general population.	• Recommended only if some other risk factor present (e.g., medical, occupational, lifestyle, travel to endemic area).

Streptococcus pneumoniae infection
 	
Vaccination schedule and dosing differ from general population:
 	
No past immunization for *streptococcus pneumonia*:
 	
If CD4 count ≥ 200:
• PCV-13 0.5 mL IM × 1. PPV23 0.5 mL IM or SQ at least 8 weeks after the PCV13 vaccine (AII).
 	
If CD4 count ≤ 200:
• PCV-13 0.5 mL IM × 1. PPV23 can be offered at least 8 weeks after receiving PCV13 (CIII) or can wait until CD4 count increased to ≥ 200 cells/µL (BIII).
 	
For individuals who have previously received PPV23:
• One dose of PCV13 should be given at least 1 year after the last receipt of PPV23. (AII)
	• PLWH have an increased risk of invasive pneumococcal disease compared to age matched controls.
	• Both PCV-13 and PPSV-23 are recommended based on past immunizations for *streptococcus pneumonia* and CD4 counts.
	• Revaccinate with PPV23 if:
	  • Age 19–64 years and ≥ 5 years since the first PPV23 dose
	  • Age ≥ 65 years, and if ≥ 5 years since the previous PPV23 dose

(continues)

TABLE 66-4 Immunizations for HIV-Infected Adults *(Continued)*

Tetanus, diphtheria, and acellular pertussis (Td/Tdap): Vaccine schedule and dosing are the same as for the general population.	• Boost every 10 years

Rating of Recommendations: A = Strong; B = Moderate; C = Optional

Rating of Evidence: I = Data from randomized controlled trials; II = Data from well-designed nonrandomized trials or observational cohort studies with long-term clinical outcomes; III = Expert opinion

Data from Centers for Disease Control and Prevention. (2015a). ACIP vaccine. Retrieved from www.cdc.gov/vaccines/hcp/acip-recs/index.html; Centers for Disease Control and Prevention. (2015e). Vaccines that might be indicated for adults based on medical and other indications. Retrieved from www.cdc.gov/vaccines/schedules/hcp/imz/adult-conditions.html; Panel on Opportunistic Infections in HIV-Infected Adults and Adolescents. (2013). *Guidelines for the prevention and treatment of opportunistic infections in HIV-infected adults and adolescents: Recommendations from the Centers for Disease Control and Prevention, the National Institutes of Health, and the HIV Medicine Association of the Infectious Diseases Society of America* (pp. Q-10, Q-11, U-2, V-1). Retrieved from https://aidsinfo.nih.gov/contentfiles/lvguidelines/Adult_OI.pdf.

    b. The U.S. Preventive Services Task Force (2013) recommends screening all patients ages 15–65 years (Grade A recommendation), with screening of younger adolescents or older adults based upon HIV risk.

2. Consent process for HIV testing: Historically, HIV testing involved separate written informed consent and extensive counseling. This process was found to be a barrier to testing and is no longer recommended (CDC, 2006). Both the CDC (2006) and the USPSTF (2013) recommend opt-out consent: a patient must specifically decline testing. Opt-out testing has been codified in the laws of many states; however, clinicians should refer to specific laws regarding consent requirements in their state of practice. A summary of these laws is available at the Clinicians Consultation Center (see Resources section).

3. Repeat screening: The CDC (2006) recommends repeat screening at least yearly for patients at high risk for HIV infection. The USPSTF (2013) states that there is insufficient evidence to make a recommendation, but it is reasonable to screen high-risk patients more frequently. Patients at high risk include:

    a. People who inject drugs and their sex partners

    b. People who exchange money or drugs for sex

    c. Anyone with an HIV-infected partner

    d. People with more than one sex partner

    e. People who have a sex partner who has multiple partners

4. Specific recommendations for MSM: Due to the high burden of HIV/AIDS in this population, the CDC (2011) recommends screening sexually active MSM every 3–6 months.

5. HIV screening in pregnancy: The CDC (2006) and the USPSTF (2013) have published specific recommendations for HIV screening in pregnancy, which are available online (see Resources).

C. Laboratory tests

1. HIV screening tests: HIV testing technology is divided into "generations," with third- or fourth-generation assays preferred for screening today. Third-generation assays detect HIV IgM antibodies, which appear about 20–23 days after infection. Fourth-generation assays (referred to as "combination," "combo," or "HIV Ab/Ag") differentiate between HIV-1 and HIV-2, as well as detect both HIV IgM antibodies and the HIV p24 antigen, which appears about 14–20 days after infection (Branson et al., 2014). These newer generations of assays are now widely available; however, clinicians may need to verify the generation of assay used at their specific clinical sites.

2. Rapid testing: Rapid testing offers the advantage of a result within 20 minutes or less. As of 2014, there are six rapid HIV antibody tests and one rapid HIV antibody/antigen combination test available in the United States (Branson et al., 2014). A rapid HIV Ab/Ag combination test is preferred, because rapid HIV antibody-only tests rely on second-generation assays that may not detect HIV for weeks to months after infection (Branson et al., 2014).

3. HIV RNA viral load testing: HIV RNA is detectable by current assays approximately 10 days after infection (Branson et al., 2014). Because of the variability of HIV viremia, RNA viral load testing is not approved by the Food and Drug Administration

for diagnosis of HIV. However, viral load testing is appropriate to identify HIV in any patient with recent HIV risk and presentation of signs and symptoms consistent with acute retroviral syndrome. During this phase of infection, when plasma HIV RNA viral loads are reliably high, viral load testing may detect evidence of HIV before antibody or antigen tests become reactive.

D. Linkage to care and partner services

Once diagnosed with HIV, immediate linkage of the patient to medical care is essential. Clinicians should also initiate conversations about partner disclosure as soon as possible. Partners of individuals with new HIV diagnoses are at particular risk for infection, and if not already infected, are prime candidates for HIV prevention services such as preexposure prophylaxis (PrEP) and postexposure prophylaxis (PEP), which are discussed in Chapters 41 and 40, respectively.

Patients may opt for self-disclosure to partners, dual disclosure (patient discloses to partners with a clinician or counselor available in the room to provide support and information), or third-party anonymous notification, in which a trained public health worker notifies partners of exposure and offers testing services without identifying the original patient. Clinicians should contact local public health authorities to check for availability of this service.

III. Database

A. Subjective

1. Medical history
   a. Obtain documentation of positive HIV antibody test. If HIV infection cannot be confirmed, repeat the HIV antibody test.
   b. Acute retroviral syndrome (ARS): review for past symptoms consistent with acute retroviral syndrome, which may help to identify approximate date of HIV infection (USDHHS, PAAGAA, 2015a)
   c. Obtain past CD4 counts (absolute and percentage), CD4 nadir, and HIV-1 viral loads.
   d. AIDS defining illnesses and HIV-related conditions: opportunistic infections (OIs), malignancies, thrush, hairy leukoplakia, herpes simplex (HSV-2), varicella zoster virus (VZV), anemia, thrombocytopenia, anal and cervical cancer.
   e. ART (in previously treated patients)
      i. Prescribed regimens: list all past regimens and antiretroviral (ARV) components of regimens, side effects, and adverse events.
      ii. Document start and stop dates for each regimen or component and changes in HIV viral load.
      iii. Document results of HIV resistance assays: genotype, phenotype, and tropism assays. Obtain past medical records to confirm information.
      iv. Review past adherence issues with ART, untreated depression or other mental illness, low health literacy, inadequate social support, active substance use, homelessness, nondisclosure of HIV status (PAGAA, 2015a).
   f. Other medications and allergies: complete a medication reconciliation of all prescribed and over-the-counter medications and complementary therapies.
   g. Transfusion of blood, platelets, or serum products between 1975 and 1985; artificial insemination from anonymous donor.
   h. Comorbid conditions: risk factors for cardiovascular disease, past history of DM, coronary artery disease, emphysema, renal insufficiency, CKD, chronic HBV or HCV, dyslipidemias, and osteoporosis.
   i. Psychiatric/behavioral: major depression or other depressive disorders, suicidal ideation or past suicide attempts, anxiety and panic disorders, posttraumatic stress disorder.
   j. Sexually transmitted diseases: history of past infections, treatment and treatment outcomes: herpes simplex-2, gonorrhea, chlamydia, chancroid, syphilis, trichomoniasis, HBV, HCV, HPV.
   k. *Mycobacterium tuberculosis* (MTB) and latent *Mycobacterium tuberculosis* infection (LTBI). Results of tuberculin skin tests (TST) or interferon gamma release assay (IGRA). If patient has a history of LTBI record date, treatment, and CXR results.
   l. Immunization status: see Table 66-4.
   m. Women: last menstrual period (LMP), previous abnormal Pap smears, genital condyloma, recurrent vaginal yeast infections, pelvic inflammatory disease (PID), gravid and para status, mammograms, bone mineral density screening.
   n. Men: genital or anal condyloma, abnormal anal Pap smear results and treatment, bone mineral density screening.

o. Foreign travel or residence in areas endemic for specific organisms (e.g., southwestern United States, coccidioidomycosis; Ohio and Indiana, histoplasmosis). Cat ownership and consumption of uncooked beef are risks for toxoplasmosis.

p. Psychiatric: mental health issues or past psychiatric care.

2. Personal and social
   a. Age, gender, gender identity, race, ethnicity.
   b. Sexual activity
      i. Number and gender(s) of partners.
      ii. Sexual practices: anal, penile–vaginal, oral.
      iii. Use of condoms or other barrier methods.
   c. Substance use: alcohol and illicit drug use.
      i. Type and mode of ingestion.
      ii. If injection drug use: injection practices and use of needle exchange programs.
      iii. Identify substance use patterns (e.g., use of drugs or alcohol with sexual activity).
   d. Cigarette smoking:
      i. Age at onset, packs per day, number of pack years.
      ii. If currently smoking, review past attempts to quit smoking and interest in smoking cessation.
   e. Social support, relationships, and housing:
      i. Patient's response to diagnosis
      ii. Disclosure of HIV status to partner(s). Partner's HIV status.
      iii. Homeless or marginally housed and without stable housing.
      iv. Referral to HIV/AIDS service organizations and support groups.
   f. Intimate partner violence (IPV) or sexual assault
   g. Past incarceration

3. Family history
   a. Malignancies, neurologic diseases, osteoporosis, atherosclerotic disease, and history of early coronary heart disease (i.e., MI in first-degree-relative before age 55 in males and before age 65 in females)

4. Review of systems
   a. General: usual body weight, fever or drenching sweats, unintentional weight loss of more than 10%, and persistent fatigue or anorexia.
   b. Dermatologic: persistent skin rashes, recurrent outbreaks of HSV, easy bruising or bleeding, red- to violet-colored papular or macular lesions, pruritic papules.
   c. Lymph nodes: rapid or asymmetrical lymph node swelling or a change in the size of a node or tender lymph nodes.
   d. Ear, nose, and throat: oral lesions or sores, periodontal disease, caries; painful or sensitive teeth.
   e. Eyes: decreased visual acuity or vision loss.
   f. Pulmonary: cough, dyspnea, and hemoptysis.
   g. Cardiac: chest pain, murmurs, palpitations.
   h. Gastrointestinal: diarrhea, nausea, emesis, bloating, rectal pain, rectal lesions or discharge, bright red blood per rectum.
   i. Genitourinary and gynecologic: genital lesions or sores, dysuria, vaginal discharge, pelvic pain, contraception, and use of barrier methods during sexual activity. Men: penile discharge, testicular pain or lumps.
   j. Anorectal: rectal pain or discharge.
   k. Musculoskeletal: weakness, arthralgia, myalgia, and risks for osteoporosis.
   l. Neurologic: persistent or severe headaches, changes in cognition, memory loss, confusion or forgetfulness, seizures, weakness, pain or numbness in hands or feet.
   m. Psychiatric: depression, anxiety, and insomnia.

5. Family history: CVD, diabetes, renal disease, alcoholism, malignancies, substance use, HIV, depression, and emotional or physical abuse.

B. Objective

1. General appearance and body habitus: wasting or unintentional weight loss, obesity, fat redistribution syndromes (dorsocervical fat pad, gynecomastia, or visceral fat accumulation), lipoatrophy (loss of subcutaneous fat in face and extremities), frailty.

2. Height, weight, blood pressure, body mass index, waist circumference, and baseline SpO_2 resting and with exercise.

3. Skin: tinea, onychomycosis, folliculitis, seborrheic dermatitis, bruising or petechiae, herpes, molluscum contagiosum, condyloma, Kaposi sarcoma lesions (purplish macular, papular, or nodular lesions; discrete and well circumscribed; do not blanch with compression)

4. Lymph nodes: completed examination for presence of lymphadenopathy defined as > 1 cm in two or more noncontiguous extrainguinal sites, one of which may be cervical. Assess for asymmetry and consistency of node.

5. Eyes: visual acuity and visual field testing. Examine for lesions on lids or sclera, funduscopic exam for hemorrhage, exudate, or cotton wool spots

6. Oropharynx: ulcerations on tongue or mucous membranes. White coating on tongue or oropharynx (oral candidiasis), fringed lesions on lateral border or dorsum of tongue (hairy leukoplakia), inflammation or receding of gingiva (periodontal disease).

7. Cardiovascular: heart exam, pulses, and presence of lower extremity edema

8. Chest: lung exam

9. Breast: nodules or nipple discharge

10. Abdomen: enlargement of spleen or liver, masses, or tenderness.

11. Gynecologic/genitourinary: external lesions, condyloma, HSV. Speculum exam: Pap smear of cervix. Men: ulcers, condyloma, testicular masses.

12. Anorectal: ulcers, fissures, digital rectal exam, anoscopy, and anal Pap smear.

13. Neurologic: screening exam, including mental status examination. Standard Mini Mental State Examination is not sensitive for detecting HIV-associated neurocognitive disorders. Montreal Cognitive Assessment (MoCA) is recommended for baseline assessments (Chartier et al., 2014).

IV. Assessment

A. Determine the diagnosis

1. HIV antibody testing

2. Plasma HIV RNA (viral load)

B. Staging of disease and HIV drug-resistance testing

1. CD4 lymphocyte count

2. Genotypic resistance assays on all ARV-naïve patients at entry into care, regardless of whether ART will be initiated immediately.

C. Motivation and ability

HIV is associated with significant stigma and disparities in healthcare outcomes. Common barriers to engaging and retaining patients in care include untreated mental illness, active substance use, nondisclosure of HIV status, transportation, childcare issues, homelessness or unstable housing, joblessness, health insurance, food insecurity, and lack of social support. During initial visits allow time to establish a therapeutic relationship, identify the patient's priorities and preferences for care, and address actual and potential barriers to care.

V. Goals of clinical management

A. Treatment Goals (USDHHS, PAAGA, 2015a)

1. Decrease HIV-associated morbidity and mortality

2. Prolong survival and increase duration and quality of life

3. Restore and preserve immunologic function

4. Durably and maximally suppress plasma HIV viral load

5. Prevent transmission of HIV

B. Healthcare maintenance

C. Support adherence to ART and retention in care

D. Prevention of new infections

VI. Plan

A. Initial laboratory and diagnostic tests

1. Order initial laboratory and diagnostic studies (**Table 66-5**).

B. Management

1. Initiate HIV-specific and routine healthcare maintenance for age and gender (Tables 66-3 and 66-4).

2. Initiate ART: Initial recommended regimens for HIV change frequently based on data from clinical trials, cohort studies, and the experience of clinicians and community members actively engaged in HIV patient care. Clinicians should review the most current treatment recommendations (https://aidsinfo.nih.gov/guidelines) and consult with an HIV expert prior to initiating an ART regimen (http://nccc.ucsf.edu).

   Recommended initial regimens are those regimens studied in randomized controlled trials and shown to be optimally effective, tolerable, and easy to use. Additional regimens are listed as "alternative" or "other" based on reduced efficacy, tolerability, and/or limited data supporting use compared to "recommended" regimens. In some cases an alternative or other regimen may be the best regimen for the patient. Current treatment recommendations include guidance on selection of initial ART based on regimen characteristics and specific clinical scenarios (PAGAA, 2015a).

3. Initiate antimicrobial prophylaxis to prevent first episode of HIV-related opportunistic infections indicated (**Table 66-6**).

TABLE 66-5 Initial Laboratory and Diagnostic Studies

Laboratory Test	Frequency and Comments
HIV-1 antibody test	• HIV infection should be confirmed in all patients entering care, either through documentation or laboratory testing (see HIV screening and testing). Repeat an HIV antibody test if HIV diagnosis has not been confirmed.
CD4 T-cell count, absolute and percentage	• At entry into care and every 3–6 months prior to initiation of ART. • Every 3–6 months after initiation of ART or if CD4 cell count < 300 cells/mm^3 • Every 6–12 months after 2 years on ART with consistently suppressed viral load (VL). Some experts recommend annual CD4 cell count if viral load durably suppressed > 2 years. • Routine monitoring of lymphocyte subsets (e.g., CD8) other than CD4 absolute and percentage not recommended.
HIV-1 RNA viral load (VL)	• Most important indicator of initial and sustained response to ART • Viral load suppression is defined as a viral load persistently below the lower limits of detection for the assay used (HIV RNA < 20 to 75 copies/mL). • Measured at entry into care, at initiation of therapy, and on a regular basis thereafter. • Repeating viral load while not on therapy is optional (C-III).
HIV resistance testing	• At entry into care and regardless of decision to initiate ART. • HIV drug resistance has been demonstrated in 6–16% of transmitted HIV-1 infection commonly to nonnucleoside reverse transcriptase inhibitors (NNRTI) and nucleoside reverse transcriptase inhibitors (NRTI). • Genotypic testing is preferred initial resistance assay to guide therapy in antiretroviral-naïve patients.
HLA-B 5701	• At entry into care or prior to starting an ART regimen containing abacavir to reduce risk of hypersensitivity reaction. • An abacavir hypersensitivity reaction (ABC HSR) is a multiorgan clinical syndrome occurring in the first few weeks of abacavir initiation in 5–8% of patients positive for haplotype HLA-B5701. • Re-challenge with abacavir following this clinical syndrome can cause a life-threatening hypersensitivity reaction. • Patients who test HLA-B 5701 positive *should not* be prescribed ABC and their positive HLA-B 5701 results should be recorded as an abacavir allergy in the medical record. (USDHHS,)
Coreceptor tropism assays	• Perform if a CCR5 antagonist is being considered as part of an ART regimen (AI). • Tropism assay screens for HIV resistance to either CCR5 and/or CXCR4 virus. • Requires HIV-1 plasma RNA of > 1,000 copies/mL. • Consult with HIV specialist prior to ordering to determine need for assay and interpretation of results.
HBV serology	• At entry into care and as clinically indicated. • Screen for anti-HBs, anti-HBc, and HBsAg. • If chronically infected with HBV (see Chapter 51 on chronic viral hepatitis), order HBeAg, anti-HBe, and HBV DNA. • If isolated anti-HBc is detected, perform an HBV DNA.
HCV serology	• At entry into care. • Screen for HCV antibody and HCV RNA. • Perform HCV genotype if HCV RNA detected (see Chapter 51 on chronic viral hepatitis).

TABLE 66-5 Initial Laboratory and Diagnostic Studies *(Continued)*

Laboratory Test	Frequency and Comments
Complete blood count with white blood count differential	• At entry into care and every 3–6 months once ART initiated and when clinically indicated. • Anemia of chronic disease, leukopenia, and thrombocytopenia are manifestations of untreated advanced HIV. • Zidovudine (ZVD) causes anemia. Follow up q 2–8 weeks after initiation of ZVD.
Basic chemistry panel	• At entry into care, every 3–6 months prior to initiation of ART, ART initiated, then every 3–6 months or as clinically indicated. • Some experts suggest monitoring the phosphorus levels of patients on tenofovir.
AST, ALT, total bilirubin	• At entry into care, q 6–12 months prior to initiation of ART, and with any ART modification. • Once on ART, every 3–6 months and as clinically indicated.
Fasting plasma glucose (FPG) or hemoglobin A1c	• At entry into care and annually if normal • At time of initiation of ART or modification of ART
Fasting lipid profile	• At entry into care, prior to initiation of ART, and as clinically indicated. • Consider q 4–5 weeks after starting new ART regimen that affects lipids.
Glucose-6-phosphate dehydrogenase (G6PD)	• Screen once at entry to care or before starting oxidant drugs. • G6PD is a genetic variation that predisposes to hemolytic anemia if oxidative drugs are prescribed. • Patients should be tested for G6PD before administration of dapsone or primaquine. An alternative agent should be used in patients found to have G6PD deficiency.
Pregnancy test	• Prior to starting ART
Toxoplasma gondii Toxo IgG	• At entry into care for exposure to *Toxoplasma gondii*. • If seronegative, counsel on prevention of new *Toxoplasma* infections. Avoid eating raw or undercooked meat. If the patient owns a cat that goes outdoors, recommend frequent litter change and thorough handwashing after changing litter box. • Retest for Toxo IgG if CD4 falls to < 100/mm^3 to determine need for primary prophylaxis for toxoplasmosis.
Urinalysis, calculated creatinine clearance (CrCl), and estimated glomerular filtration rate (eGFR)	• At entry into care • Prior to initiating or modifying ART • CrCl of ≥ 70 mL/min required for initiation of drugs containing pharmacokinetic booster cobicistat. • Some ART components require dose reduction in patients with renal insufficiency • Once ART is initiated, monitor CrCl using the Cockcroft-Gault equation and eGFR using the MDRD equation q 6 months and more frequently in patients with additional risks for renal disease.
Pregnancy Test	• Prior to initiation of ART

Data from Aberg, J. A., Gallant, J. E., Ghanem, K. G., Emmanuel, P., Zingman, B. S., & Horberg, M. A. (2014). Primary care guidelines for the management of persons infected with HIV: 2013 update by the HIV Medicine Association of the Infectious Diseases Society of America. *Clinical Infectious Diseases 58*(1): e1–34. doi:10.1093/cid/cit665; Department of Health and Human Services, Panel on Antiretroviral Guidelines for Adults and Adolescents. (2015). *Guidelines for the use of antiretroviral agents in HIV-1-infected adults and adolescents.* Retrieved from http://aidsinfo.nih.gov.

TABLE 66-6 Prophylaxis to Prevent First Episode of Opportunistic Infections in HIV-1–Infected Adults and Adolescents

Pathogen	Indication	Preferred Therapies	Alternative Therapies
Pneumocystis pneumonia (PCP)	CD4 count ≤ 200 cells/mm³ Oropharyngeal candidiasis CD4$^+$ ≤ 14% AIDS-defining illness CD4 > 200 but < 250 cells/mm³ if unable to monitor CD4 q 3 months	Trimethoprim/sulfamethoxazole (TMP-SMX) 1 double strength (DS) PO daily *or* TMP-SMX 1 single strength (SS) daily	TMP-SMX 1 DS three times weekly *or* Dapsone, 100 mg PO daily *or* Dapsone 50 mg PO BID *or* Atovaquone 1,500 mg PO daily
Toxoplasma gondii encephalitis	*Toxoplasma* IgG positive with CD4 ≤ 100/mm³ Regimens effective against toxoplasmosis also effective for PCP	TMP-SMX 1 DS PO daily	TMP-SMX three times weekly *or* TMP-SMX 1 SS daily *or* Dapsone 50 mg daily plus pyrimethamine 50 mg plus leucovorin 25 mg weekly
Disseminated *Mycobacterium avium* (MAC)	CD4 ≤ 50 cells/mm³ No evidence of active disseminated MAC disease based on clinical assessment and blood culture	Azithromycin 1,200 mg once weekly *or* Clarithromycin 500 mg BID *or* Azithromycin 600 mg PO twice weekly	Rifabutin 300 mg daily Rule out active TB before starting rifabutin
Latent *Mycobacterium tuberculosis* infection (LTBI)	Positive screening test No evidence of active TB infection No prior history of treatment for active or latent TB Close contact with person with infectious TB, regardless of screening test result for LTBI	Isoniazid (INH) 300 mg PO daily for plus pyridoxine 25 mg daily for 9 months	Rifabutin (dose adjusted based on concomitant ART) × 4 months *Dose adjustment required for ART drug interactions for some MTB regimens*
Coccidioidomycosis	A new positive IgM or IgG serologic test in patients who live in a disease-endemic area and with CD4 count < 250 cells/mm³	Fluconazole 400 mg PO daily	
Histoplasmosis capsulatum infection	CD4 count ≤ 150 cells/μL and at high risk because of occupational exposure or live in a community with a hyperendemic rate of histoplasmosis (> 10 cases/100 patient-years)	Itraconazole 200 mg PO daily	

- As of June 2015, pyrimethamine is no longer available in retail pharmacies in the United States. If there is a delay in obtaining pyrimethamine for a patient who needs this drug, refer to the specific pathogen section in the opportunistic infections guidelines for alternative drug regimens.
- TMP-SMX DS once daily also confers protection against toxoplasmosis and many respiratory bacterial infections; lower dose also likely confers protection.
- Patients should be tested for glucose-6-phosphate dehydrogenase (G6PD) before administration of dapsone or primaquine. Alternative agents should be used in patients found to have G6PD deficiency.

Modified from Panel on Opportunistic Infections in HIV-Infected Adults and Adolescents. (2013). *Guidelines for the prevention and treatment of opportunistic infections in HIV-infected adults and adolescents: recommendations from the Centers for Disease Control and Prevention, the National Institutes of Health, and the HIV Medicine Association of the Infectious Diseases Society of America.* Retrieved from http://aidsinfo.nih.gov.

4. Provide screening and counseling for prevention of HIV transmission.

5. Identify and manage chronic comorbid conditions.

6. Refer patients with illnesses of unclear etiology or evidence of HIV drug resistance to HIV specialist.

7. Refer to social worker or AIDS service organization (ASO) for case management services: housing, mental health and substance abuse treatment, health insurance, eligibility for federally funded AIDS programs, transportation to clinic appointments, childcare, and parenting needs.

C. Management issues specific to HIV-infected women

1. Reproductive counseling and contraception: Preconception counseling and referral to an HIV specialist should be provided for all women of childbearing age and their partners who desire pregnancy. The landmark AIDS Clinical Trials Group (ACTG 076) study demonstrated the safety and efficacy of ART in pregnant women for prevention of mother-to-child transmission of HIV (Connor et al., 1994). Pregnant women with HIV should be treated with ART regardless of stage of disease or CD4 cell count. Avoidance of breastfeeding in addition to the use of ART has virtually eliminated perinatal transmission of HIV in countries where access to HIV care is available. If a woman does not desire to become pregnant, provide preconception counseling and initiate discussions regarding contraception. Several protease inhibitors (PI) and nonnucleoside reverse transcriptase inhibitors (NNRTI) have drug interactions with oral contraceptives, causing changes in blood levels of ethinyl estradiol or norethindrone. Women on combined oral contraceptives (COC) and ART should use an alternative method of contraception. Progestin-only contraceptive methods seem to be effective and have no drug–drug interactions when used with currently approved ART regimens (Panel on Treatment of HIV-Infected Pregnant Women and Prevention of Perinatal Transmission, 2014). Intrauterine devices are safe to use in women with HIV and provide a reliable long-term method of contraception (World Health Organization, 2009).

2. ART regimen considerations in women: The goals of treatment for women are the same as for adults and adolescents. When constructing ART regimens for pregnant women, current recommended regimens are appropriate with some exceptions. Efavirenz should be avoided in women who are planning to become pregnant or are sexually active and not using an effective form of contraception (PAGAA, 2015a). If a woman becomes pregnant on efavirenz and has passed the first 5–6 weeks of the pregnancy, some experts recommend continuing an efavirenz-based regimen if the regimen is effective and well tolerated. Nevirapine is not recommended in treatment-naïve women with CD4 $\geq$ 250 cells/mm^3 unless risk outweighs benefits. Severe lactic acidosis is seen more commonly in women on ART and risks for lactic acidosis includes female gender, obesity, and pregnancy. Postmenopausal HIV-infected women have an increased risk of osteopenia and osteoporosis at an earlier age and an increased risk of fragility fractures. Clinicians may want to consider avoiding ART regimens that are associated with greater decrease in bone mineral density in postmenopausal women at increased risk of osteoporosis and fracture (PAGAA, 2015a).

D. Management issues specific to transgender PLWH

1. Transgender refers to individuals whose gender identity (basic sense of self as man, woman, both, or neither) or presentation is not congruent with the person's biological sex assigned at birth. Some transgender individuals may pursue surgery or use hormones to enhance feminine or masculine physical characteristics—though some may not.

2. Stigma and discrimination toward transgender individuals increases the likelihood of depression, suicide, intimate partner violence, substance use, and sexually transmitted infections other than HIV. To combat stigma, healthcare settings should affirm transgender patients through appropriate staff training, gender-inclusive registration materials and restroom facilities, and use of the patient's preferred gender when addressing or referring to the patient. Clinicians caring for transgender PLWH should make use of community agencies providing support services for transgender individuals, and refer patients to those agencies. Clinicians without experience providing hormone therapy to transgender individuals should consult with providers who have clinical expertise in this area (see Resources).

3. Healthcare maintenance for transgender PLWH is based on health risks and birth sex. In transgender women, digital rectal examinations and prostate cancer screening may be indicated based on age, other risk factors, and shared decision making by the provider and patient. In transgender men, pelvic examination, Pap smear, and mammography based on recommended guidelines should be provided.

E. Prevention of new infections

PLWH have a central role in the prevention of HIV transmission at the individual and population levels. Recognizing this role, a consortium of U.S. governmental and nonprofit HIV/AIDS service organizations has produced recommendations for HIV prevention in clinical care settings with PLWH (CDC et al., 2014). These recommendations encourage providers to consider contextual issues—individual, structural, social, ethical, and legal—when working with PLWH. In conversations with patients about HIV prevention, providers should be sensitive, respectful, culturally appropriate, and empower patients to engage in HIV prevention without blaming or shaming. Providers must acknowledge that patients have the right and responsibility to make HIV-prevention decisions for themselves.

Above all, providers must support patients in treatment adherence and engagement in care in order to achieve viral suppression, reducing infectiousness. Support includes linking patients to care; providing referrals for services such as food assistance, housing, transportation to medical visits, and medication adherence counseling; and development of healthcare systems such as the medical home model that provide patients with wraparound care.

Providers should discuss HIV risk behaviors with patients at every visit. Through education, counseling, and shared decision making, providers can support PLWH in setting realistic goals for HIV prevention using evidence-based risk reduction strategies. Providers should offer specific healthcare services that reduce the risk of HIV transmission such as condom distribution, referrals to syringe exchanges, screening for sexually transmitted infections, family planning care, and referral to treatment for substance use or psychiatric illness.

Patients often have questions and fears regarding the legal ramifications of their HIV serostatus. Laws regarding HIV serostatus disclosure vary by state. Clinicians can become familiar with these laws at the website of the Center for HIV Law and Policy (see Resources).

F. Patient education

HIV education should be conducted over several visits to provide basic information on HIV treatment, prevention of secondary transmission, and indications for ART. It is important to emphasize that HIV is a chronic manageable disease and that improved quality of life can be expected if individuals are engaged in care and motivated to take ART. There are several excellent websites that can provide resources and guidance in HIV/AIDS patient and provider education (see Resources).

VII. Resources

A. General information

1. AIDS.gov: Gateway for HIV/AIDS information and resources from the U.S. Federal government, aimed at both clinicians and patients. www.aids.gov

2. Centers for Disease Control and Prevention's HIV/AIDS Website: Basic information, statistical data, prevention tools, and clinician resources. www.cdc.gov/hiv/

3. Henry J. Kaiser Family Foundation's HIV/AIDS Website: Policy analysis, global and national HIV/AIDS data, and links to patient resources, including Spanish-language patient information. http://kff.org/hivaids/

B. Clinical management

1. AIDS*info*: Portal for HIV/AIDS clinical guidelines, education materials, and research information from the DHHS. http://aidsinfo.nih.gov/

2. AIDS Education and Training Centers (AETC): National network of HIV experts that provide guidelines, training materials, webinars, clinical consultation, and technical assistance for healthcare providers caring for PLWH. Administered by the Ryan White HIV/AIDS Program of the Human Resources and Services Administration. http://aidsetc.org/

3. U.S. Department of Health and Human Services. (2014). *HIV/AIDS Bureau Guide for HIV/AIDS Clinical Care.* http://hab.hrsa.gov/deliverhivaidscare/2014guide.pdf

4. Clinician Consultation Center (CCC): Rapid phone and online consultation on HIV/AIDS management, PEP, PrEP, perinatal HIV/AIDS, and HIV testing from HIV-expert clinicians at the University of California, San Francisco. Consultation services available nationwide. http://nccc.ucsf.edu/

5. HIV InSite: Information on HIV biology, clinical management, policy, and research, developed by the Center for HIV Information at the University of California, San Francisco. Includes *HIV InSite Knowledge Base,* a complete online textbook. http://hivinsite.ucsf.edu

6. Center of Excellence for Transgender Health: Resources and guidelines for transgender patient care from the University of California, San Francisco. http://transhealth.ucsf.edu/

7. HIVE (formerly the Bay Area Perinatal AIDS Center): Preconception and perinatal HIV/AIDS resources for patients, their partners, and healthcare providers. www.hiveonline.org/services/

8. HIV Web Study: Case-based study modules on prevention and management from the University of Washington. http://depts.washington.edu/hivaids

C. HIV medications

1. HIV InSite Database of Antiretroviral Drug Interactions: Searchable database of HIV drug interactions, provided by the University of California, San Francisco. http://arv.ucsf.edu/

2. University of Liverpool HIV Drug Interactions Portal: Searchable database of HIV drug interactions, as well as a link to a hepatitis C drug interactions database. www.hiv-druginteractions.org/

3. Stanford University HIV Drug Resistance Database: Resource for analyzing HIV drug resistance. http://hivdb.stanford.edu/

D. Patient education and advocacy

1. Project Inform: Education resources and advocacy for people living with HIV and hepatitis C. www.projectinform.org/

2. AVERT.org: Large online compendium of HIV/AIDS education materials, produced by AVERT, an international HIV/AIDS charity based in the United Kingdom. www.avert.org/

3. HIV Health Reform Website: Patient and clinician education on the Affordable Care Act and HIV/AIDS care, produced by the AIDS Foundation of Chicago and Project Inform. www.hivhealthreform.org/

4. HIV Nightline: Free, confidential emotional support and information on HIV/AIDS. Open nightly from 5 P.M. to 5 A.M. Pacific Standard Time. Nationwide toll free: 1-800-628-9240.

5. Center for HIV Law and Policy: Comprehensive resource for legal and policy issues related to HIV. www.hivlawandpolicy.org/

E. Professional organizations

1. Association of Nurses in AIDS Care (ANAC): National organization of nurses, including advanced practice nurses, dedicated to HIV/AIDS advocacy and patient care. Offers HIV specialty credentialing, presents an annual national conference, and publishes the journal *JANAC*. www.nursesinaidscare.org/

2. American Academy of HIV Medicine (AAHIVM): National organization for HIV care providers, offering membership and HIV specialty credentialing to advanced practice nurses. www.aahivm.org/

REFERENCES

Aberg, J. A., Gallant, J. E., Ghanem, K. G., Emmanuel, P., Zingman, B. S., Horberg, M. A., & Infectious Diseases Society of America. (2013). Primary care guidelines for the management of persons infected with human immunodeficiency virus: 2013 update by the HIV Medicine Association of the Infectious Diseases Society of America. *Clinical Infectious Diseases, 58*(1), e1–e34. doi: 10.1093/cid/cit665

Antiretroviral Therapy Cohort Collaborative. (2008). Life expectancy of individuals on combination antiretroviral therapy in high-income countries: A collaborative analysis of 14 cohort studies. *Lancet, 372*(9635), 293–299.

Branson, B. M., Owen, S. M., Wesolowski, L. G., Bennett, B., Werner, B. G., Wroblewski, K. E., et al. (2014). *Laboratory testing for the diagnosis of HIV infection: Updated recommendations.* Atlanta, GA: Centers for Disease Control and Prevention and Silver Spring, MD: Association of Public Health Laboratories. Retrieved from www.cdc.gov/hiv/pdf/HIV testingAlgorithmRecommendation-Final.pdf.

Brown, T. T., Cole, S. R., Kingsley, L. A., Palella, F. J., Visscher, B. R., Margolick, J. B., et al. (2005). Antiretroviral therapy and the prevalence and incidence of diabetes mellitus in the multicenter AIDS cohort study. *Archives of Internal Medicine, 165*(10), 1179–1184.

Centers for Disease Control and Prevention. (2006). Revised recommendations for HIV testing of adults, adolescents, and pregnant women in health-care settings. *MMWR, 55*(R14), 1–17. Retrieved from www.cdc.gov/mmwr/preview/mmwrhtml/rr5514a1.htm.

Centers for Disease Control and Prevention. (2010, June 25). Updated guidelines for using interferon gamma release assays to detect *Mycobacterium tuberculosis* infection in the United States, 2010. *MMWR Recommendations and Reports, 59*(RR05), 1–25. Retrieved from www.cdc.gov/mmwr/preview/mmwrhtml/rr5905a1.htm?s_cid =rr5905a1_e.

Centers for Disease Control and Prevention. (2011). HIV testing among men who have sex with men—21 cities, United States, 2008. *MMWR, 60*(21), 694–699. Retrieved from www.cdc.gov/mmwr/preview/mmwrhtml/mm6021a3.htm.

Centers for Disease Control and Prevention. (2013a). *HIV among older Americans* [Fact sheet]. Retrieved from www.cdc.gov/hiv/pdf/library_factsheet_HIV_%20AmongOlderAmericans.pdf.

Centers for Disease Control and Prevention. (2013b). *HIV among transgender people in the United States* [Fact sheet]. Retrieved from www.cdc.gov/hiv/pdf/risk_transgender.pdf.

Centers for Disease Control and Prevention. (2014a). Diagnoses of HIV infection in the United States and dependent areas, 2012. *HIV Surveillance Report, 2012, 24.* Retrieved from www.cdc.gov/hiv/pdf/statistics_2012_HIV_Surveillance_Report_vol_24.pdf.www.cdc.gov/hiv/pdf/HIV-Black-MSM-english-508.pdf.

Centers for Disease Control and Prevention. (2014b). *HIV transmission risk* [Fact sheet]. Retrieved from www.cdc.gov/hiv/pdf/policies_transmission_risk_factsheet.pdf.

Centers for Disease Control and Prevention. (2014c). Monitoring selected national HIV prevention and care objectives by using HIV surveillance data—United States and 6 dependent areas—2012. *HIV Surveillance Supplemental Report, 19*(3). Retrieved from www.cdc.gov/hiv/pdf /surveillance_report_vol_19_no_3.pdf.

Centers for Disease Control and Prevention. (2014 d). Revised surveillance case definition for HIV infection—United States, 2014. *MMWR, 63*(3), 1–10. Retrieved from www.cdc.gov/mmwr/pdf/rr/rr6303.pdf.

Centers for Disease Control and Prevention. (2014e). Vital signs: HIV diagnosis, care, and treatment among persons living with HIV—United States, 2011. *MMWR, 63*(47), 1113–1117. Retrieved from www.cdc .gov/mmwr/pdf/wk/mm6347.pdf.

Centers for Disease Control and Prevention. (2015a). ACIP vaccine. Retrieved from www.cdc.gov/vaccines/hcp/acip-recs/index.html.

Centers for Disease Control and Prevention. (2015b). *HIV among African Americans* [Fact sheet]. Retrieved from http://www.cdc.gov/hiv/pdf /HIV-AA-english-508.pdf

Centers for Disease Control and Prevention. (2015c). *HIV among gay and bisexual men* [Fact sheet]. http://www.cdc.gov/hiv/pdf/group/msm /cdc-hiv-msm.pdf.

Centers for Disease Control and Prevention. (2015d). Sexually transmitted disease treatment guidelines, 2015. *MMWR Recommendations and Reports, 64*(RR3), 1–137. Retrieved from www.cdc.gov/mmwr/preview /mmwrhtml/rr6403a1.htm.

Centers for Disease Control and Prevention. (2015e). Vaccines that might be indicated for adults based on medical and other indications. Retrieved from www.cdc.gov/vaccines/schedules/hcp/imz/adult -conditions.html.

Centers for Disease Control and Prevention, Health Resources and Services Administration, National Institutes of Health, American Academy of HIV Medicine, Association of Nurses in AIDS Care, International Association of Providers of AIDS Care, the National Minority AIDS Council, & Urban Coalition for HIV/AIDS Prevention Services. (2014). *Recommendations for HIV prevention with adults and adolescents with HIV in the United States, 2014.* Retrieved from http://stacks.cdc .gov/view/cdc/26062.

Chartier, M., Crouch, P. C., Tullis, V., Catella, S., Frawley, E., & Wong, J. K. (2014). The Montreal cognitive assessment: A pilot study of a brief screening tool for mild and moderate cognitive impairment in HIV-positive veterans. *Journal of the International Association Providers in AIDS Care.* doi: 10.1177/2325957414557270. Retrieved from http://jia .sagepub.com/content/early/2014/12/08/2325957414557270.long.

Connor, E. M., Sperling, R. S., Gelber, R. M. J., VanDyke, R., Bey, M., Shearer, W., et al. (1994). Reduction of maternal-infant transmission of human immunodeficiency virus type 1 with zidovudine treatment. *New England Journal of Medicine, 331*(18), 1173–1180.

Douek, D., Picker, L. J., & Koup, R. A. (2003). T cell dynamics in HIV-1 infection. *Annual Review of Immunology, 21,* 265–304.

Friis-Møller, N., Weber, R., Reiss, P., Thiébaut, R., Kirk, O., d'Arminio Monforte, A., et al. (2003). Cardiovascular disease risk factors in HIV patients—association with antiretroviral therapy. Results from the DAD study. *AIDS, 17*(8), 1179–1193.

Hare, C. B. (2009). Clinical overview of HIV disease. *HIV InSite Knowledge Base.* Retrieved from http://hivinsite.ucsf.edu/InSite? page=kb-00&doc=kb-03-01-01.

Henry J. Kaiser Family Foundation. (2009). *Views and experiences with HIV testing in the U.S.* [Survey brief]. Retrieved from http:// kaiserfamilyfoundation.files.wordpress.com/2013/01/7926.pdf.

Lucas, G. M., Ross, M. J., Stock, P. G., Shilipak, M. G., Wyatt, C. M., Gupta, S. K., et al. (2014). Clinical practice guideline for the management of chronic kidney disease in patients infected with HIV: 2014 update by the HIV Medicine Association of the Infectious Disease Society of America. *Clinical Infectious Diseases, 59*(9), e96–e138.

Maartens, G., Celum, C., & Lewin, S. R. (2014). HIV infection: Epidemiology, pathogenesis, treatment, and prevention. *Lancet, 384*(9939), 258–271.

Marks, G., Crepaz, N., & Janssen, R. S. (2006). Estimating sexual transmission of HIV from persons aware and unaware that they are infected with the virus in the USA. *AIDS, 20*(10), 1447–1450.

McComsey, G. A., Tebas, P., Shane, E., Yin, M. T., Huang, J. S., Aldrovandi, G. M., et al. (2010). Bone disease in HIV infection: A practical review and recommendations for HIV care providers. *Clinical Infectious Diseases, 51*(8), 937–946.

Mdodo, R., Frazier, E., Dube, S., Mattson, C., Sutton, M., Brooks, J., et al. (2015). Cigarette smoking prevalence among adults with HIV compared with the general adult population in the United States. *Annals of Internal Medicine, 162*(5), 335–343.

Monroe, A. K., Glesby, M. J., & Brown, T. (2015). Diagnosing and managing diabetes in HIV-infected patients: current concepts. *Clinical Infectious Diseases, 60*(3), 453–462.

Panel on Antiretroviral Guidelines for Adults and Adolescents. (2014, May 1). Initiating antiretroviral therapy in treatment-naïve patients. In *Guidelines for the use of antiretroviral agents in HIV-1-infected adults and adolescents* (p. E-1). U.S. Department of Health and Human Services. Retrieved from https://aidsinfo.nih.gov/contentfiles/lvguidelines /adultandadolescentgl.pdf.

Panel on Antiretroviral Guidelines for Adults and Adolescents. (2015a). *Guidelines for the use of antiretroviral agents in HIV-1-infected adults and adolescents.* U.S. Department of Health and Human Services. Retrieved from http://aidsinfo.nih.gov/contentfiles/lvguidelines /adultandadolescentgl.pdf.

Panel on Antiretroviral Guidelines for Adults and Adolescents. (2015b). *Guidelines for the use of antiretroviral agents in HIV-1-infected adults and adolescents. Considerations for antiretroviral use in patients with coinfections: hepatitis C (HCV) HIV infection.* U.S. Department of Health and Human Services. Retrieved from http://aidsinfo.nih.gov/guidelines /html/1/adult-and-adolescent-arv-guidelines/26/hiv-hcv.

Panel on Opportunistic Infections in HIV-Infected Adults and Adolescents. (2013). *Guidelines for prevention and treatment of opportunistic infections in HIV-infected adults and adolescents: Recommendations from the Centers for Disease Control and Prevention, the National Institutes of Health, and the HIV Medicine Association of the Infectious Diseases Society of America.* Retrieved from http://aidsinfo.nih.gov/contentfiles/lvguidelines/adult_oi.pdf.

Panel on Treatment of HIV-Infected Pregnant Women and Prevention of Perinatal Transmission. (2014). *Recommendations for use of antiretroviral drugs in pregnant HIV-1-infected women for maternal health and interventions to reduce perinatal HIV transmission in the United States.* Retrieved from http://aidsinfo.nih.gov/contentfiles/lvguidelines/PerinatalGL. pdf. Accessed December 23, 2015

Pretty, I. A., Anderson, G. S., & Sweet, D. J. (1999). Human bites and the risk of human immunodeficiency virus transmission. *American Journal of Forensic Medical Pathology, 20*(3), 232–239.

Purcell, D. W., Johnson, C. H., Lansky, A., Prejean, J., Stein, R., Denning, P., et al. (2012). Estimating the population size of men who have sex with men in the United States to obtain HIV and syphilis rates. *Open AIDS Journal, 6*(Suppl. 1, M6), 98–107.

Rothman, M. S., & Bessesen, M. T. (2012). HIV infection and osteoporosis: Pathophysiology, diagnosis, and treatment options. *Current Osteoporosis Report, 10*(4) 270–277.

Roukens, A. H., Visser, L. G., Leo, G., & Frank, P. (2009). A note of caution on yellow fever vaccination during maraviroc treatment: A hypothesis on a potential dangerous interaction. *AIDS, 23*(4), 542–543.

Strategies for Management of Antiretroviral Therapy (SMART) Study Group. (2006). CD4+ count-guided interruption of antiretroviral treatment. *New England Journal of Medicine, 355*(22), 2283–2296.

Tseng, A. H., Secemsky, E. A., Dowdy, D., Vittinghoff, E., Moyers, B., Wong, J. K., et al. (2012). Sudden cardiac death in patients with human immunodeficiency virus infection. *Journal of the American College of Cardiology, 59*(21), 1891–1896.

United Nations Joint Programme on HIV/AIDS. (2014). *The gap report.* Retrieved from www.unaids.org/sites/default/files/media_asset /UNAIDS_Gap_report_en.pdf.

U.S. Department of Health and Human Services. (2013). *HIV/AIDS care continuum.* Retrieved from https://www.aids.gov/federal-resources /policies/care-continuum/.

U.S. Department of Health and Human Services. (2014). *Healthy People 2020: HIV.* Retrieved from https://www.healthypeople.gov/2020 /topics-objectives/topic/hiv/.

U.S. National Institutes of Health, National Cancer Institute. (n.d.). *HIV/AIDS cancer match study.* Retrieved from www.hivmatch.cancer.gov/index.html.

U.S. Preventive Services Task Force. (2013). *Final recommendation statement: Human immunodeficiency virus (HIV) infection: Screening.* Retrieved from www .uspreventiveservicestaskforce.org/Page/Document/Recommendation StatementFinal/human-immunodeficiency-virus-hiv-infection-screening.

Young, B., Dao, C., Buchacz, K., Baker, R., Brooks, J. T., & HIV Outpatient Study (HOPS) Investigators. (2011). Increased rates of bone fracture among HIV-infected persons in the HIV Outpatient Study (HOPS) compared with the US general population, 2000–2006. *Clinical Infectious Diseases, 52*(8), 1061–1068.

Zanni, M. V., Fitch, K. V., Feldpausch, M., Han, A., Lee, H., Lu, M. T., et al. (2014). 2013 American College of Cardiology/American Heart Association and 2004 Adult Treatment Panel III cholesterol guidelines applied to HIV-infected patients with/without subclinical high-risk coronary plaque. *AIDS, 10*(28), 2061–2070.

SMOKING CESSATION

67

Kellie McNerney and Lewis Fannon

I. Introduction and background

A. The problem

Smoking is the most popular form of tobacco use worldwide. Tobacco smoking is a global epidemic responsible for 5 million preventable deaths a year (World Health Organization, 2008). Smoking "remains the leading preventable cause of premature disease and death in the United States" (U.S. Department of Health and Human Services [USDHHS], 2014, p. iii). According to the World Health Organization's 2008 MPOWER report, an anticipated 1 billion deaths will occur in this century secondary to tobacco-related illnesses. As the *Oxford Medical Companion* notes, "Tobacco is the only legally available consumer product which kills people when it is used as intended" (Walton, Barondess, & Lock, 1994, p. 908).

B. Health effects of smoking

In the United States, smoking has caused 20 million deaths over the last 50 years. Cigarette smoking kills 480,000 people each year and there are currently 16 million Americans suffering from smoking-related chronic disease conditions (USDHHS, 2014). Smoking-related deaths result from three main diseases: lung cancer, cardiovascular disease (CVD), and chronic obstructive pulmonary disease (COPD). Cigarette smoking causes 87% of lung cancer but is also responsible for 30% of all cancers, including cancer of the bladder, kidney, mouth, oral pharynx, esophagus, stomach, uterus, cervix, and pancreas as well as acute myeloid leukemia (American Cancer Society [ACS], 2014a). The direct healthcare costs of these chronic disease conditions are estimated at $132.5–175.9 billion per year (USDHHS, 2014).

C. Incidence prevalence

An estimated 40 million Americans currently smoke cigarettes (Centers for Disease Control and Prevention [CDC], 2015). The year 2014 marked the 50th anniversary of the 1964 Surgeon General Report on the harmful effects of smoking (USDHHS, 2014). Over the last 50 years, there has been a decline in the rate and incidence of smoking in the general population. There are more than 50 million former smokers—a greater number of former smokers now than actual smokers (Sanford & Goebel, 2014). The prevalence of smoking among adults has decreased from 42% in 1965 to 18% in 2012 (USDHHS, 2014). For men during this same period, the prevalence has decreased from 51.9% to around 21% (CDC, 2015; Giovino, 2002). More recently, the overall rate of smoking in the United States has declined from almost 21% of adults in 2005 to around 18% of adults in 2013 (CDC, 2015). This downward trend corresponds to the implementation of the 2009 Tobacco Control Act, which increased federal taxes on cigarettes and used that money to fund prevention and cessation policy and programs. Although rates have gone down considerably, it is important to recognize that there is variability in demographics and regions across the country. For example, smoking rates are 20.5% in the Midwest and 13.6 % in the West, are highest in West Virginia at 27.3%, and lowest in Utah at 10.3%. Smoking prevalence is higher in men than women, highest among non-Hispanic multiple race individuals and American Indians/Alaska Natives, and lowest in the Asian population (CDC, 2015). The highest rates of smoking (29.2%) are found in those living below the poverty level (CDC, 2015). To achieve the Healthy People 2020 goal of less than or equal to 12%, more needs to be done to target these groups with the highest prevalence of smoking.

D. History of tobacco, smoking, and health policy

Smoking has a long history in the United States; the earliest settlers adopted smoking from Native Americans who smoked tobacco in ritual traditions. A cigarette rolling machine invented in the late 1800s allowed the mass production of cigarettes. During World War I and World War II, tobacco was considered as indispensable as food and included in ration packets to soldiers in the field. The *Journal of the American Medical Association* (*JAMA*) and the popular media marketed cigarettes for their taste and impact on relaxation and even audaciously suggested "improved health" (Houston, 1992; Sheehan, 2004). In 1950, two British surgeons published a well-designed study linking cigarette smoking with bronchogenic carcinoma (Wynder & Graham, 1950). Despite more than 60,000 documents proving the relationship between smoking and lung cancer, the tobacco industry continued to deny and question the evidence. The tobacco industry remains a powerful lobby that prevented the Food and Drug Administration (FDA) from regulating tobacco and the sale of cigarettes. It took major litigation, congressional hearings, and 45 years before the FDA was granted the power to regulate tobacco products when President Obama signed HR 1256, Family Smoking Prevention and Tobacco Control Act in 2009 (Food and Drug Administration, 2012).

Now electronic cigarettes (e-cigarettes) are exploding on the market; e-cigarettes are being used by 6 million Americans, producing $6 billion in sales (Sanford & Goebel, 2014). First created and sold in China in 2004, they became available in the United States in 2007. E-cigarettes are not yet regulated by the FDA. Two years after becoming available in the United States, the FDA tried to ban them as unapproved drug device combination devices. Electronic cigarette manufacturers filed a lawsuit, and the court overturned the ban. In April 2014, the FDA proposed "deeming" authority, which means it has taken steps to regulate e-cigarettes and additional tobacco products such as cigars, water pipes, and gel tobacco. This would then allow them to restrict the sale to minors and put health warnings on them. As yet e-cigarettes are still not regulated (FDA, 2015; Palazzolo, 2013). E-cigarettes are small, cylindrical, battery-operated devices, colorfully marketed, often with flavor additives, that are "smoked," mimicking a cigarette. The battery heats up liquid that contains nicotine and vaporizes it so the vapor is inhaled (vaped) and not smoked. E-cigarettes are promoted as less dangerous than smoking because they are smokeless. Cigarette smoke contains 7,000 chemicals, 69 of which are known carcinogens such as benzene, arsenic and vinyl chloride to name a few. Though fewer chemicals are present in e-cigarettes than in tobacco cigarette smoke, it is not clear that they are safe just because they are smokeless (Meo & Al Asiri, 2014; Walton et al., 2015). In one brand of e-cigarettes, the liquid to vaporize nicotine was found to have diethylene glycol, an ingredient in antifreeze ("The Battle over E-Cigarettes," 2014).

It remains controversial whether e-cigarettes help people quit smoking. Current National Institutes of Health guidelines recommend further study regarding the issue (Walton et al., 2015). From a traditional harm reduction point of view, a healthcare provider may choose to work with a client using e-cigarettes to help them quit smoking. Preferably education regarding what we know and do not know about e-cigarettes is recommended along with traditional nicotine replacement products, not e-cigarettes. The perceived safety of e-cigarettes may be the most dangerous aspect of e-cigarettes and the problem in getting people not to start as well as to quit. Unfortunately, the perceived safety and the direct targeting of adolescents by the e-cigarette industry may encourage young people to start (Dutra & Glantz, 2014; McCarthy, 2014). The National Youth Tobacco Survey (NYTS) showed that e-cigarette use in junior high and high school age groups doubled from 2011 to 2012 (Dutra & Glantz, 2014). A recent *JAMA Pediatrics* article reported young people who tried e-cigarettes were six times more likely to take up smoking than those who did not try e-cigarettes (Dutra & Glantz, 2014).

E. Special populations

Those living below the poverty level, those with mental health disorders, those with other alcohol and drug use disorders, and adolescents deserve special attention as these groups remain most at risk compared to the general adult population. More research is needed to determine and overcome the barriers to effective cessation and prevention strategies in these high-use populations (Christiansen, Reeder, Hill, Baker, & Fiore, 2012).

Nicotine dependence is the most common substance use disorder among people with mental illness. Rates of smoking among people with mental health disorders are at least twice as high as in the general population and among the seriously mentally ill even higher. Cigarette use in those with schizophrenia, bipolar disorder, alcohol, and illicit drug substance use disorders are among the highest and likely account for almost half of the U.S. cigarette market. Studies of adolescents and young adults with substance use disorders find that more than 80% report current smoking behavior and daily smoking and many go on to become highly addicted long-term smokers (Hall & Prochaska, 2009).

Nicotine is the ingredient that keeps people smoking despite their desire to quit and the obvious safety hazards and known health risks of smoking. There are many reasons for the high rates of smoking co-occurring with mental health disorders, many are related to the neurobiological effects of nicotine and some are related to psychosocial factors. The reasons are multifactorial: the prioritization of mental health treatment, an individual health provider's belief that people with mental illness will not be able or willing to quit smoking, the reduced ability of the person with mental illness to cope with smoking cessation, or the lack of understanding of the health effects of smoking among mentally ill people All are cited as reasons that the mental health population has higher rates of smoking (Hall & Prochaska, 2009). Death rate among smokers over a 24-year study of long-term drug users was twice as high as that of the long-term drug users who did not smoke (Moss et al., 2010).

There is an historical connection to smoking and people with mental illness; as late as 2006, 59% of state psychiatric hospitals in the United States allowed patients to smoke. The tobacco industry even provided tax-free cigarettes to psychiatric facilities, homeless shelters, and drug treatment programs (Hall & Prochaska, 2009). Smoking in alcohol and drug treatment programs has a long intertwined history that normalized smoking behavior as a safer alternative and thus was not addressed in treatment centers despite the fact that the leading cause of substance-related death among alcohol- and drug-dependent persons is tobacco-related illnesses. Freud and both of the cofounders of Alcoholics Anonymous, Bill Wilson and Dr. Bob Smith, smoked heavily and died of tobacco-related causes. The harm reduction model was used as an explanation to allow smoking while people were quitting other drugs. Because smoking has few immediate symptoms when quitting, compared to alcohol or illicit substances, many treatment programs delayed smoking cessation or made it a low priority. The American Psychiatric Association (APA) first recommended the treatment of nicotine dependence in patients with mental health disorders and/or substance abuse in 1996, but stronger guidelines were updated in 2006 and acknowledge that, although the efforts may be more difficult and need to be more intensive, inpatient episodes can be an appropriate time to initiate smoking cessation efforts (APA, 2006; Moss et al., 2010). In 2008, Fiore's 2000 Practice Guidelines for Smoking Cessation were updated and specifically emphasized that providers need to treat all smokers with mental health and substance abuse diagnoses and that these patients be provided the same smoking cessation treatments as the general population (Fiore et al., 2008).

F. The health benefits of quitting

Stopping smoking is associated with multiple health benefits: a lowered risk for lung cancer and many other types of cancer; a reduced risk for coronary heart disease, stroke, and peripheral vascular disease; and reduced respiratory diseases such as COPD and reduced respiratory symptoms, such as coughing, wheezing, and shortness of breath. The rate of decline in lung function is slower among people who quit smoking than those who continue to smoke. For women there is a reduced risk of fertility issues and difficulty in conception, fewer miscarriages, less risk of preterm labor, fewer low-birth-weight babies, less incidence of sudden infant death syndrome (SIDS), and a reduced risk for cervical cancer (Schoendorf & Kiely, 1992; USDHHS, 2014).

G. How to get your patients to quit smoking

Around 70% of smokers say they want to quit. More than 55% of smokers have made at least one attempt to quit smoking in the past year. Most smokers try to quit "cold turkey." Relapse rates are high, less than 10% of smokers are able to quit without some form of nicotine replacement therapy (NRT) (Patel, Fencht, Reid, & Patel, 2010; USDHHS, 2014). Of those who do quit > 75% relapse within the first year. Nicotine replacement with bupropion or varenicline is the most effective way to help with cessation. Brief advice to quit smoking by the provider done routinely at each office visit increases the rates of smoking cessation (USDHHS, 2014).

Three categories of pharmacotherapy have proved helpful in smoking cessation: (a) nicotine replacement therapy, (b) bupropion, and (c) varenicline. Three nicotine replacement products are sold over the counter: (a) nicotine patches, (b) nicotine gum, and (c) nicotine lozenges. The other nicotine replacement products (the nicotine nasal spray and the nicotine inhaler) require prescriptions. There are few studies comparing which product is more efficacious than another but several studies show all nicotine products are better compared to placebo and double cessation rates. Because e-cigarettes have an unknown, unregulated nicotine content as well as other unknown, unregulated additives they are not considered a nicotine replacement product for cessation purposes, though some patients will want to use them (Meo & Al Asiri, 2014). All products also increase cessation rates when used in conjunction with a behavior modification program (Rennard & Doughton, 2014; USDHHS, 2014).

To use any nicotine replacement product the smoker is counseled to pick a quit date and start the product on the quit date. Most products are recommended for 2–3 months of use. But most providers continue the nicotine replacement as long as needed if stopping the medication means returning to smoking. The FDA is considering removing all recommendations regarding duration of use (V. Smith, personal communication, July 27, 2015). It is important to know that treatment needs to be individualized, clients may need to start before their quit date and some may require two 21 mg patches, as higher doses are required for heavier smokers. It is also considered safe to use the patch and the gum or lozenge together (Peereboom, Evers-Carey, & Leone, 2014; Rennard & Doughton, 2014). Combining nicotine replacement products is considered a safe strategy for nicotine-dependent persons trying to quit. Using a "controller" medication (patch) with a "reliever" (gum, lozenge, or inhaler) medication can be more effective to induce quitting than either medication formulation alone. The differences in pharmacology action and duration of each product make this possible. A slow-onset and long-acting product, such as the patch, can be safely combined with the use of a shorter-acting product, such as gum or lozenge (Patel et al., 2010; Peereboom et al., 2014).

Nicotine replacement is considered safe for use even in smokers with known CVD. Experts say the benefits of quitting smoking far outweigh any risk of the nicotine replacement product, although few studies exist (Fiore et al., 2008; Rennard & Doughton, 2014).

Bupropion has been available in the United States as an antidepressant since 1989. Smokers who were on bupropion recognized a decreased desire to smoke as an interesting side effect. A sustained-release form of bupropion was developed and marketed as a smoking cessation aid, Zyban®. Large studies demonstrate that the use of bupropion doubles the success rate of smoking cessation (Patel et al., 2010; Rennard & Doughton, 2014).

Varenicline (Chantix®) is hypothesized to both bind to nicotine receptors in the brain and block the nicotine in cigarette smoke from attaching to the receptor in the brain. It is hypothesized that this action reduces the rewarding sensation of nicotine, thus decreasing the desire to smoke. Multiple studies show efficacy. In February 2008 the FDA issued an alert that an increase in suicidal thinking and "aggressive and erratic behavior" was associated with patients being treated with Varenicline (FDA, 2008). Most experts recommend taking a careful psychiatric history before starting the medication and not prescribing the medication for known patients with any current or past history of unstable depression or suicidality. It is important to note that neuropsychiatric side effects have been reported even in patients with no known history. It is recommended to use with caution with careful follow-up in 1 and 2 weeks. Patients should be told to contact their provider or the office and stop the drug if they or their family notice any unusual mood or behavior symptoms.

The majority of cigarette smokers quit without using evidence-based treatments. The following treatments are evidence-based methods, shown to be effective for smokers who want help to quit. These brief clinical interventions include:

- 5 As—Ask, Advise, Assess (readiness to quit), Assist, and Arrange follow-up (Fiore et al., 2008)
- Motivational interviewing techniques (Peereboom et al., 2014)
- Individual and group classes or counseling, telephone support, Internet groups, programs to deliver treatment/support using social media and mobile phones (Fiore et al., 2008; Zhang, Yang, & Li, 2012)

H. Concluding remarks

To date, almost one in five patients smoke. Smoking remains an undertreated chronic disease well suited for clinician counseling and management. Highest risk groups are mentally ill individuals and those living in poverty or disability. The goal for the adolescent client is prevention, especially preventing use of the e-cigarette. Individualized treatments consisting of medication and counseling at every visit improve cessation rates.

II. Database

A. Subjective

1. Obtain a smoking history
   a. Ask: Do you smoke? For how long? How much do you smoke? How soon do you smoke your first cigarette in the morning? Are you interested in quitting? Have you ever quit before? What made you start again?
   b. If patient has quit, ascertain prior smoking history because recent cessation (within the year) increases the risk for relapse.

2. Past health history
   a. Medical history:
      i. Illnesses specific to cancer, such as lung, head and neck, mouth, larynx, esophagus, bladder, kidney, pancreas, brain, cervix, breast
      ii. Illnesses specific to the cardiorespiratory system, such as myocardial infarction, cardiovascular disease (CVD) or coronary artery disease (CAD), peripheral vascular disease (PVD), Reynaud's disease, hypertension (HTN), hypercholesterolemia, blood clots, COPD, bronchitis, sinusitis, pneumonia, allergies, asthma, and gastritis or peptic ulcer disease.
   b. Psychiatric disorders: prior history of depression, anxiety, or other mental health diagnosis.
   c. Substance use disorders: screen with a standardized screening tool, such as CAGE-AID or other brief screening tool, and for depression using PHQ-9 or other depression screening tool (Brown & Rounds, 1995; Spitzer, Kroenke, & Williams, 1999).
   d. Gynecological history: infertility, abnormal pap smears, low-birth-weight babies, and complications of pregnancy.
   e. Exposure history: passive smoking or asbestos.
   f. Medication history: prior use of nicotine replacement, bupropion, varenicline, or other medications related to cessation, depression, or seizures.

3. Family history: Cancer, CVD, PVD, COPD, asthma, or other respiratory symptoms.

4. Personal and social history
   a. Identify social supports and living situations in terms of other smokers.
   b. Assess coexistent stressors and coping strategies.
   c. Identify need for possible referrals.
   d. Use of alcohol and other substances.
   e. Use of telephone, Internet, or office-based support groups.

5. Review of systems
    a. Constitutional for sign or symptoms as related to cancer, infection, and CVD. Generally, no signs or symptoms present.
    b. Skin, hair, and nails: Cosmetic changes noted, such as early skin wrinkling, impaired wound healing, and finger and teeth staining.
    c. Ear, nose, mouth, and throat: allergic or irritant symptoms, postnasal drip, frequent infections, dental complaints, dysphagia or any unusual lesions on the buccal mucosa, tongue, floor of mouth.
    d. Cardiovascular: chest pain, leg pain when walking short distances, excessively cold hands, or feet with color change. Chest pain or change in activity tolerance, paroxysmal nocturnal dyspnea, or peripheral edema.
    e. Respiratory: shortness of breath, productive or nonproductive cough, postnasal drip, wheezing, decreased exercise tolerance, frequent colds, and allergy symptoms, mucus production, dyspnea, and paroxysmal nocturnal dyspnea.
    f. Gastrointestinal: abdominal burning or pain, acid indigestion, heartburn, constipation, diarrhea; frequent use of antacids; and food intolerance. Use of smoking to regulate bowels.
    g. Genitourinary: sexual or erectile dysfunction.
    h. Musculoskeletal: claudication or peripheral edema.
    i. Neurologic: paresthesias
    j. Psychiatric: screen for depression/substance abuse with CAGE-AID tool

B. **Objective**
    1. Physical examination: generally there are no signs unless an illness-related visit
        a. Vital signs: may include normal or increased heart rate or blood pressure
        b. General appearance: may appear older than stated age; clothes and hair may smell of cigarette smoke
        c. Skin, hair, nails: facial wrinkles and yellow stains on teeth and fingers
        d. Head, eyes, ears, nose, and throat: assess for periodontal disease, include bimanual examination of mouth, assess for oral lesions that may be malignant or premalignant, leukoplakia, evidence of upper respiratory irritants, infection, or allergies
        e. Lymphatic: generally, there are few findings but look for lymphadenopathy in presence of any head, eyes, ears, nose, and throat symptoms
        f. Chest: generally, there are few findings unless illness is present, but assess respiratory rate, quality of cough if observed, anteroposterior diameter, presence of adventitious sounds; office

spirometry or peak expiratory flow rates are usually normal
    g. Cardiovascular: generally, few findings are observed but evaluate cardiac rate, rhythm, extra heart sounds, and pulses
    h. Extremities: note color, temperature and pulses, note hair distribution because there is a decrease in lower extremities of those with PVD
    i. Neurologic: generally, few findings but evaluation needed if any paresthesias
    j. Psychiatric: PHQ9 and CAGE-AID tool
    2. Supporting data from relevant diagnostic tests
        a. If screening for CVD labs, CBC, blood glucose/HBA1C, lipid profile, and kidney function. If lab test abnormalities, may be able to educate client regarding effects of smoking on health.
        b. If indicated: electrocardiogram, pulmonary function tests, and chest radiograph, consider annual lung cancer screening with low dose chest CT for patients > 55 years old at higher risk for lung cancer, i.e., a 30 pack-year history or greater (Moyer, 2014; USPSTF, 2014).

III. Assessment

A. *List related ICD -10 codes (e.g., 305.1 Tobacco use disorder or V15.82 History of tobacco use)*

B. *Former, current risk of relapse*

C. *Significance of smoking history, smoking index, or pack-year in terms of disease risk*

D. *Identify comorbid illnesses or disease states*

E. *Stage of readiness to quit*

F. *Rule out concomitant physical illness*
    Examples: "Persistent and recurrent cough due to allergies versus asthma flares complicated by > 35 pack-year history of smoking in 62 yo male at high risk for lung cancer recently quit smoking 1 month ago at high risk for relapse"
    "Uncomplicated URI in young adult smoker not ready to quit"
    "New dx of cervical dysplasia in 42 yo woman ready to try to quit smoking"

IV. Goals of clinical management

Stop smoking; reduce risks for tobacco-related conditions; prevent and manage relapse; and eliminate secondhand smoke exposure.

V. Plan

A. Diagnostic

1. Pulmonary function tests are usually normal unless respiratory illness is present and are therefore not recommended.

2. Annual low-dose chest CT to rule out early lung cancer if patient is high risk, i.e., > 55 years old with 35 pack-year history, currently smoking or quit within 15 years (Moyer, 2014)

3. CVD screening lipid panel

4. Additional testing as indicated by history and physical examination

B. Treatment and management goals

1. **Advise** patient to stop smoking. If evidence of concomitant illness or sign of abnormality on examination, use this as a teachable moment, as an indication of harmful effects of tobacco and the benefit of cessation. Inform patients in a nonjudgmental way: *"Stopping smoking is the single most important thing you can do to improve your health."*

2. **Assess** patient's readiness to quit and individualize treatment plan based on assessment
   a. Precontemplative: advise to quit, acknowledge lack of readiness, state availability to assist in quitting when they are ready; evaluate readiness at every visit.
   b. Contemplative: advise to quit, acknowledge their consideration, and provide written pamphlet or resources for review. State availability to assist in quitting when ready to try or set quit date.

3. **Assist** patient to quit smoking: educate regarding medications available, OK to start ahead of quit date, help pick quit date, review behavior modification strategies, recommend nicotine replacement therapy (NRT)—both patch (at proper dose) and with gum or lozenge for back up with or without bupropion or varenicline. Know it is safe to use medications prior to anticipated quit date to reduce patient anxiety regarding abstinence for 2–4 weeks before quit date for example.

4. **Medications**
   a. Nicotine replacement products
      i. *Nicotine patch* is a transdermal system absorbed through the skin over 16–24 hours depending on the brand. It is recommended that a patient start use on their quit date, but there is evidence that pretreatment is both safe and effective in helping cessation (Peereboom

et al., 2014). Apply every morning on a dry area of upper arm, stomach, or buttock. Remove at bedtime because the nicotine may interrupt sleep. However, persons who smoke immediately on waking may find it beneficial to wear the patch during sleep. Rotate sites, reusing the same site no more frequently than every 7 days. Change every day. The different brands are generally similar in dosage. May taper over 2 months (e.g., 21 mg/day for 4 weeks, 14 mg/day for 2 weeks, and 7 mg/day for 2 weeks). The 21-mg patch is equivalent to trough concentrations (i.e., lowest level of blood nicotine) in smokers averaging one pack per day. Recognize that it is safe to use two patches at once for a two pack a day smoker, for example. And know that you may need to taper over a much longer period of time. It is considered safe to avoid deadlines for cessation. Many people require 6 months or a year of treatment with nicotine replacement, and it should be noted that the FDA is considering removing all timelines for use of the patch (www.fda.gov/downloads/ForConsumers/ConsumerUpdates/UCM346012.pdf).

NRT is well tolerated, although 50% of patch users experience some local skin irritation. It is acceptable to use topical steroid and continue use with rotation of sites. The patch can cause excessive or unusual dreams; may be removed at bedtime

      ii. *Nicotine gum* or lozenge is an oral product containing nicotine bound to a polacrilex resin. When the gum is chewed or sucked, it releases nicotine, which is absorbed through the oral mucosa. It takes 20 minutes for the nicotine level in the blood to rise. Advise the client to bite the gum slowly, not to chew, or the nicotine will be released faster than it can be absorbed and swallowed. Swallowing the nicotine causes stomach or esophageal irritation. Nicotine from the gastrointestinal tract is metabolized by the liver and essentially is ineffective. May be used with patch or after patch for "just in case." For nicotine gum, "bite and park." Bite until it tastes (radish or peppery taste) and then bite again after taste disappears. It lasts approximately 20–30 minutes. Avoid coffee and carbonated drinks for up to 20 minutes before use, because this lowers the absorption of nicotine. Use 2-mg gum for most smokers; can use 4 mg for those who smoke more than 25 cigarettes per day. Use as often as an urge occurs, up to 20 pieces per day. Taper after 6 weeks; taper one to two pieces per week. Dependence on gum is not common because the delivery system essentially acts to wean the smoker. NRT is still considered safer than smoking and may need to be used intermittently for 6–12 months or longer.

iii. For *nicotine lozenges,* do not chew; can be used for those with dentures or no teeth. Place in mouth and let dissolve for 30 minutes. Use the 2-mg dose for most smokers but 4 mg is recommended for those who smoke within 30 minutes of awakening. May use one to two per hour for the first 4–6 weeks. Consider tapering after 6 weeks; dependence issues are not likely and may need to continue for 6–12 months as needed to manage the compulsion to smoke (Peereboom et al., 2014).

iv. *Nicotine inhaler* (available only by prescription): the nicotine inhaler is a plastic mouthpiece with a nicotine cartridge placed inside. When the smoker inhales through the device, nicotine vapor, not smoke is released into the mouth and throat and absorbed through the oral mucosa. The vapor mostly does not reach the lungs and is pharmacologically more similar to gum or lozenge than a cigarette. Plasma levels of nicotine are approximately one-third that of a cigarette. May be helpful in smokers to address the behavioral and sensory aspects of cigarette smoking or in those who failed gum or lozenges. Recommended dose is 6–16 cartridges per day for the first 6–12 weeks. Taper dose over the next 6–12 weeks. Avoid or use with caution in those with a history of severe reactive airway syndromes because it may cause bronchospasm. Nicotrol inhalers differ from the e-cigarette in that the nicotine dose is a known dose and there are no additives. Studies are currently being done to compare e-cigarettes with nicotrol inhalers for smoking cessation.

v. *Nicotine nasal spray* (available only by prescription): delivers nicotine to nasal mucosa via an aqueous solution. It is more rapidly delivered with peak concentration within 10 minutes but not as rapid as a cigarette. One to two sprays per hour for the first 3 months. A high rate of nasal and throat irritation limits its use.

b. Bupropion

    i. Generally is started 1–2 weeks before quit date, but may start 4 weeks before

    ii. Start with bupropion sustained release, 150 mg once daily for 3–7 days.

    iii. Increase to twice a day for 7 days. If side effects occur on the 300-mg dose, continue at 150 mg daily.

    iv. Recommended treatment duration is 7–12 weeks, but may continue longer up to 12 months.

    v. Common side effects are insomnia, dry mouth, and headache.

    vi. Rule out bipolar affective disorder (BAD) and consult for use with patients with BAD diagnosis. There is some discussion as to whether bupropion can trigger mania especially with bipolar I (Pacchiarotti et al., 2013). Bupropion is the antidepressant of choice in BAD because it is least likely to induce mania; however, no antidepressant should be used alone in BAD treatment.

    vii. Serious side effect is seizure. Clinical trial risk of seizure is 0.1%. Contraindicated in seizure disorder or predisposition to seizures.

    viii. Rule out an anorexia-type eating disorder as bupropion has an FDA black box warning about anorexia because of its potential for appetite suppression.

c. Varenicline (Chantix®)

    i. Start 0.5 mg daily for 3 days then increase to 0.5 mg twice a day for 4 days, then 1 mg twice a day for remainder of the 12-week course, may use for longer periods up to 6–12 months.

    ii. Advise to take with food and a full glass of water to avoid the side effect of nausea.

    iii. Quit smoking 1–3 weeks after start of medication.

    iv. Common side effects are nausea, insomnia, and abnormal dreams.

    v. Because of concern regarding serious neuropsychiatric side effects, counsel patients to call office and stop medication if they or their family notice any unusual mood or behavior symptoms.

    vi. Use with caution with renal insufficiency and any history of depression.

5. **Assist and Arrange** follow-up/behavior modification and patient education

a. Encourage patient to think of quitting smoking as "learning a musical instrument or foreign language." Both efforts require practice. If a relapse occurs, encourage patient not to give up and to try again. Smoking cessation may take a while to master. It typically takes multiple attempts before a smoker stays quit for good (ACS, 2014b).

b. Encourage smokers not to feel as if they have a character defect because they did not succeed in the past. Encourage them to try again.

c. Have smokers write on a 3 × 5 file card the three most important reasons to quit, to keep this card in the same place they used to keep cigarettes, and to pull out the card and read it whenever they have an urge.

d. Have patient practice quitting a little every day, at different times of day. For example, on Monday, advise patient not to smoke from 6:00 a.m. until 9:00 a.m.; on Tuesday, not to smoke from 9:00 a.m. until 12 noon; on Wednesday, not to smoke from noon until 3:00 p.m., and so on. Once the week is completed, the smoker will learn which cigarettes were most important and then will know which cigarettes might prove to be harder to quit.

e. Or have patient keep a smoking diary, noting time of day, urge level, circumstances, and what mood or feeling was present that triggered urge.

f. Identifying what triggers smoking (this is key to determine alternate behaviors to smoking). Think of three different activities they might do instead of smoking.

g. Reward nonsmoking behaviors. Rewarded behavior is repeated.

h. Encourage patient to join a class on quitting smoking, Internet-based group, cellphone reminder group, or social media.

i. Ask patient to read as much as possible about the health effects of smoking, the benefits of quitting, and the tobacco industry.

j. Encourage plenty of rest, fresh air, exercise, and nutrition.

k. Ask patients to reach out to nonsmokers, to find a "buddy" in their quit smoking campaign. People with more social support have higher success rates.

l. Tell patient to expect a small weight gain. Bupropion may help prevent weight gain.

m. Being overweight generally is healthier than smoking.

n. Ask patient to consider walking as a way to deal with urges/triggers.

o. Advise patient to be wary of relapse. Advise patient to avoid high-risk situations initially, and to learn and practice positive imagery, meditation, or self-hypnosis techniques. Buddy up in at-risk situations.

p. Ask patient to identify other situations of success and confidence, offer strength-based support.

q. Once patient has quit for 6 months, encourage community involvement (e.g., volunteer on "former smoker" panels, teach a quit smoking class, be a buddy for other "newly quit" smokers).

r. It is helpful to have follow-up scheduled visits; to establish a quit date, quit day appointment, follow-up support at 1 week, 1 month, 3 months. Telephone calls may work as well, individualize treatment.

s. Review strategies for urge control, offer community or Internet referral sources.

t. Ask at every visit about patient's efforts.

u. Praise and congratulate any quit effort, and explore what caused any relapse.

v. If quitting is recent, offer printed self-help materials from the American Lung Association (ALA), American Cancer Society community groups, or phone, Internet, and social media sites.

w. Most of the behavior modification techniques here are part of the Freedom from Smoking Classes conducted by the ALA before there were effective medications on the market. Medications with behavior modification are the evidence-based cessation treatments of choice.

6. **Documentation**

a. Identify smoking status on problem list or vital sign record as appropriate

b. Document assessment of smoking history, readiness to quit and cessation strategies in progress notes.

c. Treatment plans—include medications/behavior modification and patient education goals, include resources for self-help and follow-up.

VI. Self-management resources

A. Online/telephone resources

1. 1-800-QUIT-NOW, a national hotline for smoking cessation

2. 1-800-NO-BUTTS, a California hotline for smoking cessation

3. 1-800-LUNGUSA, an American Lung Association phone help line

B. *Web-based support groups/social media*

1. www.ffsonline.org
2. www.quitnet.com
3. www.smokefree.gov
4. www.quitnet.com will connect user to Quit Net Forum, Quit Net Facebook, or Quit Net Twitter

VII. Consultation

A. *In patients with depression or history of depression, additional antidepressant agents other than bupropion may be required. Referral for counseling is recommended.*

B. *In pregnant patients and patients with cerebrovascular, CVD, or seizure disorder, consultation with a physician is advised before the use of pharmacologic adjuncts for smoking cessation.*

C. *Consider smoking cessation specialist.*

REFERENCES

American Cancer Society. (2014a). *Cancer facts & figures 2014.* Atlanta: American Cancer Society.

American Cancer Society. (2014b). *Guide to quitting smoking.* Retrieved from www.cancer.org/acs/groups/cid/documents/webcontent/002971-pdf.pdf.

American Psychiatric Association. (2006). *Practice guideline for the treatment of patients with substance abuse disorders* (2nd ed.). Retrieved from http://psychiatryonline.org/pb/assets/raw/sitewide/practice_guidelines/guidelines/substanceuse.pdf.

Brown, R. L., & Rounds, L. A. (1995). Conjoint screening questionnaires for alcohol and other drug abuse: Criterion validity in a primary care practice. *Wisconsin Medical Journal, 94*(3), 135–140.

Centers for Disease Control and Prevention. (2015). *Current cigarette smoking among adults in the United States.* Retrieved from www.cdc.gov/tobacco/data_statistics/fact_sheets/adult_data/cig_smoking/.

Christiansen, B., Reeder, K., Hill, M., Baker, T. B., & Fiore, M. C. (2012). Barriers to effective tobacco-dependence treatment for the very poor. *Journal of Studies on Alcohol and Drugs, 73*(6), 874–884.

Dutra, L. M., & Glantz, S. A. (2014). Electronic cigarettes and conventional cigarettes among US Adolescents: A cross sectional study. *JAMA Pediatrics, 168*(7), 610–617.

Fiore, M. C., Jaén, C. R., Baker, T. B., Bailey, W. C., Bennett, G., Neal, L., et al. (2008). *Treating tobacco use and dependence: 2008 Update. Clinical practice guideline.* Rockville, MD: U.S. Department of Health and Human Services, Public Health Service.

Food and Drug Administration. (2008). *Public health advisory: Important information on Chantix (varenicline).* Retrieved from www.fda.gov/Drugs/DrugSafety/PostmarketDrugSafetyInformationforPatientsandProviders/ucm051136.htm.

Food and Drug Administration. (2012). *HR1256: Family Smoking Prevention and Control Act.* Retrieved from www.fda.gov/TobaccoProducts/GuidanceComplianceRegulatoryInformation/ucm237092.htm.

Food and Drug Administration. (2015). *Deeming—extending authorities to additional tobacco products.* Retrieved from www.fda.gov/TobaccoProducts/Labeling/ucm388395.htm.

Giovino, G. A. (2002). Epidemiology of tobacco use in the United States. *Oncogene, 21*(48), 7326–7340.

Hall, S. M., & Prochaska, J. (2009). Treatment of smokers with co-occurring disorders: Emphasis on integration in mental health and addiction treatment Settings *Annual Review Clinical Psychology, 5,* 409–431.

Houston, T. P. (1992) Smoking cessation in office practice. *Primary Care, 19,* 493–507.

McCarthy, M. (2014). Youth exposure to e-cigarette advertising on US television soars. *British Medical Journal, 348,* 3703.

Meo, S. A., & Al Asiri, S. A. (2014). Effects of electronic cigarette smoking on human health. *European Review for Medical and Pharmacological Sciences, 18* (21), 3315–3319.

Moss, T. G., Weinberger, A. H., Vessicchio, J. C., Mancuso, V., Cushing, S. J., Pett, M., et al. (2010). A tobacco reconceptualization in psychiatry (TRIP): Towards the development of tobacco-free psychiatric facilities, *American Journal Addiction, 19*(4), 293–311.

Moyer, V. A. (2014). Screening for lung cancer: U.S. Preventive Services Task Force recommendation statement. *Annals of Internal Medicine, 160*(5), 330–338.

Pacchiarotti, I., Bond, D. J., Baldessarini, R. J., Nolen, W. A., Grunze, H., Licht, R. W., et al. (2013). The International Society for Bipolar Disorders (ISBD) task force report on antidepressant use in bipolar disorders. *American Journal of Psychiatry, 170*(11), 1249–1262.

Palazzolo, D. L. (2013). Electronic cigarettes and vaping: A new challenge in clinical medicine and public health. A literature review. *Frontiers in Public Health, 1,* 56. doi:10.3389/fpubh.2013.00056

Patel, D. R., Fencht, C., Reid, L., & Patel, N. D. (2010). Pharmacologic agents for smoking cessation. *Clinical Pharmacology, 2,* 17–29. doi:10.2147/CPAA.S8788/11/20/14

Peereboom, D., Evers-Casey, S., & Leone, F. (2014). Are you equipped to treat tobacco dependence? *Consultant, 54*(12), 903–907.

Rennard, S. I., & Daughton, D. M. (2014). Smoking cessation. *Clinics in Chest Medicine, 35*(1), 165–176.

Sanford, Z., & Goebel, L. (2014). E-cigarettes: An up to date review and discussion of the controversy. *West Virginia Medical Journal, 110*(4), 10–15.

Schoendorf, K. C., & Kiely, J. L. (1992). Relationship of sudden infant death syndrome to maternal smoking during and after pregnancy. *Pediatrics, 90*(6), 905–908.

Sheehan, K. A. (2004). Smoking cessation. In W. L. Star, L. L. Lommel, & M. T. Shannon, *Women's primary health care: Protocols for practice* (2nd ed., pp. 14-64–14-68). San Francisco: UCSF Nursing Press.

Spitzer, R. L., Kroenke, K., & Williams, J. B. W. (1999). Validation and utility of a self-report version of PRIME-MD: The PHQ primary care study. *JAMA, 282*(18), 1737–1744.

The battle over e-cigarettes. (2014, September 27). *The Week.* Retrieved from http://theweek.com/articles/443487/battle-over-ecigarettes.

U.S. Department of Health and Human Services. (2014). *The health consequences of smoking—50 years of progress: A report of the Surgeon General.* Atlanta, GA: U.S. Department of Health and Human Services, Centers for Disease Control and Prevention, National Centers for Chronic Disease Prevention and Health Promotion, Office on Smoking and Health.

U.S. Preventive Services Task Force. (2014). *Talking with your patients about screening for lung cancer.* Retrieved from www .uspreventiveservicestaskforce.org/Home/GetFileByID/796.

Walton, J., Barondess, J. A., & Lock, S. (Eds.). (1994). *The Oxford medical companion.* New York: Oxford University Press.

Walton, K. M., Abrams, D. B., Bailey, W. C., Clark, D., Connolly, G. N., Djordjevic, M. V., et al. (2015). NIH electronic cigarette workshop: Developing a research agenda. *Nicotine & Tobacco Research, 17*(2), 259–269.

World Health Organization. (2008). *WHO report on the global tobacco epidemic, 2008. The MPOWER package.* Geneva, Switzerland: Author. Retrieved from www.who.int/tobacco/mpower/mpower_report_full _2008.pdf.

Wynder, E. L., & Graham, E. A. (1950). Tobacco smoking as a possible etiological factor in bronchiogenic carcinoma. *JAMA, 143,* 329–336.

Zhang, M., Yang, C. C., & Li, J. (2012). A comparative study of smoking cessation internet programs on social media. *Lecture Notes in Computer Science, 7227,* 87–96. New York: Springer Science+Business Media LLC.

THYROID DISORDERS

JoAnne M. Saxe

CHAPTER 68

I. Introduction and general background

The adult thyroid gland is responsible for the production of hormones (L-thyroxine [T_4] and 3,5,3'-triiodothyronine [T_3]) that influence a variety of metabolic processes. Its structure and function are contingent on an intact axis between this gland and the hypothalamus and pituitary glands. Specifically, the hypothalamus secretes thyrotropin-releasing hormone, which stimulates the pituitary to produce and release thyroid-stimulating hormone (TSH). TSH triggers the production and secretion of T_3 and T_4 from the thyroid. Through a positive–negative feedback loop, these glands, when normally functioning, regulate T_3 and T_4 secretion so that metabolic homeostasis is ensured.

The thyroid gland is affected by a number of other extrathyroidal factors, such as the status of the immune system. Thus, alterations in the synthesis, secretion, and circulation of thyroid hormones may be caused by an array of primary or secondary thyroid disorders. Globally, iodine deficiency is the most common cause of thyroid dysfunction, which leads to the formation of a goiter and hypothyroidism. In regions where there is sufficient iodine supply, most thyroid disorders are due to an underlying autoimmune disease (Vanderpump, 2011). The most common thyroid conditions seen in primary care settings are primary hypothyroidism, hyperthyroidism, and thyroid nodules (Saxe, 2004).

A. Primary hypothyroidism

1. Definition and overview

   This is a condition in which there is loss of thyroid function as a result of the intrinsic thyroid pathology. Primary hypothyroidism accounts for 95% of all cases of hypothyroidism (Jameson & Weetman, 2012). The most common causes of primary hypothyroidism in the United States are:

   a. Thyroid inflammatory diseases (e.g., chronic [Hashimoto's] thyroiditis, postpartum [subacute lymphocytic] thyroiditis, and subacute thyroiditis). The initial presentation of thyroiditis, however, may have transient presentation consistent with hyperthyroidism.

   b. Radioiodine-induced or surgically induced hypothyroidism.

   c. Idiopathic thyroid atrophy (Jameson & Weetman, 2012; Saxe, 2004).

2. Prevalence and incidence

   As reported by Vanderpump (2011), a number of studies have noted the prevalence of hypothyroidism ranges from 0.6 and 12 per 1,000 in women and between 1.3 and 4.0 per 1,000 in men of the populations that were investigated. However, the prevalence of primary hypothyroidism is higher in the geriatric female population than in women under age 40 (Hollowell et al., 2002; Wang & Crapo, 1997). Additionally, in the United States, hypothyroidism has been reported to be more common in White Americans and Mexican Americans than in Black Americans (Hollowell et al., 2002).

B. Hyperthyroidism

1. Definition and overview

   Hyperfunctioning of the thyroid gland can result from a variety of diseases. The most common causes of hyperthyroidism are

   a. Diffuse toxic (hyperfunctioning) goiter (Graves' disease).

   b. Toxic multinodular goiter.

   c. Toxic uninodular goiter.

   d. Thyroid inflammatory diseases (e.g., Hashimoto's thyroiditis, postpartum thyroiditis, and subacute thyroiditis, which may cause a transient thyrotoxicosis [Saxe, 2004; Vanderpump, 2011]).

2. Prevalence and incidence

   Data from the Whickham survey and other studies indicate that the prevalence and incidence of hyperthyroidism in men are low (Vanderpump, 2011; Wang & Crapo, 1997). In women, the prevalence of overt hyperthyroidism is between 0.5% and 2% (Vanderpump, 2011). Like primary hypothyroidism, hyperthyroidism is more commonly seen in older women than in women before the fourth decade (Cooper, Greenspan, & Ladenson, 2011; Wang & Crapo, 1997), yet with significant variability in prevalence noted in different regions of the world (Vanderpump, 2011).

C. Thyroid nodules

1. Definition and overview

   Thyroid nodules may be functional (secrete thyroid hormones) or nonfunctional. The vast majority of functional and most nonfunctional thyroid nodules are benign. However, a malignancy should be suspected particularly if an individual has the following risk profile: being relatively young (< 45 years of age); previous external head or neck irradiation; a predominant nodule or recent growth of a nodule, particularly if it does not alter thyroid functions; associated hoarseness and dysphagia; and a family history of medullary cancer of the thyroid (Cooper et al., 2011; Ward, Jemal, & Chen, 2010).

2. Prevalence and incidence

   Thyroid nodules are common entities. The prevalence rates of nodules vary by detection method with rates of up to 50% of individuals who have had a thyroid ultrasound (Cooper et al., 2011). Most of the detected nodules are benign and are more commonly noted in women than in men (Cooper et al., 2011). With the exception of malignant nodules, thyroid nodules are more prevalent with increasing age as noted by incidence rates (Cooper et al., 2011; Howlader et al., 2014). Since 1980, however, there has been a rising incidence of thyroid malignancies. The age-adjusted incidence rate for invasive thyroid cancer was 4.33/100,000 in 1980 compared to 14.71/100,000 in 2011 (Howlader et al., 2014).

II. Database (may include but is not limited to)

A. Subjective

1. Primary hypothyroidism
   a. Past health history
      i. Medical illnesses: assess for autoimmune thyroid disorders that can be associated with other autoimmune diseases, such as type 1 diabetes mellitus, pernicious anemia, rheumatoid arthritis, and systemic lupus erythematosus; and secondary hypothyroidism caused by pituitary or hypothalamic diseases (low TSH and low free thyroxine [FT_4]).
      ii. Surgical history: thyroid surgery or pituitary surgery
      iii. Obstetric and gynecological history: recent pregnancy or parturition
      iv. Trauma history: brain trauma
      v. Exposure history: radiation (e.g., radioiodine therapy or external neck irradiation)
      vi. Medication history: medications or supplements that influence hormone production (e.g., amiodarone, lithium, and iodine)
   b. Family history
      i. Thyroid diseases
      ii. Other endocrinopathies
   c. Occupational and environmental history: work-related exposures to radiation or radioactive iodine
   d. Personal and social history: iodine-deficient diet (uncommon because most regions have iodination programs)
   e. Review of systems: signs and symptoms vary depending on the degree of thyroid dysfunction. The individual with subclinical hypothyroidism (a person who has abnormalities in chemical markers, an elevated thyroid-stimulating hormone and normal free levothyrotoxine hormone, yet is clinically euthyroid) or mild hypothyroidism is usually asymptomatic. Persons with moderate dysfunction often notice constitutional and skin signs and symptoms. The individual with advanced disease often has multisystem symptoms.
      i. Constitutional signs and symptoms: fatigue, weight gain, or cold intolerance
      ii. Skin, hair, and nails: dry skin, puffy and doughy skin, and coarse hair or hair loss
      iii. Ear, nose, and throat: decreased hearing, hoarseness, dysphagia, or dysarthria
      iv. Cardiac: chest pain
      v. Abdomen: constipation
      vi. Genitourinary: oligomenorrhea and menorrhagia
      vii. Musculoskeletal: joint stiffness or pain and myalgias
      viii. Neurologic: paresthesias, lethargy, less expressive at rest, depressed mood, and/or rarely ataxic gait

2. Hyperthyroidism
   a. Past health history
      i. Medical illnesses: Graves' disease, toxic uninodular or multinodular goiter, very rarely pituitary TSH-secreting tumor.
      ii. Surgical history: thyroid surgery
      iii. Obstetric and gynecological history: recent pregnancy or parturition
      iv. Medication history: medications or supplements that influence hormone production (e.g., antithyroid drug use [propylthiouracil (PTU) or methimazole], amiodarone, lithium, exogenous thyroid hormone supplements, and iodine)
   b. Family history
      i. Thyroid diseases
      ii. Other endocrinopathies
      iii. Neuroendocrine disorders
   c. Personal and social history: a recent intake of an iodine-rich diet in an individual who previously had an iodine-deficient diet (geographic regions that may not have iodination programs and that have limited access to iodine-containing foods are certain regions in South America, Africa, and Asia)
   d. Review of systems: signs and symptoms vary depending on the degree of thyroid dysfunction. The individual with subclinical and mild hyperthyroidism may be relatively asymptomatic. Persons with moderate dysfunction often notice constitutional signs and symptoms, palpitations, increased bowel motility, and neurologic signs and symptoms as depicted next. The individual with advanced disease often has multisystem symptomatology.
      i. Constitutional signs and symptoms: weakness, fatigue in the elderly, increased appetite, weight loss, insomnia, or heat intolerance
      ii. Skin: increased perspiration; pretibial myxedema in Graves' disease
      iii. Eyes: proptosis in Graves' disease
      iv. Ear, nose, and throat: hoarseness or dysphagia
      v. Pulmonary: dyspnea
      vi. Cardiac: chest pain or palpitations
      vii. Abdomen: increased bowel motility that often results in frequent bowel movements
      viii. Genitourinary: irregular menses or amenorrhea
      ix. Neurologic: tremors or nervousness and anxiety

3. Thyroid nodules
   a. Past health history
      i. Medical illnesses: thyroid disorders including thyroid cancer; and autoimmune disorders that may cause a nodular gland (e.g., Graves' disease)
      ii. Surgical history: thyroid surgery
      iii. Exposure history: radiation (e.g., radioiodine therapy or external head and neck irradiation)
      iv. Medication history: medications or supplements that influence hormone production (e.g., lithium and iodine)
   b. Family history: thyroid diseases including goitrous thyroid conditions and thyroid cancer
   c. Occupational and environmental history: work-related exposures to radiation or radioactive iodine
   d. Personal and social history
      i. Iodine-deficient diet or iodine-excessive diet (see primary hypothyroidism and hyperthyroidism for discussion)
      ii. Regular ingestion of dietary goitrogens (e.g., beets and turnips)
   e. Review of systems
      The nodules may be nonfunctional, in which case the individual is clinically euthyroid. However, the nodules or nodular gland may be hypofunctioning (resulting in signs and symptoms consistent with hypothyroidism) or autonomously functioning (resulting in signs and symptoms of hyperthyroidism). See the previous discussion on "primary hypothyroidism" or "hyperthyroidism," respectively, if an altered thyroid hormone status is suspected.
      It is important to inquire about symptoms, such as dysphagia, caused by an enlarged gland or hoarseness suggestive of malignant vocal cord infiltration (Cooper et al., 2011; Jameson & Weetman, 2012).

B. Objective

1. Physical examination findings (**Table 68-1**)
2. Supporting data from relevant diagnostic tests (**Tables 68-2** and **68-3**)

TABLE 68-1 Physical Examination Findings

Condition	Associated Findings (may or may not include):
Primary Hypothyroidism	Assess: 1. Vital signs: hypothermia and/or bradycardia 2. General appearance: flat affect and/or dull facial expressions 3. Skin/hair: dry skin (early manifestation) to pasty, rough, and spongy skin (advanced manifestation); coarse hair (early manifestation) to hair loss (advanced manifestation) 4. Eyes: periorbital edema (late manifestation) 5. Ears, nose, and throat: enlarged tongue (advanced manifestation) 6. Thyroid: nonpalpable gland to a symmetrically enlarged and smooth gland to a multinodular enlarged gland 7. Lungs: crackles (advanced manifestation) 8. Cardiovascular: (+) S_4, (+) S_3, and jugular venous distention (advanced manifestations) 9. Abdomen: diminished bowel sounds 10. Neurologic: decreased tendon reflexes or enhanced relaxation phase, depressed mood, inattentiveness, and/or somnolence
Hyperthyroidism	Assess: 1. Vital signs: tachycardia 2. General appearance: restless 3. Skin/hair: moist and warm skin; pretibial myxedema (most suggestive of Graves' disease) and/or fine and very smooth hair 4. Eyes: exophthalmos/proptosis due to Graves' disease; and/or eye signs related to sympathetic hyperstimulation (lid lag, lid retraction, diminished blinking, inability to crease the eyebrows on upward stare) 5. Thyroid: single nodule (toxic uninodular goiter); tender or painless, symmetrically enlarged gland (thyroiditis); or diffusely enlarged (Graves' disease) and/or thyroid bruit (Graves' disease) 6. Lungs: crackles 7. Cardiovascular: systolic murmur; and/or (+) S_4, (+) S_3, and jugular venous distention 8. Abdomen: enhanced bowel sounds 9. Neurologic: increased tendon reflexes and/or fine tremor of the hands and tongue
Thyroid Nodules	The associated findings are contingent upon the functional status of the thyroid: 1. Nonfunctional nodule(s): exam will be relevant only for a thyroid gland with the palpable nodule(s) 2. Hypofunctioning multinodular gland: see the Primary Hypothyroidism Associated Findings section 3. Autonomously functioning nodule(s): see the Hyperthyroidism Associated Findings section 4. Lymph nodes: assess lymph nodes of the head and neck (may suggest a malignancy)

TABLE 68-2 Common Thyroid Tests

Test	Definition	Clinical Implications	Comments
Serum-free T$_4$ (FT$_4$)	Measurement of the metabolically active T$_4$ (unbound to thyroid-binding globulin)	Decreased in primary hypothyroidism. Increased in thyrotoxicosis.	May be increased by various drugs or conditions in individuals who are clinically euthyroid.
Serum T$_3$	Measurement of bound and free serum levels of T$_3$	Increased in T$_3$ thyrotoxicosis.	May be increased by various drugs or conditions in individuals who are clinically euthyroid.
Highly sensitive thyroid-stimulating hormone (TSH)	Measurement of TSH, an anterior pituitary hormone that stimulates growth and function of thyroid cells	Sensitive and specific test for the initial assessment of thyroid dysfunction. Increased in primary hypothyroidism. Decreased in most forms of thyrotoxicosis.	Values may be altered by certain drugs (e.g., aspirin and lithium).
Serum antithyroid antibodies (e.g., antithyroid peroxidase antibodies [also known as antithyroid microsomal antibody], antithyroglobulin antibodies, and anti-TSH receptor antibodies)	Measurement of immunologic markers for autoimmune thyroid diseases	Increased antithyroid peroxidase antibodies and/or antithyroglobulin antibodies are seen in Hashimoto's thyroiditis and Graves' disease. Anti-TSH receptor antibodies and thyroid-stimulating immunoglobulin (TSI) are commonly seen in persons with Graves' disease.	May be increased in clinically euthyroid individuals. Increases in anti-TSH receptor antibodies and thyroid-stimulating immunoglobulin (TSI) are more reliably predictive of Graves' disease than the thyroidal peroxidase antibody test (Cooper et al., 2011).
Radioactive iodine uptake	Measurement of thyroid function via uptake of radioactive iodine (^{123}I) or technetium ^{99m}Tc pertechnetate (^{99m}TcO4)	Used to evaluate defects in thyroid hormone production. Low uptake of radioactive iodine noted with non–iodine-deficient hypothyroidism, thyroiditis, and factitious thyrotoxicosis. Increased uptake is often seen with Graves' disease and toxic multinodular and uninodular goiter.	Variety of medications may interfere with uptake of the radioisotope. This test is usually not necessary for the basic evaluation of most thyroid disorders. Contraindications are iodine allergy, pregnancy, and lactation.
Thyroid scintiscan	Visualization of the thyroid gland via a scintillation camera after the administration of a radioactive isotope (e.g., ^{123}I or ^{99m}TcO4)	This test provides information about the structure and function of the thyroid gland. Increased uptake of the radioactive isotope is noted in a (hot) hyperfunctioning gland or nodule (e.g., Graves' disease and toxic uninodular goiter, respectively). Decreased uptake is seen in hypothyroidism or nonfunctioning (cold) nodule (e.g., thyroid cancer).	Variety of medications may interfere with uptake of the radioisotope. This test is usually not indicated for the evaluation of primary hypothyroidism. Contraindications are iodine allergy, pregnancy, or lactation.

Reproduced from Saxe, J. M. (2004). Thyroid diseases. In W. L. Star, L. L. Lommel, & M. T. Shannon (Eds.), *Women's primary health care: Protocols for practice* (2nd ed., pp. 10-33–10-39). San Francisco, CA: UCSF Nursing Press; reassessed and adapted from Fischbach & Dunning (2014) and Jameson & Weetman (2012). Used with permission from the UCSF Nursing Press.

TABLE 68-3 Supporting Data from Other Relevant Diagnostics Studies*

Condition	Diagnostic Test	Results
Primary Hypothyroidism	• Serum sodium • Serum cholesterol • Complete blood count • Electrocardiogram and/or echocardiogram	• Decreased (advanced disease) • Increased • Mild normocytic, normochromic anemia • Changes secondary to a hypometabolic state and/or congestive heart failure
Thyrotoxicosis	• Complete blood count • Erythrocyte sedimentation rate (ESR) • Electrocardiogram and/or echocardiogram	• Elevated white blood count (WBC) with some of the thyroid inflammatory conditions (e.g., subacute thyroiditis) • Elevated ESR with some of the thyroid inflammatory conditions (e.g., subacute thyroiditis) • Changes secondary to a hypermetabolic state and/or congestive heart failure
Thyroid Nodules	• Hypofunctioning gland (see Primary Hypothyroidism) • Hyperfunctioning gland (see Thyrotoxicosis) • Fine-needle aspiration (FNA) biopsy	• Benign, malignant, or suspicious/indeterminate

*Not usually indicated for confirming the diagnosis of thyroid disease but rather for assessing target organ damage.

III. Assessment

A. Determine the diagnosis

1. Primary hypothyroidism
2. Hyperthyroidism
3. Thyroid neoplasms (benign or malignant)
4. Other conditions that may explain the patient's presentation
   a. Pituitary disease
   b. Hypothalamic disease
   c. Cardiovascular disease
   d. Extrathyroidal malignancy
   e. Psychiatric disorder

B. Severity
Assess the severity of the disease.

C. Significance and motivation

1. Assess the significance of the problem to the patient and significant others.
2. Determine the patient's willingness and ability to follow the treatment plan.

IV. Goals of clinical management

A. Screening or diagnosing thyroid disease
Choose a cost-effective approach for screening or diagnosing thyroid disease.

B. Treatment
Select a treatment plan that returns the patient to a euthyroid state in a safe and effective manner.

C. Patient adherence
Select an approach that maximizes patient adherence.

V. Plan

A. Screening
Some major authorities (Garber et al., 2012) recommend screening for high-risk populations (adults > 35 years of age, older women, individuals with autoimmune diseases or a strong family history of thyroid diseases). However, the U.S. Preventive Services Task Force (2014) has noted that there is insufficient evidence to support routine screening

TABLE 68-4 The Assessment of Thyroid Dysfunction

Order the highly sensitive thyroid-stimulating hormone (TSH) test		
↓	↓	↓
Normal TSH→ Are secondary causes of hypothyroidism suspected?	Increased TSH→ Order a serum FT_4	Decreased TSH→ Order a serum FT_4
No→ No further testing is indicated. The patient is clinically euthyroid.	Decreased FT_4—primary hypothyroidism	Increased FT_4—primary hyperthyroidism→ order anti-TSH receptor antibodies • If the antibodies are elevated, the person has an autoimmune thyroid disease (e.g. Graves' disease). • If the antibodies are normal, the patient probably has a nonimmune mediated form of thyrotoxicosis (e.g., toxic uninodular goiter). • Consult with a physician to determine the need for a thyroid scintiscan
Yes→ Order a serum FT_4	Increased FT_4—pituitary (TSH-induced) thyrotoxicosis	Normal FT_4—subclinical hyperthyroidism or a rare form of primary hyperthyroidism called T_3 toxicosis→ Does the patient have signs and symptoms consistent with thyrotoxicosis?
Decreased FT_4—Consult with a physician to determine the necessity for a thyrotropin-releasing hormone (TRH) stimulation test (a test for assessing the hypothalamic-pituitary function).	Normal FT_4—subclinical hypothyroidism→ order thyroid peroxidase antibodies. • If the antibodies are elevated, the person has compensated chronic Hashimoto's thyroiditis (subclinical hypothyroidism). • If the antibodies are normal, consult with a physician to determine the necessity for a TRH stimulation test.	Yes→ Order FT_3 • Increased FT_3—T_3 toxicosis • Consult with a physician to determine the need for a thyroid scintiscan • Normal→ Consult with a physician for other diagnostic considerations

Reproduced from Saxe, J. M. (2004). Thyroid diseases. In W. L. Star, L. Lommel, & M. Shannon (Eds.), *Women's primary health care: Protocols for practice* (2nd ed., pp. 10-33–10-39). San Francisco, CA: UCSF Nursing Press. Reassessed and adapted from Fischbach & Dunning (2014) and Jameson & Weetman (2012). Used with permission from the UCSF Nursing Press.

for thyroid disease in adults. If the clinician determines that screening for thyroid disease is indicated for an individual, the initial screening test should be the highly sensitive TSH because it is more sensitive and specific than the FT_4 and the FT_4I (Jameson & Weetman, 2012). If the highly sensitive TSH is high or low, the clinician should use the suggested diagnostic approach in **Table 68-4**.

B. Diagnostic tests

See Tables 68-2 and 68-3 for the description of relevant diagnostic studies and Table 68-4 for the suggested approach for the assessment of thyroid dysfunction.

1. Common thyroid studies may include, but are not limited to highly sensitive TSH, free T_4 (FT_4), free total T_3 (FT_3), serum antithyroid antibodies (including antithyroperoxidase antibodies and TSH receptor antibodies), radioactive iodine uptake, and thyroid scintigraphy.

2. Thyroid ultrasonography is indicated for an individual who has a neck mass of questionable thyroid origin.

3. Fine-needle aspiration is necessary to rule out a cancerous nodule.

4. Extrathyroidal diagnostic studies are warranted for assessing the status of other systems that may be affected by altered thyroid functions (Table 68-3).

C. Management (includes treatment, consultation, referral, and follow-up care)

1. Primary hypothyroidism
   a. Eliminate, if possible, medications (e.g., lithium) or exposures (work-related radiation) that may negatively affect the thyroid gland.
   b. Arrange a hospital admission for patients with severe cardiopulmonary compromise.
   c. Begin oral replacement with L-thyroxine.
      i. Suggested initial dosing for a young adult without cardiac disorders: 50–100 mcg/day.
      ii. Suggested initial dosing for an elder or an individual with heart conditions: 25 mcg/day.
   d. Increase dosage by 25–50 mcg every 4–6 weeks until the person's highly sensitive TSH is within normal parameters. The usual replacement dose is 1.6–1.7 mcg/kg/day for adults (Cooper et al., 2011).
   e. Sustain a full replacement of L-thyroxine, which is usually 100–150 mcg daily.
   f. Check the person's highly sensitive TSH every 6–12 months or as needed to assess the response to chronic therapy and to determine the need for any adjustment in daily doses (Slovik, 2014b).

2. Hyperthyroidism
   a. Reduce the intake of iodine if thought to be a contributing factor.
   b. Start the use of β-blocking agents (e.g., propranolol, 20 mg every 6 hours) to blunt the symptoms and signs of hyperthyroidism (e.g., palpitations, heat intolerance, nervousness, and tremor) (Slovik, 2014a).
   c. Consult with a physician for the use and dosing of antithyroid agents (e.g., thionamide drugs, such as methimazole, PTU, or iodide). PTU should be given to pregnant women because methimazole can cause congenital defects. It is also recommended to give PTU to lactating women because methimazole is excreted in human milk. Although the thionamide drugs have an overall low rate of serious adverse effects, hepatotoxicity, vasculitis, and agranulocytosis are the most serious adverse sequelae. PTU is more likely to cause fulminant hepatic failure and vasculitis than methimazole. Cholestatic jaundice is more likely to occur with methimazole than PTU. An autoimmune agranulocytosis can occur with both agents. Iodide is usually reserved for individuals in thyroid storm and for those being prepared for thyroid surgery (Katz, 2015).
   d. Refer the patient to a physician specialist for ablative therapy with radioactive agents (e.g., radioactive iodine) or subtotal thyroidectomy.
   e. Facilitate a hospital admission for the person with severe cardiopulmonary compromise.
   f. Assess TSH levels annually or as needed after the individual is in remission to determine the adequacy of treatment and the earliest evidence of overtreatment (evidence of hypothyroidism). If the values are abnormal, assess the FT_4 or serum T_3 levels. TSH receptor antibodies should also be obtained if the individual has Graves' disease. Consult with or refer to a physician for additional treatment if these tests are abnormal (Slovik, 2014a).
   g. Screen and treat for osteoporosis in women with hyperthyroidism.

3. Thyroid nodules
   a. Refer the patient with a solitary nodule or a dominant nodule within a multinodular gland to a physician for further diagnostic evaluation (fine-needle aspiration and possible thyroid scintigraphy) and for therapeutic interventions (e.g., L-thyroxine suppressive or replacement therapy or surgical therapy).
   b. Stop goiter-producing medications, if possible (e.g., lithium).
   c. Use the hypothyroidism treatment guidelines (see the Management section) for the person with a hypofunctioning multinodular goiter (e.g., chronic thyroiditis).
   d. Use the hyperthyroidism treatment guidelines (see the Management section) for the individual with a toxic multinodular goiter.

D. Patient education

1. Information
   Provide verbal and, preferably, written information regarding:
   a. Risk reduction and screening (e.g., stress management and relapse prevention in autoimmune-mediated hyperthyroidism, and osteoporosis screening for women with hyperthyroidism).
   b. The disease process, including signs and symptoms and underlying etiologies.
   c. Diagnostic tests that include a discussion about preparation, cost, the actual procedures, and after-care.
   d. Management (rationale, action, use, drug interactions, side effects, associated risks, and cost of therapeutic interventions; and the need for adhering to long-term treatment plans) (Saxe, 2004).

2. Counseling: preconception counseling as indicated.

VI. Self-management resources and tools

A. Patient and client education

1. American Thyroid Association

   The American Thyroid Association's (2015) website has patient and client education brochures and frequently asked question documents in English and Spanish. The documents, albeit useful and accurate, have an average grade 9–10 reading level via the Flesch-Kincaid assessment tool. Additionally, there are very few photographs, figures, or graphs to facilitate further understanding of challenging concepts.

2. Geisinger's Health Library (powered by Krames online)

   The Geisinger's Health Library (2015) includes consumer-friendly resources on common thyroid problems. The Flesch-Kincaid reading level is approximately grade 7. This educational resource includes colorful illustrations and culturally appropriate images.

B. Community support groups

1. Thyroid-Info

   Thyroid-Info has support groups postings (e.g., How to start a thyroid support group: tips on creating a support organization in your area [Shomon, 2015]).

REFERENCES

American Thyroid Association. (2015). ATA patient education. Retrieved from www.thyroid.org/patient-thyroid-information/ata-patient-education-web-brochures/.

Cooper, D. S., Greenspan, F. S., & Ladenson, P. W. (2011). The thyroid gland. In D. G. Gardner & D. Shoback (Eds.), *Greenspan's basic and clinical endocrinology* (9th ed., Chap. 7). Retrieved from http://accessmedicine.mhmedical.com/content.aspx?bookid=380&sectionid=39744038.

Fischbach, F., & Dunning, M. B., III (2014). *A manual of laboratory and diagnostic tests* (9th ed.). Philadelphia, PA: Wolters Kluwer/Lippincott Williams & Wilkins.

Garber, J. R., Cobin, R. H., Gharib, H., et al. (2012). Clinical practice guidelines for hypothyroidism in adults: Cosponsored by the American Association of Clinical Endocrinologists and the American Thyroid Association. Retrieved from www.thyroid.org/thyroid-guidelines/hypothyroidism/.

Geisinger's Health Library. (2015). Common thyroid problems. Retrieved from www.geisinger.kramesonline.com/3,S,82164.

Hollowell, J. G., Staehling, N. W., Flanders, W. D., Hannon, W. H., Gunter, E. W., Spencer, C. A., et al. (2002). Serum TSH, T, and thyroid antibodies in the United States population (1988 to 1994). National Health and Nutrition Examination Survey (NHANES III). *Journal of Clinical Endocrinology and Metabolism, 87*(2), 489–499.

Howlader, N., Noone, A. M., Krapcho, M., Garshell, J., Miller, D., Altekruse, S. F., et al. (Eds.). (2014). *SEER cancer statistics review, 1975–2011*. Bethesda, MD: National Cancer Institute. Retrieved from http://seer.cancer.gov/archive/csr/1975_2011/.

Jameson, J. L., & Weetman, A. P. (2012). Disorders of the thyroid gland. In A. S. Fauci, E. D. L. Longo, A. S. Fauci, D. L. Kasper, S. L. Hauser, J. L. Jameson, et al. (Eds.), *Harrison's principles of internal medicine* (18th ed., Chapter 341). Retrieved from http://accessmedicine.mhmedical.com/content.aspx?bookid=331&sectionid=40727146.

Katz, M. D. (2015). Thyroid disorders. In M. A. Chisholm-Burns, T. L. Schwinghammer, B. G. Wells, P. M. Malone, J. M. Kolesar, & J. T. DiPiro (Eds.), *Pharmacotherapy: Principles & practice* (3rd ed., Chapter 44). New York: McGraw-Hill Medical.

Saxe, J. M. (2004). Thyroid diseases. In W. L. Star, L. L. Lommel, & M. T. Shannon (Eds.), *Women's primary health care: Protocols for practice* (2nd ed., pp. 10-33–10-39). San Francisco, CA: UCSF Nursing Press.

Shomon, M. (2015). *How to start a thyroid support group: Tips on creating a support organization in your area*. Retrieved from www.thyroid-info.com/articles/supportgroup.htm..

Slovik, D. M. (2014a). Approach to the patient with hyperthyroidism. In A. H. Goroll & A. G. Mulley (Eds.), *Primary care medicine: Office evaluation and management of the adult patient* (7th ed., Chapter 103). Philadelphia, PA: Wolters Kluwer Health.

Slovik, D. M. (2014b). Approach to the patient with hypothyroidism. In A. H. Goroll & A. G. Mulley (Eds.), *Primary care medicine: Office evaluation and management of the adult patient* (7th ed., Chapter 104). Philadelphia, PA: Wolters Kluwer Health.

U.S. Preventive Services Task Force (2014). Evidence summary: Thyroid dysfunction screening. Retrieved from www.uspreventiveservicestaskforce.org/Page/SupportingDoc/thyroid-dysfunction-screening/evidence-summary7.

Vanderpump, M. P. J. (2011). The epidemiology of thyroid disease. *British Medical Bulletin, 99*, 39–51.

Wang, C., & Crapo, L. M. (1997). The epidemiology of thyroid disease and implications for screening. *Endocrinology and Metabolism Clinics of North America, 26*(1), 189–218.

Ward, E. M., Jemal, A., & Chen, A. (2010). Increasing incidence of thyroid cancer: Is diagnostic scrutiny the sole explanation? *Future Oncology, 6*(2), 185–188. Retrieved from http://www.futuremedicine.com/doi/pdf/10.2217/fon.09.161.

69

UPPER BACK AND NECK PAIN SYNDROMES

Rossana Segovia

I. Introduction and general background

The cervical and thoracic spine can be the source of many pain syndromes that affect the neck, the thorax, and the upper extremities. Given their anatomical proximity and the frequency of misattribution of the symptom origin, the purpose of this chapter is to focus on the most common cervical and thoracic pain syndromes.

The cervical (C) spine is a complex structure composed of vertebrae, intervertebral discs, joints, the spinal cord, nerve roots, blood vessels, muscles, and ligaments. The atlanto-occipital joints (C0–C1) are the two uppermost joints, which are responsible for flexion, extension, and side flexion. The atlantoaxial joint (C1–C2) is the most mobile joint of the spine, rotation being its primary movement. The facet joints, also known as apophyseal joints, allow flexion and extension. This mobility can cause degeneration, most often seen at the C4–C7 levels.

About 25% of the height of the cervical spine is from the intervertebral discs, which are responsible for the spine's lordotic shape. The nucleus pulposus of the disc acts as a cushion to axial compression; the disc's annulus fibrosus withstands tension within the disc. The cervical vertebrae support the weight of the head and neck (approximately 15 lb.). The vertebral arch protects the spinal cord. Cervical nerve roots are named for the vertebra below each root (e.g., the C5 nerve root is between C4 and C5 vertebrae). In the rest of the spine, the nerve root is named for the vertebra above (Magee, 2002).

Given the cervical spine's complex structure, it is vulnerable to injuries and disorders that produce pain and restrict mobility. Neck pain is generally perceived as originating from the inferior aspect of the occiput and the superior aspect of the last cervical vertebra. This forms an imaginary line that is called the "nuchal line" (Bogduk, 2003). The causes of neck pain are various and can be classified as acute (duration ≤ 3 months) or chronic (lasting ≥ 3 months).

The most common cause of neck pain is mechanical injury, often caused by everyday activities such as poor posture, repetitive movements, or nonergonomic work stations. More serious injuries, such as acute trauma or injury, can occur during sports or motor vehicle accidents (MVAs).

Nonmechanical causes of pain are less common and are often of an inflammatory or infectious nature, often presenting with "red flags" that should be considered in any differential of neck pain. Other causes of neck pain that should not be overlooked include referred pain and other visceral conditions that can present acutely. Women seem to have an increased incidence of spinal conditions, such as scoliosis in adolescence, osteoporosis with vertebral body fractures, and increased kyphosis after menopause. Men, however, have an increased incidence of kyphosis in adolescence and ankylosing spondylitis in adulthood (Green, 2001).

The anatomical arrangement provides for structural protection for the vital organs of the heart, lungs, and liver. It also forms a cavity for the lungs to expand and contract safely (Magee, 2008). The thoracic spine has very limited motion because the ribs are very firmly attached to both the posterior spine and the sternum anteriorly.

The lower three ribs do not join together anteriorly but do function to protect the vital organs while still allowing for slightly more motion. The joints between the thoracic vertebra (T12) and the lumbar vertebra (L1) allow for twisting movements from side to side. Although the thoracic spine is relatively stable due to its solid construction, this does not prevent it from being a source of radicular symptoms and pain.

Muscular thoracic pain is mostly caused by irritation or tension of the muscles, such as myofascial pain. The cause of this pain may be poor posture, mechanical injury, or referred pain from the neck. Joint dysfunction where the ribs attach to the spine can also be a source of symptoms in the thoracic spine. Genetic or injury-related conditions such as vertebral fractures, kyphosis, and scoliosis can also greatly affect the individual's well-being. Compression fractures of the vertebra at the thoracic level can be due to osteoporosis especially in the elderly.

Kyphosis and scoliosis in the thoracic area can be due to poor posture or deformity causing a great deal of chronic pain.

Some common spinal disorders, such as a herniated disc, spinal stenosis, degenerative disc disease, or spinal instability, are not as common in the thoracic spine due to the great stability of this section of the spine.

A. Mechanical spine disease (acute)

1. Definition and overview
   a. Cervical spine pain: Cervical spine problems that provoke pain account for thousands of primary care evaluations each year. Most patients suffer from acute cervical strains or osteoarthritis (OA). Neck pain can be caused by muscle strains, ligament sprains, arthritis, or nerve impingement. Most strains and sprains recover in 2–4 weeks with conservative treatment. Arthritic neck pain also often responds to medication and physical therapy in the acute phase. Acute musculoskeletal neck pain is a common problem in the general population that is frequently evaluated in emergency departments. About 71% of Americans remember at least one episode of neck pain or stiffness during their lifetimes (McReynolds & Sheridan, 2005).
   b. Thoracic spine pain: The thoracic spine has not been studied as much as the cervical or lumbar spine in regard to both genetic and epidemiologic studies. However, pain in the thoracic spine can be just as disabling, causing major physical burdens on the individual and his or her participation in the workforce (Briggs, Smith, Straker, & Bragge, 2009). Conditions such as osteoporosis, hyperkyphosis, and ankylosing spondylitis have been linked to thoracic spine pain and dysfunction (Briggs, Smith, et al., 2009). Other common conditions such as thoracic nerve impingement often correlate with the size and location of the disc herniation. Occupations and recreational activities that require prolonged sitting may predispose individuals to thoracic spinal pain. For example, there was an 8% incidence of exertional thoracic pain compared to 10% in lumbar spine pain in an army military training program. Additionally, there was a 15% prevalence of thoracic pain or chest discomfort compared to 47% of lumbar pain or stiffness in a group of sportsmen. Lastly, there was a 28% prevalence of thoracic pain in bus drivers compared to 10% in nondrivers (Manchikanti, Singh, Datta, Cohen, & Hirsch, 2009).

2. Prevalence and incidence
   a. Cervical spine pain:
      Neck pain is a common condition and the prevalence rises with age. Lifetime prevalence of neck pain is estimated at 71%. Twelve to 34% of adults experience neck pain annually. Neck pain is especially common in the middle-aged population, with the prevalence of shoulder and neck pain being highest by ages 45 to 60. Pain from the shoulder and neck region now seems to occur more frequently (Ostergren et al., 2005). According to an article in *Pain Physician* journal, the prevalence of cervical facet joint pain in patients with chronic pain after whiplash has been determined to be 54% to 60% (Manchikanti, Singh, Rivera, & Panpati, 2002).

      A study by Gordon, Trott, and Grimmer (2002) reported the prevalence of cervical pain and stiffness to be between 9.5% and 71% of the population. Furthermore, the study pointed out that one in every five patients who went to an orthopedist suffers from a cervical syndrome. In both the United States and Japan, cervical pain syndrome is the second most common cause for consultations and in pain clinics (Gordon et al., 2002).

   b. Thoracic spine pain: There is limited research on prevalence and risk factors for thoracic spine disorders, which may provoke a belief that the clinical and public health significance of thoracic spine disorders is less compared to other spinal levels. However, it has been countered in some of the literature that there is a need for research on thoracic pain and disorders especially in the young population. There is also evidence to suggest that pain or dysfunction in the thoracic spine is not uncommon in the adult population (Briggs, Smith, et al., 2009).

      There have been reports describing 3% to 23% of patients evaluated in interventional pain management settings have acute thoracic pain syndromes. A prevalence of thoracic pain was estimated in 13% of the population compared to 43% in the lumbar spine and 44% in the cervical spine during a 1-year period when this study was done (Manchikanti et al., 2009).

      A survey of factory workers found a 5% prevalence of thoracic pain, which did not show any association with age. This evaluation also showed the prevalence of cervical and lumbar pain to be 24% and 34%, respectively, with increasing prevalence with age in both cases (Manchikanti et al., 2009).

B. Cervicothoracic myofascial pain syndrome

1. Definition and overview
   Myofascial pain syndrome is also known as regional pain syndrome, which is characterized by hyperirritability areas in the body called trigger points. These

trigger points arise from taut bands in the skeletal muscle. The syndrome usually accompanies some peculiar pain pattern that is specific to the muscle area involved. Eventually, the muscle becomes weak and stiff, due to the chronicity of the symptoms, which leads to decreased range of motion. This pain is usually undertreated due to the lack of awareness of the clinicians (Jalil, Awang, & Omar, 2009).

Not all of the motor and sensory symptoms of myofascial pain syndrome have to be present in order to be clinically diagnosed. The presence of the taut band with its zone of tenderness in the muscle involved is one important feature of myofascial pain that distinguishes it from other types of muscle pain. The ability to reproduce pain in the individual while examining the tender zone and its taut band is very important (Gerwin, 2001).

a. Primary and secondary cervicothoracic myofascial pain syndrome: In an unpublished article by Gerwin (2001), it was reported that 100% of the individuals with chronic tension-type headaches and migraine symptoms of nausea and photosensitivity had active myofascial trigger point pain. Neck and shoulder muscles such as sternocleidomastoid, scalenes, levator scapulae, trapezius, suboccipital, and posterior cervical muscles can directly cause neck pain. Postural stress, such as forward head and anteriorly rotated shoulders, is a known factor causing trigger point related neck pain.

Both shoulder pain and decreased or restricted range of motion can be directly related to primary trigger point myofascial pain due to overuse of certain muscles. For example, the subscapularis muscle can be triggered by poor body posture, biomechanics, and injury.

b. Cervical whiplash: Cervical whiplash injuries can become chronic pain in 20–40% of cases and 50% of these cases are related to injury to one or more cervical facet joints (Gerwin, 2001).

c. Chronic myofascial cervical and/or thoracic pain syndrome: Chronic myofascial pain syndrome involves other muscles groups and regions because of stresses that develop along the skeletal chain.

When a muscle in this functional unit does not work effectively due to tender trigger points it becomes weak and loses its ability to lengthen, which allows for a normal range of motion. This in turn creates a chain reaction and the other muscles try to compensate for this loss and become overused and chronically shortened (Gerwin, 2001).

2. Prevalence and incidence
Unfortunately, the prevalence of myofascial pain syndrome in the general population is not known. It has been reported that separating myofascial trigger points into active and inactive states causes epidemiologic confusion. The prevalence between active and inactive clinical conditions is greater in the later. Myofascial pain studies making a distinction between these two clinical conditions are few. These studies do not usually address the prevalence of inactive clinical conditions. There are also no specific data on the prevalence among women and men (Gerwin, 2001).

C. Scalene muscle pain and thoracic outlet syndrome

1. Definition and overview
Both scalene muscle pain and thoracic outlet syndrome have been overlooked by providers due to their characteristics of symptoms mimicking cervical radiculopathy resulting from herniated discs. These have also been associated with other neuropathic diseases such as carpal tunnel syndrome and peripheral polyneuropathy due to their presentation of referred pain to the distal extremities.

a. Scalene myofascial pain syndrome: Scalene myofascial pain syndrome is a regional pain that originates over the neck area and radiates down to the arm. It may present as primary or secondary to underlying cervical pathology.

b. Thoracic oulet syndrome: Thoracic outlet syndrome is caused by compression of nerves or blood vessels in the thoracic outlet, which includes the area between the neck and the axilla including the anterior shoulders and anterior chest. An important distinction that has been identified in studies is the categorization of vascular versus neurogenic presentations (Hooper, Denton, McGalliard, Brismee, & Sizer, 2010).

2. Prevalence and incidence
a. Scalene myofascial pain syndrome: In one study it was found that 31% of patients complaining of scalene muscle pain had acute trigger points, which have been also described in all age groups and in both sexes. The syndrome most often occurs between the ages of 30 and 60 years; prevalence declines with advancing age. A study done in the 1950s studied asymptomatic Air Force recruits and found tender spots indicative of latent trigger points in 54% of the women and 45% of the men. The study also noted referred pain with palpation in 5% of the recruits (Fomby & Mellion, 1997).

b. Thoracic outlet syndrome: A survey done in 2009 on factory workers and their prevalence of thoracic pain demonstrated a 5% prevalence of thoracic pain, which was not associated with age. The same authors demonstrated a prevalence of 24% cervical pain and 34% lumbar pain, which were associated with increased age (Manchikanti et al., 2009).

Thoracic outlet syndrome is generally diagnosed between 20 and 50 years of age; however, it can be found in teenagers and most rarely in children. Neurogenic thoracic outlet syndrome is found three to four times more commonly in women compared to the vascular type, which is more equal between nonathletic women and men. This, however, is not the same in athletic individuals in whom there is a greater incidence in men than women (Hooper et al., 2010).

D. Osteoarthritis

1. Definition and overview

a. Osteoarthritis (OA) (also called degenerative joint disease or osteoarthrosis): OA is the most common form of arthritis and occurs when cartilage in the joints wears down over time. There is no cure but treatment can relieve pain and help patients maintain their activities of daily living.

Spondylosis is degeneration of the discs and vertebrae causing compression of the spinal cord in the neck. OA is the most common cause, most often affecting middle-aged and older people. This is the most common cause of spinal cord dysfunction in the older than 55 population (Steinberg, Akins, & Baran, 1999).

2. Prevalence and Incidence

In a study by Hirpara, Butler, Dolan, O'Byrne, & Poynton (2012), it was noted that the prevalence of cervical spondylosis is similar for both sexes, although the degree of severity is greater for males. Moreover, spondylotic changes in the cervical spine occurred at solitary disc space levels in about 15–40% of patients; however, in 60–85% of patients, this occurred at multiple levels. Furthermore, the discs between the third and seventh cervical vertebrae are most commonly affected. Repeated occupational trauma may also contribute to the development of cervical spondylosis. For example, there was an increased incidence in patients who carried heavy loads on their heads or shoulders as well as in dancers, gymnasts, and patients with spasmodic torticollis (Hirpara et al., 2012).

E. Strains and sprains

1. Definition and overview

Musculoskeletal strains and sprains (sports or work related) occur when there is an injury to the muscles of the neck caused by prolonged or repetitive neck extension or flexion. This is often related to poor posture at work, such as repetitive leaning or bending of the neck, and nonergonomic work stations, or during hobbies, such as knitting or crocheting. Repetition of the motion causes constant insult to the affected area and prevents healing (Steinberg et al., 1999).

2. Prevalence and incidence

According to a recent study published by Cohen, "neck pain is the fourth leading cause of disability, with an annual prevalence rate exceeding 30%" (2015, p. 284). This rate includes all types of causes of neck pain; however, most episodes of acute neck pain will resolve with or without treatment as in the case of strains. "Nearly 50% of individuals will continue to experience some degree of pain or frequent occurrences" (Cohen, 2015, p. 284).

A review article done by Briggs et al. (2009) reported the range of prevalence estimates of thoracic back pain in the general population to be very broad because of many factors, including the different types and causes as well as duration. These data ranged from 4.0–72.0% (at any one time), 0.5–51.4% (7 days), 1.4–34.8% (1 month), 4.8–7.0% (3 month), 3.5–34.8% (1 year), and 15.6–19.5% (lifetime). There was a higher prevalence for thoracic back pain in children and adolescents, especially for females. In children and adolescents, thoracic back pain was associated with female gender, postural changes associated with backpack use, backpack weight, other musculoskeletal symptoms, participation in specific sports, chair height at school, and difficulty with homework. In adults, thoracic back pain was associated with other concurrent musculoskeletal symptoms and difficulty in performing activities of daily living (Briggs et al., 2009).

F. Spinal deformities

1. Definition and overview

Spinal deformities refers to conditions in which the spine has an abnormal curvature or alignment. The two most common spinal deformities are scoliosis and hyperkyphosis.

a. Scoliosis: Scoliosis is defined as a lateral curvature of the spine that may occur in children or adults. Scoliosis may cause back pain, abnormal gait, uneven hips, and different leg lengths for adolescents and even more severe symptoms when found in adults. Most cases of scoliosis are mild, but some children develop spine deformities that continue to get more severe as they grow. Severe scoliosis can be disabling. An especially severe spinal curve can reduce the amount of space within the chest, making it difficult for the lungs to function properly. There are four types of scoliosis:

i. Congenital scoliosis, caused by a bone abnormality present at birth.

ii. Neuromuscular scoliosis is the result of abnormal muscles or nerves. Most frequently seen in people with spina bifida or cerebral palsy or in people with various conditions that are accompanied by, or result in, paralysis.

iii. Degenerative scoliosis may result from traumatic injury or illness such as bone collapse, previous major back surgery, or osteoporosis.

iv. Idiopathic scoliosis is the most common type of scoliosis and has no specific identifiable cause. There are many theories, but none have been found to be conclusive. There is, however, strong evidence that idiopathic scoliosis is inherited (National Institute of Arthritis and Musculoskeletal and Skin Diseases, 2015).

b. Hyperkyphosis: The forward bend of the spine is called kyphosis and is considered to be "failure of formation or failure of segmentation" of the front aspect of one or more vertebral bodies or discs that occurs during the embryonic development. It is usually a convex curvature of the spine that causes "hunchback" and other degrees of spinal distress depending on the degree of curvature and location in the spine. There are three types of kyphosis: congenital, developmental, and traumatic.

There are two types of congenital kyphosis. Type I deformity is the failure of formation and failure of segmentation of a portion of one or more vertebral bodies that usually worsens with growth. The deformity is usually visible at birth as a lump or bump on the infant's spine. Type II deformity is the failure of segmentation that occurs as two or more vertebrae fail to separate and to form normal discs and rectangular bones. This type of kyphosis is often more likely to be diagnosed later, after the child is walking.

i. Developmental kyphosis is defined as hyperkyphosis and classified as either postural or structural in origin.

ii. Postural kyphosis is corrected when the patient stands up straight. Patients with postural kyphosis have no abnormalities in the shape of the vertebrae.

iii. Scheuermann's kyphosis is defined as rigid (structural) kyphosis because the front sections of the vertebrae grow slower than the back sections. This occurs during a period of rapid bone growth, usually between the ages of 12 and 15 years of age in males or a few years earlier in females.

iv. Traumatic kyphosis occurs most commonly in the thoracolumbar and lumbar regions. This type of kyphosis is most common in patients with severe neurologic deficits such as quadriplegia or paraplegia.

2. Prevalence and incidence

a. Spinal deformities

A 2005 study mentioned by the Bone and Joint Initiative (BJI), USA, reported that mild to severe adult scoliosis has a prevalence as high as 68% in healthy individuals aged 60 and older (Correa & Watkins-Castillo, n.d.). Many cases of degenerative scoliosis are undiagnosed, but elderly patients often seek care because of back and leg pain that may be caused by scoliosis and associated spinal stenosis. However, the prevalence of adult spinal deformity and scoliosis is not well established, with estimates ranging from 2.5% to 25% of the population.

"According to 2010 U.S. Census Population Estimate, there were 235,205,658 people in the U.S over the age of 18 years. Prevalence of adult scoliosis cited in the literature ranges from 2.5% to 60%, depending on severity" (Correa & Watkins-Castillo, n.d., para. 2). Moreover, a conservative estimate of 2.5% of the prevalence of adult scoliosis reported yields an incidence of a minimum of 5.88 million adults in the United States with adult scoliosis. In 2010–2011 alone, there were an estimated 1.61 million of these adults who received treatment either as an inpatient or outpatient. Estimates for prevalence of kyphosis was approximated to 17% as the primary diagnosis in hospital and emergency departments (Correa & Watkins-Castillo, n.d.).

II. Database (may include but is not limited to)

Because cervical, thoracic, and/or cervicothoracic pain are usually multifactorial, it is important to determine if the pain is caused by spinal or extra spinal (soft tissue) injury or a serious infectious or inflammatory disorder.

A. Subjective

1. History of presenting illness: Description of the pain including onset; location; duration; radiation;

character, quality, and timing; and aggravating and alleviating factors. Determine modifying factors, such as rest, activity, changes in position, course of symptoms, and accompanying symptoms, such as numbness, tingling, weakness, paresthesias, and incontinence. If a traumatic injury, determine the exact mechanism of the injury.

Additional important questions: Ask if pain with inspiration or expiration or both. Is the pain affected by coughing or sneezing or straining? Is there any particular posture that intensifies or eases the pain? Is the skin in the thoracic area intact? If a traumatic injury, determine the exact mechanism of the injury.

2. Past health history
   a. Medical illnesses: cardiovascular, diabetes mellitus, carpal tunnel syndrome, cancer, osteoporosis, rheumatoid arthritis, scoliosis, OA, fibromyalgia, herpes zoster, prior neck or low back disorders (work-related or not), motor vehicle accident, risk factors for aneurysm, infection, immuno-suppressive disorder, injection drug use, or trauma.
   b. Surgical history (prior surgery to cervical, shoulder, chest or lumbar spine, recent surgery)
   c. Exposure history (e.g., recent exposure to neurotoxins if paresthesias present)
   d. Medication history: medications for the symptoms or any other disorders
   e. Allergic reactions: to medications or food

3. Family history: history of any musculoskeletal disorders (e.g., scoliosis, kyphosis, spondylosis, stenosis)

4. Occupational and environmental history: a work history is important to establish work-relatedness. If working, type of work, specific tasks, frequency of task, length of time performing same task, and length of time doing the same jobs. Note ergonomics of work station, prior jobs, prior work-related injuries, and job satisfaction.

5. Personal and social history and health-related behaviors: housing situation (alone or accompanied), support system, smoking, drinking, substance use, and sexual lifestyle

6. Review of systems
   a. Constitutional signs and symptoms: fever, chills, weight loss, and poor appetite (infectious or malignancy)
   b. Ear, nose, and throat: worsening of neck pain when swallowing (esophageal disorders), headache, visual changes, nuchal rigidity (infectious or malignancy)
   c. Skin: rash, pain, numbness or tingling, itching in area
   d. Cardiac and pulmonary: cough, dyspnea, worsening with inspiration, chest pressure, pain, arm pain, anxiety, or diaphoresis (myocardial infarction, angina, or lung cancer)
   e. Abdomen: anorexia, nausea, vomiting, heart burn, gas/flatulence, and change in bowel function or stool function (gastrointestinal disorders)
   f. Musculoskeletal: active range of motion, activities of daily living, pain with or without movement, swelling, redness, warmth, clicking, or locking.
   g. Neurologic: depressive symptoms, fatigue, headaches (multifactorial mechanical pain), numbness, tingling, weakness, vertigo, or balance disturbances.

B. Objective

1. Physical examination findings (See **Tables 69-1** through **69-3**)

TABLE 69-1 Physical Examination Findings

Inspection	Overall spinal and total body posture to determine if asymmetry contributes to problems. Check for hyperkyphosis (round back, humpback, flat back or dowager's hump) and scoliosis and the level of the deformity. Observe for breathing patterns. Observe for chest deformities such as pigeon chest, funnel chest, or barrel chest.
	Observe for scapular and clavicular symmetry and muscle atrophy. Loss of cervical lordosis is present with painful acute sprains, fractures, and infectious or neoplastic processes.
Palpation	Palpate the spinous process to define the alignment of the spine. Determine tenderness level, muscle tightness, spasms. Palpation pressure provoking paresthesias or numbness and tingling. Palpate anterior and posterior thoracic area including neck and shoulders. Palpate the spinous process to define the alignment of the spine. C7 is the most prominent spinous process. Top of thyroid cartilage is parallel to C4, and the cricoids cartilage is parallel to C6. Paraspinous muscles, trapezii, the medial border of the scapula, and sternocleidomastoid muscles palpation may provoke tenderness.

TABLE 69-1 Physical Examination Findings *(Continued)*

Range of motion (ROM) *Stabilize the trunk so motion does not occur in the thoracic spine but in the neck only.*	Flexion and extension are estimated visually in degrees. Flexion limitation can also be measured as the distance the chin lacks in touching the sternum.
	Rotation and lateral bending of neck: the degree of motion is the angle between the vertical axis and midaxis of the face. Rotation is estimated in degrees. Limited range of motion of the neck is usually common and may present in all planes. Forward flexion (normal ROM 20–45 degrees) and extension (normal ROM 25–45 degrees). Flexion limitation can also be measured with a tape measure. Measure the spine while patient is in normal standing position from C7 to T12, then ask the patient to bend forward and measure again. A 2.7-cm (1.1-inch) difference in length is considered normal.
	Lateral flexion is about 20–40 degrees to each side. A tape measure can be used to measure the distance from the floor. The distance should be equal bilaterally. Rotation is about 35–50 degrees. Ask the patient either to cross the arms in front or place the hands on opposite shoulders and then rotate to both sides. To avoid lumbar and hip rotation, the patient can be asked to perform this part of the exam while sitting. Costovertebral expansion is measured by chest expansion using a measuring tape at the level of the fourth intercostal space. The patient is asked to exhale as much as possible to take the measurement. Then the patient is asked to inhale as much as possible and hold the breath while measuring again. The normal difference between the two is 3–7.5 cm (~1–2.75 inches).
Neurologic and motor	**Assess:** **C5 Level** Deltoid—C5 axillary nerve. (Abduct the shoulder to 90 degrees. Push down on the arm to resist activity of the deltoid. True weakness of this muscle should be a uniform giving way motion.) Biceps—C5–C6 musculocutaneous nerve (ask patient to flex the elbow in the supinated position against resistance). Biceps reflex. Sensation—lateral arm: axillary nerve. **C6 Level** Wrist extensor group—C6 radial nerve. Biceps—C6 musculocutaneous nerve brachioradialis reflex. Sensation—lateral forearm: musculocutaneous nerve. **C7 Level** Triceps—C7 radial nerve (patient supine and the shoulder flexed about 90 degrees, ask the patient to extend the elbow against resistance). Wrist flexor group—C7 median and ulnar nerves. Finger extensor—C7 radial nerve. Triceps reflex. Sensation—middle finger. **C8 Level** No reflex. Examination is limited to muscle strength and sensation tests. Finger flexors (stabilize the long, index, and little fingers in extension and ask the patient to flex the fingers as you apply resistance). Sensation—ring and little fingers of the hands and distal half of the forearm ulnar side. Neurologic examination is usually normal in cervical strain. Resisted isometric movements are a gross test and subtle alterations in strength are hard to determine. If the muscles tested have been injured, contracting them will provoke pain. This exam is done while the patient is in sitting position. The examiner must be standing with one leg behind the patient's buttocks and with the arms around the patient's chest and back (hugging). Tell the patient "don't let me move you" and proceed with forward flexion, extension, side flexion (right/left), and rotation (right/left). Nerve root tested, Flexion: T6–T12 Nerve root tested, Extension: T1–T12 Nerve root tested, Rotation and Side bending: T1–T12 and L1 Nerve root tested, Elevation of the ribs: C3–C8, T1–T12, and intercostals 2–5. Nerve root tested, Depression of the ribs: T6–T12, L1–L3.

Data from Magee, D. (2008). *Orthopedic physical assessment* (5th ed.). Musculoskeletal Rehabilitation Series. St. Louis, MO: Saunders Elsevier.

TABLE 69-2 Special Tests

Spurling test	Have patient extend the neck while tilting the head to the side. This narrows the neural foramen and increases or reproduces radicular arm pain that is associated with disc herniation or cervical spondylosis (Green, 2001).
Axial Loading Test (compression test)	Push down on the patient's head. This provokes neck pain in some patients with disc problems; however, increased low back pain indicates nonorganic finding (Green, 2001).
Hoffmann Test	With the patient relaxed in supine position and the hand cradled in the clinician's hand, flick the third fingernail and look for index finger and thumb flexion. If present, it is a sign of long-tract spinal cord involvement in the neck (Green, 2001).
Distraction Test	Place one hand with palm open under the patient's chin, the other hand on the occiput, gradually lift the head to remove its weight from the neck. If the patient experiences a relief in symptom, it demonstrates the effect of neck traction, by widening the neural foramen (Hoppenfeld, 1976).
Adson Test	Take the patient's radial pulse, abduct, extend, and externally rotate the patient's arm. Ask the patient to take a deep breath and to turn his or her head toward the arm being tested. If there is compression of the subclavian artery, you will feel a marked diminution or absence of the radial pulse (Hoppenfeld, 1976).
Passive Scapular Approximation Test	Have the patient lie prone while lifting the shoulder up and back to approximate the scapulae. If pain in this area, it indicates possible T1 or T2 nerve root problem on the side of where the pain originates.
First Thoracic Nerve Root Stretch Test	Have the patient abduct and pronate the arm to 90 degrees. There should be no complaints of symptoms during this motion. Have the patient fully flex the elbow and put the hand behind the neck. This movement stretches the ulnar nerve and T1 nerve root. If pain is triggered into the scapula or arm, this is a positive test for T1 nerve root. If the patient has upper extremity symptoms at the same time as the thoracic symptoms, upper extremity tension tests should be also considered to rule out referred symptoms from the thoracic area.
Sitting Arm Lift (SAL) Test	Have the patient sit on the exam table with the hands resting on the thighs. Ask the patient to lift one arm (unaffected side) for shoulder flexion with the arm straight and the thumb up. Repeat the same with the opposite arm. Ask the patient if one arm feels heavier to lift than the other. If the answer is yes, the first part of the test is positive. Ask the patient to repeat this movement several times while palpating the spinous process along the ribs noting if there is any shifting in movements of the ribs especially at 90 degrees. If any shifting of movement is noted, it is a positive test for the second part of this test. This test can also be used to check stabilization of the scapula.
Prone Arm Lift (PAL) Test	Have the patient lie prone with the arms overhead at about 140 degrees of flexion and fully supported on the exam table. Ask the patient to lift one arm 2 cm and then lower it. Repeat on the other side. If one arm is heavier than the other, it is considered a positive for that side of the arm. Rationale: used to assess the ability of the arm to take a load in a higher angle of the shoulder flexion. Useful testing patients who do overhead work activities or who complain of problems when lifting heavy loads.
Slump Test (Sitting Dural Stretch Test)	Patient should be sitting on the exam table. Patient is asked to slump (the spine flexes forward and the shoulders sag forward) while the examiner holds the chin and head of the patient erect. If no symptoms are produced, flex the neck of the patient and hold the head down; if no symptoms are produced, passively extend one of the patient's knees; if no symptoms are produced, passively dorsiflex the foot of the same leg. Reproduction of sciatic pain or symptoms is a positive slump test. This is repeated on the other side of the leg. Rationale: this maneuver increases the stress on the intercostal nerves. The pain is usually produced at the site of the injured area.

Data from Magee, D. (2008). *Orthopedic physical assessment* (5th ed.). Musculoskeletal Rehabilitation Series. St. Louis, MO: Saunders Elsevier.

TABLE 69-3 Referred Pain Patterns

Referred Pain Pattern	Muscle Involved
Spine to the line along the medial border aspect of the scapula	Iliocostalis muscle
Adjacent to the spine	Multifidus muscle
Scapular area to posterior anterior arm down to the fifth finger	Serratus superior muscle
Medial border of the arm to medial fourth and fifth fingers	Serratus posterior muscle
Lateral chest wall to lower medial border of the scapula	Serratus anterior muscle
Medial border of the scapula	Romboids muscle
Upper thoracic spine to medial border of the scapula	Trapezius muscle
Inferior angle of the scapula to posterior shoulder and iliac crest	Latissimus dorsi muscle
Neck/shoulder angle to posterior shoulder and along medial edge of the scapula	Levator scapula muscle

Data from Magee, D. (2008). *Orthopedic physical assessment* (5th ed.). Musculoskeletal Rehabilitation Series. St. Louis, MO: Saunders Elsevier.

III. Assessment

A. Determine the cause of the neck pain, if acute or chronic.

B. Determine if the patient needs immediate referral for consultation (e.g., progressive neurologic symptoms or fracture). (See *Table 69-4* for Red Flag Conditions.)

C. Determine if the condition is work related.

D. Assess the patient's ability to perform his or her usual activities.

E. Assess the patient's pain control and coping abilities.

TABLE 69-4 Red Flag Conditions

Presentation	Etiologies	Comments
Possible cauda equina syndrome	Possible tumor, fracture, or infection	
Saddle anesthesia	Major trauma, such as MVA or fall from height	Age > 50 or < 20
Recent onset of bladder dysfunction, such as urinary retention, increased frequency, or overflow incontinence	Tumor or minor trauma (even strenuous lifting in older or potentially osteoporotic patient)	
Severe or progressive neurologic deficit in the lower extremity Pain that worsens when supine; severe nighttime pain	Spinal infection: recent bacterial infection (e.g., urinary tract infection); intravenous drug abuse; or immune suppression (from steroids, transplant, or HIV), tumor/cancer	Assess for constitutional symptoms, such as recent fever or chills or unexplained weight loss
• Unexpected laxity of the anal sphincter or perianal or perineal sensory loss • Major motor weakness: quadriceps (knee extension weakness), ankle plantar flexors, evertors, and dorsiflexors (foot drop)	Nerve root impingement	

Data from U.S. Agency for Health Care Policy and Research. (1994). *Acute low back problems in adults: Assessment and treatment. Quick reference guide for clinicians: Clinical practice guideline #14.* Rockville, MD: Author.

IV. Goals of clinical management

A. Evidence-based management of the patient's cervical and/or thoracic pain presentation

B. Cost effective plan of treatment

C. Appropriate management of the patient's condition if work related

D. Selection of management approach that maximizes the patient's adherence to the plan of care

V. Plan

A. Diagnostic criteria non–red flag conditions (see **Table 69-5**)

B. Other diagnostic tests that may be included

1. Blood tests: erythrocyte sedimentation rate, rheumatoid factor, antinuclear antibody if suspecting systemic, infectious, and inflammatory conditions; cardiac enzymes, if indicated.

2. Tuberculosis screening (tuberculin skin test or QuantiFERON®) test, if indicated.

3. Imaging: cervical/thoracic spine radiograph series, shoulder radiograph series, chest radiograph if indicated based on clinical pulmonary presentation, computerized axial tomography, or magnetic resonance imaging if patient presents with soft tissue, disc signs and symptoms, and not responding to standard treatment within expected time period.

4. Electromyelogram or nerve conduction study to rule out other structures causing the neurologic symptoms when the diagnosis is unclear.

C. Treatment (see **Table 69-6**)

D. Patient education

1. Discuss nature of condition and expected time of recovery.

2. Discuss proper posture and body mechanics.

3. Explain proper use of supportive devices such as neck pillows.

4. Discuss need for a lifelong stretching and conditioning exercise program, including use of foam roller, for maintenance and prevention of further disability.

5. Discuss stress reduction techniques.

6. Discuss medication use and compliance and other symptom relief modalities.

7. If determined to be work elated, discuss process of reporting the injury to the employer and assuming care with the employer's occupational health system.

E. Follow-up (acute and chronic)

Follow-up time frame is based on the plan of care and acuity and severity of the patient's presentation. If imaging has been ordered, follow-up should be prompt to communicate the results to the patient. If patient is taken off work, appropriate follow-up is necessary to determine whether the patient is ready to return to work and at what capacity.

TABLE 69-5 Diagnostic Criteria Non–Red Flag Conditions

Probable Diagnosis	Mechanism	Common Symptoms	Common Signs	Tests and Results
Regional neck pain	Unknown	Diffuse pain	None	None indicated
Cervical strain	Flexion–extension or rotation force, blow to the head or neck	Neck pain, difficult or decreased motion	Limited range of motion because of pain	None indicated
Cervical nerve root compression with radiculopathy	Degenerative condition, trauma	Dermatomal sensory changes, motor weakness	Specific motor, sensory, and reflex changes	None indicated for 4–6 weeks, unless progressive motor weakness
Spinal stenosis	Older patients: degenerative disc disease Younger patients: congenital stenosis	Neck, shoulder, and posterior arm pain, paresthesias in the same distribution as the pain	Weakness of the shoulder girdle and upper arms Signs worse with extension, improved with flexion of the neck	Computed tomography or magnetic resonance imaging shows spinal stenosis

Data from Glass, L. S., & Harris, J. S. (2004). *Occupational medicine practice guidelines: Evaluation and management of common health problems and functional recovery in workers* (2nd ed.). Beverly Farms, MA: OEM Press.

TABLE 69-6 Clinical Characteristics and Management of Cervicothoracic Spine Pain

Condition	Clinical Characteristics	Management
Cervical strain and sprain	Most patients can report specific mechanism of injury. May not notice pain immediately but after several hours may have tightness in the neck. Some may report nausea. Physical examination may only show mild abnormalities. May have tenderness, edema, spasms, headaches, and dizziness. With moderate injuries may present with radicular symptoms.	Diagnostic work-up: cervical radiograph to rule out fracture or dislocation if suspected. Treatment: rest in comfortable position, soft cervical collar is appropriate for 1 or 2 days if in the acute phase. Cold packs applied for 15 minutes four to six times a day, then heat. May also alternate cold and heat if combination promotes better relief. Gentle stretches of the neck and shoulders (early movements of the stable spine promote recovery). Analgesics according to symptoms especially for nighttime pain. Muscle relaxants are appropriate in the acute phase to relieve spasms and aid with nighttime sleep. Physical therapy that includes cervical traction, massage, and ultrasound can be helpful especially in the first 4 weeks. Encourage early return to normal activities, including work if appropriate.
Acute disc herniation	Pain is usually aggravated by cough, sneeze, straining, and other activities that prolong static position of the neck, especially in flexion–extension and rotation. Lifting, pushing, and pulling may also aggravate the pain. Usually, there is tenderness to palpation of the spinous process. Distraction test relieves the pain; compression test increases the pain. Usually there are associated muscle spasms and trigger point tenderness.	Diagnostic work-up: radiograph may be normal or show degenerative disc disease. May need magnetic resonance imaging (MRI), CT, or electromyogram/nerve conduction studies (EMG/NCS) if indicated based on presenting symptoms. Treatment: conservative treatment in the acute phase, absent major progressing symptoms. Rest by limiting activities, soft pillows, elevation of the head of the bed, and soft collar. Physical therapy can be helpful and may possibly include traction as well as exercises for functional range of motion and strength. Heat or cold compress to the neck for 15 minutes as tolerated can also be recommended. Nonsteroidal anti-inflammatory drugs (NSAIDs) and muscle relaxants used in the acute phase. Patients should be reassured that most disc herniations resolve without residual problems. If symptoms do not resolve within 3–6 weeks, epidural injection may be appropriate depending on presentation of symptoms and degree of limitation on activities of daily living.
Chronic disc degeneration (spondylosis or osteoarthritis)	Most common presentations are stiffness and chronic pain that worsens with upright activity. Some patients may report grinding or popping in the neck region. Referred pain to shoulder and arm, paraspinous process spasms, headaches, fatigue, and sleep disturbances. Difficulty with basic activities of daily living.	Diagnostic tests: anteroposterior and lateral radiograph shows sclerosis in the intervertebral disc area with osteophytes (bone spurs) projecting anteriorly. Osteophytes may also project posteriorly causing stenosis of the cervical canal. Anterior subluxation of one vertebra over the other may also be appreciated. Degenerative findings usually at the C5–C6 and C6–C7 levels. Treatment: usually responsive to traction. NSAIDs and muscle relaxants are helpful especially at nighttime. Cervical pillow, cervical roll, and physical therapy. Epidural injection may also be appropriate. In chronic cases without resolution of major symptoms and with radicular involvement, decompression and fusion surgery may be appropriate.

(continues)

TABLE 69-6 Clinical Characteristics and Management of Cervicothoracic Spine Pain *(Continued)*

Condition	Clinical Characteristics	Management
Cervical radiculopathy	Patients present with neck pain along with radicular pain associated with numbness and paresthesias in the upper extremity along the distribution of the nerve root involved. Muscle spasms or fasciculations may also be present in the myotomes involved. Other symptoms may be weakness, lack of coordination, difficulty with handwriting and performing fine manipulative tasks, dropping objects, and decreased strength. If stenosis of the cervical canal, patient may present with lower extremity symptoms and bowel or bladder dysfunction.	Diagnostic tests: plain radiographs may identify spondylosis or degeneration of the disc and the facet. Magnetic resonance imaging or computed tomography with intrathecal contrast confirms the diagnosis. However, this is not routine care unless progressive symptoms. Electromyelogram or nerve conduction study helps determine the location of the neurologic dysfunction and is commonly used presurgically. Treatment: in most cases, it resolves spontaneously within 6–12 weeks. Nonnarcotic analgesic is usually helpful. May also use short course of oral steroids if appropriate. Physical therapy, which may include traction, is useful in the first 2–4 weeks.
Cervical fracture	Patient may present with severe neck pain, paraspinous muscle spasms, and point tenderness to the area of fracture. Pain radiates to the shoulder or arm and may be associated with radicular symptoms if nerve root involvement is present.	Diagnostic tests: Anteroposterior, lateral, and odontoid views are the standard. Lateral radiograph should include the occiput superiorly and the top of T1 inferiorly. Swimmer's view may also be indicated to visualize the cervicothoracic junction. If no fracture is seen, it should be evaluated for instability. Treatment: immobilization of cervical spine during transportation to emergency department. Patients whose initial radiograph was negative for fracture, but continues to have pain, may use cervical collar. Repeat radiograph if symptoms persist past 7–10 days. NSAIDs and analgesics are also appropriate.
Cervicothoracic myofascial syndrome	Deep aching pain in a muscle, pain that persists or worsens Cervical spine range of motion is often limited and painful May be described as lumpiness or painful bump in the trapezius or cervical paraspinal muscles Massage is often helpful, as is superficial heat Patient's sleep may be interrupted because of pain The cervical rotation required for driving is difficult to achieve Patient may describe pain radiating into the upper extremities, accompanied by numbness and tingling, making discrimination from radiculopathy or peripheral nerve impingement difficult Dizziness or nausea may be a part of the symptomatology The patient experiences typical patterns of radiating pain referred from trigger points	Diagnostic work-up: Diagnosis is typically made after diagnosis of cervical disc prolapse has been ruled out. + Spurling's test will indicate cervical disc prolapse. Cervical radiograph and MRI can be done to assist with ruling out cervical presentation. Treatment: Manual therapy such as myofascial trigger point massage or active release therapy (Edmondston & Singer, 1997). Trigger point injections. Acupuncture. Edgelow Program has been used for neurovascular entrapment of the upper extremity but also for physical rehabilitation for posture usually recommended by physical medicine specialties NSAIDs, muscle relaxants, foam roller, and heat therapy

TABLE 69-6 Clinical Characteristics and Management of Cervicothoracic Spine Pain *(Continued)*

Condition	Clinical Characteristics	Management
Scalene muscle pain	Pain in cervical region radiating to occiput, nuchal muscles, shoulders, and upper extremities Stiffness Tenderness to the trapezius, levator scapulae, rhomboids, supraspinatus, and infraspinatus. Unilateral neck/shoulder pain.	Diagnostic work-up: Same as previously. Treatment: Same as previously.
Thoracic outlet syndrome (TOS)	Symptoms are often vague and variable. Paresthesias from the neck to the shoulder, arm, medial forearm, and fingers. If vascular, intermittent swelling and discoloration of the arm. Aching, fatigue, and weakness. Symptoms can worsen if arm is in overhead position. Tenderness.	Diagnostic work-up: Venous ultrasound studies, Doppler ultrasound and angiography in the seated position for arterial TOS, EMG/NCS Treatment: Physical therapy, Edglow Program, NSAIDs, lifestyle changes, ergonomic changes. Surgical recommendation: Depending on nature of disease.
Scoliosis	Pain localized to area of deformity. Radicular pain, if associated with compression.	Diagnostic work-up: Weight-bearing full-length PA and lateral x-rays. EMG/NCS is rare but can be done if suspecting neuropathy. NSAIDs, exercise programs, swimming, bracing in children only. Physical therapy can be helpful as well if the condition is painful.
Hyperkyphosis	Pain related to activity if poor posture	Diagnostic work-up: Weight-bearing anterior-posterior and lateral x-rays. Treatment: Observation or exercise program and physical therapy. Bracing only in noncongenital situations. Surgery depending on severity of deformity.

Data from Green, W. B. (2001). *Essentials of musculoskeletal care* (2nd ed.). Rosemont, IL: American Academy of Orthopaedic Surgeons; Griffin, L. Y. (2005). *Essentials of musculoskeletal care* (3rd ed.). Rosemont, IL: American Academy of Orthopaedic Surgeons and American Academy of Pediatrics; Steinberg, G., Akins, C., & Baran, D. (1999). *Orthopaedics in primary care* (3rd ed.). Hagerstown, MD: Lippincott Williams & Williams.

VI. Self-management resources and tools

A. Patient and client education Internet-based materials

1. OrthoInfo, www.orthoinfo.org, for spine conditioning program exercises.

2. Dynamic Chiropractic, www.dynamicchiropractic.com, for corrective exercises for thoracic kyphosis.

3. National Institute of Arthritis and Musculoskeletal and Skin Diseases (NIAMS), www.niams.nih.gov/, for back pain management and exercises.

4. Neck Injuries and Disorders (U.S. National Library of Medicine, 2015): www.nlm.nih.gov/medlineplus/neckinjuriesanddisorders.html

5. Congenital kyphosis (Scoliosis Research Society, 2015):www.srs.org/patients-and-families/conditions-and-treatments/parents/kyphosis/congenital-kyphosis

6. Neck and back: http://orthoinfo.aaos.org/menus/spine.cfm Community support groups

7. WebMD® Health Community: http://exchanges.webmd.com

8. Back Pain Support Group: http://back-pain.supportgroups.com/

9. Healia Health Communities and Support Groups: http://us.wow.com/wiki/Healia

10. eHealth Forum: http://ehealthforum.com

REFERENCES

Agency for Health Care Policy and Research. (1994). *Acute low back problems in adults: Assessment and treatment. Quick reference guide for clinicians: Clinical practice guideline #14*. Rockville, MD: Author.

Bogduk, N. (2003). The anatomy and pathophysiology of neck pain. *Physical Medicine and Rehabilitation Clinics of North America, 14*(3), 455–472.

Briggs, A. M., Bragge, P., Smith, A. J., Govil, D., & Straker, L. M. (2009). Prevalence and associated factors for thoracic spine pain in the adult working population: A literature review. *Journal of Occupational Health, 51*(3), 177–192.

Briggs, A. M., Smith, A. J., Straker, L. M., & Bragge, P. (2009). Thoracic spine pain in the general population: Prevalence, incidence and associated factors in children, adolescents and adults. A systematic review. *BMC Musculoskeletal Disorders, 10*(77). doi: 10.1186/1471-2474-10-77

Cohen, S. P. (2015). Epidemiology, diagnosis, and treatment of neck pain. *Mayo Clinic Proceedings, 90*(2), 284–299.

Correa, A., & Watkins-Castillo, S. I. (n.d.). *Prevalence of adult scoliosis: Spinal curvature*. Bone and Joint Initiative USA. Retrieved from http://www.boneandjointburden.org/2014-report/iiid21/prevalence-adult-scoliosis.

Edmondston, S. J., & Singer, K. P. (1997). Thoracic spine: Anatomical and bio-mechanical considerations for manual therapy. *Manual Therapy, 2*(3), 132–143.

Fomby, E. W., & Mellion, M. B. (1997). Identifying and treating myofascial pain syndrome. *Physician and Sports Medicine, 25*(2), 67–75.

Furman, M., & Simon, J. (2009). *Cervical disc disease*. Retrieved from http://emedicine.medscape.com/article/305720-print.

Gerwin, R. D. (2001). Classification, epidemiology, and natural history of myofascial pain syndrome. *Current Pain Headache Reports, 5*(5), 412–420.

Glass, L. S., & Harris, J. S. (2004). *Occupational medicine practice guidelines: Evaluation and management of common health problems and functional recovery in workers* (2nd ed.). Beverly Farms, MA: OEM Press.

Gordon, S. J., Trott, P., & Grimmer, K. A. (2002). Waking cervical pain and stiffness, headache, scapular or arm pain: Gender and age effects. *Australian Journal of Physiotherapy, 48*(1), 9–15.

Green, W. B. (2001). *Essentials of musculoskeletal care* (2nd ed.). Rosemont, IL: American Academy of Orthopaedic Surgeons.

Griffin, L. Y. (2005). *Essentials of musculoskeletal care* (3rd ed.). Rosemont, IL: American Academy of Orthopaedic Surgeons and American Academy of Pediatrics.

Hirpara, K. M., Butler, J. S., Dolan, R. T., O'Byrne, J. M., & Poynton, A. R. (2012). Nonoperative modalities to treat symptomatic cervical spondylosis. *Advances in Orthopedics*. Retrieved from www.hindawi.com/journals/aorth/2012/294857/.

Hooper, T. L., Denton, J., McGalliard, M. K., Brismee, J-M., & Sizer, P. S. Jr. (2010). Thoracic outlet syndrome: A controversial clinical condition. Part 1: anatomy, and clinical examination/diagnosis. *Journal of Manual & Manipulative Therapy. 18*(2), 74–83.

Hoppenfeld, S. (1976). *Physical examination of the spine and extremities*. East Norwalk, CT: Appleton-Century-Crofts.

Jalil, N. A., Sulaiman, Z., Awang, M. S., & Omar, M. (2009). Retrospective review of outcomes of a multimodal chronic pain service in a major teaching hospital: A preliminary experience in Universiti Sains Malaysia. *Malaysian Journal of Medical Sciences, 16,* 55–65.

Magee, D. J. (2002). *Orthopedic physical assessment* (4th ed.). Philadelphia, PA: W.B. Saunders.

Magee, D. J. (2008). *Orthopedic physical assessment* (5th ed). *Musculoskeletal Rehabilitation Series*. St. Louis, Missouri, Saunders Elsevier.

Manchikanti, L., Singh, V., Datta, S., Cohen, S., & Hirsch, J. (2009). Comprehensive review of epidemiology, scope, and impact of spinal pain. *Pain Physician, 12*(4), E35–E70.

Manchikanti, L., Singh, V., Rivera, J., & Pampati, V. (2002). Prevalence of cervical facet joint pain in chronic neck pain. *Pain Physician, 5*(3), 243–249.

Mantyselka, P., Kautiainen, H., & Vanhala, M. (2010). Prevalence of neck pain in subjects with metabolic syndrome—A cross-sectional population-based study. *BMC Musculoskeletal Disorders, 11*(171). doi: 10.1186/1471-2474-11-171

McReynolds, T. M., & Sheridan, B. J. (2005). Intramuscular ketorolac versus osteopathic manipulative treatment in the management of acute neck pain in the emergency department: A randomized clinical trial. *Journal of the American Osteopathic Association, 105*(2), 57–68.

National Institute of Arthritis and Musculoskeletal and Skin Diseases. (2015). What causes scoliosis. Retrieved at http://www.niams.nih.gov/Health_Info/Scoliosis/default.asp#causes

Ostergren, P. O., Hanson, B. S., Balogh, I., Ektor-Andersen, J., Isacsson, A., Orbaek, P., et al. (2005). Incidence of shoulder and neck pain in a working population: Effect modification between mechanical and psychosocial exposures at work? Results from a one year follow up of the Malmö shoulder and neck study cohort. *Journal of Epidemiology and Community Health, 59*(9), 721–728.

Steinberg, G., Akins, C., & Baran, D. (1999). *Orthopaedics in primary care* (3rd ed.). Hagerstown, MD: Lippincott Williams & Williams.

Scoliosis Research Society. (2015). *Congenital kyphosis*. Retrieved from www.srs.org/patients-and-families/conditions-and-treatments/parents/kyphosis/congenital-kyphosis.

U.S. National Library of Medicine. (2015). *Neck injuries and disorders*. Retrieved from www.nlm.nih.gov/medlineplus/neckinjuriesanddisorders.html.

CHAPTER 70

UPPER EXTREMITY TENDINOPATHY: BICIPITAL TENDINOPATHY, LATERAL EPICONDYLITIS, AND DE QUERVAIN'S TENOSYNOVITIS

Barbara J. Burgel

I. Introduction and general background

Acute and chronic injury to upper extremity tendon structures is a common health condition, often called tendonitis, which implies an inflammatory process. However, most tendon disorders are thought to be degenerative and noninflammatory involving mechanical stress to tendon structures, and are often referred to as tendinopathies (Fedorczyk, 2012; McAuliffe, 2010; Sharma & Maffulli, 2005). Inflammation may be present in tendinopathies, but it is unclear whether inflammation is the primary cause or a response to stenosis or mechanical stress (McAuliffe, 2010). Common sites of tendinopathy in the upper extremity include the shoulder (e.g., bicipital tendinopathy), the elbow (e.g., lateral epicondylitis/epicondylalgia/epicondylosis or elbow tendinopathy), and the wrist (e.g., de Quervain's tenosynovitis/tendinopathy).

Tendons connect muscles to bones and "provide the interface to transmit muscle force to bone to create joint movement" (Fedorczyk, 2012, p. 191). There are two tendon sites at risk for acute or cumulative injury: the myotendinous junction, where the muscle and tendon join, identified as the weakest point of the muscle tendon unit (Davenport, Kulig, Matharu, & Blanco, 2005; Sharma & Maffulli, 2005); and the osteotendinous junction, the site where the tendon inserts into the bone. The injury may be caused by an acute trauma or repetitive force, a chemically induced injury (e.g. fluoroquinolone antibiotics), or an infectious process (Fedorczyk, 2012). Repetitive strain at these sites, because of altered tendon loading from extrinsic forces or intrinsic factors, may cause inflammation to tendon sheaths and changes to the tendon cells (e.g., collagen disorganization and altered cell healing with adhesion formation) leading to tendon degeneration (Davenport et al., 2005; Sharma & Maffulli, 2005). Regardless of inciting trauma, there is a state of "protracted fibroplasia" and "failed healing" (Fedorczyk, 2012, p. 194) leading to persistent symptoms.

In response to this trauma, localized pain, warmth, swelling, and crepitus may occur in the affected region with associated functional impairment.

Most commonly, mechanisms of injury include extrinsic factors, many of which are the biomechanical compressive forces, including heavy loads/handling tools, repetition, overuse, awkward postures, contact stress, or cold temperature (van Rijn, Huisstede, Koes, & Burdorf, 2009). Intrinsic factors, such as anatomy (e.g., narrowed acromium space) and excessive physical training with inadequate rest periods, also contribute to injury. Treatment with fluoroquinolones (e.g., ciprofloxacin) is associated with tendinopathy and tendon rupture, thought to be caused by inhibition of tenocyte metabolism. Tenocytes are undifferentiated fibroblasts critical to the tendon healing process (Davenport et al., 2005; Sharma & Maffulli, 2005). Psychosocial work factors, such as high psychological job demands, may contribute to soft tissue complaints by increasing the speed of work or assuming a tense posture, thereby increasing extrinsic biomechanical risks (Bongers, Ijmker, van den Heuvel, & Blatter, 2006). Low job control and low social support at work are also associated with soft tissue complaints, for example, lateral epicondylitis (van Rijn et al., 2009).

A. Diagnosis: biceps tendinopathy

1. Definition and overview

    Biceps tendinopathy is defined by anterior shoulder pain, worse with overhead reaching. Tenderness is located in the bicipital groove of the proximal humerus between the greater and lesser tuberosities, where the tendon of the long head of the biceps brachii inserts at the glenoid labrum. This tendon helps to stabilize the humeral head, especially during abduction and external rotation. Risk factors for bicipital tendinopathies include

    a. Repetitive overhead motion, especially throwing sports

    b. Normal aging with degenerative changes to soft tissue and bony structures

c. Other pathology of the rotator cuff or the labrum may contribute by placing extra force on the biceps insertion site

d. Specific occupations, for example fish processing workers, have a higher prevalence of bicipital tendinopathy when compared to other occupations such as caretakers and community garden and parks workers (van Rijn, Huisstede, Koes, & Burdorf, 2010).

2. Prevalence and incidence

Due to variable case definitions, the prevalence of bicipital tendinopathy is unknown. In the general population, the 12-month prevalence of "shoulder complaints" ranges from a low of 4.7% to a high of 46.7% (van Rijn et al., 2010). In a large population-based study in the United Kingdom, the prevalence of physician-diagnosed "shoulder tendinitis" was found to be 4.5% for men and 6.1% in women, with bicipital tendinitis prevalence for both men and women documented to be 0.7% (Walker-Bone, Palmer, Reading, Coggon, & Cooper, 2004).

B. Diagnosis: lateral epicondylitis/elbow tendinopathy

1. Definition and overview

Lateral epicondylitis is defined as pain in the lateral epicondyle region of the elbow, which is provoked by extension of the wrist extensors against resistance (Walker-Bone et al., 2004). The most common risk factors for lateral epicondylitis are:

a. Repetitive and forceful movements of hands and wrists at work (Shiri, Viikari-Juntura, Varonen, & Heliovaara, 2006; van Rijn et al., 2009), including awkward postures (e.g., hands bent or twisted), handling tools weighing over 1 kg, handling vibrating tools, handling tools used to turn and screw, and frequently handling heavy loads over 20 kg more than 20 times per year at work (van Rijn et al., 2009).

b. High-impact sports, with force and repetition of the wrist in extension ("tennis elbow")

c. Former or current smoking (Shiri et al., 2006)

d. Increasing age (Shiri et al., 2006)

2. Prevalence and incidence

Physician-diagnosed lateral epicondylitis prevalence was 1.3% in a community-based sample of adults between the ages of 30 and 64 in Finland (Shiri et al., 2006). Likewise, in a large population-based study of adults in the United Kingdom, 1.3% of men and 1.1% of women were diagnosed by physical examination with lateral epicondylitis (Walker-Bone et al., 2004). Prevalence of lateral epicondylitis in workers is reported at up to 12.2% (van Rijn et al., 2009).

There is, however, variable prevalence based on case definition. For example, 12% of workers from a wide range of industries had lateral epicondylalgia if the case definition included pain only; however, when the definition included pain, tenderness, and a positive resistive maneuver, the prevalence dropped to 3.5% (Hegmann et al., 2014).

C. Diagnosis: de Quervain's tenosynovitis/ tendinopathy

1. Definition and overview

De Quervain's tenosynovitis/tendinopathy is caused by entrapment of the extensor pollicis brevis and abductor pollicis longus tendons and is characterized by pain over the radial styloid and tender swelling over the first extensor compartment, which is confirmed by pain in this location with resisted thumb extension or a positive Finkelstein's test (Fedorczyk, 2012; McAuliffe, 2010; Walker-Bone et al., 2004). Difficulty in undoing lids on jars and bottles was reported by 28.3% of those diagnosed with de Quervain's tendinopathy (Walker-Bone et al., 2004). Risk factors include:

a. Repetitive, forceful, wrist or thumb motion (American College of Occupational and Environmental Medicine [ACOEM], 2011a)

b. Direct pressure or blunt trauma, although these are less common (ACOEM, 2011a)

c. Pregnancy and lactation (Ashraf & Devadoss, 2014)

d. Persons with rheumatoid arthritis have a higher prevalence of de Quervain's tendinopathy (Ashraf & Devadoss, 2014; McAuliffe, 2010)

2. Prevalence and incidence

In a large population-based study in the United Kingdom, the prevalence of de Quervain's tenosynovitis/tendinopathy was 0.5% for men and 1.3% in women (Walker-Bone et al., 2004).

II. Database (may include but is not limited to)

A. Subjective

1. For all soft tissue complaints

a. Past health history: any prior soft tissue complaints, any past or current workers' compensation claims

b. Medical illnesses: inflammatory or degenerative arthritis, diabetes, or thyroid disorders; history of a gastrointestinal bleed and/or liver or kidney disease may assist in drug therapy choices

c. Surgical history: any prior surgery to affected area

d. Obstetric and gynecological history: current pregnancy and lactation

e. Trauma history: acute or cumulative

f. Medication history: nonsteroidal anti-inflammatory medication (oral or topical), history of cortisone injections, any allergies or sensitivity to aspirin or nonsteroidal medications

g. Family history: arthritis, thyroid disease, or diabetes

h. Occupational or environmental history (previous and current): work-related exposures

   i. Any work activity that involves repetitive or awkward postures; lifting, pushing, or pulling; contact stress; vibration; and/or cold temperature (past and current)

   ii. Computer and telephone work: ergonomic adjustment of workstation, percentage of time on computer and number of keystrokes, mouse clicks, 10-key entry; any wrist rest breaks

   iii. Psychosocial work factors: high psychological demand, low decision latitude, low coworker and low supervisor social support; rewards (esteem, respect, salary, or future job opportunities), job satisfaction; job security

   iv. Work scheduling: number of hours worked per day and per week, overtime

   v. Protective equipment used: splints or smart gloves, forearm or wrist rests

   vi. Coworkers with similar symptoms

   vii. Symptoms relieved on days away from work or made worse by certain work activities

i. Hobbies and sports

   i. Any hobby and/or sport involving repetitive or awkward postures; lifting, pushing, or pulling; contact stress; vibration; and/or cold temperature (past and current)

   ii. High-risk sports (e.g., tennis and racquetball), musical instruments, needlework (e.g., crocheting, knitting, needlepoint, or embroidery), home computer use, motorcycling and dirt biking

j. Personal and social history

   i. Functional impact of symptoms: assessment of activities of daily living to include dressing, bathing, shopping, housework, cooking, caregiving, and use of assistive devices

   ii. Substances: smoking and alcohol use; intravenous drug use (if presenting with a red, hot joint)

   iii. Sleep quality and quantity

   iv. Frequency and type of exercise (stretching and flexibility, strength, endurance conditioning, overtraining, and postural awareness)

   v. Any exposure to intimate partner violence

k. Review of systems

   i. Constitutional signs and symptoms: fatigue, fever, weight loss or gain, and night sweats

   ii. Skin, hair, and nails: erythema or warmth in affected area

   iii. Musculoskeletal: hand dominance; pain level on a 0–10 numerical or visual analogue scale; quality of pain (e.g., burning, aching, or electric shock pain); pain at rest or with activity, stiffness, limitations in motion (abrupt or chronic); presence of swelling; crepitus; locking of digits; giving way of joints; nighttime wakening with symptoms; and presence of pain in distal or proximal joints

   iv. Neurologic: paresthesias or motor weakness

B. Objective

1. Physical examination findings

a. Height and weight, overall conditioning

b. General appearance, noting pain and posture

c. Skin: erythema, warmth, bogginess, swelling, crepitus, and tenderness

d. Musculoskeletal: bony deformity, muscle atrophy, localized tenderness and pain on palpation, anatomic distribution of pain and paresthesias, range of motion, and special maneuvers (**Table 70-1**)

e. Neurologic: sensory loss mapping, motor strength, deep tendon reflexes, and special maneuvers (Table 70-1)

2. Supporting data from relevant diagnostic tests

a. Fasting blood sugar, hemoglobin A_{1C} (if suspect glucose impairment or diabetes)

b. Rheumatoid factor, antinuclear antibody, erythrocyte sedimentation rate (if suspect an inflammatory rheumatologic condition)

c. Thyroid-stimulating hormone (if suspect hypothyroidism)

d. Radiograph (e.g., for acute trauma to rule out any underlying bony fracture)

e. Nerve conduction studies (if suspect a peripheral nerve entrapment syndrome)

TABLE 70-1 Provocative Physical Examination Maneuvers for Selected Tendinopathy Diagnosis

Provocative Test—compare affected to unaffected side	Diagnosis	How To
Palpation of bicipital groove: https://meded.ucsd.edu/clinicalmed/joints2.htm	Bicipital tendinopathy	Palpate between the greater and lesser proximal humerus tuberosities with the affected arm flexed in 90 degrees; internally and externally rotate the arm while palpating; examiner will feel the tendon roll under his/her fingers. A positive test is tenderness with palpation in this region.
Yergason's test: https://meded.ucsd.edu/clinicalmed/joints2.htm	Bicipital tendinopathy	The patient's arm begins pronated and flexed by his/her side at 90 degrees. The patient then attempts to supinate arm against examiner resistance. For a positive test, pain is reproduced in the region of the long head of the biceps muscle.
Resisted wrist extension: https://meded.ucsd.edu/clinicalmed/joints4.htm	Lateral epicondylitis/elbow tendinopathy	Resisted extension of the wrist reproduces pain in the lateral epicondyle region for a positive test
Finkelstein's test: https://meded.ucsd.edu/clinicalmed/joints3.htm	de Quervain's tenosynovitis/tendinopathy	Patient makes a fist around flexed thumb and gently ulnar deviates the wrist. Pain is reported over the first extensor compartment (i.e., distal to the lateral aspect of radial styloid and proximal to the anatomic snuff box) for a positive test

f. Electromyogram (if suspect a cervical radiculopathy)

g. Ultrasound (e.g., for imaging of the biceps tendon if rupture is suspected)

h. Magnetic resonance imaging (if symptoms persist beyond 4–6 weeks of conservative treatment, and there may be a surgical intervention [e.g., a shoulder arthroscopy])

III. Assessment

A. Determine the diagnosis based on anatomic location and mechanism of injury

1. Bicipital tendinopathy
   a. Focal tenderness over long head of biceps insertion with palpation between the greater and lesser proximal humeral tuberosities (Table 70-1)
   b. Positive Yergason's test (Table 70-1)

2. Lateral epicondylitis/elbow tendinopathy
   a. Focal tenderness over lateral epicondyle of elbow
   b. Pain over lateral epicondyle with resisted wrist extension (Table 70-1)

3. de Quervain's tenosynovitis/tendinopathy
   a. Focal tenderness distal to the lateral aspect of radial styloid and proximal to the anatomic snuff box (Table 70-1)
   b. Positive Finkelstein's test (Table 70-1)

4. Other conditions that may explain the patient's presentation
   a. Referred pain from another system (e.g., Pancoast tumor in the lung with referred pain to the shoulder versus bicipital tendinopathy)
   b. Peripheral nerve entrapment (e.g., radial nerve entrapment versus lateral epicondylitis/elbow tendinopathy)
   c. Cervical radiculopathy (e.g., C6 radiculopathy versus de Quervain's tenosynovitis)
   d. Other musculoskeletal conditions (e.g., acromioclavicular joint synovitis or carpal metacarpal [thumb] arthritis)

B. Severity

1. Assess the severity of the disease, and ability to work and do activities of daily living.

2. Assess the significance of the problem in terms of health-related quality of life and impact on productivity at work and at home.

3. Screen for depression and treat if symptoms are protracted and functional recovery is delayed.

IV. Goals of clinical management

A. Diagnosing tendinopathy

In the absence of red flags, most upper extremity soft tissue disorders can be safely diagnosed with a thorough history and physical examination. After conservative treatment for 4–6 weeks, if there is no improvement, additional diagnostic studies may be ordered or specialty referral considered.

B. Treatment

Select a treatment plan that returns the client to the preinjury functional state in a safe and timely manner. Modify work and home activities to remove trigger events to prevent recurrence and also protect other coworkers, either through work redesign, tool redesign, or other ergonomic interventions. Use the worksite as part of the therapeutic treatment and rehabilitation plan. Establish a plan that minimizes disability and promotes recovery.

C. Patient adherence

Emphasizes a self-care, sports medicine approach, tailoring to lifestyle and exercise patterns. Treat all work as athletic endeavors, with need for stretching and warm-up and cool-down activities.

V. Plan

A. Diagnostic tests

1. Initial laboratory and diagnostic studies
   Most initial tendinopathy work-ups do not include diagnostic studies unless there is a history of trauma and/or there are red flags.

2. Failure of conservative therapy
   After 4–6 weeks of conservative therapy, if the patient is not showing improvement, additional diagnostics may be ordered, and/or the client is referred for specialty consultation.
   a. Imaging may be ordered sooner in the course of treatment in the presence of red flags. Red flags, in the discussion of shoulder complaints, include:
      i. History of cancer (especially lung), including pain at rest, history of immunosuppression, history of smoking
      ii. Infection, including systemic symptoms, and/or presence of immunosuppression
      iii. History of significant trauma, including prior joint dislocation, and/or presence of deformity
      iv. Progressive neurologic and/or vascular compromise (ACOEM, 2004)

B. Management

1. Therapeutic interventions
   a. For the first 4–6 weeks, if nonallergic, with normal kidney and liver function, prescribe anti-inflammatory therapeutic doses of a nonsteroidal anti-inflammatory agent, either orally or topically (ACOEM, 2011a, 2011b, 2012; Pattanittum, Turner, Green, & Buchbinder, 2013).
   b. ACOEM recommends, with strong evidence, prescribing cytoprotective medications (proton pump inhibitors and misoprostol) for anyone at an increased risk for gastrointestinal bleeding (ACOEM, 2011a, 2011b, 2012).
   c. Acetaminophen may be added for pain control and is recommended, in addition to aspirin, as initial therapy for those with cardiovascular disease risk factors.
   d. Narcotics are rarely indicated for tendinopathy, with insufficient evidence to support their use in soft tissue disorders but may be prescribed short term for acute, severe pain (ACOEM, 2011a, 2011b, 2012).
   e. ACOEM additionally recommends the consideration of topical capsicum and muscle relaxants for acute and subacute pain, and norepinephrine reuptake inhibiting antidepressants for chronic pain, although there is insufficient evidence (ACOEM, 2011b).
   f. Cortisone injections to the tendon sheath may be indicated if patient is intolerant of nonsteroidal anti-inflammatory agents, if there is one specific site of pain, or if conservative treatment is ineffective.
      i. The usual recommendation is conservative therapy for at least 3–4 weeks before cortisone injection (ACOEM, 2011a, 2011b, 2012).
      ii. Risks of cortisone injection include not only the risk of infection but also tendon rupture (Nichols, 2005).
      iii. Although cortisone injections may be appropriate for de Quervain's tendinopathy, those with lateral epicondylitis/elbow tendinopathy who receive cortisone injections have poorer long-term outcomes (Washington State Department of Labor and Industries, 2014); conservative care recommendations are the best approach for elbow disorders.

2. RICE: rest, ice, compression, and elevation
   a. Relative rest: reduce or restrict any specific motion that produces symptoms by modifying

work or sports activities (ACOEM, 2011a, 2011b, 2012; Davenport et al., 2005; Fedorczyk, 2012). There is limited evidence for rest breaks during repetitive tasks at work (e.g., 5-minute wrist rest break for every 1 hour of repetitive hand activities, or a 30-second pause for every 20 minutes of intensive work) to prevent upper extremity musculoskeletal disorders (Kennedy et al., 2010). Despite insufficient evidence, rest breaks are recommended for shoulder disorders (ACOEM, 2011b).

b. Ice: there is a consensus recommendation to use ice in the first 48 hours after initial injury to reduce inflammation and swelling, although there is currently insufficient evidence supporting this recommendation (ACOEM, 2011a, 2011b, 2012). Self-administered heat for acute, subacute, and chronic pain, despite insufficient evidence, is recommended (ACOEM 2011a, 2011b, 2012), and can be alternated with ice.

c. Compression: compression by ace wraps, taping, splints, braces, or casting aids healing by keeping the body part in neutral position and unloading specific forces to decrease pain (Davenport et al., 2005). Recommendations include beginning with more rigid and graduating to more flexible orthotic interventions, depending on patient preferences (Fedorczyk, 2012). There are, however, risks with any compressive device, including ischemia and pressure ulcers. Likewise, prolonged immobilization may lead to muscle atrophy and joint stiffness (Boyd, Benjamin, & Asplund, 2009). Short-term splint use is recommended, with patient education to include a weaning schedule for the splint over time. Splinting during sleep prevents inappropriate wrist and thumb movements, allows for long periods of rest, and may decrease overall patient resistance to splint use.

   i. For bicipital tendinopathy: shoulder immobilization may be indicated for 1–2 days only. Prolonged shoulder sling use could lead to a frozen shoulder (ACOEM, 2011b).

   ii. For lateral epicondylitis/elbow tendinopathy: splinting at the elbow with a dynamic extensor/elbow strap brace or splinting at the wrist is a consensus recommendation (although there is currently insufficient evidence) (ACOEM, 2012). Cock-up wrist splints are also recommended for elbow tendinopathies, with the goal to prevent repetitive wrist extension (ACOEM, 2012)

   iii. For de Quervain's tenosynovitis: a wrist and thumb splint is usually indicated

during the acute treatment phase (ACOEM, 2011a). A systematic review of de Quervain's tenosynovitis/tendinopathy found cortisone injections more effective than splinting alone (Ashraf & Devadoss, 2014).

d. Elevation: elevation may relieve any distal swelling.

3. Referral and consultation

   a. Referral for physical or occupational therapy to aid in return to preinjury function.

      i. Ultrasound is recommended for lateral epicondylitis (ACOEM, 2012) and for calcific shoulder tendinitis (ACOEM, 2011b) but not for de Quervain's tenosynovitis (ACOEM, 2011a)

      ii. Iontophoresis with administration of medications (e.g., corticosteroids) is recommended for lateral epicondylitis (ACOEM, 2012) and de Quervain's tenosynovitis (ACOEM, 2011a).

      iii. Myofascial release and soft tissue friction massage may be helpful, although there is insufficient evidence to support deep friction massage (ACOEM, 2012; Loew et al., 2014).

      iv. Gentle stretching during the acute treatment phase may be indicated, with introduction of a strengthening exercise program for home or work (ACOEM, 2011a, 2011b, 2012; Davenport et al., 2005; Kennedy et al., 2010). Eccentric exercise is effective in the treatment of lateral epicondylitis (Cullinane, Boocock, & Trevelyan, 2014). Postural and neuromuscular reeducation is critically important to improve function and reduce pain by identifying and modifying contributing intrinsic (e.g., postural) and extrinsic (e.g., biomechanical) factors (Davenport et al., 2005).

   b. Referral for ergonomic consultation is recommended to include workstation evaluation and adjustment with ergonomic training, rest breaks, new chairs, tool redesign to minimize forceful pinch grips, alternative keyboards, alternative pointing devices, and forearm and wrist supports (ACOEM, 2011a, 2011b, 2012; Kennedy et al., 2010). The goal is to reduce risk factors of awkward posture, force, repetition, vibration, contact stress, and cold temperature.

   c. Refer the patient to a rehabilitation or physician specialist if a more tailored rehabilitation plan or surgical intervention is needed (e.g., shoulder arthroscopy).

d. Referral for acupuncture for lateral epicondy-litis/elbow tendinopathy may be beneficial for short-term pain relief, although there remains insufficient evidence to support this recommendation (ACOEM, 2012; Washington State Department of Labor and Industries, 2014).

e. Autologous whole blood or platelet-rich plasma injections, via guided ultrasound, may enhance tissue healing by restoring "cytokine/growth factor equilibrium into the area of tendinosis" (Fedorczyk, 2012, p. 194) and has been shown to reduce pain in the short term, but not prolonged pain relief in patients with lateral epicondylitis/elbow tendinopathy (Washington State Department of Labor and Industries, 2014). The ACOEM guidelines currently recommend these therapies for chronic lateral epicondylalgia (ACOEM, 2012).

f. Return-to-work programs are particularly important (ACOEM, 2011b) to facilitate recovery, with the goal to prevent delayed recovery, associated wage loss, and potential job loss. Primary care providers need to be cautious when writing work restrictions, focusing on what the individual can do at work (for example: patient can lift up to 10 pounds; able to use left arm above shoulder, but no use of right arm above shoulder). However, removal from a specific job task that causes de Quervain's, for example, may be needed as part of the treatment plan (ACOEM, 2011a). Please note that this recommendation does not automatically translate to taking the patient off work. There may be alternate work assignments available at the workplace that can be safely done within the work restriction.

C. Client education: review

1. Self-care activities to improve overall physical conditioning include stretching, core strengthening, and postural awareness. Additionally, taking intermittent rest breaks throughout any repetitive task at work and at home is important to prevent and treat tendinopathy. Reinforce that injuries of this nature generally occur over an extended period of time and that they should not expect immediate resolution of symptoms.

2. Management plan, including medication, potential side effects, and follow-up care

3. State-specific workers' compensation procedures, including any mandatory reporting, if symptoms are caused by work activities. Support using the workplace as part of the therapeutic treatment plan, to avoid prolonged disability and wage loss, if the injury occurred at work.

4. Encourage primary prevention of injuries, including ergonomic interventions at work and at home, to prevent reinjury and injury to others.

VI. Self-management resources and tools

A. Patient and client education

1. Occupational Safety and Health Administration Ergonomics eTools
    Consumer-oriented self-help tools to reduce work-related risk factors, including an eTool for baggage handling, computer work stations, and sewing: https://www.osha.gov/dts/osta/oshasoft/index.html

2. Canadian Centre for Occupational Health and Safety www.ccohs.ca/oshanswers/diseases/tendon_disorders.html

3. National Institute of Arthritis and Musculoskeletal and Skin Diseases Clearinghouse:
    a. Bursitis and tendinitis: www.niams.nih.gov /Health_Info/Bursitis/default.asp

4. Medline Plus
    www.nlm.nih.gov/medlineplus/tendinitis.html

5. Arthritis Foundation
    www.arthritis.org/arthritis-facts/disease-center /tendinitis.php

B. Community support groups

There are online self-management and support groups for those with tendinopathies or for those who develop chronic pain from soft tissue injuries. Contact the Arthritis Foundation (www.arthritis.org/we-can-help /online-tools).

REFERENCES

American College of Occupational and Environmental Medicine. (2004). Shoulder complaints. In *Occupational medicine practice guidelines. Evaluation and management of common health problems and functional recovery in workers* (2nd ed., pp. 195–224). Elk Grove Village, IL: American College of Occupational and Environmental Medicine.

American College of Occupational and Environmental Medicine. (2011a). Hand, wrist, and forearm disorders, not including carpal tunnel syndrome. In K. T. Hegmann (Ed.), *Occupational medicine practice guidelines. Evaluation and management of common health problems and functional recovery in workers* (3rd ed.). Elk Grove Village, IL: American College of Occupational and Environmental Medicine. Retrieved from www.guideline.gov/content.aspx?id=34435.

American College of Occupational and Environmental Medicine. (2011b). Shoulder disorders. In K.T. Hegmann (Ed.), *Occupational medicine practice guidelines. Evaluation and management of common health problems and functional recovery in workers* (3rd ed.). Elk Grove Village, IL: American College of Occupational and Environmental Medicine. Retrieved from www.guideline.gov/content.aspx?id=36626.

American College of Occupational and Environmental Medicine. (2012). *Elbow disorders*. In K.T. Hegmann (Ed.), *Occupational medicine practice guidelines. Evaluation and management of common health problems and functional recovery in workers* (3rd ed.). Elk Grove Village, IL: American College of Occupational and Environmental Medicine. Retrieved from www.guideline.gov/content.aspx?id=38447.

Ashraf, M. O., & Devadoss, V. G. (2014). Systematic review and meta-analysis on steroid injection therapy for de Quervain's tenosynovitis in adults. *European Journal of Orthopaedic Surgery and Traumatology, 24*, 149–157.

Bongers, P. M., Ijmker, S., van den Heuvel, S., & Blatter, B. M. (2006). Epidemiology of work related neck and upper limb problems: Psychosocial and personal risk factors (part I) and effective interventions from a bio behavioural perspective (part II). *Journal of Occupational Rehabilitation, 16*(3), 279–302.

Boyd, A. S., Benjamin, H. J., & Asplund, C. (2009). Splints and casts: Indications and methods. *American Family Physician, 80*(5), 491–499. Retrieved from www.aafp.org/afp/2009/0901/p491.html.

Cullinane, F. L., Boocock, M. G., & Trevelyan, F. C. (2014). Is eccentric exercise an effective treatment for lateral epicondylitis? A systematic review. *Clinical Rehabilitation, 28*(1), 3–19.

Davenport, T. E., Kulig, K., Matharu, Y., & Blanco, C. E. (2005). The EdUReP model for nonsurgical management of tendinopathy. *Physical Therapy, 85*(10), 1093–1103.

Fedorczyk, J. M. (2012). Tendinopathies of the elbow, wrist, and hand: histopathology and clinical considerations. *Hand Therapy, 25*(2), 191–200.

Hegmann, K. T., Thiese, M. S., Wood, E. M., Garg, A., Kapellusch, J. M., Foster, J., et al. (2014). Impacts of differences in epidemiological case definitions on prevalence for upper-extremity musculoskeletal disorders. *Human Factors, 56*(1), 191–202.

Kennedy, C. A., Amick, B. C., Dennerlein, J. T., Brewer, S., Catli, S., Williams, R., et al. (2010). Systematic review of the role of occupational health and safety interventions in the prevention of upper extremity musculoskeletal symptoms, signs, disorders, injuries, claims and lost time. *Journal of Occupational Rehabilitation, 20*(2), 127–162.

Loew, L. M., Brosseau, L., Tugwell, P., Wells, G. A., Welch, V., et al. (2014). Deep transverse friction massage for treating lateral elbow or lateral knee tendinitis. *Cochrane Database of Systematic Reviews, 11*, CD003528.

McAuliffe, J. A. (2010). Tendon disorders of the hand and wrist. *Journal of the American Society for Surgery of the Hand, 35*(5), 846–853.

Nichols, A. W. (2005). Complications associated with the use of corticosteroids in the treatment of athletic injuries. *Clinical Journal of Sports Medicine, 15*(5), 370–375.

Pattanittum, P., Turner, T., Green, S., & Buchbinder, R. (2013). Non-steroidal anti-inflammatory drugs (NSAIDs) for treating lateral elbow pain in adults. *Cochrane Database of Systematic Reviews, 5*, CD003686.

Sharma, P., & Maffulli, N. (2005). Tendon injury and tendinopathy: Healing and repair. *Journal of Bone and Joint Surgery America, 87*, 187–202.

Shiri, R., Viikari-Juntura, E., Varonen, H., & Heliovaara, M. (2006). Prevalence and determinants of lateral and medical epicondylitis: A population study. *American Journal of Epidemiology, 164*(11), 1065–1074.

van Rijn, R. M., Huisstede, B. M., Koes, B. W., & Burdorf, A. (2009). Associations between work-related factors and specific disorders at the elbow: A systematic literature review. *Rheumatology, 48*(5), 528–536.

van Rijn, R. M., Huisstede, B. M., Koes, B. W., & Burdorf, A. (2010). Associations between work-related factors and specific disorders of the shoulder: A systematic review of the literature. *Scandinavian Journal of Work, Environment & Health, 36*(3), 189–201.

Walker-Bone, K., Palmer, K. T., Reading, I., Coggon, D., & Cooper, C. (2004). Prevalence and impact of musculoskeletal disorders of the upper limb in the general population. *Arthritis and Rheumatology, 51*(4), 642–651.

Washington State Department of Labor and Industries. (2014). Conservative care options for work-related epicondylosis. Olympia, WA: Author. Retrieved from www.guideline.gov/content.aspx?id=48216&search=epicondylosis.

WOUND CARE

CHAPTER 71

Cynthia Johnson and Patricia McCarthy-Horton

I. Introduction and general background

A wound is a break in the integrity of the skin. Wound healing is restoration of the functional and anatomic integrity of tissue (Lazarus et al., 1994). Wound healing occurs in all structures of the body. This chapter focuses on the skin and soft tissues. Burns and pressure ulcers are not included in this chapter.

There are two types of tissue injury, partial and full thickness. Partial-thickness wounds include skin damage that does not penetrate below the dermis and may be limited to the epidermal layers only. The major components of partial-thickness repair include an initial inflammatory response to injury, epithelial proliferation and migration (resurfacing), and reestablishment and differentiation of the epidermal layers to restore the barrier function of the skin. Full-thickness wounds have tissue damage involving total loss of epidermis and dermis and extending into the subcutaneous tissue and possibly into muscle or bone. Healing of full-thickness wounds occurs through the processes of hemostasis, inflammation, proliferation of new tissue, and remodeling of scar tissue (Bryant & Nix, 2012).

There are normal skin changes that occur with age. For example, there is a decrease in Langerhans cells, leading to a decreased inflammatory response and increased risk of cancer. Epidermal–dermal junction changes such as flattening of the prominent dermal papillae and rete ridges cause skin to tear more easily from mechanical trauma, including use of tape on skin. Skin elasticity decreases from changes in collagen and elastin fibers. A loss of skin barrier function occurs with less secretion of lipids to the skin along with reduction of dermal hydration. Due to these skin changes, aging skin is more fragile and wounds are acquired more easily. Wound healing is delayed and response to infection is decreased (Bryant & Nix, 2012).

Wounds are commonly divided into acute and chronic wounds. In this chapter, we discuss acute wounds and the two most common chronic wounds, venous leg ulcers and diabetic foot ulcers.

A. Acute wounds

1. Definition and overview

Acute wounds are those that have an abrupt onset with a short duration, recognizing that the duration is disease or condition specific (Lazarus et al., 1994). Acute wounds occur suddenly and move predictably through the repair process (Bryant & Nix, 2012). Surgical wounds and traumatic wounds are the most common acute wounds. Surgical wounds are deliberately made incisions. Traumatic wounds result from any foreign body impact that results in tissue damage. These include wounds caused by both blunt and penetrating trauma. Examples of traumatic wounds are crush injuries, degloving wounds, gunshot wounds, stab wounds, and lacerations. They occur abruptly, usually with significant impact, and cause tissue damage. The mechanism of injury in traumatic wounds determines the extent of damage and risk of infection. The environment of the injury and the time since injury are important factors in the development of complications including infection. A contaminated wound that is evaluated more than 6 hours after injury is at increased risk of infection.

2. Prevalence and incidence

In the United States, annually there are about 50 million incisions from elective surgeries and 50 million traumatic wounds (Franz et al., 2008). Each year trauma accounts for 41 million emergency department visits and 2.3 million hospital admissions across the nation (Centers for Disease Control and Prevention [CDC], 2014).

B. Chronic wounds

1. Definition and overview

Chronic wounds are those that fail to proceed through the healing process in an orderly and timely fashion to produce sustained functional and anatomic continuity (Lazarus et al., 1994). Chronic wounds are frequently caused by vascular compromise, chronic inflammation, or repetitive insults (Bryant & Nix, 2012). The most common types of chronic wounds are venous leg ulcers and diabetic foot ulcers.

a. Venous leg ulcer: Venous leg ulcer (VLU) is defined as an open skin lesion of the leg or foot that occurs in an area affected by venous hypertension. VLU is the most common etiology of lower extremity ulceration and accounts for 70% of all leg ulcers (O'Donnell et al., 2014).

Chronic venous disease (CVD), a debilitating condition that affects millions of individuals worldwide, is the leading cause of VLU. Both reflux and obstruction account for the pathophysiologic mechanism of CVD. The fundamental basis for CVD and venous ulceration is inflammation within the circulation that is subjected to increased hydrostatic pressure resulting in increased ambulatory pressure. Inflammation has a significant effect on the vein wall, venous valve, endothelium, and the surrounding tissue, which leads to destruction of the dermis and eventual skin changes and ulcer formation (O'Donnell et al., 2014).

More common in women and older persons, VLUs are often recurrent and can persist for weeks to several years. Severe complications include cellulitis, osteomyelitis, and malignant change (Collins & Seraj, 2010).

b. Diabetic foot ulcer: Diabetic foot ulcer (DFU) is a complex, chronic wound, which has major long-term impact on the morbidity, mortality, and quality of patients' lives (Chadwick, Edmonds, McCardle, & Armstrong, 2013). They are usually located at increased pressure points on the bottom of the feet (Yazdanpanah, Nasiri, & Adarvishi, 2015); however, neurotropic ulcers related to trauma can occur anywhere on the foot (Cleveland Clinic, 2015).

The major component of nearly all DFUs is the loss of protective sensation from peripheral neuropathy (Chadwick et al., 2013). Ninety percent of DFUs are from neuropathy and 10% from ischemia (Yazdanpanah et al., 2015). A DFU is a marker of serious disease and comorbidities. Without early and optimal intervention, the wound can rapidly deteriorate, leading to amputation of the affected limb (Chadwick et al., 2013).

A DFU is the most common complication of diabetes mellitus (DM) (Yazdanpanah et al., 2015), and DFUs are responsible for more hospitalizations than any other complication of diabetes (Rowe, 2014). Early management can prevent complications such as amputation, thus improving quality of life (Yazdanpanah et al., 2015). If infected, a DFU can increase the risk of hospitalization by nearly 56 times and amputation by nearly 155 times (Kimmel & Regler, 2011). In diabetic people with neuropathy, even if successful management results in healing of the foot ulcer, the recurrence rate is 66% (Rowe, 2014).

2. Prevalence and incidence

a. Venous leg ulcer: Approximately 7 million individuals worldwide have CVD with 3 million of those people progressing to ulceration (Wound Ostomy and Continence Nurses Society [WOCN], 2011). The overall prevalence of VLUs in the United States is estimated to be approximately 1% of the population (Collins & Seraj, 2010). Approximately 2.5 million people in the United States suffer from chronic venous insufficiency, and of those, approximately 20% will develop VLUs (O'Donnell et al., 2014). The refractory nature of these ulcers increase the risk of morbidity and mortality and have a significant impact on quality of life. The financial burden of VLUs is estimated to be $2 billion per year in the United States (Collins & Seraj, 2010).

b. Diabetic foot ulcer: In 2012, 29.1 million Americans or 9.3% of the population had diabetes. Approximately 1.25 million American children and adults have type 1 diabetes (American Diabetes Association [ADA], 2014). The percentage of Americans age 65 and older with diabetes remains high, at 25.9%, or 11.8 million seniors. Prevalence of lower extremity peripheral neuropathy is 2.4% per 100,000 of the U.S. population and increases with aging to 9%. Among diabetics, 40% have peripheral neuropathy with loss of protective sensation and 15% will develop foot ulceration (Yazdanpanah et al., 2015). According to the WOCN (2012), 14–24% will require amputation. The incidence of ulcers is 1–4.1%, and the lifetime incidence is estimated to be 25% (Wu, Driver, Wrobel, & Armstrong, 2007).

II. Database

A. Acute wounds

1. Subjective

a. Past medical history: trauma, cardiovascular disease, diabetes

b. Surgical history: recent surgery

c. Trauma history: recent trauma and mechanism of injury

d.   Family history: diabetes

e.   Social history: poor nutrition, tobacco, alcohol, and illicit substance use, homelessness

f.   Occupational history: job-related injury

g.   Medications and allergies: medications and supplements that suppress inflammation (e.g., immunosuppressive drugs, steroids, chemotherapy)

h.   Review of systems

i.   Constitutional signs and symptoms: fatigue, fever, chills, general malaise

ii.   Skin: rash, erythema, warmth, wound separation, drainage, odor, pain

iii.   Cardiac and circulatory: chest pain, edema, mottling, pallor, and cyanosis

iv.   Musculoskeletal: pain, swelling, alteration in range of motion, loss of strength

v.   Neurologic: numbness, paresthesias, gait changes

2.   Objective

a.   Physical examination findings (**Table 71-1**)

b.   Supporting data from diagnostic tests (**Table 71-2**)

B. Venous ulcers

1.   Subjective

a.   Past medical history and risk factors: advanced age, obesity, venous thromboembolism, superficial thrombophlebitis, varicose veins, venous insufficiency, leg trauma, thrombophilia, restricted range of motion of the ankle, impairment of calf muscle pump (WOCN, 2011).

Other nonvenous causes of leg ulcers should be identified. Examples include arterial insufficiency, vasculitis, lymphedema, exogenous factors, pyoderma gangrenosum, infection, neoplasia, calciphylaxis, and drug-induced causes (O'Donnell et al., 2014).

Other conditions that affect ulcer healing should be identified. Examples include DM, infection, atherosclerosis, renal failure, immune diseases, and malignancy.

b.   Surgical history: previous venous operative interventions (O'Donnell et al., 2014)

c.   Trauma history: recent or remote leg trauma

d.   Family history: venous ulcers, venous thromboembolism, varicose veins (O'Donnell et al., 2014)

e.   Social history: intravenous drug use, tobacco use, alcohol abuse, sedentary lifestyle

f.   Occupational history: prolonged standing, inability to work

g.   Medications and allergies: medications that influence immune function (corticosteroids,

chemotherapy, biologic response modifiers), recent or current antibiotics, anticoagulants, analgesics

h.   Review of systems

i.   Constitutional symptoms: fatigue, tired, heavy legs

ii.   Skin: drainage, malodor, pruritus, dry or scaly skin, hyperpigmentation

iii.   Cardiovascular: dependent or chronic edema

iv.   Musculoskeletal: pain described as burning, aching, throbbing, often exacerbated by limb dependence and relieved by elevation or rest, restless legs (O'Donnell et al., 2014)

v.   Psychiatric: depression, anxiety, social isolation

vi.   Obstetric and gynecological history: pregnancy (multiple or close together) (WOCN, 2011)

2.   Objective

a.   Physical examination findings (Table 71-1)

b.   Supporting data from diagnostic tests (Table 71-2)

C. Diabetic foot ulcers

1.   Subjective

a.   Past medical history and risk factors: diabetes, uncontrolled hyperglycemia, duration of diabetes, history of previous ulcer, blindness or visual loss, advanced age, chronic renal disease (Yazdanpanah et al., 2015), foot trauma, restricted range of motion of the ankle. Other conditions that affect ulcer healing should be identified, including DM management, infection, atherosclerosis, renal failure, immune diseases, and malignancy

b.   Surgical history: amputation with loss of part of foot or extremity

c.   Trauma history: inappropriate shoe wear, self-inflicted injury from trimming nails or calluses

d.   Family history: diabetes with DFU, amputations, venous ulcers

e.   Social history: tobacco use, alcohol abuse, illicit drug use, sedentary lifestyle, poor self-efficacy in their healthcare management, i.e., diabetes control

f.   Occupational history: prolonged standing or walking on affected foot.

g.   Medications and allergies: compliance with diabetic medications, medications that influence immune function (corticosteroids, chemotherapy, biologic response modifiers), recent or current antibiotics, anticoagulants, analgesics

TABLE 71-1 Physical Examination Findings

Condition	Associated Findings (may or may not include)
Acute wounds	Assess: 1. Vital signs: assess for changes from baseline. Assess for signs of infection and screen for sepsis. Assess for ongoing levels of pain 2. Damage to underlying soft tissue, organ, bony structures, and neurovascular bundles (compartment syndrome or occult bleeding) 3. Cardiovascular and circulatory: distal mottling, pallor, coolness, cyanosis, loss of pulses or unilateral decrease in pulse amplitude 4. Skin: tissue disrupted with open wound; note wound location, size (length, width, and depth), exudate, nature of tissue (color and consistency), odor, level of pain, uncontrolled bleeding. Assess for visualized and/or palpable underlying structures 5. Neurologic: sensory defect caused by nerve damage from trauma, compartment syndrome, and pain
Venous leg ulcers	Assess: 1. Vital signs: assess for changes from baseline. Assess for signs of infection and screen for sepsis. Assess for ongoing levels of pain 2. Skin: wound characteristics include typical location superior to medial malleolus but can occur anywhere on the lower leg; wound is often shallow with irregular wound edges; wound bed ruddy red, often with yellow fibrinous slough; exudate can be mild to heavy; may be malodorous; bleeding may or may not be present (WOCN, 2011) 3. Wound measurement: serial VLU wound measurements and documentation are important to determine baseline markers and the effect of subsequent treatment measures on healing parameters. Documentation should include number and position of ulcers on leg, the size of each ulcer, description of the wound base, wound edges, amount and type of drainage, and signs of infection (O'Donnell et al., 2014) 4. Periwound: skin may display chronic venous skin changes such as dermatitis, hyperpigmentation, hemosiderosis, lipodermatosclerosis, atrophie blanche, scarring from healed wounds (WOCN, 2011) 5. Cardiovascular: presence of lower extremity pulses (dorsalis pedis and posterior tibial), edema, varicose veins, venous cord, telangiectasia, malleolar flare, corona phlebectatica (O'Donnell et al., 2014) 6. Musculoskeletal: decrease ankle mobility (O'Donnell et al., 2014) 7. Pain increased with leg dependency and decreased with leg elevation 8. Psychiatric: anxiety and depression
Diabetic foot ulcer	Assess: 1. Vital signs: assess for changes from baseline. Assess for signs of infection and screen for sepsis. Assess for ongoing levels of pain 2. Wound measurement: Serial DFU wound measurements and documentation are important to determine baseline markers and the effect of subsequent treatment measures on healing parameters 3. General appearance: signs of poor nutrition (e.g., wasting or lethargy) 4. Skin: description of wound bed, location, presence of necrotic debris, exudate including color, amount and odor, wound edges, callus formation, periwound description, erythema, swelling, increased warmth, maceration, dry, darkened pigmentation, fissured skin dystrophic nails 5. Cardiovascular: presence of lower extremity pulses (dorsalis pedis and posterior tibial), presence of arterial or venous disease in lower extremities 6. Musculoskeletal: exam includes muscle strength, gait analysis, range of motion of the foot and ankle, as well as visual inspection for any structural deformities such as bunions, hammertoes, or charcot (Kimmel & Regler, 2011). Compare both extremities 7. Neurologic: distal symmetrical polyneuropathy with loss of protective sensation (use monofilament for testing), change in foot structure (i.e., charcot) 8. Psychiatric: anxiety and depression 9. Endocrine: glycemic control

* Assess for infection with each visit and treat aggressively. Signs of infection can be subtle in the diabetic with a foot ulcer. In addition pain, as a presenting symptom, may not be present because of the loss of protective sensation. However, it may present as a change in sensation.

TABLE 71-2 Common Wound-Related Tests

Test: Ankle-brachial index (ABI)

Definition: ABI is a ratio of Doppler-recorded systolic blood pressure in the lower and upper extremities. ABI is a noninvasive test to detect peripheral artery disease (PAD; McDermott et al., 2013).

Clinical Implications: Normal range = 1.10–1.40 (McDermott et al., 2013).

- ABI < 0.90 at rest suggests PAD. For patients with VLU and concomitant PAD, use of standard compression has been shown to be safe if ABI is 0.80 or higher. Modified compression with lower pressure ratings can be used for ABI 0.50 with close monitoring, but only after consultation with a vascular specialist (O'Donnell et al., 2014).
- ABI < 0.50 is considered to be indicative of severe arterial disease. In patients with VLU and underlying arterial disease, compression is not suggested if the ABI is 0.50 or less or if absolute ankle pressure is less than 60 mm Hg (O'Donnell et al., 2014).
- In patients with diabetes, renal insufficiency, or other diseases that cause vascular calcification, tibial vessels at the ankle become noncompressible, leading to a false elevation of the ABI. In these patients, additional noninvasive testing, such as pulse volume recordings or toe pressure measurement, should be performed to evaluate for PAD (O'Donnell et al., 2014).
- Comments: Arterial pulse examination and measurement of ABI is recommended on all patients with VLU (O'Donnell et al., 2014). ABI is critical to evaluate before applying compression in venous disease. If undiagnosed arterial disease is present, compression may result in ischemia and potentially result in ischemic limb and amputation.

Test: Color flow venous duplex ultrasound

- Definition: Used to evaluate for venous obstruction, DVT, and venous reflux and includes the following components: direct visualization of deep, superficial, and perforator venous anatomic segments; compressibility; phasic venous flow; and documentation of venous reflux with measurement of valve closure time.
- Clinical Implications: Comprehensive venous duplex ultrasound examination of the lower extremity is recommended in all patients with suspected VLU.
- Comments: Identifies patterns of venous disease that may have therapeutic implications (O'Donnell et al., 2014).

Test: Wound culture

- There is no evidence to support routine surface cultures of VLU in the absence of clinical signs of infection as these wounds are usually colonized with multiple microorganisms. If there are no clinical signs of infection and the wound is responding to treatment, there is no indication to culture the wound (O'Donnell et al., 2014).

Test: Wound biopsy

- Tissue biopsy is recommended for lower extremity ulcers that do not improve with standard therapy after 4 to 6 weeks of treatment and for all ulcers with atypical features (O'Donnell et al., 2014).

Test: Lab testing

- Standard blood work to assess for infection and glycemic control, monitor anticoagulation, and assess renal function. Laboratory evaluation for thrombophilia is suggested for patients with a history of recurrent venous thrombosis and chronic venous leg ulcers (O'Donnell et al., 2014).

Test: Simms-Weinstein monofilament

- Assess peripheral neuropathy in the foot and ankle.
- Assess the level of loss of protective sensation.

Test: Plain film x-ray

- X-ray of DFU if suspicious of osteomyelitis
- Can detect osteomyelitis, osteolysis, fractures, dislocations, arterial calcifications, soft tissue gas, foreign bodies, structural deformities, and arthritis.

h. Review of systems
 i. Constitutional symptoms: fever, chills, or malaise
 ii. Skin: callus, hyperpigmentation indicative of neuropathy or previous infection, erythema, warmth, drainage, odor, pain
 iii. Cardiovascular: dependent or chronic edema, atherosclerosis, decreased pulses
 iv. Musculoskeletal: limited joint mobility, prolonged pressure to the foot from walking without proper shoe gear, structural foot deformity, charcot, toe deformities

v. Neurologic: peripheral neuropathy with loss of protective sensation to feet, neuropathic pain

vi. Psychiatric: depression, anxiety, social isolation

vii. Endocrine: glycemic control, HgA1c

2. Objective
   a. Physical examination findings (Table 71-1)
   b. Supporting data from diagnostic tests (Table 71-2)

III. Assessment

A. Determine the diagnosis

1. Acute wound: history of surgery or trauma
2. Chronic wound: history and underlying pathology
   a. Venous ulcers
   b. Diabetic ulcers
3. Other conditions that may explain the patient's presentation especially if failure to progress or heal with appropriate therapy or if the patient has an unusual presentation or appearance
   a. Infection of bacterial or fungal origin
   b. Arterial ulcer
   c. Vasculitis
   d. Pyoderma gangrenosum
   e. Neoplasm
   f. Sickle cell ulcer
   g. Cutaneous granulomatous disease

B. Severity
Assess the severity of the disease, especially examine for infection and limb-threatening presentation (e.g., compartment syndrome or ischemia, osteomyelitis, necrotizing fasciitis).

C. Significance
How important is this problem to the patient and his/her ability to maintain lifestyle and participate in activities of daily living (e.g., mobility or function).

D. Motivation and ability of patient
Determine whether the patient has the ability and is willing to follow the plan that is developed by the provider with the patient.

IV. Goals of clinical management

A. To appropriately evaluate and diagnose the type of wound and its severity.

1. Determining the etiology will guide appropriate wound care management.

B. Develop mutually acceptable goals.

C. Select a treatment plan that promotes wound healing and minimizes the chance of complications such as infection or amputation.

1. Routinely reassess goals and plan of care and adjust treatment accordingly. If the wound has no expectation of healing, i.e., malignant tumors, then palliation may be an appropriate goal.

V. Plan

A. Diagnostic tests (See Table 71-2 for common diagnostic tests as appropriate)

B. Management

1. Acute wounds
   a. Cleanse: At each dressing change, cleanse the ulcer with a neutral, nonirritating, nontoxic solution performed with a minimum of chemical or mechanical trauma (O'Donnell et al., 2014). Water, normal saline, or a commercial wound cleanser may be used.
   b. Bite wounds and trauma wounds that are heavily contaminated can be cleansed with high-pressure irrigation (e.g., using a #18 angiocatheter with 35-mL syringe) and monitored carefully for infection.
   c. Puncture wounds are left open to heal by secondary intention. Some bite wounds can be closed after cleansing with high-pressure irrigation.
   d. Close lacerations when appropriate with adhesive glue, sutures, or staples after appropriate local analgesia is provided. Analgesia with epinephrine may result in ischemia depending on the site used (i.e., ears, nose, genitalia, fingers, and toes).
   e. Provide an optimally moist wound bed for all wounds. The choice of dressing depends on etiology, size, location, type of tissue in the wound, exudate, level of contamination, and bioburden. Avoid excessively wet dressings that result in maceration of tissues.
   f. Systemic prophylactic antibiotics are not a routine part of acute wound care but may be indicated for bite wounds or some traumatic wounds, depending on the mechanism of injury.
   g. Update tetanus immunization, if needed.
   h. Deep traumatic wounds and those that have not improved after appropriate treatment may require referral to a specialist.

2. Chronic wounds: Venous leg ulcers
   a. Cleanse: At each dressing change, cleanse the ulcer with a neutral, nonirritating, nontoxic solution performed with a minimum of chemical or mechanical trauma (O'Donnell et al., 2014). Water, normal saline, or a commercial wound cleanser may be used.
   b. Debride: VLUs should receive thorough debridement at their initial evaluation to remove obvious necrotic tissue, excessive bacterial burden, and cellular burden of dead and senescent cells. Serial wound assessment is important in determining the need for repeated debridement. A number of debridement methods are available including, sharp, enzymatic, autolytic, biologic (larval), and mechanical (O'Donnell et al., 2014). Mechanical debridement is nonselective and can be painful and therefore is not recommended.
   c. Dressing: Apply a topical dressing that will manage the ulcer exudate and maintain a moist, warm wound bed (O'Donnell et al., 2014). Dressings that absorb excess exudate include alginates, foams, cadexomer iodine, hydrocolloids, hydrocellular dressings, hydropolymers, hypertonics, and medical honey (WOCN, 2011).
   d. Adjunctive therapy: Adjunctive wound therapy options may be considered for VLUs that fail to demonstrate improvement after a minimum of 4 to 6 weeks of standard therapy. Examples are cellular therapy with allogenic bilayer skin replacements or other skin substitutes (O'Donnell et al., 2014).
   e. Periwound: Preventing periwound maceration and treating dermatitis are important measures. Skin lubricants or topical steroids may ameliorate dermatitis (O'Donnell et al., 2014).
   f. Compression: Compression therapy is the standard of care for VLUs and chronic venous insufficiency. Venous ulcers heal more quickly with compression than without compression. Compression therapy reduces edema, improves venous reflux, enhances healing of ulcers, and reduces pain (Collins & Seraj, 2010).

   The amount of therapeutic compression is typically 30–42 mm Hg at the ankle and can be provided by elastic, multilayer compression dressings (e.g., Profore) or inelastic, paste-containing bandages (e.g., Unna's boot), stockings, and boots. Antiembolism hose are not designed to provide therapeutic compression (WOCN, 2011).

   Elastic compression therapy is more effective than inelastic therapy and high compression is more effective than low compression. Multilayer bandages are more effective than single layer but require specialized training to apply. Contraindications to compression therapy include clinically significant arterial disease and uncompensated heart failure. Once an ulcer has healed, lifelong maintenance of compression therapy may reduce recurrence (Collins & Seraj, 2010).

   g. Elevation: Leg elevation is recommended and requires raising lower extremities above the level of the heart. The goal of elevation is to reduce edema, improve microcirculation and oxygen delivery, and hasten ulcer healing (Collins & Seraj, 2010). Leg elevation is most effective if performed for 30 minutes, three to four times per day (WOCN, 2011).
   h. Medications: For long-standing or large VLUs, treatment with pentoxifylline (Trental) is recommended when used in combination with compression therapy. Pentoxifylline has a powerful inhibitory effect on cytokine-mediated neutrophil activation, white cell adhesion to endothelium, and oxidative stress (O'Donnell et al., 2014). Pentoxifylline (400 mg three times per day) has been shown to be an effective adjunctive treatment for VLUs when added to compression therapy (Collins & Seraj, 2010).
   i. Pain: Wound pain related to VLUs is very common and can become chronic without proper intervention. An individualized pain management plan should be developed to meet each patient's needs. Important components include compression, leg elevation, exercise, and analgesia (WOCN, 2011). Active exercise to improve muscle pump function and to reduce pain and edema is recommended (O'Donnell, et al., 2014).
   j. Nutrition: A nutritional assessment should be performed on any patient with a VLU who has evidence of malnutrition (O'Donnell et al., 2014). Nutritional deficiencies are underdiagnosed and underreported in patients with VLUs. Protein deficiency is prevalent and caloric intake is often suboptimal (WOCN, 2011).
   k. Surgery: The role of surgery is to reduce venous reflux, hasten healing, and prevent ulcer recurrence. Surgical options for treatment of venous insufficiency include ablation of the saphenous vein; interruption of the perforating veins with subfascial endoscopic surgery; treatment of iliac vein obstruction with stenting; and removal of incompetent superficial veins with phlebectomy, stripping, sclerotherapy, or laser therapy (Collins & Seraj, 2010).

3. Chronic wounds: Diabetic foot ulcer

   a. The primary management of diabetic foot ulcers is to gain closure as quickly as possible (Yazdanpanah et al., 2015).

   b. Cleanse the wound at each dressing change with a neutral, nonirritating, nontoxic solution performed with a minimum of chemical or mechanical trauma (O'Donnell et al., 2014). Water, normal saline, or a commercial wound cleanser may be used.

   c. Off-loading, taking pressure off the wound, is the mainstay of therapy in treatment of DFUs. Peripheral neuropathy may predispose the foot to ulceration due to loss of protective sensation and is the major component of nearly all DFUs (Chadwick et al., 2013). Off-loading is the reduction of focal pressure from a specific foot site with subsequent redistribution of that pressure over the larger foot surface thus decreasing repetitive stress and pressure from shoe wear. Abnormal pressure or stress to the foot may occur from limited joint mobility and/or structural foot deformity. Unrelieved pressure impairs healing and increases the risk of complications such as infection or increased tissue damage (WOCN, 2012).

   Off-loading modalities include total contact cast (TCC), which is considered the "gold standard." However, TCC should not be used if patient has infection, poor arterial perfusion, unstable gait, fluctuating edema, or restless leg syndrome. Complete bed rest could be used to take pressure off an ulcer, however, it is not generally recommended because it could lead to debilitation (WOCN, 2012). Other choices are crutches, walkers, wheelchairs, custom shoes, depth shoes, shoe modifications, custom inserts, custom relief orthotics, diabetic boots, and forefoot and heel relief shoes.

   d. Wound debridement of nonviable tissue can be done by surgical/sharp, larval, autolytic, hydrodebridement, or ultrasonic debridement (Chadwick et al., 2013). The gold standard of debridement for DFUs is sharp debridement but should be carried out only by experienced practitioners (Chadwick et al., 2013). The nonviable tissue and callus surrounding the wound causes pressure and should be debrided at regular intervals (WOCN, 2012).

   e. Assess for and treat infection, topically or systemically depending on the level of the infection. Although approximately 56% of DFUs become infected (Chadwick et al., 2013), poor glucose control has the potential to suppress the inflammatory response thus decreasing response to infection (Yazdanpanah et al., 2015). Infection may be subtle in diabetic patients and clinical signs of infection, along with laboratory markers, may not be elevated in the presence of infection. However, antibiotic therapy should not be given as a preventive measure in the absence of signs of infection (Chadwick et al., 2013).

   Increase in drainage, swelling, necrotic tissue, abnormal granulation tissue, change in the color of the wound, purulent drainage, and increased friability can be signs of infection, along with erythema and increased warmth to the area (WOCN, 2012). For deep infected wounds, cellulitis, formation of necrotic tissue, gangrene, necrotizing fasciitis, or joint or bone involvement, intervention should be aggressive with systemic antibiotics and possible hospitalization. Culture swabs do not give an accurate account of wound bacteria and a biopsy can be done if needed (WOCN, 2012).

   f. If osteomyelitis is suspected the initial imaging should be plain films of the area, which can detect osteomyelitis, osteolysis, fractures, dislocations, arterial calcifications, soft tissue gas, foreign bodies, structural deformities, and arthritis. Magnetic resonance imaging can be done and has been called the gold standard for detection; however, tissue infection can interfere with an accurate diagnosis. A definitive diagnosis can be made through a bone biopsy with culture. Other imaging of computer tomography, or radionuclide scans can be used (Steed et al., 2006). Ideal treatment of acute osteomyelitis is surgical removal of the bone and infected tissue. If surgery is not possible, prolonged antibiotic therapy, usually for 6 weeks, is used with close follow-up and reevaluation of infection.

   g. Wound care should maintain a moist environment, promote optimal cell migration, proliferation, differentiation, and neovascularization. Dressings should be chosen to either hold moisture in a wound that has minimal exudate or to collect drainage in wounds with heavier exudate. Periwound should be kept dry and protected to prevent maceration. Choice of wound dressings should be reassessed and may change based on the evolving characteristics of the wound. Other modalities include negative pressure wound therapy (NPWT) and biological wound coverings. Both of these should be placed over a clean wound bed without any slough, biofilm, or infection.

h. Hyperbaric oxygen has been shown to be of value in reducing the amputation rate in patients with ischemic DFU.

i. Optimal glycemic control contributes to healing of the ulcer. All approaches that contribute to glycemic control should be considered.

j. Systemic evaluation and management of underlying diseases is pivotal to the management of the lifelong risk of diabetic ulcers (e.g., diabetes control, prevention of neuropathy). The goal is to prevent loss of limb through amputation.

C. Education

Written instruction should be provided to the patient and family specific to wound management. Management of the underlying disease in the chronic conditions of venous disease and diabetes requires patient and family education for a lifetime.

1. Venous ulcer (WOCN, 2011):

   a. Even after a VLU is healed, patients must commit to lifelong compression by wearing compression stockings. Not wearing stockings is associated with leg ulcer recurrence

   b. Stockings should be removed at night and applied upon rising in the morning

   c. Compression stockings should be replaced every 3–6 months

   d. Patients should be encouraged to elevate their legs several times per day

   e. Encourage optimal weight management, proper nutrition, and exercise

   f. Exercise includes brisk walking, ankle flexions, and resistance calf muscle exercises throughout the day

2. Diabetic foot ulcer

   Possibly 50% of DFUs can be prevented with effective education. Patients should be taught self-care, including (Yazdanpanah et al., 2015):

   a. Glycemic control

   b. Daily foot inspection

   c. Foot hygiene

   d. Regular podiatry visits

   e. Proper shoe wear

   f. Avoiding walking barefooted, which is discouraged even in the home

   g. Need to see primary practitioner or podiatrist immediately if foot problems occur

   Patients with diabetes require lifelong management of their chronic illness. Refer patients and their family for diabetic education. Referral should be made to a podiatrist for ongoing foot management and teaching.

REFERENCES

American Diabetes Association. (2014). Statistics about diabetes. National diabetes statistics report, 2014. Retrieved from www.diabetes.org/diabetes-basics/statistics.

Bryant, R. A., & Nix, D. P. (2012). *Acute & chronic wounds: Current management concepts*. St. Louis, MO: Mosby.

Centers for Disease Control and Prevention. (2014). Trauma statistics. Retrieved from www.nationaltraumainstitute.org/home/trauma_statistics.html.

Chadwick, P., Edmonds, M., McCardle, J., & Armstrong, D. (2013). International best practice guidelines: Wound management in diabetic foot ulcers. *Wounds International*. Retrieved from www.woundsinternational.com.

Cleveland Clinic. (2015). Lower extremity ulcers. Retrieved from http://my.clevelandclinic.org/services/heart/disorders/pad/legfootulcer.

Collins, L., & Seraj, S. (2010). Diagnosis and treatment of venous ulcers. *American Family Physician, 81,* 989–996.

Franz, M. G., Robson, M. C., Steed, D. L., Barbul, A., Brem, H., Cooper, D. M., et al. (2008). Guidelines to aid healing of acute wounds by decreasing impediments of healing. *Wound Repair and Regeneration, 16*(6), 723–748.

Kimmel, H., & Regler, J. (2011). An evidence based approach to treating diabetic foot ulcerations in a veteran population. *Journal of Diabetic Foot Complications, 3*(2), 50–54.

Lazarus, G. S., Cooper, D. M., Knighton, D. R., Margolis, D. J., Pecoraro, R. E., Rodeheaver, G., et al. (1994). Definitions and guidelines for assessment of wounds and evaluation of healing. *Archives of Dermatology, 130*(4), 489–493.

McDermott, M. M., Applegate, W. B., Bonds, D. E., Bufore, T. W., Church, T. W., Espeland, M. A., et al. (2013). Ankle brachial index values, leg symptoms, and functional performance among community-dwelling older men and women in the lifestyle interventions and independence for elders study. *Journal of the American Heart Association, 12,* 1–10.

O'Donnell, T. F., Passman, M. A., Martson, W. A., Ennis, W. J., Dalsing, M., Kistner, R. L., et al. (2014). Management of venous leg ulcers: Clinical practice guidelines of the Society for Vascular Surgery and the American Venous Forum. *Journal of Vascular Surgery, 60,* 3S–59S

Rowe, V. L. (2014). Diabetic ulcers. Medscape. Retrieved from http://emedicine.medscape.com/article/460282-overview.

Wound Ostomy and Continence Nurses Society. (2011). *Guideline for management of wounds in patients with lower-extremity venous disease.* Mount Laurel, NJ: WOCN.

Wound Ostomy and Continence Nurses Society. (2012). *Guideline for management of wounds in patients with lower-extremity neuropathic disease.* Mount Laurel, NJ: WOCN.

Wu, S. C., Driver, V. R., Wrobel, J. S., & Armstrong, D. G. (2007). Foot ulcers in the diabetic patient, prevention and treatment. *Journal of Vascular Health Risk Management, 3*(1), 65–76.

Yazdanpanah, L, Nasiri, M., & Adarvishi, S. (2015). Literature review on the management of diabetic foot ulcer. *World Journal of Diabetes, 6*(1), 37–53.

INDEX

Note: Page numbers followed by *f* or *t* represent figures or tables respectively.

A

AACAP (American Academy of Child and Adolescent Psychiatry), 83, 94, 98
AADE. *See* American Association of Diabetes Educators (AADE)
AAP. *See* American Academy of Pediatrics (AAP)
Abnormal cytology, 171
  management of, 174–176, 174–182*f*
Abnormal uterine bleeding (AUB), 140–154
  assessment of, 146–147
  clinical management goals, 147
  clinical presentations of, 140, 141*t*
  COEIN etiologies, 144–145
  databases used for, 145–146
  diagnostic testing for, 147, 148–150*t*
  etiologies of, 140, 142–143*t*
  overview of, 140, 141, 144–145
  PALM (structural) etiologies, 141, 144
  physical examination, 146
  self-management resources, 154
  treatment and management of, 147, 151–153
Abscesses, cutaneous, management of. *See* Cutaneous abscesses, management of
Abuse. *See* Maltreatment of children; Physical abuse; Substance use and abuse
ACA (Affordable Care Act), 48
ACCP (American College of Chest Physicians), 415
Acetaminophen, 482
Achenbach Child Behavior Checklist, 82
Acid inhibitors, adverse effects of, 300
ACOG. *See* American Congress of Obstetricians and Gynecologists (ACOG)
Acquired Immune Deficiency Syndrome. *See* HIV (Human immunodeficiency virus); Postexposure prophylaxis (PEP), for HIV infection
Active vs. passive immunizations, 46
Activities of daily living (ADLs), 561
Acupressure wrist bands, 296
Acute bleeding, 147, 151
Acute heart failure, 569

Acute wounds, 713, 714–715, 718
AD (Alzheimer's disease), 218, 504, 507
ADA. *See* American Diabetes Association (ADA)
Addiction. *See* Substance use and abuse
Addiction specialist, 491
Adenomyosis, 141
ADHD. *See* Attention-deficit/hyperactivity disorder (ADHD)
Adolescence, defined, 32
Adult health maintenance and promotion. *See* also specific issues
  developmental disabilities and, 345–363
  postexposure prophylaxis for HIV infection, 375–384
  transgendered individuals and, 365–372
Adult presentations. *See* also specific disorders
  anemia, 401–413
  anticoagulation therapy, oral, 415–426
  anxiety, 428–435
  asthma, 436–448
  benign prostatic hyperplasia, 449–454
  cancer survivorship, 458–466
  chronic nonmalignant pain (CNP), 477–492
  chronic obstructive pulmonary disease (COPD), 468–475
  cutaneous abscess management, 395–400
  dementia, 504–513
  depression, 514–527
  diabetes mellitus, 529–538
  epilepsy, 539–546, 541*t*
  gastroesophageal reflux disease, 547–553
  heart failure, 566–574
  herpes simplex infections, 575–581
  HIV-infected adults, primary care of, 649–669
  hypertension, 583–593
  intimate partner violence, 594–602
  irritable bowel syndrome, 605–612
  lipid disorders, 613–618
  low back pain, 619–633
  obesity, 634–647
  smoking cessation, 672–680
  thyroid disorders, 682–690

  upper back and neck pain syndromes, 691–704
  upper extremity tendinopathy, 705–711
  viral hepatitis, chronic, 494–503
  wound care, 713–721
Advanced practice nurses (APNs), 104, 107
Advisory Committee on Immunization Practices (ACIP)
  vaccination recommendations, 42, 44–45
AEDs (antiepileptic drugs), 539–540, 542–544*t*, 545
AF (atrial fibrillation), 416, 417*t*
Affordable Care Act (ACA), 48, 458
AGC (atypical glandular cells), 174
Ages and Stages Questionnaire (Squires & Bricker), 57
Agoraphobia, 431
Agreement, breaks in opiate therapy, 490
AIDS. *See* HIV (Human immunodeficiency virus); Postexposure prophylaxis (PEP), for HIV infection
Airway inflammation, 436
Alcohol consumption. *See* also Substance use and abuse
  drug use screening and, 36
  effects on INR, 418
  hypertension and, 588
Allergens
  12–21 years, 33
  asthma and, 65, 436, 441
  atopic dermatitis and, 71, 75, 76–77
  fatigue and, 82
  skin testing for, 65, 72
Allergic rhinitis, 70
Allergy & Asthma Network Mothers of Asthmatics, 69
Allergy immunotherapy, 67
α^2-Adrenergic agonists, 86
Alpha-hydroxy acid lotion, 75
Alzheimer's Association, 512, 564
Alzheimer's disease (AD), 218, 504, 507
Alzheimer's Disease Education and Referral Center, 512
Amenorrhea
  assessment of, 161

associated with pituitary dysfunction, 156–157

clinical management goals, 161

databased used for, 158, 161

diagnosis of, 161

diagnostic testing for, 161, 162, 163–164t, 165

etiologies of, 158, 159–160t, 161

hypothalamic, 156

outflow tract/uterus disorders and, 157

overview of, 156–158

PCOS and, 156–169

physical examination findings, 161, 162t

primary ovarian insufficiency and, 157

self-management resources and tools, 169

treatment and management of, 166–168

American Academy of Allergy, Asthma and Immunology, 69, 446

American Academy of Child and Adolescent Psychiatry (AACAP), 83, 94, 98

American Academy of Family Physicians, 10, 282, 578

American Academy of HIV Medicine (AAHIVM), 669

American Academy of Pain Medicine, 483

American Academy of Pediatrics (AAP)

on developmental and behavioral problems, 48

on healthy babies, 7

on parenting, 10

on post-NICU patients, 12, 17

on postpartum care, 268

American Association for the Study of Liver Diseases, 503

American Association of Clinical Endocrinologists, 226

American Association of Diabetes Educators (AADE), 310

lifestyle behaviors, 306, 308–309

American College of Cardiology Foundation, 566, 567

American College of Chest Physicians (ACCP), 415

American College of Nurse-Midwives, 252, 282

American College of Sports Medicine, 647

American Congress of Obstetricians and Gynecologists (ACOG), 190, 252

on AUB, 153

on carrier screening, 255–256, 255t

on cervical screening, 171–172

on gestational diabetes mellitus, 306

on menopause transition, 226

on postpartum care, 268

on preeclampsia, 317

on VBAC, 282

American Diabetes Association (ADA), 305, 310, 537–538

American Geriatrics Society, 564

American Geriatrics Society Beer, 564

American Heart Association (AHA), 416, 566, 567, 574, 618, 647

American Liver Foundation, 503

American Lung Association, 69, 446

American Pain Society, 483, 492

American Psychiatric Association (APA), 674

American Society for Clinical Oncology (ASCO), 458, 463

survivorship care plan template, 464–465f

American Society for Colposcopy and Cervical Pathology (ASCCP), 174

American Society for Reproductive Medicine, 154

American Society of Hematology, 413

American Society of Hypertension (ASH), 584

American Thyroid Association, 690

American Urological Association, 451, 456

Ammonium lactate, 75

Amniocentesis, 257, 258

Amphetamine salts, 84

Analgesic therapy, 397

Androgen insensitivity, 157

Anemia, 401–413

assessment of, 407, 408–410, 409t

classification of, 401, 402t

clinical management goals for, 410, 411t

databases used for, 405–407

defined, 401

differentiation of, 402t

hemolytic, 404, 406–407, 410, 412

macrocytic, 404–405, 407, 412–413

megaloblastic, 404, 407, 410, 412–413

microcytic, 402–406, 408–410

normocytic, 404, 406–407, 410, 412

overview of, 401

patient education and, 413

physical examinations for, 407, 408t

screening, 25

self-management resources and tools, 413

sideroblastic, 403, 404, 406, 410, 412

treatment of, 410, 411–413

Anemia of chronic disease (ACD), 404, 406, 410, 412

Aneuploidy, fetal, 253

Anhedonia, 90

Anorectal trauma, in children, 109

Anterior shoulder pain, 705

Anticipated early death, infants with, 15

Anticoagulation therapy. See Oral anticoagulation (OAC) therapy

Anticonvulsants, 482

Antidepressants, 94, 95, 432, 482, 522–526t

Antidepressant Skills Workbook, 527

Antiepileptic drugs (AEDs), 539–540, 542–544t, 545

Antihistamines, 66, 77–78, 296

Antimicrobial therapy, 397

Antiretroviral therapy (ART) and HIV, 385, 651–652, 653t

Anxiety, 428–435

ADHD and, 81

assessment of, 430–431

children/adolescents and, 435

database used for, 429–430

overview of, 428–429

during pregnancy, 290

psychosocial treatment, 434

special populations and, 434–435

treatment of, 431–432, 433t, 434

Anxiety Disorders Association of America, 435

APA. See American Psychiatric Association (APA)

Apgar scores, 8, 15, 100

Aphasia syndromes, 505

Apnea

fatigue and, 82

in infants, 13

APNs (advanced practice nurses), 104, 107

Arousal disorders, 226

Arthritis. See Osteoarthritis (OA)

ASB (asymptomatic bacteriuria), 323–324

ASCCP (American Society for Colposcopy and Cervical Pathology), 174

ASC-H (atypical squamous cells of undetermined significance cannot rule out high grade), 173, 180–181f

ASC-US (atypical squamous cells of undetermined significance), 173, 177f, 178f

Asherman syndrome, 157

Association of Asthma Educators, 446

Association of Nurses in AIDS Care (ANAC), 669

Association of Reproductive Health Professionals, 226

Association of Reproductive Health Professionals (ARHP), 236

Asthma, in adolescents/adults, 436–448

action plan for, 446, 447–448f

assessment of, 438

clinical management goals to control, 438

Asthma, in adolescents/adults (*cont.*)
database used for, 437–438
diagnostic screening and testing
of, 439, 441, 441*f*
etiology of, 436
management of, 441, 442–443*t*, 444
overview of, 436–437
patient education and training in,
444–446, 445–446*b*
severity/control/response to treatment,
438, 439*t*, 440*t*
Asthma, in children, 61–69
assessment of, 62
atopic dermatitis and, 70
classifying severity/control of, 62, 63–64*t*
clinical management goals in, 65
databases used for, 61–62
defined, 61
medication for, 66–67, 66*t*
overview of, 61
prevalence and incidence, 61
treatment and management of, 65
Asymptomatic bacteriuria (ASB), 323–324
Atomoxetine, 86
Atopic dermatitis (AD), 70–79
assessment of, 72
clinical management goals in, 72, 73
conditions and features associated with,
72, 74*f*
databases used for, 70–72
defined, 70
diagnostic tests for, 72, 75*t*
differential diagnoses, 72, 76*f*
etiology, 70
overview of, 70
phases of, 71, 72*f*
prevalence and incidence, 70
psychosocial and emotional support
and, 79
self-management of, 78
signs/symptoms of, 72
treatment and management of, 73, 74, 75,
76–78
triggering factors for, 71, 71*f*
Atopic eczema. *See* Atopic dermatitis (AD)
Atrial fibrillation (AF), 416, 417*t*
Attention-deficit/hyperactivity disorder
(ADHD), 80–88
assessment of, 84
database used for, 81–83
incidence and prevalence, 81
long-term issues, 87
medications for, 84, 85*t*, 86
overview of, 80–81
physical examination for, 83–84
screening tools for, 82, 82*t*

transition to adulthood, 88
treatment and management of, 84, 86–88
Attorney General opinions, 3
Atypical glandular cells (AGC), 174
Atypical squamous cells, 173
ASC-H, 173, 180–181*f*
ASC-US, 173, 177*f*, 178*f*
AUB. *See* Abnormal uterine bleeding (AUB)
Autism. *See also* Developmental delay and
autism, screening for
screening for, 48–59
Autism spectrum disorders (ASD), 347–348

B

Babies, healthy, 7–10
Back pain. *See* Low back pain (LBP)
Back Pain Support Group, 703
Bariatric surgery, 121, 645–646
Barrett's esophagus, 547
Barrier methods, contraception,
230–232, 234–235, 236
contraceptive sponge, 231
diaphragm, 231–232
female condoms, 231
FemCap, 232
male condoms, 230–231
Battering. *See* Intimate partner
violence (IPV)
BBD (bladder and bowel dysfunction),
124, 125
*Beck Depression Inventory–Primary Care
Version* (U.S. Preventive Services Task
Force), 36
Bedwetting Store, 139
Behavioral variant frontotemporal dementia
(bvFTD), 505
Behavior Assessment System for Children
(Reynolds & Kamphaus), 57
Behavior changes in adults. *See* Lifestyle
changes
Benign prostatic hyperplasia (BPH),
449–454
assessment of, 451
clinical management goals for, 451
database used for, 450–451
defined, 449
diagnostic screening and tests for, 451,
452*b*, 453*f*
impact index, 457
management and treatment of, 451–452, 454
overview of, 449
patient and family education on, 454
physical examination findings, 451
prevalence and incidence, 449–450
self-management resources
and tools, 454

symptom index, 456
Benzodiazepines, 432
β²-Agonists, 441
Beta blockers, 572*t*
Bethesda System Pap smear classification,
172–173*t*, 173–174
Beyond Blue, 527
Bicipital tendinopathy, 705–706, 708
Bioidentical hormone therapy, 222, 223
Biomarkers, 509
Bipolar affective disorder (BAD), 92, 678
Birth control. *See* Hormonal contraception;
Nonhormonal contraception
Birth Control Method Explorer, 38
Birth to 5: Watch Me Thrive! (U.S.
Departments of Health and Human
Services and Education), 48
Birth weight, 16, 16*t*
BJI (Bone and Joint Initiative), 695
"Black box" labeling, 94–95
Bladder and bowel dysfunction (BBD),
124, 125
Bladder disorders. *See* Urinary
incontinence (UI)
Bladder training, 240, 241*t*
Bladder wall muscle, 124
Bleeding
abnormal uterine bleeding. *See* Abnormal
uterine bleeding (AUB)
acute bleeding, 147, 151
breakthrough bleeding, 201
chronic bleeding, 151
withdrawal bleeding, 201
Blindness, 554
Blood pressure (BP), 583, 584, 584*t*. *See also*
Hypertension (HTN)
Blood pressure, accurate measurements,
steps for, 316*t*
Body mass index (BMI), 118, 634
Bone and Joint Initiative (BJI), 695
BPH. *See* Benign prostatic hyperplasia (BPH)
Brain imaging, 509
Breakthrough bleeding, 201
Breastfeeding, bottle feeding vs., 8, 13, 101
*Brief Infant/Toddler Social Emotional
Assessment* (Briggs-Gowan, Carter,
Irwin, Wachtel, & Cicchetti), 57
Brigance Screens II (Glascoe), 57
*Bright Futures: Guidelines for Health
Supervision of Adolescents* (American
Academy of Pediatrics and the
Maternal Child Health Bureau), 38
Bromocriptine, 166
Bronchitis, chronic. *See* Chronic obstructive
pulmonary disease (COPD)
Bronchodilators, 471

Bruises on children, 107
Bupropion, 86, 675, 678
Burns on children, 108

C

Cabergoline, 166
Calcineurin inhibitors, topical, 77
California Diabetes and Pregnancy
Program, 310
Caloric intake and absorption, 99–100
Canadian Centre for Occupational Health
and Safety, 711
Cancer screening for cervical, vaginal, and
vulvar cancers
cervical cancer in adolescents, 36
Cancer survivorship, 458–466
assessment of, 461, 462, 462f
clinical management goals, 462, 463
consultations and referrals, 466
database used for, 459–460
defined, 458
diagnostic testing and, 463
epidemiology, 459
overview of, 458
patient education on, 463
physical examination findings, 460, 461t
Cardiovascular disease (CVD), 613. See also
Heart failure
HIV and, 654
Caregivers, 511, 512, 564–565
Caregiver Strain Index (CSI), 512
Carrier screening for recessive conditions,
255–256, 255t
Cataracts, 450
Catch-up growth, 103. See also Growth
trends
CBT (cognitive behavioral therapy),
95, 97, 434
CDC. See Centers for Disease Control and
Prevention (CDC)
Cell-free fetal DNA testing, 255
Center for the Health Professions, 4
CenteringPregnancy (prenatal care model),
260, 261t
Centers for Disease Control and Prevention
(CDC), 38, 574
on asthma in children, 69
Division of Diabetes, 310
on HIV/AIDS, 649–650
on immunization schedules, 326,
327–329f
on obesity, 634
on postexposure prophylaxis for HIV, 375
sex-specific BMI-for-age growth
charts, 114

on smoking, 672
Cephalosporins, 78
Cerebral palsy (CP), 346–347
Cervical spine diseases, 692. See also Upper
back/neck pain
Cervicothoracic myofascial pain syndrome,
692–693
Cesarean deliveries, 7, 282. See also Vaginal
birth after cesarean (VBAC)
CHA2DS2-VASc score, 416, 417t
CHADS2 score, 416, 417t
Chamomile, 291
Chart reviews, 5
CHCs. See Combined hormonal
contraceptives (CHCs)
Chemoprophylaxis, USPSTF recommenda-
tions for prevention, 336t
Chest radiographs, 65
Child abuse and neglect. See Maltreatment
of children
Child Abuse Prevention and Treatment
Act, 104
Childbirth Connection, 252
Child Development Inventories (Doig, Macias,
Saylor, Craver, & Ingram), 57
Child Protective Services (CPS), 107
Children. See Pediatric health maintenance
and promotion
Children Now, 38
Children's National Medical Center, 103
Child Welfare and Information Gateway, 112
Chlamydia screening, 36
Chorionic villus sampling (CVS), 257
Chronic bleeding, 151
Chronic kidney disease (CKD), HIV
and, 654
Chronic lung disease (CLD), in infants,
12–13
Chronic neuropsychiatric conditions, 80
Chronic nonmalignant pain (CNP),
477–492
assessment of, 480, 481
clinical management goals, 481–482
databases used for, 478–480, 479f, 481f
defined, 477–478, 478f
diagnostic screening and tests, 479f, 480
management and treatment of, 482–491,
484–487f, 488–489t
overview of, 477–478, 478f
patient education, 491
physical examination findings, 480
prevalence of, 478
support resources and tools, 492
Chronic obstructive pulmonary disease
(COPD), 468–475
clinical management goals, 471

combined assessment of, 470, 470t
database used for, 469–471
defined, 468
management and treatment of, 471–475,
472t, 473–474t
overview of, 468
physical examination findings, 469, 469t
prevalence and incidence, 468
spirometric testing for, 469, 470t
Chronic pain syndrome, 477, 478
Chronic venous disease (CVD), 714
Chronic viral hepatitis, 494–503
assessment of, 498
clinical management goals, 498–499
databases used for, 495–497
diagnostic tests for, 496–498t
management and treatment of, 498–503,
501–502t
overview of, 494–495
patient education and resources on,
502–503, 502t
physical exam findings, 496, 496t
Chronic wounds, 713–714, 719–720
Cirrhosis, 494
CISA. See Clinical Immunization Safety
Assessment (CISA)
Citizens United for Research in Epilepsy
(CURE), 546
Client education. See Patient and family
education and resources
Clinical depression, 92
Clinical Immunization Safety Assessment
(CISA), 46
CNP. See Chronic nonmalignant pain (CNP)
Coagulopathy, 144
COC (combined oral contraceptives) pills,
151, 192, 200–201, 205–206
COEIN etiologies (coagulopathy, ovulatory,
endometrial, iatrogenic, not yet
classified), 144–145
Cognitive behavioral therapy (CBT),
95, 97, 434
Cold sores. See Herpes simplex virus (HSV)
infections
Collaborative practices, 4–5
Colposcopic evaluation, 174, 175
Combination therapies, 222, 223t
Combined hormonal contraceptives (CHCs)
assessment for, 205
COC pills, 151, 192, 200–201, 205–206
contraindications to start, 192, 193–199t
oral contraceptives, comparison of,
209–214t
transdermal patch, 201, 206
vaginal contraceptive ring, 201–202, 206

Combined oral contraceptives (COC) pills, 151, 192, 200–201
Common adult presentations. *See* Adult presentations
Common obstetric presentation. *See* Obstetric presentations
Common pediatric presentations. *See* Pediatric presentations
Communication with developmentally disabled adults, 348–349
Comorbidities, effect on warfarin stability, 418
Complementary and alternative medicine methods, 434
Condoms, as barrier method of contraception
    female, 231
    male, 230–231
Conduct disorder, 81
Confusion Assessment Method (CAM), 558*f*, 560
Congenital hypothyroid screening of infants, 9
Congenital scoliosis, 695
Consent, patient
    adolescents and, 32–33
    for birth choice, 285–287*f*
Constipation, 610, 611*t*
Contraception. *See* Hormonal contraception; Nonhormonal contraception
Contraceptive sponge, 231
Contraindications, for stimulants, 86–87
Controlled substances. *See* Opiates
Controller medications, 66, 441
COPD. *See* Chronic obstructive pulmonary disease (COPD)
Copper T 380-A intrauterine contraceptive, 232–235, 236
Cortical inhibitory pathway, 124
Corticosteroids, 77, 471
Counseling. *See* Patient and family education and resources
CP (cerebral palsy), 346–347
CPS (Child Protective Services), 107
CRAFFT (mnemonic), 36
CURE (Citizens United for Research in Epilepsy), 546
Current Procedural Terminology (CPT), 48
Cushing's disease, 157
Cutaneous abscesses, management of, 395–400
    assessment of, 396
    clinical management goals for, 396
    database used for, 395–396
    overview of, 395
CVS (chorionic villus sampling), 257

Cyclothymia, 92
Cystitis, 323–324
Cytology. *See* Abnormal cytology

D

Dating violence. *See* Intimate partner violence (IPV)
Daytime urinary incontinence, 125
DCM (dilated cardiomyopathy), 566
Degenerative joint disease. *See* Osteoarthritis (OA)
Degenerative scoliosis, 695
Delirium, 555–557, 560, 561, 561*t*
Dementia, 504–513
    assessment of, 509
    caregiver support and resources, 512
    causes of, 504, 505*t*
    clinical management goals for, 509
    database used for, 505, 506*t*, 507–509
    diagnostic tests for, 508–509, 509*t*
    frontotemporal, 504, 505, 507–508
    management and treatment of, 509–512, 510*t*
    mixed, 505
    overview of, 504–505, 505*t*
    vascular, 504, 507
Dementia with Lewy bodies (DLB), 504, 505, 507
Denver II Developmental Screening Test (Frankenburg, Camp, & Van Natta), 57
Depo-Provera®, 202
Depression, adults, 514–527
    assessment of, 518–519
    databases used for, 516–518, 517*t*
    definition of, 514
    diagnostic screening and tests, 515*f*, 517–519, 518*t*, 521
    management and treatment of, 521, 522–525*t*
    medications causing, 518, 518*t*
    overview of, 514–516, 515*f*, 516*f*
    patient and family education on, 521
    physical examination findings, 517
    in pregnancy, 290
    self-management resources and tools, 527
Depression, childhood, 90–98
    ADHD and, 82
    adolescent, 36
    assessment of, 94
    databases used for, 92–93
    medication for, 94–95, 96–97*t*, 97
    overview of, 90–91
    self-management resources in, 98
    treatment and management of, 94–95, 97
Depression and Bipolar Support Alliance, 527

De Quervain's tenosynovitis, 706
Dermatitis. *See* Atopic dermatitis (AD)
Detrusor muscle, 124
Developmental delay and autism, screening for, 48–59. *See also* Development and behavior appraisal
    clinician resources for, 58–59
    overview of, 48
    psychometrics, 57–58
    surveillance and screening algorithm for, 49–57, 50–51*f*, 52–56*t*
    tools for, 52–56*t*
Developmental disabilities (DDs), adults with, health maintenance for, 345–363
    assessment of, 351, 352
    databases used for, 348–351
    defined, 346
    diagnostic tests, 352, 354–361*t*
    healthcare maintenance guidelines for, 354–361*t*
    interdisciplinary healthcare teams and, 350, 351*f*
    overview of, 345–348
    physical examination considerations and, 350–351, 352*f*, 353*f*
    self-management resources and tools, 362, 363
    treatment of, 353, 362
Developmental Disabilities Assistance and Civil Rights Act of 2000, 346
Developmental kyphosis, 695
Developmental screening tools, 52–56*t*
Developmental surveillance and screening algorithm, 49–57, 50–51*f*, 52–56*t*
Development and behavior appraisal. *See also* Developmental delay and autism, screening for
    0–3 years, 19
    3–6 years, 23–24
    6–11 years, 27
    infants and, 14
    screening tests and tools, 48–50
Dextroamphetamine, 84
DFU (diabetic foot ulcer), 714, 715, 717–718, 720–721
Diabetes mellitus, 529–538. *See also* Gestational diabetes mellitus (GDM)
    assessment of, 531, 531*t*
    clinical management goals for, 532, 532*t*
    database used for, 529–530
    diagnosis screening and tests for, 530, 531*t*
    foot ulcers and, 714
    HIV and, 654
    management and treatment of, 532–537, 533*t*, 534*f*, 535–536*t*
    overview of, 529

patient and family education on, 537
self-management resources and tools,
537–538
Diabetic foot ulcer (DFU), 714, 715,
717–718, 720–721
*Diagnostic and Statistical Manual for Mental
Disorders* (DSM)
on anxiety, 430–431
on autism spectrum disorders, 347
on childhood depression, 91
on depression, 514, 518
on transgendered individuals, 365
Diagnostic screening and tests
for 0–3 years, 20–21
for 3–6 years, 24–25
for 6–11 years, 29
for 12–21 years, 36
for abscesses, 397
for ADHD, 82–83
for amenorrhea and PCOS, 161, 162,
163–165t, 165
for anemia in adults, 408–410, 409t, 411t
for asthma, 62, 65, 439, 441, 441f
for atopic dermatitis, 72, 75t
for AUB, 147, 148–150t
for benign prostatic hyperplasia, 451,
452b, 453f
for cancer screening, 179
and cancer survivorship, 463
for chronic viral hepatitis, 496–498t
for CNP, 479f, 480
for dementia, 508–509, 509t
for depression in adults, 515f,
517–519, 518t
for diabetes in pregnancy, 306, 307t
for diabetes mellitus, 530, 531t
for epilepsy, 540, 545
for FTT in infancy, 102
for GERD, 550
for heart failure, 568–569
for HIV, 657, 660–661
HIV infection and, 381, 382t
for hormonal contraception, 205
for HSV infections, 578–579
for hypertension, 586–587, 587t
for IBS, 607, 608–609t
infants and, 9
for intimate partner violence, 601
for lipid disorders, 615–616
for low back pain, 624–625
maltreatment of children and, 111
for menopause transition, 221
for nonhormonal contraception, 235
for obesity, 117–118, 637
for post-NICU patients, 16
postpartum, 272

for preeclampsia-eclampsia, 317
for preexposure prophylaxis for HIV, 388
pregnancy and, 248, 249b, 260, 262t
prenatal genetic, 253–257
for smoking, 677
for thyroid disorders, 684, 686–687t,
687, 688–689
for transgendered individuals, 367, 368t
for upper back/neck pain, 698t, 700, 700t
for upper extremity tendinopathy, 707,
708, 709
for urinary incontinence in children, 131,
132–133f, 134f
for urinary incontinence in women,
238–239, 238t
Diaphragm, 231–232
Diarrhea, 610, 611t
Diastolic heart failure, 566
Diastolic HTN, 583
Diet
history and obesity, 636
interventions and patient motivation,
638, 639–641f
Differential diagnoses
for abscesses, 396
for anemia in adults, 408–410, 409t
for asthma, 62, 438
for atopic dermatitis, 72, 76f
for heart failure, 568
for preeclampsia-eclampsia, 317
during pregnancy, 293, 295
for urinary incontinence in
women, 237, 237t
Dilated cardiomyopathy (DCM), 566
Diphtheria and tetanus toxoids and acellular
pertussis vaccine (DTaP), 42
Discomforts, of pregnancy, 290–300
musculoskeletal pain, 291–294
overview of, 290
poor quality of sleep, 290–291
Diuretic therapy, 573t
DLB (dementia with Lewy bodies), 504,
505, 507
Documentation, importance of, 1, 4–5
Domestic violence. *See* Intimate partner
violence (IPV)
Dopamine agonists, 166
Dopamine antagonists, 296, 297
Down syndrome, 348
DREAMS mnemonic, 429
Drugs and alcohol use. *See* Substance use
and abuse
DTaP vaccine, 42
Dysfunctional uterine bleeding (DUB). *See*
Abnormal uterine bleeding (AUB)
Dyslipidemia screening, 25, 29, 36

Dysmorphic features, 101
Dyspnea, 566
Dysthymia, 92–93, 514

E
Early and Periodic Screening, Diagnostic,
and Treatment (EPSDT), 48
E-cigarettes, 673
Economic abuse, 594
ECP (emergency contraception pill),
203–204, 205, 207, 230, 233
Eczema. *See* Atopic dermatitis (AD)
Education. *See* Patient and family education
and resources
Elbow tendinopathy, 706, 708
Elderly. *See* Older adults
Emergency contraception pill (ECP),
203–204, 205, 207, 230, 233.
See also Hormonal contraception
Emotional abuse, 594
Emotional or psychologic abuse. *See*
Maltreatment of children
Emotional/psychologic abuse, 105
Emphysema. *See* Chronic obstructive
pulmonary disease (COPD)
Endocervical sampling, 175
End-of-life and palliative care, 512, 573
Endometrial etiologies, 144
Endometrial sampling, 175
End-organ abnormalities, 157
Enuresis risoria, 125
Environmental history. *See* Family and
social histories
Environmental toxin exposures, 468
Epilepsy, 348, 539–546, 541t
assessment of, 540, 541
clinical management goals for, 541, 545
database used for, 539–540
defined, 539
diagnostic screening and tests for,
540, 545
overview of, 539
physical examination for, 540
referral guidelines, 545
self-management resources, 546
treatment and management of, 545, 545t
Epilepsy Therapy Project, 546
Equianalgesic tables, 488, 490
Erythropoiesis, 401
Escitalopram, 95
Esophageal carcinoma, 547
Estradiol, 218
Estrogens, 192, 200, 218, 221
Estrogen therapy, 222, 222t
Ethical concerns, 1
Ethinyl estradiol, 147

Ethnicity-based health issues
    carrier screening and, 255–256, 255*t*
    chronic viral hepatitis and, 494
    HIV and, 651
    hypertension and, 588
    PCOS and, 158
Exacerbations of COPD, 472, 474–475
Executive Function Performance Test, 508
Exercise. *See* Physical activity
External sphincter muscle, 124

F
Failure to thrive (FTT), 99–103
Fallopian tubal patency, 188
Falls, as geriatric syndromes, 555, 556, 557, 561
    prevention of, 334–335*f*
FAM (fertility awareness methods), 230, 233–234
Familial transmission of depression, 91
Family and social histories
    0–3 years, 18
    3–6 years, 23
    6–11 years, 27
    12–21 years, 33–34
    abscesses and, 395
    amenorrhea and, 158
    of anemia in adults, 405–407
    asthma and, 61, 437
    atopic dermatitis and, 71
    AUB and, 146
    benign prostatic hyperplasia and, 450
    cancer survivorship and, 460
    chronic viral hepatitis and, 495–496
    CNP and, 480
    COPD and, 469
    depression and, 90–93, 516
    of developmentally disabled adults, 350
    diabetes mellitus and, 530
    epilepsy and, 539
    FTT in children and, 100
    GERD and, 548
    heart failure and, 567
    hormonal contraception and, 204
    HSV and, 577
    hypertension and, 585
    IBS and, 606
    infants, 8
    lipid disorders and, 614
    low back pain and, 623
    maltreatment of children and, 106–107
    menopause transition and, 219
    nonhormonal contraceptives and, 234–235
    obesity and, 115, 636
    PCOS and, 161

    of post-NICU patients, 15
    postpartum care and, 269
    preeclampsia-eclampsia and, 315
    pregnancy and, 247
    smoking and, 675
    thyroid disorders and, 683–684
    transgendered individuals and, 366
    upper back/neck pain and, 696
    upper extremity tendinopathy and, 707
    wound care and, 715
Family Caregiver Alliance, 513, 564
Family education. *See* Patient and family education and resources
Family Smoking Prevention and Tobacco Control Act, 2009, 673
Fatigue. *See* Sleep
FDA. *See* U.S. Food and Drug Administration (FDA)
Female condoms, 231
Female-to-male (FTM) identities, 366, 368, 371*t*
FemCap, 232
Feminizing hormone options, 369*t*
Fertility awareness method (FAM), 230, 233–234
Fetal fibronectin (fFN), 321
Fever blisters. *See* Herpes simplex virus (HSV) infections
FHA (functional hypothalamic amenorrhea), 156
First well-baby visits, 7–10
Fluoxetine, 95
Fluvoxamine, 95
Folate (folic acid) deficiency, 405, 407, 410, 413
Food and Drug Administration. *See* U.S. Food and Drug Administration (FDA)
Forced expiratory volume (FEV), 439, 469
Forced vital capacity (FVC), 439, 469
Formal developmental assessments, infant, 14
Fractures, in children, 108–109
Frailty, 554, 556, 557, 561–562
Frontotemporal dementia (FTD), 504, 505, 507–508
FTT. *See* Failure to thrive (FTT)
Functional Activities Questionnaire, 508
Functional bowel disorder. *See* Irritable bowel syndrome (IBS)
Functional hypothalamic amenorrhea (FHA), 156

G
Gastroesophageal reflux disease (GERD), 547–553
    assessment of, 549

    clinical management goals, 550
    databases used for, 548–549
    defined, 547
    diagnostic screening and tests for, 550
    in infants, 13
    management and treatment of, 550–551, 552*t*, 553
    overview of, 547–548, 548*t*
    patient education and resources on, 553
    pregnancy and, 298–300, 299*t*
Gastrointestinal tract during pregnancy, 294–295, 295*t*, 296, 297–298, 297*t*
GCT (glucose challenge test), 306
GDM (Gestational diabetes mellitus) in pregnancy, 304–310
Geisinger's Health Library, 690
Gender identity disorder. *See* Transgendered individuals, health maintenance for
General Anxiety Disorder-7 screening tool (GAD-7), 429, 430*f*
Generalized anxiety disorder, 428, 431
Genetics
    disorders, 348
    prenatal diagnosis. *See* Prenatal genetic diagnosis
    prenatal screening. *See* Prenatal genetic screening
    transmission of depression, 91
Genital HSV, 575, 576*f*
Genitourinary syndrome of menopause (GSM), 217–218
GERD. *See* Gastroesophageal reflux disease (GERD)
Geriatric Depression Scale, 508, 512, 516
Geriatrics. *See* Older adults
Geriatric syndromes, 554–565
    assessment of, 560–561
    clinical management goals, 562
    database used for, 556–557, 560
    defined, 554
    delirium, 555–557
    diagnostic tests for, 562–564, 563*t*
    falls, 555, 556
    frailty, 554, 556
    online resources for clinicians/patients/caregivers, 564–565
    physical examinations for, 557, 558–559*f*, 560*t*
    sensory impairment, 554–555, 556
    treatment and management of, 562–564
    urinary incontinence, 555, 556
Gerontological Advanced Practice Nurses Association, 564
Gestational diabetes mellitus (GDM), in pregnancy, 304–310, 529. *See also* Diabetes mellitus

clinical management goals for, 306
defined, 305
GDM A1/A2, postpartum
    management of, 309–310
methods to diagnose, 306, 307t
overview of, 305
prevalence and incidence, 305
women with, resources for, 310
Giggle incontinence (enuresis risoria), 125
Global Consensus Statement on
    Menopausal Hormone Therapy, 221
Global Initiative for Chronic Obstructive
    Lung Disease (GOLD), 469, 471, 475
Glucose challenge test (GCT), 306
Goiter. *See* Thyroid disorders
Gonadal dysgenesis, 157
Gonadotropin-releasing hormone
    agonists, 152
Gonorrhea screening, 36
Group and family therapies, 434
Growth trends
    catch-up growth, 103
    FTT and, 101
    infants and, 8
    post-NICU patients and, 16
GSM (genitourinary syndrome of
    menopause), 217–218
Gynecology. *See also* specific issues
    abnormal uterine bleeding.
        See Abnormal uterine
        bleeding (AUB)
    amenorrhea and PCOS, 156–169
    hormonal contraception, 192–207
    lower genital tract, cancer screening for,
        171–186
    menopause transition, 217–227
    nonhormonal contraception, 230–236
    oral contraceptives, comparison of,
        209–214t
    sterilization, 188–190
    urinary incontinence, 237–244

H

H2RA (histamine-2 receptor antagonists),
    298, 300
Haemophilus influenzae Type B (Hib)
    vaccine, 42, 45
Hartford Institute for Geriatric Nursing, 565
HBV (hepatitis B virus). *See* Chronic viral
    hepatitis
HCV (hepatitis C virus). *See* Chronic viral
    hepatitis
HDL. *See* High-density lipoprotein (HDL)
Head trauma, in children, 109
Healia Health Communities and Support
    Groups, 703

Health assessment form, 349
Healthcare disparity, 345
Healthcare for Adults with Intellectual and
    Developmental Disabilities, 362
Health education. *See* Patient and family
    education and resources
Health histories
    0–3 years, 18
    3–6 years, 23
    6–11 years, 27
    12–21 years, 33
    abscesses and, 395
    ADHD in children and, 84
    of adults with developmental disabilities,
        349–350
    amenorrhea and, 158
    anemia and, 405–407
    asthma and, 61, 437
    atopic dermatitis and, 70–71
    AUB and, 145–146
    benign prostatic hyperplasia and, 450
    cancer survivorship and, 459–460
    chronic viral hepatitis and, 495–496
    CNP and, 480
    COPD and, 469
    depression and, 518
    diabetes mellitus and, 529–530
    epilepsy and, 539
    FTT in children and, 100
    heart failure and, 567
    HIV infection and, 380–381
    hormonal contraception and, 204
    HSV and, 577
    hypertension and, 585
    IBS and, 606
    of infants, 8
    lipid disorders and, 614
    low back pain and, 623
    lower genital tract cancer and, 176
    menopause transition and, 219
    obesity and, 115, 636
    PCOS and, 161
    of post-NICU patients, 15
    preeclampsia-eclampsia and, 315
    PrEP and, 386, 387
    PTB risk and, 320–321
    smoking and, 675
    sterilization and, 190
    thyroid disorders and, 683–684
    of transgendered individuals, 366
    transgendered individuals and, 366
    upper back/neck pain and, 695–696
    upper extremity tendinopathy and,
        706–707
    urinary incontinence in children,
        126, 128

urinary tract infection and, 323
wound care and, 714–715
Health maintenance and promotion, adult,
    326–343
    assessment of, 333, 335–336b
    clinical management goals for, 333
    database used for, 331, 332t, 333
    overview of, 326
Healthy People 2010 (U.S. Department of
    Health & Human Services), 634
Healthy People 2020 (U.S. Department of
    Health & Human Services), 33,
    634–635
Hearing impairment, 554–555, 556, 561
Hearing screening
    0–3 years, 9, 13–14, 20
    3–6 years, 25
    6–11 years, 29
Heartburn. *See* Gastroesophageal reflux
    disease (GERD)
Heart failure, 566–574
    assessment of, 568
    clinical management goals, 568
    database used for, 567–568
    defined, 566
    diagnostic tests for, 568–569
    overview of, 566–567
    physical examinations for, 568
    treatment and management for, 569,
        570f, 571, 571b, 573–574
HEEADSSS (mnemonic), 34
HELLP (hemolysis, elevated liver enzymes,
    and low platelets) syndrome, 295, 313
Hemiplegic cerebral palsy, 347
Hemoglobin, and hematocrit screening, 36
Hemolytic anemia, 404, 406–407, 410, 412
Hepatitis A (Hep A) vaccine, 43, 45
Hepatitis B vaccine, 42
Hepatitis B virus (HBV), 494
Hepatitis C virus (HCV), 494–495
Hepatocytes, 494
Hepcidin, 404
Herbal alternatives, for menopause
    transition, 224
Herpes Resource Center, 581
Herpes simplex virus (HSV) infections, 78,
    575–581
    assessment of, 577–578
    clinical management goals, 578
    database used for, 577
    diagnostic screening and tests for,
        578–579
    overview of, 575
    treatment and management of, 579–580,
        579–580t
    types of, 575–576

HG (hyperemesis gravidarum), 294
Hib vaccine, 42
High-density lipoprotein (HDL), 613
High-grade squamous intraepithelial lesion (HSIL), 174, 181*f*
Histamine-2 receptor antagonists (H2RA), 298, 300
HIV (Human immunodeficiency virus), 649–669. *See also* Postexposure prophylaxis (PEP), for HIV infection
  assessment of, 663
  care continuum, 652, 653–654, 653*f*, 657
  clinical management goals, 663
  database used for, 661–663
  diagnostic screening and tests, 657, 660–661
  epidemiology, 649–651, 650*t*
  immunizations for, 657, 658–660*t*
  infectious fluids, 375, 376*t*
  pathogenesis, 651–652, 653*f*
  patient education on, 668
  preexposure prophylaxis for. *See* Preexposure prophylaxis (PrEP), for HIV
  routes of exposure to, 375, 376*t*
  screening for, 36
  status, documenting, 387*f*
  treatment and management of, 663, 666*t*, 667–668
Hormonal contraception, 192–207
  alternatives to oral contraception, 215–216*t*
  assessment of, 205
  clinical management goals in, 205
  COC pills, 200–201, 205–206
  combined hormonal contraception, 192, 200–202
  contraindications to, 192, 193–199*t*
  databases used for, 204–205
  emergency contraception pill, 203–204
  oral contraceptives, comparison of, 209–214*t*
  overview of, 192
  patient adherence, 206–208
  physical examinations for, 204–205
  progestin-only contraception, 202–203
  transdermal patch, 201
  treatment and management of, 206–208
  vaginal contraceptive ring, 201–202
Hormonal gender reassignment therapy, 367
Hormone therapy (HT), 221–223
Hospital Elder Life Program, 565
Hospital for Sick Children, 294
HPV (human papillomavirus), 171
HPV DNA testing, 174

HSDD (hypoactive sexual desire disorder), 225
HSG (hysterosalpingography), 189
HSIL (high-grade squamous intraepithelial lesion), 174, 181*f*
HSV infections, 78. *See* Herpes simplex virus (HSV) infections
HT (hormone therapy), 221–223
HTN. *See* Hypertension (HTN)
Human papillomavirus (HPV), 44, 45, 171
Hydration, during pregnancy, 296
5-Hydroxytryptamine 3-receptor antagonists, 297
Hyperemesis gravidarum (HG), 294
Hyperglycemia and Adverse Pregnancy Outcomes (HAPO), 305
Hyperkyphosis, 695
Hyperprolactinemia, 157, 167
Hypertension (HTN), 583–593
  assessment of, 587
  classification of, 583
  clinical management goals, 587
  database used for, 584–587
  defined, 583
  diagnostic screening and tests for, 586–587, 587*t*
  management and treatment of, 587–588, 589*f*, 590–591*t*, 592
  patient education on, 592
  in pregnancy. *See* Preeclampsia-eclampsia
  prevalence of, 583
  substances associated with, 585, 586*t*
Hyperthyroidism, 682–683, 689
Hypertriglyceridemia, 613
Hypoactive sexual desire disorder (HSDD), 225
Hypoglycemia, 530. *See also* Diabetes mellitus
Hypothalamic amenorrhea, 156, 166. *See also* Amenorrhea; Polycystic ovarian syndrome (PCOS)
Hypothalamic-pituitary-ovarian (HPO) axis, 140, 156
Hypothyroidism, 156
Hysterectomy, 153, 188, 283
Hysterosalpingography (HSG), 189
Hysteroscopy, 189

I

IASP (International Association for the Study of Pain), 477
Iatrogenic etiologies, 144–145
IBS. *See* Irritable bowel syndrome (IBS)
Ibuprofen, 151
ID (intellectual disability), 346

Idiopathic scoliosis, 695
IFIS (intraoperative floppy iris syndrome), 450
IgE sensitization, 65, 70, 436, 441
ILAE (International League Against Epilepsy), 539
Immunizations
  0–3 years, 21
  3–6 years, 25
  6–11 years, 29
  12–21 years, 33, 37
  active vs. passive, 46
  infants, 9
  lag in, 37
  modalities, 45–46
  pediatric schedule, 42–44
  schedules, 42
Implanon®, 202
Implants, contraceptive, 202–203, 207
IN (intraepithelial neoplasia), 171
Inactivated poliovirus vaccine (IPV), 43
Incision and drainage procedure, 397, 398–400
Independent practices, 4
Independent reports on maltreatment of children, 110, 110*t*
Individuals with Disabilities Education Improvement Act (IDEA), 48
Infants, healthy, 7–10
Infectious Disease Society of America (IDSA), 649
Influenza vaccine, 43, 44
Inhaled corticosteroids (ICS), 66
Inhalers, 444–445*b*, 445
  nicotine, 678
Injectable progestin, 202, 206–207
Injuries, 106
INR. *See* International Normalized Ratio (INR)
Insomnia, during pregnancy, 291
Institute of Medicine (IOM), 458
Instrumental activities of daily living (IADLs), 561
Instrumental Activities of Daily Living Scale, 508
Insulins, 535, 536*t*
Intellectual disability (ID), 346
Interdisciplinary healthcare teams, 350, 351*f*
Intermenstrual bleeding, 219
International Association for Study of Pain (IASP), 477, 492
International Association of Diabetes and Pregnancy Study Groups (IADPSG), 305–306

International Children's Continence Society, 139

International Classification of Diseases–10 codes, 480

International League Against Epilepsy (ILAE), 539

International Normalized Ratio (INR)
managing variations in, 419, 420–421t
variables in warfarin response, 416–419, 417–418t, 419t
warfarin therapy, monitoring of, 415, 416t

International Premature Ovarian Failure Support Group, 169

International Society for Hypertension (ISH), 584

Intimate partner violence (IPV), 594–602
assessment of, 600–601, 600t
categories of, 594
client/patient education, 601
clinical management goals for, 601
consequences of, 595, 596
database used for, 598, 599t
defined, 594
diagnostic testing for, 601
overview of, 594
physical examination for, 599, 599t
prevalence and incidence, 595
self-management resources and tools, 601–602
special risk populations, 596–598t
treatment and management of, 601
victimization by race/ethnicity, 595, 595t

Intraepithelial neoplasia (IN), 171

Intraoperative floppy iris syndrome (IFIS), 450

Intrauterine contraceptive (IUC), 230, 232–233

Intravenous fluid therapy, 296

Iodine deficiency, and thyroid disorder, 682

IPV. See Intimate partner violence (IPV)

IPV (inactivated poliovirus) vaccine, 43

Iron deficiency, 20
anemia, 402, 403, 405–406, 408–409, 409t, 410, 411–412

Irritable bowel syndrome (IBS), 605–612
assessment of, 607
clinical management goals, 607
database used for, 606
defined, 605
diagnostic testing for, 607, 608–609t
epidemiology, 605–606
overview of, 605–606
pathophysiology of, 606
patient and family education on, 611
physical examination for, 606

symptoms of, 605
treatment and management of, 607, 609–611, 611t

Irritable Bowel Syndrome Association, 612

Irritants, asthma and, 66, 436

IUC (intrauterine contraceptive), 230, 232–233

J

John A. Hartford Foundation, 565

Johns Hopkins Medical School, 454

Joint National Committee on Prevention, Detection, Evaluation, and Treatment of High Blood Pressure (JNC 7), 583–584

Joslin Diabetes Center, 538

Juvenile Diabetes Research Foundation International, 538

K

Kaiser Family Foundation, 38

Kaiser Permanente Chronic Pain Program and Support Group, 492

Kyphosis, 695

L

Labor management, preterm, 320–322

Lactational amenorrhea method (LAM), 230, 234

LAM (lactational amenorrhea method), 230, 234

LARC (long-acting reversible contraception), 192, 232

Lateral epicondylitis, 706, 708

Laughter Yoga International, 492

LBP. See Low back pain (LBP)

Lead screening
0–3 years, 20
3–6 years, 25
6–11 years, 29

Learning disabilities, screening for, 83

Left ventricular heart failure, 566

Legal issues
implications of reporting child maltreatment, 110t
scope of practice, 1–5

Legislative updates, 4

Leiomyomas, 142, 144, 153

LES (lower esophageal sphincter), 547

Levonorgestrel, 192

Levonorgestrel intrauterine system (LNG-IUS), 203, 207

Life expectancy, adults with developmental disabilities, 345

Lifestyle changes
for hypertension, 587–588
and menopause transition, 224
for obesity and weight loss, 118, 120–121, 120f, 642, 643–644f, 644–645
for smoking cessation, 679

Lipid disorders, 613–618
assessment of, 615
classifications of, 613–614
clinical management goals, 615
database used for, 614–615
defined, 613
diagnostics tests for, 615–616
overview of, 613
patient education, 618
prevalence of, 613
treatment and management of, 616, 617t

Lipid profile, 0–3 years, 21

Liver diseases, 494

LNG-IUS (levonorgestrel intrauterine system), 203, 207

Long-acting reversible contraception (LARC), 192, 232

Low back pain (LBP), 619–633
assessment of, 625
causes of, 619, 619t
database used for, 619, 621t, 622–625, 622t
diagnostic screening and tests for, 624–625
management and treatment of, 626–627, 631–633
overview of, 619
patient education on, 627, 627f, 628–631f, 631–633
physical examinations for, 621t, 623–624
pregnancy and, 291–294

Lower esophageal sphincter (LES), 547

Lower genital tract, cancer screening for, 171–186
abnormal cytology, management of, 174–176, 174–182f
assessment of, 177, 178
Bethesda System Pap smear classification, 172–173t, 173–174
clinical management goals, 178, 179
database used for, 176, 177
diagnostic tests for, 179
overview of, 171–172
treatment and management of, 179, 183, 184–186f

Lower urinary tract symptoms (LUTS), 449, 450

Low-grade squamous intraepithelial lesion (LSIL), 174, 178f, 179f, 180f

Low transverse cesarean sections (LTCS), 282
Lozenge, 677–678
LSIL (low-grade squamous intraepithelial lesion), 174, 178f, 179f, 180f
LTCS (low transverse cesarean sections), 282
Lucile Packard Children's Hospital, 103
Lung disease. *See* Asthma; Chronic obstructive pulmonary disease (COPD)
LUTS (lower urinary tract symptoms), 449, 450
Lymphadenopathy, 72

M

MacArthur Initiative on Depression and Primary Care, 527
Macrocytic anemia, 404–405, 407, 412–413
Magnetic resonance imaging (MRI), 293
Major depressive disorders (MDD), 91, 92
Male condom, 230–231
Male-to-female (MTF) identities, 366, 368, 370t
Malignancy, 144
Maltreatment of children, 104–112. *See* also specific types of abuse; specific types of abuses
    assessment of, 110–111
    databases used for, 106–110
    independent report triggers for, 110, 110t
    overview of, 104
    physical examination findings in, 107–110, 108t
    safety, 110, 111
    treatment and management of, 112
Mandatory reporting, on maltreatment of children, 110–111, 110t
March of Dimes, 17, 252
Masculinizing hormone options, 370t
Mayo Clinic, 169, 553
MCV (mean cell volume), 404, 410
MDD (major depressive disorder), 91, 92
Mean cell volume (MCV), 404, 410
Measles, 40–41
Measles, mumps, rubella (MMR) vaccine, 43, 45
Medical history. *See* Health histories
Medical Nutrition Therapy (MNT), 533
Medications. *See* also Pharmacotherapy/psychotherapy; specific medications
    12–21 years, 33
    asthma and, 61
    causing depression, 518, 518t
    monitoring, 95

prescribing, supervision for, 4
    for urinary infections in pregnancy, 324t
    weight gain and, 636
Medroxyprogesterone acetate (MPA), 152, 202
Medscape eMedicine, 103
Mefenamic acid, 152
Megaloblastic anemias, 404, 407, 410, 412–413
Mended Hearts, 574
Meningococcal vaccine, 44, 45
Menometrorrhagia, 219
Menopause hormone therapy (MHT), 221
Menopause transition, 217–227
    assessment of, 220
    clinical management goals in, 220
    clinical practice guidelines for, 226–227
    database used for, 219–220
    overview of, 217
    physical examination findings, 220
    self-management resources and tools, 226
    symptoms, 217–219
    treatment and management of, 221–226
    types of, 217
Menorrhagia, 140, 219
Menstrual cycle. *See* also Amenorrhea; Polycystic ovarian syndrome (PCOS)
    disturbances in, 219, 220
    phases of, 140
Mental status examination (MSE), 93
Men who have sex with men (MSM), 385
    behavioral risk assessment, 391
    screening tool for, 392
Merck Medicus Resource Library, 454
Methicillin-resistant *Staphylococcus aureus* (MRSA), 395
MHT (menopause hormone therapy), 221
Microcytic anemias, 402–404, 408–410, 411–412
Mirena®, 203
Mixed dementia, 505
MMR vaccine. *See* Measles, mumps, rubella (MMR) vaccine
MNT (Medical Nutrition Therapy), 533
Modified British Medical Research Council Questionnaire for Assessing the Severity of Breathlessness (mMRC), 470, 470t
Monophasic COC, 152
Monosymptomatic enuresis, 126
Montreal Cognitive Assessment (MOCA), 559f, 560
Mood and cognition, menopause transition and, 218, 220, 225
Mortality/morbidity
    maternal, 283

neonatal, 283
    from preeclampsia, 314
Motherisk, 294
MPA (medroxyprogesterone acetate), 152
MRSA (methicillin-resistant *Staphylococcus aureus*), 395
MSE (mental status examination), 93
Müllerian abnormalities, 157
Multidisciplinary treatment teams. *See* Interdisciplinary healthcare teams
Multi-infarct dementia, 504
Musculoskeletal neck pain, acute, 692
Musculoskeletal pain, in pregnancy, 291–294
    differential diagnosis and management of, 291, 292t
    "red flag" symptoms, 292, 292t
    types of, 291
Musculoskeletal strains/sprains, 694
Myofascial pain syndrome, 692–693

N

NAFC (National Association for Continence), 244
NAMS (North American Menopause Society), 223, 226, 227
Naproxen sodium, 151–152
Nasal spray, nicotine, 678
National Alliance for the Mentally Ill (NAMI), 435, 527
National Association for Continence (NAFC), 244
National Association of Pediatric Nurse Practitioners, 25
National Cancer Institute (NCI), 458
National Center for Health Care Technology, 282
National Center for PTSD, 435
National Center for Transgender Equality, 372
National Center for Victims of Crime's Stalking Resource Center, 602
National Child Abuse and Neglect Data System (NCANDS), 104
National Childhood Vaccine Injury Act (NCVIA), 46
National Coalition for Cancer Survivorship (NCCS), 458
National Coalition of Anti-Violence Programs, 602
National Comprehensive Cancer Network (NCCN), 462
    survivorship baseline assessment guideline, 462f
National Diabetes Education Program, 537

National Eczema Association Support Network, 79
National Eczema Society (UK), 79
National Health and Nutrition Examination Survey (NHANES), 583, 634
National Heart, Lung, and Blood Institute, 69, 402, 446, 618
National HIV/AIDS Clinicians' Consulting Center, 384
National Institute for Diabetes, Digestive and Kidney Diseases (NIDDK), 244
National Institute for Health and Clinical Excellence (NICE), 79
National Institute of Allergy and Infectious Disease, 581
National Institute of Arthritis and Musculoskeletal and Skin Diseases (NIAMS), 703
National Institute of Child and Human Development, 282
National Institute of Diabetes and Digestive and Kidney Diseases, 503
National Institute on Aging, 565
National Institutes of Health (NIH), 10, 413, 454
 on BMI categories, 634–635
 on e-cigarettes, 673
 on GDM, 306
 on GERD, 553
 on IBS, 612
 on VBAC, 282
National Intimate Partner and Sexual Violence Survey (NISVS), 595
National Jewish Medical and Research Center, 69, 77, 79
National Online Resource Center on Violence Against Women, 602
National Sexual Violence Resource Center, 601
National Women's Health Information Center, 252
National Youth Tobacco Survey (NYTS), 673
Natural family planning (NFP), 230, 233–234, 235, 236
Nausea and vomiting of pregnancy (NVP), 294–298
 pharmacotherapy for, 297
NCANDS (National Child Abuse and Neglect Data System), 104
NCVIA. See National Childhood Vaccine Injury Act (NCVIA)
Neck pain. See Upper back/neck pain
Neglect, child, 105–106. See also Maltreatment of children
 physical examination for, 110

Nemours Children's Health Systems, 38
Neonatal intensive care unit (NICU), 12–17
Nerve impingement, 622, 622t
Neural tube defects (NTD), 253, 254–255
Neurobehavioral and sensory deficits, 13–14
Neurologic examinations, 624
Neuromuscular scoliosis, 695
Neuropsychiatric conditions, and ADHD, 83–84
Newborns, 7–10
New York Heart Association (NYHA), 566
New York State Department of Health (NYSDOH), 375, 376–377t
Nexplanon, 202
NFP (natural family planning), 230, 233–234, 235, 236
NICE (National Institute for Health and Clinical Excellence), 79
Nicotine
 addictive nature of, 673
 replacement product, 674–675, 677–678
Nicotine patch, 677
NICU patients, 12–17
NIDDK (National Institute for Diabetes, Digestive and Kidney Diseases), 244
Nighttime intermittent incontinence, 125–126
NIPT (noninvasive prenatal testing), 255
Nocturnal enuresis, 125–126
Nonhormonal contraception, 230–236
 assessment of, 235
 barrier method of contraception. See Barrier methods, contraception
 clinical management goals in, 235
 databases used for, 234–235
 overview, 230
 self-management resources and tools, 236
 treatment and management of, 235–236
Nonhormonal drugs, and menopause transition, 223–224
Noninvasive prenatal testing (NIPT), 255
Nonmalignant pain, chronic (CNP). See Chronic nonmalignant pain (CNP)
Nonmonosymptomatic enuresis, 126
Nonoccupational postexposure prophylaxis (nPEP), 377, 379f. See also Postexposure prophylaxis (PEP), for HIV infection
 risks and benefits of, 380
Nonsteroidal anti-inflammatory drugs (NSAIDs), 151–152, 482

Nonstimulant medications, and ADHD, 86
Normocytic anemia, 404, 406–407, 410, 412
North American Menopause Society (NAMS), 223, 226, 227
Not yet classified etiologies, 145
Novel antipsychotic medications and weight gain, 636
NSAIDs (nonsteroidal anti-inflammatory drugs), 151–152, 482
Nuchal line, 691
Nuchal translucency (NT), 253, 254
Nutrition
 0–3 years, 19
 3–6 years, 23
 6–11 years, 28
 FTT and, 99–103
 infants and, 8, 14
 menopause transition and, 226
 post NICU infants and, 15
 postpartum care, 270
 pregnancy and, 247, 263, 263t, 296
 and preterm labor risk, 321
 supplements use, 419
NVP. See Nausea and vomiting of pregnancy (NVP)

O

OAB (overactive bladder), 238, 238t, 240, 242t
OAC therapy. See Oral anticoagulation (OAC) therapy
Obesity, 634–647
 in adolescents, 35, 114–115
 in adults, 635
 assessment of, 118, 638
 in children, 635
 consequences of, 635
 databases used for, 115, 116f, 117–118, 636–637
 diagnostic testing for, 117–118, 637
 diet interventions and, 638, 639–641f
 in early childhood, 114
 etiology of, 635
 in infancy, 114
 mental illness and, 635–636
 overview of, 634
 patient and family education and resources on, 646–647
 in school-age children, 114
 in special populations, 115
 treatment and management of, 118, 119t, 120–121, 120f, 642, 643–644f, 644–646
 in women, 158

Obstetric health maintenance and promotion. *See also* specific issues
  medical consultation/interprofessional collaboration/transfer of care during, 277–281
  postpartum visits, 268–274
  prenatal genetic screening and diagnosis, 253–259
  prenatal visits, initial, 246–252
  prenatal visits, return, 260–266
Obstetric presentations. *See also* specific issues
  discomforts of pregnancy, 290–300
  gestational diabetes mellitus in pregnancy, 304–310
  preterm labor management, 320–322
  trial of labor vs. vaginal birth after cesarean, 282–287
  urinary tract infection in pregnancy, 323–325
Obstetrics and Gynaecology of Canada Guidelines, 227
Obstructive pulmonary disease, chronic. *See* Chronic obstructive pulmonary disease (COPD)
Occupational and environmental history, asthma and, 61
Occupational exposures (PEP). *See* Postexposure prophylaxis (PEP), for HIV infection
Office of Developmental Primary Care, University of California, 362
OGTT (oral glucose tolerance test), 305
Older adults. *See also* Dementia
  anxiety disorders and, 434–435
  individualizing screening decisions, 326, 330–331, 331*f*
  prevention of falls in, 334–335*f*
Omalizumab (Xolair), 67
Opiates
  long-acting, 488, 489*t*
  policies and protocols for, 483, 484–487*f*, 487, 488–489*t*, 490–491
  risk assessment, 480, 481*f*
  short-acting, 488, 488*t*
Oppositional defiant disorder, 81
Oral anticoagulation (OAC) therapy, 415–426
  associated risk, 416
  dosing and follow-up in, 419, 420*t*
  managing variations in INR, 419, 420–421*t*
  overview of, 415
  patient education and safety, 421, 422–424*t*
  target-specific anticoagulants, 424–425, 426*t*

  treatment duration, 416, 416*t*
  variables in warfarin response, 416–419, 417–418*t*, 419*t*
Oral contraceptives
  comparison of, 209–214*t*
  hormonal alternatives to, 215–216*t*
Oral glucose tolerance test (OGTT), 305
Oral health
  0–3 years, 19, 21
  6–11 years, 29
  12–21 years, 33
Oral systemic corticosteroids, 66
Order serum testing, 317
Osteoarthritis (OA), 694
Outflow tract/uterus disorders, and amenorrhea, 157, 167
Ovarian disorders, 167. *See also* Amenorrhea; Polycystic ovarian syndrome (PCOS)
Overactive bladder (OAB), 238, 238*t*, 240, 242*t*
Overweight. *See* Obesity
Ovulatory disorders, 144

P
Palliative care, 512, 573
PALM (polyps, adenomyosis, leiomyomas, malignancy), 141, 144
Palo Alto Medical Foundation, 38
Panic disorder, 428, 430
Pap smears
Bethesda System classification, 172–173*t*, 173–174
  evaluation techniques for, 174, 175
  screening guidelines for, 171–172
Parent-child interactions
  0–3 years, 18, 21
  3–6 years, 23
  6–11 years, 27, 30–31
  12–21 years, 32, 37
  infants, 8
  post-NICU patients and, 16
Parent education. *See* Patient and family education and resources
Parents' Evaluation of Developmental Status (Glascoe), 57
Passive vs. active immunizations, 46. *See also* Immunizations
Pathologic reflux, 13
Pathophysiology, theories for ADHD, 81
Patient and family education and resources
  0–3 years, 21
  3–6 years, 25
  6–11 years, 29–30, 30*f*
  12–21 years, 37
  on abscess infections, 400
  on ADHD, 84, 87, 88*b*

  on adults with developmental disabilities, 362, 362*f*
  on amenorrhea and PCOS, 168–169
  on anemia, 413
  on anticoagulation therapy (oral), 421, 422–424*t*
  on asthma, 67–68
  on atopic dermatitis in children, 78
  on AUB, 153–154
  on benign prostatic hyperplasia, 454
  on cancer, 183
  on cancer survivorship, 463
  on chronic nonmalignant pain, 491
  on chronic viral hepatitis, 502–503, 502*t*
  on COPD, 475
  on depression, 521
  on diabetes mellitus, 537
  on epilepsy, 545
  on FTT, 103
  on GDM, 306
  on GERD, 553
  on geriatric syndromes, 564–565
  on heart failure, 573–574
  on HIV, 668
  on HIV infection, 383
  on hormonal contraception, 205–207
  on HSV infections, 580–581*f*, 581
  on hypertension, 592
  on IBS, 611
  on infants, 10
  for intimate partner violence, 601
  on lipid disorders, 618
  on maltreatment in children, 112
  on menopause transition, 226
  for nonhormonal contraception, 236
  on obesity, 646–647
  on post-NICU patients, 17
  on postpartum care, 273–274
  on preeclampsia-eclampsia, 318
  on pregnancy, 248, 249, 250–251*f*, 263, 264–265*f*, 294, 296
  on prenatal genetic diagnosis, 259
  on PrEP, 389
  on sterilization, 190
  on tendinopathy, 711
  on thyroid disorders, 689–690
  on transgendered individuals, 372
  on upper back/neck pain, 700, 703–704
  urinary incontinence in children, 139
  on urinary incontinence in women, 244
  on wound care, 721
Patient consent. *See* Consent, patient
Patient Health Questionnaire (PHQ)-2, 516
Patient Health Questionnaire–9 (PHQ-9), 515*f*

Patient Health Questionnaire for Adolescents, 36

Patient Health Questionnaires (PHQ), 508, 512

PCOS. *See* Polycystic ovarian syndrome (PCOS)

PCV13 vaccine, 42–43, 44

PDE-4 inhibitor, 471

Peak Expiratory Flow Rate Monitoring, 444*b*, 445

Pediatric health maintenance and promotion
  0–3 years, 18–21
  3–6 years, 23–26
  6–11 years, 27–31
  12–21 years, 32–38
  developmental delay and autism, screening for, 48–59
  first well-baby visits, 7–10
  post-neonatal intensive care unit (NICU) patients, 12–17

Pediatric presentations
  asthma, 61–69
  attention-deficit/hyperactivity disorder (ADHD), 80–88
  depression, 90–98
  failure to thrive (FTT), 99–103
  maltreatment, 104–112
  urinary incontinence, 124–139

Pediatrics Symptom Checklist (Jellinek et al.), 57

Pelvic girdle pain (PGP), 291–294

Penile trauma, in children, 109

PEP. *See* Postexposure prophylaxis (PEP), for HIV infection

Percutaneous tibial nerve stimulation (PTNS), 243

Perimenopause transition, 219

Persistent abnormal vaginal bleeding, 219

Persistent depressive disorder (dysthymia), 91–92

Personal habits
  0–3 years, 19
  3–6 years, 25
  6–11 years, 28
  12–21 years, 34
  adults with developmental disabilities, 350
  and preterm birth, 320

Pertussis, 41

Pervasive Developmental Disorders Screening Test, 57

Pessaries, 243

PGP (pelvic girdle pain), 291–294

Pharmacotherapy/psychotherapy
  for anxiety disorders, 431–432, 433*t*, 434

for dementia, 510, 510*t*
for heart failure, 571, 572*b*, 573
for hypertension, 588, 590–591*t*
for smoking cessation, 674

Phenothiazines, 297

Phenylketonuria (PKU) screening, 9

Phototherapy, 78

PHQ (Patient Health Questionnaires), 508

Physical abuse, 105. *See also* Intimate partner violence (IPV); Maltreatment of children
  defined, 594
  physical examination for, 107–109, 108*t*

Physical activity
  3–6 years, 25
  6–11 years, 28
  12–21 years, 37
  asthma and, 67
  diabetes and, 533, 533*t*
  diabetes in pregnancy and, 308
  hypertension and, 588
  obesity and, 636–637
  pregnancy and, 293

Physical examinations
  0–3 years, 18–20
  3–6 years, 24
  6–11 years, 28–29
  12–21 years, 35
  for abscess assessment, 396
  for ADHD, 83–84
  of adults with developmental disabilities, 350–351, 352*f*, 353*f*
  amenorrhea and PCOS, 161, 162*t*
  for anemia, 407, 408*t*
  for anxiety, 429
  for asthma, 62, 437–438
  for atopic dermatitis, 72
  for AUB, 146
  for benign prostatic hyperplasia, 451
  for bicipital tendinopathy, 707, 708*t*
  cancer survivorship and, 460, 461*t*
  for chronic nonmalignant pain, 480
  for chronic viral hepatitis, 496, 496*t*
  for COPD, 469, 469*t*
  for depression, 517
  for epilepsy, 540
  for FTT in children, 101
  for GERD, 549
  for geriatric syndromes, 557, 558–559*f*, 560*t*
  for heart failure, 568
  for herpes simplex infections, 577
  for hormonal contraception, 204–205
  for hypertension, 585
  infants and, 8–9
  for intimate partner violence, 599, 599*t*

for irritable bowel syndrome, 606
for lipid disorders, 614–615
for low back pain, 621*t*, 623–624
for maltreatment in children, 107–110, 108*t*
for menopause transition, 220
for obesity, 117
for postexposure prophylaxis for HIV infection, 381
for post-NICU patients, 16
for preeclampsia-eclampsia, 315–316
for preexposure prophylaxis for HIV, 388
for pregnancy discomforts, 293
for prenatal visits, 248
for smoking cessation, 676
for thyroid disorders, 684, 685*t*
for transgendered individuals, 367
for upper back/neck pain, 696–699*t*
urinary incontinence in children, 128, 129–130*t*
for wound care, 716

Physiologic reflux, 13

Pituitary amenorrhea, 156–157, 166. *See also* Amenorrhea; Polycystic ovarian syndrome (PCOS)

Placenta accreta, 283

Placental growth, 294

Placental hormones, 304, 304*t*

Placenta previa, 283

Planned Parenthood, 190, 236

Plasma glucose concentrations, clinical interpretations of, 531*t*

Pneumococcal vaccine scheduling, 44, 330*f*

PNFA (progressive nonfluent aphasia), 505

POI (primary ovarian insufficiency), 157

Polio, 40

Polycystic ovarian syndrome (PCOS), 145, 156. *See also* Amenorrhea
  assessment of, 161
  databased used for, 158, 161
  defined, 157–158
  diagnostic testing for, 161, 162, 165, 165*t*
  overview, 157–158
  physical examination findings, 161, 162*t*
  self-management resources and tools, 169
  treatment and management of, 167–168

Polyps, 141, 144, 153

POP (progestin-only pill), 202, 206

Positive predictive value (PPV), of screening tests, 58

Posterior pelvic pain provocation test, 293

Postexposure prophylaxis (PEP), for HIV infection, 375–384. *See also* HIV (Human immunodeficiency virus)
  assessment of, 383
  clinician and patient resources, 383–384
  databases used for, 380–381
  diagnostic testing, 381, 382*t*
  management of, 383, 383*t*
  overview of, 375
  physical examination for, 381
  risks and recommendations, 375, 376–378*t*
Postnatal growth restriction, 13
Postnatal infection, 14
Post-neonatal intensive care unit (NICU) patients, 12–17
Postpartum care, 268–274
  assessment of, 271
  clinical management goals for, 271–272
  database used for, 269–271
  overview, 268–269
Posttraumatic stress disorder (PTSD), 428, 429, 431, 432, 433*t*
Postural kyphosis, 695
PPIs (proton pump inhibitors), 298, 300, 550
PPV (Positive predictive value), of screening tests, 58
Preeclampsia-eclampsia, 313–319
  assessment of, 316, 317
  clinical management goals for, 317
  clinical risk assessment for, 313, 315*t*
  consultation and referral, 318–319
  database used for, 315–316
  diagnostic tests, 317
  etiology of, 313
  overview of, 313–315, 314*t*
  physical examination for, 315–316
  treatment/follow-up of, 317–318
Preexposure prophylaxis (PrEP), for HIV, 385–389
  assessment of, 388
  clinical management goals for, 388
  database used for, 386, 387–388
  diagnostic screening and tests for, 388
  evidence for, 385–386
  guidance for usage, 393
  indications for, 386
  overview of, 385
  patient education and resources, 389
  treatment and management of, 388–389
Pregnancy
  abuse during, 260, 262*t*
  anxiety disorders and, 434
  complications, 277–278
  consultation and referral during, 257

dating of, 246, 247*b*
depression during, 290
diagnostic testing during, 260, 262*t*
discomforts. *See* Discomforts, of pregnancy
fetal evaluation, 265, 266*t*
gestational diabetes mellitus in, 304–310
healthcare visits, 246–252
hypertension in. *See* Preeclampsia-eclampsia
medical consultation and referral during, 278–281, 279*f*, 280*t*
medical consultation/interprofessional collaboration/transfer of care during, 277–281
nutrition and, 263, 263*t*
patient education and counseling, 263, 264–265*f*
PEP drugs during, 380, 380*t*
postterm, 265, 266*t*
urinary tract infection in, 323–325
Preimplantation genetic diagnosis, 258
Premature and late premature infants, 7, 320–322
Premature births (PTB), 320–322
Premature Ovarian Failure Support group, 169
Prenatal genetic diagnosis, 257–259
  assessment of, 258
  clinical management goals for, 258
  database used for, 258
  overview, 257
Prenatal genetic screening, 253–257
  assessment for, 256
  clinical management goals for, 256
  database used for, 256
  overview of, 253
  for trisomies/NTD/SLOS, 253–255, 254*t*
Prenatal health care visits, 246–252, 260–266
PrEP, for HIV. *See* Preexposure prophylaxis (PrEP), for HIV
Preschool and Kindergarten Behavior Scales (Allin), 57
Preschoolers. *See* Pediatric health maintenance and promotion
Prescribing medications, supervision for, 4
Preterm labor management, 320–322
Primary care setting, anxiety disorders and, 428
Primary hypothyroidism, 682, 689
Primary ovarian insufficiency (POI), 157
Professional and ethical responsibilities, 1
Professional organizations, 3–4
Progesterone, during pregnancy, 294
Progestin, 192, 200

Progestin-only contraception, 202–203. *See also* Hormonal contraception
  assessment for, 205
  implants, 202–203, 207
  injectable, 202, 206–207
  levonorgestrel intrauterine system, 203, 207
  POP pills, 202, 206
Progestogen therapy, 222, 222*t*
Progressive nonfluent aphasia (PNFA), 505
Project Health, 372
Prolactin-secreting tumors, 156–157
Prothrombin time (PT), 415
Proton pump inhibitors (PPIs), 298, 300, 550
Pruritus, 72, 78
Psychoeducation, and ADHD, 84
Psychological abuse, 594
Psychologic/emotional abuse, 105
Psychometrics, 57–58
Psychosocial and emotional support, atopic dermatitis and, 79
Psychosocial assessment and support
  12–21 years, 33–36
  atopic dermatitis in children and, 79
  interventions, 434
Psychotherapy. *See* Pharmacotherapy/ psychotherapy
PT (prothrombin time), 415
PTB (premature births), 320–322
PTNS (percutaneous tibial nerve stimulation), 243
PTSD (posttraumatic stress disorder), 428, 429, 431, 432, 433*t*
Puberty, 27, 436
Pulmonary edema, 566
PUQE (pregnancy-unique quantification of emesis/nausea) index, 295, 295*t*
Purulent exudate, 395
Pyelonephritis, 293, 323–325

Q

Quadruple (quad) marker serum examination, 254–255
Questionnaires, written, 106

R

Race. *See* Ethnicity-based health issues
RADAR mnemonic, 601
Rape, Abuse, and Incest National Network, 602
Recommended Adult Immunization Schedule, 2015, 326, 327–329*f*
Refeeding syndrome, 103
Referrals
  for anxiety disorders, 434

for cancer survivorship, 466
for diabetes, 537
for epilepsy, 545
for postpartum care, 274
for preeclampsia-eclampsia, 318–319
during pregnancy, 278–281, 279f, 280t
for pregnancy, 249, 251b, 257
for tendinopathy, 710–711
Referred neck pain, 691–692
Regional pain syndrome, 692–693
Regulations and statutes, 1–3
Regulatory agencies, 3
Reliability, of screening tests, 58
Reporting, mandatory
on maltreatment of children,
110–111, 110t
Representative samples, of screening
tests, 58
Rescue medications, 66, 441
Respiratory diseases. See Asthma; Chronic
obstructive pulmonary disease
(COPD)
Respiratory syncytial virus (RSV), 14
RICE (rest, ice, compression, elevation),
709–710
Rome III criteria, for IBS diagnosis, 605
Rotavirus vaccine (RV), 42
Rotterdam PCOS Consensus Workshop
Group (2004), 158
Roux-en-Y gastric bypass, 645–646
RSV (respiratory syncytial virus), 14
Rubella, 41
RV vaccine, 42

S

SAD PERSONS mnemonic, 515, 516t
Safety
0–3 years, 21
3–6 years, 25
6–11 years, 27–29, 30–31, 30f
12–21 years, 34, 37
infants, 10
maltreatment of children and, 110, 111
Scalene-myofascial pain syndrome, 693
Scheuermann's kyphosis, 695
Schools
3–6 years, 25
6–11 years, 28
12–21 years, 34
asthma medications and, 68–69
outcomes for FTT children, 103
Sciatica, 624
Scoliosis, 694–695
SCORAD (clinical tool), 72
Screening tests. See also specific type
accurate, characteristics of, 57–58

standardized, 48–49
Seizures. See Epilepsy
Seizure Tracker, 546
Selective serotonin reuptake inhibitors
(SSRIs), 95, 96–97t, 223–224, 432
Self-injurious behavior, 93
Self-management resources, 38
Senior citizens. See Older adults
Sensitivity, of screening tests, 57–58
Sensory impairments, 554–555, 556,
557, 561
Sequential integrated screening, 255
Serotonin-norepinephrine reuptake
inhibitors (SNRIs), 432, 482
Sertraline, 95
Serum integrated screening, 255
Sexual abuse, 105, 594. See also
Maltreatment of children
physical examination for, 109
Sexual acting out, 106
Sexual debut, 93
Sexual dysfunction, 218, 220, 225–226
Sexual functioning, 218
Sexually transmitted infections (STIs), 109,
230–231
Sexual pain disorder, 226
Sexual reassignment surgeries, 366. See also
Transgendered individuals, health
maintenance for
Short-acting β-agonists (SABA), 66
Sickle cell screening, 9
Side effects, of stimulant medications, 84
Sideroblastic anemia, 403, 404, 406, 410,
412
SIDS (Sudden Infant Death Syndrome),
674
Simon Foundation for Continence, 244
SIRS (systemic inflammatory response
syndrome), 396, 396t
Skin and soft tissue infections (SSTIs), 395
Skin disorders. See Atopic dermatitis (AD)
Skyla®, 203
Sleep
0–3 years, 19
6–11 years, 28
fatigue and, 82
FTT and, 101
medications and, 84
menopause transition and, 218–219
poor quality, during pregnancy, 290–291
Smith-Lemli-Opitz syndrome (SLOS), 253,
254–255
Smoking. See also Tobacco
and asthma, 437
benefits of quitting, 674–675
cessation, 672–680

and COPD, 469, 471, 475
health effects of, 672
and hypertension, 588
incidence/prevalence, 672
SNRIs (serotonin-norepinephrine reuptake
inhibitors), 432, 482
Social and environmental risks
6–11 years, 29
12–21 years, 33, 34–35
for asthma in children, 67
for childhood maltreatment, 106–107
for post-NICU patients, 14–15
for urinary incontinence in children, 124
Social anxiety disorder, 428, 431
Social history. See Family and social
histories
Society for the Study of Behavioural
Phenotypes, 362
Spastic diplegia, 347
Specific IgE immunoassay (in vitro), 65
Specificity, of screening tests, 58
Spermicides, 232, 234, 235
Spinal deformities, 694–695
Spirometry, 65, 439, 441, 441f, 469, 470t
Spondylosis, 694
SSHADESS (mnemonic), 34
SSRIs (selective serotonin reuptake
inhibitors), 95, 96–97t,
223–224, 432
SSTIs (skin and soft tissue infections), 395
Stages of Reproductive Aging Workshop
(STRAW), 217
Standardized screening tests, 48–49
State of California Regional Center
System, 363
State regulation of professional practice,
1–3
Statin therapy, 616, 617t
Statutes and regulations, 1–3
Sterilization, 188–190
assessment of, 190
database used for, 190
overview of, 188–190
self-management resources, 190
Stimulant medications, and ADHD, 84,
85t, 86
STIs (sexually transmitted infections), 109,
230–231
Stomach acid, 298
Strains/sprains, 694
STRAW (Stages of Reproductive Aging
Workshop), 217
Stress incontinence, 125
Stress UI (SUI), 237
Substance use and abuse, 34, 93, 477, 478f
Sudden changes in behavior, 106

Sudden death, and stimulants, 83
Sudden Infant Death Syndrome (SIDS), 674
Suicide
    12–21 years, 34
    depression and, 94
Supervision requirements, physician, 5
Supine active straight leg raise (SLR) test, 293
Surveillance, Epidemiology, and End Results
    (SEER) database, 459
Syphilis screening, 36
Systemic inflammatory response syndrome
    (SIRS), 396, 396t
Systolic heart failure, 566
Systolic HTN, 583

T

TADS (Treatment for Adolescents with
    Depression Study), 95
Target specific oral anticoagulants
    (TSOACs), 415, 424–425, 426t
Td/Tdap vaccine. See Tetanus, diphtheria,
    and acellular pertussis (Td/Tdap)
    vaccine
TE (thromboembolism), 415
Teenagers. See Pediatric health maintenance
    and promotion
Tendinopathy, 706. See Upper extremity
    tendinopathy
Tetanus, diphtheria, and acellular pertussis
    (Td/Tdap) vaccine, 44
Tetanus prophylaxis, 397
Texas Functional Living Scale, 508
Th1 and Th2 cytokines, 436
Thalassemia, 403, 403t, 406, 409, 412
Thoracic outlet syndrome, 693, 694
Thoracoabdominal trauma, in children, 109
Thromboembolism (TE), 415
Thyroid disorders, 682–690
    assessment of, 687, 688t
    clinical management goals for, 687
    databases used for, 683–684
    diagnostic screening and tests for, 684,
        686–687t, 687, 688–689
    management and treatment of, 689
    overview of, 682–683
    patient and family education and
        resources on, 689–690
Thyroid nodules, 683, 689
Thyroid-stimulating hormone (TSH), 682
Tic disorders, 83–84
Title V, Social Security Act, 48
Tobacco. See also Smoking
    and asthma, 61
    history of, 672–673
    and hypertension, 588
    mental health disorders and, 674

Tobacco Control Act, 2009, 672
Toddlers. See Pediatric health maintenance
    and promotion
Topical analgesic creams and patches, 482
Tracheal shaving, 366
Tracking medication effects, 87
Transcervical tubal occlusion, 189
Transdermal patch, 201, 206
Transgendered individuals, health
    maintenance for, 365–372
    assessment for, 367
    database used for, 366–367
    overview of, 365–366, 366f
    physical examinations, 367
    self-management resources and tools, 372
    surgical options for, 371–372, 371t
    treatment for, 367, 368–372,
        369–370t, 371t
Transgender Law Center, 372
Transsexual individuals. See Transgendered
    individuals, health maintenance for
Transvaginal ultrasound (TVUS), 153
Transvestites. See Transgendered individuals,
    health maintenance for
Traumatic kyphosis, 695
Traumatic wounds, 713
Treatment for Adolescents with Depression
    Study (TADS), 95
Trial of labor (TOL)
    contraindications for, 284, 285t
    VBAC vs., 282–287
Tricyclic antidepressants, 86, 482
Trisomies, 253, 254–255
TSOACs (target specific oral
    anticoagulants), 415, 424–425, 426t
Tubal ligation, 188–189
Tuberculosis screening
    0–3 years, 21
    3–6 years, 25
    6–11 years, 29
    12–21 years, 36
TVUS (transvaginal ultrasound), 153
Type 1 diabetes (T1D), 529. See also
    Diabetes mellitus
Type 2 diabetes (T2D), 529. See also
    Diabetes mellitus
    risk factors for, 306, 306t

U

UCSF Women's Continence Center, 244
UI. See Urinary incontinence (UI), in
    children; Urinary incontinence (UI),
    in women
Ulcers. See Wound care
Ulipristal acetate, 192
Underactive bladder, 125

United States Public Health Service
    (USPHS), 375, 376–377t, 385
University of California, San Francisco, 103
Upper back/neck pain, 691–704
    assessment of, 699, 699t
    causes of, 691
    clinical management goals for, 700
    databases used for, 695–696
    diagnostic screening and tests for, 698t,
        700, 700t
    mechanical spine disease, acute, 692
    musculoskeletal strains and sprains, 694
    myofascial pain syndrome, 692–693
    osteoarthritis, 694
    overview of, 691–692
    patient education and resources on, 700,
        703–704
    physical examination findings, 696–699t
    scalene muscle pain/thoracic outlet
        syndrome, 693–694
    treatment and management of, 701–703t
Upper extremity tendinopathy, 705–711
    assessment of, 708
    clinical management goals for, 709
    databased used for, 706–708, 708t
    diagnostic tests for, 707, 708, 709
    overview of, 705
    treatment and management of, 709–711
Upper GI (UGI) tract, 547, 548
Urge incontinence (UUI), 238, 238t,
    240, 242t
Urinalysis, 25
Urinary diary, 239, 239t
Urinary incontinence (UI), in children,
    124–139
    assessment of, 128, 130
    clinical management goals, 130–131
    databases used in, 126, 128
    daytime, 125
    defined, 124
    diagnostic tests for, 131, 132–133f, 134f
    night, 125–126
    overview of, 124–126
    physical examination findings and, 128,
        129–130t
    treatment and management of, 131,
        132–133f, 133, 134, 134f, 135–138t
    voiding and elimination history and,
        127, 127t
Urinary incontinence (UI), in women,
    237–244
    assessment of, 239–240
    clinical management goals for, 240
    initial evaluation of, 238, 238t, 239
    nonpharmacologic treatment for, 240,
        241t, 242t

overview of, 237
pharmacologic treatment for, 240,
    241t, 242t
prevalence of, 238
self-management resources
    and tools, 244
treatment and management of, 240–244
types of, 237–238, 237t
urinary diary, 239, 239t
Urinary tract infections (UTIs), 124,
    323–325
Urogenital atrophy, 220, 224
U.S. Collaborative Review of Sterilization
    (CREST), 188
U.S. Department of Health and Human
    Services (USDHHS), 649
U.S. Environmental Protection Agency, 446
U.S. Food and Drug Administration (FDA),
    94, 95, 189, 203, 223, 231, 405,
    415, 673
U.S. Preventive Services Task Force
    (USPSTF), 326, 515, 516, 565, 578
    screening/counseling recommendations,
        332t, 337t–340t
    on screening for lipid disorders, 615
Uterine bleeding. *See* Abnormal uterine
    bleeding (AUB)
Uterine ruptures, 282–283
UTIs (urinary tract infections), 124,
    323–325
UUI (urge incontinence), 238, 238t,
    240, 242t

V

Vaccinations. *See* Immunizations
Vaccine Adverse Events Reporting System
    (VAERS), 44, 46
Vaccine Injury Compensation Program
    (VICP), 46, 47
Vaccine-preventable diseases
    measles, 40–41
    pertussis, 41
    polio, 40
    rubella, 41
    varicella, 41–42
VAERS. *See* Vaccine Adverse Events
    Reporting System (VAERS)

Vaginal birth after cesarean (VBAC),
    282–287
    client information and consent,
        285–287f
    overview, 282
    success factors, 284, 284t
    success rates, 284, 284t
    trial of labor vs., 282–287
Vaginal contraceptive ring, 201–202, 206
Vaginal deliveries, 7
Vaginal/rectal electrical stimulation, 243
Vaginal reflux and postvoid dribbling, 125
Vaginal trauma, in children, 109
Validity, of screening tests, 58
Vancouver Coastal Health Clinic, 372
Varenicline, 675
Varicella vaccine, 41–42, 43, 44–45
Vascular dementia, 504, 507
Vasectomy, 188, 189–190
Vasomotor symptoms, 217, 220
VBAC. *See* Vaginal birth after cesarean
    (VBAC)
Venous leg ulcer (VLU), 714, 715
Venous thrombosis (VTE), 200, 201
VICP. *See* Vaccine Injury Compensation
    Program (VICP)
Viral hepatitis, chronic. *See* Chronic
    viral hepatitis
Vision screening
    0–3 years, 20
    3–6 years, 24
    6–11 years, 29
    infants and, 14
Visual impairment, 554–555, 556, 561
Vitamin B12 deficiency, 404–405, 407, 410,
    412–413
Vitamin K antagonists (VKA), 415. *See* also
    Oral anticoagulation (OAC) therapy
    associated risk of, 416
VKA. *See* Vitamin K antagonists (VKA)
VLU (venous leg ulcer), 714, 715
Voiding
    and elimination history, 126, 127t
    postponement, 125
    process of, 124
    von Willebrand disease (VWD), 145
VTE (venous thrombosis), 200, 201

Vulnerable child syndrome, 14
VWD (von Willebrand disease), 145

W

Warfarin therapy. *See* also Oral
    anticoagulation (OAC) therapy
    drug and nutritional supplement
        interactions with, 418–419,
        418t, 419t
    management of, 419, 420t
    monitoring of, 415, 416t
    patient education and safety with,
        421, 422
    variables affecting stability of, 420
Weight loss
    hypertension and, 588
    urinary incontinence in women and, 240
Weight-to-height ratio, 101
Well babies visits, 7–10
Wet-wrap dressings, 77
Whiplash, 693
Withdrawal bleeding, 201
Women. *See* also Pregnancy
    obesity in, 158
    urinary incontinence. *See* Urinary
        incontinence (UI) in women
Women's Health Initiative (WHI), 218, 221
Workplace modification during
    pregnancy, 293
World Federation of Societies of Biological
    Psychiatry (WFSBP), 521
World Health Organization (WHO), 118,
    200, 306, 401, 583, 672
World Professional Association for
    Transgender Health, 372
Wound care, 713–721
    assessment of, 718
    clinical management goals for, 718
    database used for, 714–715, 717–718
    diagnostic screening and tests for, 717t
    overview of, 713

Z

Zoster vaccine, 45